AORTIC STENOSIS

Collected Reprints (1963-2020)

By

William C. Roberts, MD

and

Colleagues

ISBN: 979-8-88862-153-0
Printed in the United States of America on acid-free paper.

Table of Contents

*Articles are numbered based on WCR's CV.

Aortic Stenosis: Physiological, Pathological, and Clinical Concepts

Combined Clinical Staff Conference at the National Institutes of Health

Moderator: EUGENE BRAUNWALD, M.D., F.A.C.P.
Discussants: WILLIAM C. ROBERTS, M.D., ALLAN GOLDBLATT, M.D., MAURICE M. AYGEN, M.D., S. DAVID ROCKOFF, M.D., and JOSEPH W. GILBERT, M.D.

Bethesda, Maryland

DR. EUGENE BRAUNWALD: The region of the aortic valve is the last point passed by the blood in its course through the heart and lungs. As long as the functions of the left ventricle and left atrium are well maintained, obstruction to left ventricular outflow may be extremely severe without the clinical manifestations of heart failure, which tend to occur earlier in the course of the disease, when the obstruction exists at a point upstream to the aortic valve. As a consequence, the relationships between the physiological and clinical abnormalities that exist in patients with obstruction to left ventricular outflow differ distinctly from those occurring in other forms of heart disease. It is the purpose of this conference to review some of the pertinent pathologic, physiologic, clinical, and surgical features of aortic stenosis.

Obstruction to left ventricular outflow may occur at sites above and below the aortic valve, as well as at the valve itself. Since there are considerable differences in the anatomic lesions and in the surgical treatment of obstruction at each of these specific sites, the term "aortic stenosis" is probably best used only in a general sense, and should be preceded by the designations "valvular," "supravalvular," or by the prefix "sub" depending on the site of obstruction. Dr. Roberts will now review some of the pathologic features of the various forms of obstruction to left ventricular outflow.

DR. WILLIAM C. ROBERTS: In all types of aortic stenosis, there is concentric hypertrophy of the left ventricular wall with a decrease in left ventricular chamber size (Figure 1). In the supravalvular variety (Figure 1a) the ascending aorta is usually hypoplastic; whereas, in the valvular type (Figure 1b) the ascending aorta is usually dilated, and in the idiopathic hypertrophic subvalvular type (Figure 1d) the ascending

Received December 5, 1962; accepted for publication December 26, 1962.

This is an edited transcription of a combined clinical staff conference at the Clinical Center, Bethesda, Maryland, by the National Heart Institute, National Institutes of Health, Public Health Service, Department of Health, Education, and Welfare.

Requests for reprints should be addressed to Eugene Braunwald, M.D., Cardiology Branch, National Heart Institute, Bethesda 14, Maryland.

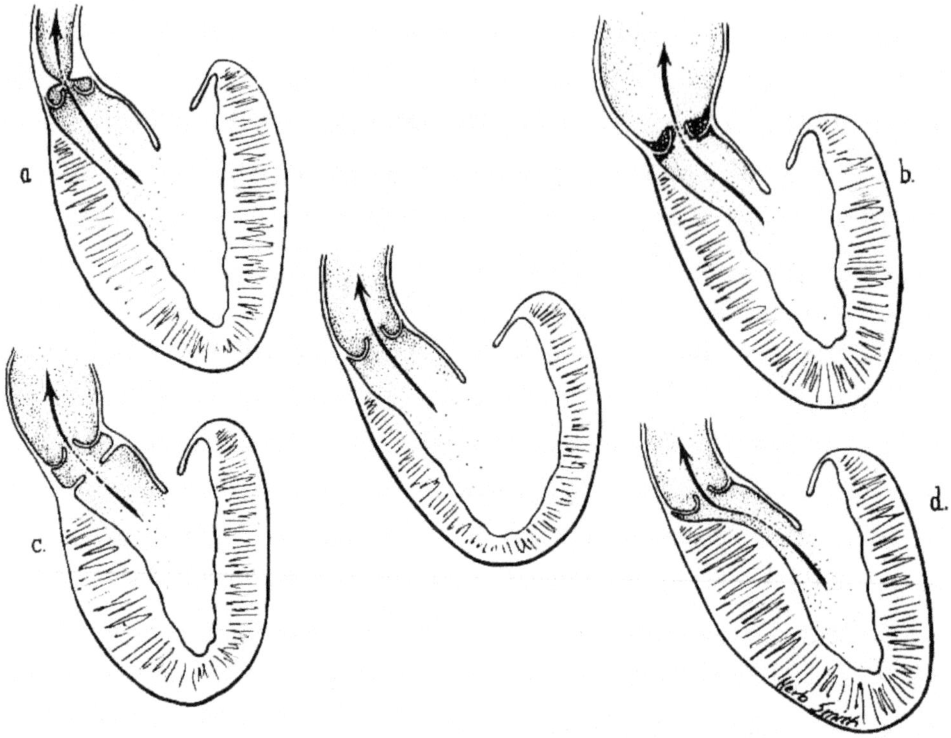

FIGURE 1. Diagram illustrating the 4 forms of obstruction to left ventricular outflow. The central figure represents the normal heart. In all forms of obstruction the left ventricular wall is hypertrophied and its cavity is relatively small. The size of the ascending aorta is variable, depending primarily on the location of the obstruction. *a.* Supravalvular aortic stenosis. The site of the obstruction is immediately above the aortic valve. *b.* Valvular aortic stenosis. Calcium deposits are present on the cusps. *c.* and *d.* Subvalvular aortic stenosis. In *c.* the subvalvular obstruction is discrete, being produced by a fibrous band located usually approximately 1 cm below the aortic valve. In *d.* the subvalvular obstruction is produced by marked hypertrophy of the upper portion of the muscular ventricular septum.

aorta is normal or smaller than normal in size. In discrete subvalvular stenosis (Figure 1c) the ascending aorta may be small or normal, but most often it is dilated. The presence or absence of aortic dilatation is an important diagnostic sign, and when the ascending aorta is not dilated, a search should be made for the presence of one of the rarer forms of aortic stenosis.

The least common form of "aortic" stenosis is the supravalvular variety which was described initially only 32 years ago (1). There are necropsy data in the literature from only 11 patients (8 males, 3 females) with this malformation (2–5), including the 2 patients studied both clinically and pathologically at the Clinical Center. There are at least 3 forms of supravalvular stenosis; in one type the obstruction is produced by an inwardly protruding annular constriction involving the entire circumference of the aorta at the upper margins of the sinuses of Valsalva. The infolding is due to a combination of intimal fibrous proliferation and medial hypertrophy. In the second type the obstruction is due to a "tube-like" narrowing of the ascending aorta beginning immediately above the aortic valve and usually extending up to the transverse aorta. In this instance the narrowing is produced primarily by uniform thickening of the aortic media with little intimal proliferation. In the third and probably the least common type of supravalvular aortic stenosis, the obstruction is due to a thin membrane with a central opening located just above the aortic valve.

Valvular aortic stenosis is a common disease and is either congenital or acquired in etiology. The calcification of the valve cusps is always acquired, and represents a complication of either congenital or acquired stenosis. The valve may be deformed at birth; it may be dome-shaped and contain no commissures (Figure 2); it may be dome-shaped and contain one commissure (the unicommissural valve of Edwards (6); it may contain only 2 cusps, or as many as 4 cusps. The dome-shaped valves, which are in actuality unicuspid valves, are intrinsically stenotic, but the bicuspid valve is intrinsically regurgitant and becomes stenotic only as it becomes calcified (7). The calcification in these instances tends to involve each cusp uniformly and appears to be the result of wear and tear on a deformed valve.

There is strong evidence that, with rare exception, acquired aortic stenosis is the result of antecedent rheumatic endocarditis, most commonly producing fusion of 2 of the 3 cusps at one of the commissures. The fusion is believed to be the result of healing of the active rheumatic endocarditis. The usual site of fusion is the commissure between the right and left anterior cusps (8). The conjoined leaflet

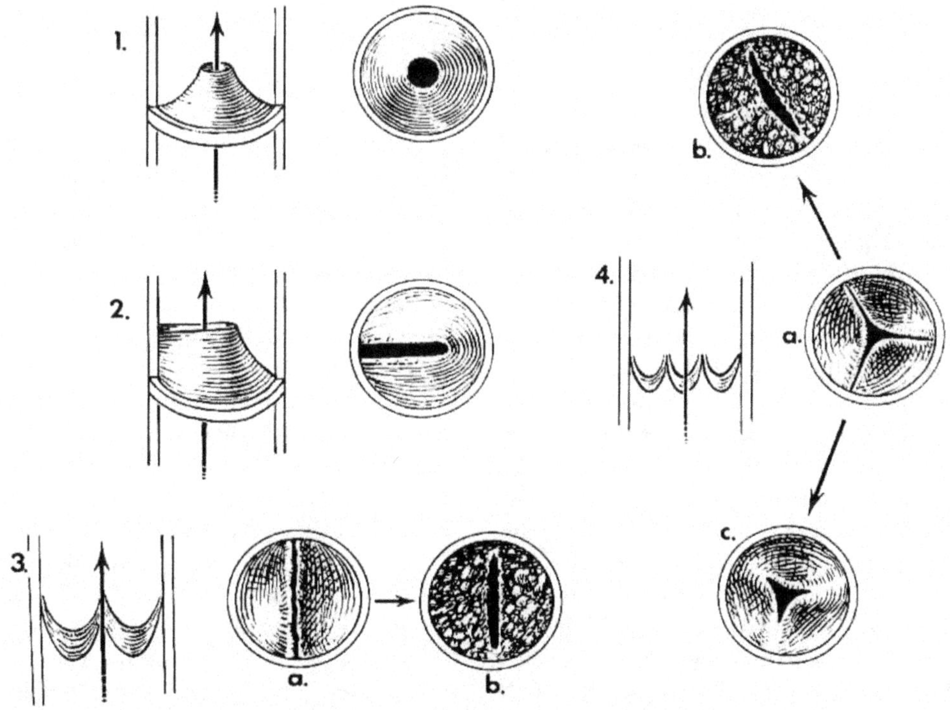

FIGURE 2. Diagram illustrating the various forms of valvular aortic stenosis. In *1* and *2* the stenosis is produced by dome-shaped valves. Each of these valves is intrinsically stenotic. In *1* the valve has no lateral attachments to the wall of the ascending aorta. The orifice is centrally located. In *2* the valve has one lateral attachment (commissure) and its orifice is eccentrically located. *3*. A congenitally bicuspid valve is shown. This bicuspid semilunar valve is not intrinsically stenotic but becomes stenotic only as it becomes calcified. The calcification in this instance is usually uniformly distributed. *4*. A tri-cuspid aortic valve is shown (*a*.). When rheumatic fever attacks this valve, one of the commissures is usually fused, and the valve becomes bicuspid. Later, calcium deposition occurs and stenosis appears (*b*.). Rarely, all 3 commissures are fused (*c*.) and the valve becomes stenotic in the absence of calcium deposition.

undergoes heavy calcification and later may become fixed to the wall of the aorta. The only significant valve action that remains is that of the posterior cusp, which acts as a flap valve. Eventually the posterior cusp becomes heavily calcified, its mobility considerably reduced, and stenosis becomes severe. When more than one commissure is fused, the movement of the posterior cusp is even more restricted. Usually when this occurs there is some retraction of cuspal tissue so that the aortic orifice tends to be more or less the same size throughout the cardiac cycle; thus, an element of valvular regurgitation is added to that of stenosis. On rare occasions the rheumatic aortic valve may be stenotic but not calcified. This results from fusion of all 3 cusps and is considered to be a direct result of rheumatic endocarditis.

The aortic valve may be calcified without fusion of its commissures. This situation usually occurs in the elderly person with calcification of the aortic valve but a normal-size heart. The calcium in these valves is deposited uniformly and usually only within the sinuses of Valsalva. Since there is no fusion of the commissures, restriction of valvular function results only from the rigidity imparted to the leaflets by the calcium. The etiology of the aortic valve calcification which is seen in the elderly person is debatable, but since there usually is no history of rheumatic fever and since the mitral valve is normal, the process appears not to be related to rheumatic fever. Various forms of valvular aortic stenosis are illustrated in Figure 3.

There may be numerous complications of valvular aortic stenosis, several of which are listed in Table 1. Hypertrophic muscular subaortic stenosis occasionally occurs as a result of the valvular obstruction. Interstitial myocardial fibrosis is a common finding in patients with long-standing aortic stenosis. In 1885, Sir William Osler pointed out the susceptibility of congenitally deformed and sclerotic valves to bacterial endocarditis (9). Active bacterial or fungal endocarditis can itself produce aortic stenosis in addition to being a complication of aortic stenosis. We have recently observed several patients with fungal vegetations on a calcified aortic valve (10). McKusick, Logue, and Bahnson (11) first reported the occurrence of cystic medial necrosis in the ascending aortas of several patients with valvular aortic stenosis and marked post-stenotic dilatation, a finding which has been amply confirmed (12). Rarely a fleck of calcium becomes dislodged from a calcified aortic valve; indeed embolization of calcium is a recognized complication of aortic valve surgery. Calcium may extend from the aortic valve to adjacent structures; extension down the anterior mitral leaflet may lead to mitral regurgitation in an otherwise normal mitral valve, while extension into the bundle of His may lead to heart block. The lumen of the coronary arterial ostia may be compromised by the calcific process, occasionally leading to acute myocardial infarction when the coronary arteries themselves are free of significant atheromata.

TABLE 1. Complications of Valvular Aortic Stenosis

I. Muscular subaortic stenosis.
II. Interstitial myocardial fibrosis.
III. Congestive heart failure.
IV. Bacterial or fungal endocarditis.
V. Medial cystic necrosis, aorta.
VI. Dislodgment of calcium from valve → embolus.
VII. Extension of calcium to adjacent structures
    A. Anterior mitral leaflet → mitral insufficiency
    B. Bundle of His → heart block
    C. Ostia of coronary arteries → coronary insufficiency
    D. Pulmonary trunk or rt. atrium → arterio-venous fistula.

Subaortic stenosis is more common than was once believed. It may be localized, being produced by a discrete fibrous band or "tunnel," or it may be diffuse. In the discrete form a membrane or diaphragm is present, usually a centimeter below the base of the aortic valve. Not infrequently the outflow tract of the left ventricle is

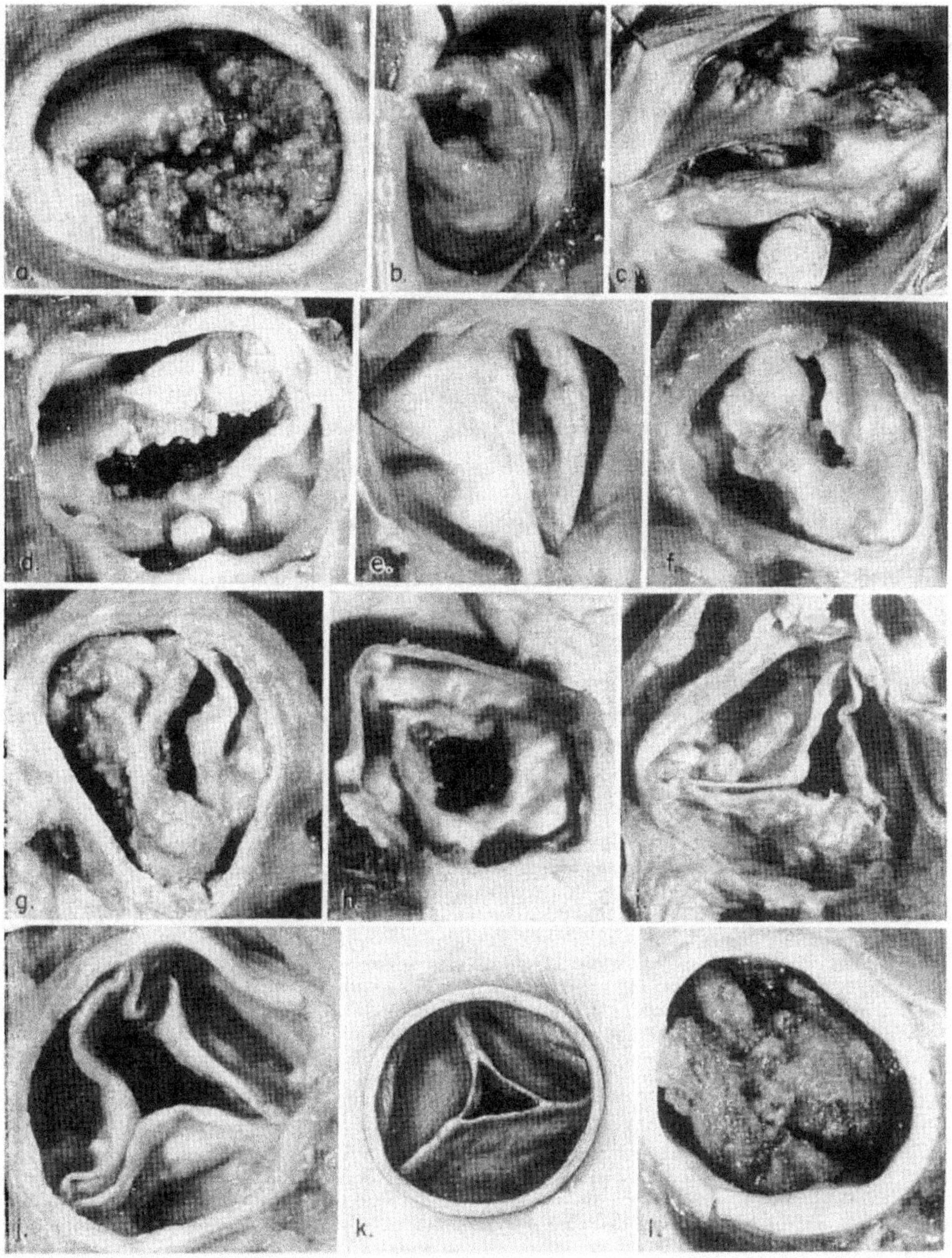

FIGURE 3. The aortic valve as seen from above is shown in 12 patients who died of valvular aortic stenosis. In *a.* to *c.* the valve was congenitally deformed; *a.* and *b.* are dome-shaped, unicuspid, unicommissural valves. The patient whose valve is shown in *a.* was a 32-year-old woman with a known cardiac murmur since the age of 5 years and a peak systolic aortic valve gradient of 90 mm Hg. The patient whose aortic valve is shown in *b.* was a 16-year-old boy, who had a cardiac murmur from birth and a peak systolic aortic valvular gradient of 125 mm Hg. The bicuspid valve shown in *c.* is from a 40-year-old woman with a known cardiac murmur since the age of 6 years and a peak systolic aortic valvular gradient of 70 mm Hg. The bicuspid valve shown in *d.* is from a 37-year-old man with a known cardiac murmur since the age of 19 years. The valve shown in Figure *e.* came from a 34-year-old man with a known cardiac murmur since the age of 5 years and a peak systolic aortic valvular gradient of 90 mm Hg.

narrowed for a distance of 1 to 3 centimeters (tunnel-like narrowing). When the latter type of obstruction occurs, the subvalvular fibrous process usually extends onto the aortic valve cusps and almost always makes contact with the ventricular aspects of the anterior mitral leaflet at its base. In the hearts of patients who have persistent common atrioventricular canal, there are usually accessory chordae tendineae extending from the anterior mitral leaflet to the base of the ventricular septum. These anomalous chordae may produce an obstruction in the outflow tract of the left ventricle. The diffuse form of subaortic stenosis is a muscle disease which results in severe hypertrophy of the myocardium in the left ventricular outflow tract. When primary, it has been termed "idiopathic hypertrophic subaortic stenosis" (13) (Figure 1d). Secondary hypertrophy of the more superior portion of the ventricular septum occurs in a number of conditions, including discrete fibrous subaortic stenosis, as well as the valvular and supravalvular forms of aortic stenosis. In some patients with obstruction to right ventricular outflow associated hypertrophic subaortic stenosis is sometimes also seen (14, 15).

DR. EUGENE BRAUNWALD: Dr. Goldblatt will now discuss the clinical features in one of the forms of obstruction to left ventricular outflow just presented. He will summarize the results of a study of 100 patients with congenital aortic stenosis, in all of whom the diagnosis has been firmly established, and in all of whom the severity of obstruction was assessed by measuring the systolic pressure gradient between the left ventricle and brachial artery. These findings will be presented in greater detail elsewhere (16, 17).

DR. ALLAN GOLDBLATT: In our patients the sex ratio was 4 to 1 in favor of the males, a finding which is consistent with other reports in the literature (18–20). Sixty-five of the patients had valvular aortic stenosis, 5 patients had supravalvular aortic stenosis, and there were 20 patients with discrete subvalvular aortic stenosis. In 10 patients the site of obstruc-

Although the finding was not readily apparent, this valve contained many calcium deposits. The precise structure of the valves shown in *f.* and *g.* is obliterated by extensive deposits of calcium, but each of these valves was probably congenitally bicuspid. The valve shown in *f.* is from a 39-year-old man with a peak systolic gradient across the aortic valve of 75 mm Hg. The valve shown in *g.* is from a 54-year-old man who had a 130-mm Hg peak systolic aortic valvular gradient. Note that the sinuses of Valsalva are completely filled with calcium. The mitral valve was normal. In *h.* and *i.* the valve disease appears definitely to have resulted from an acquired process. The valve shown in *h.* has a fixed central orifice as contrasted to the fixed eccentrically placed orifices of the valves shown in *f.* and *g.* In these instances the aortic valve orifice tends to be more or less the same size throughout the cardiac cycle and therefore the valve is incompetent as well as stenotic. Thus, in each of the 3 patients whose valves are shown in *f.*, *g.*, and *h.*, a murmur of aortic regurgitation was audible in addition to the one of aortic stenosis. The patient whose valve is shown in *i.* was a 67-year-old man with rheumatic aortic stenosis. There is no fusion of the valvular commissures and the calcium deposits lie only within the sinuses of Valsalva. No calcium is deposited on the ventricular aspects of the aortic valve cusps. This distribution of the aortic valve calcium and the lack of commissural fusion is commonly observed in patients who also have rheumatic mitral disease. The valve shown in *j.* is similar to the one shown in *i.* except that the calcium deposition is not quite as extensive. Here again there is no fusion of the commissures, but in this case the mitral valve was normal. This was the aortic valve of a 77-year-old man who died of leukemia. A loud basal precordial systolic murmur had been present. Since there was no fusion of the commissures and the calcium deposits were not extensive, function of this valve was probably insignificantly altered. The valve illustrated in *k.* is from a 28-year-old man with rheumatic mitral and aortic disease. There is partial fusion of all 3 commissures without calcium deposition. The valve shown in *i.*, which came from the heart of a heroin addict who previously had had a normal aortic valve, is obscured by a large vegetation. The endocarditis in this instance was caused by *Candida parapsilosis*, and this valve is shown to point out that endocarditis when active can produce obstruction to left ventricular outflow.

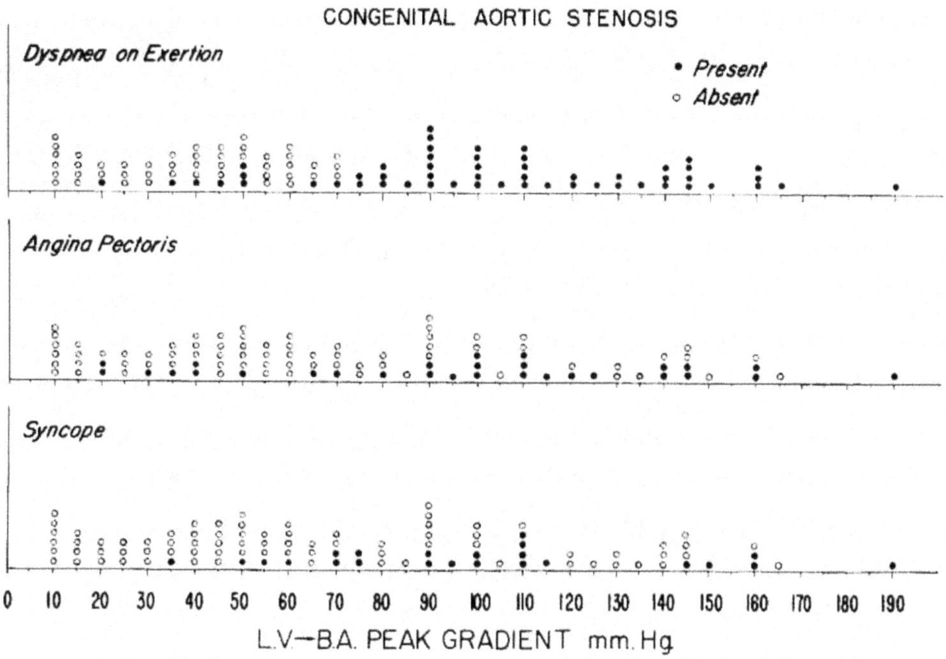

FIGURE 4. Relationship between the presence or absence of 3 symptoms and the systolic pressure gradient in each of the 100 patients with congenital aortic stenosis.

tion has not yet been localized. Patients with idiopathic hypertrophic subaortic stenosis were not included in this analysis. Left heart catheterization, usually carried out by the transseptal technique (21), was utilized to establish the diagnosis of obstruction to left ventricular outflow. The diagnoses of supravalvular aortic stenosis as well as subvalvular aortic stenosis were confirmed by retrograde left ventricular catheterization and selective angiography. In addition, in 56 patients the diagnoses were confirmed at operation and in 4 patients at post-mortem examination.

These patients ranged in age from 2 to 38 years, with an average age of 14 years. Eight patients had an associated patent ductus arteriosus, 5 had associated coarctation of the aorta, 2 had ventricular septal defect, 2 had pulmonic stenosis, one had an associated aorticopulmonary window, one an atrioventricular canal, and one congenital heart block. The frequent association of patent ductus, and of coarctation of the aorta with congenital aortic stenosis, has been noted previously (22, 23).

When the most common symptoms that occur in congenital aortic stenosis, *i.e.*, exertional dyspnea, angina pectoris, and syncope, were related to the left ventricular-brachial artery peak systolic gradient, it was noted that every patient whose gradient was above 70 mm Hg exhibited dyspnea on exertion. However, in 8 patients whose gradients were equal to or less than 70 mm Hg dyspnea on exertion was a prominent symptom as well. Six of these patients had associated congenital cardiac lesions, and the other 2 patients were adults, 32 and 34 years of age, with calcific congenital aortic stenosis. It is apparent, therefore, that in patients with congenital aortic stenosis without associated anomalies, clear-cut dyspnea usually indicates the presence of severe stenosis (Figure 4). The frequency of angina pectoris and syncope was also greater in patients with high gradients, but there were a number of patients with severe stenosis who did not have these symptoms and, conversely, several patients with mild stenosis in whom a history of angina or syncope could be elicited (Figure 4).

A left ventricular lift and precordial thrill were noted in all patients whose gradients exceeded 30 mm Hg. However, several patients with gradients below 30 mm Hg exhibited a thrill and left ventricular lift as well (Figure 5). Although the appreciation of a left ventricular lift and precordial thrill depends to some extent on the size and the build of the patient, it seems clear that in the majority of patients the presence of a lift and a precordial thrill indicate that there is hemodynamically significant, but not necessarily severe, obstruction to left ventricular emptying. Conversely, the absence of a left ventricular lift and precordial thrill indicates the presence of mild aortic stenosis. An early systolic sound (ejection sound) was audible at the base of the heart in 59 of the 100 patients. This sound was heard more frequently in patients with lower gradients than in those with higher gradients (Figure 5).

In a review of the findings obtained at right heart catheterization in these 100 patients, 16 were found to have elevations of the pulmonary artery pressure, *i.e.*, a systolic pressure exceeding 30 mm Hg and a mean pressure exceeding 20 mm Hg. Eight of these 16 patients had associated left-to-right shunts and the other 8 patients had left ventricular-brachial artery gradients ranging from 90 mm Hg to 188 mm Hg, with an average gradient of 114 mm Hg. Four of these 8 patients with severe aortic stenosis and pulmonary hypertension showed signs of left heart failure, and in 6 of these 8 patients the effective orifice size (24) was found to range from 0.21 square centimeter to 0.57 square centimeter, with an average of 0.40 square centimeter. Thus, it appears that pulmonary hypertension in a patient with congenital

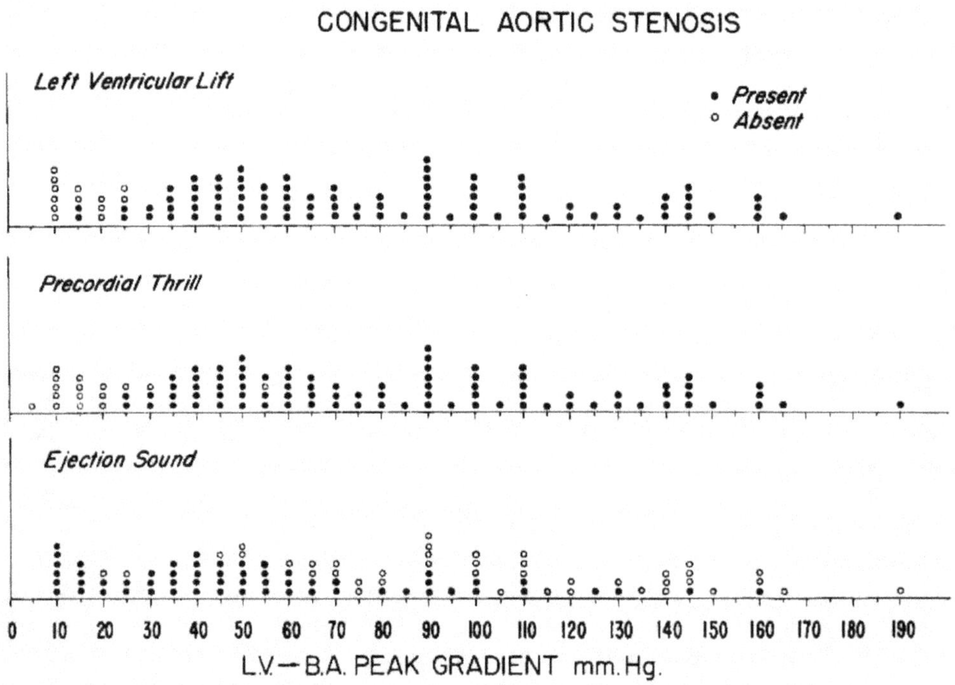

FIGURE 5. Relationship between the presence or absence of each of 3 physical findings and the systolic pressure gradient in the patients with congenital aortic stenosis.

aortic stenosis is a significant finding and denotes either the presence of an associated lesion or of severe obstruction.

No differences were observed in the presenting symptoms between patients with valvular and those with discrete subvalvular aortic stenosis, but some differences in physical findings are noted. The incidence of an aortic diastolic murmur was greater in the discrete subvalvular type (55 per cent) than in the valvular form (13 per cent), and the frequency of the ejection sound was significantly higher in the patients with valvular aortic stenosis.

It is generally considered that the electrocardiogram is an extremely reliable tool in assessing the severity of obstruction in patients with congenital aortic stenosis, and it has been employed frequently as an important aid in reaching decisions regarding the necessity for left heart catheterization or operation, or both. Accordingly, the electrocardiographic findings were correlated with the hemodynamic data in our 100 patients. When the S wave in V_1 was related to the left ventricular-brachial artery gradient, as well as to the left ventricular systolic pressure, some correlation was observed in patients under 10 years of age, but none was seen in patients above 10 years of age. Although no patient under 10 years of age with a gradient above 80 mm Hg had an S wave in V_1 which was less than 20 millimeters, the converse was not the case (Figure 6). In patients under 10 years of age, some correlation between the height of the R wave in V_5 and the gradient was present, while none existed in older patients. No patient under 10 years of age with a gradient above 50 mm Hg had an R wave less than 20 millimeters, but, again, the converse was not true (Figure 7). In relating the R/S ratio in V-1 and in V-5, as well as the sum of the S V-1 and R V-5, to the systolic pressure gradient, no improvement of the correlations was observed. When the height of the T wave in left precordial leads was related to the systolic pressure gradient there again was considerable scatter, with upright T waves present in patients who had gradients as high as 110 mm Hg, and inverted T waves present in patients with gradients as low as 30 mm Hg.

Although congenital aortic stenosis is associated with characteristic symptoms, physical signs, and electrocardiographic changes, these findings do not always correlate sufficiently closely with the hemodynamic evidence of obstruction to left ventricular outflow to permit physicians to evaluate the severity of the lesion with

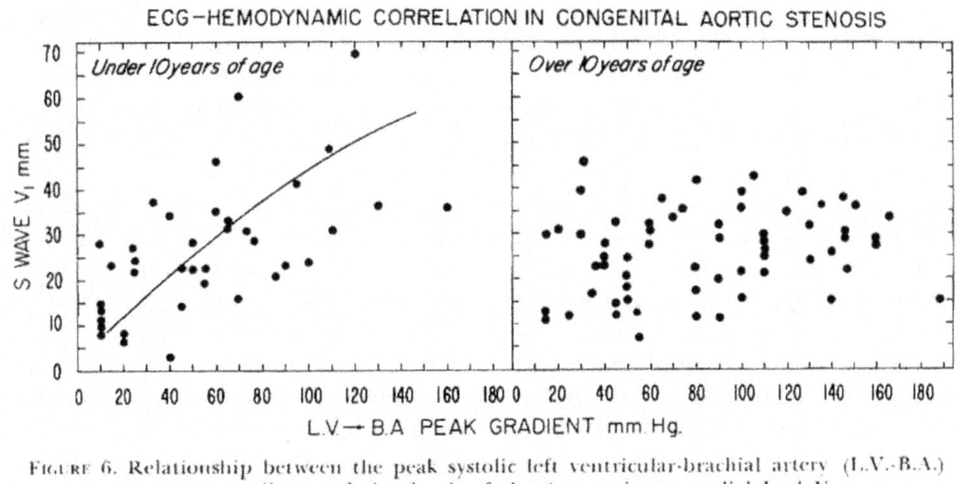

FIGURE 6. Relationship between the peak systolic left ventricular-brachial artery (L.V.-B.A.) pressure gradient and the depth of the S wave in precordial lead V_1.

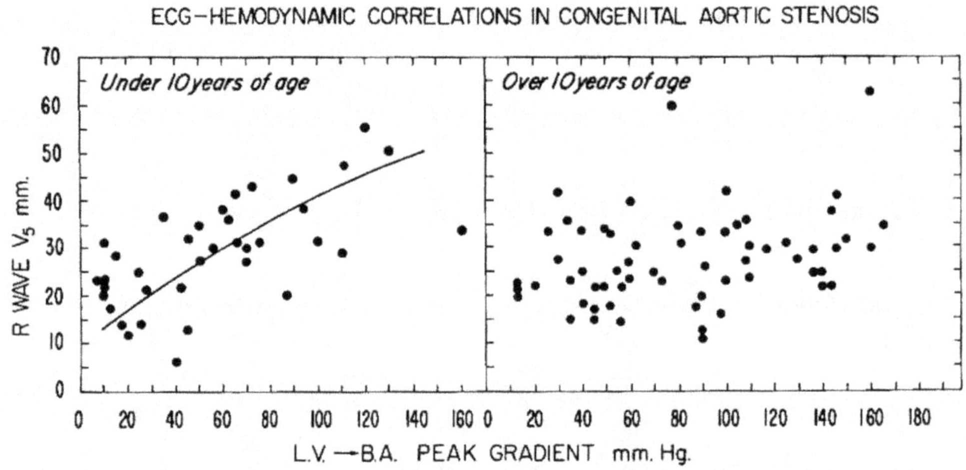

FIGURE 7. Relationship between the peak systolic left ventricular-brachial artery (L.V.-B.A.) pressure gradient and the height of the R wave in precordial lead V_5.

confidence in all patients without the aid of left heart catheterization.

DR. EUGENE BRAUNWALD: Considerable information concerning the localization and severity of obstruction in patients with the various forms of aortic stenosis can be obtained by means of detailed analysis of the phonocardiogram, the indirect jugular phlebogram, the indirect carotid arterial pulse, and the apex cardiogram. These graphic methods constitute relatively simple and objective methods of study. In order to determine their value, Dr. Maurice Aygen analyzed the records of 157 patients with acquired or congenital aortic stenosis and correlated the findings with physiologic, radiologic, and operative data.

DR. MAURICE M. AYGEN: The indirect carotid pulse contour of normal subjects shows an uninterrupted anacrotic rise to a primary peak or to a high anacrotic shoulder followed by a more gradual rise to a peak. The arterial pulse contour of patients with aortic stenosis revealed an anacrotic rise interrupted at varying levels by an anacrotic notch or shoulder (Figure 8). The anacrotic notch was followed either by a very slow ascent to a delayed peak or by a plateau. Systolic vibrations were frequently superimposed upon the pulse curve (Figure 9) and the incisura was usually delayed. The pulse contour of patients with idiopathic hypertrophic subaortic stenosis (Figure 10) usually demonstrated a percussion wave with a steep anacrotic rise followed by a lower, rounded hump ending in a sharp and delayed incisura. None of the patients with this type of obstruction had systolic vibrations superimposed on the pressure pulse curve.

Weissler, Peeler, and Roehll (25) found close agreement between measurements of ejection time as determined from the intra-arterial central aortic pressure pulse and the indirect carotid or subclavian pulse tracings. These authors also demonstrated a prolonged ejection time relative to stroke volume in patients with aortic stenosis. The ejection period (time interval from the onset of the anacrotic rise to the incisura), the upstroke time (time interval from the onset of the anacrotic rise to the highest peak), and the half upstroke time (time required for the pressure pulse to attain half of its peak value) were measured in 25 normal subjects and in patients with various forms of aortic stenosis. In comparison with the values obtained from the normal subjects, the average values of these 3 variables were markedly increased in patients with valvular and discrete subvalvular obstruction, but not in the patients with idiopathic hypertrophic subaortic stenosis (Table 2). The latter demonstrated a prolonged ejection period but short upstroke and half upstroke times. None of these 3 variables correlated well with the magnitude of the aortic gradient, the left ventricular systolic pressure, or the aortic valve area. Twelve of 13 (92 per cent) patients with discrete subvalvular stenosis and 51 of 90 (50 per cent) patients with valvular stenosis exhibited a carotid shudder. However, the presence or absence of the carotid shudder did not correlate with the gradient or the left ventricular systolic pressure.

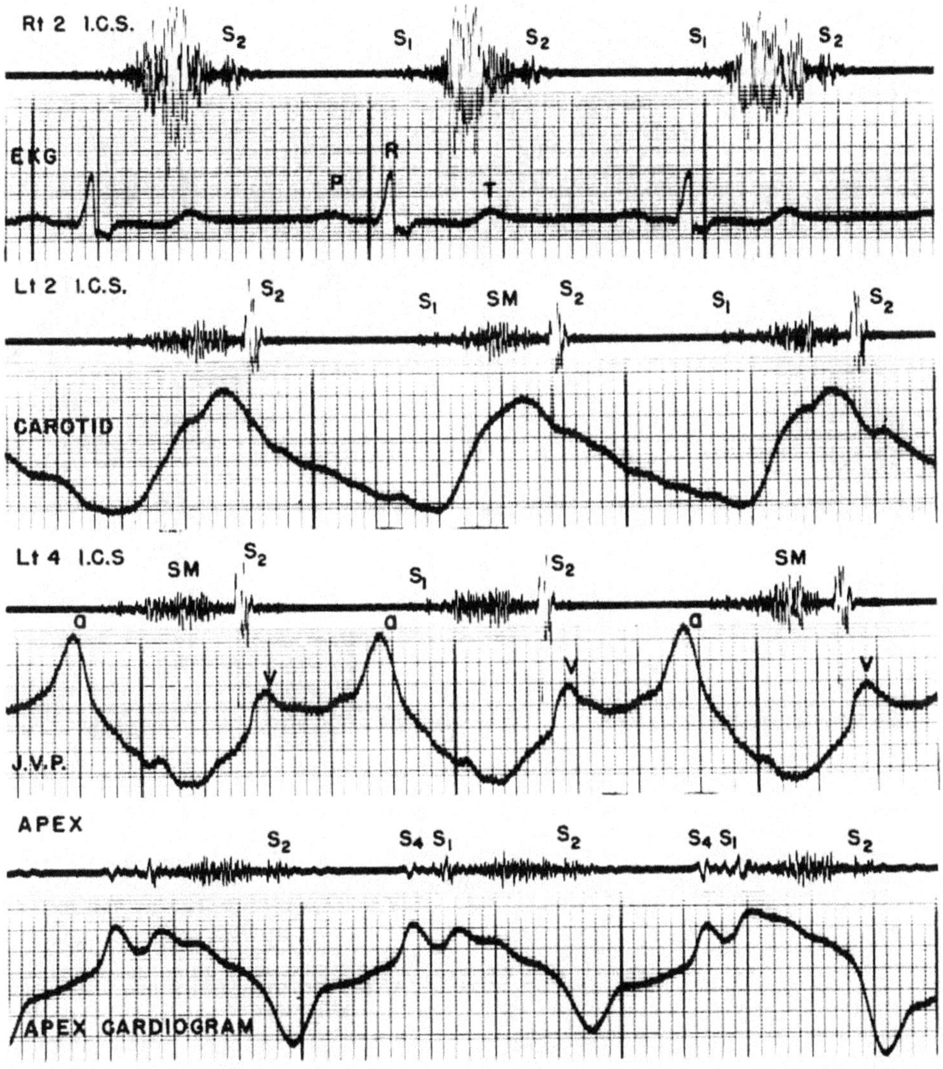

FIGURE 8. The phonocardiogram, indirect carotid pressure pulse, jugular venous pulse (J.V.P.), and the apex cardiogram in a 56-year-old male with a gradient of 110 mm Hg across the aortic valve. A diamond-shaped systolic murmur (S.M.) was best recorded at the aortic area and a prominent atrial sound (S_4) was recorded at the apex. The carotid pulse showed an anacrotic shoulder. There was a prominent *a* wave in the J.V.P. and a prominent presystolic wave in the apex cardiogram.

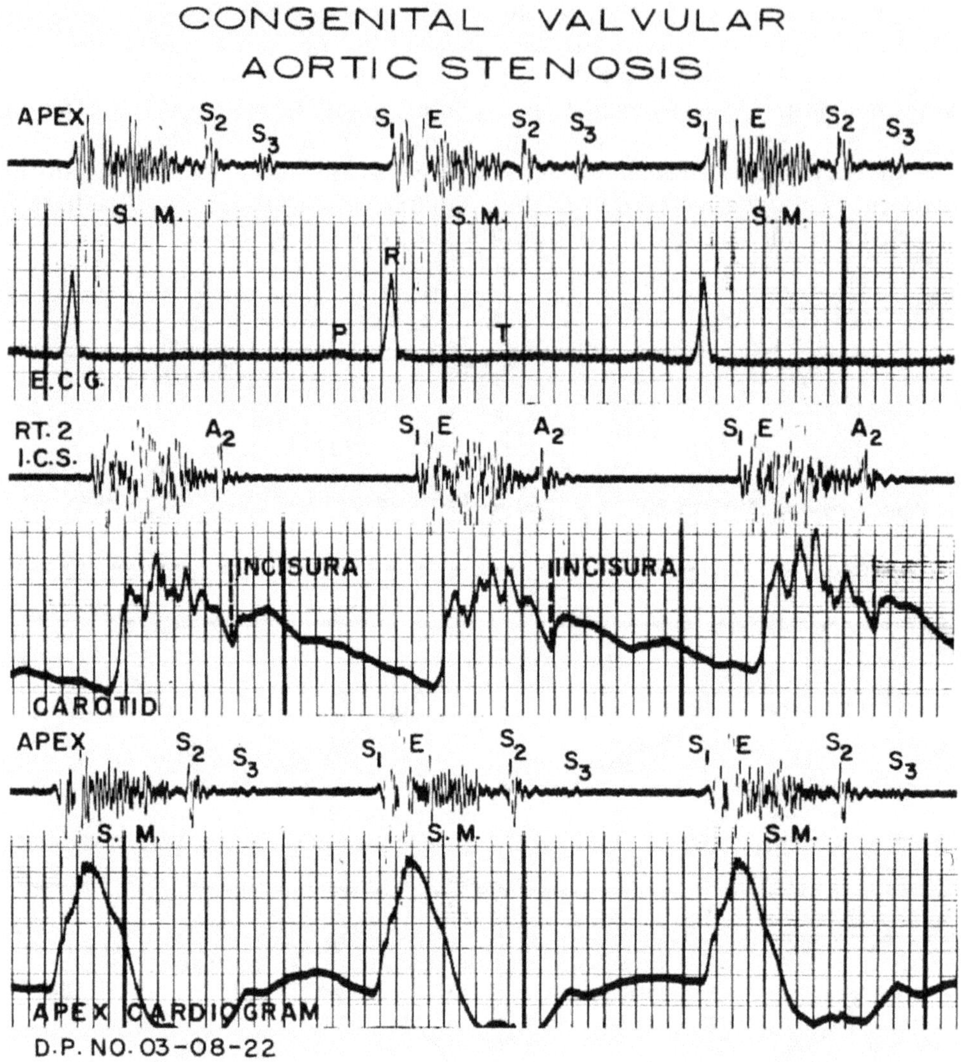

FIGURE 9. Phonocardiogram, indirect carotid pressure pulse, and the apex cardiogram of a 15-year-old boy with congenital valvular aortic stenosis who had a peak systolic gradient of 50 mm Hg across the aortic valve. The phonocardiogram revealed a prominent ejection sound (E), an ejection type of early systolic murmur (S.M.), and a third heart sound (S_3). There are systolic vibrations on the carotid pulse tracing and the apex cardiogram revealed only a prominent systolic wave.

The jugular venous pulse usually reveals a prominent *a* wave when aortic stenosis is associated with pulmonary hypertension or it may exhibit a dominant *v* wave with an abrupt *y* descent in the presence of associated right ventricular failure. In addition, mild to moderate increases in the magnitude of the *a* wave in the jugular venous pulse occur in a considerable number of patients with aortic stenosis even in the absence of pulmonary hypertension (Figure 8). This finding suggests that in these patients there is an increased resistance to right atrial emptying, the cause of which is not clear. It might be due to bulging of the hypertrophied septum into

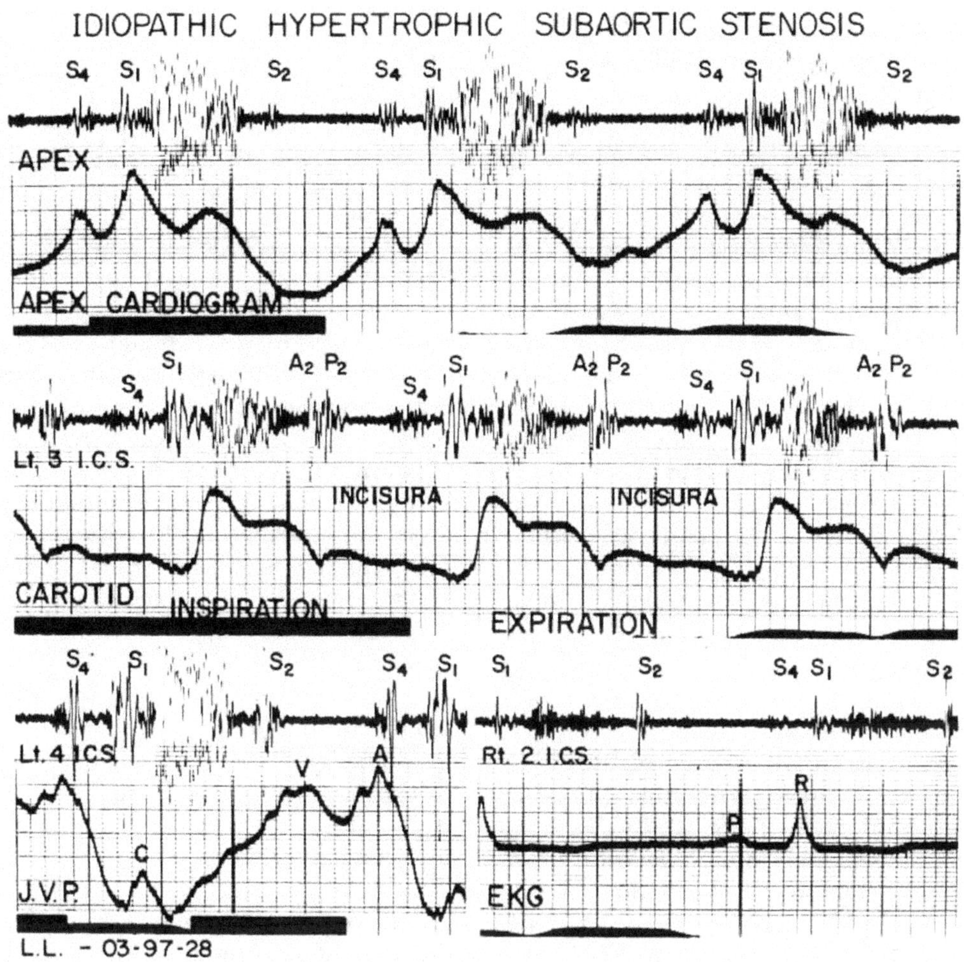

FIGURE 10. The phonocardiogram, apex cardiogram, indirect carotid pressure pulse, and the jugular venous pulse of a 37-year-old female with idiopathic hypertrophic subaortic stenosis and a gradient of 60 mm Hg in the subvalvular region. The phonocardiogram shows a prominent atrial sound (S_4), a diamond-shaped systolic murmur best recorded at the apex and faint at the aortic area, and normal splitting of the second heart sound. The apex cardiogram revealed a very prominent presystolic wave. The carotid tracing showed a primary wave followed by a second hump during systole. The jugular venous pulse was unremarkable.

TABLE 2. Average Durations of Ejection Period, Upstroke Times, and Incidence of Carotid Shudder as Determined From the Indirect Carotid Pressure Pulse

Diagnosis	Number of Patients	Ejection Period*	U.T.	½ U.T.	Carotid Shudder Present
Normal	25	257	51	25	0%
Valvular	90	340	150	55	56%
Subvalvular (discrete)	13	310	120	50	92%
Subvalvular (hypertrophic)	20	310	50	23	0%

* The durations of the ejection period, of the upstroke time (U.T.), and of the one-half upstroke time (½ U.T) are presented in milliseconds.

the right ventricular cavity causing an increased resistance to passive right ventricular filling.

Sixty-nine of the 145 patients with aortic stenosis exhibited an aortic ejection sound (Figure 9). This sound was identified and differentiated from tricuspid closure and from the pulmonic ejection sounds by its prominence at the apex, its temporal relationship to the mitral closure sound and to the onset of the carotid upstroke, as well as by its failure to show respiratory variations in intensity. The incidence of an aortic ejection sound in various forms of aortic stenosis is demonstrated in Table 3. Half of the patients with rheumatic stenosis, 31 of the 35 (88 per cent) patients with congenital valvular and 5 of 14 patients with discrete subvalvular aortic stenosis exhibited an ejection sound. On the other hand, an ejection sound was heard or recorded in only one patient with hypertrophic subaortic stenosis. An ejection sound was recorded in 11 of 19 (58 per cent) patients without detectable dilatation of the aorta and in 35 of 42 (83 per cent) patients with post-stenotic dilatation.

The mechanism of production of the ejection sound in patients with aortic stenosis is still under debate. Wolferth and Margolies (26) and Hancock (27) have subscribed to the view that the ejection sound in aortic stenosis represents an opening snap of the aortic valve. Others have attributed it to sudden distention of the dilated aorta after the onset of ejection (28). In 46 patients with congenital aortic stenosis the time interval between the onset of the carotid upstroke and the ejection sound ranged from 0 to 60 milliseconds. Correction for the delay in the carotid tracing was made in each individual by determining the time interval from the onset of the aortic closure sound to the nadir of the incisura in the carotid pulse. In 38 of the 46 patients with congenital aortic stenosis, in whom ejection sounds were recorded, the corrected time interval between the upstroke of the carotid pressure pulse and the ejection sound exceeded 20 milliseconds. From these data it is therefore unlikely that this sound is a direct result of aortic valve opening.

A rhomboid-shaped systolic murmur which ends before the aortic component of the second heart sound was the most consistent auscultatory and phonocardiographic sign of aortic stenosis. This harsh murmur was usually associated with a thrill, and was maximal in the aortic area and radiated along the neck vessels. In none of the patients with idiopathic hypertrophic subaortic stenosis was a thrill palpated in the aortic area. In these patients the systolic murmurs were always most prominent to the left of the sternum or at the apex, and they were barely or not audible in the second right intercostal space and in the neck. In patients with hypertrophic subaortic stenosis and severe obstruction the murmur was usually associated with an apical or with a left precordial thrill. In contrast, the differentiation between valvular and discrete subvalvular aortic stenosis could not be made on the basis of the location of the murmur. The patients with supravalvular aortic stenosis had disproportionately prominent thrills and murmurs in the neck.

The absolute length of the murmur and the ratio of murmur length to the duration of left ventricular systole were plotted

TABLE 3. Incidence of Ejection Sound in Patients with Obstruction to Left Ventricular Outflow

	Number of Patients	Ejection Sound Present	%
Rheumatic A. S.	66	33	50
Congenital valvular A. S.	35	31	88
Congenital discrete subvalvular A. S.	14	5	36
Congenital (site undetermined)	12	10	81
Idiopathic hypertrophic subaortic stenosis	30	1	3

against the left ventricular pressure, the aortic valve gradient, and the aortic valve area. Although the murmurs tended to be longer with higher left ventricular pressures and gradients, the correlation was poor. It was found that in no patient with a gradient of more than 70 mm Hg did the systolic murmur peak during the first 40 per cent of systole. However, there were a number of patients with mild aortic stenosis who had murmurs which peaked in mid or late systole.

Contraction of the atrium causes active rapid filling of the ventricles. When the compliance of the left ventricle is decreased by ventricular hypertrophy, the contribution of left atrial contraction to left ventricular filling is increased. Inspection of the heart during operation shows a sudden expansion of the ventricle during vigorous contraction of the atrium (29). This sudden expansion of the left ventricle during the presystolic period can be appreciated by the clinician's hands placed over the apex and can be recorded by various methods. The atrial contraction precedes the major systolic positive wave and causes a double apical pulsation. Children and young adults without heart disease or patients with mild aortic stenosis not infrequently had small presystolic waves recorded in their apex cardiograms, but these impulses were usually not appreciated by palpation. A palpable presystolic pulsation was almost always associated with a severe degree of aortic stenosis (Figure 8). Although there does not appear to be any direct causal connection between the atrial contraction wave and the aortic stenosis *per se*, the atrial contribution to ventricular filling probably reflects the degree of compensatory hypertrophy of the left ventricle and left atrium which is present in patients with severe degrees of obstruction. All patients with idiopathic hypertrophic subaortic stenosis had a double apical impulse regardless of the severity of outflow tract obstruction (Figure 10).

Atrial contraction and active rapid ventricular filling are also manifested as the fourth heart sound (Figure 8). The presystolic filling sound is frequently audible in normal children and in subjects with prolonged P-R intervals in the electrocardiogram. After all patients below the age of 13 years and those with prolonged P-R intervals were excluded, the phonocardiograms of 52 patients with valvular and discrete subvalvular forms of aortic stenosis were correlated with the hemodynamic findings (30). A fourth heart sound was usually associated with aortic gradients exceeding 70 mm Hg, an *a* wave peak in the left atrial pressure pulse exceeding 13 mm Hg, and a left ventricular end-diastolic pressure greater than 11 mm Hg (Figure 11). Again, as with the apical presystolic pulsation, the correlation between the degree of stenosis and the presence of a presystolic filling sound is indirect and probably reflects the degree of left ventricular and atrial hypertrophy. An atrial sound is frequently audible in patients with systemic hypertension, ischemic heart disease, and cardiomyopathies. All patients with idiopathic hypertrophic subaortic stenosis had prominent filling sounds regardless of the severity of the obstruction (Figure 10).

In a large percentage of patients with aortic stenosis the behavior of the second heart sound differs from that which we have observed in the normal (31). In normal subjects, the aortic closure sound (A_2) during expiration is synchronous with or precedes the sound of pulmonary valve closure (P_2) by a number of milliseconds, resulting in a single or a closely split second heart sound on auscultation. During inspiration, shortening of left and prolongation of right ventricular systole result in a net augmentation of the interval between the 2 components of the second sound. In 67 normal subjects, the A_2–P_2 interval during expiration ranged from 0 to 40 milliseconds, and with inspiration

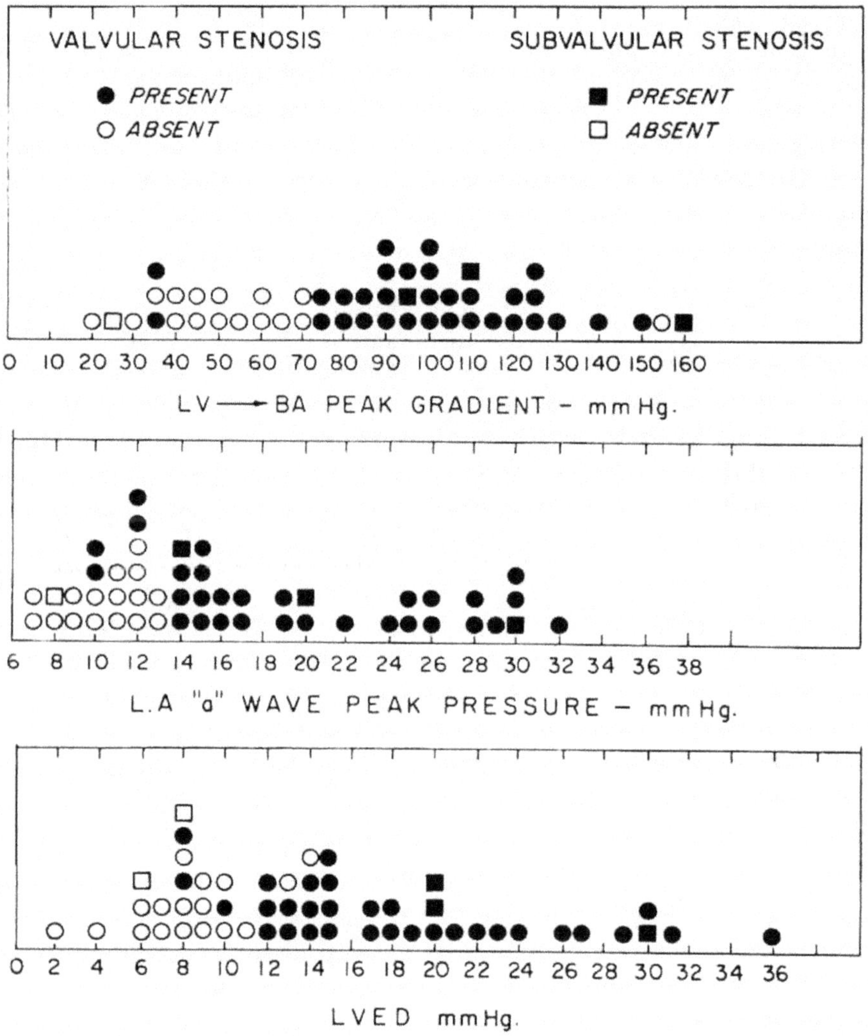

FIGURE 11. Top: Relationship between peak systolic ventricular-brachial artery pressure gradient and the presence or absence of a fourth heart sound. Center: Relationship between left atrial "a" wave peak pressure and the presence or absence of a fourth heart sound. Bottom: Relationship between left ventricular end-diastolic pressure and the presence or absence of a fourth heart sound.

this interval increased by increments from 0 to 60 milliseconds (Figure 12). Three patterns were observed in the patients with aortic stenosis. Twenty-one patients exhibited a pattern indistinguishable from the normal. The mean aortic gradient in these 21 patients was 50 mm Hg, and only 20 per cent of them had gradients larger than 70 mm Hg. The second group, which consisted of 95 patients, had a single second sound during expiration and either no increase or a subnormal increase during inspiration. The average gradient in these patients was 95 mm Hg. and 80 per cent had gradients exceeding 70 mm Hg. The remaining 18 patients exhibited paradoxical splitting in the absence of left bundle branch block. In this group the aortic closure sound followed the pulmonic sound by 20 to 70 milliseconds, and the interval decreased by increments from 0 to 60 milliseconds during inspiration. All patients in this group had peak gradients greater than 70 mm Hg, and the average gradient was 98 mm Hg.

An explanation for the abnormal behavior of the second heart sound in aortic stenosis is provided by the data in Figure 13. The time intervals from the onset of ventricular depolarization to aortic valve closure (Q-A_2) during expiration are plotted against the heart rate, in normal subjects and in patients with aortic stenosis. As anticipated, there was an inverse relationship between heart rate and the Q-A_2 intervals in both groups, but 97 out of the 135 patients with aortic stenosis had values of Q-A_2 which were greater than those observed in normal subjects with similar heart rates. The time interval between the onset of ventricular depolarization and closure of the aortic valve represents the sum of the electromechanical latent interval, the duration of isometric contraction, and the duration of the left ventricular ejection period. The first 2 of these components did not show any significant differences in patients with obstruction to left ventricular outflow and in normal subjects, except for a slight increase in the electromechanical latent interval in patients with idiopathic hypertrophic subaortic stenosis. Thus the delay of the aortic components of the second heart sound which occurs in the majority of patients with aortic stenosis is the result of prolongation of the ejection period, presumably due to the increased resistance to left ventricular emptying.

DR. EUGENE BRAUNWALD: I think that it should be stressed that most of the findings described by Dr. Aygen can be elicited by careful physical examination, and that the graphic techniques merely serve to confirm and to help in the quantification of these findings. The other major techniques which are commonly employed in the study of patients with obstruction to left ventricular

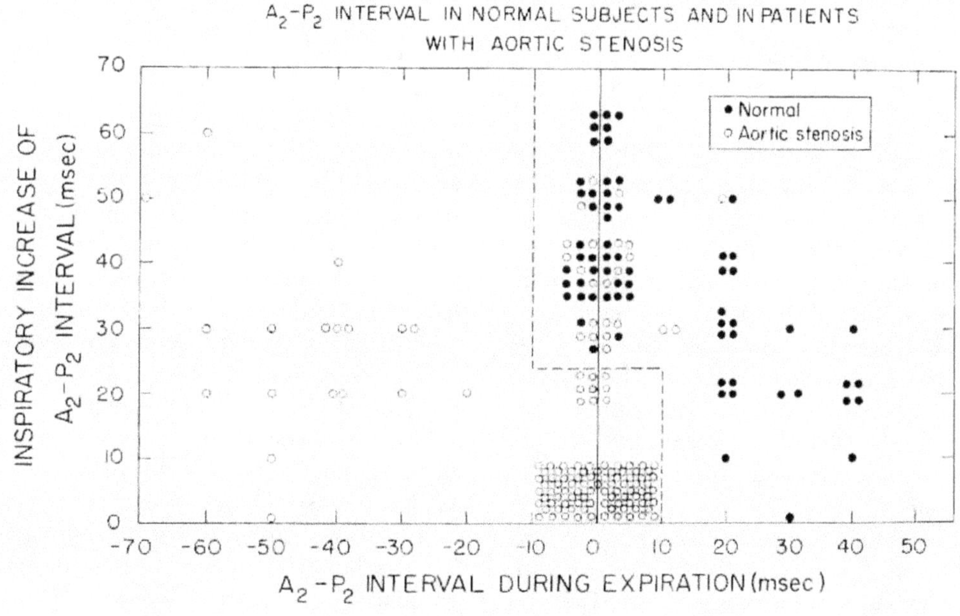

FIGURE 12. Time interval between aortic valve closure (A_2) and pulmonic valve closure (P_2) during expiration, and the increase of this interval during inspiration in normal subjects and in patients with aortic stenosis. When A_2 followed P_2, the A_2-P_2 interval was considered to be negative. All values to the left and below the broken line were outside of the normal range.

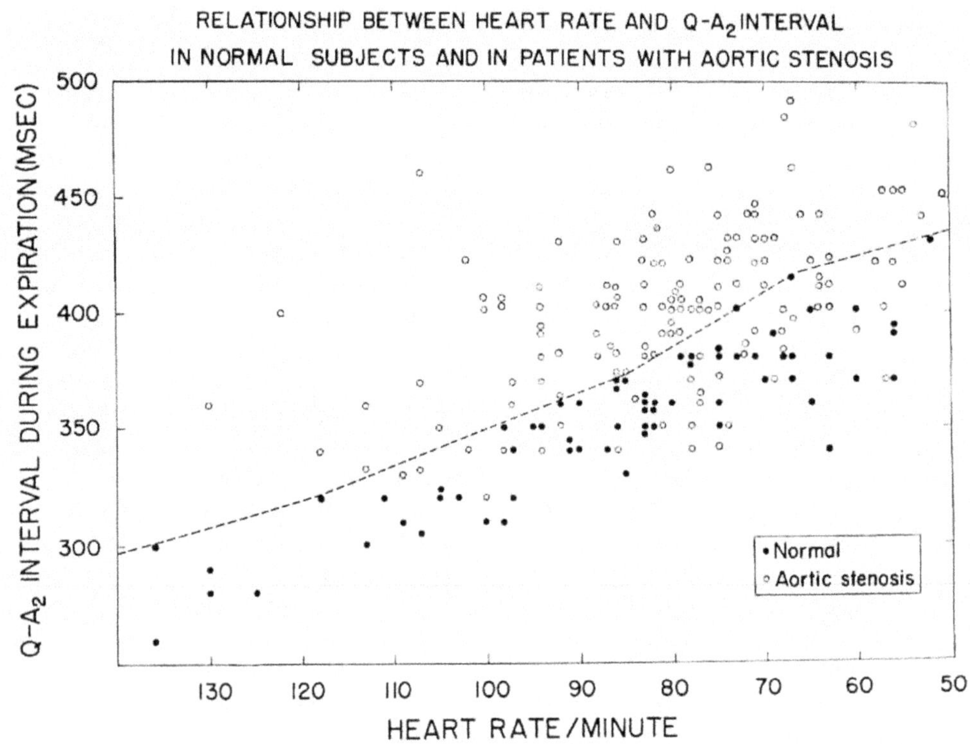

FIGURE 13. Relationship between heart rate and the interval between the onset of electrical depolarization and aortic valve closure (Q-A_2) recorded during expiration in normal subjects and in patients with aortic stenosis.

outflow are the radiological methods. These will now be discussed by Dr. S. David Rockoff.

DR. S. DAVID ROCKOFF: In order to determine the radiological changes in the cardiovascular silhouette due to congenital aortic stenosis, the preoperative roentgenograms of the patients with congenital aortic stenosis presented by Dr. Goldblatt were analyzed, after exclusion of patients with associated cardiovascular lesions. Left atrial and left ventricular size and aortic tortuosity and dilatation were classified as 0 to 3 +, indicating normal to markedly abnormal.

Analysis of plain roentgenograms revealed that the general heart size in congenital valvular stenosis was normal in the majority of patients. However, 80 per cent of the patients with subvalvular aortic stenosis showed some enlargement of the overall heart size. No cardiac silhouettes were noted that were considered to be markedly enlarged. The left ventricle, on the other hand, was usually enlarged in both congenital valvular and subvalvular aortic stenosis. As is shown in Figure 14, moderate or marked enlargement of the left ventricle tended to occur somewhat more frequently in the subvalvular than in the valvular form of the disease. No correlation was present between the radiographic size of the left ventricle in congenital aortic stenosis and the aortic valvular orifice size, the left ventricular systolic pressure, or the peak aortic systolic gradient.

Tortuosity and dilatation of the aorta occurred in the majority of patients with congenital aortic valvular and subvalvular stenosis. Poststenotic dilatation of the ascending aorta was present in 68 per cent of the patients with valvular stenosis and was at least moderate in severity in 42 per cent. In contrast, although dilatation of the ascending aorta was present in 60 per cent of the patients with subvalvular stenosis, it was of moderate severity in only 7 per cent. No correlation existed between the presence or degree of aortic tortuosity or dilatation and the peak aortic systolic gradient or the aortic valvular orifice size.

Radiological evidence of left atrial enlargement was found in only 9 per cent of the patients with congenital aortic stenosis. This was usually slight in degree and, in all but one patient, was associated with a peak aortic systolic gradient of greater than 90 mm Hg. A calcified aortic valve on radiologic examination occurred in 18 per cent of the patients in this series. As expected, no radiological calcifications of the aortic valve were noted in the patients with subvalvular obstruction. In the patients with valvular obstruction, calcification was noted in 9 of the 15 patients above the age of 20 years who were studied, and in only one of the 39 patients under the age of 20 years.

Angiography is a very useful means of localizing the obstruction to left ventricular outflow. The films obtained after injection of the contrast material intravenously, into the right side of the heart or into the pulmonary artery have been very disappointing, since by the time the contrast material reaches the left side of the heart, it has become so dilute that identification of the details necessary to make the diagnosis is frequently impossible. The retrograde placement of a catheter into the left ventricle is of limited value since it is frequently difficult to pass the catheter through the stenotic aortic valves.

Angiography performed through percutaneous left ventricular puncture has been

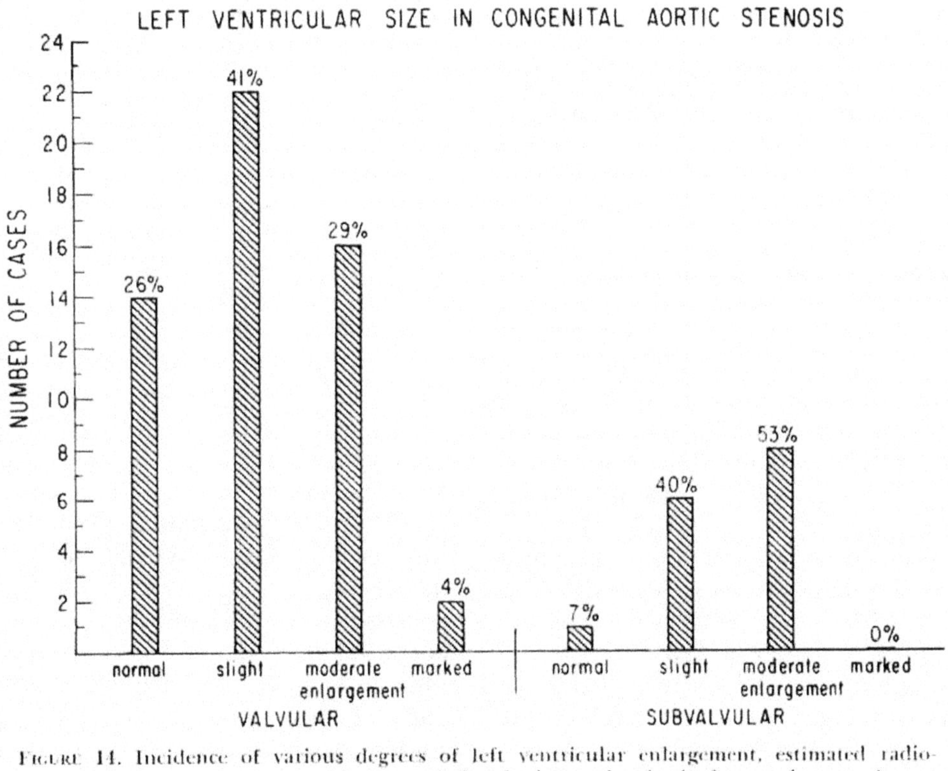

FIGURE 11. Incidence of various degrees of left ventricular enlargement, estimated radiographically, in patients with congenital valvular and subvalvular aortic stenosis.

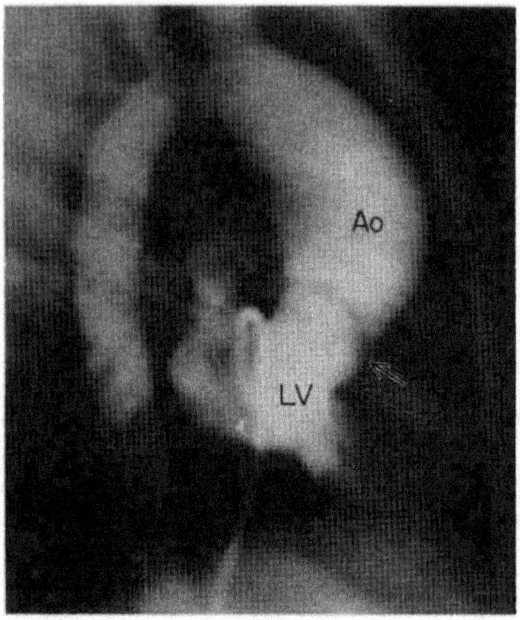

FIGURE 15. Left ventricular angiocardiogram, performed by the transseptal method, in a patient with congenital valvular aortic stenosis. Ao. = post-stenotic dilatation of the aorta. L.V. = left ventricle. The oblique arrows denote the thickened valve cusps.

associated with considerable hazard, making routine use of this procedure undesirable. The development of the transseptal technique of left ventricular angiography has therefore been found to be helpful in the radiological study of aortic stenosis (32). Figure 15 shows a film obtained during a transseptal left ventricular angiocardiogram performed on a patient with congenital aortic valvular stenosis; the thickened, domed, aortic valvular leaflets and post-stenotic dilatation of the ascending aorta are evident. The subvalvular region is widely patent. From this study, the diagnosis of aortic valvular stenosis can be made. Figure 16 was reproduced from a retrograde aortogram performed on a patient with supravalvular aortic stenosis. The caliber of the aortic arch distal to the supravalvular narrowing is very small. In this case, the right coronary artery appears to arise from above the sinuses of Valsalva, and it is not as dilated as the left coronary artery. This is because the right coronary artery arises from above the area of stenosis in the aorta. Even the left coronary artery in this patient is not as dilated as it is frequently in supravalvular aortic stenosis.

In an analysis of 50 patients with acquired aortic stenosis (33), it was found that in 90 per cent some degree of left ventricular enlargement was present. Thirteen per cent had markedly enlarged left ventricles. Marked enlargement of the left ventricle, on the other hand, was uncommon in our patients with congenital stenosis. Post-stenotic dilatation of the ascending aorta was present to some degree in 90 per cent of the patients with acquired aortic stenosis, which is somewhat more frequent than in the patients with congenital aortic stenosis. Radiological enlargement of the left atrium was noted in 30 per cent of the cases with acquired stenosis as compared with 9 per cent in the congenital cases. Radiologic evidence of calcification of the aortic valves was noted in 78 per cent of the patients with acquired disease and in only 18 per cent of those with congenital aortic stenosis.

While it is apparent from the preceding discussion that, in general, patients with acquired aortic valvular stenosis have larger left ventricles, more dilatation of the ascending aorta, a higher incidence of enlarged left atria, and a much higher incidence of calcification of the aortic valves than do patients with congenital aortic stenosis, it must be remembered that the average age (46 years) of patients with the acquired form of the disease was about 30 years greater than in the group of patients with the congenital form. It is not unreasonable to assume that many of the differences between the radiological appearances of congenital and acquired aortic valvular stenosis are due to the great difference in age between the 2 groups.

DR. EUGENE BRAUNWALD: The previous speakers have already referred to idiopathic hypertrophic subaortic stenosis. This con-

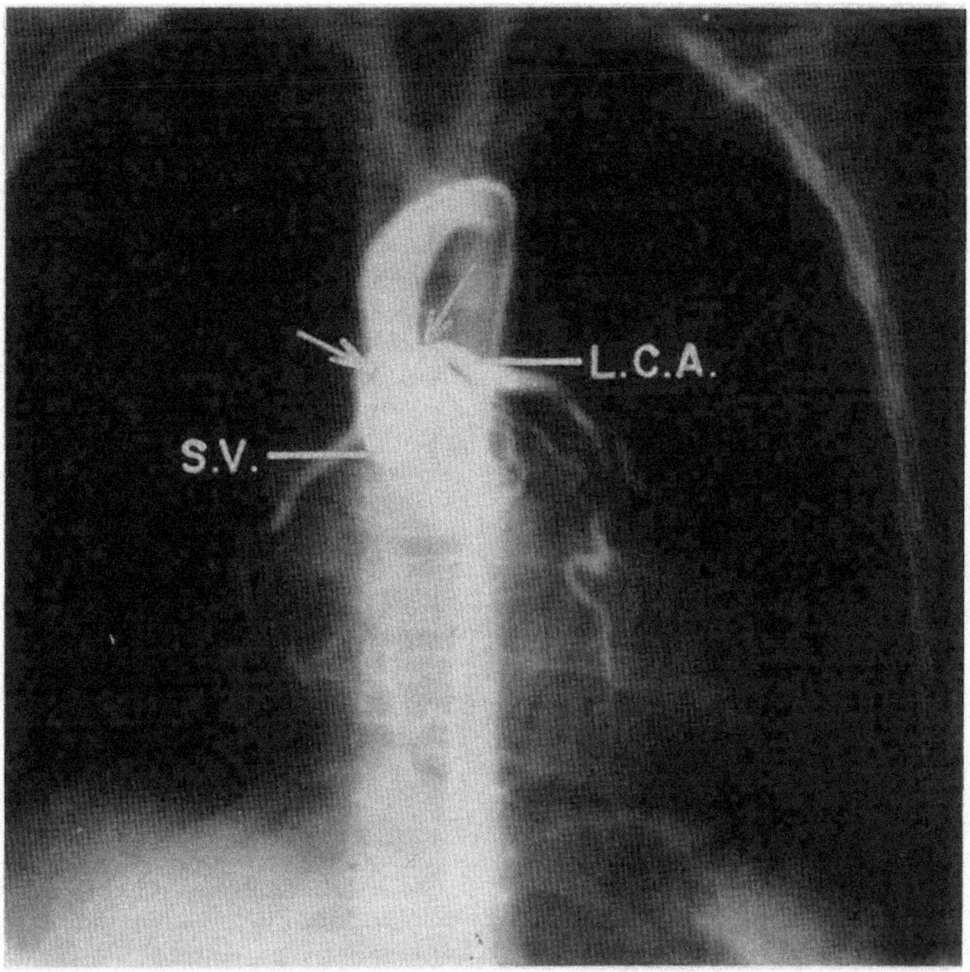

FIGURE 16. Retrograde thoracic aortogram in a patient with supravalvular aortic stenosis, in the frontal projection. S.V. = dilated sinus of Valsalva. L.C.A. = dilated left coronary artery. The oblique arrows denote the supravalvular constriction.

dition, which is being recognized with increasing frequency, can be classified as one of the cardiomyopathies of unexplained etiology (34). Pathologically, ventricular hypertrophy is diffuse, but the interventricular septum is usually disproportionately thickened. The obstruction to left ventricular outflow results from systolic narrowing of the hypertrophied left ventricular outflow tract.

One of the most intriguing aspects of this disease is the variability of the obstruction that it produces (35). In patients with hypertrophic subaortic stenosis, obstruction is not uniform throughout all of ventricular ejection, as it is in the other forms of aortic stenosis. The sharp upstroke of the systemic arterial pulse suggests that ejection is not impeded during the first portion of ventricular systole, and the sharp cutoff in the pulse during mid-systole indicates that the obstruction becomes manifest later in the course of ejection. In our early experience with this condition it was noted that selective angiocardiograms of the left ventricle revealed an inverted cone, which was considered to be characteristic of hypertrophic subaortic stenosis (13); the apex of the cone was thought to represent the site of obstruction. However, more recent cineangiographic observations have suggested that the inverted cone is not pathognomonic for hypertrophic subaortic stenosis, and that in some instances the cone is more prominent during early diastole rather than during systole. Presumably, the septal leaflet of the mitral valve contributes to the appearance of the inverted cone. Although not absolutely specific, we still consider that this radiologic sign, when taken together with the irregular encroachment on the left ventricular cavity by the asymmetric muscular hypertrophy, is of aid in the diagnosis of idiopathic hypertrophic subaortic stenosis.

Obstruction to left ventricular outflow varies not only during the course of one systole, but varies from moment to moment, depending on the force of ventricular contraction. Thus, the augmented contraction which characterizes the beat following a premature contraction results in a paradoxical decline in the arterial pulse pressure. The latter presumably represents a reduced stroke volume consequent to the excessive narrowing of the ventricular outflow tract during the more vigorous contraction (36). Similarly, augmentation of the force of contraction by digitalis glycosides (37) and by isoproterenol (Isuprel) (38) tends to increase the severity of obstruction. It is likely that both of these drugs resulted in a diminished end-systolic residual volume, and that the latter is associated with accentuated narrowing of the left ventricular outflow tract. Aggravation of obstruction has also been noted when alterations in intraventricular conduction occur (38). This finding supports the hypothesis that the precise sequence of left ventricular excitation and contraction can modify the obstructive process. The administration of methoxamine (Vasoxyl) reduces or even eliminates the systolic intraventricular pressure gradient (38) (Figure 17). The mechanism of this effect is presumably opposite to that of isoproterenol; thus it may involve an increase of the ventricle's end-systolic volume and a consequent increase in the cross-section of the obstructive orifice.

Spontaneous changes in the severity of obstruction have been noted repeatedly. Thus, even large gradients have been found to disappear completely when the same patients were recatheterized (35). It is also of interest to note that while the majority of patients have obstruction to left ventricular outflow, other affected members of their families may present with involvement of both the left and the right ventricular outflow tracts, while in some instances only the right ventricular outflow tract shows significant obstruction. Finally, in the familial form of hypertrophic subaortic stenosis, one member of the family may have all the typical features of the disease without a detectable intraventricular pressure gradient, while the others present the classical form of the disease with obstruction to left ventricular outflow.

It may also be of interest to consider the relationship between idiopathic hypertrophic subaortic stenosis and idiopathic myocardial hypertrophy without obstruction to left ventricular outflow. We have recently studied 11 patients with idiopathic myocardial hypertrophy (39). These patients were either asymptomatic or their symptoms showed little if any progression over many years. None had congestive heart failure, cardiac dilatation, arrhythmias, or evidence of embolization, features which have been considered characteristic of cardiomyopathies. Instead, the clinical findings of a brisk arterial pulse, a loud fourth heart sound, ejection systolic murmur, and evidence of left ventricular hypertrophy on clinical, electrocardiographic, roentgenologic, and angiocardiographic examinations were similar to the findings in patients with idiopathic hypertrophic subaortic stenosis. In contrast, however,

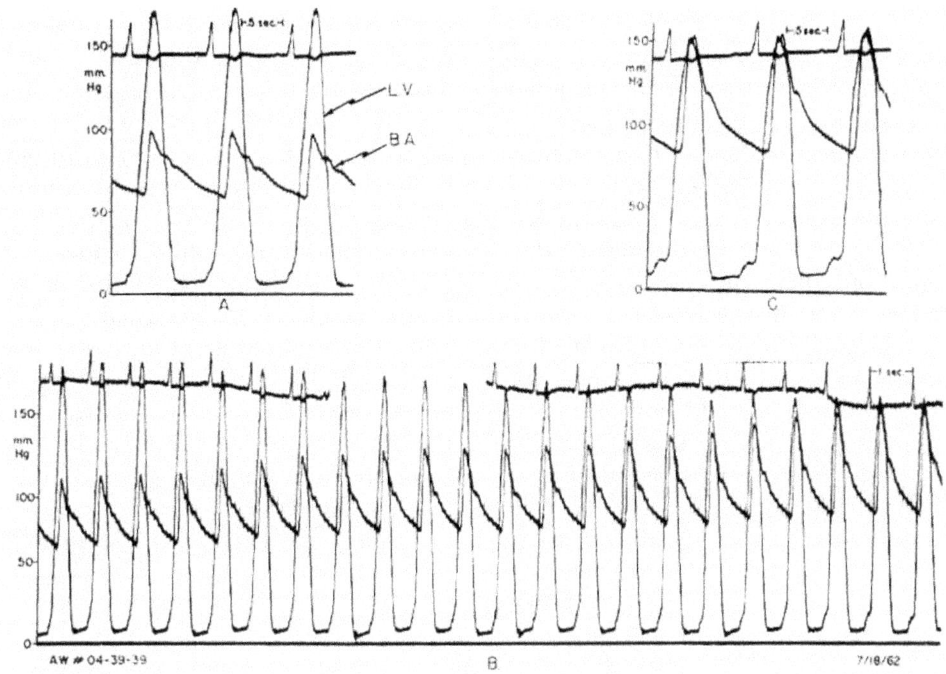

FIGURE 17. Effects of 2 mg methoxamine on the pressure gradient between the left ventricle (L.V.) and the brachial artery (B.A.) in a patient with idiopathic hypertrophic subaortic stenosis. A. = Control pressure tracings, prior to the injection of the drug. The cardiac output, measured by the indicator dilution method, equaled 2.79 liters/min/m² at this time. B. = Continuous tracing recorded as the arterial pressure rose and the left ventricular pressure fell, *i.e.*, as the gradient disappeared, immediately after the administration of methoxamine. C. = Pressure tracings taken after the gradient had disappeared. The cardiac output equaled 2.89 liters/min/m² this time.

none of these 11 patients exhibited any hemodynamic evidence of obstruction to blood flow during the control state. The close relationship between the patients with idiopathic hypertrophic subaortic stenosis and those with idiopathic left ventricular hypertrophy without hemodynamic evidence of obstruction to left ventricular outflow is demonstrated by the tracings reproduced in Figure 18. No pressure gradient was evident during the control tracing. However, a large gradient could be provoked repeatedly by the administration of isoproterenol (Isuprel). It is therefore suggested that the basic disease process in some patients with idiopathic left ventricular hypertrophy without obstruction to ventricular outflow is similar to that which occurs in patients with hypertrophic subaortic stenosis. It seems reasonable to suggest that the presence or absence of the pressure gradient in some of the patients with idiopathic left ventricular hypertrophy is dependent upon the precise localization and severity of the muscular hypertrophy.

The techniques and results of surgical treatment of the various forms of obstruction to left ventricular outflow will now be discussed by Dr. Joseph W. Gilbert.

DR. JOSEPH W. GILBERT: The cardiopulmonary bypass techniques that permit direct-vision operation upon the aortic valve are now familiar to all. Certain maneuvers peculiar to operations performed in this region are, however, noteworthy (17). The heart is exposed through a median sternotomy incision and the right ventricle is cannulated either directly or through the right atrial appendage. A decompression cannula or vent, passed through a stab-wound into the left ventricle, prevents dilatation of this chamber during perfusion. Arterialized blood is returned via a heat-exchanger to a common femoral artery. Tourniquet occlusion of the main pulmonary artery excludes the lungs and the left side of the heart from the circulation; then the aorta is clamped proximal to the arch vessels and is opened. Coronary circulation is maintained during the period in which the valve is exposed by means of an additional arterial line supplying cannulae placed in the coronary ostia. Continuous aspiration of the left ventricle by means of the vent cannula enhances exposure of the valve by obviating the need for a suction tip in the field. Following the institution of cardiopulmonary bypass, total body temperature is reduced promptly to the range of 28 C to 30 C, and commissurotomy, debridement, or replacement procedures are performed as indicated by the pathology encountered. Individual leaflets are replaced as necessary with cusps of Teflon® fabric of the type designed by Bahnson (40). The Muller prosthesis (41) has been employed for total replacement of the aortic valve. Great care is taken to assure the removal of air and calcific material from the left ventricle prior to release of aortic occlusion.

Twenty patients with acquired calcific

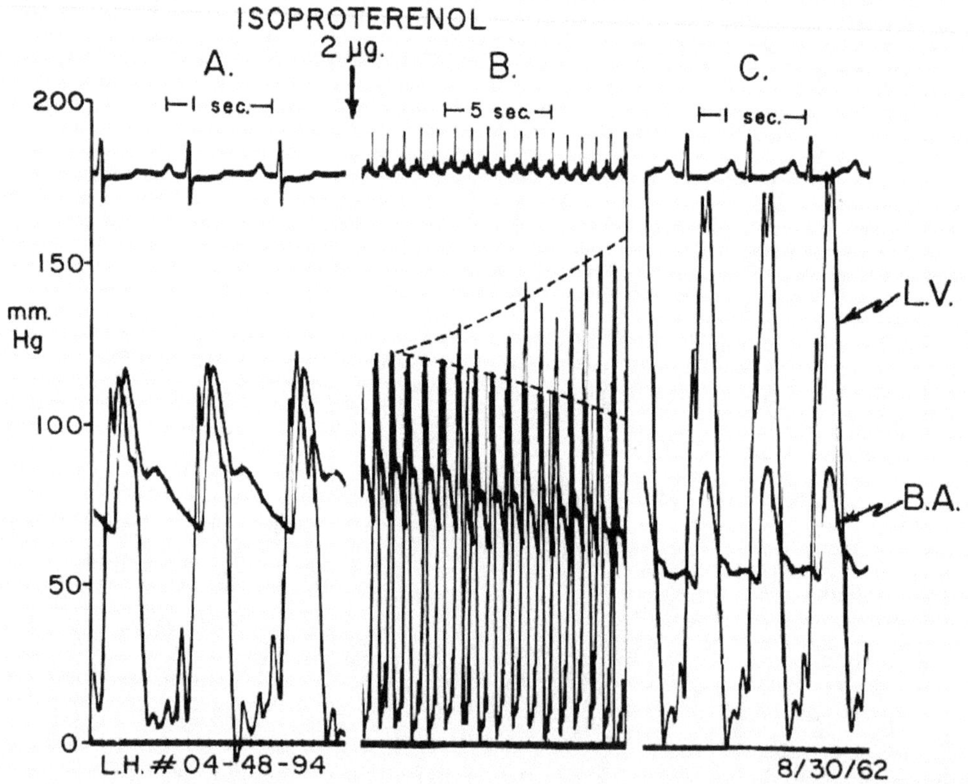

FIGURE 18. Effects of 2 μg isoproterenol on the pressure gradient in a patient with idiopathic left ventricular hypertrophy. The pressure gradient is not present at A., prior to the injection of the drug, at which time the cardiac output equaled 3.05 liter/min/m². The development of a gradient is seen in panel B, recorded at a slower paper speed, immediately after the isoproterenol was given. Panel C shows a large gradient between the left ventricle (L.V.) and brachial artery (B.A.) at the height of the drug effect. The cardiac output equaled 3.31 liters/min/m² at this time.

aortic stenosis were operated upon at the National Heart Institute in 1961 and have been described in detail elsewhere (42). This group consisted of 18 men and 2 women; their average age was 47 years. Incapacitating dyspnea or exercise intolerance (19 patients), angina (14 patients), and syncope (6 patients) constituted the most frequent complaints, and 9 patients had been treated for cardiac failure over a period of 2 to 24 months prior to operation. The classical physical, electrocardiographic, and X-ray findings were present in each patient, and calcification in the region of the aortic valve was demonstrated by fluoroscopy in 12 patients.

The peak systolic gradient across the aortic valve, as determined by transseptal left heart catheterization or percutaneous puncture of the left ventricle, ranged from 50 mm Hg to 132 mm Hg. Effective aortic valve orifices, calculated in 16 patients, ranged from 0.5 cm² per m² BSA to 0.86 cm² per m² BSA. In general, we consider that a peak systolic gradient across the aortic valve of 50 mm Hg or more, under conditions prevail'ng at the time of cardiac catheterization with local anesthesia, or an effective orifice below 0.5 cm² per m² BSA to 0.75 cm² per m² BSA reflects severe obstruction. Although indications for operations must be individualized, such severe obstruction is usually accompanied by serious disability and supports the need for operation.

With use of the techniques described, these procedures were performed: commissurotomy and leaflet debridement in 15 patients, leaflet replacement in 4, and total valve replacement in one patient. Four operative deaths occurred, all in severely ill patients. Irreversible ventricular fibrillation occurred in one patient in the operating room prior to thoracotomy. Coronary embolization of calcific debris accounted for another operating room fatality. One patient died in the recovery room as a consequence of hemorrhage, and another of intractable cardiac failure.

The surgical results as determined by operating room pressure determinations (Figure 19) were judged satisfactory in all but one patient, in whom a systolic gradient of 50 mm Hg across the aortic valve persisted. The pulse pressure, measured by arterial puncture, indicated the presence of significant aortic regurgitation in 3 patients having diastolic pressures below 60 mm Hg. One late death occurred. Although the postoperative interval has been too brief to permit fair evaluation, angina and syncope have been relieved in every instance, and all patients have professed substantial increase in exercise tolerance and general subjective improvement.

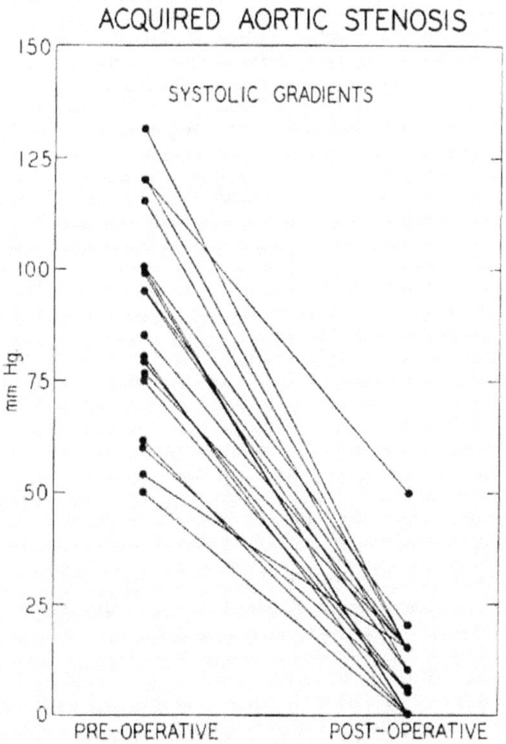

FIGURE 19. Peak systolic left ventricular-brachial artery pressure gradients, as determined by left heart catheterization before operation, and by needle puncture at the operating table immediately after operation, in patients with acquired aortic stenosis.

Dr. Goldblatt has dealt in detail with the relationships between the clinical and hemodynamic findings in 100 patients with congenital aortic stenosis. Fifty-six of these have been subjected to operation, 41 with the aid of cardiopulmonary bypass. These experiences have been presented in detail elsewhere (17). This group consisted of 25 males and 16 females, averaging 15 years of age. The most common complaints were dyspnea (31 patients), fatigability (29 patients), syncope (14 patients), and angina (12 patients). Two patients with congenital aortic stenosis were asymptomatic. The systolic pressure gradients between the left ventricle and a systemic artery ranged from 50 mm Hg to 165 mm Hg. The calculated orifice sizes ranged from 0.32 cm^2 per m^2 BSA to 1.02 cm^2 per m^2 BSA. It is difficult to specify categorical indications for operations in patients with congenital aortic stenosis. For the reasons which have been elaborated by Dr. Goldblatt, however, hemodynamic data are of critical importance in the management of patients in this group. This fact is supported by the recognized incidence of sudden death in carefully followed series (43). Operation has thus been recommended in asymptomatic patients having systolic gradients of 50 mm Hg or more across the aortic valve or aortic valve orifices of 0.5 cm^2 per m^2 BSA or smaller.

At operation the site of obstruction was identified as valvular in 30 patients, 15 of whom had bicuspid valves. In 9 a subvalvular diaphragm was present, and in one patient valvular and subvalvular stenoses were coexistent. Calcification was present in 3 patients. The fused commissures were opened as widely as leaflet competency was judged to permit; this is very difficult to ascertain in patients having bicuspid valves. Rudimentary commissures were opened only partially, if at all. Debridement was performed as necessary, and in one patient in this group leaflet replacement was carried out. Subvalvular diaphragms were

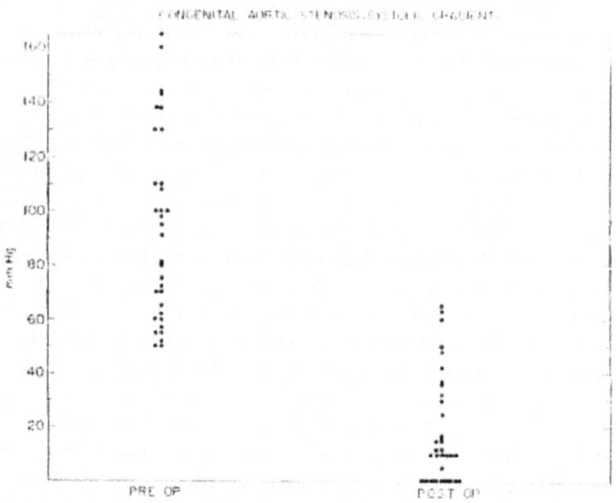

FIGURE 20. Peak systolic left ventricular-brachial artery pressure gradients determined at left heart catheterization both preoperatively and postoperatively in patients with congenital aortic stenosis.

resected as completely as possible. Supravalvular aortic stenosis in 2 patients was managed by the insertion of a diamond-shaped patch in the narrowed valve ring.

Four operative deaths occurred in this group. In 2 patients operated upon early in this experience, satisfactory cardiac action could not be restored following elective potassium citrate asystole. One patient died postoperatively as a consequence of diffuse hemorrhage, and another of renal failure.

The results, as represented by preoperative and postoperative pressure gradients, are shown in Figure 20. Satisfactory relief of the stenotic lesion was obtained in all but 4 patients. Significant aortic incompetence was produced in only 4 patients. The resection of subvalvular diaphragms resulted in mitral incompetence due to damage to the anterior leaflet of this valve in 2 patients. This was satisfactorily corrected in both.

Operative experience with idiopathic hypertrophic subaortic stenosis has been reported recently by Morrow and Brockenbrough (44). Operations have now been performed upon 5 patients. The hypertrophic myocardium was incised from the apex of the left ventricle to the aortic annulus, and more recently resection of portions of the hypertrophied myocardium has also been performed. Postoperative pressure measurements have disclosed the abolition or substantial reduction of the obstruction.

It is apparent from this review of recent experience that considerable progress has been realized in the surgical treatment of the various forms of aortic stenosis. Several questions do, however, remain to be answered: What will be the natural history of patients in whom calcific aortic valves have been reconstituted by debridement and commissurotomy? What will be the ultimate fate of the various types of prosthetic leaflets and valves which have been employed? The solution of such problems and the further evolution of operative correction of aortic stenosis will depend upon the continuing assessment of results over long periods.

Summario in Interlingua

In le hic-reportate conferentia, le characteristicas clinic, pathologic, hemodynamic, radiologic, e chirurgic del varie formas de obstruction del effluxo sinistro-ventricular esseva revistate. Stenosis aortic supravalvular—que es, inter le formas de obstruction discutite, le plus rar—resimila congenite stenosis de valvula aortic in su manifestationes clinic sed pote esser definitivemente diagnosticate per aortographia thoracic. Le tractamento chirurgic de iste anormalitate es usualmente plus difficile que le tractamento de congenite stenosis de valvula aortic. Quando congenite stenosis del valvula aortic o discrete congenite stenosis subvalvular es sever, illo es usualmente associate con dyspnea in effortio, sed angina de pectore e syncope non se monstrava strictemente correlationate con le presentia de sever grados de stenosis. Le electrocardiogramma es possibilemente de adjuta in identificar juveniles de minus que 10 annos de etate con congenite stenosis aortic e leve grados de obstruction, sed illo es alteremente de pauco assistentia in estimar le magnitude del gradiente de pression. Del altere latere, le presentia o absentia del quarte sono cardiac e le comportamento del secunde sono cardiac provide importante indicios relative al severitate del obstruction. In le ultime analyse, le datos obtenite al tempore del catheterismo sinistro-cardiac e del selective angiocardiographia se monstrava del plus grande importantia in le evalutation de patientes con stenosis aortic.

Esseva presentate datos corroboratori pro le existentia de un variabile obstruction del effluxo sinistro-ventricular in patientes con idiopathic hypertrophic stenosis subaortic. Le administration de isoproterenol intensificava le gradiente, durante que methoxamina reduceva o mesmo aboliva le gradiente. Le intime relation inter idiopathic hypertrophia myocardial sin obstruction del effluxo sinistro-ventricular e idiopathic hypertrophic stenosis subaortic esseva sublineate.

Le characteristicas radiologic del varie formas de obstruction del effluxo sinistro-ventricular esseva revistate. Le dimension del corde o del ventriculo sinistre, como illo pote esser estimate roentgenographicamente, provide pauc information in re le sito del stenosis o le severitate del obstruction. Tamen, le presentia de calcification valvular indica que le obstruction se trova al nivello valvular, durante que absentia de dilatation post-stenotic del aorta suggere le presentia de hypertrophic stenosis subaortic o de stenosis aortic supravalvular.

Le technicas chirurgic pro le correction de stenosis aortic e le resultatos del therapia per intervention chirurgic esseva revistate. Sever obstruction, con un gradiente de pression systolic in excesso de 50 mm de Hg inter le ventriculo sinistre e le arteria brachial (con le patiente in stato basal) deberea esser presente ante le effectuation de un operation chirurgic in patientes con ulle del formas de obstruction del effluxo sinistro-ventricular. Juveniles con congenite stenosis valvular o congenite discrete stenosis subvalvular es operate quando illes es asymptomatic, sed patientes con acquirite stenosis aortic e hypertrophic stenosis subaortic debe manifestar significative symptomas e sever grados de obstruction ante que un intervention chirurgic pote esser recommendate.

References

1. Mencarelli, L.: Stenosi sopravalvolare aortica ad anello. *Arch. Ital. Anat. Path.* 1: 829, 1930.
2. Denie, J. J., Verheugt, A. P.: Supravalvular aortic stenosis. *Circulation* 18: 902, 1958.
3. Morrow, A. G., Waldhausen, J. A., Peters, R. L., Bloodwell, R. D., Braunwald, E.: Supravalvular aortic stenosis. Clinical, hemodynamic and pathologic observations. *Circulation* 20: 1003, 1959.
4. Perou, M. L.: Congenital supravalvular aortic stenosis. *Arch. Path.* 71: 453, 1961.

5. Wooley, C. F., Hosier, D. M., Booth, R. W., Molnar, W., Sirak, H. D., Ryan, J. M.: Supravalvular aortic stenosis: clinical experiences with four patients including familial occurrence. *Amer. J. Med.* 31: 717, 1961.
6. Edwards, J. E.: Pathologic aspects of cardiac valvular insufficiencies. *Arch. Surg.* 77: 634, 1958.
7. Edwards, J. E.: Editorial. The congenital bicuspid aortic valve. *Circulation* 23: 485, 1961.
8. Edwards, J. E.: Calcific aortic stenosis: pathologic features. *Proc. Mayo Clin.* 36: 444, 1961.
9. Osler, W.: The Gulstonian Lectures on malignant endocarditis. *Brit. Med. J.* 1: 522, 1885.
10. Andriole, V. T., Kravetz, H. M., Roberts, W. C., Utz, J. P.: Candida endocarditis: clinical and pathological studies. *Amer. J. Med.* 32: 251, 1962.
11. McKusick, V. A., Logue, R. B., Bahnson, H. T.: Association of aortic valvular disease and cystic medial necrosis of the ascending aorta. Report of four instances. *Circulation* 16: 188, 1957.
12. Heath, D., Edwards, J. E., Smith, L. A.: The rheologic significance of medial necrosis and dissecting aneurysm of the ascending aorta in association with calcific aortic stenosis. *Proc. Mayo Clin.* 33: 228, 1958.
13. Braunwald, E., Morrow, A. G., Cornell, W. P., Aygen, M. M., Hilbish, T. F.: Idiopathic hypertrophic subaortic stenosis. Clinical, hemodynamic and angiographic manifestations. *Amer. J. Med.* 29: 924, 1960.
14. Neufeld, H. N., Ongley, P. A., Edwards, J. E.: Combined congenital subaortic stenosis and infundibular pulmonary stenosis. *Brit. Heart J.* 22: 686, 1960.
15. Brachfeld, N., Gorlin, R.: Subaortic stenosis. A revised concept of the disease. *Medicine* 38: 415, 1959.
16. Braunwald, E., Goldblatt, A., Aygen, M. M., Rockoff, S. D., Morrow, A. G.: Congenital aortic stenosis. I. Clinical and hemodynamic findings in 100 patients. *Circulation.* In press.
17. Morrow, A. G., Goldblatt, A., Braunwald, E.: Congenital aortic stenosis II. Surgical treatment and the results of operation. *Circulation.* In press.
18. Taussig, H. B.: *Congenital Malformations of the Heart*, 2d Ed., Harvard University Press, Cambridge, 1960, Vol. II, p. 835.
19. Ongley, P. A., Nadas, A. S., Paul, M. H., Rudolph, A. M., Starkey, G. W. B.: Aortic stenosis in infants and children. *Pediatrics* 21: 207, 1958.
20. Spencer, F. C., Neill, C. A., Sank, L., Bahnson, H. T.: Anatomical variations in 46 patients with congenital aortic stenosis. *Amer. Surg.* 26: 204, 1960.
21. Brockenbrough, E. C., Braunwald, E., Ross, J., Jr.: Transseptal left heart catheterization: a review of 450 studies and description of an improved technic. *Circulation* 25: 15, 1962.
22. Mark, H., Jacobson, B., Young, D.: Coexistence of patent ductus arteriosus and congenital aortic valvular disease. *Circulation* 17: 359, 1958.
23. Ellis, F. H., Jr., Kirklin, J. W.: Congenital valvular aortic stenosis: anatomic findings and surgical technique. *J. Thor. Cardiov. Surg.* 43: 199, 1962.
24. Gorlin, R., Gorlin, S. G.: Hydraulic formula for calculation of the area of the stenotic mitral valve, other cardiac valves, and central circulatory shunts. I. *Amer. Heart J.* 41: 1, 1951.
25. Weissler, A. M., Peeler, R. G., Roehll, W. H., Jr.: Relationships between left ventricular ejection time, stroke volume, and heart rate in normal individuals and patients with cardiovascular disease. *Amer. Heart J.* 62: 367, 1961.
26. Wolferth, C. C., Margolies, A.: *Heart Sounds in Diagnosis and Treatment of Cardiovascular Diseases*, ed. by Stroud, W. D., and Stroud, M. W., 5th ed., F. A. Davis Company, Philadelphia, 1957, p. 33.
27. Hancock, E. W. Differentiation of valvar, subvalvar and supravalvar aortic stenosis. *Guy's Hosp. Rep.* 110: 1, 1961.
28. Leatham, A., Vogelpoel, L.: The early systolic sound in dilatation of the pulmonary artery. *Brit. Heart J.* 16: 21, 1954.
29. Mounsey, P.: Praecordial pulsations in relation to cardiac movement and sounds. *Brit. Heart J.* 21: 457, 1959.
30. Goldblatt, A., Aygen, M. M., Braunwald, E.: Hemodynamic-phonocardiographic correlations of the fourth heart sound in aortic stenosis. *Circulation* 26: 92, 1962.
31. Aygen, M. M., Braunwald, E.: The splitting of the second heart sound in normal subjects and in patients with congenital heart disease. *Circulation* 25: 328, 1962.
32. Braunwald, E., Brockenbrough, E. C., Talbert, J. L., Folse, J. R., Rockoff, S. D.: Selective left heart angiocardiography by the transseptal route. *Amer. J. Med.* 33: 213, 1962.
33. Rockoff, S. D., Austen, W. G.: The hemodynamic significance of the radiological changes in acquired aortic stenosis. *Amer. Heart J.* In press.
34. Goodwin, J. F., Gordon, H., Hallman, A., Bishop, M. B.: Clinical aspects of cardiomyopathy. *Brit. Med. J.* 1: 69, 1961.
35. Braunwald, E., Brockenbrough, E. C., Morrow, A. G.: Editorial. Hypertrophic subaortic stenosis—a broadened concept. *Circulation* 26: 161, 1962.
36. Brockenbrough, E. C., Braunwald, E., Morrow, A. G.: A hemodynamic technic for the detection of hypertrophic subaortic stenosis. *Circulation* 23: 189, 1961.
37. Braunwald, E., Brockenbrough, E. C., Frye, R. L.: Studies on digitalis: V. Comparison

of the effects of ouabain on left ventricular dynamics in valvular aortic stenosis and hypertrophic subaortic stenosis. *Circulation* 26: 166, 1962.

38. Braunwald, E., Ebert, P. A.: Hemodynamic alterations in idiopathic hypertrophic subaortic stenosis induced by sympathomimetic drugs. *Amer. J. Cardiol.* 10: 489, 1962.

39. Braunwald, E., Aygen, M. M.: Idiopathic myocardial hypertrophy without congestive heart failure or obstruction to blood flow: clinical, hemodynamic, and angiocardiographic studies in eleven patients. *Amer. J. Med.* In press.

40. Bahnson, H. T., Spencer, F. C., Busse, E. F. G., Davis, F. W., Jr.: Cusp replacement and coronary artery perfusion in open operations on the aortic valve. *Ann. Surg.* 152: 494, 1960.

41. Muller, W. H., Jr., Littlefield, J. G., Dummann, J. F., Jr.: "Subcoronary Prosthetic Replacement of the Aortic Valve," in *Prosthetic Valves for Cardiac Surgery,* Charles C Thomas, Springfield, Illinois, 1961, p. 403.

42. Morrow, A. G., Austen, W. G., Braunwald, E.: The surgical treatment of calcific aortic stenosis: operative methods and the results of pre- and postoperative hemodynamic assessments. *Ann. Surg.* In press.

43. Braverman, I. B., Gibson, S.: The outlook for children with congenital aortic stenosis. *Amer. Heart J.* 53: 487, 1957.

44. Morrow, A. G., Brockenbrough, E. C.: Surgical treatment of idiopathic hypertrophic subaortic stenosis. *Ann. Surg.* 154: 181, 1961.

CONGENITAL AORTIC STENOSIS PRODUCED BY A UNICOMMISSURAL VALVE

BY

WILLIAM C. ROBERTS AND ANDREW G. MORROW

From the Clinic of Surgery, National Heart Institute, National Institutes of Health, Bethesda, Maryland, U.S.A.

Received September 25, 1964

At the National Heart Institute we have studied a large number of patients in whom obstruction to left ventricular outflow resulted from a congenital malformation of the aortic valve. In each, the congenital basis of the stenotic lesion was established by a history of a præcordial murmur before the age of 5 years and/or by the structure of the valve as determined at open operation or at necropsy. In 4 of these patients, the valve was proved to consist of only a single cusp and a single commissure. This report summarizes the clinical and pathological findings in these 4 patients, and calls attention to the importance of recognizing this unusual form of valvular aortic stenosis when operative treatment is undertaken.

Case Reports

Case 1. A 28-year-old mechanic grew and developed normally. A præcordial murmur was discovered during a routine examination when he was 17 years of age. He was asymptomatic until 5 months before admission when he developed dyspnœa on exertion, orthopnœa, hæmoptysis, hepatomegaly, and œdema of the ankles. On examination, the blood pressure was 100/80 mm. Hg. A grade 2/6 ejection-type systolic murmur and a grade 2/6 blowing diastolic murmur were heard at the base of the heart and along the left sternal border. A third heart sound was audible at the cardiac apex. The electrocardiogram disclosed left bundle-branch block. The chest radiograph showed considerable cardiomegaly with particular prominence of the left ventricle and left atrium. The patient died one month after admission while being treated for severe congestive cardiac failure.

Case 2. A 16-year-old boy had been found to have a præcordial murmur at birth, but his growth and development were normal. At the age of 11 years, he first noted occasional substernal chest pain and, in subsequent years, mild exertional dyspnœa and easy fatiguability developed. On examination, a grade 5/6 ejection-type systolic murmur was heard at the base of the heart and over the carotid arteries. No diastolic murmur was audible. The electrocardiogram showed left ventricular hypertrophy and a left ventricular conduction delay. Radiographic examinations revealed moderate left ventricular enlargement. At left heart catheterization the mean left atrial pressure was 17 mm. Hg, the left ventricular pressure 230/8 mm. Hg, and the brachial arterial pressure, measured simultaneously, 105/75 mm. Hg. The peak systolic pressure gradient was 125 mm. Hg. The evening before a scheduled operation the patient suddenly developed ventricular fibrillation and died.

Case 3. A 9-year-old boy was found to have a præcordial murmur at birth. Growth and development were normal and he was entirely asymptomatic. Examination disclosed a grade 4/6 ejection-type systolic murmur at the base of the heart, which was referred over the entire præcordium and into the neck. No diastolic murmur was audible. The electrocardiogram was interpreted as normal, and chest radiograph disclosed only mild left ventricular enlargement. Cardiac catheterization disclosed normal pressures in the right-sided cardiac chambers. The pressures in the left ventricle (percutaneous puncture) and brachial artery were 190/11 and 104/50 mm. Hg, respectively, giving a peak systolic pressure gradient of 86 mm. Hg.

On August 8, 1958, aortic valvulotomy was performed during extracorporeal circulation and a period of elective cardiac arrest induced with potassium citrate. The orifice of the aortic valve was eccentric and the valve appeared to be of the usual bicuspid type with fusion of the posterior of the two commissures. Accordingly, the valve was incised posteriorly from the orifice to the aortic wall. When circulation was restored, there was evidence of severe aortic regurgitation; the left ventricle was dilated, and a diastolic thrill was palpable in the aorta and left ventricle. After operation, the patient bled excessively and was returned to the operating room for evacuation of a hæmothorax. Cardiac standstill occurred during this procedure and resuscitation was unsuccessful.

Case 4. A 32-year-old housewife had been found to have a præcordial murmur at the age of 5 years. Growth and development were normal and she was asymptomatic until age 29 when she developed streptococcal endocarditis, which responded to treatment with penicillin. Thereafter, she was well until 5 months before admission when angina pectoris and signs and symptoms of right- and left-sided congestive cardiac failure developed. On examination, a grade 3/6 ejection-type systolic murmur was heard at the base of the heart and over the carotid arteries. No diastolic murmur was audible. The electrocardiogram indicated a previous anterior myocardial infarct, left ventricular and left atrial hypertrophy, and S–T segment changes compatible with subendocardial injury. A percutaneous left ventricular puncture revealed a left ventricular pressure of 176/26 mm. Hg; simultaneous brachial arterial pressure was 82/66 mm. Hg; the peak systolic pressure gradient was 90 mm. Hg. The patient's cardiac failure was refractory to treatment, and she died one month after admission.

The relevant clinical data concerning each of the patients are summarized in the Table.

TABLE

CLINICAL AND PATHOLOGICAL FEATURES IN 4 PATIENTS WITH UNICOMMISSURAL AORTIC VALVULAR STENOSIS

Case No.	Age (yr.) at death, and sex	Age (yr.) præcordial murmur first detected	Age (yr.) cardiac signs or symptoms appeared	Angina pectoris	Syncope	Congestive heart failure	Murmur of aortic regurgitation	Electrocardiogram	Peak systolic aorta-LV gradient (mm. Hg)	Calcium in aortic valve	Weight of heart (g.)
1	28 M	16	27	0	0	++++	+	Left BBB	—	++++	600
2	16 M	At birth	9	0	0	+	0	LVH, LVS	125	++	650
3	9* M	At birth	Asymptomatic	0	0	0	0	Normal	86	0	200†
4	32 M	5	29	+	0	++++	0	Old myocardial infarct LVH, LAH	90	++++	500

* Died following aortic valvulotomy.
† Average weight for normal heart in 9-year-old boy is 115 g.
LV, left ventricle; BBB, bundle-branch block; LVH, left ventricular hypertrophy; LVS, left ventricular strain; LAH, left atrial hypertrophy.

PATHOLOGICAL FINDINGS

The aortic valve in each of the 4 patients consisted of only one cusp and one commissure and was severely stenotic. The appearance of each valve is illustrated in Fig. 1. The single cusp was diffusely fibrotic in all four patients and calcified in three of them. In Case 1 the valve was completely rigid and, since the leaflet could not move during either phase of the cardiac cycle, the valve was regurgitant as well as stenotic. The hearts of all 4 patients demonstrated hypertrophy, predominantly of the left ventricle; in the 3 older patients they weighed 500 to 650 g., and the heart of the child weighed 200 g. (normal 115 g.). The tricuspid, pulmonary, and mitral valves and the coronary arteries were normal in all 4 patients. The heart of Case 4 was placed in a pulse-duplicator (Davila *et al.*, 1956) and the aortic valve was visualized as it functioned (Fig. 2). It was observed that during ventricular diastole the mass of calcium in the valve was pushed against the aortic wall at the sites of the coronary ostia. The relation of the calcified valve to the coronary ostia is also shown in Fig. 3 and 4. This patient had several healed infarcts in the left ventricle and ventricular septum, but the coronary arteries were widely patent and free of atheroma. This combination of findings indicated that infarction had resulted from intermittent occlusion of the coronary ostia by the calcareous mass. Histological examination of the left ventricle of Case 3 revealed extensive areas of acute myocardial necrosis, a finding subsequently proved to result from the use of potassium citrate to induce cardiac arrest (McFarland *et al.*, 1960).

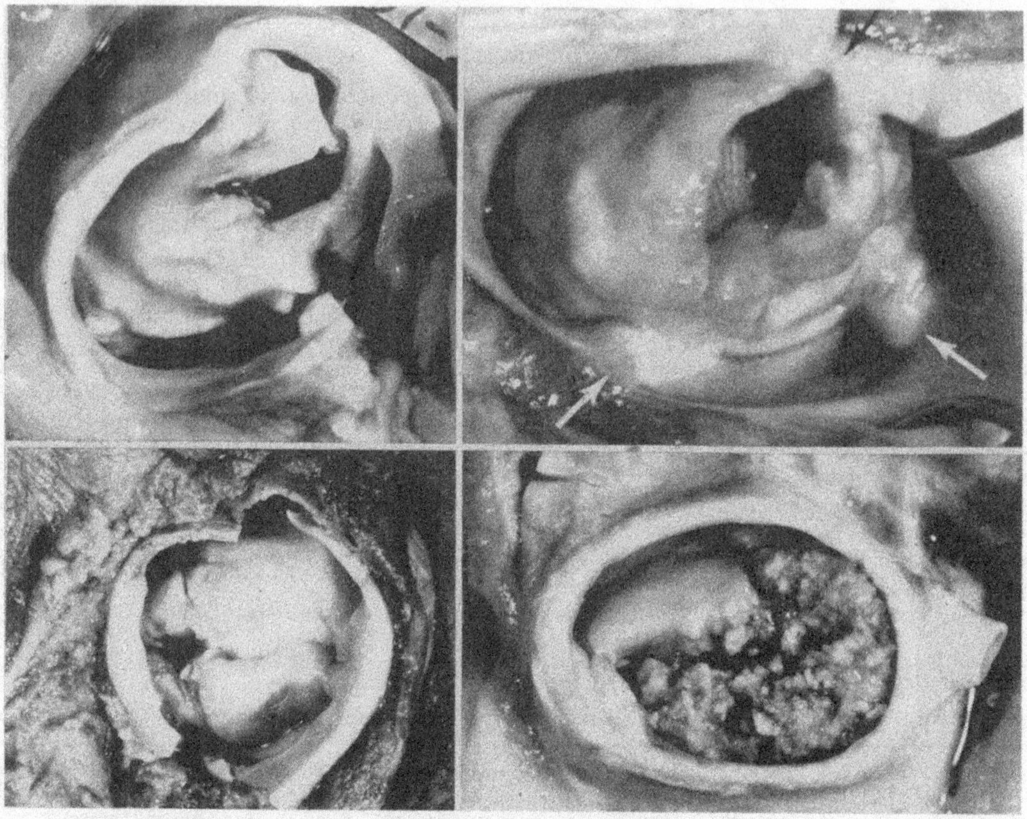

FIG. 1.—Photographs of the aortic valve from above in the four patients. *Upper left:* Case 1. *Upper right:* Case 2. *Lower left:* Case 3. *Lower right:* Case 4. The arrows in the upper right photograph indicate the true commissure (black arrow) and false commissures or raphes (white arrows).

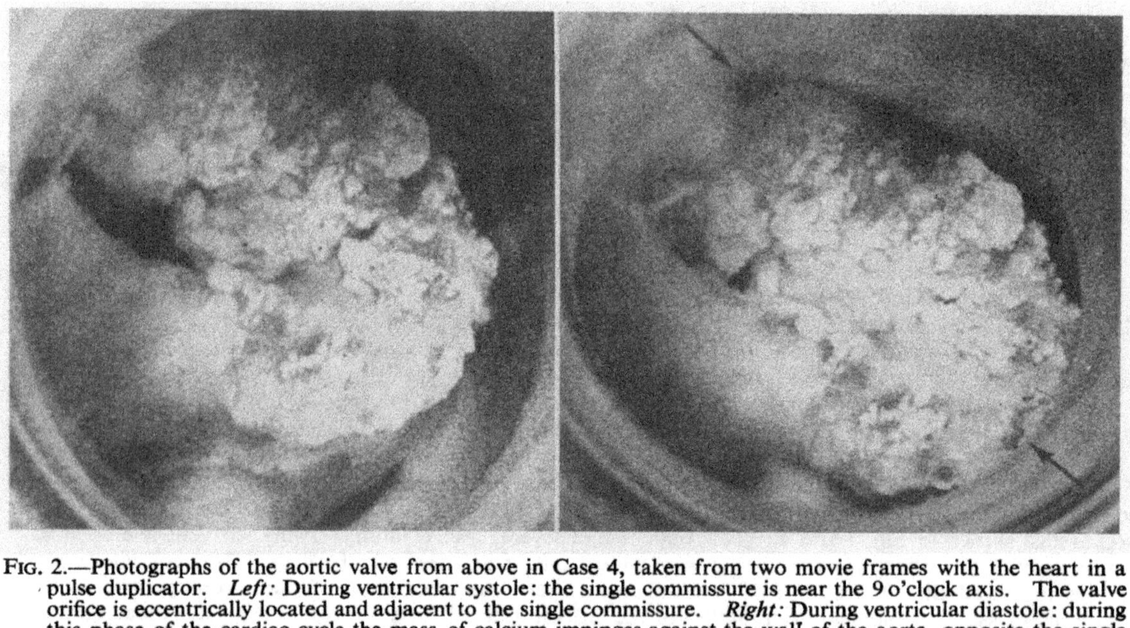

FIG. 2.—Photographs of the aortic valve from above in Case 4, taken from two movie frames with the heart in a pulse duplicator. *Left:* During ventricular systole: the single commissure is near the 9 o'clock axis. The valve orifice is eccentrically located and adjacent to the single commissure. *Right:* During ventricular diastole: during this phase of the cardiac cycle the mass of calcium impinges against the wall of the aorta, opposite the single commissure. The locations of the coronary arterial ostia are indicated by the arrows. In this patient, angina pectoris and myocardial infarction apparently resulted from partial obstruction of the coronary ostia during ventricular diastole by the mass of calcium in the aortic valve.

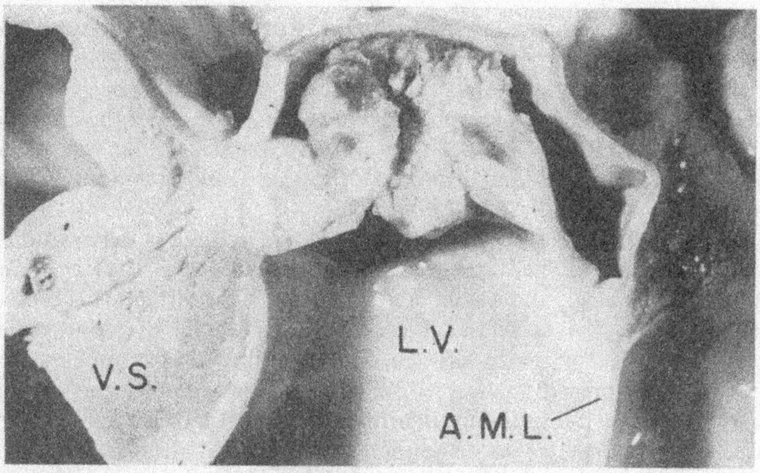

Fig. 3.—Photograph illustrating the aortic valve of Case 4 following removal of its anterior half. The dome-shaped configuration of the valve is apparent. L.V.=left ventricle; V.S.=ventricular septum; A.M.L.=anterior mitral leaflet.

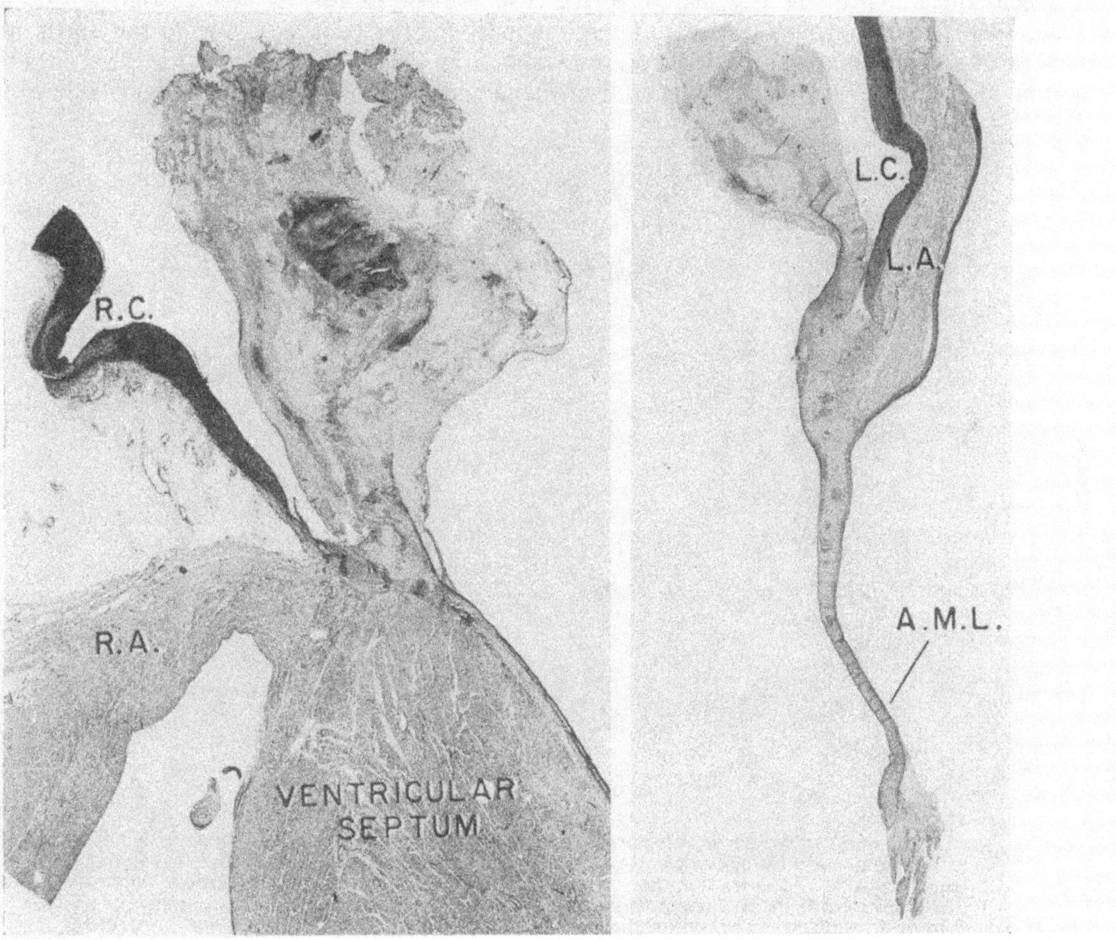

Fig. 4.—Photomicrographs of the fibrotic and calcified aortic valve cusp in Case 4. *Left:* The ostium of the right coronary artery (R.C.) is shown. *Right:* The ostium of the left coronary artery (L.C.) is demonstrated. The ostia of both coronary arteries, particularly the left one, were compromised during ventricular diastole by the large calcified mass contacting the aortic wall. R.A.=right atrial wall; L.A.=left atrial wall; A.M.L.=anterior mitral leaflet. (Verhoeff-van Gieson elastic tissue stains; magnification ×5 *left*, ×3 *right*.)

Comment

Several anatomically different congenital malformations of the aortic valve producing obstruction to left ventricular outflow have been encountered at open operation. Spencer *et al.* (1960) found in the majority of their 27 patients that the valve was essentially bicuspid, but a third commissure was often evident. This type of bicuspid valve was present in 29 of the 33 patients described by Ellis and Kirklin (1962), and it also has been the most frequent valvular malformation encountered in this clinic (Morrow, Goldblatt, and Braunwald, 1963). Less commonly, three well-formed leaflets and commissures are present.

Edwards (1958) described the appearance of the aortic valves in three patients studied at necropsy. In each, the valve was dome-shaped, had an eccentrically located orifice (having the appearance of an exclamation point), a single cusp, and a single commissure. He termed this type of valve "unicommissural dome stenosis". Valves of this type, as illustrated by the four patients described above, produce considerable obstruction to left ventricular outflow, but it appears that they cannot be identified pre-operatively by present methods of clinical, hæmodynamic, and angiographic study. Even at operation or necropsy, the unicommissural domed aortic valve may be mistaken for a bicuspid valve, since frequently one or more raphes are present at the base of the aortic wall at some point away from the true commissure. On careful gross examination such raphes may be distinguished from true commissures since they do not extend far from the base of the leaflet toward its free edge; that is, they fail to reach as high on the aortic wall as the true commissure, the height of which equals that of the free margin of the cusp. These raphes, as pointed out by Edwards (1958, 1960), do not provide adequate lateral support for the valvular tissue to the aortic wall. Incision of a unicommissural aortic valve, as illustrated in Case 3 (Fig. 5), produces two flaps that have no attachment to the aortic wall, and overwhelming aortic regurgitation is an inevitable sequel.

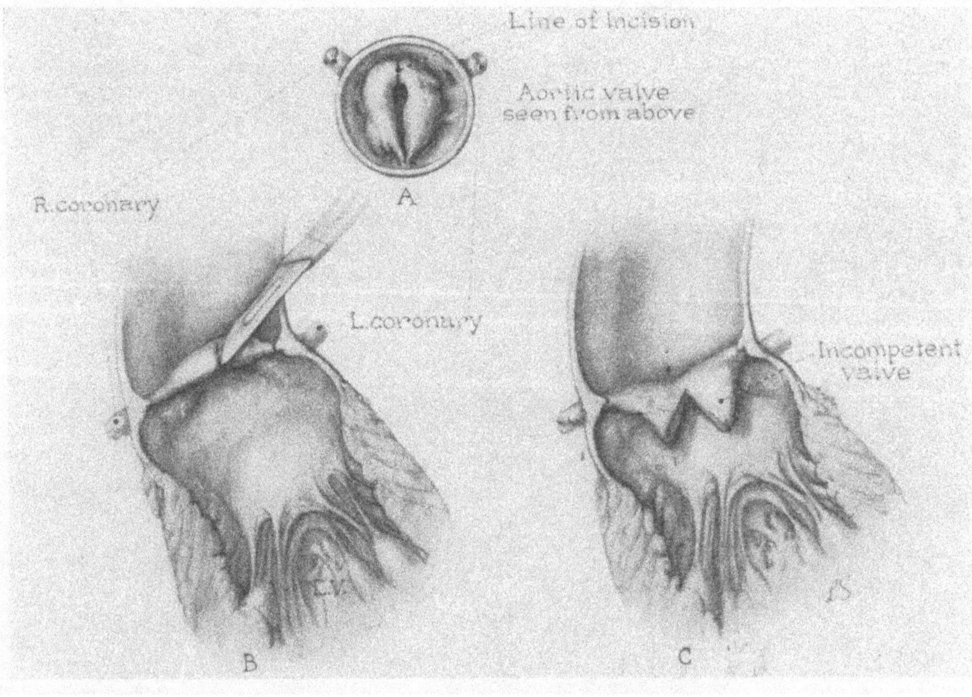

Fig. 5.—Drawings of the aortic valve before and after valvulotomy, Case 3. The true commissure is located at the 6 o'clock axis and two raphes are also present (A). The valve was free of calcium deposits. At operation, the valve was judged to be bicuspid and an incision was made in the cusp opposite the true commissure (B). The incision resulted in two flaps, neither of which had an attachment to the wall of the aorta, and massive aortic regurgitation was produced (C).

Unicommissural valves were present in two of the patients reported by Ellis and Kirklin (1962), and valvulotomy was performed in each of them. Severe aortic regurgitation did not result, but they do not state whether or not stenosis was relieved. The pathological findings in the present four patients indicate that when left ventricular outflow obstruction is found to be caused by a unicommissural aortic valve, simple valvulotomy is contraindicated and that excision and prosthetic replacement of the valve is the only means by which effective hæmodynamic function can be restored.

Summary

Four patients are described in whom severe left ventricular outflow obstruction resulted from a congenitally malformed aortic valve which consisted of only a single cusp and a single commissure. The clinical and hæmodynamic examinations did not differ from those seen in patients with the more common types of congenital valvular aortic stenosis. The pathological findings indicate that when this malformation is encountered at operation simple valvulotomy is contraindicated, since massive aortic regurgitation will almost certainly result. The only effective method of surgical treatment appears to be prosthetic replacement of the unicommissural valve.

References

Davila, J. C., Trout, R. G., Sunner, J. E., and Glover, R. P. (1956). A simple mechanical pulse duplicator for cinematography of cardiac valves in action. *Ann. Surg.*, **143**, 544.

Edwards, J. E. (1958). Pathologic aspects of cardiac valvular insufficiencies. *Arch. Surg.*, **77**, 634.

—— (1960). Congenital malformations of the heart and great vessels. Malformations of the valves. In *Pathology of the Heart*, ed. S. E. Gould, 2nd ed., p. 409. Charles C Thomas, Springfield, Illinois.

Ellis, F. H., and Kirklin, J. W. (1962). Congenital valvular aortic stenosis: Anatomic findings and surgical technique. *J. thorac. cardiovasc. Surg.*, **43**, 199.

McFarland, J. A., Thomas, L. B., Gilbert, J. W., and Morrow, A. G. (1960). Myocardial necrosis following elective cardiac arrest induced with potassium citrate. *J. thorac. cardiovasc. Surg.*, **40**, 200.

Morrow, A. G., Goldblatt, A., and Braunwald, E. (1963). Congenital aortic stenosis. II. Surgical treatment and the results of operation. *Circulation*, **27**, 450.

Spencer, F. C., Neill, C. A., Sank, L., and Bahnson, H. T. (1960). Anatomical variations in 46 patients with congenital aortic stenosis. *Amer. Surg.*, **26**, 204.

Cardiac Valves and the Surgical Pathologist

WILLIAM C. ROBERTS, MD, AND ANDREW G. MORROW, MD, BETHESDA, MD

The excised cardiac valve should not be processed as a "routine surgical specimen." The most precise pathologic diagnosis will probably result from careful gross inspection of the valve, and not from histologic examination of sections of it. Photographs of the valve provide the most effective record of the pathologic findings, and permit correlations between the anatomic malformation and the clinical, hemodynamic, and operative findings.

Accepted for publication June 29, 1966.

From the Clinic of Surgery, National Heart Institute, National Institutes of Health, Bethesda, Md.

Reprint requests to Laboratory of Pathology, Clinic of Surgery, National Heart Institute, National Institutes of Health, Bethesda, Md 20014 (Dr. Roberts).

COINCIDENT with the development and widespread clinical use of prosthetic heart valves, the surgical pathologist has been introduced to a new type of specimen, the cardiac valve. Prior to the modern era of intracardiac surgery, valves were seen by the pathologist only at autopsy, but in many medical centers one or more cardiac valves now appear in the pathological laboratory almost daily. Classically, the surgical pathologist's examination of excised tissue consists of gross inspection and description, followed by sectioning of the specimen for histologic study; with most tissues the diagnosis will

Fig 1.—Mitral valve (S63-2480) in a 46-year-old woman with severe mitral regurgitation (left ventricular cineangiocardiogram) and moderate mitral stenosis (10 mm Hg left atrial to left ventricular mean diastolic pressure gradient). *Top left,* A view from left atrial aspect. *Top right,* Anterior mitral leaflet is depicted here demonstrating that the leaflets insert almost directly into the papillary muscles. *Bottom left,* A view from left ventricular aspect. *Bottom right,* Radiograph showing minimal calcium deposits.

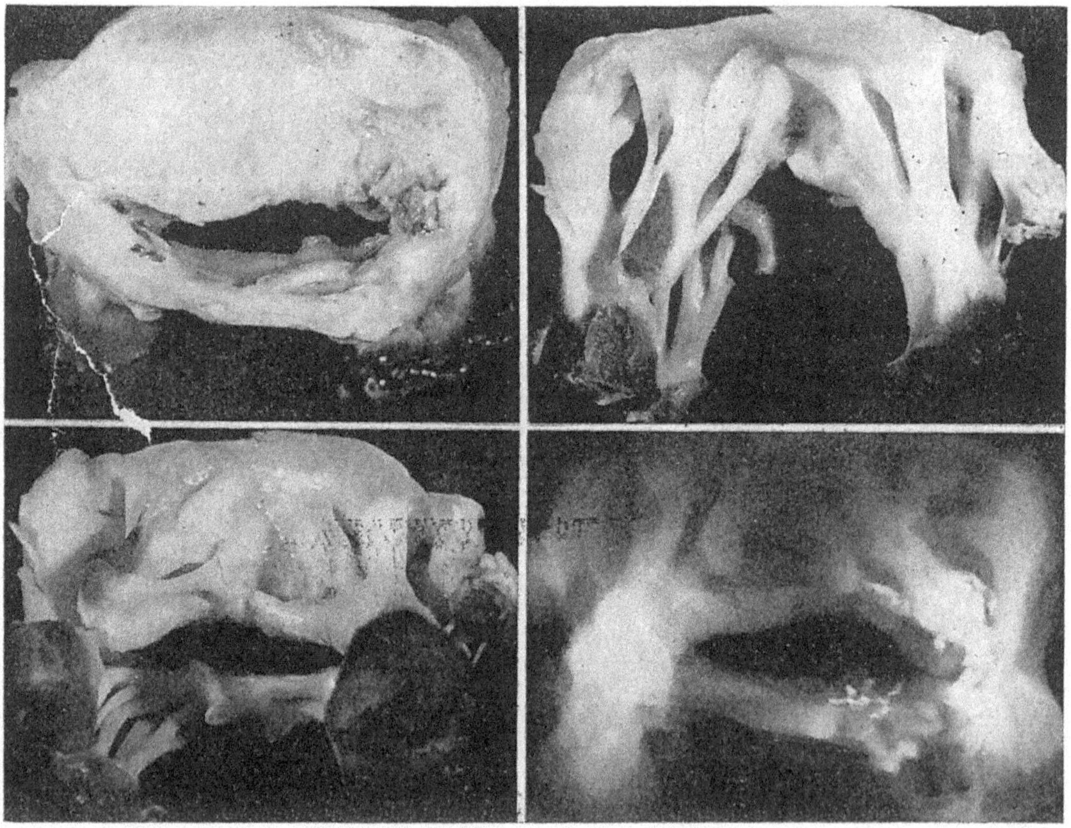

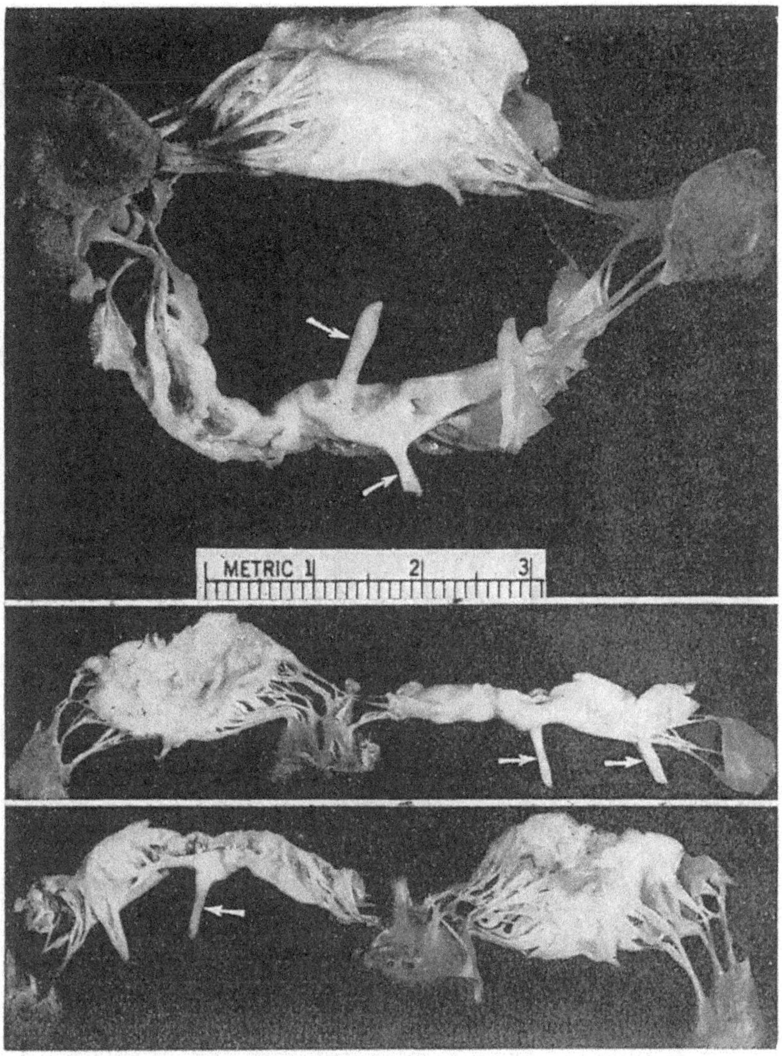

Fig 2.—Mitral valve (S66-1050) of a 64-year-old man who at catheterization was shown to have such massive mitral regurgitation that blood in the left atrium refluxed back into the main right and left pulmonary arteries during ventricular systole. This patient had no history of rheumatic fever, and had been well until about two years before operation. The mean left atrial pressure preoperatively was 28 mm Hg (normal ≦ 12 mm Hg) with v-waves to 70 mm Hg (normal ≦ 21 mm Hg), and the cardiac index was only 1.1 liters/min/sq m (normal = 2.5 to 3.5 liters/min/sq m). *Top,* The intact valve as viewed from the left ventricular aspect. Regurgitation was the consequence of ruptured chordae tendineae (*arrows*) from the posterior mitral leaflet. *Center,* The opened valve shows its atrial surface. *Bottom,* Ventricular surface.

depend primarily upon the microscopic findings. Such methods of examination, however, which are adhered to almost ritualistically in many laboratories, are not likely to provide the most meaningful information concerning an excised cardiac valve. The present comments suggest alternate procedures which have been found effective in relating the valvular malformation to the clinical, hemodynamic, and operative findings.

Ideally a cardiac valve should be removed intact, and the responsibility for this important initial step rests with the surgeon. The mitral or tricuspid leaflets are detached circumferentially from the valve ring, and the papillary muscles are then divided at their origins from the ventricular walls, thus preserving the attachments of the chordae tendineae to both the leaflets and papillary muscles. Most diseased aortic valves, whether

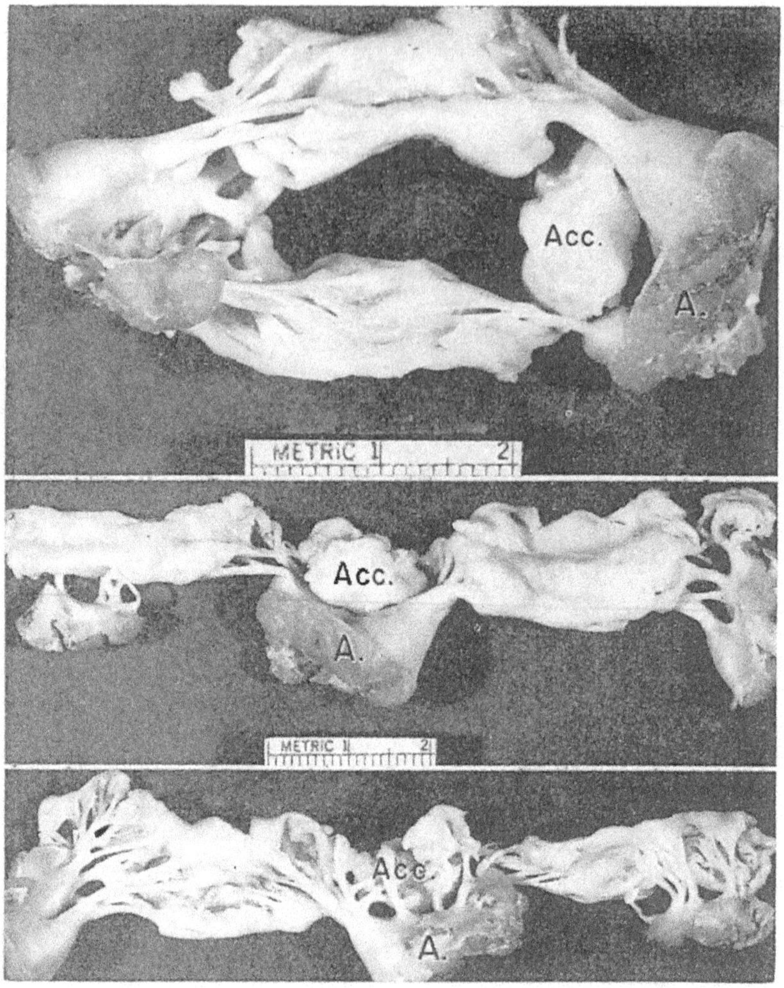

Fig 3.—Mitral valve (S65-3398) of a 6-year-old boy who had massive mitral regurgitation four years following closure of a ventricular septal defect. At operation, endocardial fibroelastosis involving the left ventricle also was observed. *Top,* Intact mitral valve showing an accessory leaflet (*Acc.*) adjacent to the anterolateral. (*A.*) papillary muscle. *Center* and *Bottom,* The atrial and ventricular aspects of the opened valve. Margins of all the leaflets are thickened and rolled. Presence of the accessory leaflet indicates that the valve is congenitally malformed.

stenotic or regurgitant, fibrotic or calcific, also can be excised intact, although en bloc removal of the aortic valve is, of course, facilitated when the commissures are fused.

When the valve is examined by the surgical pathologist he must first describe it accurately and informatively. In the case of an atrioventricular valve mention should be made in the description of all its components. Are the leaflets fibrotic, calcified, or normal? Is the fibrosis or calcification focal or diffuse; how is it distributed on the leaflets, only at their margins, on one surface or both? Are the leaflets immobile, shortened, stretched, or normal? Are the commissures fused, and to what extent? Are the chordae tendineae intact, ruptured, shortened, elongated, fused, or normal? Are the papillary muscles normal in number, scarred, hypertrophied, or elongated? Is the valve incompetent, stenotic, or both? If the valve appears incompetent an answer as to why should be sought. Is the incompetency due in whole or in part to an inadequate amount of valvular tissue, to a dilated annulus, to ruptured chordae, or to a ruptured, scarred, or shortened papillary muscle?

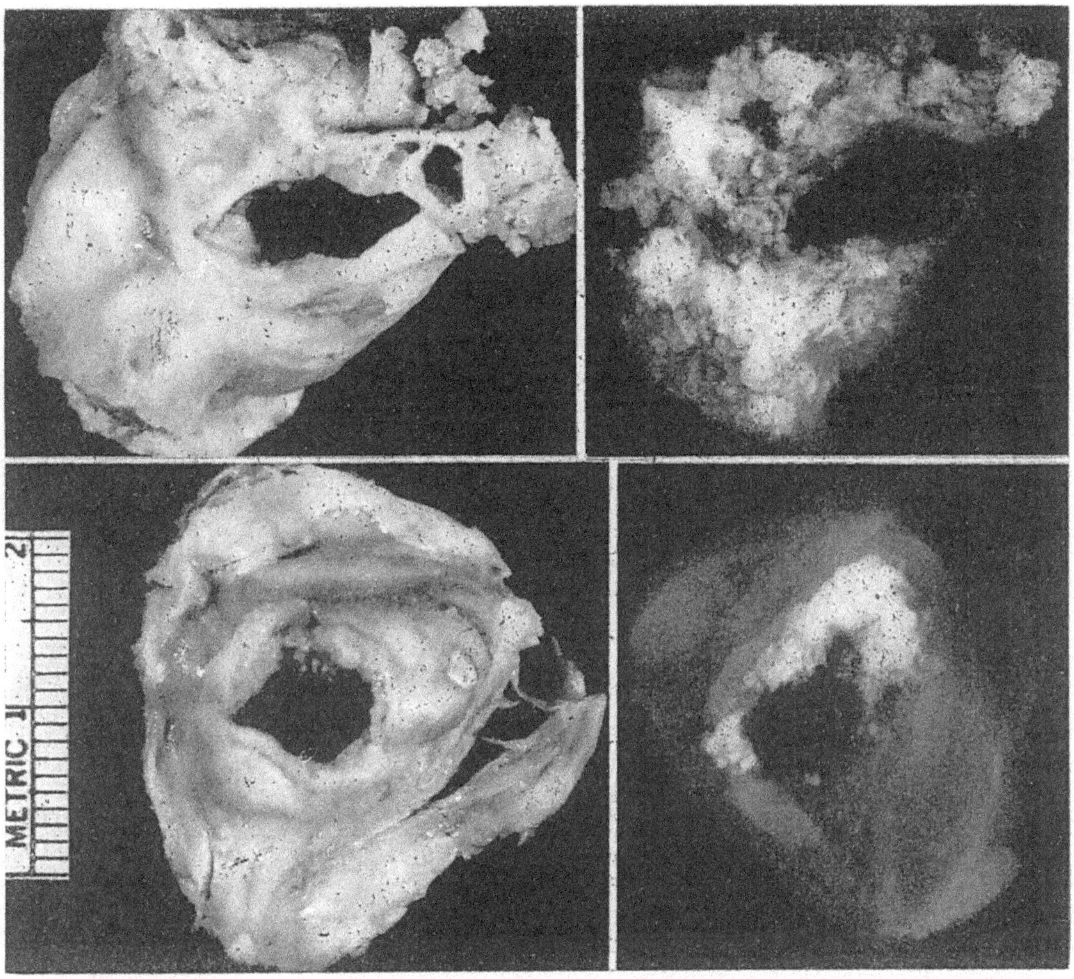

Fig 4.—*Top,* S63-2268; *Bottom,* S65-4170. Aortic valves in two patients viewed from the aortic aspect with accompanying radiographs. The valve at top has an eccentric orifice and consists of a massively calcified single cusp (unicuspid or unicommissural) which probably was stenotic from birth.[1] The peak systolic pressure gradient across it was 80 mm Hg, and the cardiac index was 3.2 liters/min/sq m. The valve at bottom has a centrally located orifice, and contains relatively small deposits of calcium. This 51-year-old woman had acute rheumatic fever in childhood and associated mitral stenosis (11 mm Hg left atrial to left ventricular mean diastolic pressure gradient). The peak systolic pressure gradient across the aortic valve was 130 mm Hg, and the cardiac index, 2.0 liters/min/sq m. This valve probably was normal at birth.

The structure of the semilunar valves is less complex than that of the atrioventricular valves, but most of the questions concerning the atrioventricular leaflets, commissures, and orifices also are applicable to the excised aortic valve. In addition, special attention should be directed to the size and number of the valve cusps. Are three cusps present, or does the valve consist of only one cusp (unicuspid or unicommissural) or two cusps (bicuspid) ; if two or three cusps are present are they of equal or unequal size?

Following inspection and description of the excised valve, it is photographed. In the case of an atrioventricular valve, both the atrial aspect and the ventricular aspect are shown (Fig 1-3). The former view better illustrates the relative size of the valve orifice in comparison to the circumference of the valve annulus, while the latter demonstrates the chordae tendineae and also the ventricular surface of the leaflets. An aortic valve is preferably photographed from both aortic and ventricular aspects, the view from above being the most informative one (Fig 4). When more than one cardiac valve is removed from the same patient, it is preferable to photograph them together.

Almost always the final anatomic diagnosis is best made from gross inspection of the valve. Although most mitral valves seen by the surgical pathologist are from patients with rheumatic heart disease, he should be alert to anatomic features which might indicate a congenital or other nonrheumatic etiology. This caution should especially be observed when applying an etiological diagnosis to the excised, diffusely calcified and stenotic aortic valve, which is usually not of rheumatic origin, but is more often related to a congenital malformation.

After describing and photographing the excised valve, the surgical pathologist may then, and only then, consider the advisability of sectioning the valve for histologic study. He should be aware, however, that examination of histologic sections is rarely helpful in providing either an anatomic or an etiologic diagnosis. For example, the microscopic appeareance of a calcified, nonrheumatic bicuspid aortic valve is likely to be indistinguishable from that of a calcified, rheumatic, tricuspid aortic valve. In this situation the microscope reveals only the end-stage of a disease process, and information as to etiology is now nearly impossible to obtain. In determining whether or not to section a valve, the pathologist must decide whether the possible value of the microscopic study justifies destruction of the valve structure. If sectioned, later studies correlating the valvular pathology to preoperative clinical, hemodynamic, and radiographic findings will be impossible.

In summary, the excised cardiac valve should not be processed as a routine surgical specimen. The most precise pathologic diagnosis will probably result from careful gross inspection of the valve, and not from histologic examination of sections of it. Photographs of the valve provide the most effective record of the pathologic findings, and permit correlations between the anatomic malformation and the clinical, hemodynamic, and operative findings.

REFERENCE

1. Roberts, W.C., and Morrow, A.G.: Congenital Aortic Stenosis Produced by a Unicommissural Valve, *Brit Heart J* **27**:505-510, 1965.

Obstruction to Left Ventricular Outflow

Current Concepts of Management and Operative Treatment

Moderator: ANDREW G. MORROW, M.D. *Discussants:* WILLIAM C. ROBERTS, M.D., JOHN ROSS, JR., M.D., R. DARRYL FISHER, M.D., DOUGLAS M. BEHRENDT, M.D., DEAN T. MASON, M.D., and EUGENE BRAUNWALD, M.D.

Bethesda, Maryland

DR. ANDREW G. MORROW: Since the clinical program of the National Heart Institute was initiated in 1953, a continuing interest in both the Cardiology and Surgery Branches has been the study and treatment of patients with the congenital or acquired malformations that result in obstruction to left ventricular outflow, that is, aortic stenosis in its various forms. In 1963 an NIH Clinical Staff Conference was devoted to the subject of aortic stenosis (1). In the ensuing 5 years our understanding of the physiologic, pathologic, and hemodynamic characteristics of these malformations has increased manyfold, and the techniques and the results of operative treatment have altered radically. This Conference provides a current reassessment of the clinical problems involved in managing patients with the various forms of aortic stenosis.

The most common site at which obstruction to left ventricular outflow occurs is the aortic valve.

PATHOLOGIC ANATOMY OF THE STENOTIC AORTIC VALVE

DR. WILLIAM C. ROBERTS*: I would like to make two points in this presentation: [1] that anatomically isolated aortic valve disease is rarely if ever the consequence of acute rheumatic fever, chorea, or rheumatic heart disease, and [2] that anatomically isolated aortic valve disease most often results from acquired changes in a congenitally malformed aortic valve.

These two conclusions were reached after the examination at necropsy of the hearts of 371 patients over 14 years of age who had severe valvular heart disease (Table 1). In 285 of the 371 patients the aortic valve was anatomically abnormal. Of the remaining 86 patients, 78 had anatomic disease of the mitral valve only, 6 had anatomic involvement of the mitral and tricuspid valves, and 2 had anatomic disease limited to the tricuspid valve. (Patients with carcinoid heart disease were not included in this study.) All 371 patients had symptoms of cardiac dysfunction, and most of them were in functional classes III and IV (New York Heart Association classification (NYHA)). Patients who had no symptoms of cardiac dysfunction (functional class I) were excluded. Cardiac operations (valvulotomy, valvuloplasty, or valve replacement) had been performed in 155 of the 371 patients.

* Chief, Section on Pathology, Surgery Branch, National Heart Institute.

Received September 20, 1968; accepted October 9, 1968.

This is an edited transcription of a Combined Clinical Staff Conference at the Clinical Center, Bethesda, Md., by the National Heart Institute, National Institutes of Health, U. S. Department of Health, Education, and Welfare.

Requests for reprints should be addressed to Andrew G. Morrow, M.D., Chief, Clinic of Surgery, National Heart Institute, Bldg. 10, Rm. 6-N-252, National Institutes of Health, Bethesda, Md. 20014.

TABLE 1. Cardiac Valvular Disease: Summary of 371 Autopsy Patients over 14 Years Old

Valve Involved Anatomically*	Number of Patients	Males	Clearly Nonrheumatic Cause	Rheumatic Cause	History of Acute Rheumatic Fever or Chorea	History of Acute Rheumatic Fever or Chorea
		%	no.		no.	%
1. Aortic only	155	83	135	?20	18	11
a. AS with or without AR	100	76	100	0	3†	3
b. Pure AR	35	91	31	? 4	4	12
c. AS or pure AR, diffusely thickened mitral leaflets but normal chordae	20	100	4†	?16	10	50
2. Aortic and mitral	98	63	3‡	95	75	79
a. Clinically AS or AR *and* MS or MR	66	70	3	63	52	83
b. Clinically MS and/or MR only	24	46	0	24	17	71
c. Clinically AS and/or AR only	8	62	0	8	6	75
3. Aortic, mitral, and tricuspid§	32	41	1‖	31	23	74
a. Clinically AS or AR, MS or MR, *and* TS** or TR	9					
b. Clinically AS *and* MS or MR	8					
c. Clinically MS or MR only	6					
d. Clinically MS or MR and TS** or TR	6					
e. Clinically AS or AR only	3					
4. Mitral only	78	36	21††	57	40	70
5. Mitral and tricuspid	6	17	0	6	5	83
6. Tricuspid only	2	0	2‡‡	0	0	0
Totals	371	63	182§§ (49%)	189 (51%)	142	75

* AS = aortic stenosis; AR = aortic regurgitation; MS = mitral stenosis; MR = mitral regurgitation; TS = tricuspid stenosis; TR = tricuspid regurgitation.

† Each had a congenitally bicuspid aortic valve.

‡ Two patients had the Marfan syndrome and the other, congenital malformations of both valves.

§ Two patients also had focal thickening of the pulmonic valve cusps without functional disturbance.

‖ Patient had rheumatoid arthritis with rheumatoid heart disease.

** Three patients.

†† Each had pure mitral regurgitation. Cause: congenital, 5; ruptured chordae mainly from infection, 10; ? Marfan's, 4; calcified annulus, 1; cause uncertain, 1.

‡‡ Each had pure tricuspid regurgitation secondary to infective endocarditis. Each was a heroin addict.

§§ The 20 patients in the *aortic only* group with a ? rheumatic cause are included in this figure.

Table 1 shows that a history of acute rheumatic fever or chorea is *unusual* in patients with anatomically isolated aortic valve disease, but that it is *usual* in patients in whom the mitral valve is anatomically involved, with or without involvement of other cardiac valves. Only 3 of 100 patients with anatomically isolated aortic valve disease causing stenosis, with or without associated regurgitation, had histories of acute rheumatic fever or chorea, and each of them at autopsy was found to have a congenitally bicuspid aortic valve. In contrast, 142 of 189 patients (75%) with anatomic disease of the mitral valve, with or without anatomic disease of other valves, had histories of acute rheumatic fever or chorea.

Thus, a history of acute rheumatic fever or chorea was virtually never obtained in patients with isolated aortic stenosis but was obtained in 29 of 44 necropsied patients (66%) with isolated mitral stenosis. Also included in the *aortic only* group (Table 1) are 20 patients

TABLE 2. Valve Structure in Anatomically Isolated Aortic Valvular Disease: Summary of 155 Autopsy Patients over Age 14

	Number of Patients	Males	Unicuspid	Bicuspid	Tricuspid	Structure Uncertain	Congenitally Malformed
		%		no.			%
1a. Aortic stenosis with or without aortic regurgitation	100	76	14	49	31*	6	63†
1b. Pure aortic regurgitation	35	91	0	10‡	25	0	29
1c. Clinically aortic stenosis or aortic regurgitation§ but thickened mitral leaflets and normal chordae tendineae	20	100	0	4‖	16**		20
Totals	155	83					

* In three patients the cusps were of unequal size, and one of them also had a congenitally bicuspid pulmonic valve.

† This percentage rises to *71%* if the "uncertain" category is either included in or excluded from the congenitally malformed group and if the three patients with unequal sized tricuspid aortic valves are included in the congenitally malformed group.

‡ In eight patients infective endocarditis caused the valve to be incompetent.

§ Three of the 20 patients had pure aortic regurgitation. The other 17 had aortic stenosis with or without regurgitation.

‖ In two patients the valvulvar orifice was severely stenotic, and in two it was only mildly stenotic (18 mm Hg and 24 mm Hg peak systolic pressure gradients, respectively) but severely incompetent.

** In 11 patients the valve was severely stenotic, in 1 patient mildly stenotic and severely incompetent, and in 3 subjects the valve was purely incompetent.

with aortic stenosis, or regurgitation, or both, in whom there was also diffuse fibrous thickening of the mitral leaflets but in whom the chordae tendineae were normal. There is probably some overlap between this group (Table 1, 1-c), and those included in the *aortic plus mitral* group (Table 1, 2) since the prevalence of a history of acute rheumatic fever or chorea in patients in group 1-c approaches that of patients in group 2 (50% compared with 79%). In group 2, however, the mitral chordae were always abnormal, and frequently the mitral leaflets were calcified. The fibrous thickening of the mitral leaflets without chordal thickening or shortening (group 1-c) may have resulted from excessive trauma to the mitral leaflets by increased left ventricular pressures.

SEX DIFFERENCES

The sex of patients with anatomically isolated mitral disease differs strikingly from that of subjects with anatomically isolated aortic valve disease: 128 of the 155 autopsied patients (83%) with isolated aortic valve involvement were males, whereas only 28 of 78 patients (36%) with isolated mitral valve disease were males. Interestingly, when both mitral and aortic valves were anatomically abnormal, males also predominated (63%).

ANATOMICAL FEATURES

Of the 371 patients with valvular heart disease, only 12 had Aschoff bodies in their

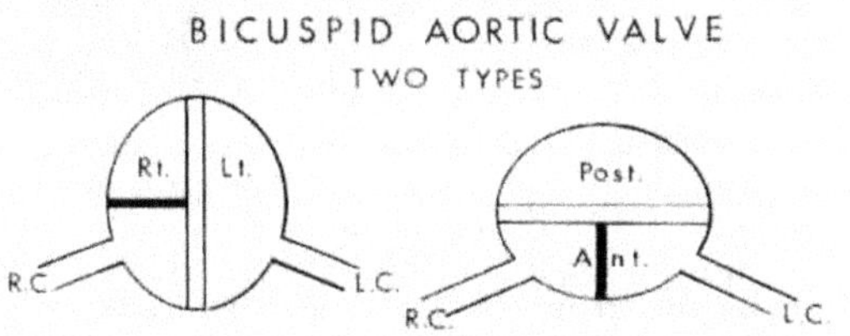

FIGURE 1. The two basic types of congenitally bicuspid aortic valves. When the cusps are located right and left the commissures are anterior and posterior, and a coronary artery arises from behind each cusp. When the cusps are located anteriorly and posteriorly the commissures are right and left, and both coronary arteries arise from the aortic root in front of the anterior cusp. When false raphes (*black bars*) are present they are located in the right cusp or the anterior cusp.

hearts at necropsy, but such nodules were never observed in the 155 subjects with anatomically isolated aortic valve disease. In contrast, each of the 12 patients with Aschoff bodies had anatomic mitral valve involvement, and 11 of them had other valves involved as well. It seems probable that *rheumatic heart disease always results in anatomic involvement of the mitral valve*, although other valves may also be involved. Anatomic disease of a cardiac valve, in general, corresponds with functional involvement, but there are exceptions to this general rule. For example, a patient with a history of acute rheumatic fever or chorea may present clinical signs and symptoms of isolated aortic valve disease. The history is the tip-off, however.

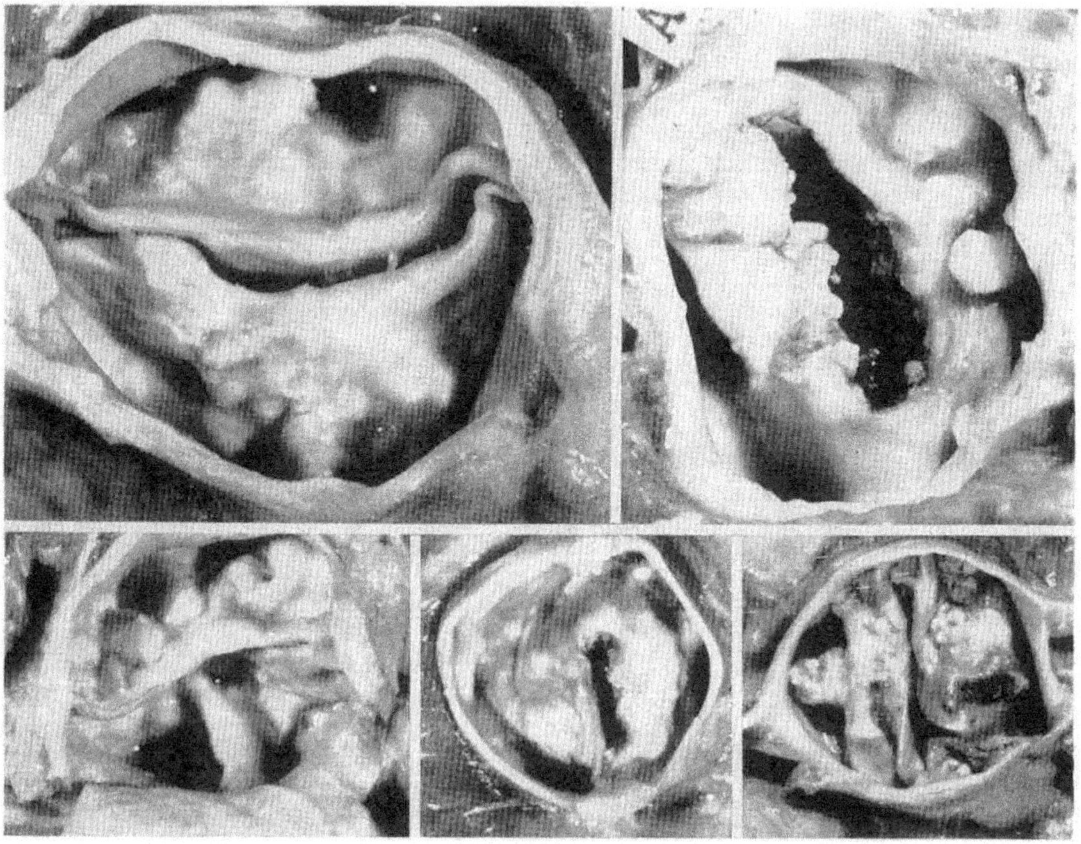

FIGURE 2. Calcified, stenotic, congenitally bicuspid aortic valves in five patients. In two patients (*upper left* and *lower left*) the cusps are located anteriorly and posteriorly, respectively, and a false raphe is present in each of the anterior cusps. In the other three patients the cusps are situated right and left, respectively, and a false raphe is visible in only one (*lower right*), but is present in two. Upper left: The valve of a 59-year-old man. The peak systolic gradient across the valve was 45 mm Hg, and he had complete heart block secondary to destruction of the atrioventricular bundle by calcium, which presumedly had extended down from the aortic valve cusps. Lower left: The valve of a 60-year-old man who suddenly collapsed on the street. Electrocardiogram recorded in the emergency room showed left bundle branch block. His only symptom of cardiac disease previously had been mild exertional dyspnea. Upper right: The valve of a 37-year-old man who also had left bundle branch block and died of progressive congestive heart failure. Lower middle: The valve of a 34-year-old man who also died of progressive congestive heart failure. The more posterior of the two commissures is fused. Lower right: The valve of a 79-year-old woman who was asymptomatic until 2 years earlier when signs and symptoms of congestive heart failure appeared. The false raphe in the right cusp is calcified. The heart weighed 700 g.

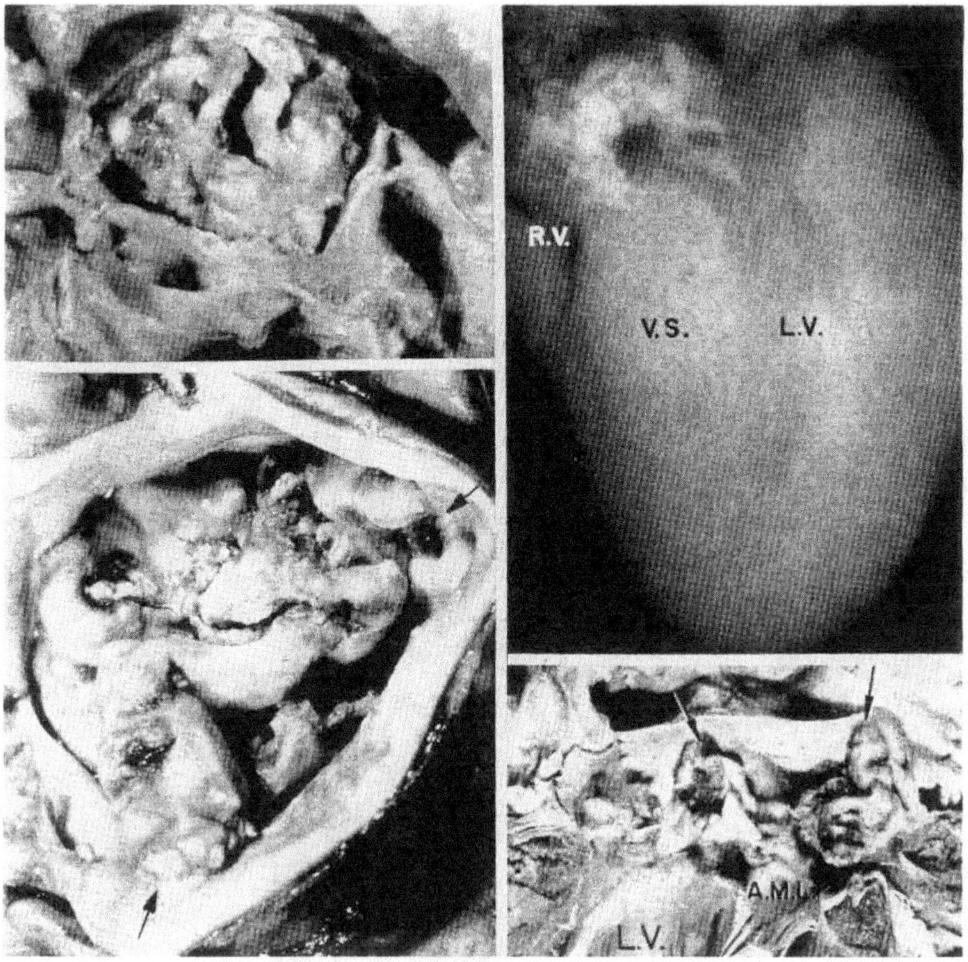

FIGURE 3. Extremely heavily calcified congenitally bicuspid aortic valves. This degree of calcium deposition is unusual. Upper left: The valve of a 54-year-old man who had the onset of mild heart failure 9 years earlier. A peak systolic pressure gradient of 129 mm Hg was measured across the aortic valve shortly before death. A roentgenogram of the heart specimen is shown in the upper right. The aortic valve is severely calcified and the ventricular septum (*V.S.*) severely hypertrophied. R.V. = right ventricle; L.V. = left ventricle. Lower left: The valve of a 63-year-old man who died during transventricular aortic valvulotomy in 1959. The two arrows designate the two commissures that are also seen in the photograph of the opened aortic valve (*lower right*). A 90 mm Hg peak systolic pressure gradient was measured across this valve preoperatively. This patient also had left bundle branch block. A.M.L. = anterior mitral leaflet.

that almost certainly the mitral valve is *anatomically* abnormal. The mitral lesion may cause no functional derangement, but, on the other hand, the functional disturbance may be severe, although obscured by the aortic valve lesion. Indeed, the only clinical clue to "silent mitral stenosis" may be a positive history of acute rheumatic fever or chorea.

Further evidence that anatomically isolated aortic valve disease is not of rheumatic origin is gained by examination of the structure of this valve in these patients. Table 2 shows that 49 of 100 patients with isolated aortic stenosis, with or without regurgitation, had congenitally bicuspid aortic valves; another 14 had congenitally unicuspid or unicommissural valves (that

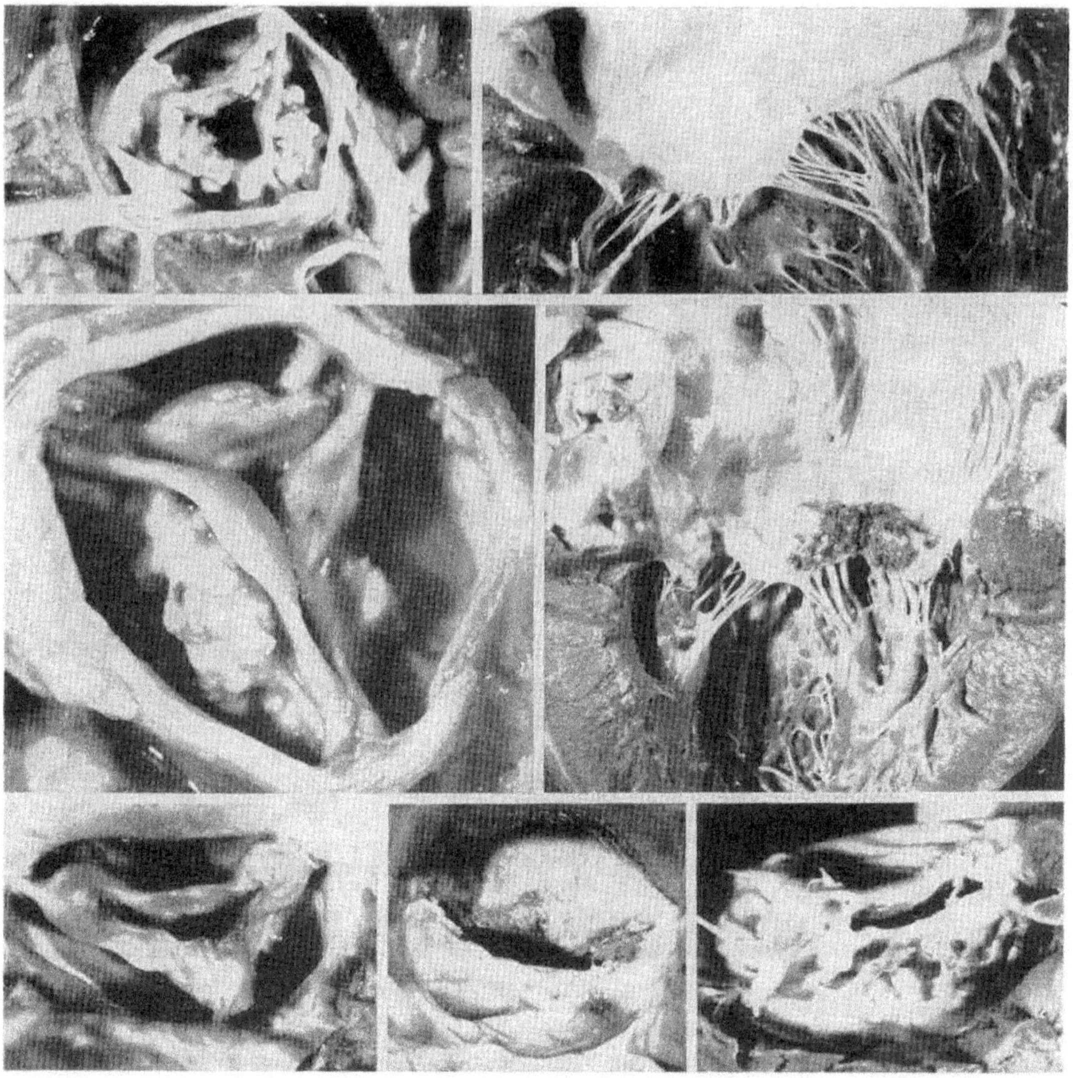

FIGURE 4. Three cuspid stenotic aortic valves. Left upper: Aortic valve of a 42-year-old man, functionally class IV, who died of severe congestive heart failure. The valve orifice is triangular in shape, stenotic, and incompetent. His opened mitral valve is shown in the right upper photograph. The mitral leaflets are mildly but diffusely thickened, but the chordae tendineae are normal. Thus, this patient is classified in group 1-c, Table 1. Whether the mild mitral leaflet thickening was the result of rheumatic disease in the past or the result of excessive trauma secondary to the elevated left ventricular systolic pressure is uncertain. This patient did have a history of acute rheumatic fever.

Left middle: Aortic valve of a 61-year-old man with angina pectoris and congestive heart failure for 3 years. He died suddenly while shaving. On chest roentgenograms the heart was of normal size, but at necropsy it weighed 500 g. Deposits of calcium are present on the aortic aspects of each of the three aortic cusps, but none of the commissures are fused. His mitral valve (*right middle*) is diffusely fibrotic and heavily calcified. He had no history of acute rheumatic fever.

Left lower: Aortic valve of a 59-year-old woman, functionally class IV, with combined aortic and mitral stenosis. Each of the three aortic valvular commissures is fused and, although the cusps are calcified, the calcific deposits are covered by smooth endocardium. Her mitral valve as seen from the left atrial aspect is shown in the lower middle photograph, and as seen from the left ventricular aspect in the lower right photograph. She had no history of acute rheumatic fever.

is, valves consisting of only 1 cusp and 1 commissure), and in at least 3 patients with 3-cuspid aortic valves the cusps were of unequal size. In 6 patients the valves were so deformed that the underlying structure was not discernible, but it is strongly suspected that these valves were also congenitally malformed. Thus, in approximately 70% of the 100 patients with isolated aortic stenosis the valve was congenitally malformed. In contrast, the aortic valve was 3-cuspid in all of the 132 patients who had anatomic disease of the mitral valve as well as aortic valve disease. The anatomic features of these valves are illustrated in Figures 1 to 6.

Dr. Morrow: When one considers the advisability of operative treatment in a patient with acquired aortic valve disease, he must try to judge the extent to which operation may or may not affect the natural history of the disease. Data concerning the natural history of malformations that are amenable to operation are exceedingly difficult to acquire in this era of cardiac surgery. However, Dr. John Ross has compiled information concerning this important problem.

Natural History of Severe Aortic Stenosis in Adults

Dr. John Ross, Jr.*: There is an important need for accurate information concerning the natural history of patients with

* Chief, Section on Cardiovascular Diagnosis, Cardiology Branch, National Heart Institute.

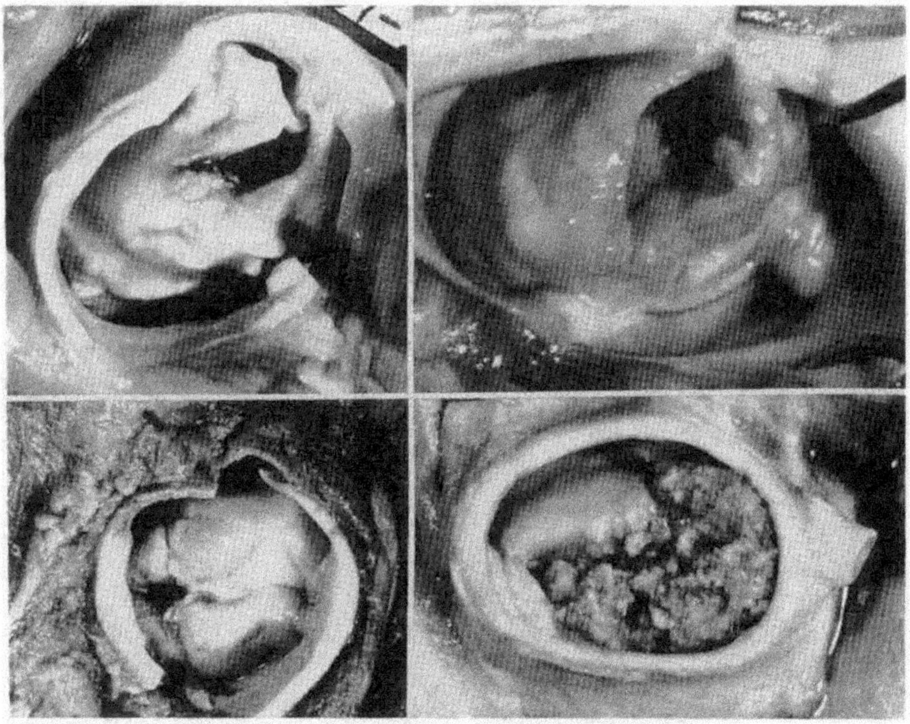

Figure 5. Congenitally unicuspid, unicommissural aortic valves in four patients. Upper left: A 28-year-old man with cardiac symptoms for 5 months. He had severe heart failure and left bundle branch block. Upper right: A 16-year-old boy with mild symptoms of heart failure for 7 years. A 125 mm Hg peak systolic gradient (PSG) was measured across the valve. Lower left: A 9-year-old boy who died of severe aortic regurgitation after valvulotomy. The PSG across the valve preoperatively was 86 mm Hg. Lower right: This 32-year-old woman was asymptomatic until 3 years earlier when streptococcal endocarditis occurred. The cardiac infection was cured, but symptoms of heart failure persisted thereafter. The PSG across the valve was 90 mm Hg.

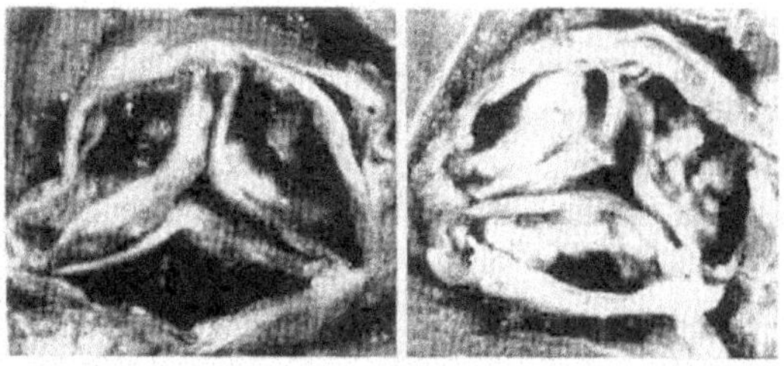

FIGURE 6. Aortic valve calcification in the elderly. This common entity appears to result from wear and tear of the cusps over many years. Calcium deposits occur as a rule only on the aortic aspects of the cusps, and the commissures are not fused. Usually no ventricular hypertrophy results since the deposits are not large enough to prevent adequate movement of the cusps. The valves shown here in two patients, however, are exceptions to this general rule. One (*left*) was in an 88-year-old man who died suddenly and unexpectedly. A precordial murmur had not been recorded. The heart weighed 440 g. The other valve shown (*right*) was from an 85-year-old woman who died of congestive cardiac failure. A murmur typical of aortic stenosis had been audible, and the electrocardiogram had shown left ventricular hypertrophy. The heart weighed 500 g.

cardiac lesions that are potentially correctable by operation. This is particularly true in relation to adult patients with aortic stenosis, not only because of the unique problem of sudden death associated with this disease, but because of the serious prognosis that accompanies the onset of symptoms and an operative mortality that continues to be relatively high. Accurate information concerning the natural history of aortic stenosis has been difficult to obtain, however, largely because the development of objective means for the assessment of its severity by left heart catheterization arrived on the scene almost simultaneously with the advent of surgical treatment. Thus, interruption of the natural course by operation has led to a lack of prospective information concerning the outlook for patients with obstruction of known hemodynamic severity.

I shall review the natural course of valvular aortic stenosis in the adult, using information assembled largely from retrospective clinical and postmortem analyses published before 1955 (2) and discuss some more recent studies supported by hemodynamic data. I shall then compare in a general way the current results of operation for correction of valvular aortic stenosis in the adult with the predicted natural mortality. Within the term "acquired" aortic stenosis are included patients who have developed stenosis of a congenitally deformed valve, as discussed by Dr. Roberts.

CLINICAL COURSE

In postmortem studies (2–5), about three quarters of the patients with aortic stenosis were males, and the average age at death of the male patients was 63 years. The average duration of symptoms was short, a history of angina pectoris having been present for an average of 3 years, syncope for 3 years, and congestive heart failure for 1.5 to 2 years. Figure 7 summarizes the course of the average patient with valvular aortic stenosis, as determined from postmortem data. There is a relatively long latent period, presumably marked by increasing obstruction, or increasing myocardial disease due to long-standing overload on the left ventricle, or both. The average age at the onset of symptoms typically occurs in the sixth decade, and the average life expectancy after the onset of severe symptoms is about 4 years. When data were summarized from clinical rather than postmortem stud-

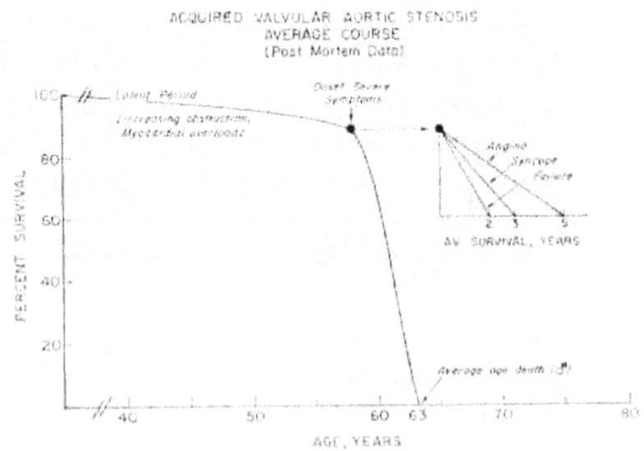

FIGURE 7. The average natural course of aortic stenosis in adult patients, assembled from postmortem data. AV. = average.

ies, the patients were first seen somewhat earlier in their course; their average age was 48 years (2, 3, 5, 6). A history of angina pectoris, when present, averaged 5 years in duration, congestive heart failure about 2 years, and a history of syncope encompassed a range of 1 to 18 years. Again, however, on the average the history of symptoms was relatively short.

What about the problem of sudden death in adult patients with valvular aortic stenosis? Death is sudden in about 15% of all patients dying with valvular aortic stenosis (4). However, from 65 to 80% of these patients have significant symptoms of angina pectoris, syncope, or heart failure before death, and, therefore, only 3 to 5% of deaths occur suddenly in patients without symptoms.

In the analysis of these retrospective data, a number of problems appear. First, the selection of patients was extremely variable. Many patients had significant associated aortic regurgitation, or even predominant aortic regurgitation; others had associated mitral valve disease, recognized or unrecognized; some died of subacute bacterial endocarditis or heart failure, complications that could probably have been modified or prevented by more modern therapeutic methods. In addition, in the early studies the hemodynamic severity of stenosis was unknown.

Dr. Stuart Frank of the Cardiology Branch and I identified, among the patients with aortic stenosis seen at the National Heart Institute over the last 12 years, a group of 15 patients with valvular aortic stenosis of severe degree, documented hemodynamically, who did not undergo operation and in whom a long follow-up could be obtained. Some patients refused operation, others were considered too ill for operation, and in some symptoms were not sufficiently severe to warrant operation. When these patients were first seen their ages ranged from 32 to 59 years, and there were 12 men and 3 women. All had severe aortic stenosis, with a pressure gradient between left ventricle and brachial artery of more than 50 mm Hg or a valve orifice area index ≤ 0.70 cm²/M² body surface area (BSA), or both. No associated mitral valve disease was detected nor was there significant aortic regurgitation in any patient.

The 15 patients were followed for periods up to 12 years after initial hemodynamic study. The average age at onset of symptoms was 48 years, and the average life expectancy after the onset of symptoms was less than 4 years. Ten of the 15 patients were dead at the end of the follow-up period. There were no hemodynamic differences between patients who survived and those who died, and there were no important differences in the incidence of symptoms in the survivors and nonsurvivors. At the end of 4½ years 50% of the patients were dead, and at the end of 8 years 80% were dead. It also is of interest that the clinical course after the onset of significant symptoms in each of the patients who died was not influenced by the age at which symptoms began; it was rapid at any age. Three of the five patients who were alive at the termination of the study had symptoms, although symptoms had been present for only 1 to 4 years.

SURGICAL RESULTS

How does this rather grim outlook compare with the results of surgical treatment? Data were recently summarized from the published results of several surgical centers in the United States (2). The follow-up period in patients who had had replacement of the aortic valve with a ball-valve prosthesis ranged from 1 to 5 years. The average early plus late mortality after these operations ranged from 16 to 30% and averaged 23%. Specific data concerning the patients operated upon here by Dr. Morrow and his associates will be presented later.

The average effects of operation on the course of adult patients with severe valvular aortic stenosis are contrasted with the aver-

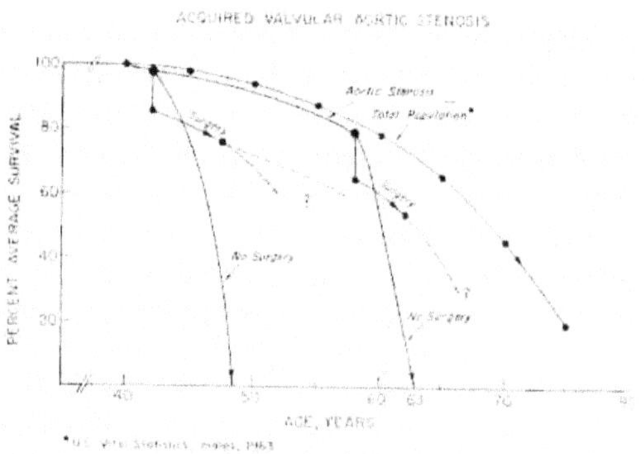

FIGURE 8. The effect of operation on the course of adult patients with aortic stenosis. The upper curve represents the total male U.S. population. The lower curves represent the average course when severe symptoms began in the fifth and in the sixth decades (no surgery), the course being brief at either age. The immediate operative mortality trend is indicated by the vertical lines, and the mortality derived from initial postoperative studies is indicated.

age course in patients not operated upon, in Figure 8. With operative treatment, there is a 5 to 15% early mortality and a 5 to 15% late mortality. During the initial 5-year period of follow-up, the percent survival after the initial operative mortality appears in general to parallel the trend of the total male population. Whether or not this trend will continue is, of course, uncertain. In younger patients who undergo operation, it sems likely that as longer periods of postoperative follow-up are obtained, the course may deviate downward from that parallel to the total male population of comparable age.

CHOICE OF VALVE REPLACEMENT

From this brief review it may be concluded that when symptoms of angina pectoris, syncope, or left ventricular decompensation develop in adult patients with hemodynamically severe aortic stenosis, the immediate outlook is exceedingly poor but can be improved substantially by replacement of the aortic valve. Thus, the risk of operation in this group of patients is considerably lower than the risk of nonoperative treatment. In addition, the clinical improvement in most of the survivors has been remarkable. The problem of whether or not to recommend operation in patients without symptoms but with severe aortic stenosis remains unresolved. However, at present the risk of operation appears to be appreciably higher than the risk of sudden death in such patients. The influence of aortic valve replacement on long-term survival and disability is not yet established, nor is it certain whether or not the incidence of complications observed during these initial years after the advent of valve replacement will continue. The answers to these questions will be forthcoming only when prospective studies are carried out in patients who have no symptoms but stenosis of known hemodynamic severity and when detailed long-range studies of operative results become available.

DR. MORROW: Past and sometimes bitter experience has shown us that reconstructive operations are ineffective for the relief of acquired aortic stenosis or regurgitation. Thus, when operative treatment is undertaken in the adult patient with aortic valve disease, aortic valve replacement will almost always be necessary.

AORTIC VALVE REPLACEMENT

DR. R. DARRYL FISHER*: Between February 1963 and April 1967 isolated aortic valve replacement was carried out in 133 patients at the National Heart Institute. The Starr-Edwards prosthetic valve was utilized in all patients. Other patients who had an operation on the mitral valve in addition to aortic valve replacement are not included in the analysis.

The ages of the 133 patients ranged from 16 to 68 years, and the mean age was 47 years; there were 98 men and 35 women. Fifty-six patients gave unequivocal histories of rheumatic fever and at operation were found to have symmetrical tricuspid aortic valves characteristic of rheumatic valvulitis. In 38 patients without his-

* Clinical Associate, Surgery Branch, National Heart Institute.

tories of rheumatic fever the anatomy of the valve was obscured by calcium, and no cause of the valve disease could be established. Thirty-five patients had congenitally deformed, usually bicuspid, valves. In three patients the valve had been destroyed by bacterial endocarditis, and one patient had syphilitic aortic regurgitation.

On the basis of the preoperative hemodynamic and angiographic findings, 59 patients were considered to have pure or predominant aortic stenosis, 40 to have pure or predominant aortic regurgitation, and 34 to have mixed aortic stenosis and regurgitation.

Twelve patients were in functional class IV (NYHA), and 86 patients were in class III. The remaining 35 patients had only episodes of angina and syncope as their main symptoms, and the classificaiton system specifies their placement in class II. All of the patients complained of fatigue; 81% had angina, and nearly half of the entire group experienced angina at least daily. Symptoms of left ventricular failure were present in two thirds, and symptoms of right ventricular failure were present in 27%. One third of the patients had had one or more frank syncopal attacks, and many others had experienced exertional vertigo. In a significant number of the patients associated diseases were evident: in 12% coronary arteriosclerosis, or myocardial scarring, or both, was evident at operation; chronic lung disease was present in 8%; impaired renal function in 7%; and mitral disease not requiring surgical intervention was present in 5%.

By electrocardiographic criteria, 87% of the group had left ventricular hyperthrophy, and ST-T wave abnormalities were evident in 77%. Electrocardiographic evidences of previous myocardial infarction were present in 12%. Two patients were in atrial fibrillation; the other 131 were in sinus rhythm, and 21 had first- or second-degree heart block. Nearly all of the patients had gross cardiomegaly apparent roentgenographically, and pulmonary vascular engorgement was evident in 18 patients.

SURGICAL MANAGEMENT

When congestive heart failure was evident preoperatively, patients were treated with digoxin, sodium restriction, bed rest, and diuretics. Immediately before operation, however, diuretics were omitted for 3 days, and digoxin for 24 to 48 hr.

At operation, the heart was exposed through a median sternotomy, and cardiopulmonary bypass was established. The left coronary artery was perfused uninterruptedly during the operation, and mild (30°) general body hypothermia was used. After excision of the diseased valve, a Starr-Edwards prosthesis was selected that could be freely accommodated in the aortic annulus and aorta. The prosthetic valve was fixed with approximately 15 figure-of-eight dacron sutures in the aortic annulus, and both ends of the suture passed through the fabric sewing ring.

Postoperatively, in most patients the endotracheal tube was left in place overnight, and assisted ventilation was provided; the morning after operation, the tube was either removed or replaced by tracheostomy if assisted ventilation were still required. Ventricular arrhythmias were relatively frequent but were usually controlled with potassium chloride infusion, or intravenous lidocaine, or both. Oliguria usually responded to a fluid load; but if it persisted, mannitol or ethacrynic acid was used. Anticoagulation with warfarin has been initiated during the first postoperative week since 1965, and it is continued indefinitely unless individually contraindicated.

EARLY DEATHS AND COMPLICATIONS

Twenty-one patients died in the hospital after aortic valve replacement was performed. Five patients died in the operating room as a result of technical problems; these included irreparable damage to a coronary artery by the perfusion cannula, obstruction of the right coronary ostium by the fabric sewing ring, aortic dissection, and incomplete seating of the ball due to calcific aortic deposits. These technical difficulties were encountered early in the series, and none has occurred in the past 2 years. Two patients could not become independent of extracorporeal support after placement of the prosthesis. Four patients died of postoperative ventricular arrhythmias and three of the low cardiac output syn-

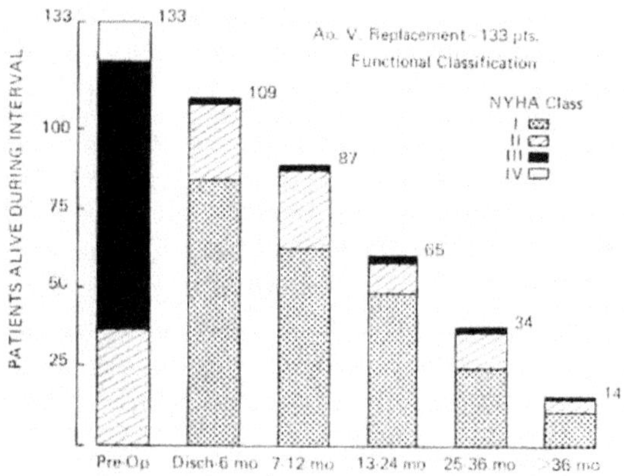

FIGURE 9. Functional classification (New York Heart Association (*NYHA*)) preoperatively and at successive postoperative intervals of 133 patients in whom aortic valve (*Ao.V.*) replacement was performed. The number of patients under observation during each interval is indicated by the figure at the top of the respective bar.

drome, presumably related to improper prosthesis size or to myocardial disease. Two deaths were sudden and unexplained. Cerebral hemorrhage, infected aortotomy, renal failure, respiratory insufficiency, and hyperkalemia caused death in one patient each.

Early, nonfatal complications occurred during postoperative convalescence in nearly 70% of all patients. Atrial arrhythmias occurred in 30 patients and usually converted to sinus rhythm with the administration of additional digoxin. Nineteen patients required reoperation for evacuation of hemothorax or for control of intrathoracic hemorrhage. Permanent complete heart block was sustained by one patient. Nine patients developed acute renal failure. Nine patients had ventricular fibrillation with successful conversion. Five patients developed superificial wound infections, and four sustained postoperative myocardial infarctions. Four patients developed gastrointestinal hemorrhage.

DR. DOUGLAS M. BEHRENDT *: Nonfatal complications after discharge from the hospital tended to occur early in the postoperative period. Twenty-seven patients developed hepatitis, and hemorrhage related to anticoagulant therapy occurred in six patients. A degenerated silastic ball was successfully replaced in one patient at another hospital. Twenty-two episodes of thromboembolism have affected 19 patients; 3 patients have had 2 embolic episodes, and 1 patient has had 3 episodes. Only one patient, however, has significant neurologic sequels. Since the institution of warfarin anticoagulation on a routine basis, the incidence of embolic episodes has been reduced.

Eight patients have died suddenly in the late postoperative period after evidencing both clinical and hemodynamic improvement. Six of these eight patients had associated myocardial disease. Fatal coronary artery emboli originated from the metal cage struts in two patients. Two patients died of documented myocardial infarctions. Subdural hematoma, fulminant hepatitis, intractable myocardial failure, and aortic dissection caused death in four additional patients. One case of endocarditis has occurred; the source of infection was never identified in this patient, and he died of massive aortic regurgitation 3 months after operation. Fatal degeneration of the silastic ball occurred in three patients in this 4-year period. The total mortality in the entire group of 133 patients during the 4-year period may be summarized as: operative mortality, 16%; late mortality, 15%; and 69% of the patients operated on are surviving.

RESULTS OF OPERATION

Detailed clinical and hemodynamic reassessments have been carried out in all surviving patients on one or more occasions. At the time of postoperative study virtually all patients have described substantial symptomatic improvement. The changes in functional classification after valve replacement are shown graphically in Figure 9. Before operation, most patients were severely limited and were in class III

* Clinical Associate, Surgery Branch, National Heart Institute.

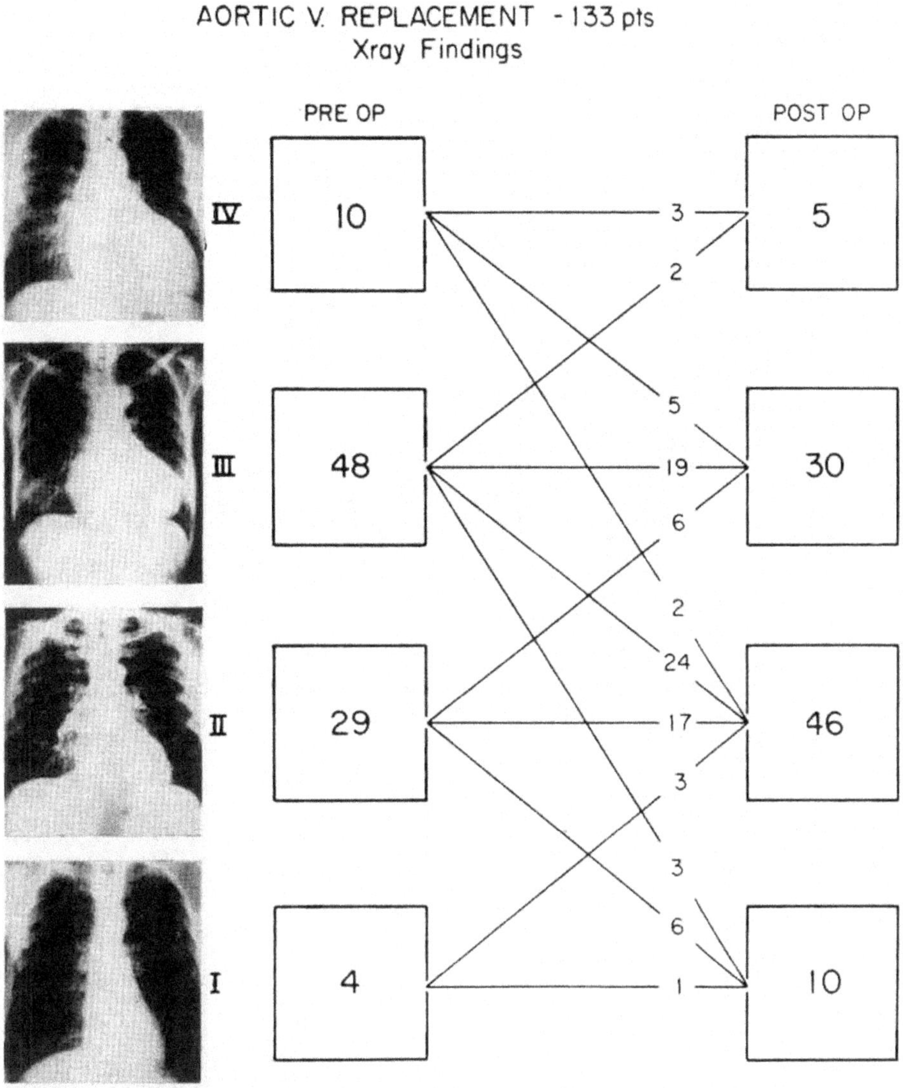

FIGURE 10. Changes in heart size that followed aortic valve replacement in 91 of 133 patients who survived at least 6 months. The extent of cardiomegaly was graded on a scale of I (least) to IV (most), as illustrated by the chest roentgenograms.

or class IV, while at succesive periods of follow-up most patients were asymptomatic or only mildly limited. These data may be interpreted in another manner; of the 112 patients who survived operation, each has thus far been furnished with approximately 2 years of class I or class II existence that he would not otherwise have had.

Changes in the size of the cardiac silhouette after operation are illustrated in Figure 10. The extent of cardiac enlargement pre- and postoperatively was arbitrarily graded I (none) to IV (most), and chest roentgenograms representative of these four categories are shown. Of 87 patients in whom cardiac enlargement was evident preoperatively, the size of the heart was distinctly smaller postoperatively in 40, and in 39 remained unchanged.

Hemodynamic studies have been carried out from 6 to 12 months after operation in 71 of the surviving patients, and compari-

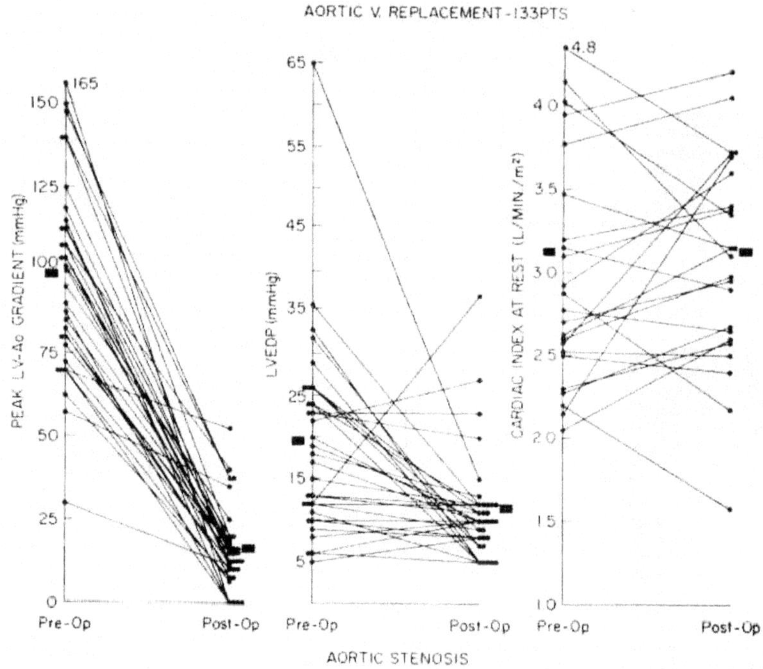

Figure 11. Measurements of the peak systolic pressure gradient, left ventricular end-diastolic pressure, and cardiac index determined pre- and postoperatively in patients in whom aortic stenosis was the predominant lesion.

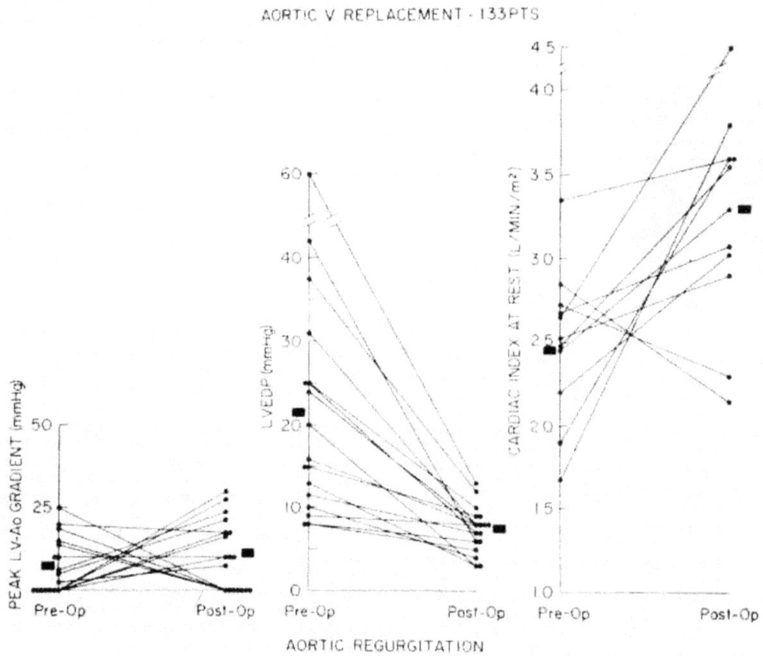

Figure 12. Measurements of the peak systolic pressure (*LV-Ao*) gradient, left ventricular end-diastolic pressure (*LVEDP*), and cardiac index determined pre- and postoperatively in patients in whom aortic regurgitation was the predominant lesion.

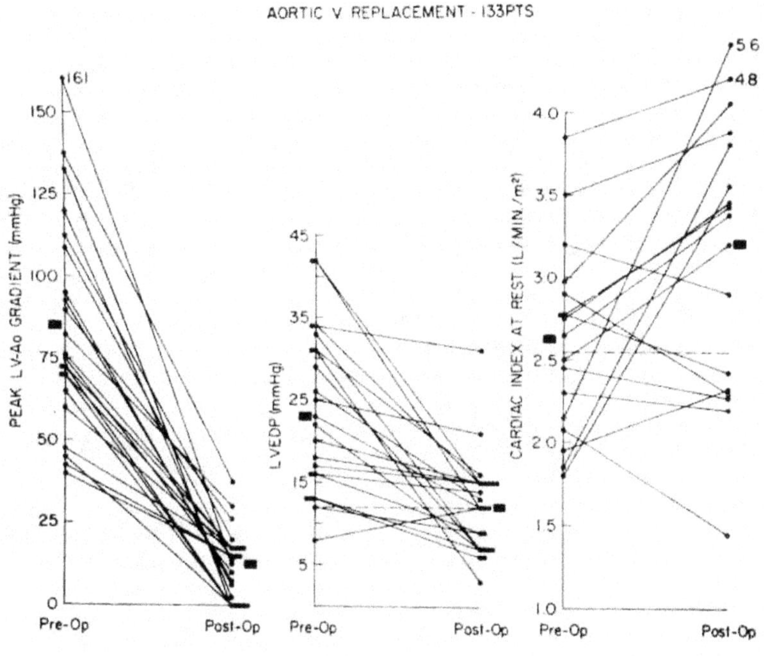

FIGURE 13. Measurements of the peak systolic pressure (*LV-Ao*) gradient, left ventricular end-diastolic pressure (*LVEDP*), and cardiac index determined pre- and postoperatively in patients with combined aortic stenosis (*AS*) and regurgitation (*AR*).

sons of pre- and postoperative values are shown in Figures 11 to 13. The usual gradient across the prosthesis was 10 to 15 mm Hg, occasionally as high as 30 mm Hg. In the vast majority of patients the left ventricular end-diastolic pressure was normal after operation; the changes in cardiac index were not consistent.

In summary, our experience would indicate that aortic valve replacement can be carried out with an acceptable operative risk, even in patients severely ill with cardiac disease and often with other coexistent diseases. Clinical improvement after aortic valve replacement is almost always gratifying, and most patients have been able to return to their former occupations. Importantly, symptomatic improvement has been paralleled by prompt return of the intracardiac pressures to normal or near normal levels. Initially it appeared that the major problem after aortic valve replacement would be thromboembolism, but anticoagulation has reduced this risk, and the recent development of a fabric-covered prosthesis that allows autologous tissue ingrowth may completely eliminate it. It now seems that the greatest hazard is late sudden death among patients who have achieved excellent clinical and hemodynamic improvement. Some of these deaths are attributable to myocardial or coronary arterial disease and are probably inevitable. Others, however, have resulted from degeneration of the silastic ball. The fabric-covered valve being evaluated at the Institute has a metallic ball and, hopefully, this new design will eliminate the problem of late ball variance.

Questions

Dr. Morrow: I think we might pause and contemplate some of the problems of acquired aortic valve disease, if there are questions or comments from those in the audience.

Question: I noticed that in your operative series of 133 patients, there were 56 patients who were thought to have rheumatic aortic valve disease, and only 5% of these had other valve involvement. This would suggest that there was quite a high prevalence of isolated aortic valve disease of rheumatic origin among the patients operated on.

Dr. Roberts: The group of patients that I discussed were those in whom all of the cardiac valves were examined at autopsy. I believe that if we had an opportunity to see the mitral valves of a number of the patients you refer to, they would be found anatomically abnormal. You must remember, however, that a valve may be abnormal anatomically but function normally.

Question: Would you elaborate on antibiotic prophylaxis for later operative procedures in patients who have had a prosthetic valve inserted?

Dr. Morrow: We are concerned about the problem of antibiotic prophylaxis for the reasons that have been emphasized. When these patients undergo valve replacement, they receive penicillin and streptomycin intramuscularly, beginning the night before operation and continuing for 6 days thereafter; on rare occasions methicillin is added to this regimen. There has been no case of endocarditis occurring as an intraoperative infection. When these patients undergo later operations that are "clean" by a surgeon's definition, that is an infected or contaminated field will not be crossed, we feel that penicillin and streptomycin will suffice. Further problems arise, however, when the patient has to undergo a urologic or gynecologic procedure, or an intestinal anastomosis, when the field is likely to be contaminated. Under these circumstances we give a combination of penicillin, streptomycin, and methicillin, and usually give the penicillin intravenously.

For outpatient treatment, the regimen of prophylaxis outlined is obviously impossible, but effective prophylaxis is mandatory; for example, for dental procedures that involve the soft tissues. In talking with dentists in this and other communities it seems easiest to have the patient receive the initial priming dose of antibiotics parenterally, not necessarily intravenously, an hour or two before the procedure. The antibiotics then are continued orally for 3 to 5 days.

The problems in the management of children and young adults with the discrete forms of congenital aortic stenosis differ in a number of respects from those of other patients with acquired aortic valvular disease.

Results of Operative Treatment in Congenital Aortic Stenosis

Dr. Dean T. Mason*: The most common congenital forms of obstruction to left ventricular outflow are valvular aortic stenosis, the discrete type of congenital subaortic stenosis, and supravalvular narrowing of the ascending aorta. These malformations are ordinarily recognized during childhood or adolescence and for these reasons a detailed description of the results of operative treatment in young patients will be considered. It is appreciated that a certain number of adult patients with calcific aortic stenosis have congenitally deformed valves, but the operative management of these patients ordinarily involves valve replacement, which has already been discussed.

A total of 45 patients with congenital aortic stenosis, operated upon consecutively between 1961 and 1967, form the basis for this report. The prevalence of each of the various forms of congenital aortic stenosis, and the ages of the patients are shown in Figure 14.

Patients with hypertrophic subaortic stenosis are not included, since a detailed description of the operative experience with this lesion will be examined separately. Of the total group of 45 patients, 18 were female and 27 were male.

* Cardiology Branch, National Heart Institute.

The majority of patients with valvular and supravalvular aortic stenosis were boys, while most of the patients with subvalvular stenosis were girls. Two patients with subvalvular stenosis also had patent ductus arteriosus, and 4 patients had other types of congenital cardiovascular anomalies. In the patients with patent ductus arteriosus or coarctation of the aorta, these malformations were corrected at separate operations, before the operation for relief of aortic stenosis. In the remaining patients the associated cardiac lesion was corrected at the time of the relief of aortic stenosis. All operations for congenital aortic stenosis are carried out during cardiopulmonary bypass, and detailed descriptions of the operative methods have been presented elsewhere (7, 8).

ANATOMICAL FEATURES

In 26 patients the site of obstruction was the aortic valve, and most frequently valvular stenosis resulted from a bicuspid valve. Such valves consist of two leaflets of nearly equal size, with the commissures oriented anteroposteriorly. Most often there is fusion of the anterior commissure and an eccentric stenotic orifice. Relief of this form of stenosis is accomplished by making a precise incision of the fused commissure nearly to the aortic wall. A third rudimentary commissure or raphe in the left leaflet can usually be identified; it is important that division of this incomplete commissure should not be carried out, since the two halves of this leaflet are then improperly suspended, and severe valvular incompetence results. When a stenotic tricuspid valve is found all three of the fused commissures may be divided, and, in contrast to the bicuspid valve, complete relief of obstruction is often achieved. The unicommissural aortic valve, found in one patient, consists of only a single cusp, a single commissure, and there is an eccentric, comma-shaped, stenotic orifice. Fortunately the unicommissural valve is encountered only rarely, since effective relief of obstruction cannot be achieved except by valve replacement; incision of the single leaflet opposite the commissure results in massive aortic incompetence. The combined or "tunnel" form of valvular and subvalvular aortic stenosis, encountered in three patients, is characterized by hypoplasia of the aortic valve ring and distal left ventricular outflow tract, long and thickened valve leaflets, and an underdeveloped ascending aorta. This malformation is also infrequently encountered, but poses a difficult problem since effective correction of stenosis often cannot be achieved by simple incision.

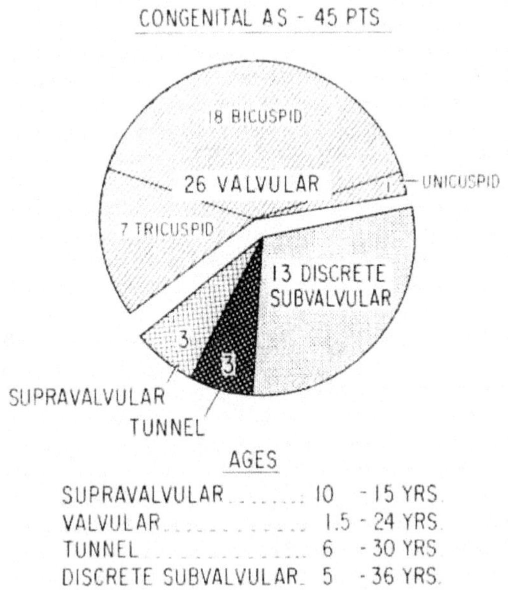

FIGURE 14. Anatomic site and type of obstruction and age range in 45 patients with congenital aortic stenosis (*AS*) in whom operative treatment was carried out.

Thirteen patients had the discrete form of congenital subaortic stenosis. In this malformation, obstruction results from a crescent-shaped fibrous membrane across the anterior two thirds of the outflow tract immediately below the aortic annulus; the membrane inserts at either end into the anterior leaflet of the mitral valve. The subaortic membrane is exposed by retracting the valve leaflets and is excised with a knife. The aortic valve leaflets are often traumatized by the jet of blood impinging upon them from below, and mild aortic

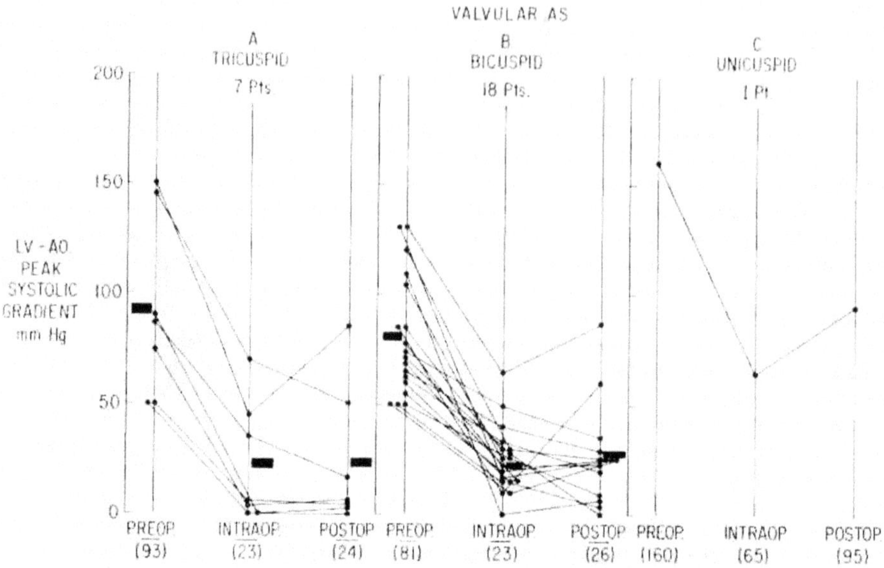

FIGURE 15. Measurements of peak systolic pressure gradients between the left ventricle (*LV*) and the aorta or brachial artery (*AO*) in patients with valvular aortic stenosis, recorded preoperatively (*preop*), at the conclusion of the operative procedure (*intraop*), and at the time of postoperative catheterization (*postop*). In panel A are data obtained from patients with tricuspid valves, in B from patients with bicuspid valves, and in C from the patient with a unicuspid valve. Average values are shown in parentheses at the bottom.

regurgitation frequently accompanies discrete subvalvular stenosis.

Congenital supravalvular aortic stenosis is a relatively uncommon anomaly, and surgical experience with its correction is limited. The effectiveness of operation is largely based on the extent and nature of the obstruction in the ascending aorta. When the narrowed segment is discrete a vertical incision is extended across the deformity into the noncoronary sinus; the stenotic area is then enlarged by the insertion of an elliptical patch-graft into the aortic wall. With diffuse hypoplasia of the aorta and marked intimal proliferation, the prosthesis may have to extend the entire length of the ascending aorta, and in spite of this relief of stenosis may be incomplete.

SURGICAL RESULTS AND HEMODYNAMICS

Forty-one of the 45 patients operated on are living. One operative death occurred in a patient with the tunnel type of stenosis, and three patients have died in the late postoperative period; one each had had valvular, subvalvular, and supravalvular stenosis. Two patients with valvular aortic stenosis have severe aortic regurgitation after operation, and in one child complete heart block followed operation for discrete subaortic stenosis; he has an implanted pacemaker. All but four surviving patients are asymptomatic; two are those with aortic regurgitation noted above. The other two patients are symptomatic because of incomplete relief of stenosis; one had a unicommissural valve; the other, discrete subaortic obstruction.

The severity of aortic stenosis was assessed preoperatively in every patient by means of left heart catheterization. At the conclusion of the operation, before the thoracotomy was closed, left ventricular pressure was measured by direct puncture. Thirty-four patients have returned for postoperative left heart catheterization at intervals ranging from 6 months to 5 years after operation, the average interval being 18

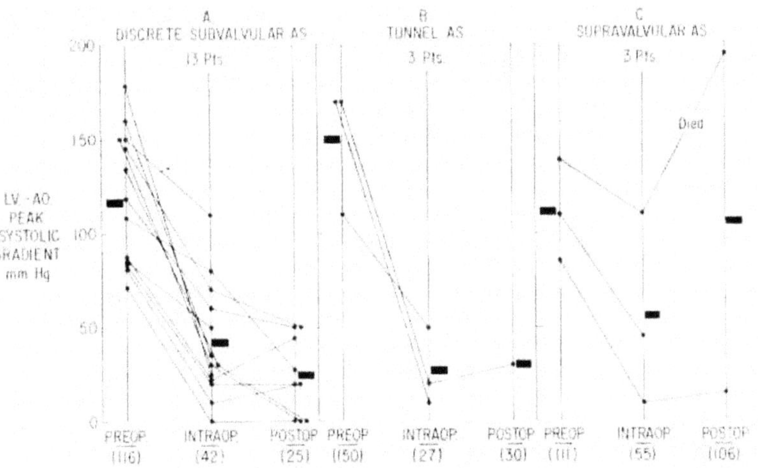

FIGURE 16. Peak systolic pressure gradients between the left ventricle (*LV.*) and brachial artery (*AO.*) in patients wth discrete subvalvular stenosis (*A*), tunnel stenosis (*B*), and supravalvular stenosis (C). The preoperative, intraoperative, and postoperative measurements are designated as in Figure 15.

months. The measurements of the peak systolic pressure gradient between the left ventricle and brachial artery recorded preoperatively, at the conclusion of the operative procedure, and at the time of postoperative catheterization are illustrated in Figure 15 for the 26 patients with valvular aortic stenosis. A substantial immediate reduction in the gradient was achieved in every patient, and in 18 of the 26 the intraoperative gradient was less than 30 mm Hg. In general, the gradients recorded at postoperative catheterization were higher than those measured in the operating room, probably due to the lower cardiac output in the latter setting. The systolic pressure gradient was below 30 mm Hg in 16 of the 22 patients studied late postoperatively. A less satisfactory but acceptable result was achieved in two additional patients in whom residual gradients of 30 to 50 mm Hg were recorded postoperatively. Thus, the postoperative gradient exceeded 50 mm Hg, the value often used in selecting operative candidates, in only four patients; two of these patients had bicuspid valves, one a tricuspid valve, and the other was the single patient with a unicuspid valve.

The preoperative, intraoperative, and late postoperative left ventriculoarterial peak systolic pressure gradients in patients with discrete subvalvular stenosis, tunnel aortic stenosis, and supravalvular aortic stenosis are plotted in Figure 16. In all, reduction of the gradient was evident at completion of the operation. Thirteen patients with discrete subvalvular stenosis under-

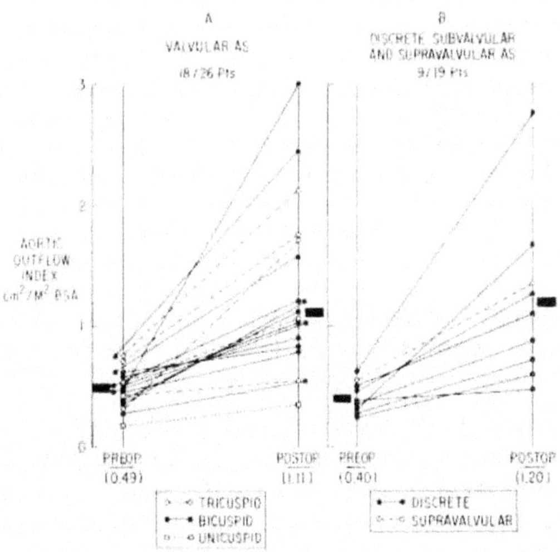

FIGURE 17. Effective left ventricular outflow orifice indices calculated preoperatively and at late postoperative catheterization in patients with valvular stenosis (*A*) and with discrete subvalvular or supravalvular stenosis (*B*). Average values are shown in parentheses.

TABLE 3. Data in 11 Autopsied Patients with

Patient	Age, Sex	Family History Heart Disease	Electrocardiogram*	Length of Symptoms	Functional Class*	Associated Lesions‡	Clinical Diagnosis§
	yr			*yr*			
A56-43	54, M	0	LVH, LVS	8	III	Hypertension	AS
A61-127	26, F	+	AF, LVH, LVS	8	IV	MR	MR
A63-77	40, F	+	AF, LAD	3	IV	MR, aneurysm PT	MR
A63-90	27, F	0	LVH, LVS	12	III	—	IHSS
A64-19	53, M	+	LVH, LAE, LAD, 1° HB, AF††	3	III	—	IHSS
A65-217	12, M	+	LVH, LVS, LAE	4	II	—	IHSS
A65-236	33, F	+	LBBB, LAE, 1° HB	0	II	—	IHSS
A66-212	74, F	—	Old MI	3	II	Calcified MV ring, hypertension	IHSS
A67-70	35, F	+	LBBB, LAE, 1° HB	18	III	—	IHSS
A67-72	41, F	—	LVH, LVS, 1° and 2° HB	9	III	Hypertension	IHSS
A67-121	36, F	+	Bilateral BBB, 1° HB, LAD	4	III	Fibromas LV, MV, AV	IHSS

* LVH = left ventricular hypertrophy; LVS = left ventricular strain; AF = atrial fibrillation; LAD = left deviation; LAE = left atrial enlargement; 1° HB = first-degree heart block (PR interval > 0.20 sec); LBBB = left bundle branch block; MI = myocardial infarction; 2° HB = second-degree heart block; BBB = bundle branch block.

† New York Heart Association classification.

went late postoperative study; six had residual gradients of less than 30 mm Hg, and none was greater than 50 mm Hg. In each of the patients with tunnel aortic stenosis the intraoperative gradient was 50 mm Hg or less, and in the single patient studied late it was 30 mm Hg. Two of the three patients with supravalvular stenosis were studied late postoperatively; in one the gradient was reduced to 15 mm Hg; in the other patient no relief of stenosis was evident, and he later died.

The cardiac index was normal (> 2.5 liters/min per M^2 BSA) in all of the patients both before and after operation, and the average cardiac index was not altered significantly after operation. The cardiac output was determined simultaneously with the outflow gradient in 27 patients both pre- and postoperatively, and the effective orifice areas could thus be calculated (Figure 17). In 12 of 18 patients with valvular stenosis the effective aortic outflow index was greater than 1 cm^2/M^2 BSA and was

Idiopathic Hypertrophic Subaortic Stenosis (IHSS)

Hemodynamics, *mm Hg*				Cause of Death**	Cardiac Pathology		
Left Ventricle (LV)	Systemic Artery (SH)	LV-SA PSG‖ at Rest	PA-RV PSG‖ at Rest		Heart Weight	Endocardial Plaque Ventricular Septum	Abnormal Mitral Valve
					g		
265/22	110/70	155	—	Sudden	650	+	+
103/2	95/55	8	10	CHF	380	+	+
125/12	130/85	0	0	Operation	470	+	+
230/7	100/60	130	25	Cardiac catheterization	490	+	+
210/10	100/60	110	55	Operation	800	+	+
138/8	118/80	20	8	Cardiac catheterization	250	0	0
100/30	100/60	0	—	Suicide	350	+	+
—	—	—	—	Pneumonia	650	+	+
108/34	114/64	0	0	Sudden	430	0	+
200/7	195/105	5	—	Sudden	730	+	+
160/18	85/50	75	0	Sudden	450	+	+

‡ MR = mitral regurgitation; PT = pulmonary trunk; MV = mitral valve; LV = left ventricle; AV = aortic valve.

§ AS = aortic stenosis.

‖ PSG = peak systolic gradient.

** CHF = congestive heart failure.

‡‡ Atrial fibrillation appeared postoperatively.

more than 0.75 cm^2/M^2 BSA in three additional patients. In five of the nine patients with subvalvular or supravalvular stenosis studied postoperatively, the orifice index was above 1 cm^2/M^2 BSA, while a less satisfactory result was achieved in the others.

The left ventricular end-diastolic pressure was recorded both pre- and postoperatively in 31 patients. In 7 of the 16 patients who had abnormally elevated end-diastolic pressure preoperatively (> 12 mm Hg) the pressure returned to normal postoperatively.

The information provided by the present patients indicates that in all of the various forms of congenital aortic stenosis effective relief of obstruction to left ventricular outflow can usually be accomplished at minimal risk. Exceptions to this general statement are evident in certain patients with the tunnel form of stenosis and in others with diffuse supravalvular obstruction. It seems likely, however, that improved operative methods will evolve and lead to more satisfactory results in these groups. Regardless of the site of obstruction, operations for congenital aortic stenosis are usually performed during childhood or adolescence, and the long-term results of the various procedures must await careful and continued clinical and hemodynamic evaluations.

Dr. Morrow: We will now move to a consideration of that entity in which we have a rather paternal interest here at the National Heart Institute. The disease is now relatively well understood, but as yet there is not agreement on a proper name for it. Idiopathic hypertrophic subaortic stenosis (IHSS) is our favorite term, because we invented it, but obstructive cardiomyopathy, diffuse subvalvular aortic stenosis, muscular subaortic stenosis, and functional aortic stenosis are all used. To engage the subject of IHSS, Dr. Roberts will tell us something about his anatomic observations.

Anatomic Studies in Idiopathic Hypertrophic Subaortic Stenosis

Dr. William C. Roberts: We have studied at necropsy 11 patients who fall into the general category of idiopathic hypertrophic subaortic stenosis. Pertinent clinical and pathologic features of these patients are summarized in Table 3.

The 11 patients ranged in age from 12 to 74 years (average: 39), and 8 were females. In seven patients one or more members of their families had a similar form of heart disease. One patient (Patient 7, Table 3) was asymptomatic; symptoms of cardiac dysfunction had been present for 3 to 18 years (average: 7.2) in the other 10 patients. Two patients had been in functional class IV, six in class III, three in class II, and one in class I. Cardiac catheterization had been performed in 10 patients, and pertinent hemodynamic data are included in Table 3. Systolic pressure gradients between the left ventricle and a systemic artery were recorded in seven patients, and five patients had gradients within the right ventricular outflow tract. Three patients had labile systemic hypertension. On chest roentgenograms all 11 patients had evidence of left ventricular enlargement. The electrocardiograms of six patients showed left ventricular hypertrophy, and five of them had the strain pattern as well. Three patients had atrial fibrillation; two had left bundle-branch-block; and one, bilateral bundle-branch-block; five had first- or second-degree heart block, or both; at least five patients had had premature ventricular contractions recorded; and five patients had evidence of left atrial enlargement.

Death in six patients resulted from the disease; while in five, other factors were operative: one patient died 7 days after what had been considered a successful left ventricular myotomy; one died 4 days after cardiotomy for planned mitral replacement; but the valve was considered normal at operation (the correct diagnosis of IHSS was apparent only at autopsy); two died of complications of cardiac catheterization; and one patient, the only one who was asymptomatic, committed suicide. Five of the remaining six patients died suddenly and unexpectedly, and three of them had had large (75 to 155 mm Hg) gradients within the left ventricle. The remaining patient (Patient 2, Table 3) died of progressive congestive heart failure. The clinical diagnosis in eight patients was IHSS; in two patients, mitral regurgitation; and in one patient, aortic stenosis.

At necropsy, the hearts of the 10 adult patients ranged in weight from 350 to 800 g (average: 530 g). All 11 patients had hypertrophy of the cephalad portion of the ventricular septum far out of proportion to that of the free wall of the left ventricle. In nine patients the endocardium in the left ventricular outflow tract was thickened; and in 10 patients the mitral valve, mainly the anterior leaflet, was abnormal. None of the patients had significant coronary arterial narrowing. These anatomic features are illustrated in Figures 18 to 20.

Thus, the three major anatomic findings in the heart in IHSS are as follows: [1] disproportionate septal hypertrophy; [2] thickened endocardium in the left ventricular outflow tract opposite the anterior mitral leaflet; and, [3] an abnormal mitral valve, with fibrous thickening and some degree of contracture of the anterior leaflet and the

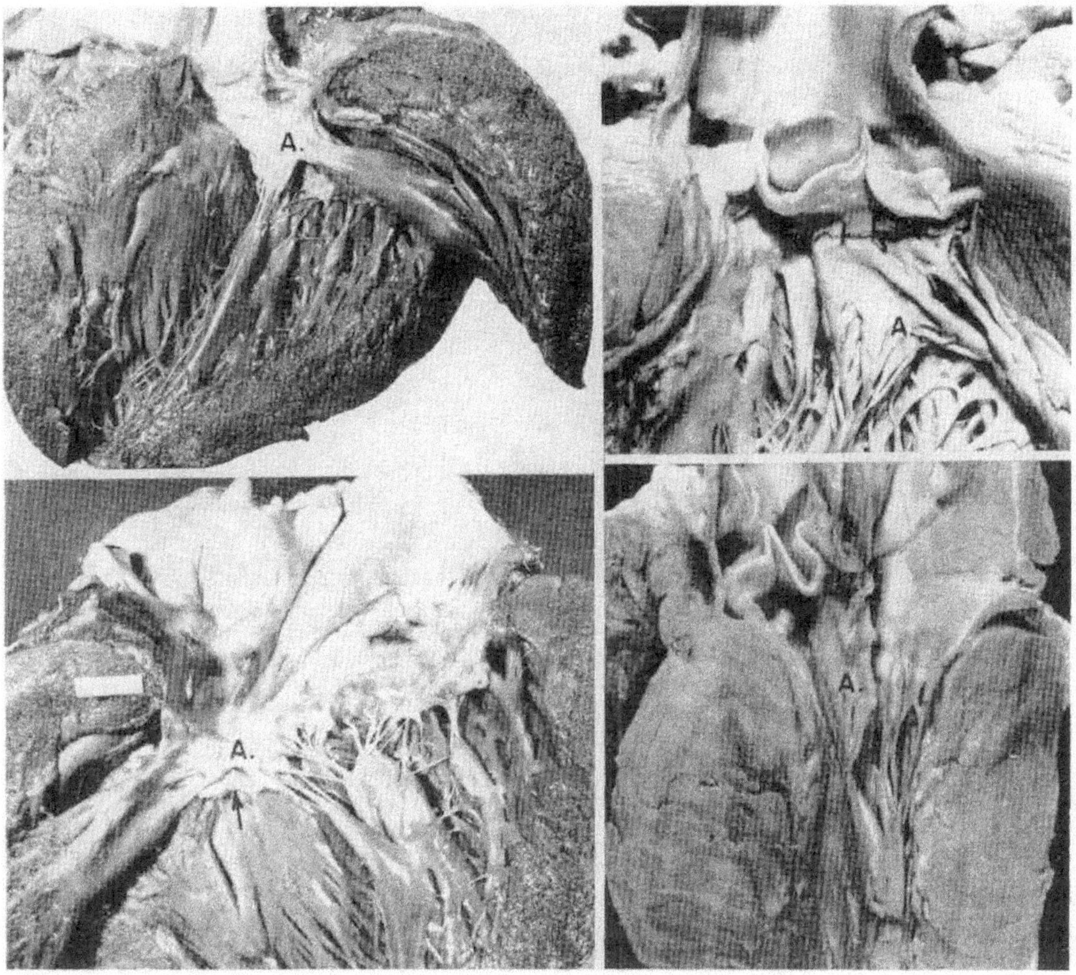

FIGURE 18. Idiopathic hypertrophic subaortic stenosis (*IHSS*) with large (155 and 130 mm Hg) peak systolic pressure gradients between the left ventricle and a systemic artery.

Left panel. Patient 1, Table 3. Upper left: opened left ventricle, aortic valve, and aorta. There is severe hypertrophy of the left ventricular wall with disproportionate hypertrophy of the ventricular septum. The endocardium of the ventricular septum (septal endocardial plaque) opposite the anterior mitral leaflet (*A.*) is thickened, as is the anterior mitral leaflet and the chordae tendineae attached to it. Lower left: opened left atrium, mitral valve, and left ventricle. The anterior mitral leaflet (*A.*) is thickened and the septal endocardial plaque, which is visible, contacts this leaflet (*arrow*).

Right panel. Patient 4, Table 3. Upper right: opened left ventricular outflow tract, aortic valve, and aorta. The septal endocardial plaque and the thickened anterior mitral leaflet (*A.*) are visible. Lower right: longitudinal section through the heart showing the relative small size of the left ventricular cavity and the disproportionate hyperthrophy of the ventricular septum. The anterior mitral leaflet (*A.*) is indicated and illustrates how it is possible for the anterior mitral leaflet to contact the endocardium of the cephalad portion of the ventricular septum during ventricular systole.

chordae tendineae attached to it. The mitral leaflet thickening also corresponds to the thickening of the endocardium in the left ventricular outflow tract. In addition, the three cusps of the aortic valve are normal or nearly normal, and the left atrium may be dilated to a mild to moderate degree.

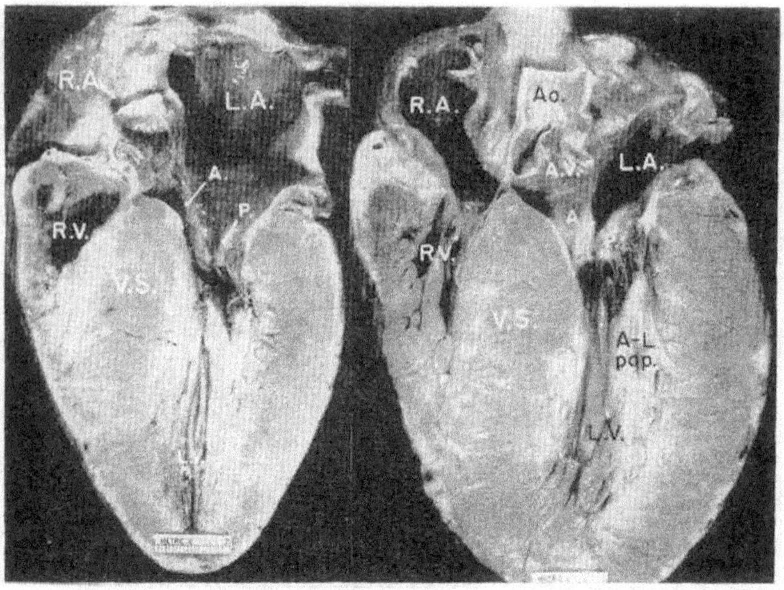

FIGURE 19. Hearts of two patients (Patients 11 and 10, Table 3). Each is anatomically similar, yet one (*left*) had a 75 mm Hg peak systolic pressure gradient at rest, and the other patient (*right*) had only a 5 mm Hg gradient at rest. Each heart has been sectioned longitudinally. In each, the ventricular septum (*V.S.*) is severely hypertrophied, and the thickening is much greater than that of the free walls of the ventricles. Each has a septal endocardial plaque opposite the anterior mitral leaflet (*A.*). The ventricular cavities are relatively small. R.A. = right atrium; R.V. = right ventricle; L.A. = left atrium; P = posterior mitral leaflet; A-L pap = anterolateral papillary muscle; L.V. = left ventricle.

PATHOGENESIS OF ANATOMICAL FEATURES

Of the three major anatomic features of IHSS it appears reasonable to believe that only the disproportionate septal hypertrophy is present at birth and that the thickening of the wall of the left ventricular outflow tract and the mitral valve are acquired lesions. Evidence that this is the case is suggested by the 12-year-old boy (Patient 6, Table 3) who was the only one of 11 patients who had an entirely normal mitral valve and no endocardial plaque in the left ventricular outflow tract; the cephalad portion of the ventricular septum, however, was severely hypertrophied. It is speculated that the endocardial thickening in the left ventricular outflow tract and the thickening of the anterior mitral leaflet are due to trauma from contact of these structures during ventricular systole. The anatomic site of the systolic pressure differential in IHSS is probably the distal margin of the anterior mitral leaflet, and this distal margin in turn corresponds with the most caudal border of the endocardial mural plaque in the ventricular septal portion of the outflow tract.

If these speculations concerning the mechanism of the endocardial thickening in the left ventricular outflow tract and of the site of the maximal pressure differential are correct, it might then follow that the endocardial thickening is simply an anatomic expression of left ventricular outflow obstruction. This was not necessarily the case, however, since five patients with valvular and mural left ventricular outflow endocardial thickening had no or only minimal pressure gradients (5 and 8 mm Hg) within the left ventricle. In two of these patients (Patients 7 and 9, Table 3) the ventricular septum was extensively

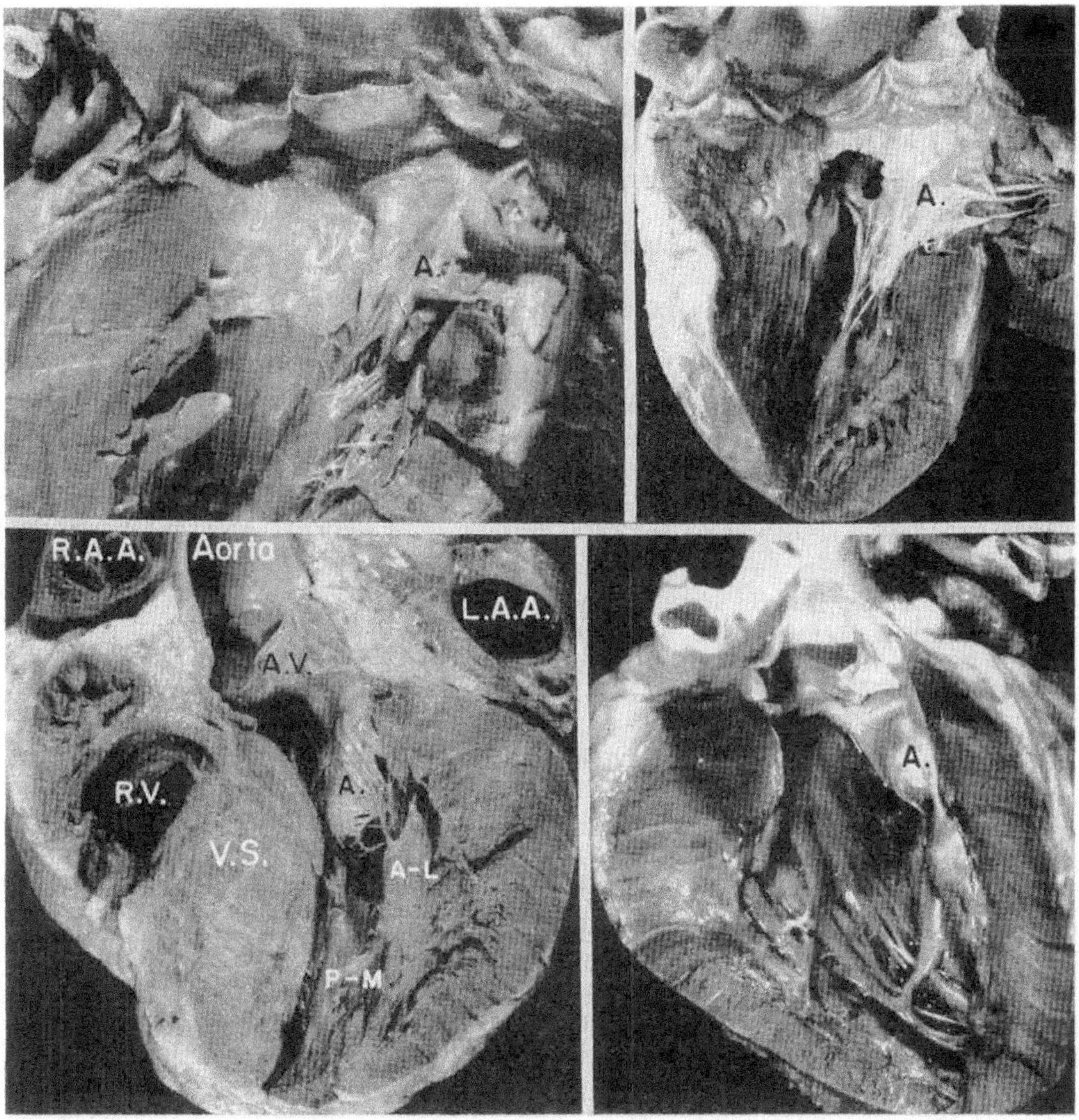

FIGURE 20. Opened left ventricles, aortic valves, and aortas in four patients with idiopathic hypertrophic subaortic stenosis (*IHSS*) without significant (0 to 20 mm Hg) systolic pressure gradients within the left ventricle. Upper left: Patient 3, Table 3. Clinically this patient was considered to have severe rheumatic mitral regurgitation and underwent atriotomy for the purpose of replacing the mitral valve. The valve, however, was normal, and replacement was not carried out. The patient died of an acute myocardial infarct 4 days later. At necropsy, the anterior mitral leaflet (*A.*) was thickened, the posterior mitral leaflet was normal, the cephalad portion of the ventricular septum was hypertrophied, and a septal endocardial plaque was present opposite anterior mitral leaflet.

Upper right: Patient 7, Table 3. Again a large, thick, septal endocardial plaque is present, but in addition the ventricular septum is extensively scarred and vascularized. The septum, however, is considerably thicker than the free wall of the left ventricle.

Lower left: Patient 9, Table 3. Longitudinal section of heart showing the very thick ventricular septum (*V.S.*). The ventricular surface of the anterior mitral leaflet is only minimally thickened, and no septal endocardial plaque is present.

Lower right: Patient 6, Table 3. This 12-year-old boy had a severely hypertrophied left ventricle, and a 20 mm Hg peak systolic pressure gradient between the left ventricle and a systemic artery. The mitral valve is normal, and no septal endocardial plaque is present.

scarred and contained numerous, relatively large, intramural coronary arteries. It is possible that a large systolic pressure gradient had been present at one time within the left ventricular outflow tract, but the gradient disappeared as the ventricular septum became extensively scarred. Also, the septal fibrosis led to some contracture of the ventricular septum. Similar scarring was not present in the left ventricular free walls of either patient.

In two other patients (Patients 2 and 3, Table 3) who had left ventricular outflow endocardial thickening without significant pressure gradients it is possible that the severe mitral regurgitation, which was present in each, prevented the development of left ventricular outflow obstruction. Clinically, both of these patients were considered to have pure mitral regurgitation of rheumatic origin, and one of them (Patient 3, Table 3) underwent cardiotomy for planned mitral valve replacement. The mitral valve, however, was normal when visualized at operation, and no procedure was carried out. The diagnosis of IHSS in each of these two patients was apparent only at necropsy when the three anatomic components of IHSS were evident. The ventricular septum of the remaining patient (Patient 5, Table 3) with left ventricular outflow endocardial thickening and an insignificant systolic pressure gradient was far more hypertrophied than the other four patients, and the septal hypertrophy was of the magnitude seen in the four patients (Patients 1, 4, 5, and 11; Table 3) with large outflow gradients. It is probable that a large left ventricular outflow pressure gradient was present in him at sometime and, indeed, a pressure gradient of 34 mm Hg was produced by the Valsalva maneuver.

In summary, three anatomic criteria of IHSS are described. Disproportionate hypertrophy of the interventricular septum is the major and primary anatomic finding, and thickening of the endocardium in the left ventricular outflow tract and thickening of the anterior mitral leaflet appear to be acquired lesions. By application of these anatomic criteria, two patients who clinically appeared to have pure rheumatic mitral regurgitation were found at autopsy to have IHSS.

The Natural History of Idiopathic Hypertrophic Subaortic Stenosis

Dr. Eugene Braunwald*: As the experience with IHSS evolved, attention was first directed towards a description of the hemodynamic features characteristic of the disease and the development of clinical and laboratory techniques that permit its diagnosis (9); more recently, medical and surgical forms of treatment have received major attention. Our experience with IHSS was reviewed in detail in one of these conferences in 1963 (1). At that time two major unresolved questions remained: the first was the elucidation of the cause or causes of the disease, and the second, to which this presentation is directed, was an understanding of the natural history of IHSS. By the end of 1966 we had studied a total of 126 patients at the National Heart Institute, and the majority of them have been reexamined or restudied at intervals for periods of up to 12 years. Dr. Stuart Frank and I recently analyzed the data obtained from these studies (10), and I will now summarize the results of this analysis.

Follow-up information is available on 98 of the 126 patients. Fourteen patients were seen on only one occasion, and surgical treatment was undertaken in the other 14 at the time of the first admission. Of these 126 patients, 101 had an outflow pressure gradient in the basal state—that is, a pressure difference between the left ventricular cavity and the subvalvular region (Figure 21). Another 18 patients developed a gradient only with provocation (9); 7 patients had no pressure gradient, but we consid-

* Clinical Director and Chief, Cardiology Branch, National Heart Institute.

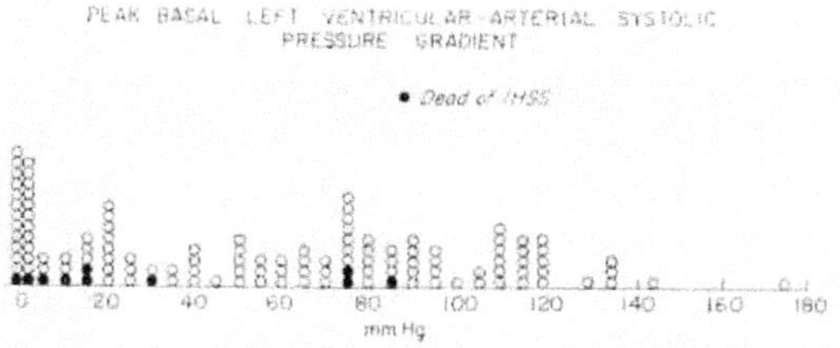

FIGURE 21. Peak basal left ventriculoarterial systolic pressure gradient at the time of the initial catheterization. Only 3 of the 10 patients who died of idiopathic hypertrophic subaortic stenosis (*IHSS*) had a systolic pressure gradient exceeding 30 mm Hg.

ered them to have IHSS because of a positive family history and evidence of left ventricular hypertrophy.

FUNCTIONAL CLASS AND AGE

When the patients first entered the study those with most severe symptoms, that is, those in functional classes III and IV, were older than those patients in classes I and II. On first consideration this observation suggests that the seriously symptomatic patients were merely further along in the course of their disease. However, the interval between the discovery of a murmur or the development of symptoms and the patient's entry into the study was similar in patients in all functional classes. These observations suggest that the patients who were more severely disabled did not merely come under observation at a later stage of the disease than those who were asymptomatic. Instead, they are more consonant with the possibility that patients with IHSS are composed of two different populations: a younger group of patients who are asymptomatic or mildly disabled and tend to remain so, and an older group in whom the clinical manifestations develop later in life and who become progressively more disabled.

Forty-two patients who entered the study in class I have been followed for an average of 38 months, 40 patients who entered in class I for 33 months, and 16 patients in classes III or IV have been followed for an average of 31 months (Figure 22). The condition of the majority of patients who were in class I at the time they entered the study has remained stable, at least for the limited period of time during which we have followed them. On the other hand, approximately half of the patients who were in class II and only one third of the patients who were in classes III or IV at the time of entry into the study have remained in a stable condition. Substantial fractions of the symptomatic patients have died or have shown symptomatic deterioration during observation. On the other hand, it is interesting that 6 of the 16 patients who entered the study in classes III or IV have demonstrated spontaneous improvement. Thus, it appears that the majority of the patients in class I have thus far exhibited a stable course, but there has been considerable deterioration or fluctuation in the courses of the patients who were already symptomatic at the time they were first observed.

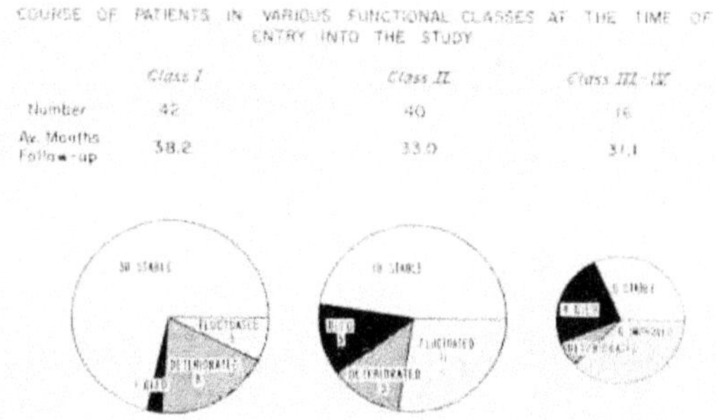

FIGURE 22. The clinical course of patients in various functional classifications at the time of entry into the study. The patients in class I tended to remain stable, whereas those who were more disabled (classes II–IV) tended to pursue a more variable course.

FAMILIAL AND SPORADIC CASES

We were particularly interested in the question of differences between the familial and sporadic forms of the disease. In Figure 23 each patient is represented by a separate symbol. Approximately one third of the patients clearly have familial IHSS,

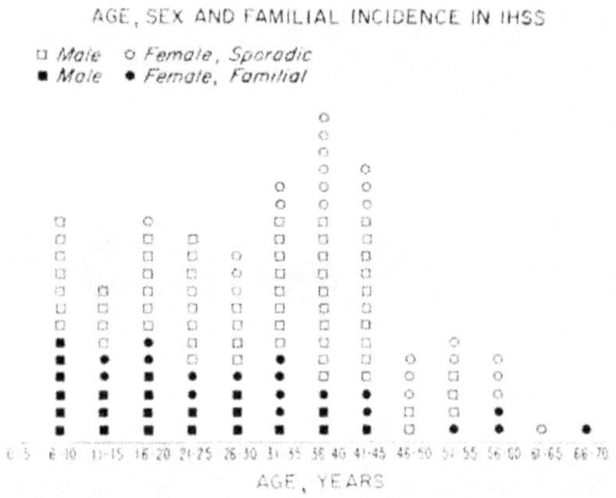

FIGURE 23. The age, sex, and family incidence in idiopathic hypertrophic subaortic stenosis (*IHSS*). Each symbol denotes one patient. Note the relative infrequency of young females with sporadic IHSS, and of older males with familial IHSS.

and the others have the sporadic form. The patients with the familial form constitute a higher percentage among the younger patients and the sporadic cases, a higher percentage among the older patients. Also, the male-to-female sex ratio differs in the two groups; the sexes were distributed approximately equally in the patients with familial IHSS, but only one fourth of the patients with the sporadic form of the disease were females; the sporadic form was uncommon in girls and young women, while familial IHSS was rare in older men. As we ascend in age, we deal with a progressively larger fraction of patients with the sporadic form of the disease and a progressively smaller fraction with the familial form. Similarly, as we go from patients in class I to those in classes III and IV, there are progressively greater fractions of patients with the sporadic form of the disease. Thus, the older and more symptomatic patients tend to have sporadic IHSS while the younger patients and the least symptomatic group more frequently have the familial form.

There are also some differences in the hemodynamics between these two forms of the disease. Only 10 of 86 patients with the sporadic form had no obstruction to left ventricular outflow in the basal state, yet a third with familial IHSS had no obstruction; the average cardiac index was essentially the same in the two groups. The left ventricular-aortic pressure gradient in the patients with the sporadic form of IHSS (average = 60 mm Hg) was significantly greater than that observed in the familial group (average = 42 mm Hg).

EVOLUTION AND DEATHS

Ten of our patients have died as a consequence of IHSS. These patients do not necessarily correspond to those just described by Dr. Roberts because he had the opportunity to examine the hearts of some patients whom we did not study clinically. Only 3 of these 10 patients had significant obstruction in the basal state, with gradients exceeding 30 mm Hg, while the other 7 had no or only mild obstruction (Figure 21). Five patients had familial IHSS and the other five, the sporadic form of the disease. Six of the patients died suddenly, and five of these six had been symptomatic before death. The other four patients showed progressive symptomatic deterioration before their death. The average age at death for the entire group was 30 years. The five patients with familial IHSS who died were significantly younger than were the patients with the sporadic form.

In order to determine whether any changes occurred in the severity of obstruction to left ventricular outflow during the follow-up period, 23 patients were studied on at least 2 occasions at an average interval of 3 years. Thirteen of 23 patients showed no significant change in the pressure gradient during this period. In general, there was little correlation between the change in the hemodynamic severity of obstruction and the patient's clinical condition. Six of the 23 patients have shown a reduction in their gradients by more than 30 mm Hg, and 4 have shown a distinct increase in their gradients. All four of the latter patients have exhibited evidence of clinical deterioration. On the other hand, five patients have shown deterioration without a change in obstruction.

In Figure 21 the solid symbols represent patients who have died as a consequence of IHSS. Only 3 of these 10 patients would be classified as having severe obstruction at rest. One hears a great deal of discussion about prophylactic operation in patients with IHSS, particularly in patients with the familial form of the disease and whose close relatives have died suddenly. I presume that in such patients operation is carried out in order to prevent severe obstruction, which is thought to lead to sudden death. There appears to be little if any evidence that the majority of the patients who die actually have severe obstruction, and for this reason we do not recommend prophylactic operations in patients with mild obstruction.

In addition to the data concerning the natural history of IHSS, review of these 126 patients has provided some interesting information not previously available. Forty-two percent of our 126 patients had a precordial thrill, and in them the systolic pressure gradient was higher (average = 74 mm Hg) than in those without a thrill (average = 41 mm Hg). Of even greater significance is the fact that only 1 of the 25 patients without a gradient in the basal state had a thrill. Sixty-five percent of the patients had normal splitting of the second heart sound during respiration, and 11% had a single second heart sound; in these patients obstruction tended to be less severe (average gradient = 49 mm Hg) than in those with paradoxical splitting (average gradient = 77 mm Hg). Two thirds of the patients with IHSS exhibited a bifid indirect carotid pressure tracing. In these patients the average pressure gradient (66 mm Hg) was much higher than in the patients with a normal carotid pulse contour (average = 23 mm Hg).

In conclusion, careful observation of an increasing number of patients with IHSS has confirmed the earlier impression that this is not an uncommon form of heart disease, that it is relatively simple to recognize, and that the severity of obstruction to left ventricular outflow can often be estimated by careful clinical examinations.

Operative Treatment in Hypertrophic Subaortic Stenosis

Dr. Andrew G. Morrow: As Dr. Braunwald has indicated, the diagnosis of IHSS has been established in nearly 150 patients studied at the Clinical Center. Operations designed to relieve obstruction to left ventricular outflow have now been carried out in 25 patients of this group, and I will briefly summarize the clinical and hemodynamic results of these operations.

Fifteen of the 25 patients were men or boys, 10 were women. At the time of operation their ages ranged from 10 to 64 years, and 5 of them were considered to have the familial form of the disease. Essentially all described dyspnea with effort; two thirds had angina, and it was usually of limiting severity. Half of the patients had been hospitalized for the treatment of congestive heart failure, and half experienced frank syncope. Twelve patients had orthopnea; 10, nocturnal dyspnea; and in 7 symptoms were grossly exaggerated by paroxysmal arrhythmia, usually supraventricular. Six patients had the classic triad of angina, syncope, and congestive heart failure. I will not comment in detail upon the physical, roentgenographic, and electrocardiographic findings, except to say they were those usually associated with IHSS.

Hemodynamics

Hemodynamic studies were carried out in all patients preoperatively and usually on more than one occasion. In all, pressure gradients within the outflow tract of the left ventricle were demonstrated. The gradients, measured at rest, ranged from 26 to 175 mm Hg, and the average was 102 mm Hg. The left ventricular end-diastolic pressure was abnormally elevated in all but 4 patients, the average value being 19 mm Hg. The calculated area of the stenotic orifice ranged from 0.33 to 1.5 cm², and the average was 0.65 cm². All but one of the patients demonstrated abnormal postextrasystolic augmentation of the arterial pulse pressure. Six of the 25 had severe pulmonary hypertension, the systolic pressures in the pulmonary artery exceeding 40 mm Hg. Four patients had significant gradients within the outflow tract of the right ventricle ranging as high as 60 mm Hg.

OPERATIVE METHODS

The operative methods we use in IHSS have been described in detail elsewhere (11).

A median sternotomy is used, and mild general hypothermia is induced during cardiopulmonary bypass. A vertical incision in the aorta is made, extending down to the noncoronary sinus of Valsalva, and the left coronary artery is perfused. The aortic valve leaflets are uniformly found to be normal, and when the leaflets are retracted the uppermost portion of a mass of thickened and hypertrophied muscle can be seen; it occupies the region of the interventricular septum and the left lateral free wall of the ventricle. With a double-bladed knife or with a malleable mitral valvulotome introduced through the aorta, two incisions are made over the prominence of the mass of hypertrophic muscle. The first incision is oriented approximately to the commissure between the left and right coronary leaflets of the aortic valve. A second incision is made parallel to the first one, and about 1 cm to the right of the first one. These incisions are carried through the endocardium and the superficial muscle layers only. After the incisions have been made, a finger is introduced from the aorta, and with digital pressure the deeper muscle layers are split. In the thickest part of the muscle mass the myotomies are 1.5 to 2.0 cm in depth. The bridge of tissue between the two myotomies is then resected with an angled rongeur, which is introduced both from the aorta and from the stab wound at the left ventricular apex.

OPERATIVE RESULTS

Twenty-three of the 25 patients operated upon are living. One died suddenly on the eighth postoperative day, undoubtedly of arrhythmia. He had developed atrial fibrillation on the second postoperative day, and at that time we did not appreciate the deleterious effect of this arrhythmia in patients with IHSS.

One 61-year-old patient died at home 8 months after operation. In the early postoperative period she evidenced some left ventricular failure but made a satisfactory recovery and did well for 6 months. She was then admitted to her local hospital in cardiac failure and shortly thereafter developed hemiparesis, apparently the result of cerebral thrombosis. She remained paralyzed and died shortly thereafter. Unfortunately, facilities for an autopsy were not available.

Important complications of operation occurred in three patients. In two, operated upon early in the series, complete heart blocks resulted from making the myotomy and resection too far clockwise, toward the membranous portion of interventricular septum. This, of course, is an avoidable complication, and if the resection is oriented to the area between the left and right coronary leaflets the conduction system will not be endangered. In one of the patients in whom heart block was produced, a small interventricular septal defect was also created. No attempt was made to close the defect, and subsequent studies have shown that the shunt through it is trivial. Both of these patients are living, and have implanted pacemakers. Another patient became comatose about the tenth postoperative day and was found to have a cerebral hemorrhage. He made a full recovery, and the relationship of this complication to the operation is obscure.

Twenty-one of the 23 surviving patients have been followed for at least 1 year, and the mean duration of follow-up in the entire group is 4 years. The functional classifications of the patients preoperatively and at the time of most recent study are compared graphically in Figure 24. Specifically,

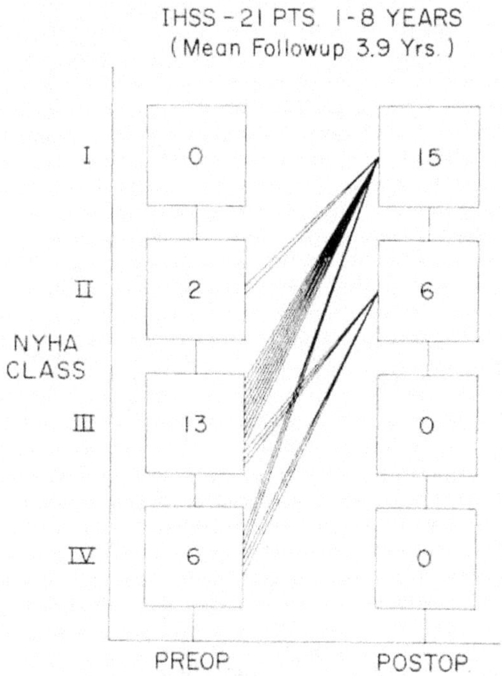

FIGURE 24. Functional classifications (New York Heart Association) of 21 patients with idiopathic hypertrophic subaortic stenosis (*IHSS*) before and after operation. Duration of follow-up was 1 to 8 years. The number within each box indicates the number of patients in that class.

no patient has had syncope, orthopnea, congestive heart failure, or paroxysmal nocturnal dyspnea after operation, and, with one possible exception, none has limiting angina pectoris.

POSTOPERATIVE HEMODYNAMICS

All of the patients have returned on one or more occasions for postoperative hemodynamic assessment. In Figure 25 the peak systolic pressure gradients recorded preoperatively and at the time of most recent postoperative study are compared. In 19 of the 21 patients, no gradient was evident within the left ventricle under resting conditions; in the other 2 gradients of 8 and 11 mm Hg were recorded. The left ventricular end-diastolic pressures measured pre- and postoperatively are compared in Figure 26. All but two of the patients in whom the end-diastolic pressure was abnor-

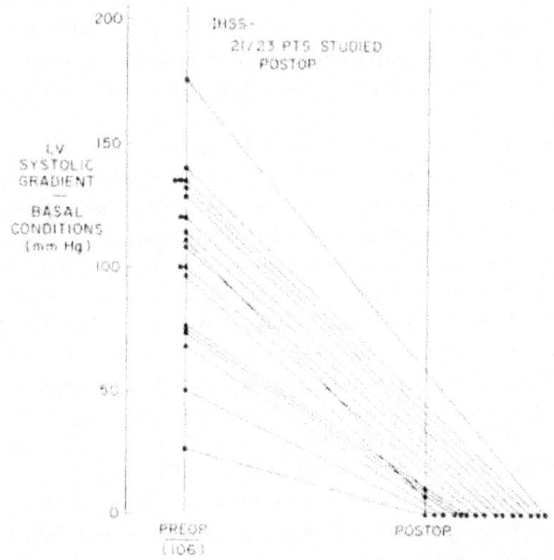

FIGURE 25. Peak systolic pressure gradients between the left ventricle (*LV*) and the aorta or a peripheral artery recorded under resting basal conditions in 21 patients with idiopathic hypertrophic subaortic stenosis (*IHSS*) studied pre- and postoperatively.

mal preoperatively showed striking reductions in this pressure. Preoperatively, the mean value was 20 mm Hg, and postoperatively, it was normal, 11 mm Hg. No systematic changes in cardiac index were observed; most measurements were normal

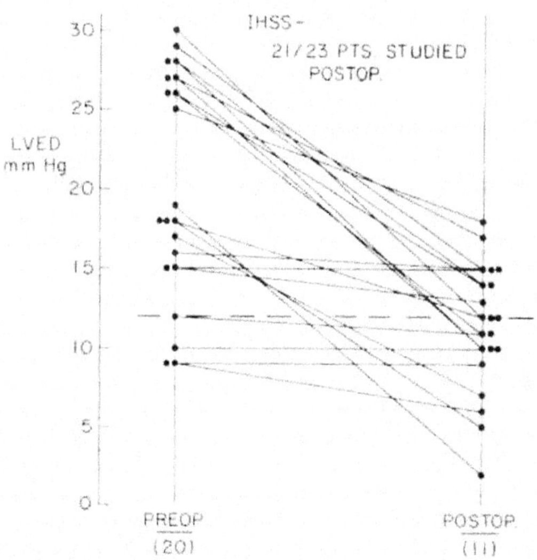

FIGURE 26. Measurements of left ventricular end-diastolic pressure (*LVED*) made in 21 patients with idiopathic hypertrophic subaortic stenosis (*IHSS*) pre- and postoperatively. The mean values of each group of values are indicated in parentheses.

both pre- and postoperatively. Normal postextrasystolic responses in the arterial pulse pressure were observed in 17 of the 21 patients after operation.

The abnormal contour of indirect carotid tracing, present in all patients preoperatively, disappeared in all postoperatively. Also, in patients who had fourth heart sounds preoperatively, these have not been detected afterward.

In patients with hypertrophic subaortic stenosis relief of obstruction can be achieved at a mortality and morbidity comparable with that associated with the operative treatment of the more common forms of aortic stenosis; secondly, in all surviving patients distinct symptomatic improvement has occurred, and parallel to the symptomatic improvement has been a return of intracardiac pressures to normal or near normal levels.

Acknowledgments

Figures 7, 8, and 21 through 26 are reproduced by permission of the American Heart Association, Inc., New York, N. Y. Figures 7 and 8 from Ross and Braunwald (2). Figures 21 through 23 from Frank and Braunwald (10). Figures 24 through 26 from Morrow, Fogarty, Hannah, and Braunwald (11).

References

1. Braunwald, E., Roberts, W. C., Goldblatt, A., Aygen, M. M., Rockoff, S. D., Gilbert, J. W.: Aortic stenosis: physiological, pathological, and clinical concepts. Combined Clinical Staff Conference at the National Institutes of Health. *Ann. Intern. Med.* 58: 494, 1963.
2. Ross, J., Braunwald, E.: The influence of corrective operations on the natural history of aortic stenosis. *Circulation.* In press, 1968.
3. Mitchell, A. M., Sackett, C. H., Hunzicker, W. J., Levine, S. A.: The clinical features of aortic stenosis. *Amer. Heart J.* 48: 684, 1954.
4. Kumpe, C. W., Bean, W. B.: Aortic stenosis: a study of the clinical and pathologic aspects of 107 proved cases. *Medicine (Balt.)* 27: 139, 1948.
5. Bergeron, J., Adelmann, W. H., Vazquez-Milan, H., Ellis, L. B.: Aortic stenosis—clinical manifestations and course of the disease. *Arch. Intern. Med. (Chicago)* 94: 911, 1954.
6. Wood, P.: Aortic stenosis. *Amer. J. Cardiol.* 1: 553, 1958.
7. Morrow, A. G., Goldblatt, A., Braunwald, E.: Congenital aortic stenosis. II. Surgical treatment and the results of operation. *Circulation* 27: 450, 1963.
8. Morrow, A. G.: Congenital and acquired malformations of the aortic valve and left ventricular outflow tract, in *Modern Trends in Cardiac Surgery*, edited by Wooler, G. H., Aberdeen, E., Butterworth & Co., Publishers, Ltd., London, in press, 1968.
9. Braunwald, E., Lambrew, C. T., Rockoff, S. D., Ross, J., Jr., Morrow, A. G.: Idiopathic hypertrophic subaortic stenosis: I. A description of the disease based upon an analysis of 64 patients. *Circulation* 30 (suppl. 4): 3, 1964.
10. Frank, S., Braunwald, E.: Idiopathic hypertrophic subaortic stenosis. A clinical analysis of 126 patients with emphasis on natural history. *Circulation.* In press, 1968.
11. Morrow, A. G., Fogarty, T. J., Hannah, H., III, Braunwald, E.: Operative treatment in idiopathic hypertrophic subaortic stenosis: techniques, and the results of preoperative and postoperative clinical and hemodynamic assessments. *Circulation* 37: 589, 1968.

LESIONS COMPLICATING THE CONGENITALLY BICUSPID AORTIC VALVE

Anatomic and Radiographic Features

WILLIAM C. ROBERTS, M.D.

Chief, Section of Pathology, National Heart Institute, National Institutes of Health, Bethesda, Maryland

LARRY P. ELLIOTT, M.D.

Professor of Radiology, Department of Radiology, University of Florida College of Medicine, Gainesville, Florida

In 1886 William Osler[8] pointed out the susceptibility of a congenitally bicuspid aortic valve to infection. Since that time it has become clear that not only is this type of malformed valve frequently involved by infective endocarditis, but that it also is the most common structure of the aortic valve seen in patients with anatomically isolated aortic stenosis with or without regurgitation.

PATHOLOGIC FINDINGS

Two basic types of congenitally bicuspid aortic valves have been observed at necropsy (Fig. 1). In this series, each type occurred with equal frequency. Approximately 50 per cent of patients with congenitally bicuspid aortic valves have so-called false raphes (Figs. 1 and 2). This ridge of tissue, which partially divides one of the two major cusps into two segments, lies vertically in the wall of the aortic sinus (Fig. 2).

Supported by National Institutes of Health Cardiovascular Radiology Training Grant No. HE-05856-01.

Among 371 patients over age 14 years with functionally severe (usually classes III and IV, New York Heart Association) valvular cardiac disease studied at necropsy at the National Heart Institute, 100 had anatomically isolated aortic valvular disease causing stenosis with or without associated regurgitation. In 49 of them, the aortic valve was congenitally bicuspid, in 31 tricuspid, in 14 congenitally unicuspid, and in six the structure was uncertain. Thus, in virtually 50 per cent of patients with anatomically isolated aortic stenosis with or without associated regurgitation, the aortic valve was congenitally bicuspid. Among 35 patients over age 14 with anatomically isolated aortic valve disease causing pure regurgitation, the aortic valve was congenitally bicuspid in 10, congenitally unicuspid in none, and tricuspid in 25. The aortic regurgitation in 8 of the 10 patients with congenitally bicuspid aortic valves was the result of *infective endocarditis* causing destruction of cuspal tissue. In addition to these 59 patients with congenitally bicuspid aortic valves causing severe stenosis or regurgitation, 11 subjects with normally functioning congenitally bicuspid aortic valves

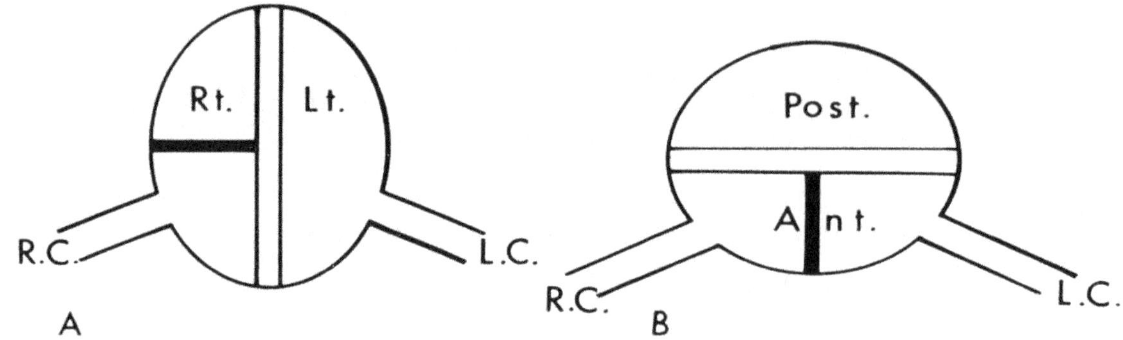

Figure 1. Diagram of the two basic types of congenitally bicuspid aortic valves. *a,* When the cusps are located right and left, the commissures are anterior and posterior and a coronary artery arises from behind each cusp. *b,* When the cusps are located anteriorly and posteriorly, the commissures are right and left and both coronary arteries arise from the aortic root in front of the anterior cusp. When false raphes (black bars) are present, they are located in the right cusp or the anterior cusp.

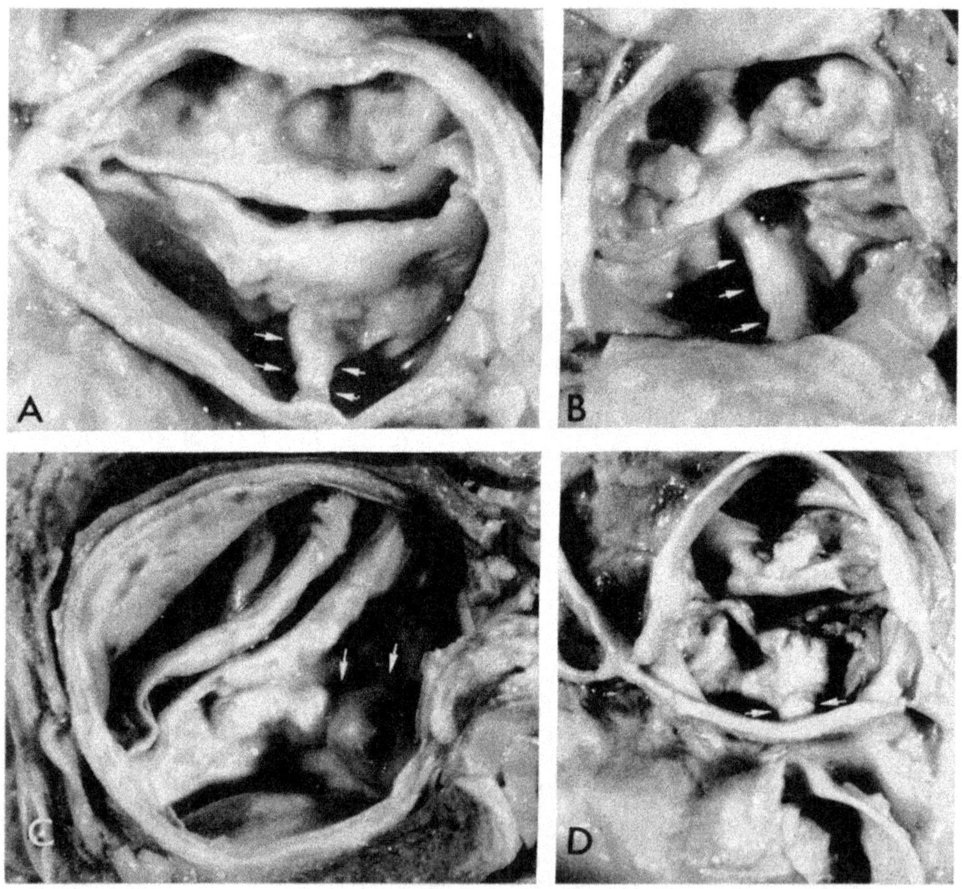

Figure 2. Calcified, stenotic, congenitally bicuspid aortic valves in four patients. The cusps in each are situated anteriorly and posteriorly and the commissures right and left, respectively. Each of the valves has a false raphe (white arrows) in the anterior cusp. *a,* The valve of a 59-year-old man. The peak systolic gradient (PSG) across the valve was 45 mm. Hg, and he had complete heart block secondary to destruction of the atrioventricular bundle by calcium, which presumedly had extended down from the aortic valvular cusps. *b,* The valve of a 60-year-old man who suddenly collapsed on the street. Electrocardiogram recorded in the emergency room showed left bundle branch block. His only symptom of cardiac dysfunction previously was mild exertional dyspnea. *c,* The valve of a 75-year-old man who died after resection of an asymptomatic abdominal

(*Legend continued on facing page.*)

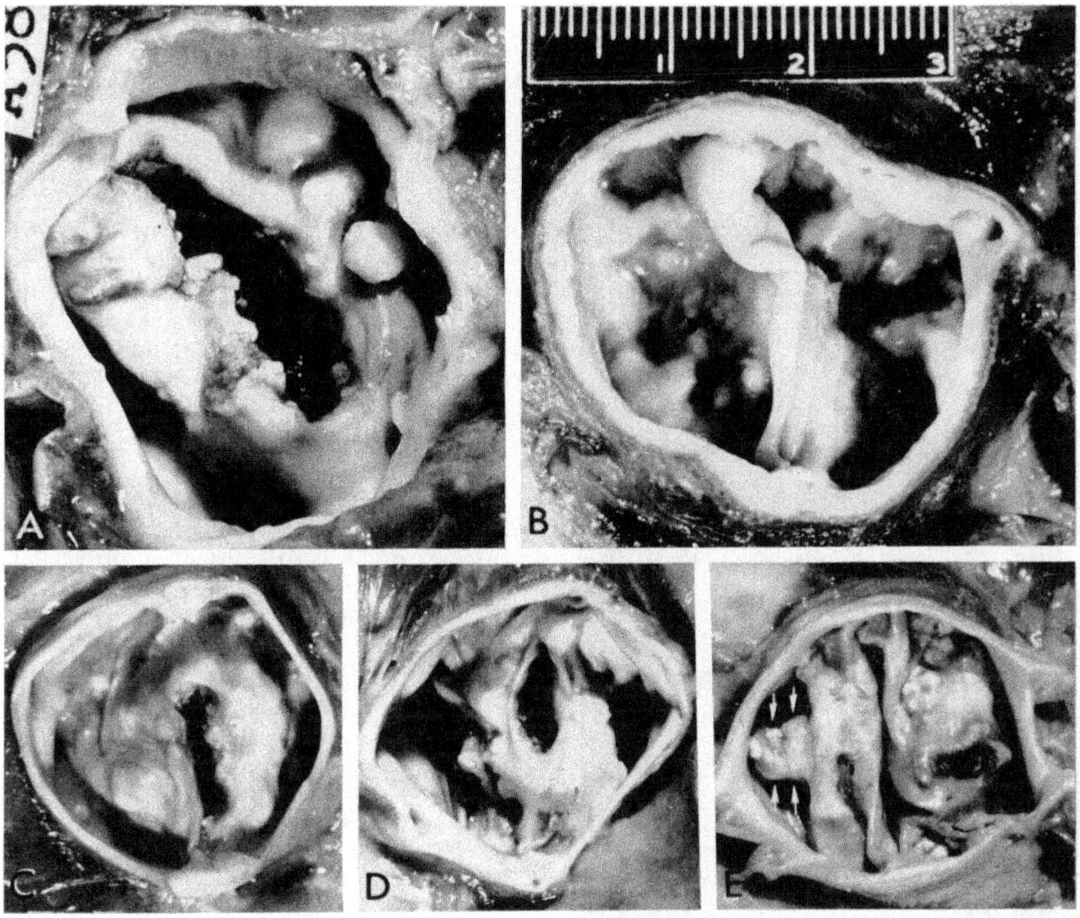

Figure 3. Calcified, stenotic, congenitally bicuspid aortic valves in five patients. In each the cusps are located right and left and the commissures anteriorly and posteriorly, respectively. In only one patient (*e*) can a false raphe (arrows) be definitely identified. In three of the five patients one of the two commissures is partially fused. *a,* The valve of a 37-year-old man who died of progressive cardiac failure. He also had left bundle branch block. *b,* The valve of a 54-year-old man who died during aortic valvuloplasty. The PSG across the valve was 70 mm. Hg. *c,* The valve of a 34-year-old man who died of progressive congestive cardiac failure. *d,* The valve of a 54-year-old man who died of progressive cardiac failure and had a massive pulmonary embolus terminally. He had had symptoms of cardiac dysfunction for 6 years. *e,* The valve of a 79-year-old woman who had been asymptomatic until 2 years earlier, when manifestations of cardiac failure appeared. The heart weighed 700 gm.

were studied at autopsy. The 11 patients ranged in age from 23 to 59 years (average 45), each died from a noncardiac disease, each had a normal-sized heart, and none had a precordial murmur during life. Thus, some congenitally bicuspid aortic valves may function normally for a full lifetime without the development of stenosis, regurgitation, or infection.

Valvular stenosis, therefore, is the most frequent complication of a congenitally bicuspid aortic valve; valvular regurgitation is next, and the latter lesion is most frequently the result of its being the site of infective endocarditis. Why one congenitally bicuspid aortic valve becomes stenotic, another incompetent, and another the site of infective endocarditis is unknown. It appears,

Figure 2. Continued.
aortic aneurysm, which had been discovered during a routine physical examination. A grade 3/6 murmur consistent with aortic stenosis had been heard, but he had no symptoms of cardiac dysfunction. The heart weighed 600 gm. *d,* The valve of a 51-year-old man. The PSG across this valve was only 18 mm. Hg, but the valve was severely incompetent, and the heart weighed 800 gm. Electrocardiogram showed left bundle branch block.

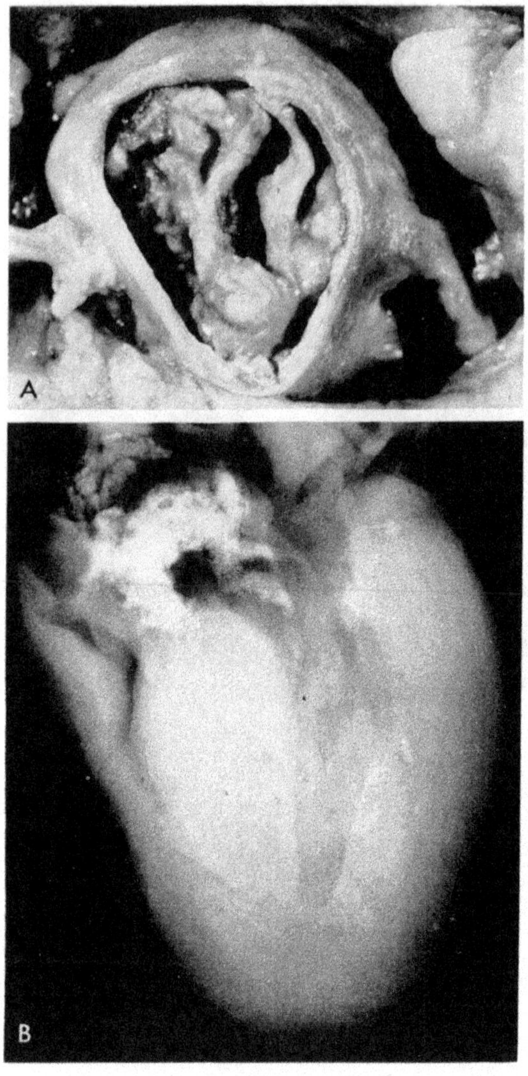

Figure 4. Heavily calcified, severely stenotic, congenitally bicuspid aortic valve (*a*) and radiograph of the heart specimen (*b*) of a 54-year-old man. The peak systolic pressure gradient across the valve was 129 mm. Hg. The calcium deposits extend down the anterior mitral leaflet on one side and through the wall of the aorta on the other side at the level of the pulmonic valve. The ventricular septum is severely hypertrophied; this observation is common in patients with severe valvular aortic stenosis.

however, that stenosis, regurgitation, and infection are *complications* of a congenitally bicuspid aortic valve and none of them are present at birth. A congenitally bicuspid aortic valve becomes stenotic only as its cusps become fibrotic and calcified.

Among a total of 75 patients* aged 15 to 79 years (59 male and 16 female) with congenitally bicuspid aortic valves studied at autopsy at the National Heart Institute, 54 had some degree of stenosis with or without regurgitation, 10 had pure regurgitation, and 11 had normally functioning valves. Heavy deposits of calcium were present in the aortic valve in 52 of the 54 patients with aortic stenosis, but none of the ten patients with pure aortic regurgitation had more than one or two small focal deposits of calcium in the valves and most had none. None of the 11 patients with functionally normal aortic valves had grossly visible calcific deposits on them. Calcific deposits on congenitally bicuspid aortic valves tend to involve each cusp uniformly, so that each cusp contains similar amounts of calcium. Gross calcium deposits are distinctly unusual before the age of 20 years in patients with stenotic congenitally bicuspid aortic valves, and stenotic congenitally bicuspid aortic valves in adults without calcium deposits, as indicated, are rare. Development of infective endocarditis on a heavily calcified valve also is rare. Two of the 54 patients with stenotic congenitally bicuspid aortic valves had a history of infective endocarditis: one had heavy deposits of calcium on his valve before the infection, and the second never had calcium. As mentioned, of the 10 patients with pure aortic regurgitation, infective endocarditis was the cause of the valvular incompetency in eight, and none of these patients had significant aortic valvular calcification. Other anatomic features of the stenotic or incompetent congenitally bicuspid aortic valve are illustrated in Figures 1 to 6.

The mechanism by which a congenitally bicuspid aortic valve becomes stenotic or incompetent is uncertain. There is no evidence to indicate that the valve is stenotic or incompetent at birth. Likewise, there is no evidence to indicate that superimposed rheumatic fever or rheumatic heart disease is the cause of the stenosis or incompetency.

Among 100 autopsied patients with anatomically isolated aortic valve disease causing stenosis studied at the National Heart Institute, only five gave a history of acute

* Five of these patients also had anatomic abnormalities of the mitral valve, either congenital in origin or secondary to hemodynamic alterations.

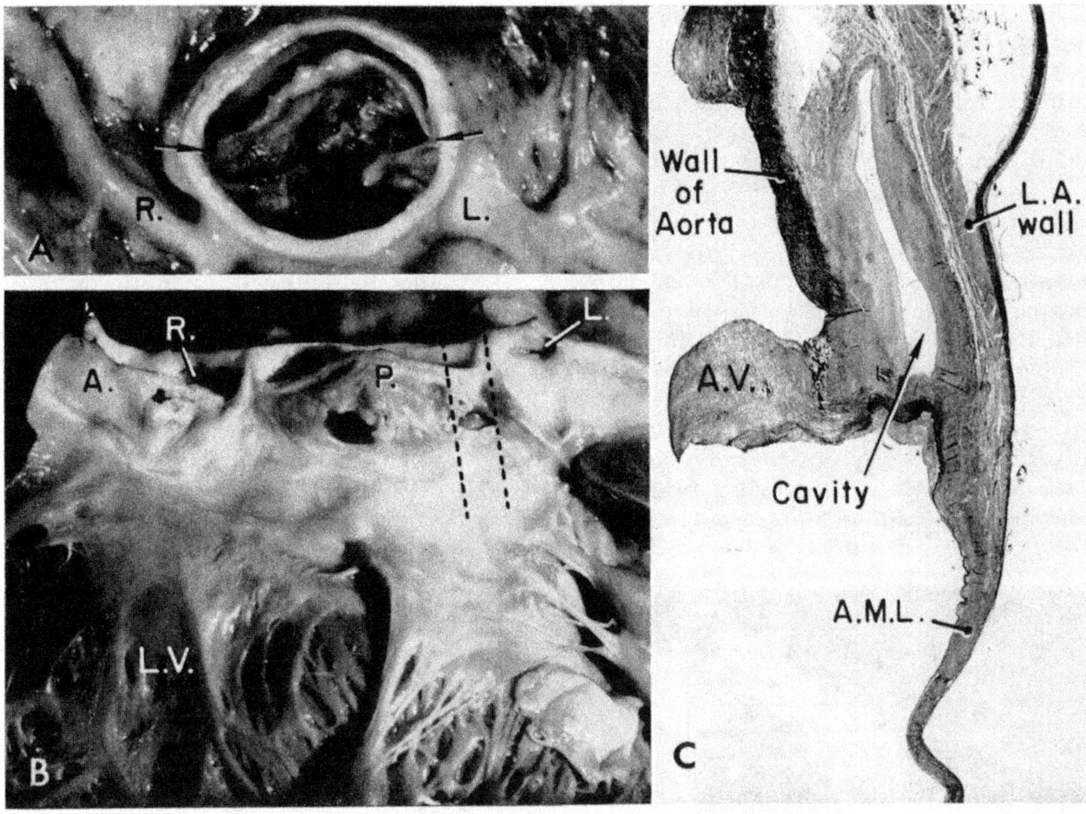

Figure 5. Aortic valve in a 55-year-old woman with Staphylococcus aureus endocarditis on a congenitally bicuspid aortic valve. She had been entirely well without signs or symptoms of cardiac disease until the onset of infective endocarditis 4½ months before death. Although the organism was sensitive to antibiotics in vitro, eradication of the organism never occurred in vivo, massive aortic regurgitation developed, and she died. *a*, Aortic valve from above. The arrows designate the two commissures. L, Left coronary artery; R, right coronary artery. *b*, Opened aortic valve demonstrating perforations in each of the cusps. A, Anterior cusp; P, posterior cusp; L. V., left ventricle; R and L. ostium of right and left coronary artery, respectively. *c*, The photomicrograph includes the area between the two dashed parallel lines. A healed mycotic aneurysm, labelled cavity, is located between the walls of the aorta and left atrium (L. A.). A. V., aortic valve cusp; A.M.L., anterior mitral leaflet. Hematoxylin and eosin stain; × 4½.

rheumatic fever or chorea, and four of them had congenitally bicuspid aortic valves, indicating that the history was probably fallacious. In contrast, of 78 patients with anatomic disease limited to the mitral valve, the percentage with a history of acute rheumatic fever or chorea was 70 per cent, and in the 98 in whom both mitral and aortic valves were anatomically involved, the percentage rose to 79 per cent. Furthermore, none of the patients with anatomically isolated aortic valvular disease had Aschoff bodies in their hearts at necropsy. Aschoff bodies, however, were found in the hearts of 12 of the remaining 271 patients without isolated aortic valve disease causing stenosis. Each had anatomic mitral valve disease, and 11 of them had involvement of the aortic valve as well.

Since superimposed rheumatic fever or rheumatic heart disease is clearly not the cause of the stenosis or incompetency of a congenitally bicuspid aortic valve, other causes must be searched for. The explanation advanced by Edwards[1, 2, 4] is attractive. He proposes that it is not mechanically possible for a congenitally bicuspid valve to open and close properly. The free margin of a normal tricuspid aortic valve is a curved line, and its actual length is greater than the straight-line distance between its ends. This extra length allows the cusps to move freely during opening and closing of the valve. In contrast, the free margin of the cusp of a congenitally bicuspid aortic valve approaches a straight line. If each of these margins were exactly a straight line, it would not be possible for the valve to open during ventricular systole; consequently, one of the cusps is larger than the other, and both may be oversize. This excessive length of either or both cusps produces abnormal contact between the two cusps, which results in focal fibrous thickening that in time becomes diffuse. Subsequently, dystrophic calcification occurs. Thus, stenosis of a congenitally bicuspid aortic valve is simply the result of *trauma* to these cusps produced by their abnormal contact with one another. Although this explanation is appealing, it does not explain why one congenitally bicuspid valve becomes stenotic, another becomes entirely incompetent, and another develops no complications at all.

ROENTGENOLOGIC FINDINGS

Among patients with stenotic or incompetent congenitally bicuspid aortic valves, the plain film signs nearly always indicate an abnormal left ventricle. In the frontal projection, the heart almost invariably assumes the so-called left ventricular (LV) configuration (Figs. 7 and 8*a*). The likelihood of a congenitally bicuspid aortic valve producing some other type of cardiac silhouette

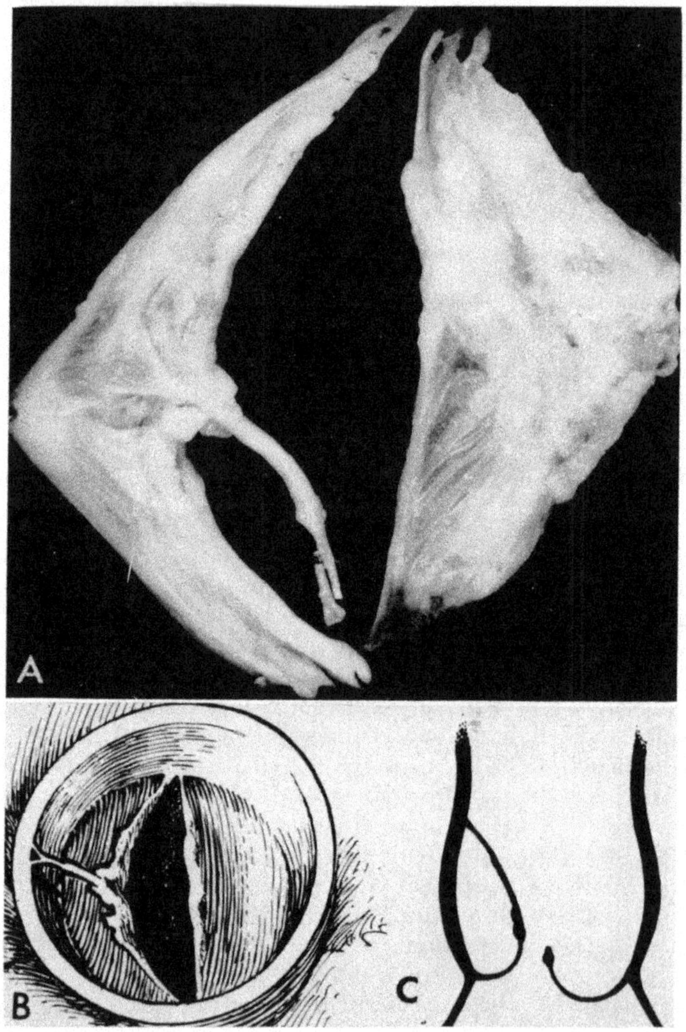

Figure 6. *a*, Excised congenitally bicuspid aortic valve in a 27-year-old man with pure aortic regurgitation. Preoperatively, the left ventricular pressure was 125/25 and the brachial arterial pressure, 126/54 mm. Hg. Aortic root angiocardiogram disclosed severe (4+) aortic regurgitation. In addition, there was a right-sided aortic arch. He died suddenly and unexpectedly 13 months after aortic valve replacement. At necropsy the heart weighed 800 gm. One of the aortic valve cusps is larger than the other and a supporting bandlike brace connected the free margin of one cusp to the aortic wall as illustrated in the lower drawings (*b* and *c*). No calcium deposits were present in this purely incompetent valve.

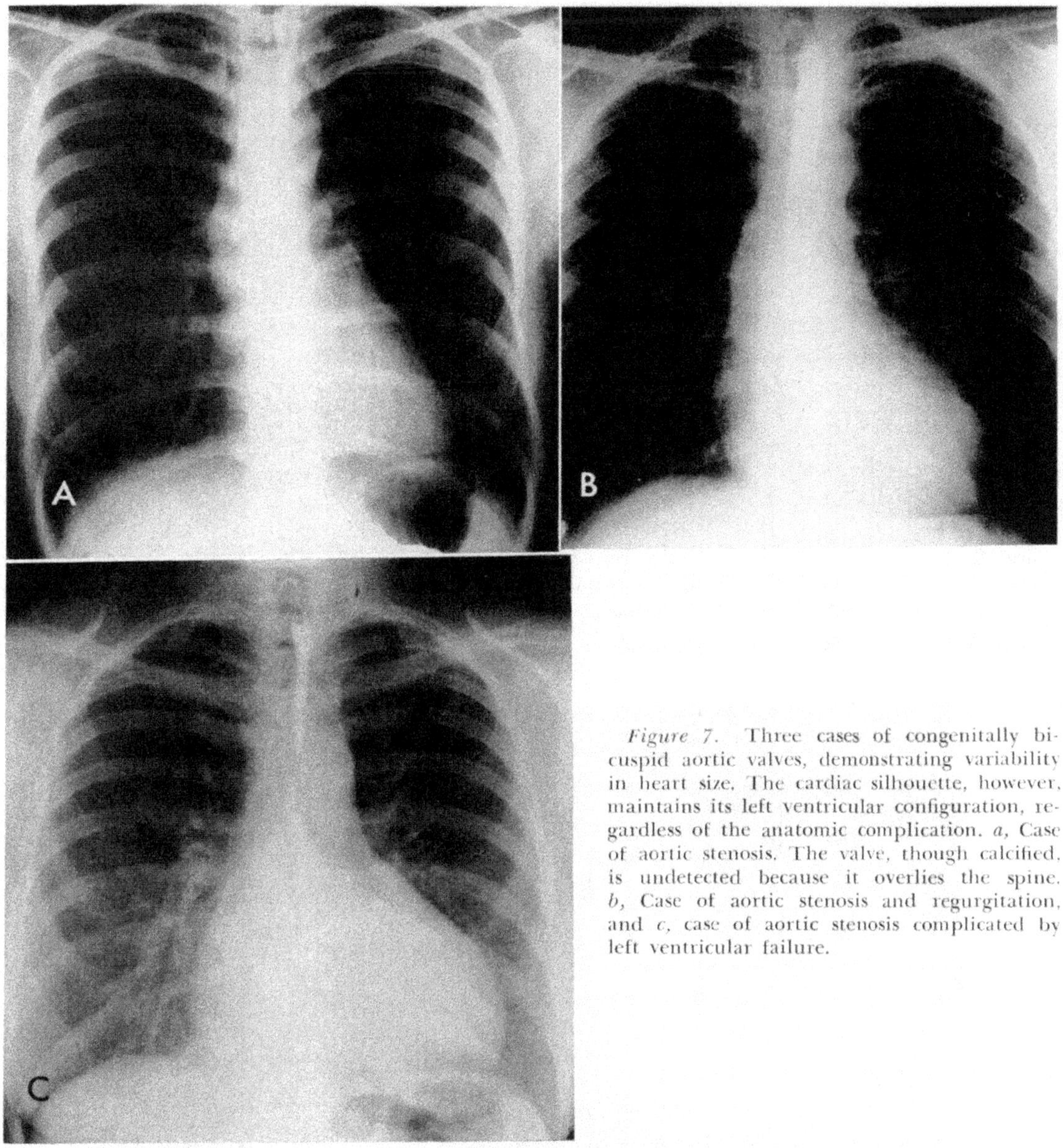

Figure 7. Three cases of congenitally bicuspid aortic valves, demonstrating variability in heart size. The cardiac silhouette, however, maintains its left ventricular configuration, regardless of the anatomic complication. *a,* Case of aortic stenosis. The valve, though calcified, is undetected because it overlies the spine. *b,* Case of aortic stenosis and regurgitation, and *c,* case of aortic stenosis complicated by left ventricular failure.

is remote. The left anterior oblique and lateral views confirm the roentgen signs of essentially pure left ventricular involvement.

In patients with congenitally bicuspid aortic valves, the heart may be normal in size or enlarged (Fig. 7). Heart size, additional signs indicating a failing left ventricle, secondary mitral valve incompetence, etc., will obviously depend upon the *type* and *severity* of the valve lesion. To reiterate, there may be pure aortic valve stenosis (Fig. 7*a*) or stenosis with regurgitation (Fig. 7*b*; each showing a high incidence of calcification) or pure regurgitation.

The most reliable roentgenologic indication of a congenitally bicuspid aortic valve is the presence of calcium in the valve itself (Fig. 9). This finding, together with no history of acute rheumatic fever or chorea, and no physical or roentgenologic signs of organic mitral valve disease (especially stenosis), strongly suggests that the aortic valve is *congenitally malformed.* Statistically, the most common lesion is the congenitally bicuspid valve.

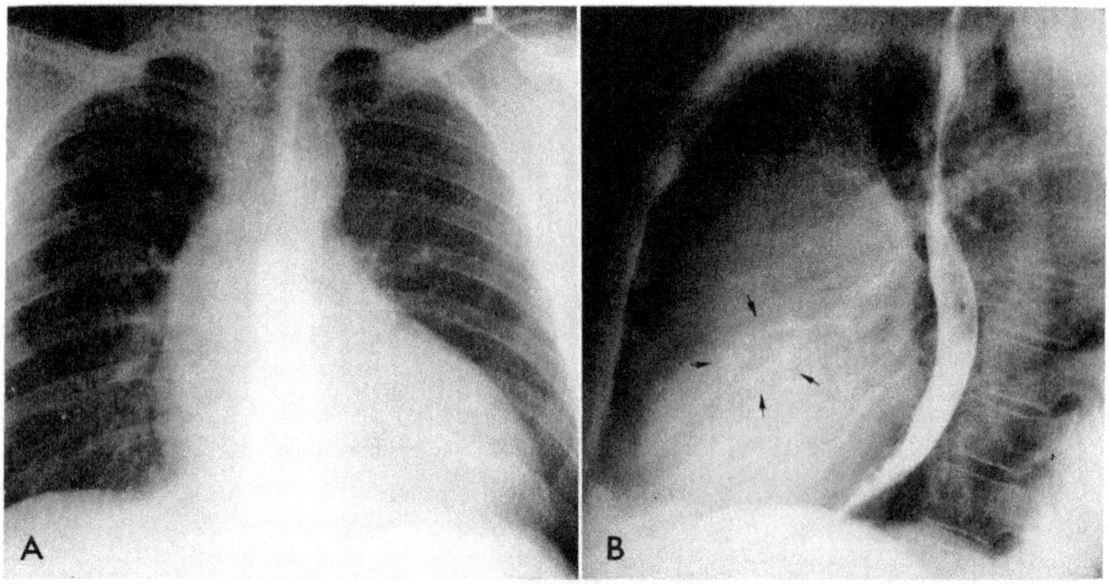

Figure 8. Case of congenitally bicuspid aortic valve stenosis complicated further by calcification (arrows) and regurgitation. *a*, Posteroanterior view and *b*, lateral view. There is evidence of a moderate degree of left atrial enlargement and overt signs of calcification (arrows). Mitral valve incompetence in this case was secondary to left ventricular dilatation, rather than rheumatic endocarditis.

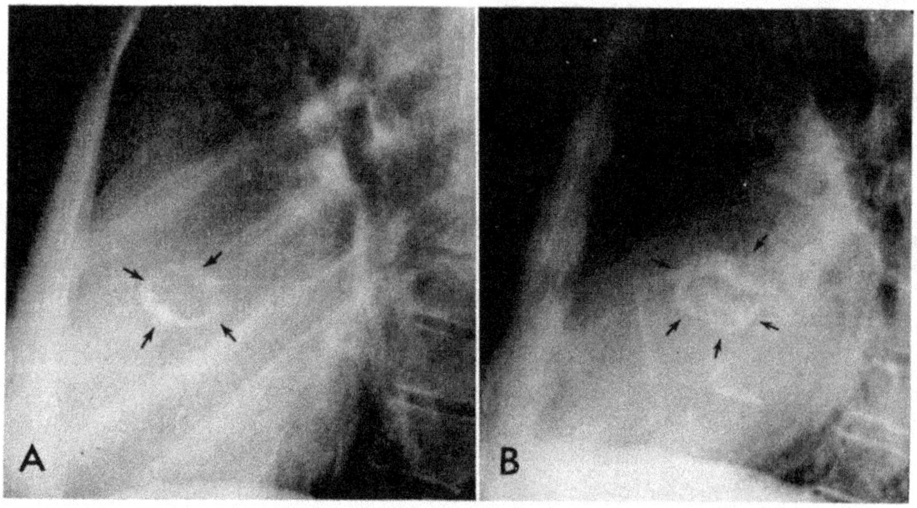

Figure 9. Lateral views of two cases of congenitally bicuspid aortic valves with severe degrees of calcification. All cases with this degree of valvular calcification exhibit aortic regurgitation. In *b*, both cusps are well outlined.

Once a patient with a congenitally bicuspid aortic valve develops LV failure, pulmonary venous congesion and varying degrees of left atrial enlargement usually occur (Fig. 8). The differential diagnosis obviously becomes extensive, because any number of disease processes which affect or stress primarily the left ventricle (systemic hypertension, atherosclerotic ischemic heart disease, diseases of the muscle, etc.) may ultimately result in LV failure and present in this manner. The one redeeming factor from a diagnostic viewpoint is that most patients with congenitally bicuspid aortic valves, by the time LV failure is established, will exhibit an overtly calcified valve.

On occasion, the calcium cannot be accurately detected on plain films in sick patients with large hearts and congested lung fields. Herein lies the value of image intensification fluoroscopy in the adult with heart disease.

Considerable difficulty may arise in distinguishing patients with congenitally bicuspid aortic valves and secondary mitral valve disease or LV failure (Fig. 8) from cases with *combined* rheumatic mitral and aortic valve disease. The heart in a patient with *secondary* or functional mitral valve incompetence owing to LV dilatation, infarction or fibrosis of papillary muscles, etc., retains its LV configuration in spite of the development of left atrial enlargement and pulmonary venous obstruction (Fig. 8). Patients with significant *rheumatic* or organic mitral valve disease, with or without associated aortic valve disease, usually exhibit a triangular or "mitral configuration" cardiac silhouette of varying size. This difference in cardiac contour resides, for the most part, in the fact that patients with organic mitral valve disease have a larger left atrial appendage and pulmonary trunk than patients with functional mitral valve disease. Unfortunately, there are exceptions to these rules.

With this general background, the plain film findings of each major complication of the congenitally bicuspid aortic valve will be discussed.

Bicuspid Aortic Valve with Abnormal Murmur and Normal Hemodynamics. It is unknown how many patients harbor a bicuspid valve. There are a small number of patients who exhibit a low-intensity murmur of aortic stenosis, a left ventricular type configuration of normal size with a prominent ascending aorta on plain films, and a normal electrocardiogram. Although thoracic aortography may demonstrate a bicuspid aortic valve as well as poststenotic dilatation of the ascending aorta, there is no systolic pressure difference across the aortic valve. Therefore, should these patients be considered as normal variants or as having mild anatomic aortic valve "stenosis"? Although a valve orifice must be reduced at least 50 per cent before a systolic pressure difference occurs, the valve orifice in these patients is narrow enough to produce a "jet" of high velocity blood with the ultimate development of poststenotic dilatation of the ascending aorta. The important point is that these patients should be followed because of the possible development of bacterial endocarditis or real valve stenosis.

Bicuspid Aortic Valve with Pure Stenosis. In these patients, the cardiac silhouette is of the left ventricular configuration type (Fig. 7*a*). The heart size and pulmonary vascularity are normal as long as the left ventricle maintains compensation. When these patients have overt cardiomegaly, the additional complications of aortic valve regurgitation or left ventricular failure are present (Fig. 7*c*). The majority of these patients will exhibit roentgen evidence of a calcified aortic valve by 40 years of age. The ascending aorta is prominent, especially in the left anterior oblique (LAO) view.

There is a distinct tendency for the stenotic bicuspid aortic valve to occur in males, a fact which is consistent with other forms of aortic stenosis as well.

Bicuspid Aortic Valve with Stenosis and Regurgitation. The valves in these patients are almost always calcified (Fig. 8). These are patients who begin with predominant aortic stenosis. As in patients with pure stenosis, the ascending aorta is usually quite prominent, especially in the LAO view.

These patients present with an enlarged heart of the left ventricular configuration type (Figs. 7*b* and 8). Signs of pulmonary venous obstruction are almost invariably present, as well as signs of secondary mitral valve disease. The cause of the secondary mitral valve disease is not certain, but is probably related to dilatation of the left ventricle with widening of the mitral annulus and stretching of the papillary muscles or to fibrosis of the papillary muscles. Papillary muscle fibrosis occurs in a high percentage of patients with aortic stenosis.[7]

Bicuspid Aortic Valve with Pure Aortic Regurgitation. This has been uncommon in the experience of both authors. Patients with pure aortic valve incompetence usually show an enlarged left ventricular configuration and rarely have valve calcification. The ascending aorta in patients with pure regurgitation owing to intrinsic aortic valve disease is not as prominent as in patients with aortic stenosis or conditions of the ascending aorta producing aortic valve incompetence.[6] This is because the aorta is rarely as dilated as in conditions of the ascending aorta, which in themselves cause aortic valve incompetence.

In any patient with roentgenologic and clinical signs of pure aortic regurgitation, diagnosis of a congenitally bicuspid aortic valve is strongly suggested if there are no clinical or roentgen signs of rheumatic mitral valve disease, and if conditions of the ascending aorta which in themselves cause aortic regurgitation are ruled out.[6] Once the diagnosis of congenitally bicuspid aortic valve is probable, pathologic studies (W. C. R.) indicate a strong tendency for the additional complication of infectious endocarditis.

Calcific Aortic and Mitral Valve Disease. The tendency is to regard isolated aortic valve calcification as congenital in etiology and combined aortic and mitral valve calcification as secondary to rheumatic endocarditis. There is, however, a small number of patients with a calcified congenitally bicuspid aortic valve with calcification of the mitral valve as well. The latter phenomenon is not caused by rheumatic endocarditis, but is simply an extension or migration of the aortic valve calcific deposits inferiorly to involve the anterior leaflet of the mitral valve (Fig. 4*b*).

If this secondary extension involves the major portion of the anterior mitral valve leaflet, it can often be detected on plain films or fluoroscopy (especially in the lateral and right anterior oblique projections). These patients, besides presenting with aortic valve disease, may exhibit signs of mitral valve dysfunction as well.

There is another group of patients with a calcified congenitally bicuspid aortic valve and roentgenologic evidence of a calcified mitral valve annulus. Since the latter has a distinct radiographic appearance, it should not be confused with calcified valve leaflets. The calcified mitral valve annulus is not abnormal per se and usually occurs in women over age 70. Earlier calcium deposition in this area may be a manifestation of abnormal left ventricular hemodynamics. The important points to realize are (1) not all examples of combined aortic and mitral valve calcification are rheumatic in origin, and (2) when the aortic valve is diffusely calcified and the mitral valve calcification is limited to the anterior leaflet or the valve annulus, a congenitally bicuspid aortic valve should be suspected.

Bicuspid Aortic Valve and Coarctation of the Aorta. There is a strong tendency for coarctation of the aorta (CoA) to occur in association with congenitally bicuspid aortic valves. Approximately 85 per cent of cases of coarctation will demonstrate this valvular anomaly, regardless of the severity of the aortic coarctation.[5] The bicuspid aortic valve in CoA is prone to the same complications as occur in patients without CoA. The valve is most prone to stenosis. Moreover, the incidence of a normally functioning aortic valve in patients with CoA is relatively low. This conclusion is based upon the results of aortography (L.P.E.) in 30 patients with CoA before operation. In these 30 patients, the aortic valve was bicuspid in 24, deformed but tricuspid in four (possibly a partially bicuspid aortic valve), and normally tricuspid in two. Only five of the 30 patients showed a normally functioning valve, and three of these had congenitally bicuspid aortic valves. It is probable that the associated left ventricle and aortic hypertension in CoA may accelerate the fibrosis and calcification of the aortic valve in these patients. Because of this experience, we recommend evaluation of the aortic valve by thoracic aortography in almost all patients with CoA.

Complications of the Calcium Per Se. In calcified aortic valves, the calcium is distributed throughout the valve, and the primary hemodynamic abnormality is related to the rigidity created by these deposits. However, it is not uncommon for secondary extensions of calcific material to involve other structures.[3] Calcium deposits may encroach upon or obstruct the ostia of the coronary arteries, and signs of coronary insufficiency will be superimposed upon an already complex clinical situation.

Calcific material may extend inferiorly into the left ventricle and involve the left branch of the bundle of His. Involvement of the anterior leaflet of the mitral valve has been discussed. These secondary extensions of calcium may be difficult to detect roentgenologically, since the additional deposits

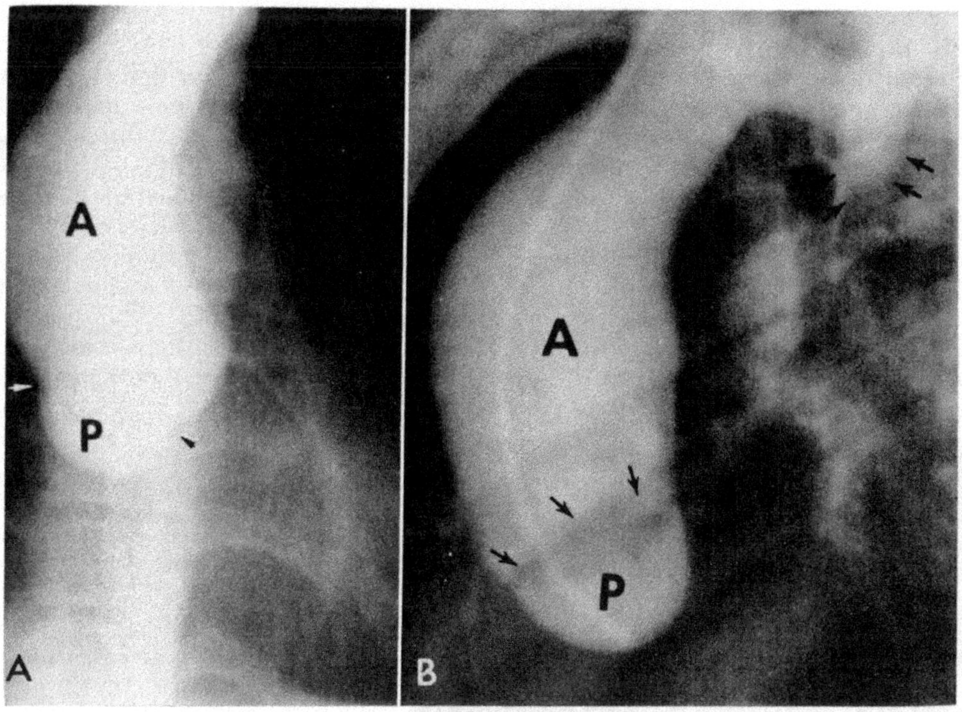

Figure 10. Thoracic aortogram in case of aortic coarctation associated with a congenitally bicuspid aortic valve. *a,* Anteroposterior view and *b,* lateral view. In *b,* the posterior cusp (P) is enlarged and forms one component of the bicuspid valve. It encompasses the entire width of the aortic root. The vertical arrows indicate the nondescript fused right and left cusps. In *a,* the posterior cusp (P) is enlarged (arrows) and its lower margin is situated more inferior than the normal. A, ascending aorta.

may overlie the valve or lie so close to the valve that they are interpreted as a part of the valve itself.

Angiocardiographic Features

To better understand the angiocardiographic findings, a review of the embryologic development of the aortic valve seems appropriate.[9] In formation of the normally tricuspid aortic and pulmonary valves (semilunar valves), two cusps of each semilunar valve are formed from the so-called truncal swellings. The third cusp of each semilunar valve is formed from another type of tissue, the intercalated valve swelling. Both types of tissue are located at the distal end of the truncus. The truncal swellings develop into the right (anterior) and left aortic valve cusps, whereas the noncoronary or posterior aortic valve cusp is formed from the intercalated valve swelling. Developmentally, therefore, it seems reasonable to expect that the majority of cases of congenitally bicuspid aortic valves would have one component represented by the posterior cusp (intercalated valve swelling) and the other component represented by the fused right and left cusps (truncal swellings). This view is supported angiocardiographically, because this type of bicuspid aortic valve is the most common one seen at thoracic aortography —a fact that does not alter the pathologic classification presented earlier.

The angiocardiographic features of this type of bicuspid aortic valve are characteristic, and are best shown in the lateral view (Figs. 10*b* and 11*b*). In this view, the posterior cusp is overtly enlarged and forms the entire valvular component between the anterior and posterior extremities of the aortic root. In the normal tricuspid aortic valve, the posterior cusp does not encompass the entire width of the aortic root (Fig. 11*a*). Also, discrete right and left cusps are not seen. In many patients, the fused or conjoined right and left cusps in the lateral view produce an irregular radiolucent band the width of the aortic root at the projected level of the commissures (Fig. 10*b*).

The false raphe, when present, is extremely difficult to detect. It may result in a valve that appears to be tricuspid at thoracic aortography. One sign is a slight indentation in the mid aspect of the aforementioned radiolucent band. The indentation is caused by the insertion of the raphe itself.

In patients with severe calcification, the anatomic features may be so distorted (Fig. 12), that visualization of two cusps is not possible.

The anteroposterior view is less helpful. The posterior cusp often appears enlarged and redundant, and its inferior margin is situated in an abnormally low position (Fig. 10*a*). Passage of a catheter in a retrograde manner through a calcified aortic valve is extremely difficult. Under these circumstances, the left ventricle may be entered by transseptal (atrial septum) techniques or, as a last resort, transthoracic puncture of the left ventricle. The latter should be performed

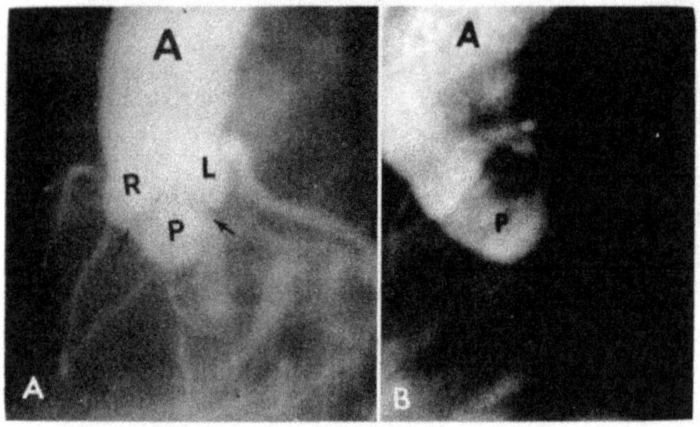

Figure 11. Lateral views of a tricuspid aortic valve (*a*) and congenitally bicuspid aortic valve (*b*). In *a*, the valve shows three distinct cusps: R, right or anterior cusp; P, posterior or noncoronary cusp; and L, left cusp. Note the size and relationship of the posterior cusp in (*a*) as compared with (*b*). A, ascending aorta.

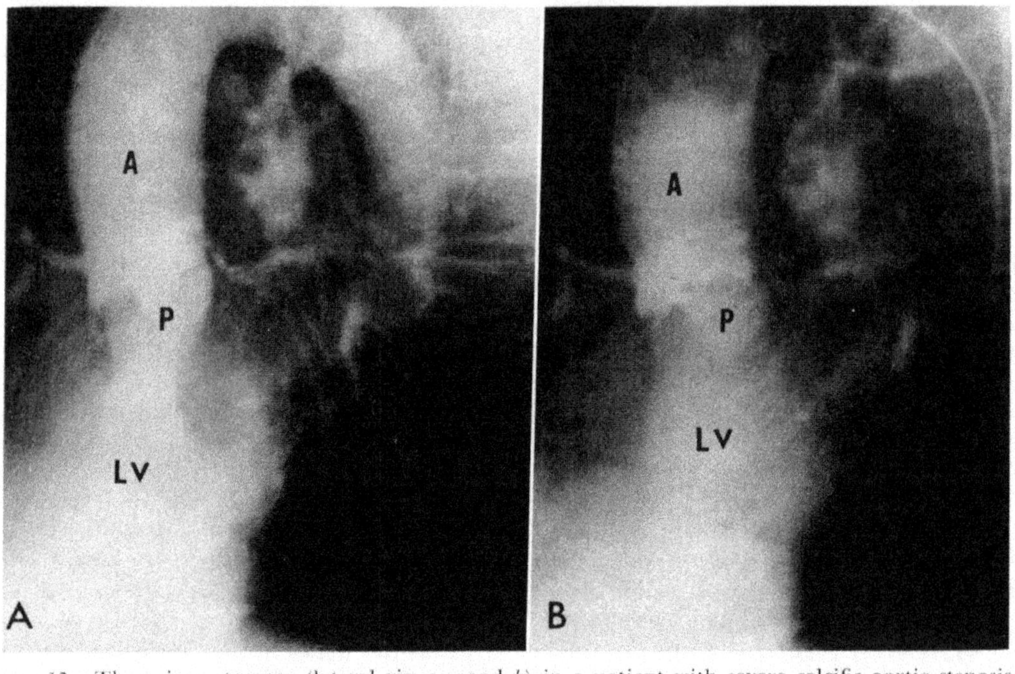

Figure 12. Thoracic aortogram (lateral views *a* and *b*) in a patient with severe calcific aortic stenosis and regurgitation. The usual bicuspid valve anatomy is distorted by the calcific deposits. There is a large calcium deposit producing a filling defect in the anterior aspect of the posterior aortic cusp (p). Note the extreme opacification of the left ventricle (LV) after the ascending aorta (A) injection.

with a Teflon needle, so that angiocardiography may be performed.

CONCLUSIONS AND SUMMARY

1. Congenitally bicuspid aortic valves are neither stenotic nor incompetent at birth.

2. Stenosis, incompetency, and infection are *complications* of congenitally bicuspid aortic valves. This is an extremely common condition often misinterpreted as rheumatic heart disease.

3. Congenitally bicuspid stenotic aortic valves are nearly always heavily calcified. Significant calcification on this valve is rare under age 20.

4. Infective endocarditis is by far the most common cause of pure incompetency of a congenitally bicuspid aortic valve.

5. The cusps of the purely incompetent bicuspid aortic valve are usually not calcified.

6. The bicuspid condition of the aortic valve does not necessarily mean that the valve will become stenotic or incompetent. Congenitally bicuspid aortic valves are seen occasionally in elderly patients in whom there was no evidence of cardiac dysfunction, precordial murmur, or cardiomegaly.

7. The natural history of a congenitally bicuspid aortic valve is unknown. The percentage of individuals born with bicuspid aortic valves who develop stenosis, incompetency, or infection at this site, and the percentage who never develop any of these complications during an entire lifetime is also unknown.

8. Because of the extreme variability in type and severity of the anatomic-hemodynamic abnormalities of the bicuspid aortic valve, the plain film findings regarding heart size, pulmonary vascularity, etc., are variable. Regardless of the functional state of the aortic valve, the cardiac silhouette almost invariably assumes a LV configuration in the frontal projection and shows signs of pure left ventricular involvement in the other views.

9. The roentgen hallmark of the congenital bicuspid aortic valve is calcification. Calcification of the aortic valve among patients without additional signs of rheumatic mitral valve disease usually means that the aortic valve is congenitally malformed. At least 50 per cent of these patients will harbor a congenitally bicuspid aortic valve.

10. Approximately 85 per cent of patients with CoA have congenitally bicuspid aortic valves. Among patients with CoA and a tricuspid aortic valve, there is still a high incidence of valve abnormality. Some of these tricuspid valves are in reality partially bicuspid valves.

11. The angiocardiographic features of the bicuspid valve are characteristic. When the valve is heavily calcified, the characteristic angiocardiographic features are distorted.

REFERENCES

1. Edwards, J. E.: Calcific aortic stenosis: Pathologic features. Proc. Staff Meet. Mayo Clin., *36*:444-451, 1961.
2. Edwards, J. E.: The congenital bicuspid aortic valve. Circulation, *23*:485-488, 1961.
3. Edwards, J. E.: An Atlas of Acquired Diseases of the Heart and Great Vessels. Vol. I. Diseases of the Valves and Pericardium. Philadelphia, W. B. Saunders Co., 1961.
4. Edwards, J. E.: On the etiology of calcific aortic stenosis. Circulation, *26*:817-818, 1962.
5. Edwards, J. E., Carey, L. S., Neufeld, H. N., and Lester, R. G.: Congenital Heart Disease. Correlation of Pathologic Anatomy and Angiocardiography. Philadelphia, W. B. Saunders Co., 1965, p. 684.
6. Elliott, L. P., and Eliot, R. S.: Roentgenologic findings in conditions of the ascending aorta simulating aortic valvular insufficiency. Amer. J. Roentgenol., *97*:390-410, 1966.
7. Moller, J. H., Nakib, A., and Edwards, J. E.: Infarction of papillary muscles and mitral insufficiency associated with congenital aortic stenosis. Circulation, *34*:87-91, 1966.
8. Osler, W.: The bicuspid condition of the aortic valves. Trans. Assoc. Amer. Physicians, *1*:185-192, 1886.
9. Van Mierop, L. H. S.: Anatomy of the heart, embryology of the heart and congenital heart disease. In CIBA Collection of Medical Illustrations, Vol. 5, Circulatory System, Part I. In press.

National Heart Institute
National Institutes of Health
Bethesda, Maryland 20014

The Structure of the Aortic Valve in Clinically Isolated Aortic Stenosis

An Autopsy Study of 162 Patients Over 15 Years of Age

By William C. Roberts, M.D.

SUMMARY

The structure of the aortic valve at autopsy is described in 162 patients over 15 years of age with clinically isolated, severe valvular aortic stenosis with or without aortic regurgitation. The valves were congenitally unicuspid, unicommissural in 17 patients, congenitally bicuspid in 67, tricuspid in 71, and in seven the structure was uncertain. Thus, in at least 84 (52%) of the patients the valve was congenitally malformed at birth. It is proposed that minor aortic valvular cuspal inequality, also present from birth, may be an underlying malformation in some of the patients with tricuspid stenotic aortic valves. Degeneration or wear-and-tear from aging almost certainly explains aortic stenosis in most of the elderly patients. Although no patient had clinical evidence of mitral valvular dysfunction, the mitral leaflets were diffusely thickened by fibrous tissue in 26 of the 162 patients. Rheumatic disease is believed to be the cause of the valve involvement in 22 of them (the other four had congenitally bicuspid aortic valves). Rheumatic disease did not appear to be the cause of the aortic stenosis in the other 136 patients with anatomically normal mitral valves.

Additional Indexing Words:

Bicuspid aortic valve	Cardiac calcification	Congenital heart disease
Mitral valvular dysfunction	Rheumatic heart disease	Unicuspid aortic valve

RECENTLY, the aortic valve has been shown to be congenitally bicuspid in a high percentage of patients with valvular aortic stenosis,[1] and other factors[2] have indicated that anatomically isolated aortic valvular disease is usually not rheumatic in origin. In the present postmortem study the hearts of 162 patients who presented clinically with isolated aortic stenosis with or without aortic regurgitation were reviewed. The prime purpose was to determine how often the aortic valve was congenitally malformed and how often the functionally normal mitral valve was anatomically abnormal.

From the Section of Pathology, National Heart and Lung Institute, National Institutes of Health, Bethesda, Maryland.

Received February 27, 1970; accepted for publication March 12, 1970.

Patients Studied

Observations in the 162 patients are summarized in table 1. Clinically, each was in functional class III or IV (New York Heart Association classification). Patients less than age 16 years were excluded. The average age was 52 years; 34 patients were older than 60 years of age and 16 were older than 70 years of age. Aortic valve operation (valvuloplasty or partial or total replacement) was performed in 106 patients; the average age of death in them was 49 years. The average age at death of the 56 patients on whom no cardiac operation was performed was 57 years, but 16 of the 20 who were older than 65 years of age were included in this group. The three patients without grossly visible calcific deposits in the aortic valve were aged 16, 24, and 33 years, and the peak systolic pressure gradients between the left ventricle and a

Table 1

Data in Patients with Clinically Isolated Valvular Aortic Stenosis

Valve structure	No. of patients	Age range (av)	No. of patients older than 65 yr	Sex M	Sex F	History of ARF or chorea	LV-SA PSG (mm Hg)	Aortic valvular calcium (g)	Heart wt. (g) Range (av)
Unicommissural	17	16-62 (44)	0	13	4	1	10-158 (78)*	17	400-880 (616)
Biscuspid	67	16-79 (49)	2	48	19	5	12-165 (93)†	64	295-1000 (600)
Tricuspid	71	21-90 (57)	18	53	18	14	20-160 (84)‡	71	380-1050 (643)
MV normal	49	28-90 (59)	16	34	15	1	20-160 (93)	49	380-1000 (595)
MV leaflets thick; CT normal	16	39-76 (53)	2	14	2	9	25-120 (70)	16	480-900 (717)
MV leaflets and CT thick	6	21-61 (46)	0	5	1	4	20-90 (61)	6	530-1050 (731)
Uncertain	7	41-58 (52)	0	7	0	0	52-105 (81)§	7	400-880 (600)
Total	162	16-90 (52)	20	122 (75%)	41 (25%)	20 (13%)	10-165 (87)	159	295-1050 (619)

*10 patients; PSG < 50 mm Hg in two.
†52 patients; PSG < 50 mm Hg in six.
‡49 patients; PSG < 50 mm Hg in seven.
§5 patients; PSG < 50 mm Hg in none.
Abbreviations: ARF = acute rheumatic fever; CT = chordae tendineae; LV = left ventricle; MV = mitral valve; PSG = peak systolic gradient; SA = systemic artery.

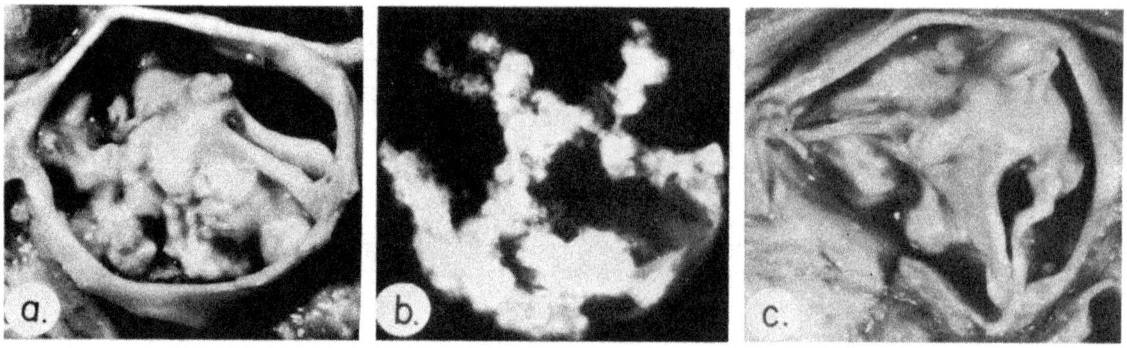

Figure 1

Stenotic unicommissural unicuspid aortic valves from above in two patients. (a) The valve in this 48-year-old man (A68-101) is severely stenotic and heavily calcified. (b) Same patient as a. The heart weighed 750 g. (c) The valve in this 62-year-old man (A69-276) also is severely stenotic, but the heart weighed 400 g. In contrast to the valve shown in a, two false commissures are present in addition to the one true commissure.

systemic artery in them were 80, 150, and 160 mm Hg, respectively.

The 162 patients were divided into four groups depending on the structure of the aortic valve. Representative valves are illustrated in figures 1 to 3. The excised valves in all patients who had undergone valve replacement also were re-examined (most had been removed intact). The prosthetic aortic valve in each, however, was removed so that the number of lateral attachments (commissures) of the cusps to the aorta could be determined.

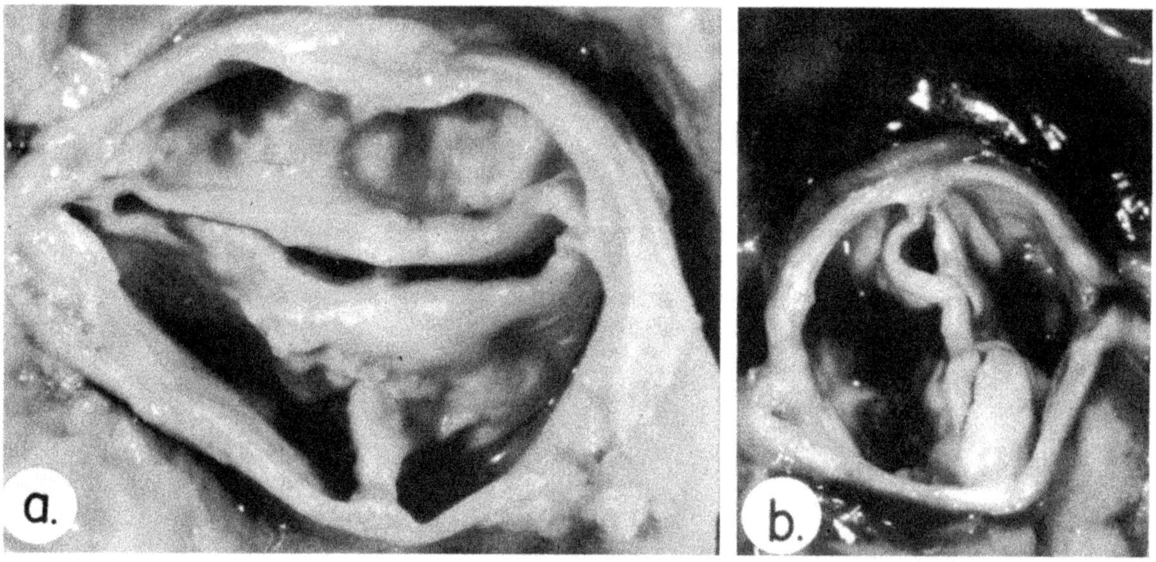

Figure 2

Stenotic congenitally bicuspid aortic valves from above in two patients. (a) The valve in this 61-year-old man (A64-155) contains a raphe in the anterior cusp. The peak systolic left ventricular-to-systemic arterial pressure gradient across this valve 2 years before death was 45 mm Hg. The heart weighed 700 g. (b) The valve in this 56-year-old woman (A70-6) was operatively debrided of calcific deposits a day before death. The peak systolic pressure gradient across the valve preoperatively was 47 mm Hg. The cusps are located on the right and the left, respectively. The heart weighed only 295 g.

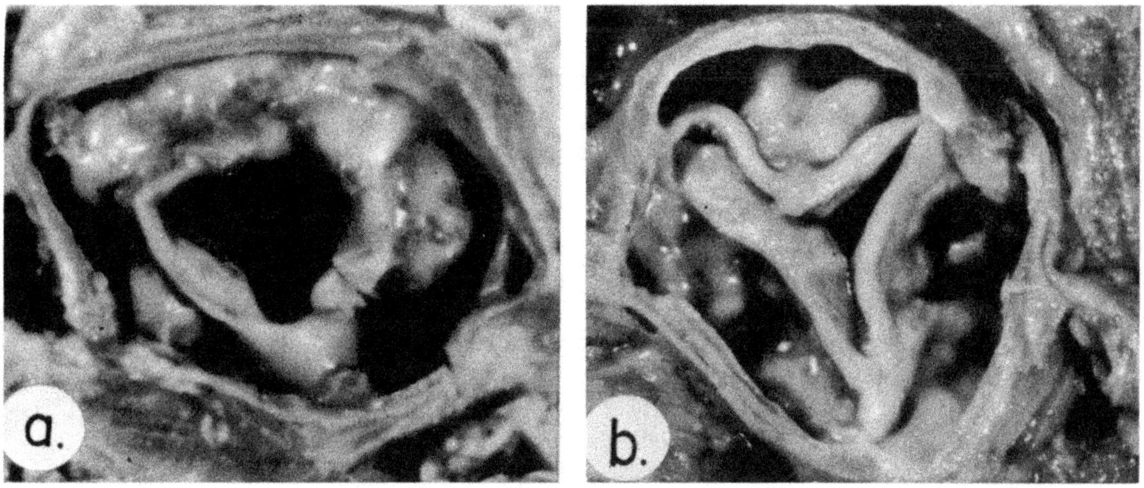

Figure 3

Stenotic three-cuspid aortic valves in two patients. (a) Each of the three commissures are fused in this stenotic and incompetent valve of a 49-year-old man (A58-19). The peak systolic pressure gradient across the valve was 74 mm Hg and the heart weighed 600 g. (b) This valve is from an 80-year-old woman who had clinical features of severe aortic stenosis. One commissure is fused but only minimally. The cusps are made relatively immobile by calcific deposits only. The heart weighed 400 g.

In 17 patients the aortic valve was unicommissural and unicuspid. In a few of the 17, two raphes (false commissures) were visible, but in most no raphe was present.

In 67 patients the aortic valve was congenitally bicuspid. Two basic types of bicuspid valves were seen: (1) In 54% of subjects the two cusps were located right and left, the commissures anteriorly and posteriorly, and a coronary artery arose from behind each cusp. (2) In 46% of the patients the two cusps were located anteriorly and posteriorly, the commissures, on the right and left, and both coronary arteries arose in front of the anterior cusp. Raphes were clearly visible in half the valves. When the cusps were located on the right and the left, the false commissures were always in the right cusp; when the cusps were located anteriorly and posteriorly, the raphe was always in the anterior cusp. In several patients with congenitally bicuspid aortic valves one true commissure was fused, producing in essence an acquired unicommissural aortic valve. The valves were divided, however, according to their original structure.

The 71 patients with tricuspid aortic valves were subdivided according to whether the mitral leaflets and chordae tendineae were normal or thickened by fibrous tissue. In 49 patients (69%), the mitral leaflets and chordae were entirely normal. Sixteen (33%) of these 49 patients were over 65 years of age whereas only four (4%) of the remaining 113 with aortic stenosis were over 65 years of age. In at least three of the 49 patients the aortic valve cusps were unequal in size and one of them also had a congenitally bicuspid pulmonic valve. In 16 of the 71 patients with tricuspid aortic valves the mitral valve leaflets were diffusely although mildly thickened and the mitral chordae tendineae were normal. Nine of these 16 patients had positive histories of acute rheumatic fever or chorea whereas only one of the 49 with tricuspid aortic valves and normal mitral valves had positive histories. In six of the 71 patients with tricuspid aortic valves the mitral chordae tendineae as well as the mitral leaflets were diffusely but mildly thickened, and four of them had positive histories of acute rheumatic fever or chorea. (The mitral valve was normal in each of the 17 patients with unicommissural aortic valves and in 62 of the 66 with congenitally bicuspid valves. In the other four, the leaflets were diffusely but mildly thickened, and the chordae were normal. In each of the seven patients in whom aortic valve structure was uncertain the mitral valve was normal.)

In seven of the 162 patients the underlying structure of the aortic valve was uncertain. Each of these patients had heavily calcified valves, and each had been excised and replaced by a prosthesis. The valves in them were not excised intact, and the number of commissures on the wall of the aortic root was unclear after removing the prosthesis.

At least four histologic sections of myocardium were examined in all 162 patients, and none had Aschoff bodies.

Discussion

The data show that among adults with clinically isolated valvular aortic stenosis with or without aortic regurgitation the aortic valve is congenitally bicuspid in 43%, tricuspid in 46%, and congenitally unicommissural, unicuspid in 11%. Thus, 54% of the patients in whom the aortic valve structure was discernible had congenitally bicuspid or unicuspid aortic valves. The mitral valves were normal in 136 (84%) and thickened in 26 (16%). Of the 136 patients with normal mitral valves, seven (5%) had positive histories of acute rheumatic fever or chorea whereas 13 (50%) of the 26 with thickened mitral valves (including four with congenitally bicuspid aortic valves) had positive histories.

Although the structure of the aortic valves in 96% of the described patients was clear, the cause of the valvular obstruction in most of them is less clear. Without question a congenital malformation was the underlying valve disturbance in the 17 patients with unicommissural valves, in the 67 with bicuspid valves, and probably also in the seven whose valve structure was uncertain. Although the valvular *malformation* was congenital, the valvular *obstruction* may or may not have been present from the time of birth. Edwards[3] has stated that the congenitally unicommissural aortic valve is inherently stenotic and that the unicuspid valve is the only type of valve stenotic at the time of birth. Of the 17 patients with congenitally unicommissural aortic valves described herein, each was stenotic, none was purely incompetent, and only one patient had had a history of infective endocarditis. Edwards[4] has contended that the congenitally bicuspid valve, in contrast to the unicuspid one, is not stenotic at birth but becomes stenotic only as it becomes fibrotic and calcified. In contrast to the congenitally unicommissural aortic valve, however, the congenitally bicuspid aortic valve may be

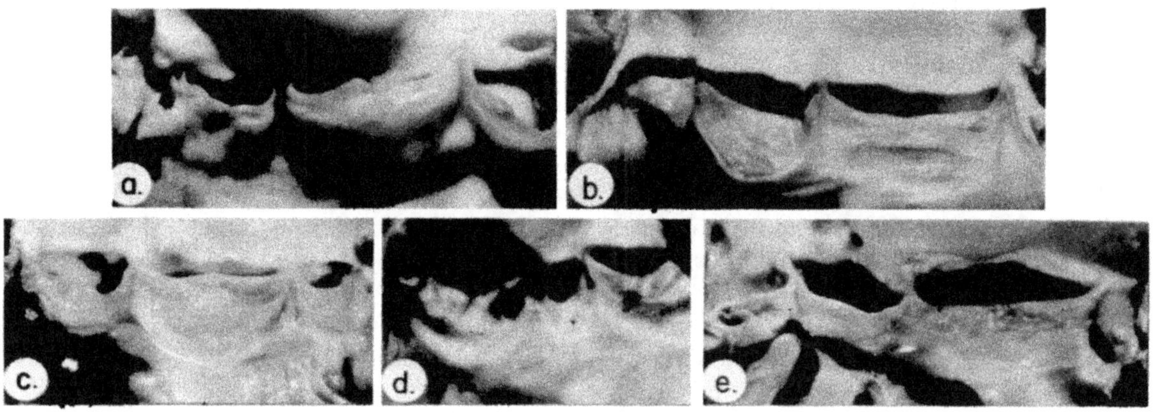

Figure 4

Shown here are opened, functionally normal aortic valves in five patients with unequal-sized cusps. Note the differing distances between the commissures in the patients. (a) Age 4 years. (b) Age 21 years. (c) Age 7 years. (d) Age 36 years. (e) Age 60 years. All five patients died of noncardiac conditions (leukemia [a and c], lymphoma [d and e], and cystic fibrosis of pancreas [b]).

The Three-cuspid Aortic Valve

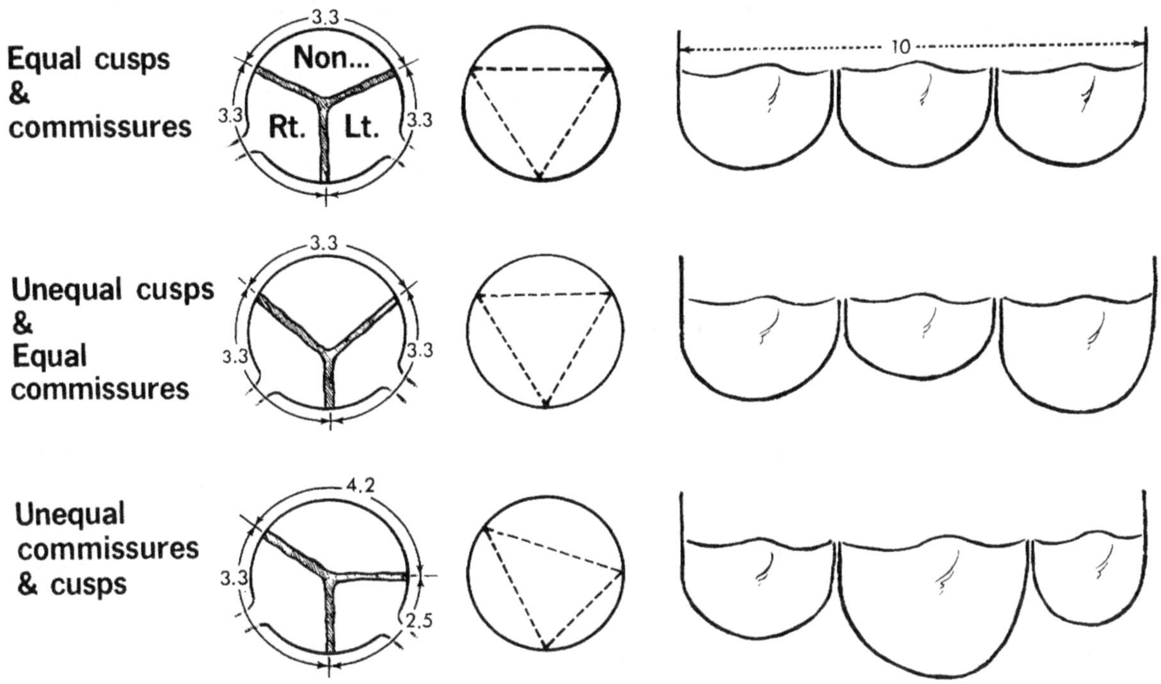

Figure 5

Diagrammatic portrayal of equal and unequal-sized aortic valve cusps. (Top row) *The cusps of the aortic valve are equal in size and the circumferential distances between the commissures are equal. The straight-line distances between the commissures (as indicated by the dashed lines in the center circle) also are equal. On the right the aortic valve is opened.* (Middle row) *Here the cusps are of unequal size, and they are made unequal by differing cephalocaudal lengths of the individual cusps. The distances between the commissures circumferentially around the aorta and the straight-line distances within the lumen of the aorta are similar to the normal shown in the top panel.* (Lower row) *Here not only are the cephalocaudal lengths of the individual cusps different, but the circumferential distances around the aorta and the straight-line distances within the lumen of the aorta between the commissures (lateral attachments) are different.*

purely incompetent, may be more often the site of infective endocarditis, and may function normally for an entire lifetime without developing any complication (stenosis, incompetence, or infection).[1]

The cause of the aortic stenosis in many of the 71 patients with tricuspid aortic valves is speculative. It is reasonable to believe that the etiology is rheumatic in most or all of the 22 patients with associated anatomic disease of the mitral valve. In addition to the anatomic mitral valvular involvement, the incidence of positive histories of acute rheumatic fever in them was high (60%). The cause of the aortic stenosis in the 49 patients with tricuspid aortic valves and normal mitral valves is almost certainly not rheumatic. Only one of the 49 patients had a positive history of acute rheumatic fever or chorea. Healed infective endocarditis likewise seems unlikely from anatomic study of the valves and from the lack of a positive history of infective endocarditis in any patient. No patient had a recorded history of, or anatomic evidence of, brucellosis.[5] Could the aortic valve be tricuspid and still congenitally malformed? At least three of the 49 patients clearly had aortic valve cusps of unequal size. The pulmonic valvular cusps are of slightly unequal size in most normal subjects.[6] Cuspal inequality in the low pressure right side of the heart is obviously of no consequence. Similar inequality of cuspal size in the high pressure left side of the heart, however, may be far more important. Unequal-sized aortic valve cusps are occasionally observed at autopsy in individuals dying of noncardiac conditions (fig. 4). When the cusps become severely fibrotic, nodular, calcified, or focally contracted, however, cuspal inequality probably is difficult to appreciate. This thesis of minor aortic cuspal inequality as an underlying congenital malformation in adults with valvular aortic stenosis is expanded in figure 5.

Fibrosis and calcification of the three aortic valve cusps as a consequence of aging (wear-and-tear) is almost certainly the explanation of the aortic stenosis in a significant percentage of the subjects with three-cuspid aortic valves and intrinsically normal mitral valves. Sixteen of the 49 patients with aortic stenosis, three-cuspid aortic valves, and normal (except for expected age changes) mitral valves were over 65 years of age. In addition to heavy calcific deposits in the aortic valve in these 16 patients, 14 also had calcific deposits in the mitral annulus and subvalvular angle beneath the posterior mitral leaflet, and all 16 had calcific deposits in the walls of one or more of the three major extramural coronary arteries. Commissural fusion in the older patients was unusual. None had positive histories of acute rheumatic fever or chorea. It seems most reasonable to believe that the aortic valvular calcification and stenosis in these 16 patients is on the basis of aging or degeneration.

Acknowledgment

I am enormously indebted to my present and past associates, particularly Dr. Andrew G. Morrow and Dr. Eugene Braunwald, for free access to clinical information on the patients discussed herein.

References

1. Roberts WC: The congenitally bicuspid aortic valve: A study of 85 autopsy patients. Amer J Cardiol. In press
2. Roberts WC: Anatomically-isolated aortic valvular disease: The case against its being of rheumatic etiology. Amer J Med In press
3. Edwards JE: Calcific aortic stenosis: Pathologic features. Proc Mayo Clin 36: 444, 1961
4. Edwards JE: The congenital bicuspid aortic valve. Circulation 23: 485, 1961
5. Peery TM: Brucellosis and heart disease: IV. Etiology of calcific aortic stenosis. JAMA 166: 1123, 1958
6. Roberts WC: Examination of the heart and precordium. Chest In press

The Congenitally Bicuspid Aortic Valve

A Study of 85 Autopsy Cases

WILLIAM C. ROBERTS, MD, FACC

Bethesda, Maryland

Clinical and necropsy observations are described in 85 autopsy cases in which the subjects had congenitally bicuspid aortic valves. Sixty-one subjects had aortic stenosis with or without aortic regurgitation; 11, pure aortic regurgitation; and 13, unexpectedly, had a congenitally bicuspid aortic valve that apparently had functioned normally. The average age at death in patients with stenotic valves was 49 years, and in those with pure regurgitation, 31 years. Aortic valvular calcific deposits occurred in 59 of 61 patients with stenosis but was minimal or absent in the patients with pure regurgitation or normally functioning valves. Infective endocarditis appeared responsible for incompetency in 8 of 11 patients with pure regurgitation. Five of 61 patients with stenosis had had infective endocarditis, but infection occurred on a previously heavily calcified valve in only 1 patient.

Sixty-nine of the 72 patients with functionally abnormal valves were observed in a study of 400 autopsy cases; all subjects were over age 14 years, with severe valvular cardiac disease. The 13 functionally normal valves were found during study of 1,440 necropsy cases in which the subjects were free of other valvular or septal defects. The bicuspid aortic valve is the most frequent congenital malformation of the heart or great vessels. It occurs in over 50 percent of patients with anatomically isolated aortic stenosis and in about 25 percent of patients with clinically pure aortic regurgitation. It is not certain why 1 congenitally bicuspid valve becomes severely scarred, calcified and stenotic, another only mildly scarred and incompetent, another the site of infection, and why another remains free of these complications during life.

In 1844 Paget[1] called attention to the peculiar liability of congenitally bicuspid aortic valves to disease, but their importance as something other than a pathologic curiosity was not appreciated. In 1858 Peacock[2] pointed out that bicuspid aortic valves tended to become "thick . . . ossified . . . inducing first obstruction . . . and then incompetency." Osler[3] in 1886 first described the abnormal liability of the bicuspid aortic valve to develop infective endocarditis. Since that time the tendency of this malformed valve to be the site of infection generally has been recognized, but only in the past 20 years has it become appreciated that the congenitally bicuspid aortic valve is a common cause of isolated calcareous aortic stenosis.[4–6]

The natural history of the congenitally bicuspid aortic valve is unknown. The percentage of individuals born with bicuspid aortic valves in whom stenosis, incompetency or infection develops at this site and the percentage who never have any of these complications

From the Section of Pathology, National Heart and Lung Institute, National Institutes of Health, Bethesda, Md. Manuscript received April 21, 1969, accepted September 23, 1969.

Address for reprints: William C. Roberts, MD, Section of Pathology, National Heart and Lung Institute, National Institutes of Health, Bethesda, Md. 20014.

TABLE I
Eighty-Five Cases of Congenitally Bicuspid Aortic Valve

Patients (no.)	Age (yr) at Death [Range & (Average)]	Sex M	Sex F	Infective Endocarditis	Precordial Murmur Systolic	Precordial Murmur Diastolic	LV-SA PSG [Range & (Average)] (mm Hg)	Aortic Valve Calcium Deposits	Heart Weight (g) [Range & (Average)]
Group 1. Aortic Stenosis With or Without Aortic Regurgitation									
61	16–79(49)[a]	45	16	5[c]	61	25	12–165(92)[f]	59[h]	330–1000(605)
Group 2. Pure Aortic Regurgitation									
11	15–55(31)[b]	9	2	8[d]	6	9	0–0 (0)[g]	2[i]	240–950(573)
Group 3. Functionally Normal Valve									
13	23–59(45)	7	6	0	5[e]	0	—	4[i]	200–320(270)[j]
Totals									
85	15–79(46)	61 (72%)	24 (28%)	13 (15%)				65 (76%)	

[a] Average age of death in 21 patients without operation 53 years; in 40 patients with operation 46 years.
[b] Average age of death in 8 patients without operation 34 years; in the 3 patients with operation 26 years.
[c] Healed in each.
[d] Healed in 1; active in 7. Infective endocarditis was the cause of aortic regurgitation in all 8 patients.
[e] In 3 patients the murmur was at the apex; in 2 it was at the base. In 3 patients the murmur was grade 2/6 intensity; in 1, grade 3/6; and 1, grade 1/6. All 5 subjects were over 45 years of age, and 3 were anemic.
[f] Cardiac catheterizations in 48 patients. Only 5 patients had gradients less than 50 mm Hg.
[g] Cardiac catheterizations in 3 patients.
[h] Large in each.
[i] Small focal deposits in each and not roentgenographically visible.
[j] Excludes 3 patients who had systemic hypertension.
LV = left ventricle; SA = systemic artery (aorta, brachial or femoral); PSG = peak systolic gradient.

during an entire lifetime is unknown. To obtain information in this regard, clinical and necropsy findings were reviewed in 85 patients who were found at autopsy to have congenitally bicuspid aortic valves.

Results

Observations in the 85 autopsy cases are summarized in Table I. Subjects 14 years old and under were excluded.

Group 1. Aortic Stenosis With or Without Regurgitation

Sixty-one patients (Fig. 1 to 5) had some degree of aortic stenosis. Accurate heart weights,[7] available in 56 of the 61 patients, ranged from 330 to 1,000 g (average 605 g); in 42 men the heart weights averaged 651 g, and in 14 women, 466 g. The presence of a diastolic precordial murmur typical of aortic regurgitation also altered cardiac weights; in 5 women with murmurs of aortic regurgitation in addition to murmurs of aortic stenosis the heart weights averaged 516 g, whereas in 9 women without murmurs of regurgitation the hearts averaged 438 g; in 20 men with murmurs of aortic regurgitation the hearts averaged 702 g, whereas in 22 men without murmurs of regurgitation the hearts averaged 601 g. Although there was a significant difference in heart weights depending on sex and on the presence or absence of murmurs of aortic regurgitation, neither of these factors tended to alter consistently the peak systolic pressure gradient between the left ventricle and a systemic artery. This gradient in 34 men averaged 91 mm Hg and in 14 women, 97 mm Hg. In 5 women with murmurs of aortic regurgitation the peak systolic gradient averaged 94 mm Hg (the gradient was only 12 mm Hg in 1 patient), and in 7 women without murmurs of regurgitation the gradient averaged 100 mm Hg. Fifteen men with murmurs of aortic regurgitation had a lower peak systolic gradient (average 83 mm Hg) than the 20 men without murmurs of regurgitation (average 97 mm Hg).

Grossly visible deposits of calcium were present on each of the 2 aortic valve cusps in 59 of the 61 patients in Group 1. Of the 2 patients with no aortic valvular calcific deposits 1 was a 16 year old girl with

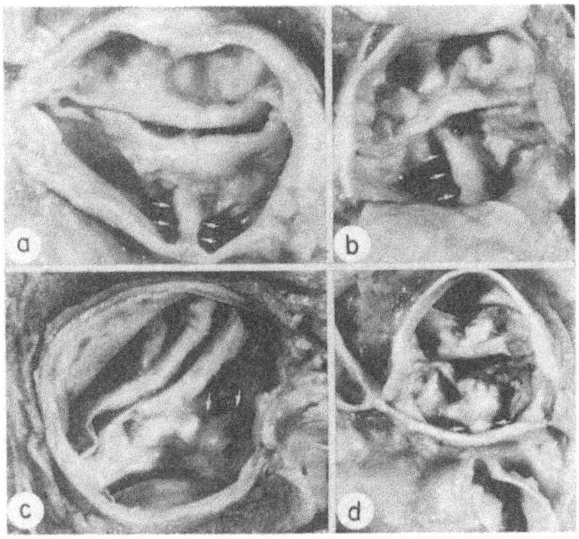

Figure 1. Calcified, stenotic, congenitally bicuspid aortic valves in 4 patients. The cusps in each are situated anteriorly and posteriorly and the commissures right and left, respectively. Each of the valves has a raphe **(white arrows)** in the anterior cusp. **a,** valve of a 61 year old man. At catheterization 2 years before death, the peak systolic gradient across the valve was 45 mm Hg when the cardiac index was 2.6 liters/min per m^2. **b,** valve of a 60 year old man who suddenly collapsed on the street. Electrocardiogram recorded in the emergency room showed left bundle branch block. His only symptom of cardiac dysfunction previously was mild exertional dyspnea. **c,** valve of a 75 year old man who died after resection of an asymptomatic abdominal aortic aneurysm that had been discovered during a routine physical examination. He had no symptoms of cardiac dysfunction. **d,** valve of a 51 year old man. The peak systolic gradient across this valve was 18 mm Hg, but the valve was severely incompetent.

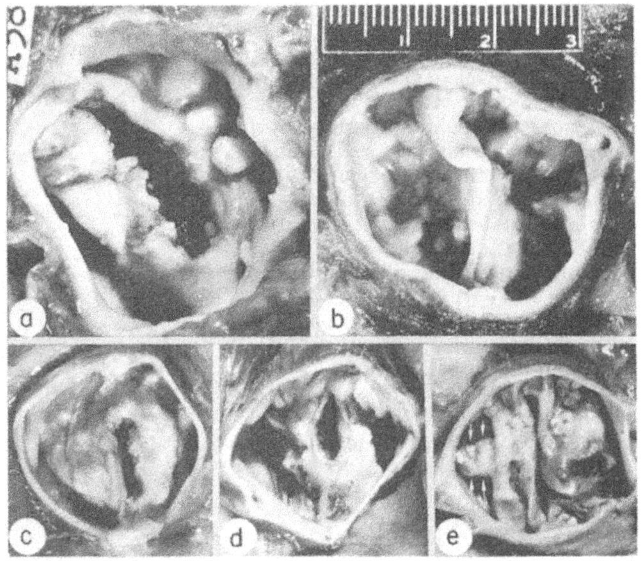

Figure 2. Calcified, stenotic, congenitally bicuspid aortic valves in 5 patients. In each the cusps are located right and left and the commissures, anteriorly and posteriorly. In valve **e** a false commissure is identifiable. In 3 of the 5 patients 1 of the 2 true commissures is partially fused. **a,** valve of a 37 year old man who died of progressive cardiac failure. **b,** valve of a 54 year old man who died during aortic valvuloplasty. The peak systolic gradient across the valve was 70 mm Hg. **c,** valve of a 34 year old man who died of progressive congestive cardiac failure. The peak systolic gradient across the valve was 92 mm Hg. **d,** valve of a 54 year old man who had progressive cardiac failure and, terminally, a massive pulmonary embolus. He had had symptoms of cardiac dysfunction for 6 years. **e,** valve of a 79 year old woman who had been asymptomatic until 2 years earlier when manifestations of cardiac failure appeared. The heart weighed 700 g.

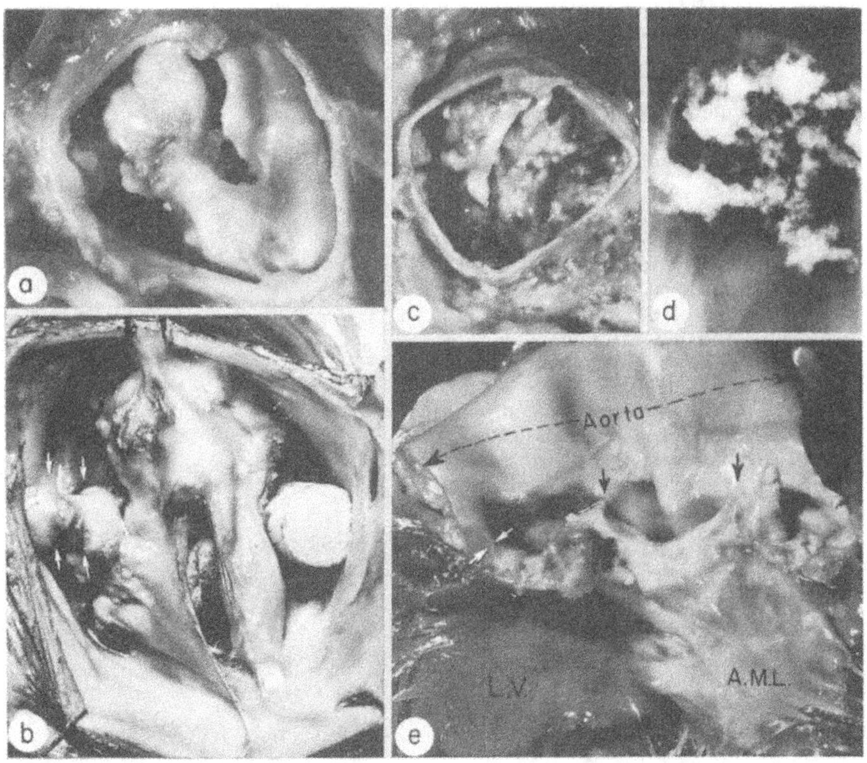

Figure 3. Calcified, stenotic, congenitally bicuspid aortic valves in 4 patients. In 3 the cusps are located right and left, and the commissures anteriorly and posteriorly. One commissure in each is fused. **a,** valve of a 39 year old man who experienced congestive cardiac failure 3 years earlier. He died during thoracotomy. Catheterization disclosed a 75 mm Hg peak systolic gradient across the valve when the cardiac index was 2.2 liters/min per m^2. **b,** valve of a 40 year old woman who died during valvulotomy which caused perforations of the left cusp (stick protruding through the perforation). Preoperatively, the peak systolic gradient across the valve was 70 mm Hg. The heart weighed only 400 g. The raphe is designated by **arrows. c,** valve of a 53 year old man who died suddenly and unexpectedly 77 months after valvuloplasty. Before operation at age 46 the peak systolic gradient across the valve had been 63 mm Hg when the cardiac index was 3.0 liters/min per m^2 and no aortic regurgitation was present. Catheterization 4 months after operation disclosed no systolic gradient, and catheterization 60 months after operation showed a 36 mm Hg peak systolic gradient across the valve when the cardiac index was 2.3 liters/min per m^2. **d,** radiograph of the valve shown in **c** showing large calcific deposits. **e,** opened valve of a 56 year old man who died suddenly and unexpectedly 1 month before scheduled aortic valve replacement. At catheterization 2 months before death the peak systolic gradient across the valve was 87 mm Hg when the cardiac index was 2.6 liters/min per m^2. The 2 commissures are designated by **vertical arrows,** and a small raphe, by **horizontal arrows.** A.M.L. = anterior mitral leaflet, L.V. = left ventricle.

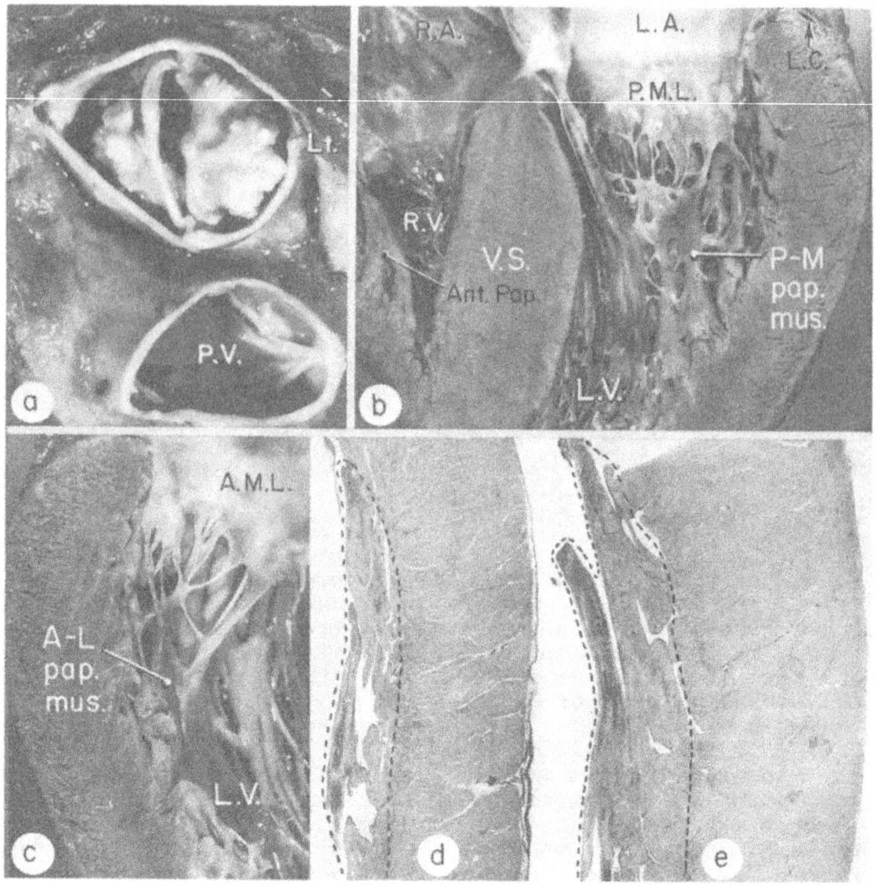

Figure 4. Stenotic, congenitally bicuspid aortic valve and atrophied and scarred papillary muscles in a 52 year old woman. This patient had symptoms of cardiac dysfunction for 3 years and a precordial murmur typical of mitral regurgitation in addition to murmurs of aortic stenosis and regurgitation. At catheterization, the peak systolic gradient across the aortic valve was 130 mm Hg (left ventricle 230/30 and aorta 100/70 mm Hg). The pulmonary arterial wedge mean pressure was 36 with **v** waves of 46 mm Hg, and the mean diastolic gradient between pulmonary arterial wedge and left ventricle was 12 mm Hg. The pulmonary arterial pressure was 75/40 mm Hg. Cardiac index was 2.1 liters/min per m^2. Aortic root and left ventricular cineangiocardiograms confirmed aortic regurgitation (3+/4+) and mitral regurgitation (2+/4+). Shortly after catheterization she experienced various atrial arrhythmias and irreversible overt congestive cardiac failure.

a, aortic and pulmonic (P.V.) valves from above showing the heavily calcified bicuspid aortic valve. The anterior commissure is partially fused. Lt. = left coronary artery. All coronary arteries were widely patent. **b,** longitudinal section of heart showing portions of all 4 cardiac chambers. The posteromedial (P-M) left ventricular papillary muscle is atrophied and scarred, and the anterior (ant.) right ventricular papillary (pap.) muscle is focally scarred. The left ventricular cavity is dilated, but the mitral annulus is not dilated. P.M.L. = posterior mitral leaflet; V.S. = ventricular septum; L.C. = left circumflex coronary artery. **c,** section of left ventricle (L.V.) showing severe atrophy of anterolateral (A-L) papillary muscle. The mitral leaflets are normal. A.M.L. = anterior mitral leaflet. **d** and **e,** photomicrographs of section of anterolateral **(d)** and posteromedial **(e)** left ventricular papillary muscles. Both are scarred and the anterolateral papillary muscle is extremely atrophied. The mitral regurgitation in this patient probably resulted from scarring and atrophy of the papillary muscles.

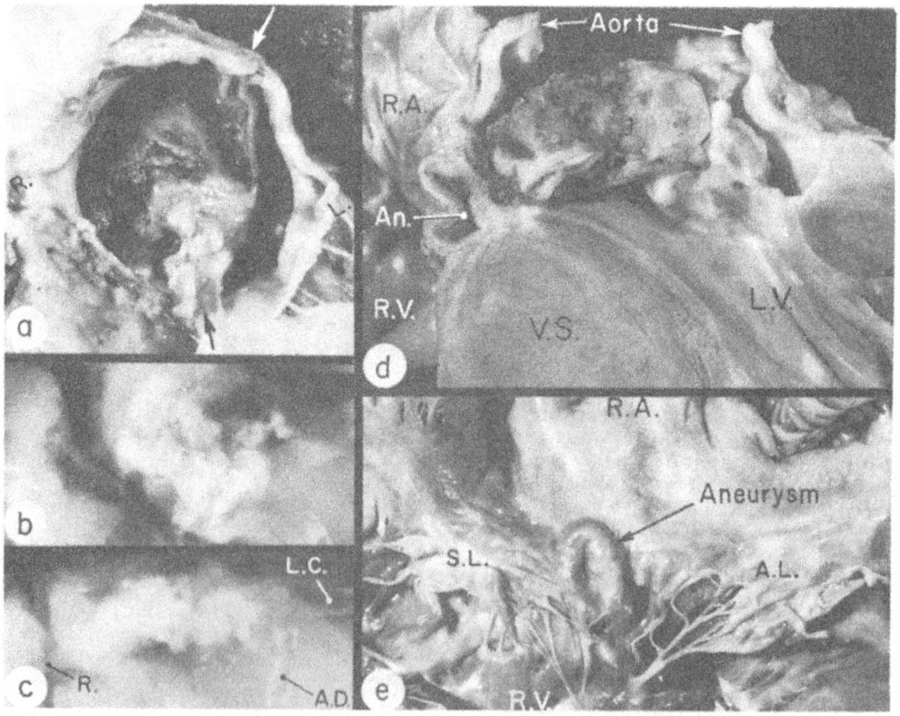

Figure 5. Infective endocarditis in a heavily calcified, congenitally bicuspid, aortic valve of a 63 year old man with features of congestive cardiac failure for at least 3 years. Fever, chills, alteration in intensity of the precordial murmurs, and prolonged P-R interval were noted 3½ months before death and Streptococcus viridans was cultured from the blood. He received penicillin and streptomycin for 1 month, the fever disappeared, and blood cultures became negative. Nevertheless, he fainted twice and complete heart block and atrial fibrillation developed. The congestive cardiac failure worsened, and he died.

The heart weighed 700 g and the aortic valve orifice was tiny **(a).** The anterior commissure **(black arrow)** was fused and only a small posteriorly-located orifice remained. R. = right coronary and L. = left coronary artery. The valve was heavily calcified **(b** and **c).** A radiograph of the valve from above is shown in **b,** and a lateral view, in **c.** All 3 major coronary arteries also are calcified. R. = right, L.C. = left circumflex, and A.D. = anterior descending coronary arteries. **d,** longitudinal section of aortic valve, left ventricular (L.V.) outflow tract, and ventricular septum (V.S.). A large lump of necrotic debris is present in the aortic valve which communicates with an aneurysm (An.) which bulges from the root of the aorta into the right atrium (R.A.), better seen in **e.** The aneurysm is believed to represent a healed "mycotic" aneurysm. No organisms were seen in histologic sections of the valve or aneurysm. S.L. = septal leaflet and A.L. = anterior leaflet of tricuspid valve. This patient thus had infective endocarditis superimposed on a previously heavily calcified valve, a rare circumstance.

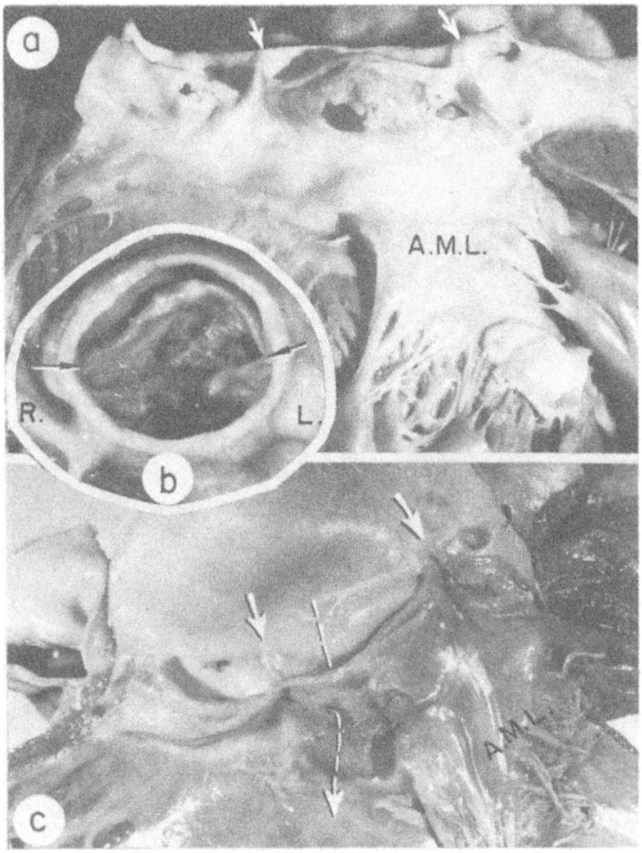

Figure 6. Infective endocarditis on previously functionally normal, congenitally bicuspid aortic valves causing fatal aortic regurgitation. **a,** opened aortic valve of a 55 year old woman. She had no signs or symptoms of cardiac disease until the onset of Staphylococcus aureus endocarditis 4½ months before death. Eradication of the organisms never was successful, the cusps perforated, and massive aortic regurgitation developed. A.M.L. = anterior mitral leaflet. The insert **(b)** shows the valve before it was opened. The **arrows** designate the true commissures. **c,** opened perforated aortic valve of a 33 year old man who developed Streptococcus viridans endocarditis after a tooth extraction and died of heart failure 2 months later. Before the extraction he had had no symptoms or signs of cardiac dysfunction. The **solid arrows** designate the true commissures and the **dashed irregular arrow,** the site of cuspal rupture.

an 80 mm Hg peak systolic gradient between the left ventricle and brachial artery, and the second was a 24 year old man with associated arthrogryposis multiplex congenita and a 150 mm Hg peak systolic gradient across the valve.[8] Two patients, a 53 year old woman and a 25 year old man, had only small focal calcific deposits on their aortic valves, but each had minimal stenosis (peak systolic gradient 12 and 30 mm Hg, respectively). The remaining 57 patients had large calcific deposits on the aortic valve, and all were over 30 years of age.

Group 2. Pure Aortic Regurgitation

In 8 of the 11 patients with pure aortic regurgitation (Fig. 6 and 7) the regurgitation was secondary to infective endocarditis. In 7 of these 8 patients precordial murmurs were absent or not mentioned until the valves became the site of infection. In 7 of the 8 patients with infective endocarditis, 1 or both cusps were perforated and partially destroyed by the inflammatory process. The eighth patient had large vegetations containing Histoplasma capsulatum on his biscuspid aortic valve, but neither cusp was perforated. This 35 year old man had generalized systemic histoplasmosis during his last 20 months of life, but an antemortum diagnosis of histoplasma endocarditis was never established despite 20 blood cultures for fungi. In 2 patients murmurs of the aortic regurgitation type were not heard, but in neither of the patients was infective endocarditis suspected clinically; 1, the 35 year old man just mentioned, had systemic histoplasmosis, and the second was asymptomatic until a day before death when unilateral hemiplegia suddenly appeared. The latter patient had ulcerated aortic cusps at autopsy although the heart weighed only 270 g. In the 3 patients with pure aortic regurgitation without historical or anatomic evidence of infective endocarditis, their aortic valve cusps at necropsy were mildly fibrotic and contracted, and symptoms of cardiac dysfunction had been present for 2 to 7 years before death. Each had associated congenital malformations: patent ductus arteriosus in 1, coarctation of the aorta in 1, and right aortic arch in 1 patient.

Group 3. Functionally Normal Valves

In each of the 13 patients in this group (Fig. 8 and 9) a congenitally bicuspid aortic valve was an incidental finding at necropsy, and in each the valve is believed to have functioned normally during life. Seven died of neoplasms, 1 of coronary heart disease, 1 of chronic parenchymal pulmonary disease, 1 of aplastic anemia, 1 of renal disease and 2 of acute dissecting aortic aneurysms with rupture. The aortic valve cusps in all 13 patients were slightly but focally thickened and in 4 contained small foci of calcium. However, in all patients the aortic valve cusps were freely movable, and in none did the valve orifice appear stenotic or incompetent.

Associated congenital cardiovascular malformations: These occurred in 11 of the 85 patients (13 percent) (Table II).

Positive histories of acute rheumatic fever or chorea: These were present in 5 of the 85 patients. Each had severe aortic stenosis, and 3 were men.

The mitral valves: These valves were normal in 79 of the 85 patients. Of the remaining 6 patients, 4 had mitral valve leaflets that were diffusely thickened by fibrous tissue, but their chordae tendineae

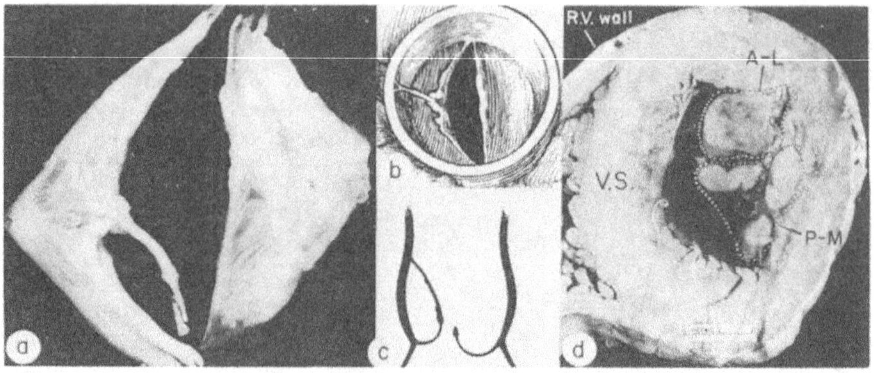

Figure 7. Pure aortic regurgitation complicating a congenitally bicuspid aortic valve without a history of infective endocarditis. The 27 year old man whose aortic valve and portion of left ventricle are illustrated here was found to have aortic regurgitation at age 17, but was asymptomatic until age 25 when moderate exertional dyspnea appeared. At catheterization shortly before valve replacement, the left ventricular pressure was 125/25 and the brachial arterial pressure, 126/54 mm Hg when the cardiac index (Fick method) was 2.2 liters/min per m². He died suddenly and unexpectedly 13 months after valve replacement. The heart weighed 800 g. The aortic arch coursed over the right bronchus. **a**, the excised aortic valve. A supporting fibrous band stretched from the margin in the mid portion of one cusp to the aortic wall above the sinuses of Valsalva as shown in **b** and **c**. **d**, a transverse section across the left ventricle (L.V.) showing atrophy of the posteromedial papillary muscle but no atrophy of the anterolateral papillary muscle. The coronary arteries were widely patent.

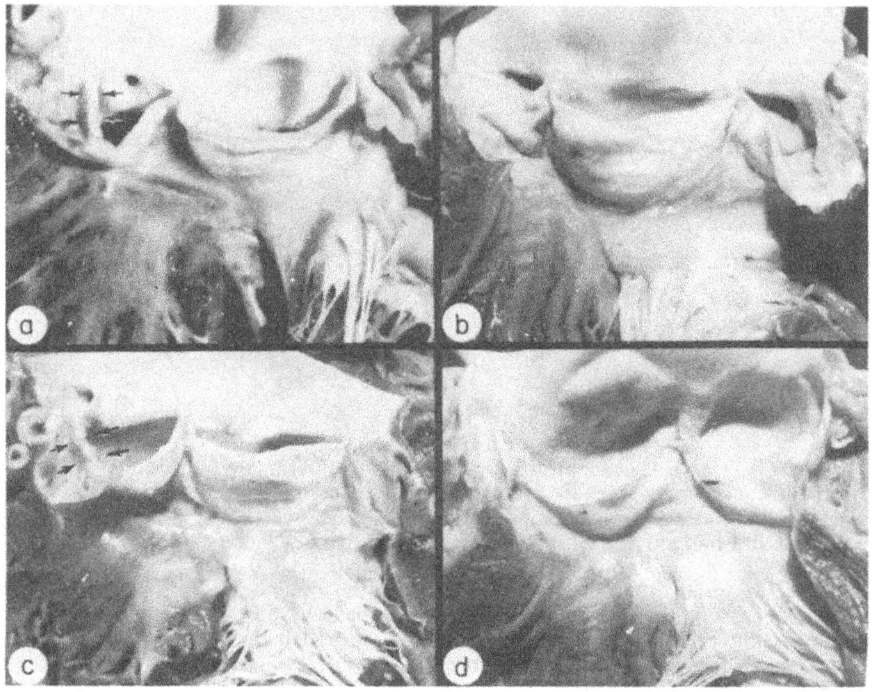

Figure 8. Functionally normal congenitally bicuspid aortic valves in 4 patients. The valve, aorta and left ventricle are opened. Three patients **(a, b, c)** died of leukemia and 1 **(d)** of lymphosarcoma. None of the patients (3 men, 1 woman; ages 23 to 47 years) had signs or symptoms of cardiac disease, and the heart weights ranged from 230 to 290 g. Raphes, designated by **horizontal arrows,** are visible in **a** and **c.**

were normal and there was no clinical evidence of mitral valve dysfunction. A fifth patient, mentioned earlier (Table II), had a congenitally malformed mitral valve. The sixth patient, a 20 year old man who also had the Marfan syndrome, had elongated "floppy" mitral leaflets that contained excessive acid-mucopolysaccharide material and fibrous tissue.

Location of aortic valve cusps: Information regarding the location of each of the 2 aortic valve cusps and the presence or absence of raphes was ascertainable in 59 patients. In some patients who had undergone aortic valve replacement this information was not precise and was therefore omitted. Of the patients who had undergone aortic valve replacement, the valves in most had been excised intact,[9] and each was re-examined. In addition, the prosthetic valves were removed from the hearts at autopsy; this permitted accurate determination of the number of aortic valve cusps and commissures that had been present. In 28 of 59 patients (47.5 percent) 1 cusp was located anteriorly, the second posteriorly and the commissures to the right and left, respectively (Fig. 10). In each of the 28 patients both coronary arteries arose in front of the anterior cusp, and a raphe, present in 16 of the 28 subjects, was always located in the anterior cusp. In 31 of the 59 patients (52.5 percent) the cusps were situated right and left with the 2 commissures situated anteriorly and posteriorly, respectively. When this relation was present the right coronary artery arose from behind the right cusp and the left coronary artery from behind the left cusp. A raphe, present in 14 of the 31 patients, was always located in the right cusp. Raphes were observed in 30 of 59 patients (51 percent). However, their presence in 10 of 13 patients with normally functioning valves, that is, those in

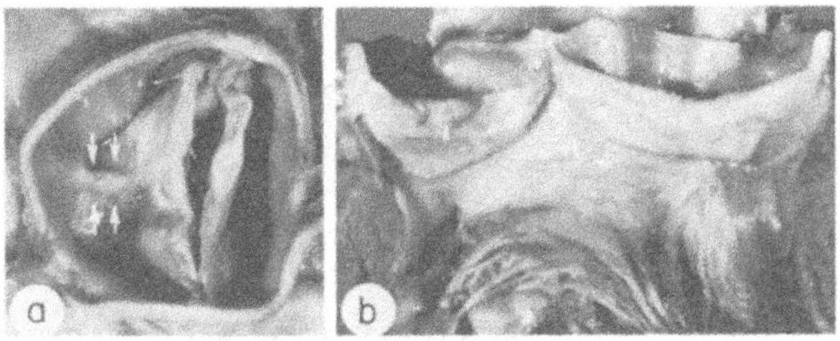

Figure 9. Functionally normal aortic valve with unequal-sized cusps. A raphe (arrows) is present in the right cusp. **a**, valve from above; **b**, valve opened.

whom the valve architecture was best preserved, suggests that some raphes were obscured by heavy deposits of calcium.

Comments

Incidence in general population: The 13 normally functioning congenitally bicuspid aortic valves described were observed by me during examination of the hearts of 1,440 patients who had no other cardiac valvular, septal or great vessel abnormality. The bicuspid condition of the aortic valve was specifically looked for. Since this anomaly otherwise may escape notice, information about its frequency obtained by scanning postmortem records is unreliable. This incidence of 0.90 percent is similar to that reported by others who examined hearts specifically for the presence or absence of congenitally bicuspid aortic valves. Osler[10] found 7 apparently normally functioning congenitally bicuspid aortic valves in 800 autopsies (750 of which were performed by him), an incidence of 1.3 percent. Eight additional patients had infective endocarditis involving congenitally bicuspid aortic valves. Thus, 18 of 800 (2 percent) had either normally functioning or infected congenitally bicuspid aortic valves. Lewis and Grant[11] found 3 apparently normally functioning congenitally bicuspid aortic valves among 215 consecutive autopsies. Grant et al.[12] found apparently normally functioning congenitally bicuspid aortic valves in 12 of 1,350 (0.89 percent) autopsy cases. Neither Osler, Lewis nor Grant et al. appear to have appreciated that the bicuspid condition of this valve may underlie severe stenosis or calcification at this site. Bonnabeau et al.[13] observed at necropsy 5 apparently normally functioning congenitally bicuspid aortic valves in a period during which they also observed 20 severely stenotic congenitally bicuspid aortic valves. The oldest of the 13 patients with normally functioning bicuspid aortic valves described herein was 59 years of age.

TABLE II

Congenital Malformations Associated With Congenitally Bicuspid Aortic Valves Among 85 Patients Over 14 Years of Age

Coarctation of aorta	5
Patent ductus arteriosus	1
Congenital mitral regurgitation	1
Ebstein malformation, tricuspid valve*	1
Right aortic arch*	1
Biscuspid pulmonic valve*	1
Spontaneously-closed ventricular septal defect*	1
TOTAL 11† in 85 patients (13%)	

* Did not cause functional disturbance

† No patient had more than 1 associated congenital anomaly. In addition, 2 men, aged 46 and 57 years, respectively, died of dissecting aortic aneurysms.

Thus, if congenitally bicuspid aortic valves that develop complications (stenosis, incompetency with or without infection) are added to those which function normally during an entire lifetime, the frequency of congenitally bicuspid aortic valves may approach 2 percent of the population. It appears that the bicuspid aortic valve is the most common congenital malformation of the heart or great vessels.

Incidence in patients with aortic valvular disease: Sixty-nine of the 72 patients described herein with abnormally functioning congenitally bicuspid aortic valves were observed during study at necropsy of 400 patients over age 14 years with functionally severe cardiac valvular disease (classes III and IV, New York Heart Association classification).[14] Of the 105 patients with anatomic disease limited to the aortic valve causing stenosis with or without regurgitation, 54 had congenitally bicuspid valves, 13 had congenitally unicommissural, unicuspid valves, 32 had tricuspid valves (3 with distinctly unequal-sized cusps) and 6 had valves so scarred, calcified and deformed that their basic structure was not discernible. It is strongly suspected that these latter 6 patients also had congenitally malformed valves. Thus, over 50 percent of patients studied at autopsy by the author with anatomically isolated aortic stenosis had congenitally bicuspid aortic valves, and over 70 percent had congenitally malformed valves of various types. Campbell,[15] in reviewing a coroner's necropsy records, found bicuspid aortic valves described in 9 of 60 patients (15 percent) with calcific aortic stenosis. Ninety percent of the patients were over 50 years of age. In my necropsy study of 34 patients with clinically pure aortic regurgitation 9 (26.5 percent) had congenitally bicuspid aortic valves. The valves in 7 of the 9 patients were made incompetent by superimposed infective endocarditis. Of the remaining 6 of 69 patients with abnormally functioning congenitally bicuspid aortic valves, 4 had diffuse fibrous thickening of the mitral leaflets but normal chordae tendineae. None of the 4 had evidence of mitral valve dysfunction, and all had aortic stenosis with or without regurgitation. One patient with a congenitally bicuspid stenotic and incompetent aortic valve had a severely incompetent congenitally malformed mitral valve, and another with a congenitally incompetent bicuspid aortic valve had a "floppy" incompetent mitral valve and the Marfan syndrome. Thus, among 173 patients with anatomically abnormal mitral and aortic valves, 6 had congenitally bicuspid aortic valves. However, 4 of the 6 were among 24 patients with fibrous thickening of the mitral leaflets but normal chordae and normal mitral function.

Incidence of valvular stenosis, regurgitation and infection: Valvular stenosis is the most frequent complication of a congenitally bicuspid aortic valve; valvular regurgitation is next, and the latter lesion is most frequently the result of its being the site of infective endocarditis. The reason 1 congenitally bicuspid aortic valve becomes stenotic, another incompetent, and another the site of infective endocarditis is unknown. However, it is clear that stenosis, regurgitation and infection are complications of the bicuspid condition of the aortic valve and none of them are present at birth. It appears likely that a congenitally bicuspid aortic valve becomes stenotic only as its cusps become fibrotic and calcified; neither cusp of a congenitally bicuspid aortic valve is fibrotic or calcified at the time of birth.

The frequency of development of stenosis or incompetency at the site of a congenitally bicuspid aortic valve also is unknown. Lewis and Grant[11] concluded that vegetations develop at these sites in 23 percent of adults (16 of 69) with congenitally bicuspid aortic valves. More information is available regarding the incidence of congenitally bicuspid valves in patients with infective endocarditis involving the aortic valve. Of 31 patients with "subacute infective endocarditis" studied at autopsy by Lewis and Grant,[11] 8 had congenitally bicuspid aortic valves. Four of 13 patients with infective endocarditis involving the aortic valve studied at autopsy by Starling,[16] 2 of 22 patients studied at autopsy by Fulton and Levine[17] and 3 of 20 patients studied at autopsy by Bayles and Lewis[18] had congenitally bicuspid aortic valves. None of these investigators apparently were aware that a congenitally bicuspid aortic valve also could become stenotic.

Valve calcification: Of the 61 patients with congenitally bicuspid stenotic aortic valves, 59 had calcific deposits in the valve. Of the 57 patients over 30 years of age all had large calcific deposits in the valve cusps; of the 4 under 30 years of age 2 had no calcific deposits, and 2 had only small focal ones. None of the 11 patients with pure aortic regurgitation had more than 1 or 2 small focal deposits of calcium in the valves, and most had none. Of the 13 patients with functionally normal aortic valves, 4 had small focal calcific deposits in them. Thus, large calcific deposits on congenitally bicuspid aortic valves are unusual before the age of 30 years, and stenotic congenitally bicuspid aortic valves without calcific deposits are rare in persons over 30 years of age. Heavy deposits of calcium do not occur in purely incompetent congenitally bicuspid aortic valves; valvular stenosis appears to be prerequisite for the development of heavy deposits of calcium at this site. Development of infective endocarditis on a heavily calcified valve also is rare. Of 5 patients with stenotic congenitally bicuspid aortic valves only 1 had heavy deposits of calcium on his valve before the onset of the infection. Of the 11 patients with pure aortic regurgitation, infective endocarditis was the cause of the valvular incompetency in 8, and none had significant valvular calcific deposits.

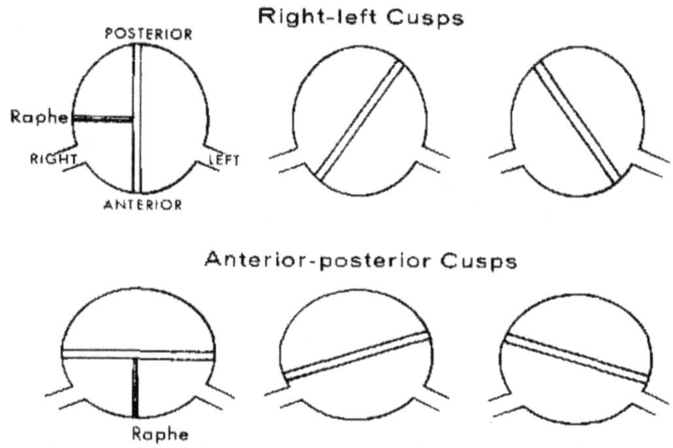

Figure 10. Diagram showing the 2 basic types of congenitally bicuspid aortic valves. See text for explanation.

Mechanism of valvular stenosis and regurgitation: The mechanism by which a congenitally bicuspid aortic valve becomes stenotic or incompetent is uncertain. There is no evidence to indicate that the valve is stenotic or incompetent at birth. Likewise, there is no evidence to indicate that superimposed rheumatic fever or rheumatic heart disease is the cause of the stenosis or incompetency. Five of the 85 patients (6 percent) described herein had histories of acute rheumatic fever or chorea. However, it is suspected that their illness had been inaccurately diagnosed as acute rheumatic fever. All 5 patients had aortic stenosis, and many patients with this valvular lesion have precordial murmurs during childhood. The presence of a febrile illness in a child with a precordial murmur tends to be diagnosed as acute rheumatic fever when this may not be the case. In contrast to its low incidence in the patients with anatomically isolated aortic valvular disease, a his-

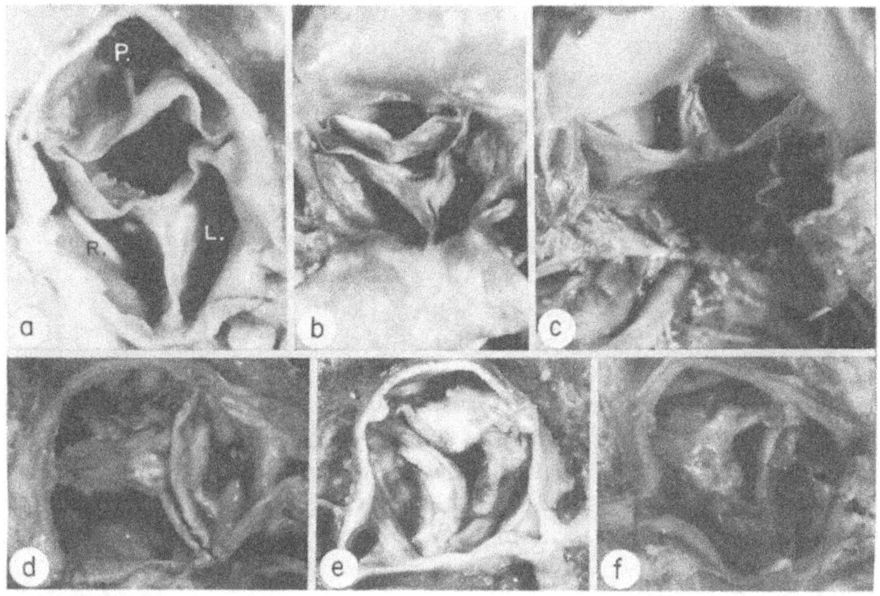

Figure 11. Acquired bicuspid aortic valves (viewed from above) in 6 patients. **a,** valve of a 54 year old man who died of bronchogenic carcinoma. Unexpected findings at necropsy were a left atrial myxoma and fibrous fusion of 1 of 3 commissures of the aortic valve. This valve caused no known cardiac dysfunction during life. The mitral valve leaflets were focally thickened. **b,** valve of a 76 year old man who had systemic hypertension but no other evidence of cardiac dysfunction. The mitral valve was normal. **c,** opened valve in a 30 year old man with Fallot's tetrad. Fusion of the commissure between the left and posterior cusps was an incidental necropsy finding.[24] The mitral valve was normal. **d,** valve in a 68 year old man who had shown clinical features of acute rheumatic fever 1 month before death and at autopsy had numerous myocardial Aschoff bodies. The commissure between the right and posterior cusps is completely fused. The mitral leaflets were diffusely thickened and focally calcified. **e,** valve of a 70 year old woman who died of gastric carcinoma but during life was believed to have mitral regurgitation. The mitral leaflets and chordae were anatomically normal, but the aortic cusps were fibrotic, calcified and rigid and the commissure between the left and posterior cusps was fused. **f,** valve of a 50 year old woman who had a history of acute rheumatic fever at age 7 years and on examination shortly before death was believed to have mitral and tricuspid regurgitation. The tricuspid valve leaflets were mildly thickened, the mitral leaflets were diffusely fibrotic and calcified, and the aortic cusps were diffusely fibrotic, focally calcified, and the commissure between the right and posterior cusps was completely fused.

Fusion occurred in 1 of the 3 commissures of the aortic valve in each of these 6 patients. The circumferential distances between a fused and a nonfused commissure were similar to the distances between the 2 nonfused commissures in all patients. The most cephalad margin of the fused commissures in each patient was on the same horizontal level as the most cephalad margins of the nonfused commissures. In 2 patients **(d and f)** the cause of the commissural fusion was rheumatic since both had extensive mitral valvular scarring. The cause of the commissural fusion in the other 4 subjects is unknown, but in only 1 **(e)** of them did the commissural fusion cause functional disturbance. Histologic sections of the fused commissures illustrated showed that they were devoid of elastic fibrils, evidence that the fusion was acquired.

tory of acute rheumatic fever or chorea was present in nearly 70 percent of 256 patients with anatomic disease of the mitral valve with or without anatomic involvement of the aortic valve studied at autopsy by me.[19] Further evidence supporting the theory that superimposed rheumatic heart disease is not the cause of stenosis or incompetency of the congenitally bicuspid aortic valve is that no patient with anatomically isolated aortic valvular disease had Aschoff bodies in the heart at necropsy. These lesions were found in the hearts of 11 of the 256 patients over 14 years of age with anatomic mitral valvular disease, and 10 of them had anatomic involvement of other valves as well.

Since superimposed rheumatic heart disease is clearly not the cause of the stenosis or incompetence of a congenitally bicuspid aortic valve, a search for other causes is necessary. The explanation advanced by Edwards[20] is attractive. He proposed that it is not mechanically possible for a congenitally bicuspid aortic valve to open and close properly. The distances between lateral attachments of normal aortic valvular cusps along their free margins are curved lines. The extra lengths allow the cusps to move freely during opening and closing of the valves. In contrast, the distances between lateral attachments of congenitally bicuspid aortic valves along their free margins approach straight lines. If these distances were exactly straight lines, the valves could not open during ventricular systole. Consequently, at least 1 cusp is larger than the other. The excessive length of 1 or both cusps of a congenitally bicuspid aortic valve produces abnormal contact between the cusps. This abnormal contact, in turn, causes focal fibrous thickening that with time becomes diffuse, and dystrophic calcification thereafter occurs. Thus, stenosis of a congenitally bicuspid aortic valve may be the result of trauma to these cusps produced by their abnormal contact with each other. Although this explanation is appealing, it does not explain why 1 congenitally bicuspid valve becomes stenotic, another becomes entirely incompetent, and another remains free of complications.

Differentiation of congenital and acquired bicuspid valve: Criteria for differentiating a bicuspid valve of congenital origin from a bicuspid valve of acquired origin (Fig. 11) have been debated. No controversy has arisen in distinguishing a congenitally bicuspid aortic valve devoid of a raphe (false commissure or ridge) and of complications (stenosis, incompetency or infection) from a tricuspid aortic valve also devoid of similar complications. Controversy has existed about the means of differentiating a congenitally bicuspid aortic valve with a raphe from an acquired bicuspid aortic valve resulting from fusion of 2 cusps at 1 true commissure.* Osler,[3] from the study of 18 hearts (15 adults), listed the following characteristics, all recognizable by gross observation, of the congenitally bicuspid aortic valve: (1) The raphe is located where normally the true commissure would be, between the right and left anterior aortic valve cusps; (2) the length of the free margin of the cusp containing no raphe is slightly shorter (by an average of 12 percent in his measurements on 7 hearts) than the length of the margin of the cusp containing a raphe, the "conjoint" cusp; (3) the free border of the conjoint cusp is straight or curled and free of nodular thickenings indicative of corpus Arantii; (4) the border of attachment of the conjoint cusp, as viewed from the ventricular aspect, presents either the contour of a single semilunar cusp or a shallow groove, indicative of the junction of 2 cusps; (5) the raphe may be located on the aortic wall alone or may extend onto the cusp for variable distances, but in either case it usually divides the sinus of Valsalva into equal-sized units.

In 1923 Lewis and Grant[11] clarified several gross features of unequivocally congenitally bicuspid aortic valves and presented histologic criteria for differentiating bicuspid valves of "congenital" origin from those of "inflammatory" origin. In contrast to Osler, these authors found that fusion could occur not only between right and left anterior cusps but also between right anterior and posterior cusps. A raphe, dividing one of the 2 cusps, was observed "in about half the cases." The 2 cusps could be equal or unequal in size, but usually the conjoined cusp was larger, but not twice the size of the undivided cusp. Or, "the subdivided cusp is larger than 1 normal cusp but smaller than 2 normal cusps." However, Lewis and Grant considered gross distinction between congenital and acquired bicuspid aortic valves unreliable. Elastic tissue stains of transverse sections of congenital raphes disclosed them to consist mainly of elastic fibers; thus the raphe histologically was similar to the media of the aorta. In contrast, transverse sections of 2 fused cusps at a true commissure disclosed that the fused commissure was devoid of elastic fibers and consisted of fibrous valvular tissue. Other investigators[21,22] confirmed these histologic criteria. Koletsky[22] also pointed out that congenital raphes were devoid of vascular channels and of inflammatory cells whereas both were seen in acquired, fused commissures. Since Lewis and Grant described these histologic features, many pathologists have been reluctant to distinguish between congenital and acquired bicuspid aortic valves without microscopic examination of raphes. However, these histologic criteria are helpful but not specific (Fig. 12).

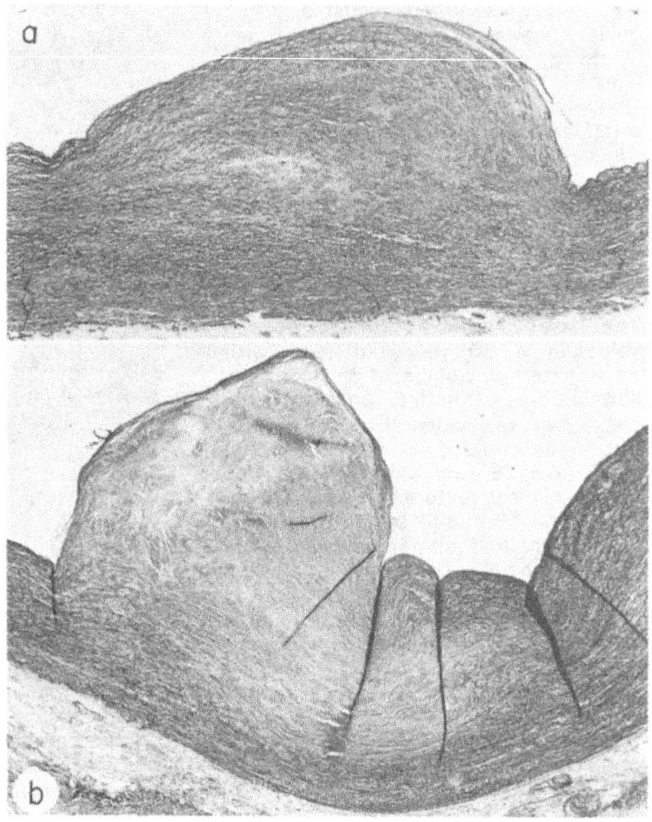

Figure 12. Photomicrographs of transverse sections of raphes in 2 patients with congenitally bicuspid aortic valves, each stained for elastic fibers (elastic Van Gieson method). **a,** characteristic appearance of raphe showing many elastic fibers, similar to aortic media. **b,** raphe from patient whose valve is illustrated in Figure 2**d.** The raphe is devoid of elastic fibers, but the valve grossly is unequivocally congenitally bicuspid. The raphe, although difficult to see in Figure 2**d,** is in the right cusp. Original magnification × 27 **(a),** × 24 **(b);** reduced by 25 percent.

* The definition of a commissure differs depending on whether a semilunar or an atrioventricular (A–V) cardiac valve is under consideration. The aortic valve commissure is the space between 2 lateral attachments on the aortic wall. Normally each aortic valve cusp is an independent similar-sized unit and adherence of one cusp with another at the narrow space (commissure) between the 2 cusps is abnormal. In contrast to a semilunar valve, the leaflets of an atrioventricular valve are continuous one with another. Thus, the commissures of the A–V valves are the sites of attachment between the unequal-sized leaflets, not the spaces between the cusps as in the case of the semilunar valves.

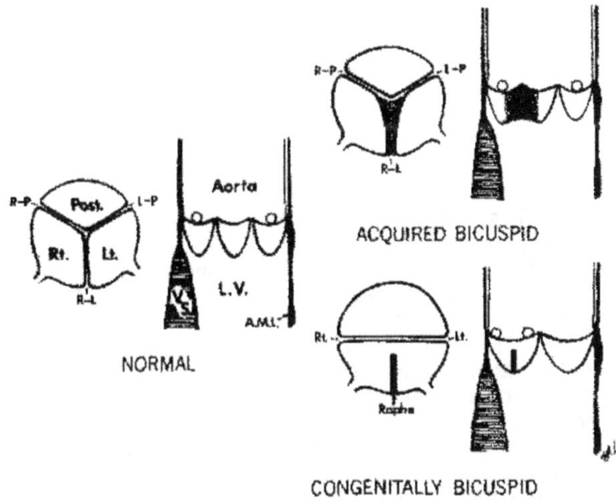

Figure 13. Diagram illustrating differences between bicuspid aortic valves of acquired and of congenital origins as compared to the normal valve. The circumferential distances between each of the 3 commissures in a normally formed valve are similar. L-P = left-posterior, R-L = right-left, and R-P = right-posterior commissures; Rt. = right, Lt. = left, and Post. = posterior cusps; V.S. = ventricular septum; L.V. = left ventricular outflow tract; and A.M.L. = anterior mitral leaflet. **In the acquired bicuspid valve** the circumferential distance between the commissures remains equal, as in the normal. The fused commissure is wide, the distal margins of each of the 2 fused cusps are still usually visible, and the most cephalad margin of the fused commissure is on the same horizontal level as the most cephalad margins of the 2 nonfused commissures. **In the congenitally bicuspid valve** the raphe is generally narrow and rarely extends to the free margin of the conjoined cusp or to the cephalad level reached by the 2 true commissures. The circumferential distance between the 2 true commissures is greater than the circumferential distances between either true commissure and the raphe. The circumferential distance between the true commissures around the conjoined cusp, that is, the cusp that has the raphe, is equal to or slightly greater than the circumferential distance between the true commissures around the cusp devoid of the raphe.

In patients in whom some sections of a raphe show a structure like that of the aortic media, other sections of the same raphe may show only fibrous tissue. Also, the congenital raphe may lose its elastic fibers as the valvular cusps become fibrotic and calcified. The raphe may be the first portion of a congenitally bicuspid aortic valve to calcify, and these deposits destroy existing elastic fibers. Interestingly, Lewis and Grant and others who emphasized the importance of histologic distinction between congenital raphes and fused true commissures were unaware that calcific stenosis was a consequence of a congenitally bicuspid aortic valve. Once the valve is extensively scarred and calcified, histologic examination of the raphe is often fruitless. Furthermore, as Edwards[24] pointed out, in an occasional patient with a bicuspid aortic valve that must be assumed to be congenital, as in infants with aortic coarctation, the raphe not only may be fibrous, but may grossly display features suggesting fusion of 2 distinguishable, separate cusps.

Useful features to distinguish between bicuspid aortic valves of acquired and of congenital origin are summarized in Figure 13. Emphasis is placed on obvious gross differences between fused true commissures and raphes.

Acknowledgment

I am indebted to my past and present colleagues, particularly Drs. Andrew G. Morrow and Eugene Braunwald, for free access to the clinical data on the patients described in this study.

References

1. **Paget J:** On obstructions of the branches of the pulmonary artery. Med-Chir Trans 27:162–188, 1844
2. **Peacock TB:** On Malformations of the Human Heart, second edition. London, Churchill, 1866, p 204
3. **Osler W:** The bicuspid condition of the aortic valves. Trans Ass Amer Physicians 2:185–192, 1886
4. **Campbell M, Kauntze R:** Congenital aortic valvular stenosis. Brit Heart J 15:179–194, 1953
5. **Smith DE, Matthews MB:** Aortic valvular stenosis with coarctation of the aorta. With special reference to the development of aortic stenosis upon congenital bicuspid valves. Brit Heart J 17:198–206, 1955
6. **Bacon APC, Matthews MB:** Congenital bicuspid aortic valves and the aetiology of isolated aortic valvular stenosis. Quart J Med 28:545–560, 1959
7. **Roberts, WC:** Examining the precordium and the heart. Chest, in press
8. **Friedman WF, Mason DT, Braunwald E:** Arthrogryposis multiplex congenita associated with congenital aortic stenosis. J Pediat 67:682–685, 1965
9. **Roberts WC, Morrow AG:** Cardiac valves and the surgical pathologist. Arch Path (Chicago) 82:309–313, 1966
10. **Osler W:** On the condition of fusion of two segments of the semilunar valves. Montreal Gen Hosp Reports 1:233, 1880
11. **Lewis T, Grant RT:** Observations relating to subacute infective endocarditis. Heart 10:21–99, 1923
12. **Grant RT, Wood JE Jr, Jones TD:** Heart valve irregularities in relation to subacute bacterial endocarditis. Heart 14:247–255, 1928
13. **Bonnabeau RC Jr, Lillehei CW, Edwards JE:** Relationship of the congenital bicuspid aortic valve to calcific aortic stenosis (abstr). Circulation 29, 30: Suppl III:51, 1964
14. **Roberts WC:** Severe valvular cardiac disease. A study

of 400 autopsy patients over 14 years of age. In preparation
15. **Campbell M:** Calcific aortic stenosis and congenital bicuspid aortic valves. Brit Heart J 30:606–616, 1968
16. **Starling HJ:** Endocarditis lenta. Quart J Med 16:263–281, 1923
17. **Fulton MN, Levine SA:** Subacute bacterial endocarditis, with special reference to the valvular lesions and previous history. Amer J Med Sci 183:60–77, 1932
18. **Bayles TB, Lewis WH Jr:** Subacute bacterial endocarditis in older people. Ann Intern Med 13:2154–2163, 1940
19. **Roberts WC:** Anatomically isolated aortic valve disease. The case against its being of rheumatic etiology. Amer J Med, in press.
20. **Edwards JE:** The congenital bicuspid aortic valve. Circulation 23:485–488, 1961
21. **Bishop LF Jr, Trubek M:** Bicuspid aortic valve: a differential study between inflammatory and congenital origin. J Tech Meth 15:111–131, 1936
22. **Koletsky S:** Congenital bicuspid aortic valves. Arch Intern Med (Chicago) 67:129–176, 1941
23. **Edwards JE:** Congenital malformations of the heart and great vessels. C. Malformations of the valves. In, Pathology of the Heart and Blood Vessels, third edition (Gould SE, ed). Springfield, Ill., Charles C Thomas, 1968 p 341
24. **Glancy DL, Morrow AG, Roberts WC:** Malformations of the aortic valve in patients with the tetralogy of Fallot. Amer Heart J 76:755–759, 1968

Anatomically Isolated Aortic Valvular Disease

The Case Against Its Being of Rheumatic Etiology

WILLIAM C. ROBERTS, M.D.
Bethesda, Maryland

Data are presented in 400 autopsy patients, each over fourteen years of age (average age, forty-five years) with functionally severe valvular cardiac disease. Of 139 patients with anatomically isolated aortic valvular disease (aortic stenosis [AS] in 105 and pure aortic regurgitation [AR] in thirty-four), 6 per cent had positive histories of acute rheumatic fever (ARF) or chorea, none had Aschoff bodies, nearly all had histologically normal atrial walls, and 72 per cent of the 105 patients with AS and 26.5 per cent of the thirty-four patients with pure AR had congenitally malformed aortic valves. In contrast, of 235 patients with anatomic mitral disease with or without anatomic involvement of other valves, 68 per cent had positive histories of ARF or chorea, twelve (5 per cent) had Aschoff bodies, nearly all had histologically abnormal left atrial walls, and only two patients (<1 per cent) had congenitally malformed valves. It is concluded that anatomically isolated aortic valve disease is of nonrheumatic etiology and most frequently the consequence of a congenital malformation.

Considerable evidence indicates that isolated mitral stenosis is nearly always of rheumatic etiology. Likewise, combined anatomic disease of both mitral and aortic valves is generally rheumatic in origin. Anatomically isolated aortic valvular disease causing stenosis or regurgitation or both also has been considered by numerous investigators generally to be of rheumatic etiology. Study of 400 autopsy patients with various forms of functionally severe valvular cardiac disease, however, has convinced me that anatomically isolated aortic valvular disease is not rheumatic in origin. Observations on these 400 patients which allowed this conclusion are described.

PATIENTS STUDIED AND RESULTS

Data in the 400 patients studied at necropsy are summarized in Table I. Each patient died between 1953 and 1968 inclusive: 331 had been studied clinically at the National Heart Institute, and sixty-nine were studied clinically at other institutions and their hearts submitted to me for examination. Clinical data were available in all patients. Cardiac catheterization had been performed in 315 patients, and cardiac valvular operation (commissurotomy, valvuloplasty or replacement) had been performed in 280 patients, a few of whom had never undergone cardiac catheterization. Each of the 400 patients was over fourteen years of age (range fifteen to eighty-eight years; average forty-five years); twelve were over seventy and thirty-seven were under thirty years of age at death. Each had been considered to be in functional classes III or IV (New York Heart Association Classification). Patients with carcinoid heart disease [1,2] and left ventricular papillary muscle dysfunction, fibrosis or necrosis [3] were excluded. The hospital charts of all 400 patients

From the Section of Pathology, National Heart and Lung Institute, National Institutes of Health, Bethesda, Maryland 20014. Requests for reprints should be addressed to Dr. William C. Roberts. Manuscript received September 11, 1969.

TABLE I Data in 400 Autopsy Patients Over Fourteen Years of Age with Valvular Cardiac Disease

Group	Valve Involved Anatomically	No. Patients	% of Total	Age (yr) Range	Age (yr) Average	Sex (No.) Male	Sex (No.) Female	Sex (%) Male	Sex (%) Female	Nonrheumatic Etiology No.	Nonrheumatic Etiology %	Rheumatic Etiology No.	Rheumatic Etiology %	History of ARF or Chorea (No.)	Rheumatic Subjects with History of ARF or Chorea (%)	Total with History of ARF or Chorea (%)
I	Aortic only	163	41	15–88	48	134	29	82	18	141	87	?22	?13	21	. . .	13
	a. AS with or without AR	105	26	16–88	50	80	25	76	24	105	100	0	0	6*	0	6
	b. Pure AR	34	9	15–69	40	31	3	91	9	32	89	?4	11	2†	0	6
	c. Clinically AS or pure AR but thickened mitral leaflets and normal chordae tendineae	24‡	6	34–74	50	23	1	96	4	4§	17	20	83	13	65	54
II	Mitral + aortic	116	29	20–85	45	75	41	65	35	4	3	112	97	87	78	75
III	Mitral only	75	19	15–78	42	27	48	36	64	18¶	24	57#	76	40	70	53
IV	Mitral + aortic + tricuspid‖	38	9	18–65	41	16	22	42	58	1	3	37	97	27	73	71
V	Mitral + tricuspid	6	1.5	30–57	47	1	5	17	83	0	0	6	100	5	83	83
VI	Tricuspid only	2¶	0.5	31–65	48	1	1	50	50	2	100	0	0	0	0	0
	Totals	400	100	15–88	45	254	146	63.5	36.5	166	41.5	234	58.5	180	77**	45

* Five had congenitally bicuspid aortic valves.
† One had ankylosing spondylitis.
‡ Five patients had pure AR; nineteen had some degree of AS.
§ Each had congenitally bicuspid aortic valves; none had a positive history of ARF.
¶ Each had pure mitral regurgitation.
\# Each had mitral stenosis with or without regurgitation.
‖ Two also had focally thickened but functionally normal pulmonic valve cusps.
** If group I were excluded this percentage would be 75 instead of 77.

were reviewed. A history of acute rheumatic fever (ARF) was considered positive if the patient stated that he had been told that he had ARF in the past or if he described a febrile illness during childhood characterized by signs or symptoms of arthritis necessitating rest in bed. Most of the latter patients were told that they had heart murmurs during their febrile illnesses. Electrocardiographic, roentgenographic, hemodynamic and autopsy observations were recorded. The heart of each patient was examined on at least two occasions by me. The patients were divided according to which cardiac valve or valves were involved anatomically (Table I).

The aortic valve only was involved in 163 patients. (group I). Aortic stenosis (AS) with or without aortic regurgitation (AR) (group Ia) occurred in 105 of them: eighty (76 per cent) were male, twenty-five (24 per cent) female; six (6 per cent) had a history of acute rheumatic fever (ARF) or chorea, but five of the six had congenitally bicuspid aortic valves. The diagnosis of ARF in these five therefore is probably fallacious. Left heart catheterization was performed in seventy-four of the 105 patients with isolated AS. The peak systolic pressure gradients between the left ventricle and a systemic artery ranged from 18 to 165 mm Hg (average 97 mm Hg). In only three patients were these pressure gradients less than 50 mm Hg. Of the thirty-four patients with pure AR, thirty-one (91 per cent) were male, and two (6 per cent) had a history of ARF or chorea. The various causes of AR in these thirty-four patients are summarized in Table II. Cardiac catheterization in nineteen patients with pure AR showed zero or negative systolic pressure gradients between the left ventricle and a systemic artery in each. In addition to the 105 patients with AS and the thirty-four with pure AR, twenty-four other subjects are included in the "aortic only" group since they also had AS or AR or both. In contrast to the other 139 patients in group I, however, their mitral leaflets also were diffusely thickened (Fig. 1). Their mitral chordae tendineae, however, were normal, and the valves functioned normally. It is suspected that thickening of the mitral leaflets in some of them resulted from the elevated left ventricular pressures, but others probably belong in the mitral plus aortic category (group II), especially since thirteen (54 per cent) had a positive history of ARF or chorea. If the four patients with congenitally bicuspid aortic valves, none of whom had a positive history of ARF, are excluded, this percentage rises to 65 per cent. Cardiac catheterization was performed in twenty of the twenty-four patients in group Ic. Of the fifteen with AS, the peak systolic pressure gradients between the left ventricle and a systemic artery ranged from 18 to 120 mm Hg (average 65 mm Hg). No pressure gradient between the left ventricle and a systemic artery occurred in any of the five patients with pure AR.

Accurate heart weights were available in 146 of the 163 patients in group I. The heart weight ranged from 330 to 1,100 gm (average 650 gm). The heart weight of ninety-two patients with isolated AS ranged from 330 to 1,000 gm (average 608 gm). The weight depended more on the sex than the degree of obstruction across the aortic valve: in the twenty women the heart weight averaged 477 gm (range 330 to 700 gm) and in the seventy-two men 645 gm (range 400 to 1,000 gm). In ten (all women) of the ninety-two patients with accurately weighed hearts in group I, the heart weight was 400 gm or less; and in the six in whom cardiac catheterization was performed, the peak systolic pressure gradients between the left ventricle and a systemic artery ranged from 70 to 145 mm Hg (average 98 mm Hg). Of thirty-one patients with pure AR the heart weight ranged from 390 to 1,100 gm (average 691 gm). Of thirty-three patients in group Ic (Table I) the heart weight ranged from 530 to 1,050 gm (average 754 gm). In none of the patients in group Ic did the heart weigh 400 gm or less, but in one man in group Ib in whom infective endocarditis caused acute fatal AR, the heart weighed 390 gm.

In contrast to its low incidence (6 per cent) in the 139 patients with anatomically isolated AS (group Ia) and pure AR (group Ib), the incidence of a positive history of ARF or chorea in the 235 patients with anatomic mitral valvular involvement (groups II through V, Table I) ranged from 53 to 83 per cent (average 68 per cent). The latter average rises to 74 per cent if the twenty-three patients with clearly nonrheumatic valvular disease in groups II through V are eliminated. Although male subjects predominated (65 per cent) in the 116 patients with anatomic disease of both mitral and aortic valves (group II), female subjects predominated (63 per cent) in the other 119 patients with involvement in the mitral valve, whether alone (group III), in combination with both aortic and tricuspid valves (group IV) or in combination with the tricuspid valve (group V). In twenty-three of the 235 patients with mitral valvular disease the etiology was clearly nonrheumatic. Eighteen had isolated mitral involvement with pure regurgitation resulting from rupture of chordae tendineae (infective endocarditis) in previously normal valves [4] (ten patients), "floppy" mitral leaflets [5] (four patients), congenital malformations (two patients), probably secondary to mitral annular calcification (one patient) and uncertain etiology [6] (one patient). Each of the four patients with combined mitral and aortic involvement of nonrheumatic etiology had severe mitral and aortic regurgitation, and one had mild (30 mm Hg peak systolic pressure gradient) AS in addition. The latter patient had a congenitally bicuspid aortic valve and a congenitally malformed mitral valve. Two of the other patients had the Marfan syndrome, and the third had Marfan-type diseased valves without the clinical syndrome **(forme fruste).** The only patient with three-valve involvement of nonrheumatic nature had rheumatoid heart disease [7]. Anatomically isolated tricuspid valve disease is nonrheumatic; each of the two patients (group VI, Table I) studied by me was a heroin addict with infective endocarditis superimposed on previously normal valves [8].

The structure of the aortic valve in the 163 patients with anatomically isolated aortic valvular disease is summarized in Table III. Of the 105 patients with

TABLE II Etiology of Pure Aortic Regurgitation. Thirty-Four Patients > Age Fourteen Years with Anatomically Isolated Aortic Valve Disease*

Etiology	No. of Patients
Infective endocarditis	9†
Syphilis	9‡
Medial cystic necrosis of aorta	5§
Ankylosing spondylitis	5
Congenital	2#
Trauma	1
Juvenile rheumatoid arthritis	1
Chronic dissecting aortic aneurysm	1
Etiology undetermined	1¶
	34

* Eight other patients among the 400 studied also had clinically pure aortic regurgitation (AR), but the mitral valve was anatomically abnormal in each, although three were in class 1c. The etiology in each is considered rheumatic.

† Seven and possibly eight had congenitally bicuspid aortic valves, and none had evidence of AR until manifestations of the cardiac infection appeared.

‡ Serologic test for syphilis positive in only three patients; histologic changes in ascending aorta consistent with syphilis in each.

§ Four had the Marfan syndrome.

\# Each had congenitally bicuspid aortic valves which were intrinsically incompetent and neither patient ever had clinical or anatomic evidence of infective endocarditis.

¶ Patient was stated to have "had acute rheumatic fever at age ten years."

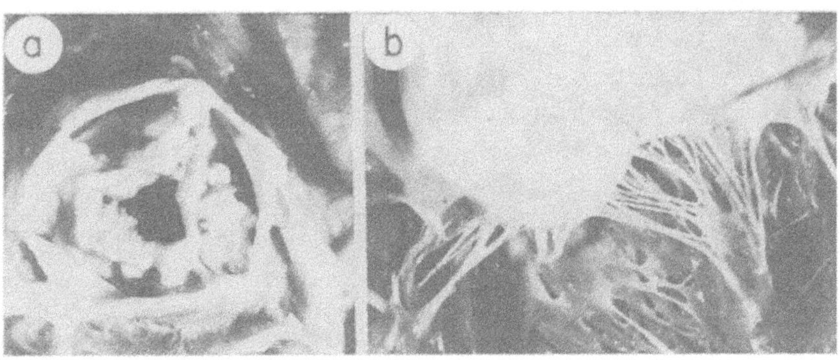

Fig. 1. *Aortic valve from above (a) and opened mitral valve (b) in a forty-one year old man (A66-136) with a positive history of acute rheumatic fever and severe aortic stenosis and regurgitation. The aortic valve is three-cuspid but each of the three commissures is partially fused, producing a central triangular shaped orifice. The two mitral leaflets are diffusely thickened but the chordae tendineae are normal. Thus, this case is in group Ic (Table I).*

TABLE III Valve Structure in Anatomically Isolated Aortic Valvular Disease. Summary of 163 Autopsy Patients Over Age Fourteen

Group	Functional Lesion	No. Patients	Unicuspid	Bicuspid	Tricuspid	Structure Uncertain	Per Cent Congenitally Malformed
1a	AS with or without AR	105	13	54	32*	6	64†
1b	Pure AR	34	0	9‡	25	0	26.5
1c	Clinically AS or AR but thickened mitral leaflets and normal chordae tendineae	24	0	4§	20#	0	17
	Totals	163	13	67	77	. . .	49

* In three patients the cusps were of unequal size, and one of them also had a congenitally bicuspid pulmonic valve.
† This percentage rises to 72 per cent if the "uncertain" category is either included in or excluded from the congenitally malformed group and if the three patients with unequal sized three-cuspid aortic valves are included in the congenitally malformed group.
‡ In seven of the nine patients infective endocarditis caused the valve to be incompetent.
§ In two patients the valvular orifice was severely stenotic, and in two it was only mildly stenotic (18 and 24 mm Hg peak systolic pressure gradients, respectively) but severely incompetent.
\# In fourteen patients the valve orifice was severely stenotic, in one patient mildly stenotic and severely incompetent, and in five subjects purely incompetent.

AS with or without AR, thirteen had congenitally unicuspid unicommissural aortic valves [9,10] (Fig. 2), fifty-four had congenitally bicuspid valves [11] (Fig. 3), thirty-two had three-cuspid valves (Fig. 4), and in six the valves were so deformed, scarred and calcified that the structure was not discernible. Thus, 64 per cent had congenitally malformed valves. It is likely that the six patients in whom the valve structure was uncertain also had congenitally malformed valves (either bicuspid or unicommissural) since tricuspid aortic valves are relatively easily delineated. In three of the thirty-two patients with tricuspid aortic valves the cusps were clearly unequal in size. Thus, if the "structure-uncertain" group (Table III) and the three subjects with unequal sized three-cuspid valves were included with the sixty-seven patients with congenitally unicommissural or bicuspid valves, the number of patients with congenitally malformed valves rises to seventy-six (72 per cent). Of the thirty-four patients with pure AR, nine (26.5 per cent) had malformed valves, and each was congenitally bicuspid.

In each of the 400 patients studied at least one section from the wall of each cardiac chamber was examined histologically. An average of seven histologic sections of heart were studied in each patient; Aschoff bodies were found in twelve patients. In only five of the twelve patients, however, were Aschoff bodies plentiful and unequivocal; Aschoff bodies were rare and equivocal in the other seven. None was found in the 163 patients with anatomically isolated aortic valve disease. All twelve patients had anatomic involvement of the mitral valve, eleven also had aortic valve involvement, and five also had tricuspid valve involvement.

Histologic sections of the walls of the right and left atria were examined in all patients. Some myocardial fiber degeneration or atrophy with or without interstitial myocardial fibrosis was observed in the sections of left atrial walls and often also of right atrial wall in nearly all patients with anatomic mitral valvular disease (groups II through V) (Fig. 5). In contrast, myocardial fiber degeneration or interstitial fibrosis was nearly always absent in sections of left and right atrial walls in the patients with anatomically isolated aortic valvular disease. In both groups, however, the myocardial fibers of the atrial walls and the smooth muscle fibers of

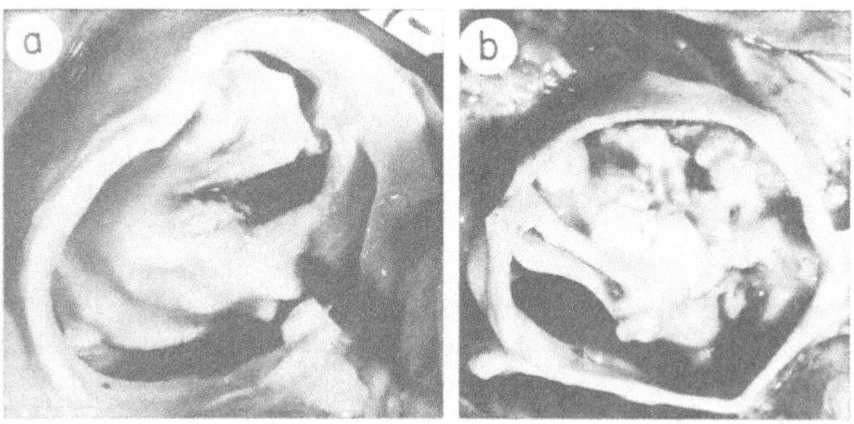

Fig. 2. *Congenitally unicuspid, unicommissural aortic valves from above in two men (A57-59 and A68-109), aged twenty-eight (a) and aged forty-eight years (b). Congenitally unicommissural aortic valves are always stenotic.*

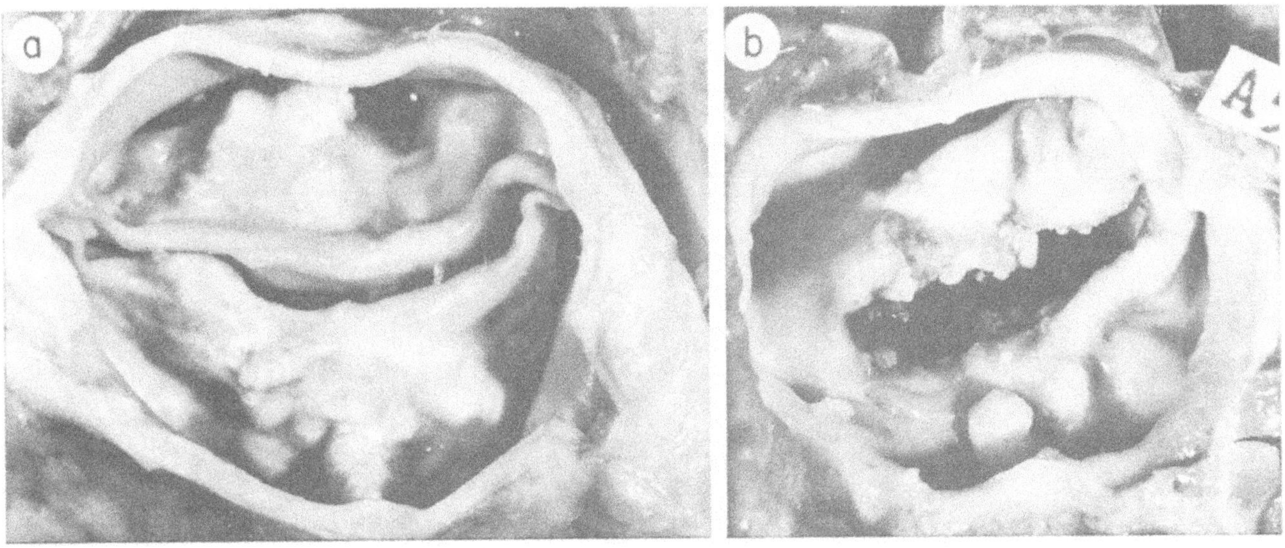

Fig. 3. *Congenitally bicuspid aortic valves in two men (A64-155 and A58-219), aged sixty-one (a) and thirty-seven years (b), respectively. Each is severely stenotic.*

the left atrial endocardium were nearly always hypertrophied.

COMMENTS

These findings in 400 autopsy patients with functionally severe valvular cardiac disease indicate that anatomically isolated aortic valvular disease is nonrheumatic in etiology. Four factors allow this conclusion: (1) the low incidence (6 per cent) of a history of ARF or chorea in the subjects with anatomically isolated aortic valvular disease (groups Ia and Ib, Table I) compared to the high incidence (68 per cent) of a positive history in the patients with anatomic mitral valvular disease with or without involvement of other cardiac valves; (2) the absence of Aschoff bodies in any of the 163 patients with anatomically isolated aortic valvular disease compared to the presence of the pathognomonic bodies in twelve of 235 patients (5 per cent) with mitral valvular disease; (3) the absence of interstitial fibrosis and myocardial fiber degeneration in the left atrial walls of patients with anatomically isolated aortic valvular disease compared to the nearly universal presence of these lesions in patients with mitral valvular disease; (4) the high incidence (72 per cent) of congenitally malformed valves in the patients with anatomically isolated aortic valvular disease causing stenosis compared to a zero incidence in the patients with anatomically isolated mitral valvular disease causing stenosis.

Although a similar incidence has been reported [12–15] in patients with isolated aortic valvular disease and in patients with mitral valvular disease with and without other valvular involvement, positive histories of ARF or chorea have been found by most observers infrequently in patients with isolated aortic valvular disease or at least far less frequently than in subjects with mitral or multivalvular disease. Of forty-two autopsy patients with "calcareous aortic valvular disease" described by Margolis and associates [16], three (7 per cent) had a history of ARF or chorea. Nineteen of seventy-three autopsy patients (26 per cent) with isolated aortic stenosis and thirty-seven of fifty autopsy patients (74 per cent) with combined mitral and aortic stenosis reported by McGinn and White [17] had a posi-

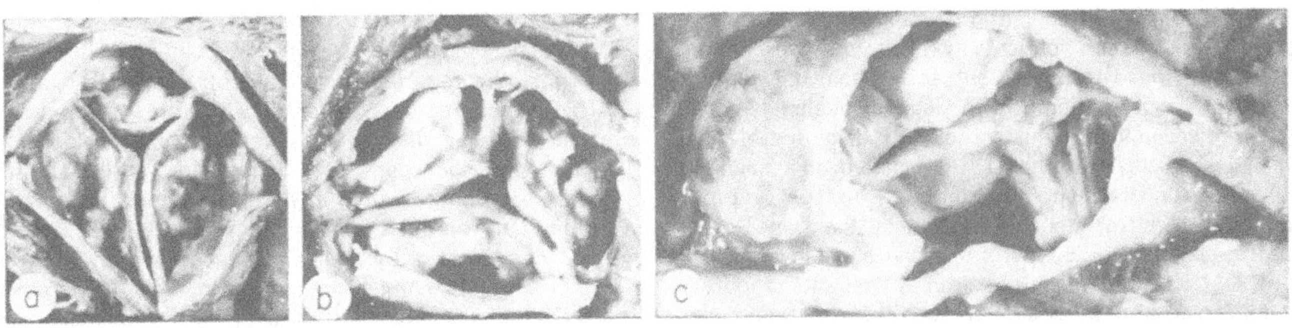

Fig. 4. *Heavily calcified, stenotic tricuspid aortic valves seen from above, in three patients. The mitral valves in each were normal except for focal aging changes. a, the three cusps are of unequal size in this eighty year old man. b, the three cusps are of similar size in this eighty-five year old man. c, one of the three commissures is completely fused in the aortic valve of this fifty-two year old man. The peak systolic pressure gradient across this valve was 85 mm Hg and the calculated valve area was 0.35 cu cm.*

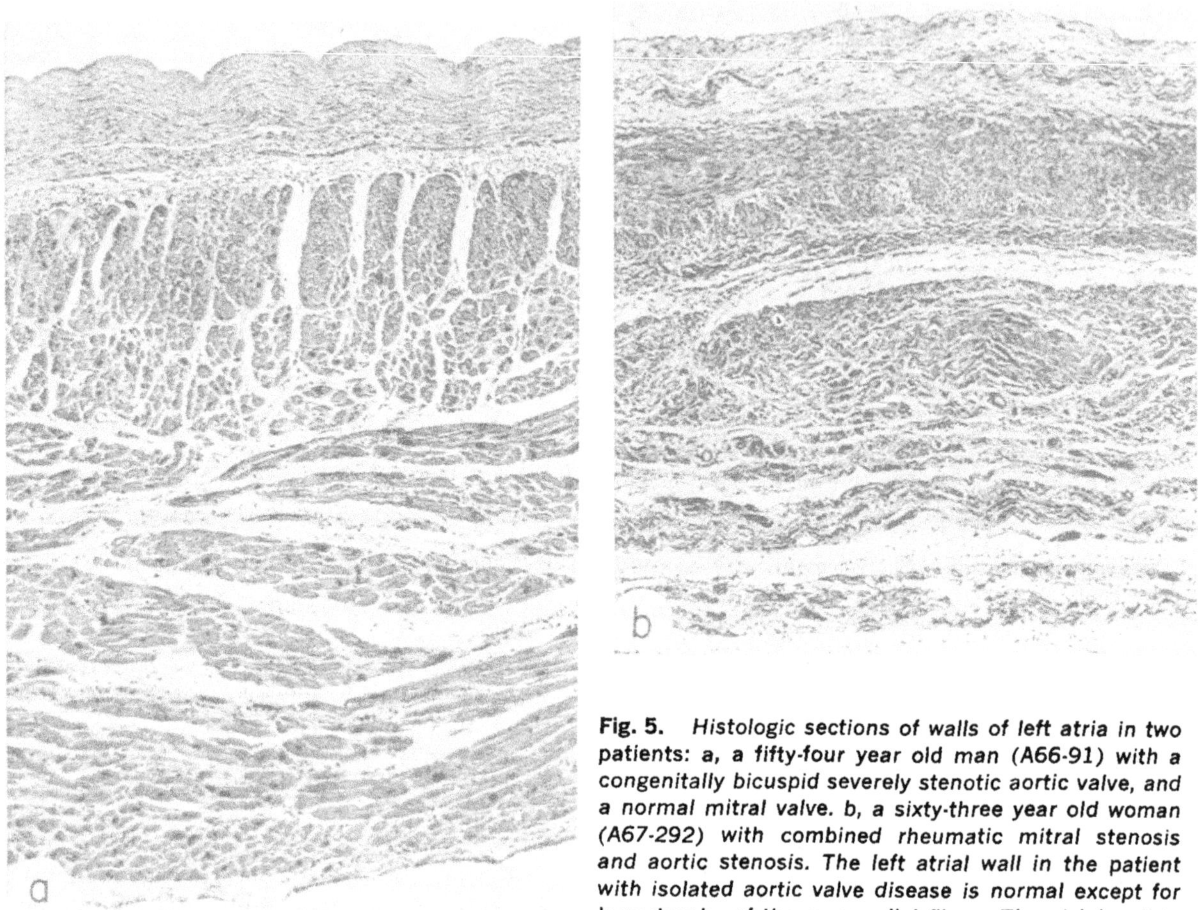

Fig. 5. *Histologic sections of walls of left atria in two patients: a, a fifty-four year old man (A66-91) with a congenitally bicuspid severely stenotic aortic valve, and a normal mitral valve. b, a sixty-three year old woman (A67-292) with combined rheumatic mitral stenosis and aortic stenosis. The left atrial wall in the patient with isolated aortic valve disease is normal except for hypertrophy of the myocardial fibers. The atrial wall in the patient with combined mitral and aortic valve disease contains severely degenerated myocardial fibers and extensive interstitial and replacement myocardial fibrosis. Hematoxylin and eosin stains; original magnification × 55 (a) and × 60 (b).*

tive history of ARF. Of 200 autopsy patients with "the calcified nodular deformity of the aortic valve" studied by Clawson and associates [18] seventy (35 per cent) had a positive history of ARF but eighty-nine of the 200 patients had associated mitral valvular disease. Of 106 autopsy patients with calcified aortic valves studied by Dry and Willius [19], sixteen (15 per cent) had a history of ARF; thirty-two of the 106 patients, however, had associated mitral valvular disease, and fifteen of the sixteen patients with a positive history were among these thirty-two subjects. Thus, only one of the seventy-four patients with isolated calcific aortic valvular disease had a history of ARF, and in this patient it is not clear whether it was isolated or associated with mitral involvement. In contrast, of 106 autopsy patients with mitral stenosis studied by the same investigators, sixty-seven (63 per cent) had a positive history of ARF. None of the nine autopsy patients reported by Cohen et al. [20], five of twenty-two autopsy patients (23 per cent) studied by Reich [21], twenty-one of 100 autopsy patients (21 per cent) studied by Horan and Barnes [22] and thirteen of forty-nine autopsy patients (27 per cent) studied by Anderson and associates [23] with calcific aortic "stenosis" had a positive history of ARF or chorea. Among 200 autopsy patients with "calcific disease of the aortic valve" studied by Karsner and Koletsky [24] thirty-five (18 per cent) had a positive history of migratory polyarthritis or chorea. Of the 109 patients with isolated aortic valvular disease, however, only three (2.8 per cent) had a history of ARF or chorea, whereas thirty-two of ninety-one patients (35 per cent) with multivalvular disease (aortic plus mitral with or without involvement of the tricuspid or pulmonic valve) had a positive history.

Thus, the reported incidences of a positive history of ARF or chorea in patients with presumed isolated aortic valvular disease has varied from possibly zero [19] to 67 per cent [15]. The wide spread between these percentages probably results from lack of discrimination between isolated aortic valve disease and that complicated by mitral disease. Willius and Dry [19], and later Anderson and associates [23], emphasized that separating patients with isolated aortic valve disease from those with mitral or multivalvular involvement could lead to missing a rheumatic etiology in the former group. As early as 1909, however, Allbutt [25] stated: "to understand [cardiac valvular] stenosis we must study it in its unmixed form." Kumpe and

Bean [15] in 1948 again emphasized this point. Another cause of disagreement in reported incidences of a positive history of ARF or chorea in patients with various cardiac valvular diseases is that the anatomic data in nearly all previous studies has been obtained by review of autopsy protocols and not by re-examination of hearts by an investigator seeking preplanned specific information. The latter method, however, is the only reliable one. The heart of each of the 400 patients included in the present study was examined by me on at least two occasions, the second without knowledge of how the heart had been classified on the initial examination.

The relatively low incidences of a positive history of ARF or chorea in patients with anatomically isolated aortic valvular disease have not deterred most investigators from attributing this valvular lesion to a rheumatic etiology. Their reasoning has been as follows: The episodes of ARF in the patients with isolated aortic disease were so **mild** or **atypical** that their true nature went unrecognized. Since the attack of ARF in them was mild, the mitral value and myocardium escaped with minimal or no injury. Or, since the patients with isolated aortic valvular disease are **older** than the subjects with mitral disease, the episode of ARF was forgotten or occurred in an era when ARF was not well recognized.

Although some investigators recorded a similar incidence of histories of ARF or chorea in patients with apparently isolated aortic valvular disease and in those with isolated mitral disease, a striking difference in **sex** and **age** among those two groups was universally recognized. Cabot [12] explained the age difference by reasoning that the "heart and circulatory system accommodates itself more easily to a pure aortic lesion than to any of the other valve lesions or combinations of such," and as a result the patients live into old age. Cabot found no explanation for the sex difference but Willius and Dry [26] reasoned that "although the incidence of rheumatic fever is about the same in the two sexes, women apparently do not have the same **relative immunity** to serious and widespread cardiac involvement by the disease as men."

Koletsky [27] and others have listed several gross and histologic "unequivocal stigmas of rheumatic heart disease," but none of them is specific except the Aschoff body. It is present in the heart of two-thirds of the patients who die of ARF or chorea [28]. Of 190 autopsy patients with ARF or chorea collected by Clawson by combining studies of several investigators, 127 (67 per cent) had Aschoff bodies in their heart [28]. Aschoff bodies also are reported to occur frequently in operatively excised atrial appendages, the incidence ranging from 18 to 74 per cent (average 33 per cent) in 1,180 patients tabulated by Tedeschi, Wagner and Pani [29]. In contrast, the incidence of Aschoff bodies in autopsy patients with rheumatic heart disease is relatively low. Clawson [18] found myocardial Aschoff nodules in seven of fifty-four patients (13 per cent) with isolated calcareous aortic "stenosis," and in nine of sixty-eight autopsy patients (13 per cent) in whom "other" valves were involved. Hall and Ichioka [14] reported Aschoff bodies in nine of nineteen autopsy patients (47 per cent) with isolated aortic valvular disease, and in seven of twelve autopsy patients (58 per cent) with mitral plus aortic valvular disease. It is apparent, however, that they used loose histologic criteria for diagnosing Aschoff bodies. Interestingly, eight of their nineteen patients with isolated aortic valvular disease had bicuspid valves, whereas none of their twelve patients with combined valvular disease had bicuspid valves. Karsner and Koletsky [24] reported myocardial Aschoff bodies in only three of 119 autopsy patients (2.5 per cent) with isolated "calcific disease of the aortic valve" and in seventeen of ninety-one autopsy patients (19 per cent) with mitral and aortic disease with or without associated tricuspid or pulmonic valvular involvement. These investigators explained the frequent absence of cardiac Aschoff bodies in their patients "by the fact that the specimens all represent chronic or healed stages of disease." In the present study no Aschoff bodies were found in the hearts of the 163 patients with isolated aortic valvular disease, whereas they were observed in twelve of the 235 patients (5 per cent) with mitral valvular disease with or without involvement of other cardiac valves. The criteria I use for defining an Aschoff body are those initially described by Aschoff and summarized by Saphir [30].

Study of the walls of the atria, particularly the left one, is useful in arriving at an etiologic diagnosis in patients with valvular cardiac disease. Gross [31] in 1935 described histologic abnormalities in the left atrial walls in each of eighty-seven patients with rheumatic disease: sixty-seven had active rheumatic fever with Aschoff bodies, and twenty had chronic valvular scarring and no Aschoff bodies. The atrial histologic changes observed other than Aschoff bodies included small lymphocytic infiltrates, distorted, concentrated and reduplicated elastica, increased and irregular smooth muscle in the endocardium and thickened, fibrotic and abnormally vascularized subendocardium; marked fiber hypertrophy, lymphocytic infiltrates and fibrosis in the myocardium; and inflammation and/or fibrosis in the pericardium. Gross considered these atrial changes to be evidence of rheumatic disease, and a year later he and Sohval [32] reported their presence in thirteen autopsy patients with multivalvular heart disease and their absence in nineteen patients with isolated calcific sclerosis of the aortic valve. In the present study a difference also was noted in the histologic, and often also in the gross appearance of the left atrial walls in patients with anatomically isolated aortic valvular stenosis or regurgitation or both and in patients with isolated mitral or combined mitral and aortic disease. The histologic changes in the left atrial wall appear to result at least in part from rheumatic involvement of the wall itself and not entirely from altered left atrial hemodynamics produced by the mitral valve lesion. In subjects with anatomic (rheumatic) involvement of both mitral and aortic valves causing dysfunction of only the aortic valve, these histologic changes occur. Furthermore, in subjects with severe mitral regurgitation secondary to ruptured chordae tendineae in otherwise normal valves, i.e., nonrheumatic etiology, no changes have been noted in the left atria histologically other than hypertrophy of the myocardial fibers [4]. Virtually none of the 163 patients with anatomically isolated aortic valvular disease had degeneration or distortion of myocardial fibers, interstitial myocardial fibrosis or abnormal fibrous thickening of the endocardium or subendocardium. In contrast, these lesions were observed histologically in the sections of atria of nearly all subjects studied with isolated rheumatic mitral or combined mitral and aortic disease.

The factor most against a rheumatic etiology of anatomically isolated aortic valvular disease causing stenosis is the high incidence of congenital malformations of this valve. In the present study fifty-four of the 105 patients with isolated aortic stenosis with or without regurgitation had congenitally bicuspid valves [11], thirteen had congenitally unicommissural unicuspid valves, six had probable congenitally malformed valves, and thirty-two had three-cuspid valves. Nine of the thirty-four patients with pure aortic regurgitation had congenitally bicuspid valves, and in seven the regurgitation was secondary to infective endocarditis partially destroying one or both of its cusps. Although it has been appreciated for nearly ninety years that congenitally bicuspid aortic valves are frequently the site of infective endocarditis, only during the past few years has it become widely recognized that congenitally bicuspid aortic valves become stenotic [11,33–38]. Paget [39], however, in 1844 had suggested that bicuspid aortic valves, because of their defective development, peculiar shape and imperfect tissue were "very liable to disease," and Peacock [40] fourteen years later had pointed out that bicuspid aortic valves could become thick, rigid, ossified, obstructed and finally incompetent. Although he emphasized their frequency and their liability to subacute infective endocarditis, Osler apparently was unaware that a congenitally bicuspid aortic valve could become the site of stenosis [41]. Likewise, Lewis and Grant [42], who in 1923 reviewed all cases of congenitally bicuspid aortic valves reported up to that time and established histologic criteria for distinguishing between congenital and acquired aortic valve deformities, were apparently unaware that this malformed valve could become stenotic although they mentioned "calcific sclerosis" in one of their eleven personally studied cases. Of twenty-eight autopsy patients with calcific aortic stenosis described by Cabot [12] in 1926, no mention is made of the possibility of congenital malformation of this valve although one of two valves illustrated (Fig. 39, p. 224) almost surely is congenitally bicuspid. Christian [13] in 1931 did not consider the possibility of a congenital origin of aortic stenosis. Libman [43], however, the same year stated that calcareous deposits may be superimposed on a congenitally bicuspid aortic valve. McGinn and White [17] in 1934 mentioned congenitally bicuspid aortic valves in four of 123 autopsy patients with aortic stenosis (fifty also had mitral stenosis), but in none of the 123 patients did they consider the stenosis to be of congenital origin. Four of their fifty patients (8 per cent) with combined mitral and aortic disease and twenty-six of seventy-three patients (36 per cent) with presumably isolated aortic stenosis, however, had "fusion of two aortic cusps giving a bicuspid arrangement." One of nine autopsy patients described by Cohen and associates [20] and nine of nineteen autopsy subjects with isolated calcific aortic stenosis reported by Hall and Ichioka [14] had bicuspid aortic valves. Twenty-three of the 200 patients with calcareous disease of the aortic valve reported by Karsner and Koletsky [24] in 1947 had bicuspid aortic valves. The latter investigators considered only two of the twenty-three to be congenitally malformed. This view is debatable. The aortic valve illustrated in their Figure 7 is labeled "acquired bicuspid aortic valve with stenosis" but to me it is a classic congenitally bicuspid valve.

Nearly one third of the 105 patients with anatomically isolated aortic stenosis had three-cuspid aortic valves. The cause of the valvular stenosis in them is uncertain but probably variable. Congenital malformation may be possible in a few. In at least three of the thirty-two patients with isolated aortic stenosis and three-cuspid valves, the circumferential distances between the lateral attachments of the cusps were variable. In the other twenty-nine patients the circumferential distances between the lateral cuspal attachments appeared similar. The cusps, however, may vary in size even though the distances, measured along the aortic root at the most cephalad margins of the commissures between the lateral attachments, are identical. One or more cusps may be elongated. In this case the distances along the cuspal margins vary. When the cusps are fibrotic and calcified, however, it is usually difficult to appreciate inequality of cuspal size. Unequal sized cusps are common in the pulmonic valve but cause no cuspal scarring or apparent hemodynamic consequence in this low pressure circuit. But when aortic valve cusps are of unequal size it is possible that the usual wear and tear on these cusps in this high pressure circuit may be exaggerated. Congenitally unequally sized cusps almost certainly do not contact one another properly during ventricular diastole and the prolonged abnormal contact or trauma in the systemic circulation may lead to fibrous thickening of the cusps and eventually to calcification and valvular stenosis.

Calcific deposits on aortic valve cusps are extremely common in elderly persons. Although these aortic valve calcific deposits may produce murmurs characteristic of "aortic stenosis," true obstruction is usually not present as judged by the lack of left ventricular hypertrophy either at autopsy or on the electrocardiogram. Of the 105 patients described with isolated aortic stenosis (group Ia), five were over seventy years of age; three had tricuspid and two had bicuspid aortic valves. Thus, this degenerative process is probably not the explanation for the stenosis in the patients with three-cuspid aortic valves described here.

REFERENCES

1. Roberts WC, Sjoerdsma A: The cardiac disease associated with the carcinoid syndrome (carcinoid heart disease). Amer J Med 36: 5, 1964.
2. Roberts WC, Mason DT, Wright LD Jr: The nondistensible right atrium of carcinoid disease of the heart. Amer J Clin Path 44: 627, 1965.
3. Cohen LS, Roberts WC: The clinical and pathologic spectrum of mitral regurgitation caused by malformation of the papillary muscles of fibrosis of the left ventricular free wall. Circulation 37, 38 (supp): VI-57, 1968.
4. Roberts WC, Braunwald E, Morrow AG: Acute severe mitral regurgitation secondary to ruptured chordae tendineae. Clinical, hemodynamic, and pathologic considerations. Circulation 33: 58, 1966.
5. Read RC, Thal AP, Wendt VE: Symptomatic valvular myxomatous transformation (the floppy valve syndrome). A possible forme fruste of the Marfan syndrome. Circulation 32: 897, 1965.
6. Roberts WC, Ross RC, Eggleston JC, Massumi RA: Chronic mitral regurgitation of unresolved etiology in the elderly. A clinico-pathologic study of two patients. Johns Hopkins Med J 122: 26, 1968.
7. Carpenter DF, Golden A, Roberts WC: Quadrivalvular rheumatoid heart disease associated with left bundle branch block. Amer J Med 43: 922, 1967.
8. Glancy DL, Marcus FI, Cuadra M, Ewy GA, Roberts WC: Isolated organic tricuspid valvular regurgitation: causes and consequences. Amer J Med 46: 989, 1969.
9. Edwards JE: Pathologic aspects of cardiac valvular insufficiencies. Arch Surg 77: 634, 1958.
10. Roberts WC, Morrow AG: Congenital aortic stenosis produced by a unicommissural valve. Brit Heart J 27: 505, 1965.
11. Roberts WC: The congenitally bicuspid aortic valve. A study of 85 autopsy patients. Amer J Cardiol (in press).
12. Cabot RC: Facts on Heart Disease, Philadelphia, W. B. Saunders Company, 1926, p 205.
13. Christian HA: Aortic stenosis with calcification of the cusps. JAMA 97: 158, 1931.
14. Hall EM, Ichioka T: Etiology of calcified nodular aortic stenosis. Amer J Path 16: 761, 1940.
15. Kumpe CW, Bean WB: Aortic stenosis: a study of the clinical and pathologic aspects of 107 proved cases. Medicine 27: 139, 1948.
16. Margolis HM, Ziellessen FO, Barnes AR: Calcareous aortic valvular disease. Amer Heart J 6: 349, 1931.
17. McGinn S, White PD: Clinical observations on aortic stenosis. Amer J Med Sci 188: 1, 1934.
18. Clawson BJ, Noble JF, Lufkin NH: The calcified nodular deformity of the aortic valve. Amer Heart J 15: 58, 1938.
19. Dry TJ, Willius FA: Calcareous disease of the aortic valve. A study of two hundred twenty-eight cases. Amer Heart J 17: 138, 1939.
20. Cohen L, Gray I, Nash PI, Fink H: Calcareous aortic stenosis; report of nine cases with autopsy findings. Ann Intern Med 13: 2091, 1940.
21. Reich NE: Calcific aortic valve stenosis: a clinico-pathologic correlation of 22 cases. Ann Intern Med 22: 234, 1945.
22. Horan MJ, Barnes AR: Calcareous aortic stenosis and coronary artery disease. Amer J Med Sci 215: 451, 1948.
23. Anderson MW, Kelsey JR Jr, Edwards JE: Clinical and pathological considerations in cases of calcific aortic stenosis. JAMA 149: 9, 1952.
24. Karsner HT, Koletsky S: Calcific Disease of the Aortic Valve, Philadelphia, J. B. Lippincott Company, 1947.
25. Allbutt C: Diseases of the aortic area of the heart, A System of Medicine by Many Writers, vol 6. Diseases of the Heart and Blood Vessels. (Allbutt C, Rolleston HD, eds) London, MacMillan & Company, Ltd., 1909, p 444.
26. Willius FA, Dry TJ: Cardiac clinics. LVIII. A talk on the etiology of calcareous stenosis of the aortic valve. Proc Staff Meet Mayo Clinic 14: 245, 1939.
27. Koletsky S: Bicuspid aortic valves and endocarditis. Amer Heart J 26: 343, 1943.
28. Clawson BJ: The Aschoff nodule. Arch Path 8: 664, 1929.
29. Tedeschi CG, Wagner BM, Pani KC: Studies in rheumatic fever. I. The clinical significance of the Aschoff body based on morphologic observations. Arch Path 60: 408, 1955.
30. Saphir O: The Aschoff nodule. Amer J Clin Path 31: 534, 1959.
31. Gross L: Lesions of the left auricle in rheumatic fever. Amer J Path 11: 711, 1935.
32. Sohval AR, Gross L: Calcific sclerosis of the aortic valve (Mönckeberg type). Arch Path 22: 477, 1936.
33. Campbell M, Kauntze R: Congenital aortic valvular stenosis. Brit Heart J 15: 179, 1953.
34. Smith DE, Matthews MB: Aortic valvular stenosis with coarctation of the aorta. With special reference to the development of aortic stenosis upon congenital bicuspid valves. Brit Heart J 17: 198, 1955.
35. Bacon APC, Matthews MB: Congenital bicuspid aortic valves and the aetiology of isolated aortic valvular stenosis. Quart J Med 28 (n.s.): 545, 1959.
36. Edwards JE: Calcific aortic stenosis: pathologic features. Proc Staff Meet Mayo Clinic 36: 444, 1961.
37. Morrow AG, Goldblatt A, Braunwald E: Congenital aortic stenosis. II. Surgical treatment and results of operation. Circulation 37: 450, 1963.
38. Campbell M: Calcific aortic stenosis and congenital bicuspid aortic valves. Brit Heart J 30: 606, 1968.
39. Paget J: On obstructions of the branches of the pulmonary artery. Trans Royal Med Chir Soc, London 27: 162, 1844.
40. Peacock TB: On Malformations of the Human Heart, 2nd ed, London, J Churchill & Sons, 1866.
41. Osler W: The bicuspid condition of the aortic valves. Trans Ass Amer Physicians 2: 185, 1886.
42. Lewis T, Grant RT: Observations relating to subacute infective endocarditis. Heart 10: 21, 1923.
43. Libman E: Discussion of paper by Christian, H. A. Trans Ass Amer Physicians 46: 103, 1931.

Severe Valvular Aortic Stenosis in Patients Over 65 Years of Age

A Clinicopathologic Study

WILLIAM C. ROBERTS, MD, FACC
JOSEPH K. PERLOFF, MD, FACC
THOMAS COSTANTINO, MD

Bethesda, Maryland
Washington, D. C.

Clinical and anatomic data are presented in 21 autopsy cases of patients over 65 years of age with severe valvular aortic stenosis. Attention is called to the unusual nature of the valvular lesion in the elderly compared to its manifestations in younger adults. The degree of aortic stenosis even in the very elderly may be extreme. The aortic valve in 2 patients was congenitally bicuspid, and in 19, tricuspid. The latter valves usually were characterized by the uniform distribution of nodular calcific deposits on the aortic aspects of the cusps and by the lack or near lack of commissural fusion. Calcification of the mitral annulus occurred in 16 of the 21 patients. Clinically, aortic stenosis in the elderly is characterized by several features that are either absent or more prominent than in younger subjects with this valvular lesion: The systemic arterial pulse pressure may be increased due to systolic hypertension; a harsh right basal systolic murmur may be relatively inconspicuous, whereas a pure musical systolic murmur may be prominent at the apex; a coexisting apical systolic murmur of mitral regurgitation may be related to mitral annular calcification and not to left ventricular failure; and systemic systolic hypertension can result in a comparatively small pressure gradient despite severe left ventricular outflow obstruction.

It has long been appreciated that aortic systolic murmurs and aortic valvular calcific deposits are common in older people. Although these murmurs in older patients may be prominent, they are usually not considered indicative of significant aortic valvular obstruction.[1] Indeed, Hancock et al.[2] referred to this condition as "aortic stenosis of no physiologic significance." It is less well known that the same pathologic process can result in extensive valvular calcification and severe aortic stenosis.[3] The true incidence of valvular aortic stenosis in elderly persons is unknown for several reasons. The lesion may be missed since its clinical signs are not necessarily those occurring in younger individuals with valvular aortic stenosis; relatively few hemodynamic studies have been performed; and mild degrees of obstruction may be overlooked at necropsy. During the past 4 years we have assembled clinical and necropsy information on 21 patients over 65 years of age with severe valvular aortic stenosis. Five underwent left heart catheterization. This report summarizes clinical, hemodynamic and autopsy observations in these patients and provides evidence that the valvular lesion in the elderly is unique, often severe, and amenable to operative repair.

Observations in Patients Studied

Clinical and autopsy data from the 21 patients are summarized in Table I. Their ages ranged from 66 to 90 years (average 78); 12

From the Section of Pathology, National Heart and Lung Institute, National Institutes of Health, Bethesda, Md., and the Department of Medicine, Georgetown University School of Medicine, Division of Cardiology, Georgetown University Hospital, Washington, D. C. This study was supported in part by U. S. Public Health Service Research Career Program Award HE 14009 and the Eric T. Paglin Memorial Fund for Cardiovascular Teaching and Research. Manuscript received April 27, 1970, accepted July 28, 1970.

Address for reprints: William C. Roberts, MD, Section of Pathology, National Heart and Lung Institute, National Institutes of Health, Bethesda, Md. 20014.

TABLE I
Valvular Aortic Stenosis in Patients More than 65 Years of Age

Case no.	Age (yr) & Sex	Chronic CHF	Angina Pectoris	Syncope	Murmurs: Basal Systolic	Murmurs: Apical Systolic	Murmurs: Basal Diastolic	AF by ECG	LVH by ECG	Aortic Stenosis Diagnosed During Life	Aortic Valve: no. of Cusps	Aortic Valve: Commissural Fusion	Mitral Valve Annular Calcium	Coronary Artery Calcium	Coronary Artery Luminal Narrowing (%)	Left Ventricle: Dilation	Left Ventricle: Scarring	Left Ventricle: Necrosis	Heart Weight (g)
1	79F	+	0	0	+	+	0	0	0	+	2	0	0	0	<25	+	+	0	700
2	75M	+	0	0	+	+	0	0	+	0	2	0	0	+	>75	+	+	0	600
3	69M	+	0	0	+	0	0	+	+	+	3	0	+	0	<25	0	+	0	510
4	70M	0	0	0	+	0	0	0	+	0	3	0	0	+	<50	+	0	0	480
5	80M	+	0	0	+	+	+	0	0	0	3	0	+	+	<50	+	0	0	660
6	89M	0	+	0	+	0	0	+	0	0	3	0	0	+	<50	0	0	0	440
7	85F	+	0	0	+	+	0	0	+	0	3	0	+	+	>75	+	+	+	...
8	80M	+	0	0	+	+	0	0	0	0	3	0	+	+	>75	+	+	?	400
9	66M	+	0	0	+	0	0	+	0	0	3	+	+	+	<50	+	+	0	800
10	70F	+	0	0	+	+	0	0	0	0	3	+	+	+	<50	+	+	0	550
11	76F	0	+	+	+	0	+	0	+	+	3	0	+	+	<25	0	+	0	480
12	82M	+	+	+	+	0	0	0	+	+	3	+	+	+	>75	+	+	0	450
13	71M	+	0	0	+	+	0	0	+	0	3	+	+	+	>75	+	+	+	650
14	75F	0	+	+	+	0	+	0	+	+	3	+	+	+	>75	0	+	...	390
15	90F	+	0	+	+	+	0	+	+	+	3	0	+	+	>75	+	0	+	550
16	83F	0	0	+	+	+	0	+	0	+	3	0	+	+	>75	0	0	+	380
17	80F	0	0	0	+	+	0	0	0	0	3	+	+	+	>50	0	+	+	390
18	81F	0	+	0	+	+	0	0	+	+	3	0	+	+	>75	0	0	0	400
19	74F	+	0	0	+	+	+	+	0	+	3	0	+	0	<25	+	0	0	530
20	76F	+	0	0	+	0	+	+	0	+	3	+	+	+	<25	+	0	0	480
21	73F	+	0	0	+	0	0	0	+	0	3	0	+	+	<50	+	0	0	530

AF = atrial fibrillation; CHF = congestive heart failure; LVH = left ventricular hypertrophy.

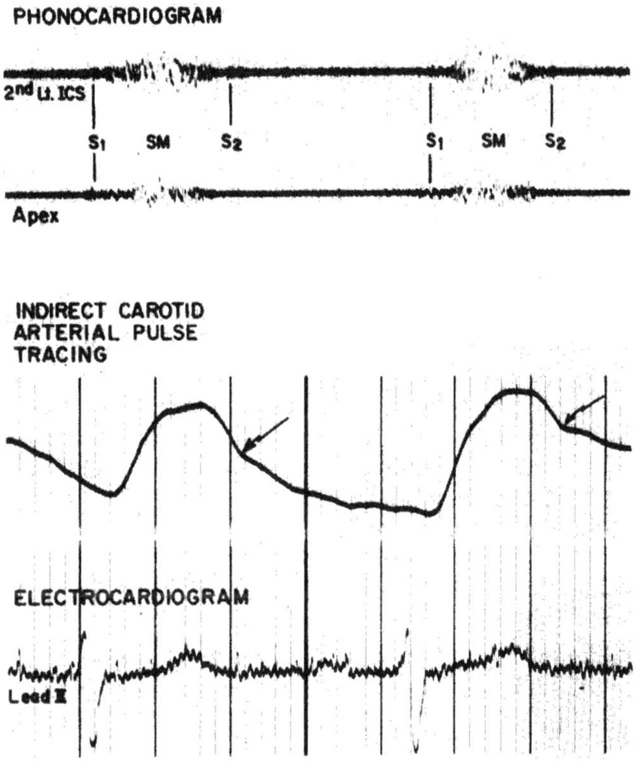

Figure 1. Case 16. Chest wall phonocardiogram with indirect carotid arterial pulse tracing and lead II of the electrocardiogram. A crescendo-decrescendo systolic murmur (SM) is equally well recorded at both base and apex. The indirect carotid arterial pulse tracing shows marked retardation of the rate of rise and slurred dicrotic notch (**arrow**).

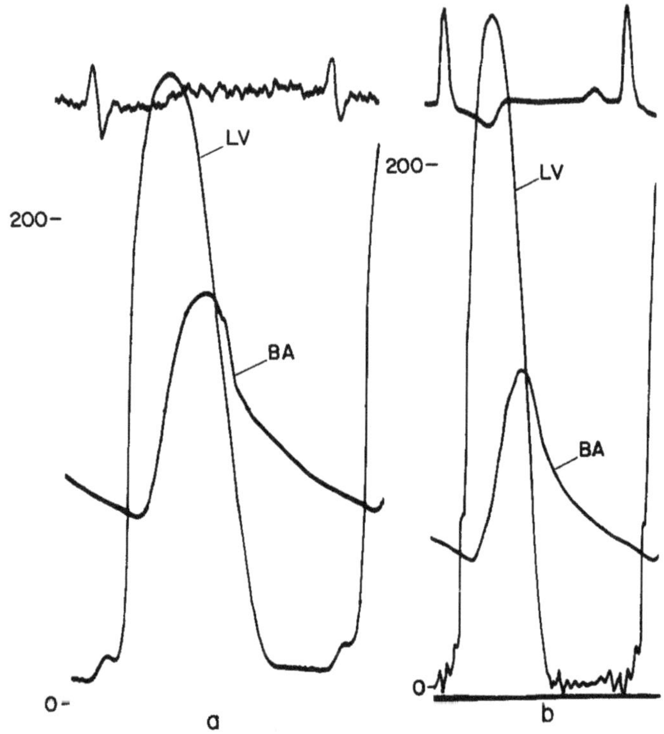

Figure 2. Simultaneous left ventricular (LV) and brachial arterial (BA) pressure tracings of 2 patients. **a,** Case 18, age 81 years. Although the LV systolic pressure is 265 mm Hg, the peak systolic pressure gradient across the aortic valve is only 93 mm Hg since the BA systolic pressure is elevated (172 mm Hg). **b,** Case 11, age 76 years. The LV systolic pressure in this patient is 256 mm Hg, slightly lower than that of Patient 18, but the peak systolic pressure gradient is much higher (160 mm Hg) since the BA systolic pressure is much lower (126 mm Hg).

were women and 9 were men. None had a history of rheumatic fever, chorea, brucellosis or infective endocarditis. All patients had evidence of cardiac dysfunction for various periods: 14 manifested chronic congestive cardiac failure, 5 angina pectoris, and 5 syncope. In addition, 3 patients had had myocardial infarcts, 4 had a history of systemic hypertension, and 3, mild diabetes mellitus.

Clinical findings: All patients had precordial systolic murmurs ranging from grade 2/6 to 4/6 (Fig. 1). Harsh midsystolic murmurs of varying intensity were uniformly present at the right base. In 11 patients high frequency, occasionally musical cooing, apical systolic murmurs of equal or greater intensity were present (Fig. 1). The apical murmurs were usually midsystolic but occasionally holosystolic. Five patients had high frequency early diastolic murmurs considered to represent aortic incompetence, minimal in 3, and moderate in 2.

TABLE II

Hemodynamic Findings in 5 Patients

Case no.	Pressures (mm Hg) RV	LV	BA	Gradient (mm Hg) LV-BA Peak Systolic	Mean	CO	CI	Aortic Valve Area (cm²)
11	30/8	256/12	126/55	130	102	2.0	1.4	0.2
14	...	280/8	120/50	160	...	2.2	1.7	0.2
16	23/4	180/4	115/40	65	55	3.6	...	0.5
18	48/9	265/25	172/78	93	59	...	...	...
19	...	205/20	135/44	70	55	1.8	1.1	0.3

BA = brachial artery; CI = cardiac index (liters/min per m²); CO = cardiac output (liters/min); LV = left ventricle; RV = right ventricle.

Chest roentgenograms showed evidence of left ventricular enlargement in 15 patients, but the heart was of normal size in the posteroanterior projection in 6 patients. Aortic valve calcific deposits were identified in 15 patients. Electrocardiograms showed left ventricular hypertrophy in 11 patients, atrial fibrillation in 7, complete left bundle branch block in 1, complete right bundle branch block in 1, and transient complete heart block in 3.

Catheterization of the left side of the heart was performed in 5 patients. The hemodynamic data are summarized in Table II, and a pressure tracing from 2 patients is shown in Figure 2.

Clinical diagnoses of aortic stenosis were made in 10 of the 21 patients; correct clinical diagnoses were achieved in only 3 of the first 10 patients studied.

An operation on the aortic valve was carried out in 3 patients. The 2 patients (Cases 11 and 19) with an aortic prosthesis (Hufnagel discoid type) survived 2 and 15 months, respectively, after operation; 1 patient died of infection at the site of the prosthesis, and the second, of aortic regurgitation secondary to a peribasilar leak. The third patient (Case 14) underwent aortic valve debridement but during this procedure 1 cusp was inadvertently perforated and she died 6 months later of severe, operatively induced aortic regurgitation.

The 18 patients unoperated on died of various causes: 5 of acute myocardial infarction; 7 of acute (2 patients) or progressive (5 patients) congestive cardiac failure; 4 of noncardiac conditions (gastric carcinoma in 2, complications of portal cirrhosis in 1, and immediately after operative resection of an abdominal aortic aneurysm in 1; each of these patients, however, had evidence of congestive cardiac failure); 1 died suddenly of un-

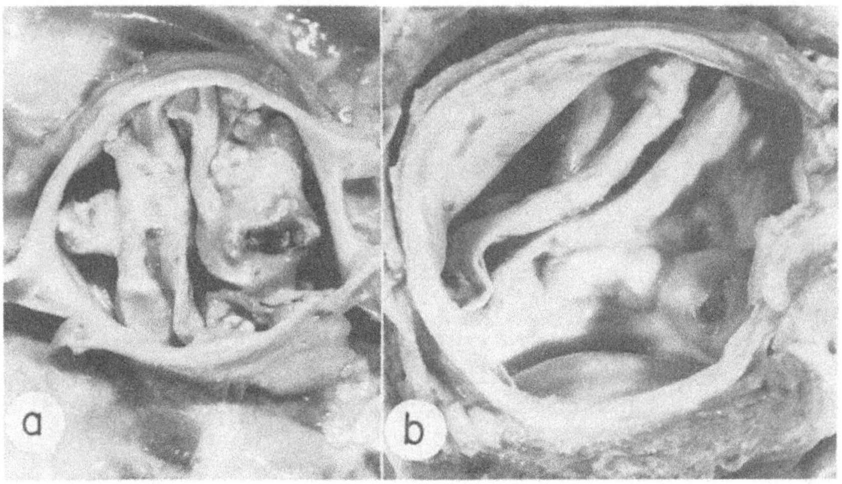

Figure 3. Congenitally bicuspid aortic valves in 2 patients. **a**, Case 1; **b**, Case 2. In both, the valves are heavily calcified and severely stenotic. In neither are the commissures fused. Calcified raphes (false commissures) are present in 1 cusp of each valve.

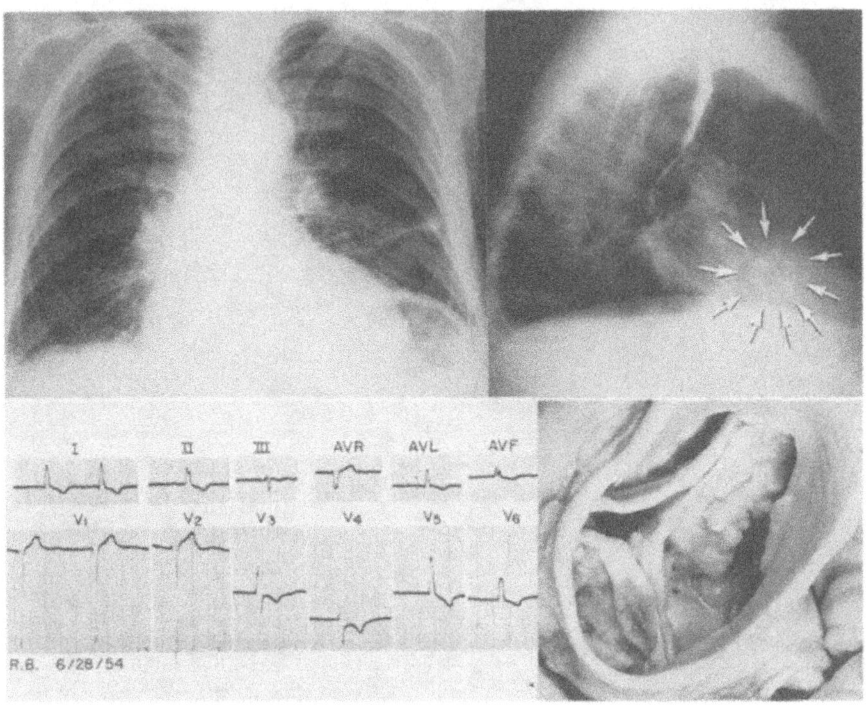

Figure 4. Case 3. Chest roentgenograms, electrocardiogram and aortic valve. The heart is enlarged on X-ray. On the lateral view a heavy ring of calcium (**arrows**) is present in the aortic valve. The electrocardiogram shows left ventricular hypertrophy with strain. Heavy deposits of calcium are present on the aortic aspects of each aortic valve cusp. None of the 3 aortic valve commissures is fused.

determined cause; and 1 died of cardiac tamponade shortly after cardiac catheterization performed by left ventricular puncture.

Autopsy findings: The left ventricular wall in all 21 patients was hypertrophied (greater than 1.5 cm thick). The left ventricular cavity was considered normal in size in 7 patients and mildly to moderately dilated in 14. The hearts weighed from 380 to 800 g (average 524). Two of the 3 patients whose hearts weighed less than 400 g had undergone cardiac catheterization; the peak left ventricular to systemic arterial systolic pressure gradient in 1 was 65 and in the second, 160 mm Hg. The aortic valves in all 21 patients (including the excised valves in 2 patients who had undergone aortic valve replacement) were severely stenotic,

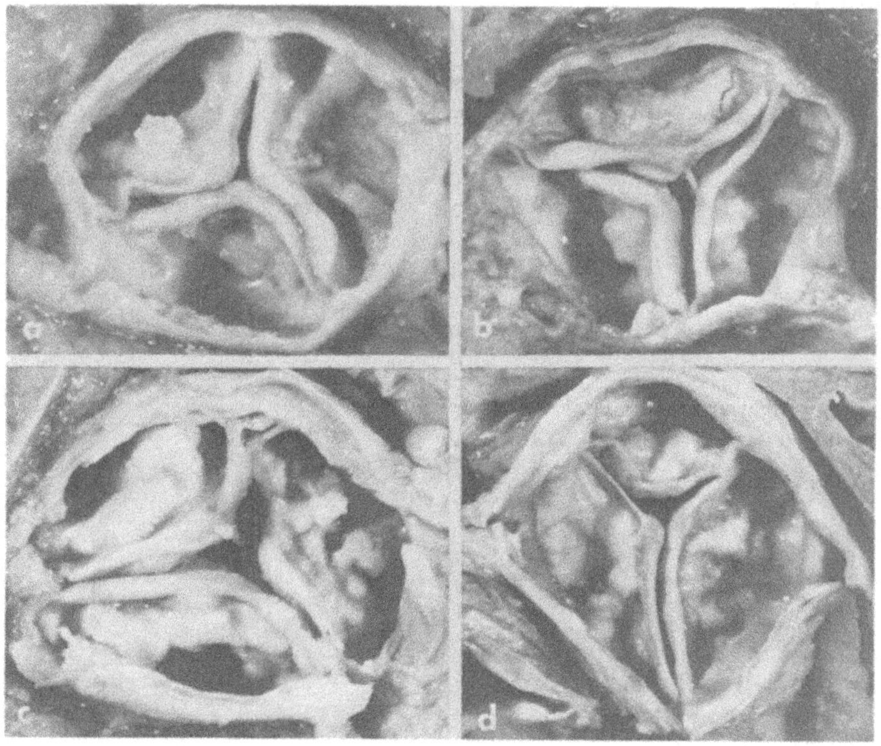

Figure 5. Aortic valves in 4 patients. **a,** Case 16; **b,** Case 18; **c,** Case 7; **d,** Case 8. One commissure in the valves shown in **c** and **d** is slightly fused. All other commissures are open. The cusps in **d** are of unequal size.

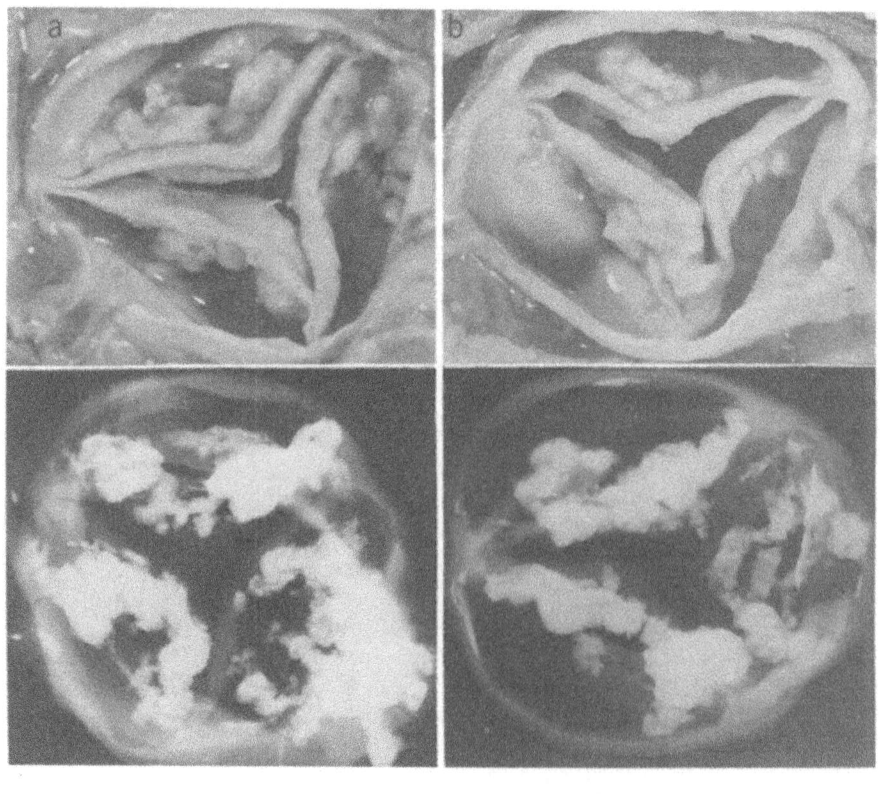

Figure 6. Aortic valves with radiographs below in 2 patients. **a,** Case 15; **b,** Case 21. The cusps of both valves are heavily calcified. One of the 3 commissures in **b** is fused.

and in 5 patients aortic regurgitation of mild degree also was present. In 2 patients the aortic valve was congenitally bicuspid (Fig. 3) and in the other 19 patients the valve was tricuspid (Fig. 4 to 10). No commissural fusion occurred in 12 of the 19 patients with tricuspid aortic valves or in the 2 patients with congenitally bicuspid valves; in 4 others the commissural fusion was minimal and involved only 1 of 3 commissures; and in 3 patients commissural fusion was significant, involving 1

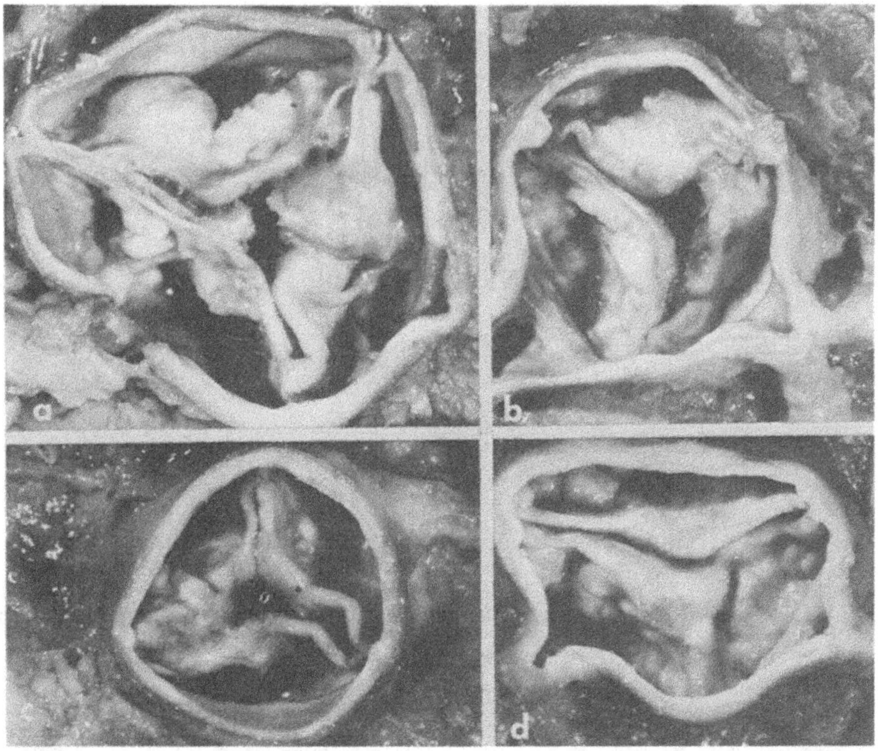

Figure 7. Aortic valves in 4 patients. In 3 (**b** to **d**) 1 commissure is fused, and in 1 (**a**) 2 commissures are fused. Each valve is severely stenotic and heavily calcified. **a,** Case 9; **b,** Case 10; **c,** Case 20; **d,** Case 12.

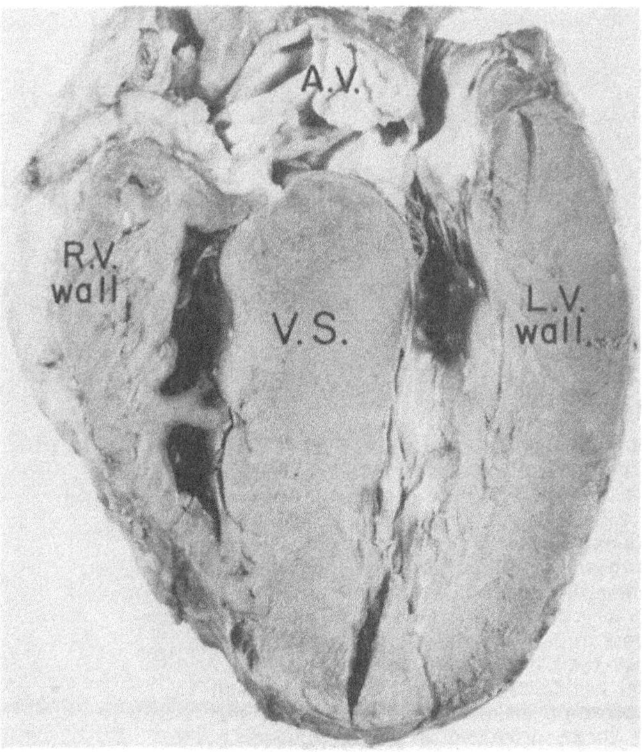

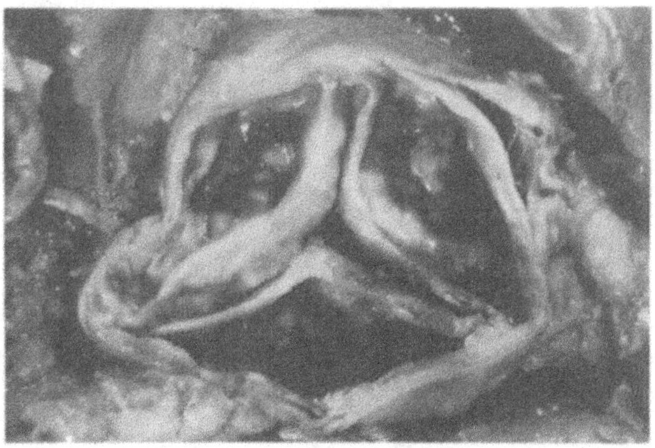

Figure 8. Case 6. Aortic valve (A.V.) **(left)** and longitudinal section of heart **(right)**. The valve is heavily calcified, severely stenotic, but free of commissural fusion. The longitudinal section shows that the cephalad portion of the ventricular septum (V.S.) is thicker than the free wall of the left ventricle (L.V.). The septum beneath the aortic valve bulges toward the mitral valve, giving the septum a sigmoid shape. This sigmoid configuration commonly occurs in persons over age 50 years but is rare in hearts weighing over 400 g.[16] The heart shown weighed 440 g. The sigmoid septum also is unusual in hearts with a dilated left ventricular cavity[4], and the chamber of the heart shown here is of normal size or small. R.V. = right ventricular.

commissure in 2 patients and 2 commissures in 1 patient. In all 21 patients the aortic valves were heavily calcified. The calcific deposits were located on the aortic aspects of the cusps in all patients, but in 3 the calcified deposits also extended a short distance down the ventricular aspect of the anterior mitral leaflets. The cusps were made rigid by the calcific deposits, and the stenoses were attributable to the rigidity of the cusps which contacted or nearly contacted one another when the valves were viewed from either above or below.

In addition to the calcific deposits in the aortic valves of all 21 patients, calcific deposits were present in the coronary arteries in 18 patients and in the annulus and subleaflet area of the posterior mitral leaflet in 17 patients. The deposits in the

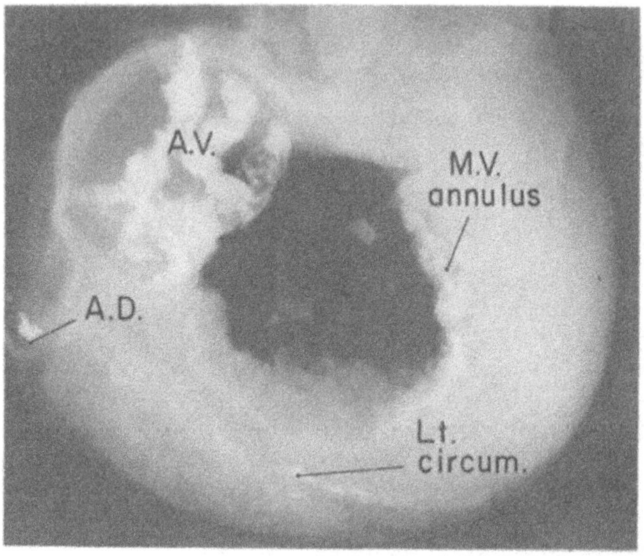

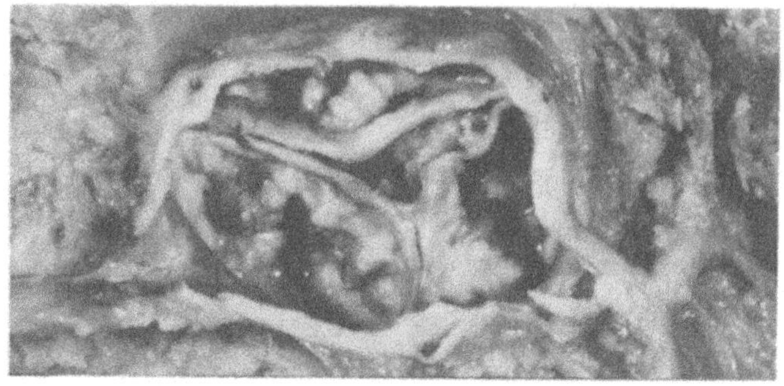

Figure 9. Case 13. Aortic valve and roentgenogram of heart specimen **at left.** Two of the 3 aortic valve (A.V.) commissures are fused. Calcific deposits are present in the mitral (M.V.) annulus and coronary arteries as well as in the aortic valve. Calcific deposits were observed in the mitral valve annulus or coronary arteries, or both, in 20 of the 21 patients studied. A.D. = anterior descending coronary artery; Lt. circum. = left circumflex coronary artery.

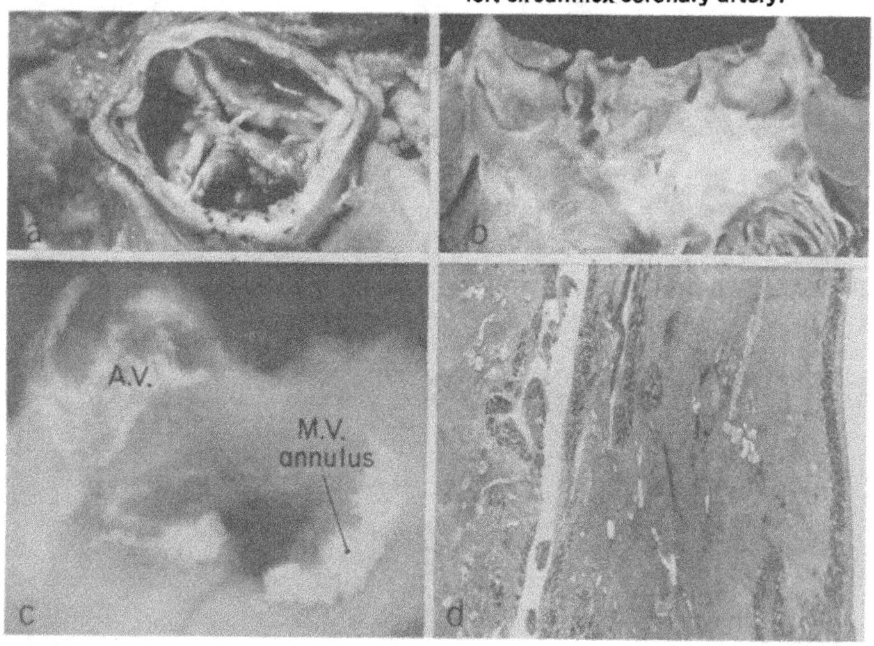

Figure 10. Case 14. Aortic valve, radiograph of heart, and portion of left ventricular papillary muscle. A 160 mm Hg peak systolic pressure gradient was recorded between the left ventricle and the brachial artery before aortic valve debridement 6 months before death. None of the 3 valve commissures is fused. The opened valve (**b**) shows no calcific deposits on the ventricular aspects of the cusps. The radiograph (**c**) shows heavy calcific deposits in the aortic valve cusps despite the absence of nodules of calcium on either the aortic (**a**) or ventricular (**b**) aspects of the cusps. Also, large deposits of calcium are present in the mitral annulus and submitral area (**c**) and in the coronary arteries. Both papillary muscles and left ventricular free walls beneath their bases were severely scarred. A portion of one is shown in **d.** Mitral annular calcification and left ventricular papillary muscle scarring, both of which are common lesions in elderly people, may present auscultatory features simulating those produced in older patients by valvular aortic stenosis alone.

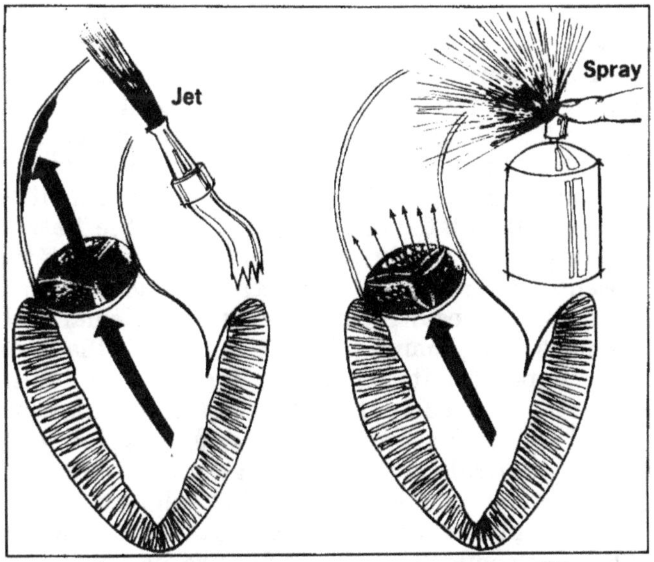

Figure 11. Diagram illustrating the auscultatory differences between fixed orifice (**left**) and non-fixed orifice (**right**) valvular aortic stenosis. A jet lesion appears to occur when severe fixed stenosis is present but is not apparent when there is a spray effect in non-fixed stenosis.

coronary arteries and mitral annuli were grossly visible and confirmed by either radiograph of the specimen or by histologic section. The mitral valve leaflets and chordae tendineae were intrinsically normal in 19 patients and thickened by fibrous tissue in 2; however, all mitral valves showed mild aging changes.[5] The tricuspid and pulmonic valves were normal in all 21 patients. The lumens of 1 or more of the 3 major extramural coronary arteries were narrowed by more than 50 percent in 10 patients and by less than 50 percent in 11 patients. Eleven patients had foci of myocardial fibrosis involving the left ventricular free wall with or without papillary muscle scarring, and 4 others had papillary muscle scarring only. Unequivocal atrophy of the left ventricular papillary muscles occurred in 2 patients. Five subjects had anatomic evidence of acute myocardial infarction (necrosis). At least 1 histologic section from the wall of each cardiac chamber was examined, and no Aschoff bodies were found in the sections from any of the 21 patients.

Comments

Differences between older and younger patients with aortic stenosis: Comparison of certain clinical and anatomic features in these 21 autopsy patients over 65 years of age with 119 autopsy patients between 16 and 65 years of age who had clinically isolated severe valvular aortic stenosis (described in detail elsewhere[6]) discloses several striking differences. First, the aortic valve *structure* is often different. It was tricuspid in approximately 90 percent and congenitally bicuspid in 10 percent of the 21 elderly patients; in contrast, the aortic valve was tricuspid in 45 percent, congenitally bicuspid in 45 percent, congenitally unicommissural unicuspid in 10 percent of the 119 younger patients. In addition to differences in basic valvular configuration, *commissural fusion* was unusual in older patients but common in the younger subjects. Second, the *origin* of the valvular lesion was different in the 2 age groups. Congenital malformations were the commonest causes of isolated aortic stenosis in the younger age group,[6–8] whereas simple degeneration or wear and tear was believed to be the most frequent cause in the older patient. Third, the *clinical diagnosis* of aortic stenosis in older patients may be overlooked because of peculiarities of the intensity and frequency composition of the systolic murmurs and because the systemic arterial pulse is likely to have a normal rate of rise and a normal or increased pulse pressure.[9,10] Fourth, *sex* in the 2 groups is different: Women were more frequent (57 percent) among the older patients, whereas 80 percent of the younger patients were men. Fifth, the *method of operative repair* may differ in the 2 groups: Valve debridement may prove useful in older patients, whereas valve replacement will usually be necessary in the younger adult. However, valve debridement was carried out in only 9 of 70 older surgical patients with aortic stenosis (age range 57 to 80 years, average 64) studied by Finegan and associates.[3]

Auscultatory signs: Certain auscultatory signs that accompany aortic stenosis in the elderly require explanation. Ejection sounds are characteristically absent, presumably because the cusps remain as individual units (since commissural fusion is absent) and the valve does not move abruptly as a single unit. Atrial sounds (fourth heart sounds), useful for judging the severity of aortic stenosis in the younger adult, are of little diagnostic help in the elderly since these sounds occur in elderly persons without aortic stenosis due to the decreased left ventricular compliance with age. Ordinarily, the murmur of valvular aortic stenosis is harsh, rough, grunting and loudest at the right base with radiation upward and to the right. In elderly patients with aortic stenosis, the harsh murmur at the right base may persist but with appreciably less intensity, and auscultation may be dominated instead by a loud, pure frequency musical systolic murmur maximal at or near the cardiac apex. At least 3 reasons account for these patterns: (1) Older persons tend to have increased upper thoracic chest dimensions which soften the basal murmurs.[10] (2) The morphology of the stenotic aortic valve differs in the 2 age groups. A rigid, calcified valve *with* commissural fusion provides a suitable mechanism for a high velocity jet into the ascending aorta (Fig. 11); the noisy murmur at the right base appears to originate within the ascending aorta because of turbulence caused by the high velocity jet.[10] A calcified, stenotic trileaflet aortic valve *without* commissural fusion, the most common type in the elderly, appears to behave differently. Ejection into the ascending aorta may take the form of a "spray" instead of a jet (Fig. 11), so that the harsh murmur at the right base may be comparatively inconspicuous. Since the cusps are not fused, each may vibrate during ventricular ejection. The accompanying pure frequency, musical cooing murmur probably results from these periodic vibrations.[10] Such murmurs are recordable within the left ventricular cavity and therefore are transmitted best to the chest wall overlying the left ventricle, that is, the cardiac apex. (3) Calcification of the mitral annulus, itself a producer of precordial murmurs, frequently accompanies calcification of the aortic valve in elderly patients. Mitral regurgitation can result from inability of the calcified annulus to decrease its circumference during ventricular contraction.[11] Accordingly, the holosystolic murmur of mitral regurgitation may be present at the apex and may be difficult to distinguish from the coexisting pure frequency aortic stenotic apical murmur. Seventeen of the 21 elderly patients described herein had calcified mitral annuli, and in 10 of them the deposits were "massive." These large deposits at the annulus and beneath the posterior mitral leaflet may well have prevented this valve from closing completely during ventricular systole. Although mitral annular calcification tends to complicate the auscultatory diagnosis of aortic stenosis, its radiologic identification is useful since it implies that coexisting aortic stenosis is likely to be caused by calcific deposits on a trileaflet valve without commissural fusion.

Systolic hypertension: The degree of left ventricular systolic hypertension in elderly patients may be considerably higher than that occurring in younger subjects with similar degrees of aortic stenosis since the peripheral systolic systemic pressure usually increases with age.[12] The degree of systolic hypertension which the left ventricle in the elderly is capable of achieving can be astonishingly high, particularly since this chamber seldom maintains a systolic pressure in excess of 250 mm Hg even in younger subjects.[13] In Patient 18 (Table II) the left ventricular systolic pressure was 265 mm Hg, but the peak systolic pressure gradient across the valve was only 93 mm Hg since the peripheral systemic systolic pressure was elevated (172 mm Hg) (Fig. 2). Thus, systemic hypertension may reduce the aortic gradient, and the degree of obstruction may be underestimated in these elderly patients if the systolic pressure difference is taken as the only index of severity. As the gradient diminishes in the presence of systemic systolic hypertension, the murmur at the right base may soften and shorten. Even if this auscultatory change does not occur with systemic hypertension, the modification of the systemic arterial pulse may be misleading since the rate of rise can be relatively normal and the pulse pressure increased despite severe obstruction to left ventricular outflow.

Atrial fibrillation: Another important clinical feature was the presence of atrial fibrillation in 7 of the 21 patients presented. It is recognized that this arrhythmia is common in elderly persons without valvular cardiac disease. The left atrial cavities were mildly dilated in all 21 patients, but left atrial dilatation commonly accompanies old age in the absence of functionally significant valvular lesions. It is also appreciated that the left ventricular wall becomes less compliant with age and that the superimposed left ventricular hypertrophy (without left ventricular dilatation) of aortic stenosis may further impede left atrial emptying. In addition, the mitral orifice may be narrowed by annular or subleaflet calcific deposits that might slow left atrial emptying and result in left atrial dilatation. The only common anatomic feature in elderly patients with atrial fibrillation is left atrial dilatation.[14] The combination of atrial fibrillation, a long apical systolic murmur and left atrial dilatation can obscure the diagnosis of aortic stenosis and lead to a mistaken diagnosis of isolated mitral regurgitation. Furthermore, atrial fibrillation is especially undesirable in aortic stenosis since the left ventricle requires the help of augmented left atrial contraction which increases end-diastolic fiber length and permits the left ventricle to contract with greater force.

Etiology: The cause of the aortic stenosis in elderly patients is uncertain, but simple wear and tear or degeneration appears to be the most reasonable explanation.[15] The presence in the same hearts of other wear and tear lesions such as calcified mitral annuli, calcified coronary arteries and focal thickening of other valve leaflets supports this contention. Certainly there is nothing to support a rheumatic origin—none of the patients had a history of acute rheumatic fever or chorea, none had Aschoff bodies, and all but 2 had intrinsically normal mitral valves.[7]

Addendum

During the 10 month interval from submission of this manuscript to receipt of the galleys severe valvular aortic stenosis was seen at necropsy by us in 11 additional patients aged 68 to 87 years (average 76). Seven were men, 4 women. All 11 patients had precordial systolic murmurs and evidence of congestive cardiac failure. Only 1 patient underwent cardiac catheterization, and she had a peak systolic pressure gradient of 100 mm Hg between the left ventricle and a systemic artery. At necropsy, the heart weight in the 11 patients ranged from 400 to 770 g (average 536). Ten patients had tricuspid aortic valves. In 8 no commissural fusion was present, and in 2 patients, 1 of 3 commissures was slightly fused. The eleventh patient had a congenitally bicuspid aortic valve.

References

1. **Bruns DL, Van der Hauwaert LG:** The aortic systolic murmur developing with increasing age. Brit Heart J 20:370–378, 1958
2. **Hancock EW, Madison WM Jr, Proctor MH, et al:** Aortic stenosis of no physiologic significance. New Eng J Med 258:305–312, 1958
3. **Finegan RE, Gianelly RE, Harrison DC:** Aortic stenosis in the elderly: relevance of age to diagnosis and treatment. New Eng J Med 281:1261–1264, 1969
4. **Goor D, Lillehei CW, Edwards JE:** The "sigmoid septum." Variation in the contour of the left ventricular outlet. Amer J Roentgen 107:366–376, 1969
5. **Sell S, Scully RE:** Aging changes in the aortic and mitral valves. Histologic and histochemical studies, with observations on the pathogenesis of calcific aortic stenosis and calcification of the mitral annulus. Amer J Path 46: 345–365, 1965
6. **Roberts WC:** The structure of the aortic valve in clinically isolated aortic stenosis. An autopsy study of 162 patients over 15 years of age. Circulation 42:91–97, 1970
7. **Roberts WC:** Anatomically isolated aortic valvular disease. The case against its being of rheumatic etiology. Amer J Med 151–159, 1970
8. **Roberts WC:** The congenitally bicuspid aortic valve. A study of 85 autopsy cases. Amer J Cardiol 26:72–83, 1970
9. **Perloff JK, Binnion PF, Caulfield WH, et al:** The use of angiotensin in the assessment of left ventricular function in fixed orifice aortic stenosis. Circulation 35:347–357, 1967
10. **Perloff JK:** Clinical recognition of aortic stenosis. The physical signs and differential diagnoses of the various forms of obstruction to left ventricular outflow. Progr Cardiovasc Dis 10:323–348, 1968
11. **Korn D, DeSanctis RW, Sell S:** Massive calcification of the mitral annulus. A clinicopathological study of fourteen cases. New Eng J Med 267:900–909, 1962
12. **Colandrea MA, Friedman GD, Nichaman MZ, et al:** Systolic hypertension in the elderly. An epidemiologic assessment. Circulation 41:239–245, 1970
13. **Gorlin R, McMillan IKR, Medd WE, et al:** Dynamics of the circulation in aortic valvular disease. Amer J Med 18:855–870, 1955
14. **Neufeld HN, Wagenvoort CA, Burchell HB, et al:** Idiopathic atrial fibrillation. Amer J Cardiol 8:193–197, 1961
15. **Hultgren HN:** Calcific disease of the aortic valve. Arch Path (Chicago) 45:694–706, 1948

Congenital Aortic Stenosis Resulting From a Unicommissural Valve

Clinical and Anatomic Features in Twenty-one Adult Patients

By M. WAYNE FALCONE, M.D., WILLIAM C. ROBERTS, M.D., ANDREW G. MORROW, M.D., AND JOSEPH K. PERLOFF, M.D.

SUMMARY

Clinical, electrocardiographic, phonocardiographic, radiographic, hemodynamic, and anatomic findings are presented in 21 adult patients with stenotic unicommissural aortic valves. Distinction between congenitally unicuspid and bicuspid aortic valves before operation or autopsy was not possible. Although the basic structure of the valve may render it inherently stenotic, the age at which a murmur was first noted (average, 19 years), the duration of a known murmur (average, 25 years), and the age of onset of first symptoms of left ventricular outflow obstruction (average, 41 years) strongly suggest that stenosis at least in part is acquired. The relationship of the true and false commissures to the coronary arterial ostia could be determined with certainty in 12 patients. The basic division of the aortic valve into left, right, and noncoronary cusps is maintained, but the raphes do not extend to the valve orifice. Because the aortic valve is attached to the ascending aorta at only one point (the true commissure), which is at the level of the orifice, valvotomy is hazardous, and valve replacement appears indicated when operative treatment becomes necessary in the adult patient with a stenotic unicommissural aortic valve.

Additional Indexing Words:

Aortic regurgitation
Aortic valve surgery
Bicuspid aortic valve
Infective endocarditis
Papillary muscle dysfunction

A CONGENITAL malformation of the aortic valve is the most common cause of anatomically isolated aortic stenosis.[1, 2] Usually the stenotic valve is found to be congenital-

From the Section of Pathology and Clinic of Surgery, National Heart and Lung Institute, National Institutes of Health, Bethesda, Maryland, and the Departments of Medicine and Pediatrics, Georgetown University School of Medicine, Division of Cardiology, Georgetown University Hospital, Washington, D. C.

Address for reprints: William C. Roberts, M.D., Section of Pathology, National Heart and Lung Institute, National Institutes of Health, Bethesda, Maryland 20014.

Received February 11, 1971; accepted for publication March 23, 1971.

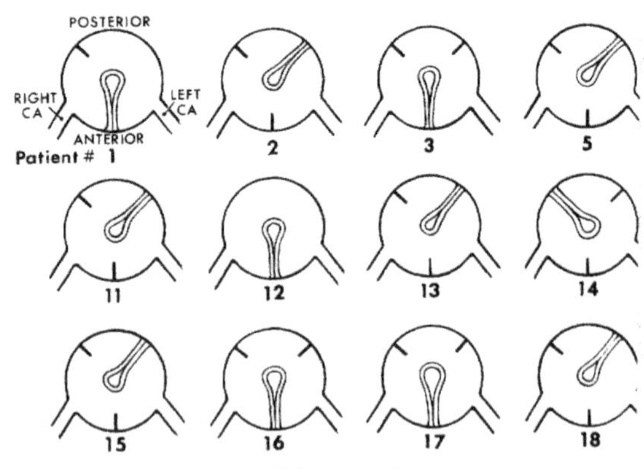

Figure 1

Schematic representation of the positions of the tr commissure and raphes in 12 patients with congenit ly unicommissural aortic valves. CA = coronary arte ly bicuspid,[3] but not infrequently stenosis may result from a congenitally unicuspid aortic valve, two forms of which are recognized.[4] Both have a dome shape: one has no commissures or lateral attachments to the aorta at the level of the orifice (*acommissural*); the second has one lateral attachment to the aorta at the level of the orifice (*unicommissural*). The dome-shaped valves are reported to be stenotic from birth,[4] and constitute the major cause of symptomatic valvular aortic stenosis in the first year of life.[5] Unicommissural aortic valves are known to cause severe aortic stenosis in childhood, but relatively little attention has been paid to the occurrence of this aortic valvular malformation in adults. This report describes the clinical, hemodynamic, and anatomic findings in 21 adult patients in whom isolated aortic stenosis resulted from a unicommissural valve.

Patients Studied

Among 543 patients over 14 years of age with severe (functional classes III and IV, New York Heart Association classification) valvular cardiac disease, studied at autopsy, 182 or 34% had isolated aortic stenosis, with or without associated aortic regurgitation. Of these 182 patients, 27

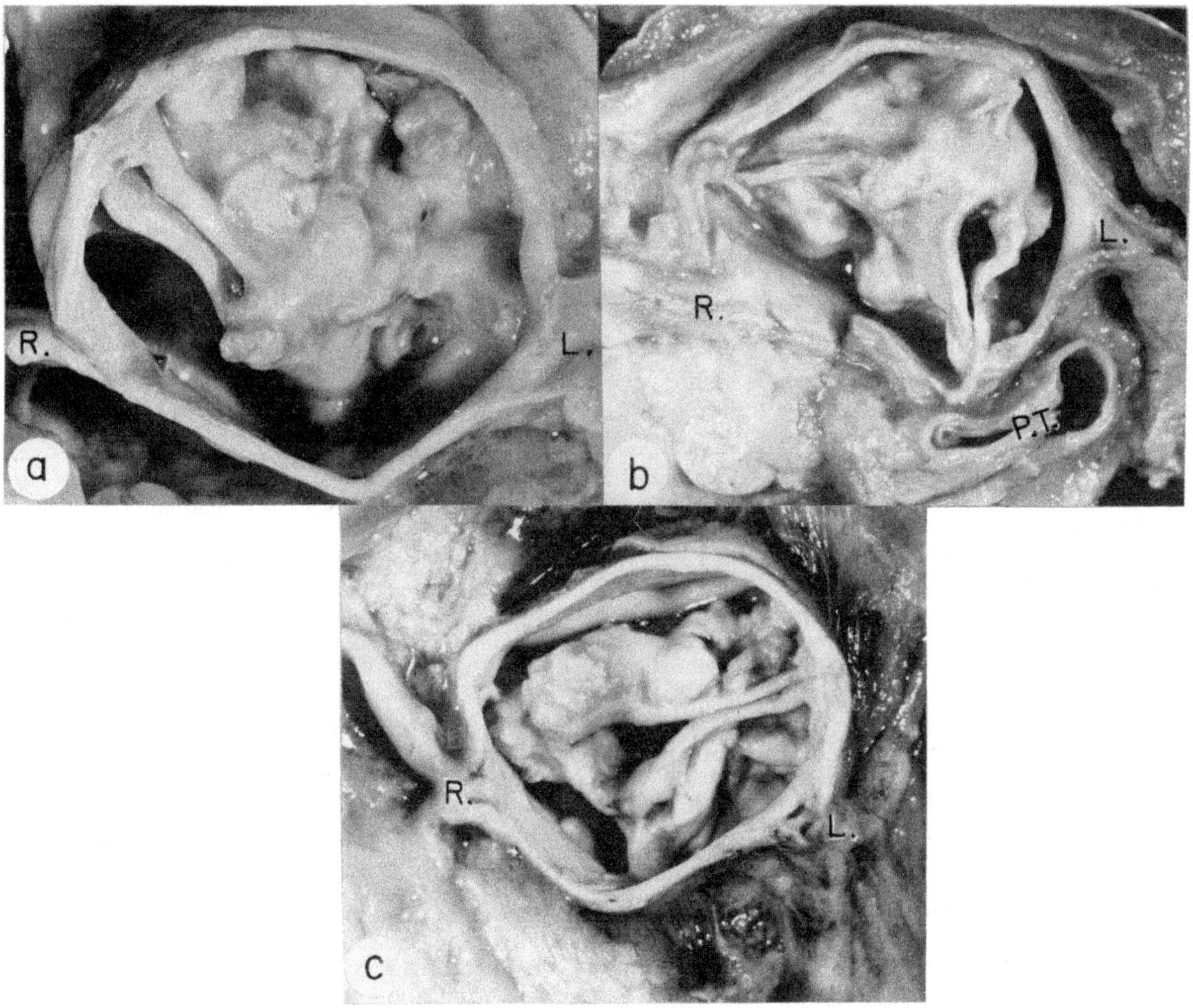

Figure 2

Photographs of in situ congenitally unicommissural aortic valves in three patients. (a) Patient No. 14. (b) Patient No. 17. (c) Patient No. 15. L. = left coronary artery; P.T. = pulmonary trunk; R. = right coronary artery.

Table 1

Clinical and Morphologic Data in Twenty-One Adult Patients with Stenotic Congenitally Unicommissural Aortic Valves

Pt.	Age at death (yr)	Sex	Age murmur first heard (yr)	Hx of ARF	Duration of CHF (yr)	Angina	Syncope	AR
1	47	F	32	0	2	+	0	+
2	16	M	Birth	0	7	+	0	0
3	40	F	Infancy	0	6/12	+	+	+
4	32	F	5	0	6/12	+	0	0
5	57	M	35	0	3	0	0	0
6	50	M	47	0	8/12	+	0	+
7	19	F	17	0	2	+	+	+
8	37	M	7	0	6	+	0	+
9	55	M	12	+	0	0	0	+
10	61	M	13	+	2	0	0	+
11	31	M	5	0	3/12	0	0	+†
12	28	M	16	0	1 6/12	0	0	+
13	57	M	55	0	1	+	0	+
14	48	M	10	0	11	0	0	0
15	59	M	58	+	1	0	+	+
16	52	M	13	+	2	0	0	+
17	62	M	6	0	1	+	0	+
18	35	M	18	+	1/12	0	0	+
19	41	M	4	0	4	+	+	+
20	53	M	12	0	6	+	0	+
21	47	M	27	0	1	+	+	0
Total no. of patients		17 M 4 F		5		12	5	16
Range	16–62		Birth–58		1½–11			
Average	44		19		2 ½			

*Cardiac catheterization in each patient was performed within 1 month of death.

†The predominant functional lesion was AR. AR was mild in 12 of the 16 patients wih AR murmurs.

Abbreviations: ARF = acute rheumatic fever; AR = aortic regurgitation; AV = aortic valve; CHF = congestive heart failure; CI = cardiac index; ECG = electrocardiogram; F = female; Hx = history; IE = infective endocarditis; IPO = immediate postoperative period; LAD = left axis deviation; LBBB = left bundle-branch block; LPO = late postoperative period (> 2 years postop.); LVH = left ventricular hypertrophy; LVI = left ventricular ischemia; LV PAP fibrosis = left ventricular papillary muscle fibrosis; LV-SA PSG = left ventricle-systemic arterial peak systolic gradient; M = male; NC = noncardiac; op. = operation; SUD = sudden, unexpected death.

were older than age 65 (average, 78 years), and 25 had tricuspid and two had bicuspid aortic valves. Of the remaining 155 patients, aged 15 to 65 years (average, 46 years), 18 (12%) had congenitally unicommissural valves, 72 (46%) had congenitally bicuspid valves, 57 (37%) had tricuspid aortic valves, and in eight (5%) the basic structure of the stenotic aortic valve was not discernible.

In addition to the 18 patients with congenitally unicommissural aortic valves studied at autopsy, congenitally unicommissural aortic valves were excised at operation in three additional living patients. Table 1 summarizes the clinical and necropsy findings in these 21 patients. In each, only one aortic valve commissure was attached to the aortic wall at the level of the valve orifice, which, when viewed from above, had an exclamation-point configuration (figs. 1–3). Raphes (false commissures), extending only part way from the base of the valve toward its free edge, also were present in most patients. All had midsystolic murmurs characteristic of aortic stenosis, and 16 also had murmurs of aortic regurgitation (fig. 4). Three patients (nos. 10, 11, and 15) had holosystolic, blowing apical murmurs indicating mitral regurgitation; each patient was in terminal congestive cardiac failure, and two (nos. 11 and 15) also had murmurs of tricuspid regurgitation. Two patients (nos. 4 and 18) had histories of infective endocarditis. Of 13 patients in whom phonocardiograms were ob-

ECG	LV-SA* PSG (mm Hg)	CI* (liters/min/m²)	AV op.	Cause of death	Heart weight (g)	Calcium AV (0–4+)	LV PAP fibrosis (0–4+)
LVH	150	3.0	+	IPO	400	4+	1+
LVH	90	—	0	SUD	600	2+	1+
LVH	158	2.8	+	IPO	550	4+	1+
LVH	90	—	0	CHF	500	4+	0
LAD; LVI	82	2.4	0	CHF	630	4+	—
LVH	80	3.2	+	LPO	700	4+	3+
LVH; LBBB	105	2.9	+	IPO	500	4+	4+
LBBB	29	3.0	+	LPO	860	4+	4+
LVH	104	2.3	+	NC	400	4+	3+
LAD; LVH	18	2.0	+	IPO	620	2+	3+
LAD; LVH	15†	—	0	CHF	880	3+	1+
LAD; LBBB	—	—	0	SUD	640	4+	0
LAD; LVH	—	—	0	CHF	760	3+	1+
LVH	—	—	0	SUD	750	4+	1+
LAD; LBBB	—	—	0	SUD	650	3+	1+
LVH	—	—	0	CHF	640	2+	—
LVH	—	—	0	NC	400	4+	2+
LVH	—	—	0	IE	550	2+	1+
LVH	150	—	+	(Living)	—	4+	—
LVH	—	—	+	(Living)	—	4+	—
LVH	65	—	+	(Living)	—	4+	—
17 LVH 6 LAD 4 LBBB			10			21/21	14/16
	15–158	2.0–3.2			400–800		
	87	2.7			590		

tained, unequivocal ejection sounds were present in two (nos. 7 and 15), and questionable ones in two others (nos. 2 and 4) (fig. 4). Representative electrocardiograms and chest roentgenograms are illustrated in figures 5 and 6, respectively, and atrophied left ventricular papillary muscles are shown in figure 7.

Comments

It is apparently impossible to determine before operation or autopsy the presence of a stenotic unicommissural unicuspid aortic valve in an adult. The frequency of congestive cardiac failure, angina pectoris, syncope, left ventricular hypertrophy, aortic regurgitation, aortic valvular calcification, aortic ejection sound, and infective endocarditis are similar among patients with stenotic congenitally unicuspid and bicuspid aortic valves.

Edwards[4] believes that the unicuspid aortic valve is intrinsically stenotic from birth, and Moller and associates[5] found congenitally unicommissural aortic valves in nine of 11 children less than 1 year of age who had symptomatic aortic stenosis. Their patients exhibited gross enlargement of all four cardiac chambers. Left ventricular endocardial fibroelastosis also was present in eight of these 11 patients. In all five patients in whom left ventricular angiocardiograms were obtained mitral regurgitation was evident and presumed to be the result of papillary muscle infarction.[5]

Of our 21 patients, a precordial murmur was discovered in infancy in two, by age 7 in five, between ages 7 and 30 in nine, and after 30 years of age in five. The duration of a known murmur ranged from birth to 56 years (average, 25 years), and the age at onset of symptoms referable to left ventricular outflow

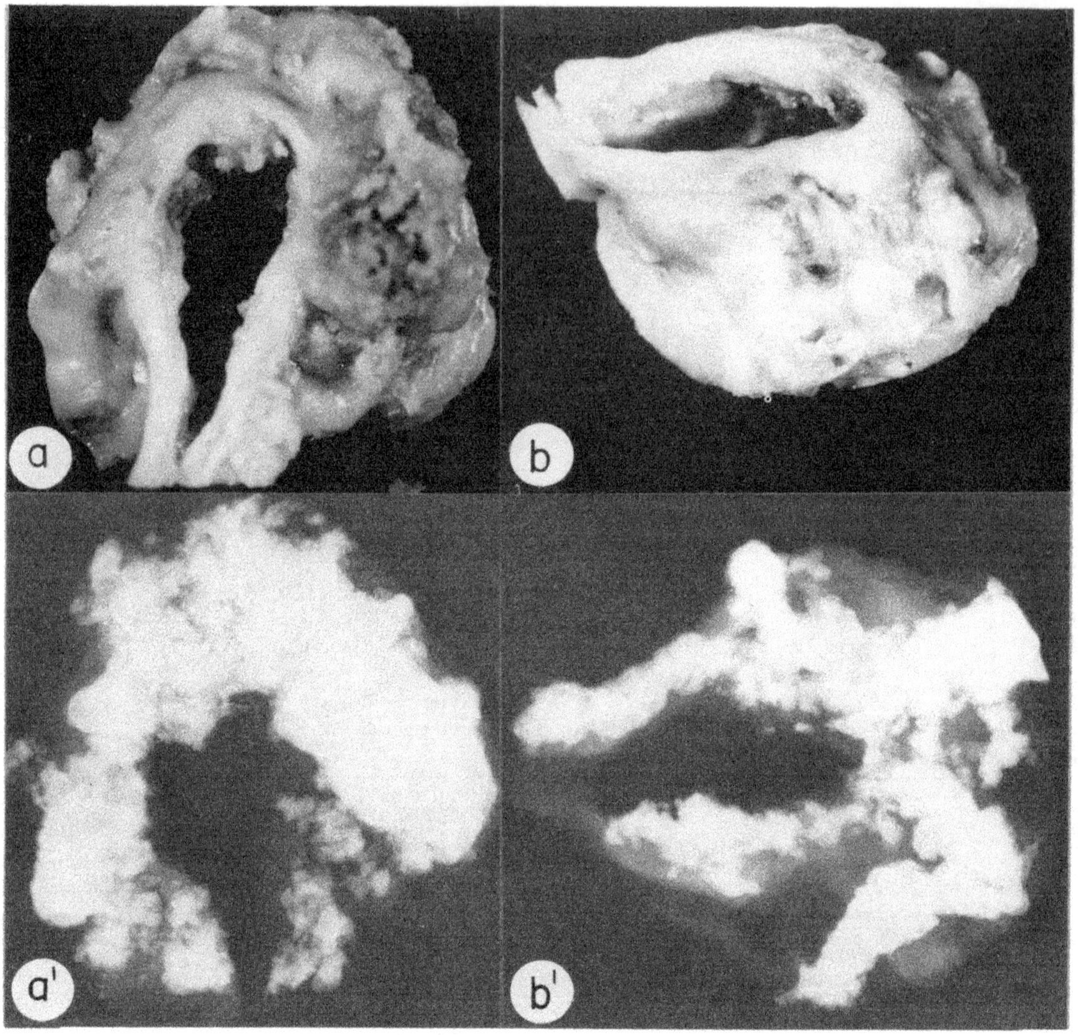

Figure 3

Photographs (a and b) and radiographs (a^1 and b^1) of congenitally unicommissural aortic valves excised at operation in patient No. 20 (a and a^1) and patient No 19 (b and b^1). Both valves are heavily calcified.

Figure 4

Phonocardiograms in four patients. (a) Patient No. 10. Crescendo-decrescendo systolic murmur (SM) with delayed upstroke of carotid pulse tracing. (b) Patient No. 7. Aortic ejection sound (E) timing with onset of carotid upstroke. (c) Patient No. 15. Severe delay of carotid upstroke accompanied by left bundle-branch block. Left axis deviation and paradoxical splitting of S_2. (d) Patient No. 11. Crescendo-decrescendo systolic murmur with high frequency early diastolic murmur (EDM), low frequency middiastolic murmur (MDM) (Austin-Flint murmur), and third heart sound (S_3). Abbreviations: 2 RICS = second right intercostal space; A_2 = aortic component of second heart sound; P_2 = pulmonic component of second heart sound; S_1 = first heart sound; S_2 = second heart sound; 2 LICS and 4 LICS = second and fourth left intercostal spaces, respectively.

obstruction ranged from 9–61 years (average, 41 years). Apparently some patients with congenitally unicommissural aortic valves have evidence of left ventricular outflow obstruction at birth, while in others obstruction does not appear until adulthood. It seems likely that in the latter patients stenosis is gradually acquired as the result of fibrosis and

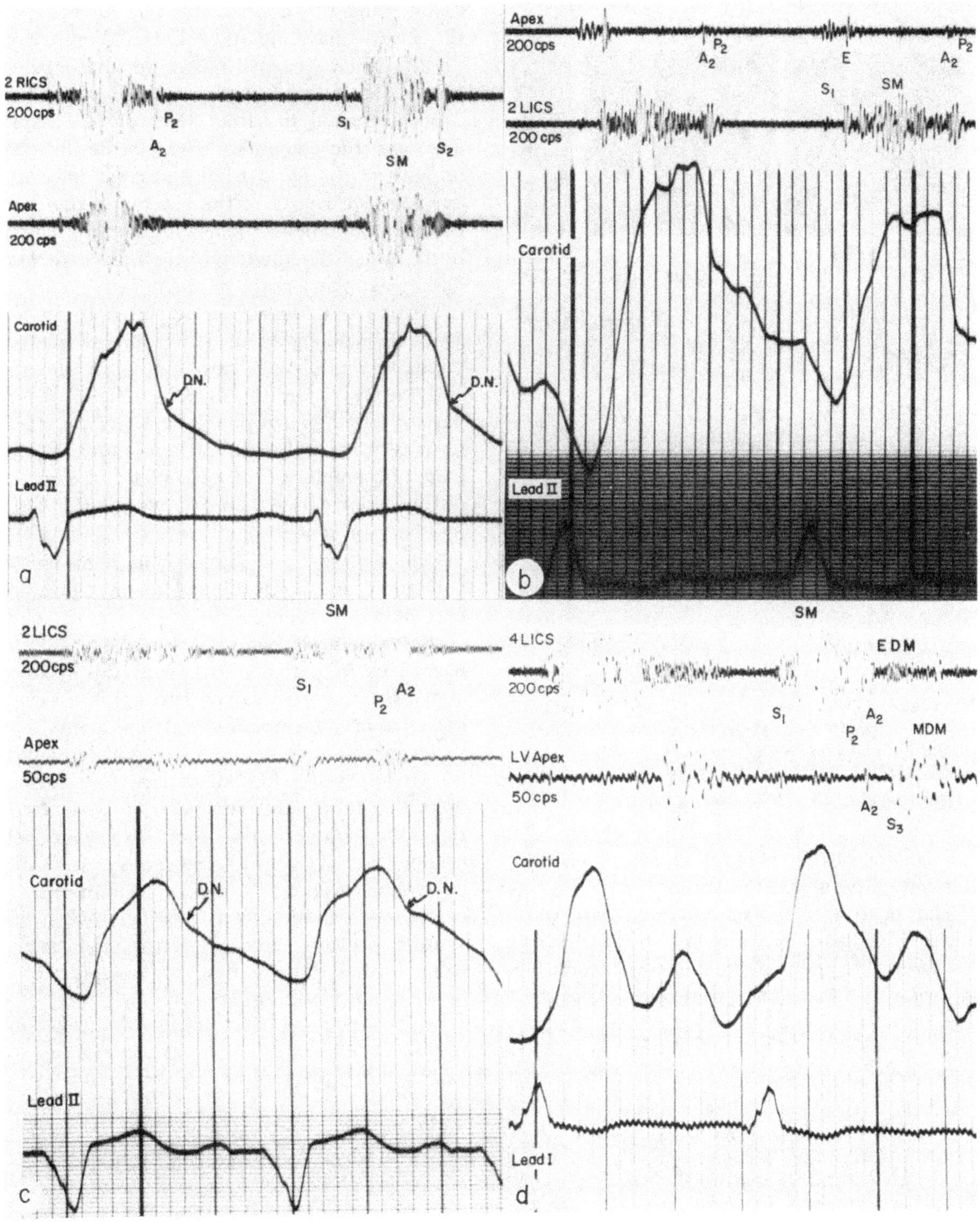

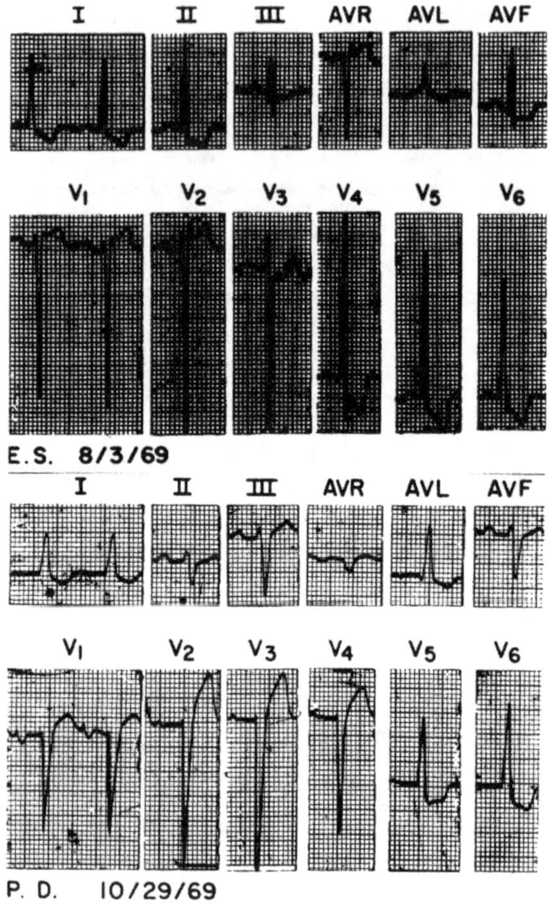

Figure 5

Electrocardiograms in patient No. 17 (top) and patient No. 11 (bottom). Both show left ventricular hypertrophy with repolarization abnormalities. In addition, patient No. 11 (P.D.) has left axis deviation and an intraventricular conduction delay.

calcification of the valve rather than from the inherent structure of the valve.

The location of the single commissure was noted in 12 hearts in which it was possible to determine the anatomic relations with certainty (fig. 1). Two raphes were present in ten patients, one in one patient, and none in one patient. The distances between the true and false commissures, when present, were essentially equal, dividing the valve into thirds, and maintaining the normal anatomic division of the aortic valve into right, left, and posterior (noncoronary) cusps. There was no separation of the "cusps," however, and none of the raphes reached the free edges of the cusps. The one true commissure was located at the junction of the normal left and right coronary cusps in five hearts, at the junction of the left coronary and noncoronary (posterior) cusps in six, and at the junction of the right coronary and noncoronary cusps in one.

Despite left ventricular hypertrophy in all 18 autopsied patients, the posteromedial papillary muscle was atrophied in 11 hearts and severely fibrotic in five (fig. 7). No patient had hypertrophied papillary muscles. Four patients had focal thickening of the free edge of the anterior mitral leaflet, but in each of these four patients aortic regurgitation also had been present.

Only one patient (no. 2) had an aortic valvotomy, and he developed aortic regurgitation postoperatively; nine other patients had aortic valve replacement. Aortic valvotomy is hazardous in patients with congenitally unicommissural aortic valves because the valve has a lateral attachment at only one point.[7] Of seven infants undergoing valvotomy reported by Moller et al.,[5] four died during operation or in the immediate postoperative period. Of the three who survived from 2 to 6 years, all retained loud systolic murmurs, and all developed grade 2/6 diastolic murmurs of aortic regurgitation. One patient with no systolic pressure gradient across the aortic valve postoperatively had angiographic evidence of aortic regurgitation.

Figure 6

Chest roentgenograms in four patients. (a and a¹) Patient No. 7. (b and b¹) Patient No. 17. Large calcific deposits (arrows) are present in the aortic valve of both patients. (c) Patient No. 15. (d) Patient No. 11. Both latter patients have very large hearts and pulmonary venous congestion. When the (c) and (d) roentgenograms were taken both patients were in terminal congestive cardiac failure and had the murmurs of mitral and tricuspid regurgitation also.

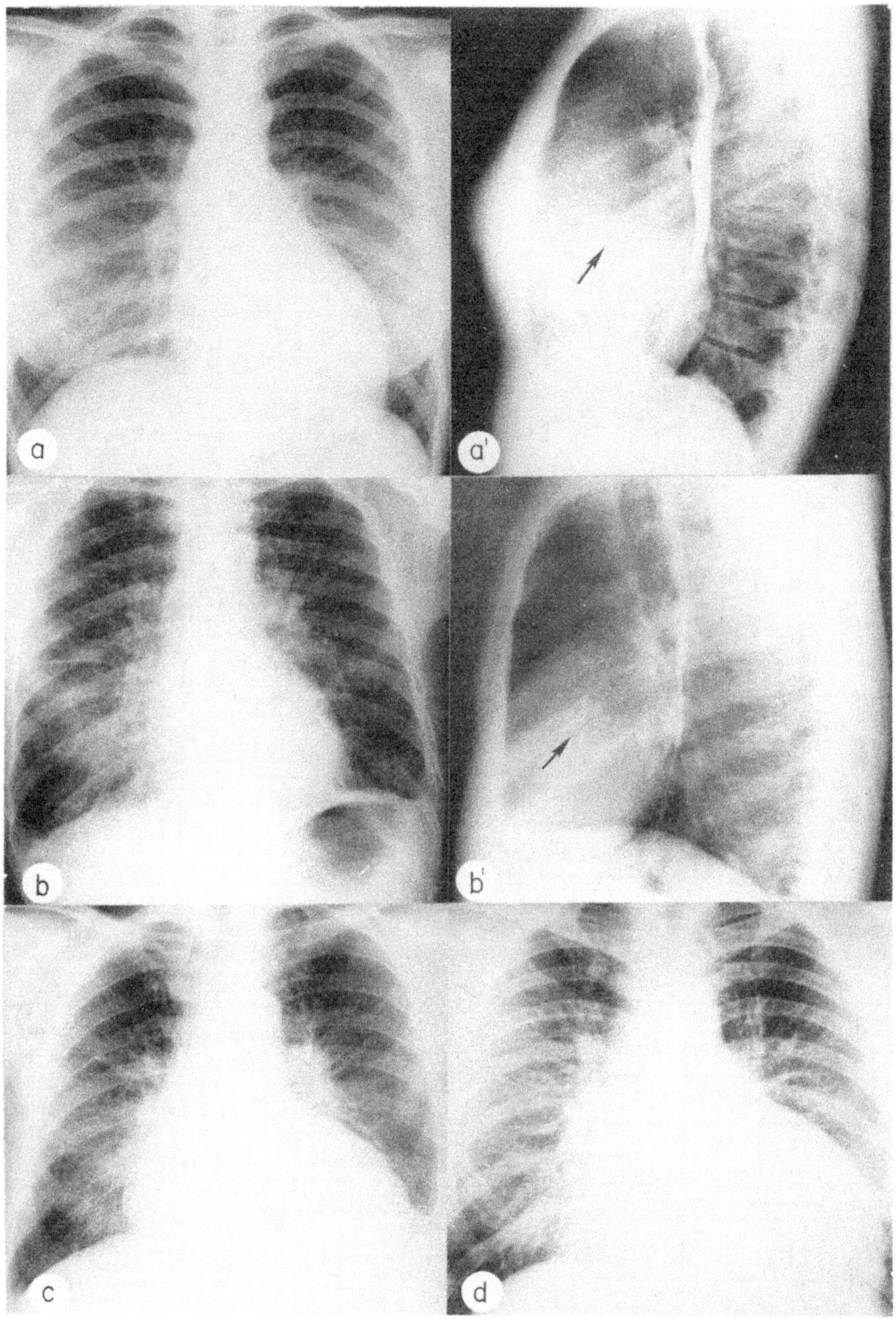

a
a'
b
b'
c
d

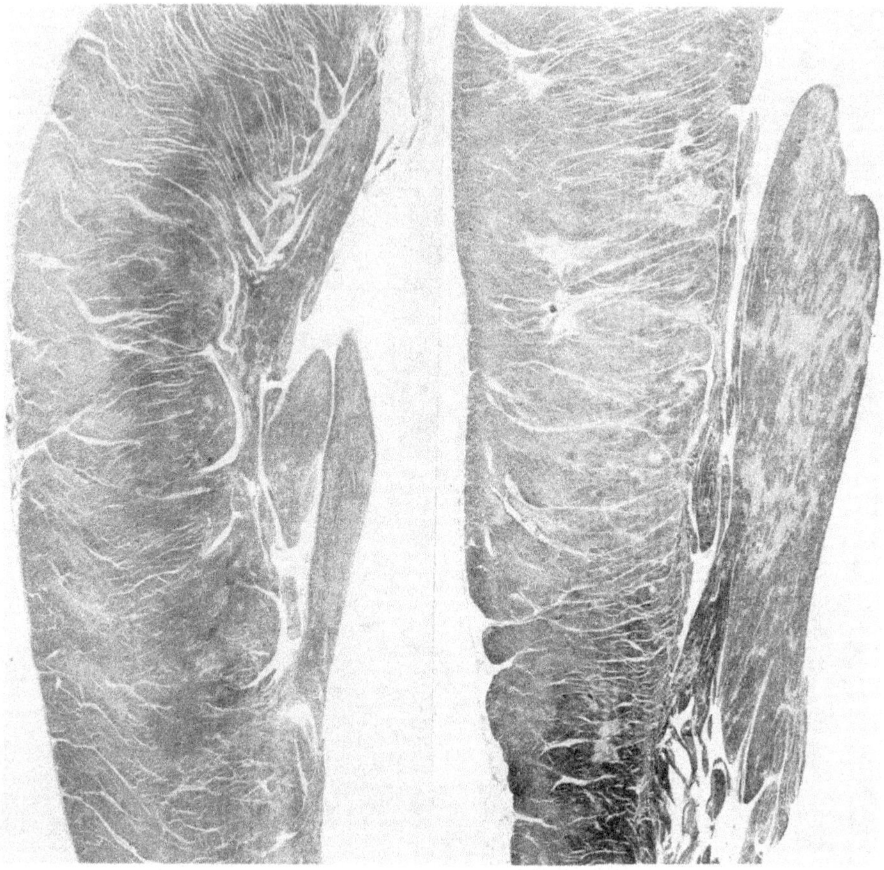

Figure 7

Longitudinal sections of posteromedial left ventricular papillary muscles in two patients with congenitally unicommissural aortic valves. (Left) Patient No. 7. The papillary muscle is severely scarred and atrophied. (Right) Patient No. 6. The papillary muscle is focally fibrotic and only minimally atrophied. Hematoxylin and eosin stains; each × 2.

References

1. Roberts WC: The structure of the aortic valve in clinically-isolated aortic stenosis. A study of 162 autopsy patients over 15 years of age. Circulation **42:** 91, 1970
2. Roberts WC: Anatomically isolated aortic valvular disease. The case against its being of rheumatic etiology. Amer J Med **49:** 151, 1970
3. Roberts WC: The congenitally bicuspid aortic valve. A study of 85 autopsy patients. Amer J Cardiol **26:** 72, 1970
4. Edwards JE: Pathologic aspects of cardiac valvular insufficiencies. Arch Surg (Chicago) **77:** 634, 1958
5. Moller JH, Nakib A, Eliot RS, Edwards JE: Symptomatic congenital aortic stenosis in the first year of life. J Pediat **69:** 728, 1966
6. Moller JH, Nakib A, Edwards JE: Infarction of papillary muscles and mitral insufficiency in association with congenital aortic stenosis. Circulation **34:** 87, 1966
7. Roberts WC, Morrow AG: Congenital aortic stenosis produced by a unicommissural valve. Brit Heart J **27:** 505, 1965

Valvular, Subvalvular, and Supravalvular Aortic Stenosis: Morphologic Features

William C. Roberts, M. D.

Obstruction to left ventricular outflow may occur at, below, or above the aortic valve. Clinical features of five adult patients with obstructions at these sites are summarized below.

Patient 1

G.I., a 48-year-old man, was asymptomatic until 7 months before death when congestive cardiac failure and episodes of lightheadedness appeared. He had been told of a precordial murmur when he was 9 years old. He never had evidence of acute rheumatic fever. By one month before death he was functionally class IV (New York Heart Association). He had a grade 4/6 ejection-type systolic murmur (with thrill), loudest over the cardiac base with good radiation into the neck but not into the axilla. A grade 1/6 diastolic murmur was heard at the cardiac base. Electrocardiogram showed sinus rhythm and left ventricular hypertrophy with strain. Chest radiograph showed cardiomegaly with left ventricular prominence, dilatation of the ascending aorta, and heavy deposits of calcium in the region of the aortic valve. The cardiac failure worsened, pneumonia appeared, and he died.

Patient 2

M.A., an 85-year-old woman, was healthy until six months before death when congestive cardiac failure appeared. She never had evidence of rheumatic fever. On examination, two days before death, she was cachectic. The blood pressure was 140/60 mm.Hg. The heart was large and the left ventricular impulse, sustained. A grade 3/6 ejection-type, midsystolic murmur was present over the aortic area with radiation into the neck. A different grade 3/6 blowing pansystolic murmur was heard over the cardiac apex. Subcutaneous dependent edema was evident. Electrocardiogram showed sinus rhythm and left ventricular hypertrophy. Chest radiograph showed cardiomegaly with left ventricular prominence, and dilatation of the ascending aorta, but no calcific deposits were seen. Cardiac failure progressed and she died.

Patient 3

D.W., a 36-year-old woman, was well until age 32, four years before death, when evidence of congestive cardiac failure appeared during her second pregnancy. Despite digitalization, diuretics and salt restriction, the cardiac failure gradually progressed. Angina pectoris and lightheadedness appeared periodically beginning at age 34. On examination at age 35, one year before death, a grade 3/6 holosystolic precordial murmur (without thrill) was present, maximal over the cardiac apex. No diastolic murmur was heard. Third and fourth heart sounds were audible. Electrocardiogram showed sinus rhythm, prolonged (0.23 second) P–R interval, left axis deviation, and right bundle branch block. Chest radiograph showed cardiomegaly, with left ventricular and left atrial prominence, no enlargement of the ascending aorta, and no calcific deposits. Episodes of rapid heart action, primarily paroxysmal atrial tachycardia, appeared three months before death. Fatal acute pulmonary edema developed during one of these episodes of tachycardia.

Patient 4

J.M., a 28-year-old man, who was known to have had a precordial murmur since early childhood but never evidence of acute rheumatic fever, was asymptomatic until six months before death when exertional dyspnea and pedal edema appeared and he began losing weight. He was improved transiently by digitalis and diuretics. Three weeks before death malaise, headache, fever, and productive cough appeared, exertional dyspnea worsened, and he was hospitalized. He was thin but not acutely ill. The blood pressure was 120/70 mm. Hg. Basal pulmonary rales and hepatomegaly were present. The heart was enlarged. A grade 3/6 midsystolic ejection-type murmur (with thrill) was present over the cardiac base and it radiated into the neck. A grade 2/6 diastolic blowing murmur was heard along the left sternal border. The blood hematocrit was 34 per cent. Electrocardiogram showed sinus tachycardia, left ventricular hypertrophy, and marked clockwise rotation. Chest roentgenogram showed cardiomegaly with prominence of the left ventricle, no calcific deposits, and no dilatation of the ascending aorta. Eighteen hours after admission he suddenly developed supraventricular tachycardia followed quickly by fatal acute pulmonary edema.

Patient 5

E.B., an 18-year-old boy, was found to have a precordial murmur when about 1 year of age. At age 3, examination disclosed a systolic thrill and murmur over the cardiac base, a normal-sized heart by chest roentgenogram, and inverted T waves in electrocardiographic leads II and III. At age 7 he had pneumococcal endocarditis which was cured by penicillin. By age 10 the heart was enlarged by radiograph, and electrocardiogram showed complete left bundle branch block. By age 13 the left radial pulse was noted to be diminished as compared to the right one. Chest roentgenogram at age 16 disclosed an aneurysm in the ascending aorta with calcific deposits. He was hospitalized for workup one week before death. He had always been asymptomatic except for occasional bilateral intermittent claudication after running a block, and one episode of precordial chest pain 15 months before death. A 3-year-old sister also had a murmur consistent with "aortic stenosis." On examination, he was well developed. His heart was enlarged. A systolic thrill and grade 5/6 midsystolic ejection-type murmur was heard over the precordium, loudest over the second right intercostal space and with radiation into the back. No diastolic murmur was heard. The left radial and both femoral arterial pulses were diminished. He died during cardiac operation.

Comments

Patients 1 and 2 had valvular aortic stenosis. Patient 1 had a congenitally unicommissural aortic valve (Fig. 1)[1,2] and patient 2 had a three-cuspid aortic valve of the type seen in the elderly (Fig. 2).[3] Patient 3 had hypertrophic cardiomyopathy with subaortic stenosis (idiopathic hypertrophic subaortic steno-

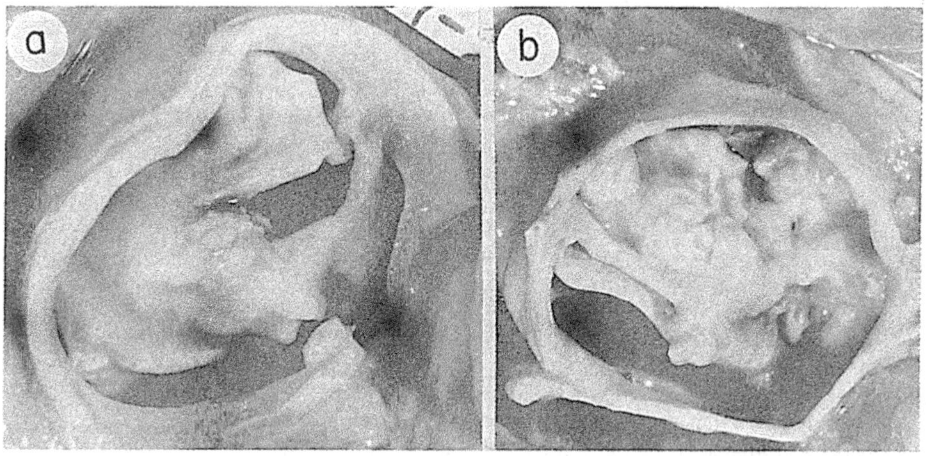

Figure 1. Stenotic unicommissural unicuspid aortic valves viewed from above in two men aged 28 (a) and aged 48 (b).

Table 1. Left ventricular outflow obstruction

Site of obstruction	*Number (%) patients < age 15 years*	*Number (%) patients age 15 to 65 years*	*Number (%) patients > 65 years*
Valve	169 (71)	170 (85)	25 (83)
Discrete subvalvular	26 (11)	5 (3)	0 (0)
Diffuse subvalvular*	12 (5)	22 (11)	5 (17)
Supravalvular	11 (5)	1 (0.5)	0 (0)
Complicated†	19 (8)	1 (0.5)	0 (0)
	237 (100)‡	199 (100)§	30 (100)§

* Also called *hypertrophic cardiomyopathy with or without subaortic stenosis* and *idiopathic hypertrophic subaortic stenosis.*

† Includes patients with diffuse left ventricular endocardial fibroelastosis, hypoplastic left ventricle (excluding aortic atresia), severe abnormalities of the mitral valve, and combined valvular, subvalvular with or without supravalvular aortic stenosis.

‡ These 237 patients were studied clinically by Lambert and associates[6] at the Children's Hospital of Buffalo. A few of the patients were aged 15 to 17 years.

§ These patients were studied at necropsy by the author at the National Heart and Lung Institute.

sis) (Fig. 3). Patient 4 had congenitally discrete subaortic stenosis complicated by alpha hemolytic endocarditis (Fig. 4).[4] Patient 5 had congenital supravalvular aortic stenosis with aneurysmal formation in the ascending aorta (Figs. 5, 6).[5]

The sites of left ventricular outflow obstruction in two large series of patients, one in subjects up to age 15 years studied by Lambert[6] and the other in patients 14 years and older studied at necropsy by the author, are summarized in Table 1. If aortic atresia were included in Lambert's age group, the "complicated group" would form a much higher percentage. The remainder of this paper will discuss the obstructions at the specific levels.

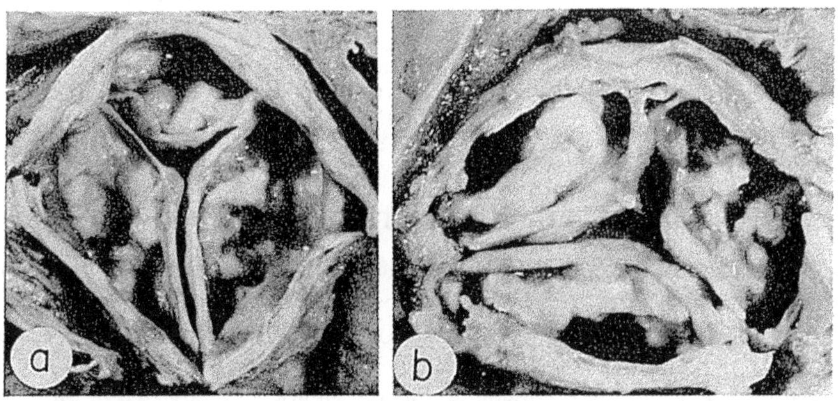

Figure 2. Stenotic tricuspid aortic valves in two elderly patients. a, Eighty-year-old man. b, Eighty-five-year-old woman. Aortic stenosis in the elderly is characterized by calcific deposits on the aortic surfaces of the cusps and typically no commissural fusion. One of the three commissures in each valve shown here is slightly fused.

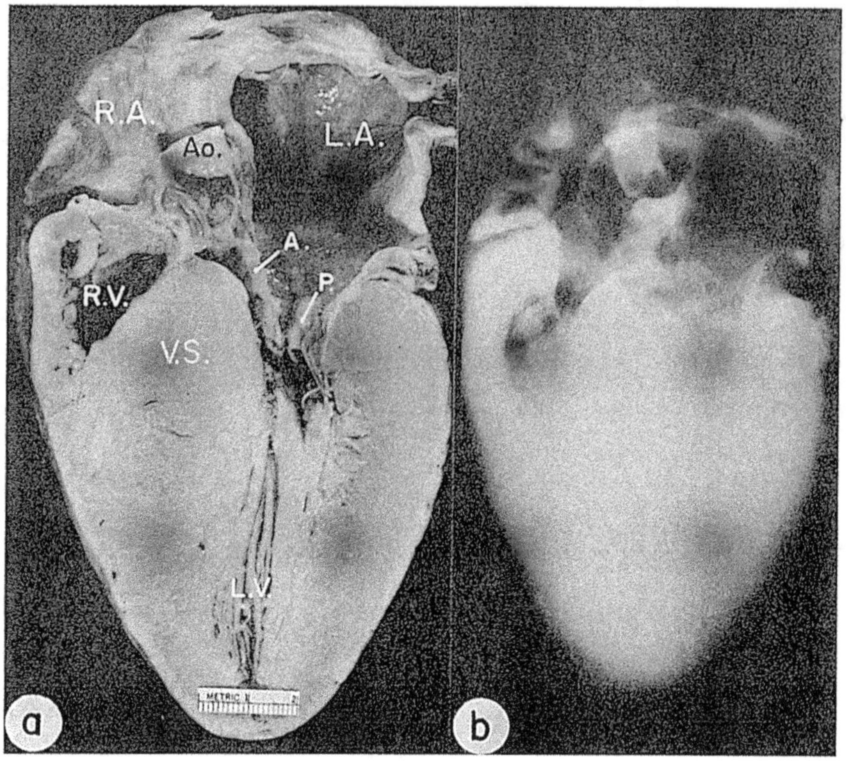

Figure 3. Longitudinal section (a) through right ventricle (R.V.), ventricular septum (V.S.), left ventricle (L.V.), and left atrium (L.A.), and radiograph of heart (b) in the 36-year-old woman described as patient 3. This patient had hypertrophic cardiomyopathy with subaortic stenosis documented during life by left heart catheterization and left ventricular angiography. At rest, the peak systolic pressure gradient between left ventricle and femoral artery was 75 mm. Hg when the cardiac index was 2.0 L./min./m^2. With provocation (Valsalva) this gradient rose to 125 mm. Hg.

The left ventricular cavity is minute. The ventricular septum is much thicker than the left ventricular free wall. Fibromas (contact lesions) are present on the mitral and aortic valves and on mural endocardium of the left ventricle. The radiograph further demonstrates the huge amount of left ventricular myocardium compared to the small left ventricular cavity. R.A. = right atrium. Ao. = aorta. A. and P. = anterior and posterior mitral leaflets, respectively.

VALVULAR AORTIC STENOSIS

Obstruction at the level of the aortic valve is by far the most common cause of left ventricular outflow tract obstruction. Classically, valvular aortic stenosis has been divided into two types: congenital and acquired. Although malformation of the aortic valve is the most common major congenital anomaly of the heart or great vessels,[7] congenital aortic stenosis is not a common lesion. The reason lies in the fact that most congenitally malformed aortic valves are not stenotic at birth. The stenosis most commonly is acquired and due to fibrosis and calcification of the malformed cusps. Thus, acquired valvular aortic stenosis

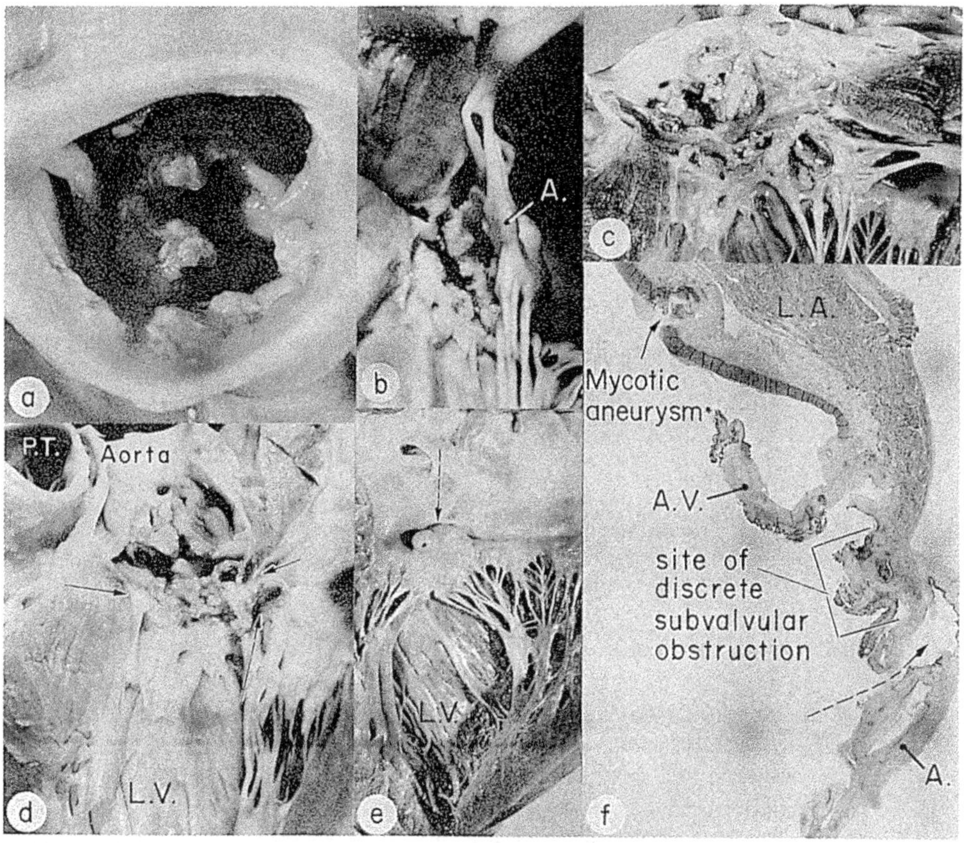

Figure 4. Alpha hemolytic streptococcus endocarditis complicating congenitally discrete subaortic stenosis in a 28-year-old man. The infection, which appeared about nine months before death, produced severe valvular aortic regurgitation. a, Aortic valve as viewed from above. b, Left ventricular outflow tract viewed from below showing vegetative material on the subvalvular "membrane" adjacent to the anterior mitral leaflet (A.). c, Opened left ventricular outflow tract showing vegetations on each aortic cusp, and on the subvalvular "membrane" and ventricular surface of anterior mitral leaflet. d, Longitudinal section showing the left ventricular outflow tract. The area of subaortic stenosis is well seen (between the solid arrows) and a mycotic aneurysm (dashed arrow) is seen in the anterior mitral leaflet. The mitral aneurysm is in the high pressure portion of the left ventricle (L.V.), i.e., below the discrete subvalvular obstruction. P.T. = pulmonary trunk. e, Opened mitral valve showing atrial aspect of the mycotic aneurysm (dashed arrow) on the anterior leaflet. f, Photomicrograph of section through aorta, left atrium (L.A.) aortic valve (A.V.) cusp. subvalvular "membrane," and anterior mitral leaflet (A.). A mycotic aneurysm is present in the ascending aorta as well as in the anterior mitral leaflet (dashed arrow). Vegetations are present on the aortic valve cusp and on the subvalvular membrane. (Hematoxylin-eosin, reduced 35% from × 3.2.)

is also of two types: (1) that involving a previously congenitally malformed but initially functionally-normal valve, and (2) that involving a previously normally-formed valve.

Several types of congenitally malformed aortic valves have been described. Each type is determined by its number of cusps and commissures. At least two *unicuspid* aortic valves exist (Fig. 7). In one the orifice is located in the center

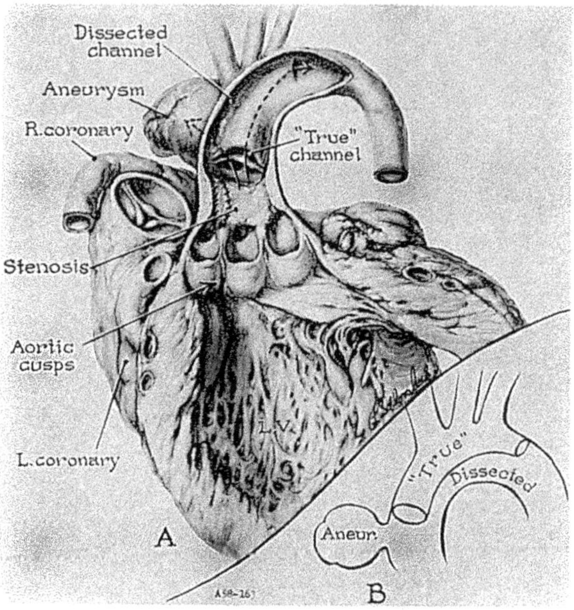

Figure 5. Supravalvular aortic stenosis of the hourglass type in an 18-year-old boy. In addition to the narrowing of the aorta just above the aortic valve, a large saccular aneurysm is present in the ascending aorta and a healed dissecting aneurysm is present in the ascending aorta. The diameters of the coronary arteries proximally are nearly as large as the descending thoracic aorta.

of the leaflet and there are no lateral attachments to the wall of the aorta. Edwards[8] has referred to this valve as the *simple-dome* type. It also may be considered an *acommissural* valve. It is often the type observed in the pulmonic area in patients with valvular pulmonic stenosis. Often three remnants of commissures are observed in this valve, and the undeveloped "commissures" have caused it to be confused with tricuspid aortic valves. A second type of unicuspid valve is the *unicommissural* one (see Fig. 1). This valve, described by Edwards in 1958,[8] is characterized by an eccentrically located orifice and only one lateral attachment to the aortic wall at the level of the orifice. From above, this valve has the appearance of an exclamation mark. Remnants of undeveloped commissures also are present in the unicommissural valve.[1]

The most frequent malformation of the aortic valve is the presence of only two cusps. The *bicuspid* valve is basically of two types (Figs. 8–10)[7]: (1) the cusps are located right and left, the commissures anteriorly and posteriorly, a raphe or false commissure, if present, is always in the right cusp, and a coronary artery arises from behind each cusp; (2) the cusps are located anteriorly and posteriorly, the commissures right and left, a raphe, if present, is always in the anterior cusp, and both coronary arteries arise in front of the anterior cusp. These two types are divided about equally among patients with congenitally bicuspid aortic valves.[7]

Occasionally a *tricuspid* aortic valve is malformed. When this occurs the cusps are of unequal size. Minor differences in cuspal size are frequent, but major differences appear to constitute a congenital malformation. There may be some basis for believing that contact of unequal-sized cusps with one another can lead to focal cuspal fibrosis with eventual calcification and stenosis.[9] A *quadricuspid* aortic valve on rare occasion may be stenotic.[10] Most quadricuspid

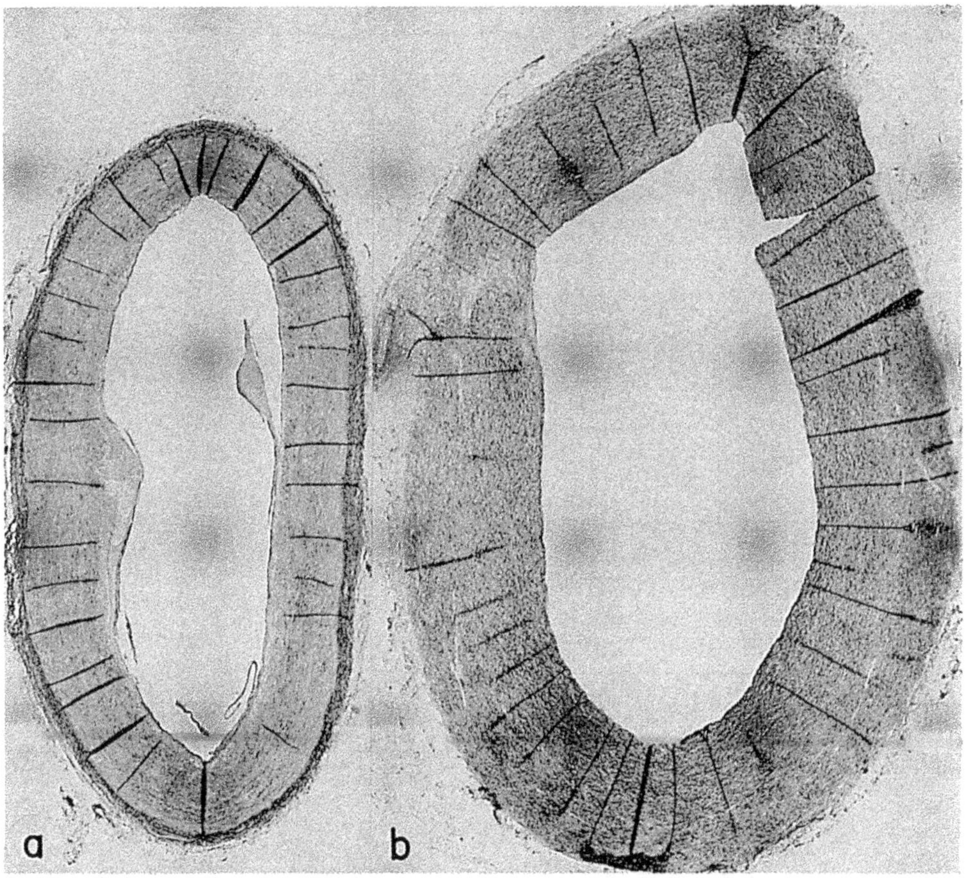

Figure 6. Histologic sections of right coronary artery (a) and descending thoracic aorta (b) in the patient described in Figure 5 and as patient 5. The lumens of these two arteries are comparable since each was taken at the same magnification. The coronary artery is thick-walled and contains more elastic fibers than normally but certainly not nearly as many as does the aorta. (Elastic tissue stains, reduced 5% from × 10.)

valves, however, function normally. An occasional one may be purely incompetent.[11] Although six-cuspid valves may occur, particularly in persistent truncus arteriosus, stenosis of these multicuspid valves is rare.

Function of the malformed aortic valves at birth is variable. The fewer the number of cusps and commissures the greater the likelihood that the valve is stenotic at birth. Edwards[8,12] has emphasized that the acommissural and unicommissural unicuspid valves are stenotic from birth. The orifices of these valves are small and there is little opportunity for the valvular orifice to alter its size during either phase of the cardiac cycle; most patients dying in the first year or so of life from congenital aortic stenosis have unicuspid valves.[12] Most patients with unicuspid aortic valves have precordial murmurs from birth, whereas this is probably not the case in most patients with congenitally bicuspid aortic valves.

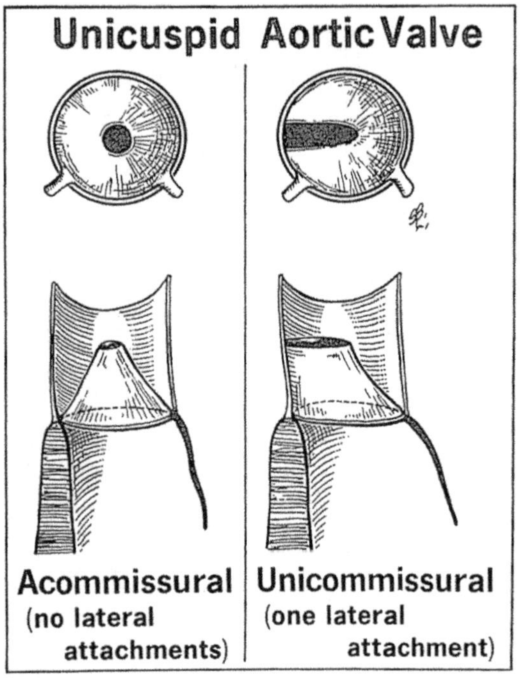

Figure 7. Diagram depicting the two types of unicuspid aortic valves: the simple dome or acommissural (left) and unicommissural (right).

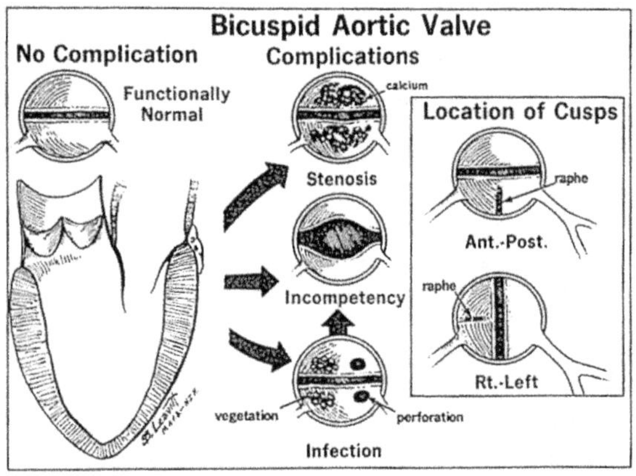

Figure 8. The congenitally bicuspid aortic valve. The location of the cusps and raphes and the acquired complications of this congenital malformation are depicted.

According to Edwards,[13] the bicuspid aortic valve is usually not stenotic at birth; it becomes stenotic only as it thickens and calcifies. This view, however, is not a universal one. Many surgeons, for example, describe stenotic aortic valves in children at operation as being bicuspid. Among 30 patients, mostly children, with congenital valvular aortic stenosis operated upon by Morrow,[14] 18 had bicuspid valves, 11 tricuspid, and 1 a unicommissural unicuspid valve. Unicommissural valves, however, may well be called bicuspid at operation. Unicommissural valves are the most frequent ones found in fatal congenital aortic valve stenosis in early life.[12]

Tricuspid aortic valves rarely appear to be stenotic at birth. If stenosis is present at birth and the aortic valve is three-cuspid, the stenosis is more usually

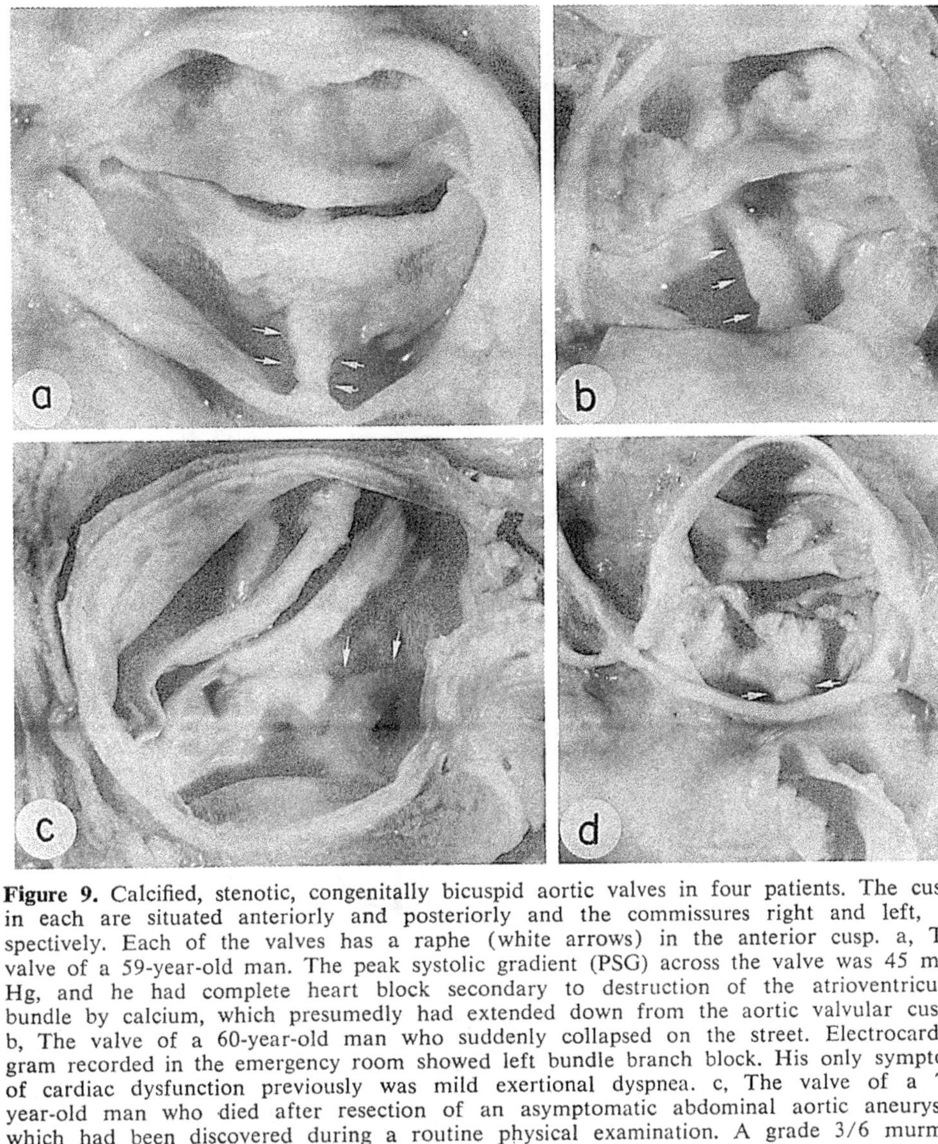

Figure 9. Calcified, stenotic, congenitally bicuspid aortic valves in four patients. The cusps in each are situated anteriorly and posteriorly and the commissures right and left, respectively. Each of the valves has a raphe (white arrows) in the anterior cusp. a, The valve of a 59-year-old man. The peak systolic gradient (PSG) across the valve was 45 mm. Hg, and he had complete heart block secondary to destruction of the atrioventricular bundle by calcium, which presumedly had extended down from the aortic valvular cusps. b, The valve of a 60-year-old man who suddenly collapsed on the street. Electrocardiogram recorded in the emergency room showed left bundle branch block. His only symptom of cardiac dysfunction previously was mild exertional dyspnea. c, The valve of a 75-year-old man who died after resection of an asymptomatic abdominal aortic aneurysm, which had been discovered during a routine physical examination. A grade 3/6 murmur consistent with aortic stenosis had been heard, but he had no symptoms of cardiac dysfunction. The heart weighed 600 gm. d, The valve of a 51-year-old man. The PSG across this valve was only 18 mm. Hg, but the valve was severely incompetent, and the heart weighed 800 gm. Electrocardiogram showed left bundle branch block.

the result of a very small aortic "annulus" rather than the result of fusion of the cusps. Acquired stenosis of a three-cuspid aortic valve, in contrast, is very common (Fig. 11). Of the 168 patients, aged 15 to 65 years, with clinically isolated aortic stenosis (with or without regurgitation) studied by me at necropsy (Table 2), 59 (35 per cent) had tricuspid valves, and among the 27 patients

Table 2. Structure of aortic valve in valvular aortic stenosis

Valve structure	*Number (%) patients < age 15 years*	*Number (%) patients age 15 to 56 years*	*Number (%) patients > age 65 years*	*Totals*
Unicuspid	*			
Acommissural		0	0	0
Unicommissural		19 (12)	0	19 (10)
Bicuspid	*	79 (47)	2 (7)	81 (41)
Tricuspid	*	59 (35)	25 (93)	84 (43)
Uncertain	*	11 (6)	0	11 (6)
Totals		168 (100)	27 (100)	195 (100)

* Information not available.

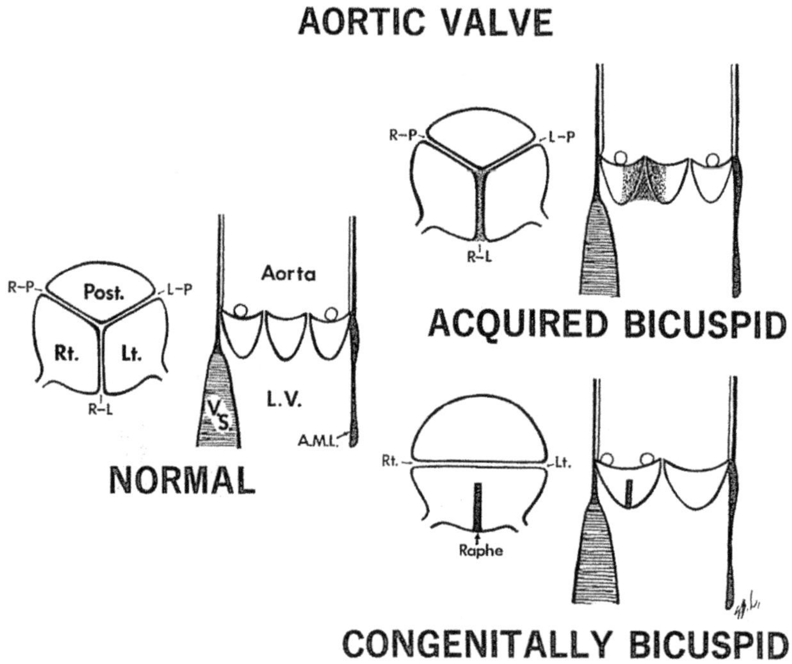

Figure 10. Diagram illustrating differences between bicuspid aortic valves of acquired and congenital origins as compared to the normal valve. The circumferential distances between each of the three commissures in a normally formed valve are similar. L-P = left-posterior, R-L = right-left, and R-P = right-posterior commissures; Rt. = right, Lt. = left, and Post. = posterior cusps; V.S. = ventricular septum; L.V. = left ventricular outflow tract; and A.M.L. = anterior mitral leaflet. In the acquired bicuspid valve the circumferential distances between the commissures remain equal, as in the normal. The fused commissure is wide, the distal margins of each of the two fused cusps are still usually visible, and the most cephalad margin of the fused commissure is on the same horizontal level as the most cephalad margins of the two nonfused commissures. In the congenitally bicuspid valve the raphe (false commissure) is generally narrow and rarely extends to the free margin of the conjoined cusp or to the cephalad level reached by the two true commissures. The circumferential distance between the two true commissures is greater than the circumferential distances between either true commissure and the raphe. The circumferential distance between the true commissures around the conjoined cusp, i.e., the one containing the raphe, is equal to or slightly greater than the circumferential distance between the true commissures around the cusp devoid of the raphe.

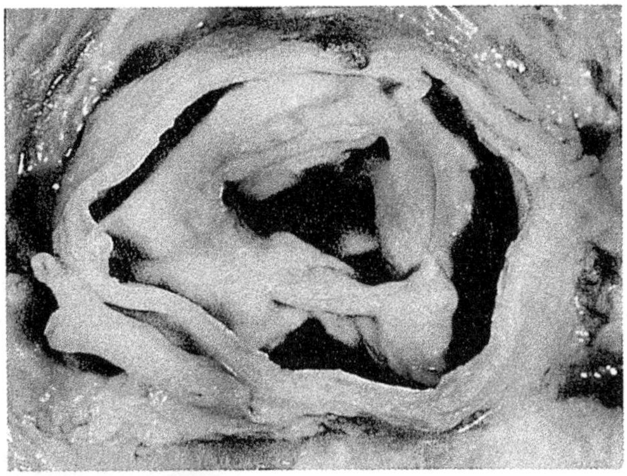

Figure 11. Stenotic tricuspid aortic valve in a 55-year-old man. Each of the three commissures is fused producing a triangular-shaped fixed central orifice which is both stenotic and incompetent.

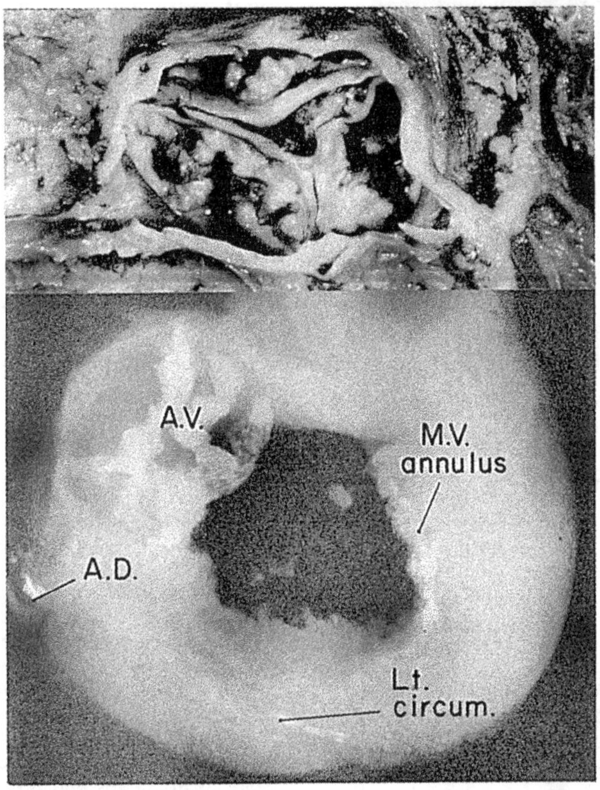

Figure 12. Stenotic three-cuspid aortic valve and radiograph of heart in a 71-year-old man who died of severe congestive cardiac failure. In addition to heavy aortic valvular (A.V.) calcific deposits, similar deposits are present in the mitral valve (M.V.) annulus and in the anterior descending (A.D.) and left (Lt.) circumflex coronary arteries. The aortic valve is severely stenotic. In contrast to the usual type stenotic aortic valve observed in older patients, one of the 3 commissures is completely fused.

over age 65, 25 (93 per cent) had tricuspid valves. In the 15 to 65-year age group, about half of the 59 patients with clinically isolated aortic stenosis had diffuse fibrous thickening of the mitral leaflets as well. The associated diffuse mitral leaflet thickening in them is strong evidence that the etiology of the stenosis in this group is rheumatic.[14] Also, about 70 per cent of this group had positive histories of acute rheumatic fever, whereas only 6 per cent of the other group (i.e., those with anatomically normal mitral valves) with valvular aortic stenosis had positive histories.[14] The etiology of the aortic stenosis in the patients with anatomically normal mitral valves is unsolved. Possibly, as mentioned earlier, minor abnormalities in the sizes of the aortic valve cusps from birth set the stage for abnormal contact of the leaflets with one another with resultant fibrosis and finally stenosis.[9]

Stenosis of the aortic valve in patients over age 65 years is usually characteristic (Figs. 2,12,13).[3] The valves are tricuspid; nodular calcific deposits are rather uniformly distributed on the aortic aspects of the cusps; and the commissures are not fused. Obstruction is due entirely to the presence of large calcific deposits which prevent the cusps from retracting adequately during ventricular systole. Because the commissures are usually not fused, associated aortic regurgitation is infrequent.

Clinically, aortic stenosis in the elderly is characterized by several features which are either absent or more prominent than in younger subjects with this valvular lesion: (1) the systemic arterial pulse pressure may be increased due to systolic hypertension; (2) a harsh right basal systolic murmur may be relatively inconspicuous while a pure musical systolic murmur may be prominent at the apex; (3) a coexisting apical systolic murmur of mitral regurgitation may be related to mitral annular calcification and not to left ventricular failure; and (4) systemic systolic hypertension can result in a comparatively small pressure gradient despite severe left ventricular outflow obstruction.

Certain auscultatory signs that accompany aortic stenosis in the elderly require explanation.[3] Ejection sounds are characteristically absent since the cusps are rigid and ejection sounds depend upon abrupt movement of mobile valves. Atrial sounds (fourth heart sounds) are useful signs for judging the severity of aortic stenosis in the younger adult but are of little help in this regard in the elderly patient since they may occur normally in the older age group.

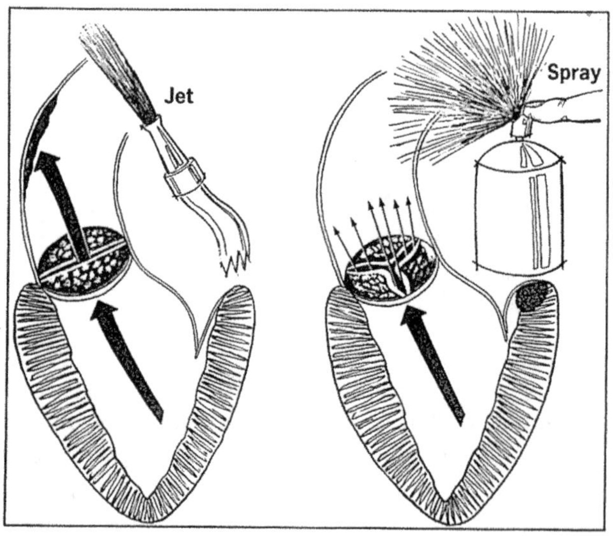

Figure 13. Diagram illustrating anatomic and auscultatory differences between aortic stenosis in younger patients (left) and in elderly patients (right). A jet lesion appears to occur when severe fixed stenosis is present and the valve structure in this situation is most commonly congenitally bicuspid. In the older patients with stenotic tricuspid aortic valves and little or no commissural fusion, the stenosis is probably not fixed and a spray effect may occur. Mitral annular calcification also is usually present in the elderly patients with valvular aortic stenosis.

Ordinarily, the systolic murmur of valvular aortic stenosis is harsh, rough, grunting, and loudest at the right base with radiation upward and to the right. In elderly patients with aortic stenosis, the harsh murmur at the right base may persist but be of less intensity, and auscultation may be dominated instead by a loud, pure frequency, musical systolic murmur maximal at or near the cardiac apex. At least three reasons account for these patterns. First, older persons tend to have increased upper thoracic chest dimensions which soften the basal murmurs. Second is the effect of the morphology of the stenotic aortic valve. A rigid, calcified valve *with* commissural fusion provides a suitable mechanism for a high velocity jet into the ascending aorta (see Fig. 13); the noisy murmur at the right base appears to originate within the ascending aorta because of turbulence caused by the high velocity jet. A calcified, stenotic, trileaflet aortic value *without* commissural fusion, the most common type in the elderly, behaves differently. Ejection into the ascending aorta may take the form of a "spray" instead of a jet (see Fig. 13), so that the harsh murmur at the right base may be comparatively inconspicuous. Since the cusps are not fused, they may vibrate during ventricular ejection and the latter may account for the pure frequency, musical cooing murmur recordable within the left ventricle. Third, calcification of the mitral annulus, itself a producer of precordial murmurs, in elderly patients frequently accompanies calcification of the aortic valve. Mitral regurgitation can result from inability of the calcified annulus to decrease its circumference during ventricular contraction. Accordingly, the holosystolic murmur of mitral regurgitation may be present at the apex and may be difficult to distinguish from the coexisting pure frequency aortic stenotic apical murmur. Although mitral annular calcification tends to complicate the auscultatory diagnosis of aortic stenosis, the radiologic identification of these calcific deposits implies that coexisting aortic stenosis is likely to be caused by calcific deposits on a trileaflet valve without commissural fusion.

The degree of left ventricular systolic hypertension in elderly patients may be considerably higher than that occurring in younger subjects with similar degrees of aortic stenosis, since the peripheral systolic systemic pressure usually rises with age. The degree of systolic hypertension which the elderly left ventricle is capable of achieving can be astonishingly high, particularly since this chamber seldom maintains a systolic pressure in excess of 250 mm. Hg even in younger subjects. Systemic hypertension may reduce the aortic gradient, and the degree of obstruction may be underestimated in the elderly patients if the peak systolic pressure difference is taken as the only index of severity. As the gradient diminishes in the presence of systemic systolic hypertension, the murmur at the right base may soften and shorten. Even if this auscultatory change does not occur with systemic hypertension, the modification of the systemic arterial pulse may be misleading since the rate of rise can be relatively normal and the pulse pressure increased despite severe obstruction to the left ventricular outflow.

Another important clinical feature in elderly patients with aortic stenosis is the presence of atrial fibrillation in about one third of them. This arrhythmia, however, is common in elderly persons without valvular cardiac disease. The left atrial cavities are mildly dilated in patients with aortic stenosis, but left atrial dilatation commonly accompanies old age in the absence of functionally significant valvular lesions. The left ventricular wall becomes less compliant with age, and the superimposed left ventricular hypertrophy (without left ventricular dilatation) of aortic stenosis may further impede left atrial emptying. The only common anatomic feature in elderly patients with atrial fibrillation is left atrial dilatation.[15a] The combination of atrial fibrillation, a long apical systolic murmur, and left atrial dilatation can obscure the diagnosis of aortic stenosis and lead to a mistaken diagnosis of isolated mitral regurgitation. Atrial fibrillation is especially undesirable in aortic stenosis since the left ventricle requires the help of augmented left atrial contraction which increases end-diastolic fiber length and permits the left ventricle to contract with greater force.

The cause of the aortic stenosis in elderly patients in uncertain, but simple wear-and-tear or degeneration appears to be the most reasonable explanation. The presence in the same hearts of other wear-and-tear lesions such as calcified mitral annuli, calcified coronary arteries, and focal thickening of other valve leaflets supports this contention. Certainly there is nothing to support a rheumatic etiology.

Although relatively few patients with valvular aortic stenosis have positive histories of acute rheumatic fever, the occurrence of a positive history in a patient presenting clinically with apparently pure aortic stenosis (with or without regurgitation) should caution the examining physician to the possibility of accompanying mitral valvular disease. Usually in this situation the mitral leaflets are diffusely, although mildly, thickened but mitral valvular function is normal. On rare occasions, however, mitral stenosis may be an accompanying lesion and of such severity that it is clinically silent (Figs. 14, 15). Mitral stenosis should be ruled out, however, before operative therapy is undertaken in any patient presenting with apparently isolated valvular aortic stenosis (with or without regurgitation) and a positive history of acute rheumatic fever.

HYPERTROPHIC (ASYMMETRIC) CARDIOMYOPATHY WITH OR WITHOUT SUBAORTIC STENOSIS (IDIOPATHIC HYPERTROPHIC SUBAORTIC STENOSIS [IHSS]

This section will summarize observations in 32 patients with hypertrophic cardiomyopathy studied at necropsy by the author. Findings in some of these patients have been described previously.[16-19] The 32 patients ranged in age from 12 to 78 years (avg. 46): 20 were women, 12 were males. Other family members of 13 patients had similar cardiac conditions. Ten patients had systemic hypertension; 5, anemia (blood hematocrit $<$ 35 per cent); 8, atrial fibrillation; 9, bundle branch block (left in 3, indeterminate in 5, and bilateral in 1); and 1, complete heart block. The latter was preceded by left bundle branch block. Thirteen patients died naturally of the cardiac condition (8, suddenly; 5, progressive congestive cardiac failure); 7, after a cardiac operation; 3 of complications of cardiac catheterization; and 9 from noncardiac causes.

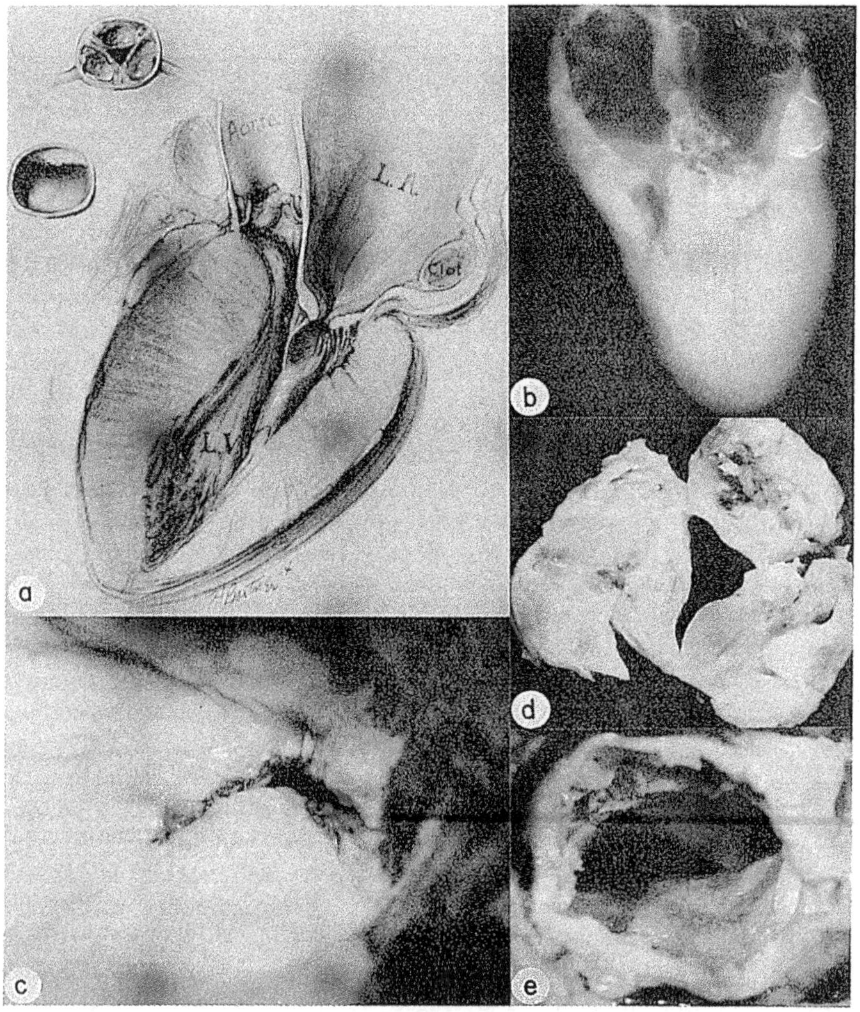

Figure 14. Heart of a 59-year-old woman with severe but clinically silent mitral stenosis associated with severe and clinically apparent valvular aortic stenosis. This patient had a positive history of acute rheumatic fever when she was 12 years old. She developed mild exertional dyspnea and atrial fibrillation at age 45 and, at age 56, angina pectoris and syncope appeared. On admission several days before death, she was functionally class IV (New York Heart Association). In addition to atrial fibrillation she had episodic complete heart block. A grade 4/6 systolic ejection murmur consistent with aortic stenosis and a grade 1/6 blowing diastolic murmur consistent with aortic regurgitation were heard. No diastolic apical rumble was audible. The left ventricular pressure (obtained by percutaneous left ventricular puncture) was 263/25 and the brachial arterial pressure was 195/60, yielding a 68 mm. Hg peak systolic pressure gradient. The cardiac index was 1.45 L./min./m^2. Aortic valve replacement was attempted but she died in the operating room.

The findings at necropsy are summarized in (a). The mitral valve was found to be severely stenotic. The left ventricular cavity and ascending aorta were small, and a thrombus was found in the body of the left atrium. The ventricular septum bulged into the left ventricular outflow tract and it contacted calcific deposits on the anterior mitral leaflet. The ventricular septum, however, was not thicker than was the left ventricular free wall (b). Calcium was present in the mitral and aortic valves, left atrial thrombus and coronary arteries. c, Stenotic mitral valve from left atrium. d, Excised three-cuspid stenotic aortic valve. e, Left ventricular outflow tract with aortic valve excised showing the ventricular septum protruding toward the anterior mitral leaflet.

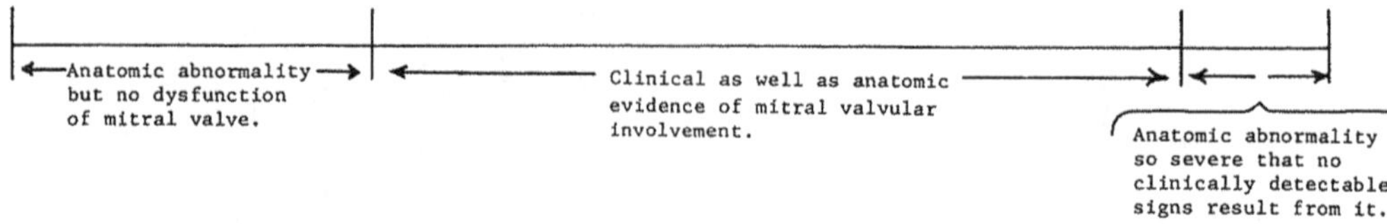

Figure 15. Spectrum of mitral valvular disease in patients with clinical evidence of aortic valvular disease and a positive history of acute rheumatic fever or chorea.

The 32 patients were divided into three groups (Table 3) on the basis of documentation by cardiac catheterization of the presence or absence of peak systolic pressure gradient (PSG) at rest between left ventricle and a systemic artery. Fourteen patients had subaortic stenosis with PSG at rest from 20 to 162 mm. Hg (average 93) (Group I). Eleven patients who had zero pressure gradients at rest comprise Group II; in 8 of them, however, gradients (range 10 to 150 mm. Hg) occurred with provocation. The seven patients in whom cardiac catheterization was not performed comprise Group III. Diagnosis of IHSS was established preoperatively in 13 of 14 patients in Group I, in 9 of 11 patients in Group II, and in only 2 of 7 patients in Group III. The fourteenth patient in Group I was studied in 1956 before IHSS was recognized as a distinct entity. The other two patients in Group II clinically had pure mitral regurgitation believed to be on a rheumatic basis. At mitral valve replacement in one, the left ventricular wall was found to be thick, and the cavity small; IHSS, therefore, was suspected and later confirmed at postoperative catheterization. The clue to proper diagnosis of IHSS in each of the two patients in Group III was rapidly rising systemic arterial pulses. An additional clue in one patient was increased intensity of the precordial systolic murmur during the beats following premature ventricular contractions.[17] Diagnosis of IHSS in each of the eight patients in whom this diagnosis was not established or strongly suspected clinically was made at necropsy by observing anatomic cardiac findings identical to those in patients in whom the diagnosis was established by clinical means. Six of the eight clinically nondiagnosed patients were in Group III.

The 14 patients in Group I averaged 45 years of age; the 11 in Group II, 34 years; and the seven in Group III, 67 years. All patients in Group I had symptoms of cardiac dysfunction; one patient in Group II and four in Group III were asymptomatic. Whereas only four patients in Group I had histories of similar heart disease in other family members, all nine patients in Group II in whom this information was available had positive histories. Precordial systolic murmurs ranging in intensity from grade 3/6 to 5/6 were present at some time in all 14 patients in Group I. In one patient, however, a grade 3/6 systolic precordial murmur was audible eight years before death when the PSG was 70 mm Hg, but when examined during the last year of life, no precordial murmur was audible. Similar murmurs occurred in 10 of 11 patients in Group II but their intensity was less (grade 3/6 in three patients; grade 2/6 in four; grade 1/6 in three). Systolic murmurs were audible in six (grade 4/6 in one; grade 3/6 in four) of seven patients in Group III. Three of 14 patients in Group I, 4 of 11 in Group II, and 1 of 7 in Group III had atrial

Table 3. Clinical and necropsy observations in hypertrophic cardiomyopathy: 32 necropsy patients

Groups	No. patients	Positive family history of heart disease	Ages (years) Range (avg.)	Sex No. F	Sex No. M	Length of symptoms (years) Range (avg.)	Hyper-tension*	LV–SA PSG (mm. Hg) (rest)	LV–SA PSG (mm. Hg) (provocation)	Heart wt. (grams) Range (avg.)	VS > LVFW	"Small" or normal RV and LV cavities	Endocardial plaque LVO	Thick mitral valve	Dilated left atrium	Normal aortic valve	No. of patients with CA > 50% narrowed
I With subaortic stenosis	14	4	18–70 (45)	9	5	4 mo.–25 (9)	4	20–162 (93)	80–140† (104)	390–800 (580)	11	14	14	14	13	11	6‡
II Without subaortic stenosis	11	9§	12–55 (34)	6	5	0–18 (7)	1	0	0–150‖	350–1020¶ (563)	10	10	6	6	10	11	0
III No catheterization	7	0	49–78 (67)	5	2	0–20** (3)	5	–	–	430–710 (518)	6	7	4	4	7	7	0
TOTALS	32	13	12–78 (46)	20	12	0–25 (7)	10	0–162	0–150	350–1020¶ (582)	27	31	24	24	30	29	6‡

* Systemic blood pressure by cuff > 140 systolic or > 90 mm. Hg diastolic or both.

† The PSG increased in each of the seven patients provoked (by isoproterenol or Valsalva maneuver).

‡ Only one of the total 32 patients had left ventricular or ventricular septal scarring which extended through the entire wall (transmural).

§ No information available in two patients.

‖ Of ten patients provoked, PSG remained zero in two and increased 10 to 150 mm. Hg in eight. In only one of the eight, however, was the PSG with provocation > 32 mm. Hg.

¶ Heart in a child, aged 12, not included in this total. His heart weighed 250 gm.

** Five of the seven patients had no symptoms of cardiac dysfunction.

ABBREVIATIONS: CA = coronary artery; LV = left ventricle; LVFW = left ventricular free wall; LVO = left ventricular outflow tract; PSG = peak systolic gradient; RV = right ventricle; SA = systemic artery; VS = ventricular septum.

fibrillation. Of 10 patients in Group I in whom left ventricular angiographic studies were performed, four had mitral regurgitation. Six patients in Group I and four in Group II had systolic pressure gradients between right ventricle and pulmonary artery. One of the latter patients had a 128 mm. Hg PSG between right ventricular body and pulmonary artery and no PSG between left ventricle and systemic artery. His brother, however, had typical left-sided IHSS. Two patients in Group I and three in Group II had pulmonary hypertension; in only one patient (Group I) was the pulmonary systolic pressure more than 50 mm. Hg. Three of six patients in Group I and five of seven patients in Group II had elevated left atrial pressures; all eight patients with elevated left atrial pressures had either mitral regurgitation or elevated left ventricular end-diastolic pressures. Nine patients in Group I and seven in Group II had elevated ($\geqq$ 12 mm. Hg) left ventricular end-diastolic pressures.

Necropsy cardiac observations in 32 patients are summarized in Table 3. The heart weights of the 31 adult patients ranged from 350 to 1020 gm. (avg. 582); the hearts of the 20 women averaged 511 gm., and those of the 11 adult men, 662 gm. In 27 patients, the ventricular septa were unequivocally thicker than the left ventricular free walls and in 31 patients both ventricular cavities appeared smaller than normal or normal in size. In only one patient were the ventricular cavities unequivocally dilated. The mural endocardium of the left ventricular outflow tract in apposition to the anterior mitral leaflet was thickened in 24 patients. The mitral valve leaflets, particularly the anterior ones, were thickened by fibrous tissue in 24 patients. Both left and right atria were dilated in 30 patients. Except for fibromas in two patients and mild diffuse thickening in one, the aortic valve cusps were normal. Foci of fibrosis were observed grossly in the left ventricular papillary muscles in 31 patients and these structures appeared smaller than normal in all of them. Other subendocardial scars were present grossly in a number of patients. Only one had transmural fibrosis and it was small. Except for several patients who died after cardiac operations, no foci of myocardial necrosis were present. Histologic examination of sections of left ventricular free wall and ventricular septum disclosed interstitial and perivascular fibrosis of varying degrees in all patients and usually foci of replacement fibrosis as well. Varying degrees of disorientation of myocardial fibers were observed in histologic sections of the ventricular septa in all 32 patients. A marked prominence of intramural coronary arteries in the ventricular septa was observed in one patient.

The myocardium in the left ventricular outflow tract of patients with IHSS is distinctive by light and electron microscopy. Ferrans and coworkers[20] studied by electron microscope the operatively-excised left ventricular outflow tract muscle in 14 patients with IHSS. Distinctive abnormalities were found in each patient. Bundles of muscle cells were severely disorganized with cells running in different directions instead of parallel. Muscle cells were wider and shorter than in hypertrophy due to other causes and showed increased cellular branching, extensive side-to-side intercellular junctions, widened Z bands, and evidence of formation of new sarcomeres. Some myofibrils were oriented obliquely or perpendicular to the longitudinal axes of the cells, and some myofilaments that originated from a single Z band inserted into Z bands of other myofibrils. Examination of left ventricular apical myocardium in 2 of the 14 patients disclosed hypertrophied but normally arranged muscle cells. The abnormal architecture of the muscle cells appears to be the basic morphologic feature of hypertrophic cardiomyopathy.

Study of the above-described patients with hypertrophic cardiomyopathy allows delineation of characteristic anatomic features of this entity: (1) disproportional hypertrophy of the ventricular septum; (2) small or normal-sized left and right ventricular cavities; (3) endocardial mural plaque, left ventricular outflow tract; (4) thickened mitral valve; (5) dilated left and right atria; (6) hypertrophied free walls of all four cardiac chambers; (7) normal or nearly-normal aortic valve cusps; (8) normal-sized ascending aorta; (9) severe abnormalities involving the organization of muscle cell bundles and the arrangement and orientation of myofibrils and myofilaments of individual muscle cells in the ventricular septum (Fig. 16).

The major gross anatomic feature of hypertrophic cardiomyopathy is disproportional hypertrophy of the ventricular septum, i.e., the ventricular septum is thicker than the left ventricular free wall. Normally, at all ages, the ventricular septum and left ventricular free wall are equal in thickness. Disproportional or asymmetric septal hypertrophy is the characteristic anatomic feature of hypertrophic cardiomyopathy. Disproportional septal hypertrophy and disorganization of the septal muscle fibers are probably the only anatomic features of hypertrophic cardiomyopathy present from birth. The other features appear secondary to these basic defects and are acquired later. Originally, it was believed that the thickest portion of the ventricular septum in this condition was that portion just below the aortic valve. Study of our 32 necropsy patients, however, clearly demonstrates that the thickest portion of the septum is about midway between the base of the aortic valve cusps and the apex of the left ventricle. The thickest portion of the septum also is usually just opposite the apex of the right ventricle. Thus, an adequate myotomy or myectomy in IHSS must include interruption or excision of myocardium located in the middle one third of the septum and not just that portion close to the aortic valve.

If asymmetric septal hypertrophy is considered nearly a sine qua non of hypertrophic cardiomyopathy, an explanation is required for the inclusion of five among the 32 patients in whom this feature did not occur. In all five the septum and free wall were of equal thickness. One patient, a 50-year-old woman, had undergone left ventricular outflow myotomy and myectomy 31 months earlier with total obliteration of the systolic pressure gradient. This patient clearly had disproportional septal hypertrophy before operation. Two other patients, both women, age 33 and 46 years, respectively, had severe scarring of the ventricular septum without significant scarring of the free wall. It is probable that the scarring caused contracture of the septum in them. Furthermore, one patient had no pressure gradient at rest; the other one who eight years earlier had had a 70 mm. Hg peak systolic pressure gradient between left ventricle and a systemic artery and a loud precordial murmur, had no murmur when examined during her last months of life. The cause of the lack of disproportional septal

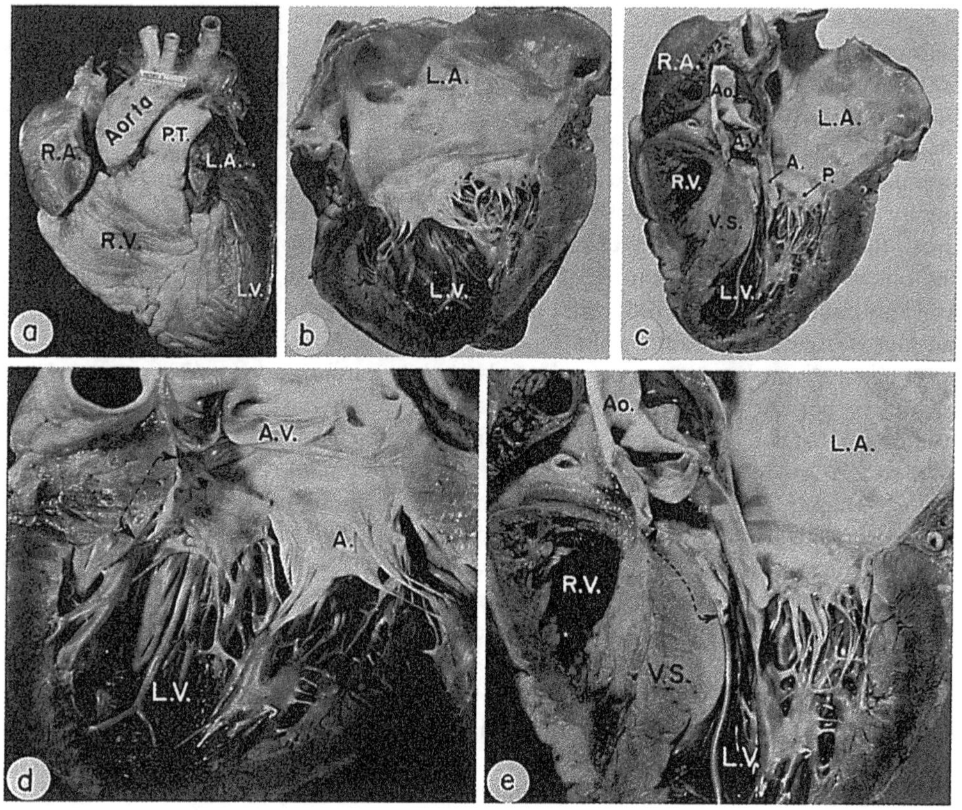

Figure 16. Heart of a 26-year-old man with familial hypertrophic cardiomyopathy and subaortic stenosis. At catheterization three years before death, a 30 mm. Hg peak systolic pressure gradient was present between left ventricle and brachial artery and the gradient increased to 85 mm. Hg with provocation (ouabain). The cardiac index was 2.1 L./min./m^2. At repeat catheterization six days before sudden death, this gradient at rest was zero and it rose to only 33 mm. Hg when provoked by isoproterenol. The cardiac index was 2.0 L./min./m^2.

The anatomic features of hypertrophic cardiomyopathy are demonstrated in these photographs. a, Exterior view. Both right (R.A.) and left (L.A.) atrium are dilated. P.T. = pulmonary trunk. R.V. = right ventricle. L.V. = left ventricle. b, Opened left atrium, mitral valve and left ventricle showing focal thickening of the mitral leaflets and chordae. c, Coronal section. The ventricular septum (V.S.) is thicker than the left ventricular free wall. Ao. = aorta. A. = anterior. P. = posterior mitral leaflets. A close-up view of the outflow tract is shown in (e). The left ventricular mural endocardial plaque opposite the anterior mitral leaflet is designated in (e). d, Opened aorta, aortic valve (A.V.) and left ventricle. The thickening of mural endocardium corresponds to the thickening of the anterior (A.) mitral leaflet. The aortic valve is normal.

hypertrophy in the fourth patient, a 65-year-old woman, is unclear. She was asymptomatic and never had evidence of cardiac dysfunction. Although she did not undergo cardiac catheterization, it is probable that she had no pressure gradient. The fifth patient, a 54-year-old woman had no left ventricular outflow gradient at rest and a 25 mm. Hg PSG with provocation. She was the only patient with dilated ventricular cavities and she did not have an outflow mural plaque or a thickened mitral valve. Four of her children, however, had catheterization-documented IHSS. The hearts in the five patients ranged from 370 to 500 gm. (avg. 437), smaller average weights than those in the other 27 patients with disproportional septal hypertrophy.

The small systolic pressure gradients between right ventricular body and pulmonary trunk which occur in many patients with hypertrophic cardiomyopathy almost certainly result from severe hypertrophy of the ventricular septum, since these gradients often disappear after left ventricular myotomy with or without myectomy. The cause of the hypertrophy of the right ventricular free wall in patients with IHSS without right ventricular systolic hypertension or outflow obstruction is uncertain.

The left ventricular cavity in hypertrophic cardiomyopathy is smaller than normal or normal in size. Most commonly, the cavity is slitlike with an S-shaped configuration. The papillary muscles actually contact one another during ventricular systole as do the anterior mitral leaflet and the mural endocardium of the left ventricular outflow tract. Fibromas, which appear to result from abnormal contact of surfaces together during ventricular contraction, were present in two of our patients. In one patient, a 19-year-old girl with a 162 mm. Hg left ventricular outflow tract pressure gradient, a saccular aneurysm was present at the apex of the left ventricle. It consisted entirely of myocardium but its thickness was considerably less than that of the wall in other areas.

The small left ventricular cavity appears to be responsible for the thickening of the mural endocardium in the left ventricular outflow tract and also for the fibrous thickening of the mitral leaflets. It is important to recall that the mitral valve resides in the left ventricle, which being relatively small in IHSS, causes abnormal contact of the leaflets with themselves and causes the anterior leaflet to contact the mural endocardial plaque in the left ventricular outflow tract. The caudal margin of the mural endocardial plaque corresponds precisely to the distal margin of the anterior mitral leaflet. The focal fibrous thickening of the posterior mitral leaflet probably results from contact of the mitral leaflets during ventricular systole, since there is not enough room in the left ventricular cavity to accommodate the leaflets and chordae easily. The ventricle and mitral leaflets in this respect may be regarded as being similar to an accordion. The mitral leaflet thickening in IHSS is somewhat analogous to that which occurs normally as a consequence of aging. With aging, the left ventricular cavity becomes smaller, presumably in response to the lowered cardiac output; the mitral leaflets, thicker; the left ventricular muscle, less compliant; and the left atrium dilates in response to increased work required to fill the small left ventricle. Similar mechanisms appear to be accelerated in IHSS.

Most patients with IHSS have some degree of mitral regurgitation. It is not related to annular dilatation since the mitral annulus in this condition is smaller than normal. Furthermore, the leaflet thickening in and of itself, is not extensive enough to cause valvular regurgitation. The most likely explanation appears to be abnormal bending of the papillary muscles, particularly the anterolateral one.[21] These structures may be bent abnormally by the bulging ventricular septum with resulting excessive tension on the chordae tendineae preventing closure of the mitral orifice. Although they are usually present in the papillary muscles in IHSS, focal scars cannot account for the regurgitation. Although it is usually mild in IHSS, mitral regurgitation may be the predominant clinical feature of this condition. Mitral valve replacement in IHSS is hazardous since the small left ventricular cavity is rarely capable of freely accommodating a prosthesis.

DISCRETE SUBAORTIC STENOSIS

Five adults, aged 17 to 47 years (avg. 28) with discrete subaortic stenosis (DSS), have been studied at necropsy by the author. Three were males, two, females. All five patients had precordial diastolic murmurs (grade 1–3/6 intensity) typical of aortic regurgitation, in addition to loud (grade 2–5/6) systolic murmurs typical of "aortic" stenosis. Left ventricular to systemic arterial peak systolic pressure gradients in four patients ranged from 70 to 170 mm. Hg (avg. 120) and pressure tracings in each indicated discrete obstruction in the subvalvular region. The left ventricular systolic pressures ranged from 156 to 270 mm. Hg (avg. 222). Four patients underwent operative resection of the subaortic membrane; three died within one month of operation, and one, six years later from degeneration of the silicone rubber of the caged ball prosthesis.[4] The one unoperated patient died at age 28 of undiagnosed alpha streptococcal endocarditis of the aortic valve.

In four patients DSS was the only congenital lesion present, but two of them developed infective endocarditis on the aortic valve producing severe aortic regurgitation.[4] The fifth patient had a large patent ductus arteriosus and mild isthmic aortic coarctation. In no patient was the ascending aorta dilated.

The subaortic membrane had been excised at operation in four patients and was still present at necropsy in only one (see Fig. 4). In each patient, however, the discrete membrane was or had been located in circumferential fashion on a plane corresponding with the ventricular aspect of the basal attachment of the anterior mitral leaflet. The membranes consisted of dense fibrous tissue. The aortic valves were three-cuspid in each patient, and their ventricular aspects in each were thickened by fibrous tissue. In none was the aortic valve narrowed or its "annulus" small. One was the site of active infective endocarditis (see Fig. 4. The hearts weighed 480 to 620 gm. (avg. 543). The left ventricles were severely hypertrophied in each patient but dilated in none. The left atria were normal in size in each patient. The left ventricular papillary muscles were the sites of focal scarring in all five patients.

A major purpose of summarizing the necropsy findings in these five patients with DSS is to emphasize the frequency of acquired lesions of the aortic valve in patients with this congenital malformation. All five patients had thickened aortic valve cusps and each had precordial murmurs of aortic regurgitation in addition to murmurs of "aortic" stenosis. The thickening and incompetence of the aortic valves in most or all of these subjects almost certainly resulted from contact of blood ejected through the narrowed subaortic orifice under high pressure onto the aortic cusps. The resulting jet lesions are highly susceptible to infection, and bacterial endocarditis occurred in two of the five patients. The patients were 28 and 41 years old, respectively, when the aortic valvular infective endocarditis appeared. It produced severe aortic regurgitation in each.

Several anatomic differences between DSS and IHSS need amplifying (Fig. 17). In both conditions, mural endocardial thickening occurs in the left ventricular outflow tract. In DSS, however, the endocardial thickening consists of a fibrous ridge on a plane corresponding with the annulus fibrosis of the anterior mitral leaflet. This fibrous band is located about 1 cm. caudal to the base of the aortic valve cusps. Just caudal to the fibrous band the mural endocardium may be thickened in a plaquelike fashion as in IHSS, but this flat mural thickening has an irregular longitudinal extension caudally and does not have a clear cutoff point corresponding to the distal margin of the anterior mitral leaflet as in IHSS. In IHSS no discrete circumferential fibrous membrane is present in the left ventricular outflow tract. In DSS, the mitral leaflets, except for the most basal portion of the ventricular aspect of the anterior mitral leaflet, are normal, in contrast to IHSS. Disproportional hypertrophy of the ventricular septum appears unique to IHSS, but functionally residual subaortic obstruction may remain transiently after excision of the left ventricular outflow membrane in DSS. Fibrous thickening of the aortic valve cusps is an expected complication of DSS, whereas it is uncommon in IHSS. The aortic valve cusps in DSS even may develop calcific deposits. Aortic regurgitation is common in DSS but nearly unheard of in IHSS. Infective endocarditis, likewise, is rare in IHSS but common in DSS. Left atrial dilatation, common in IHSS, is uncommon in DSS.

Although most patients with IHSS or DSS can be clearly distinguished from one another, these two conditions appear to overlap on occasion (Fig. 18). Whether DSS can be transformed into "IHSS" or whether the overlap group begins life as such is unclear. Also, the anatomic and clinical features of patients with hypoplastic ascending aortae and aortic valve "annuli" with and without

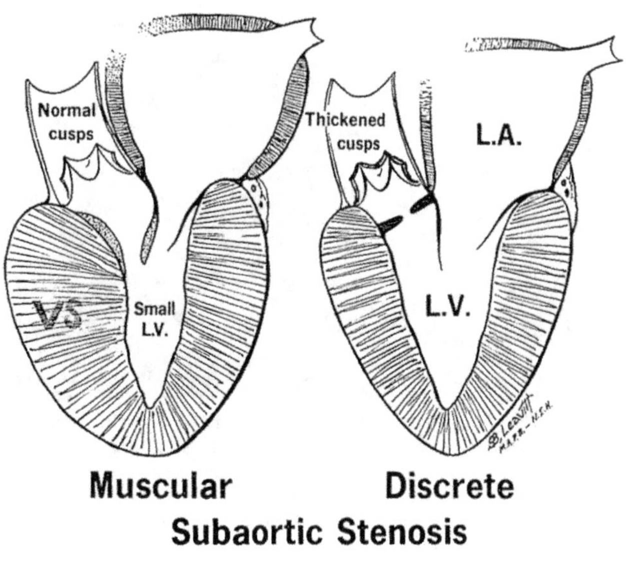

Figure 17. Diagram depicting the major anatomic differences between discrete and muscular subaortic stenosis.

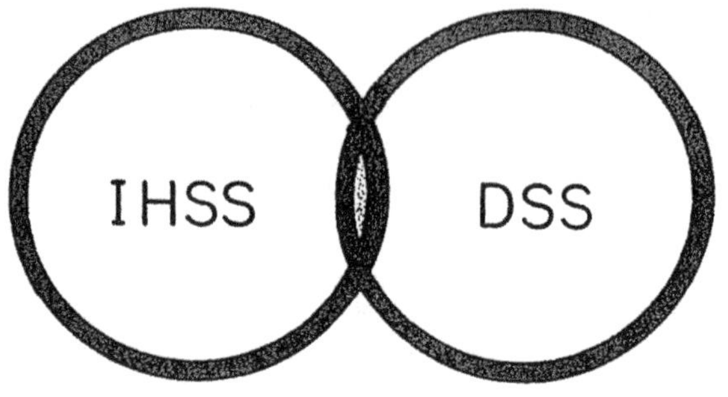

Figure 18. Diagram depicting a small overlap group between hypertrophic cardiomyopathy with diffuse subaortic stenosis (IHSS) and discrete subaortic stenosis (DSS).

actual aortic valve stenosis in association with subaortic obstruction, so-called *tunnel aortic stenosis,* are not yet clearly defined, but this condition is not uncommon and operative results in these patients are poor in contrast to the expected good results in patients with DSS and IHSS.[22]

Other conditions on occasion may be associated with varying degrees of discrete subaortic stenosis.[23] In all patients with partial A–V canal (endocardial cushion defect), chordae tendineae from the cleft anterior mitral leaflet insert onto the crest of the ventricular septum (Fig. 19). These anomalous chordae are responsible for the gooseneck type deformity in the left ventricular outflow tract on angiography. On rare occasion, these anomalous chordae may narrow the outflow tract to such an extent that actual subaortic stenosis is the result.[24] Of approximately 40 patients with partial A–V canal examined at necropsy

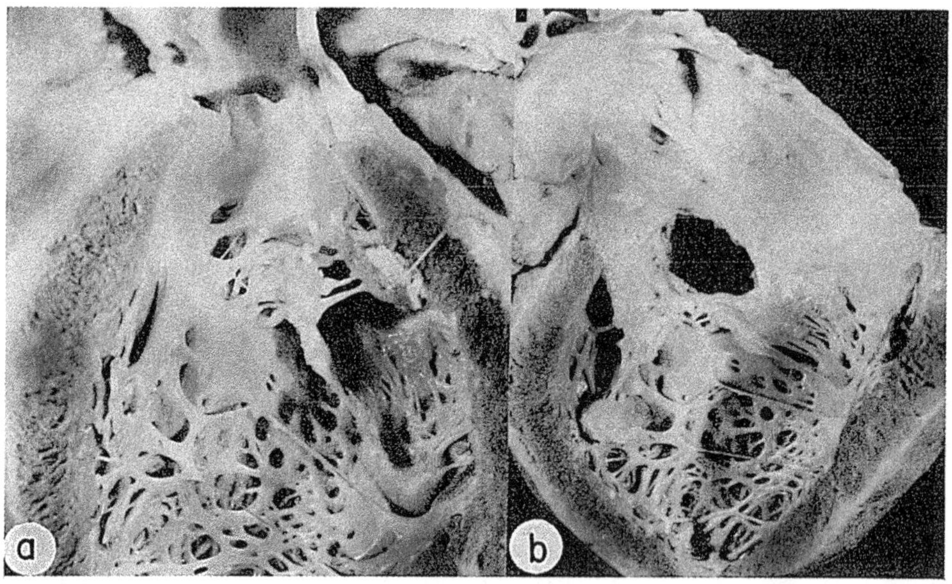

Figure 19. The heart of a 5-year-old boy with partial atrioventricular canal. a, Opened aorta, aortic valve and left ventricle showing anomalous chordae tendineae from the anterior mitral leaflet inserting onto the ventricular septum. b, Opened left atrium, mitral valve and left ventricle disclosing a defect in the lowermost portion of the atrial septum (ostium primum type defect) and a cleft in the anterior mitral leaflet. The anomalously inserting chordae tendineae arise from the margins of the cleft in the anterior leaflet.

by the author, clear anatomic obstruction by this mechanism was present in only one.

In the condition, combined ventricular septal defect and aortic regurgitation, a discrete membrane may be located just below the defect in the left ventricular outflow tract (Fig. 20). Of six patients with combined ventricular septal defect and aortic regurgitation studied at necropsy by the author, two had had small (20 and 30 mm. Hg) systolic pressure gradients at this location during life. The obstruction resulted from discrete fibrous thickening in this region.

Although diffuse muscular subaortic stenosis has been described in patients with single left ventricular papillary muscles, and indeed forms a part of the parachute mitral valve syndrome,[25] discrete subaortic stenosis may occur instead of the diffuse variety of left ventricular outflow obstruction (Fig. 21).[26]

SUPRAVALVULAR AORTIC STENOSIS

The least common variety of obstruction to left ventricular outflow is that which is due to narrowing of the ascending aorta, either discretely (just above the aortic valve and coronary ostia) or diffusely (involving its entire length). This malformation in some patients is inherited as an autosomal dominant trait.[27] In others, it is part of a more generalized disorder usually associated with hypercalcemia of infancy,[28] and indeed may be produced experimentally in newborn rabbits by hypervitaminosis D in their mothers.[29] A third group of

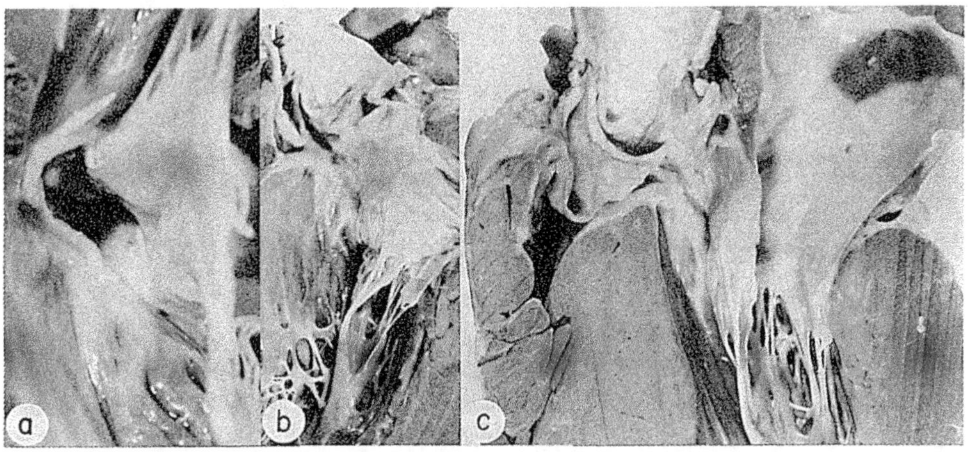

Figure 20. Fibrous membrane type discrete subaortic stenosis associated with combined congenital ventricular septal defect and aortic regurgitation in a 16-year-old boy. A 30 mm. Hg peak systolic pressure gradient was present between left ventricle and brachial artery. The pulmonary to systemic flow ratio was 1.3 to 1. This patient died suddenly one night before planned cardiac operation. a, Left ventricular outflow tract from below showing a discrete membrane on the mural endocardium. b, Opened aorta, aortic valve and left ventricle further delineating the fibrous membrane just below the aortic valve. c, Longitudinal section exposing right ventricle, ventricular septum, left ventricle, mitral and aortic valves, and left atrium. The right anterior aortic valve cusp has prolapsed into the right ventricle. The fibrous membrane is on the left ventricular aspect of the caudal margin of the ventricular septal defect.

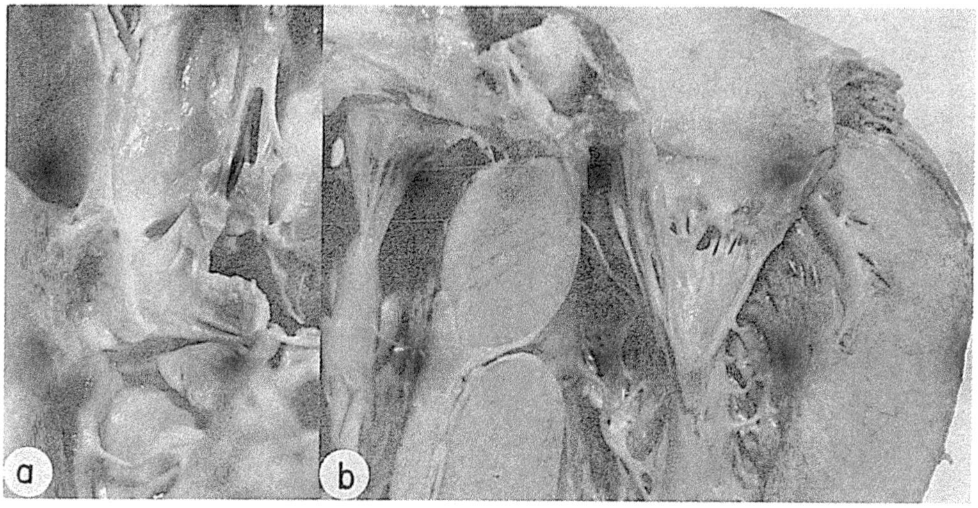

Figure 21. Discrete subaortic stenosis associated with valvular aortic stenosis superimposed on a congenitally bicuspid aortic valve, coarctation of the aorta, parachute mitral valve (single left ventricular papillary muscle) and spontaneously closed ventricular septal defect in a 14-year-old boy. This boy had congestive cardiac failure during his first twc months of life but thereafter was well until age 13 (one year before death) when congestive heart failure appeared again. Before that time he had participated in vigorous activities. Catheterization at age 5 years had disclosed a 90 mm. Hg peak systolic pressure gradient between left ventricle and a systemic artery, and restudy at age 13 disclosed an 80 mm. Hg gradient. Operation (Dr. Charles Hufnagel) was performed at age 6 years; the ascending aorta was found to be small and the aortic valve to be bicuspid with a small "annulus." It was not possible to widen the aortic valve area. He died in severe congestive cardiac failure eight years later. a, Left ventricular outflow tract from below disclosing discrete subaortic obstruction. b, Longitudinal section through left ventricular outflow tract showing a very small aortic root. The mitral valve has a parachute configuration. A spontaneously closed ventricular septal defect is apparent. Mitral valve function apparently was normal. The left ventricular outflow tract obstruction falls into the *tunnel* group.

patients with supravalvular aortic stenosis (SAS) has neither a family history of this anomaly nor any stigmata of infantile hypercalcemia.

Three anatomic types of SAS have been described by Edwards and his associates[23,30]: (1) an hourglass type of narrowing (66 per cent of 68 cases analyzed[30]) which is associated with severe thickening of aortic media and usually with superimposed fibrous intimal proliferation; (2) a fibrous membranous type with a central opening and a more normal-sized aorta (13 per cent); and (3) a hypoplastic type characterized by diffuse hypoplasia of the ascending aorta (21 per cent). The hourglass type occurred in each of the two patients with supravalvular aortic stenosis studied at necropsy by the author (see Fig. 5).[5] The area of obstruction in each patient was several millimeters in length, and the true lumen of the entire ascending aorta distal to the focal obstruction was smaller than normal.

In about 30 per cent[30] of patients with supravalvular aortic stenosis the aortic valve cusps are thickened, and at times the upper margin of one or more aortic valve cusps is adherent to the aortic wall at the site of the supravalvular obstruction, as occurred in one patient studied by the author. Rarely, this attachment of a valve cusp completely separates an aortic sinus and its coronary arterial ostium from the aortic lumen. The aortic valvular abnormalities are occasionally responsible for mild aortic regurgitation.

An intriguing aspect of SAS is the exposure of the coronary arteries to the extremely elevated left ventricular systolic pressure.[31] This situation is brought about by the location of the coronary ostia below the site of obstruction and as a consequence these vessels must be perfused mainly during systole, not during diastole. As a result, the coronary arteries become dilated and extremely thick-walled. At times the lumen of a major coronary artery in this condition may be as large as the aorta itself (in its nonobstructed portion) (see Fig. 6). These vessels elongate and become tortuous also. Interestingly, although they are also proximal to the obstruction, the aortic sinuses of Valsalva are usually not dilated but are normal in size.

Not only is the ascending aorta narrowed in SAS, but arteries arising from the aortic arch and pulmonary arteries also may be narrowed. When the ascending aortic obstruction is of the hypoplastic type, the obstructions in the branches of the arch and possibly also those involving the pulmonary arteries are of the hypoplastic type.[30] Likewise, aortic arch branch stenosis associated with hourglass type obstruction of the ascending aorta also tends to be of the hourglass variety.[30] Peripheral pulmonary arterial stenosis is exceedingly common in patients with SAS.[27,28,30,32]

Infective aortitis is a complication of SAS, but this infection appears to be proportionally far less frequent than is infective endocarditis complicating discrete subaortic stenosis. Intravascular infection in SAS generally is located in the ascending aorta at the site of obstruction.

Although it is nearly always congenital in origin, SAS on rare occasion may be acquired. Healing of an aortotomy incision may constrict the aorta. An obstruction (30 mm. Hg peak systolic pressure gradient) appeared to have been produced by this means in the ascending aorta in a patient, studied by the author, who died many months after aortic valve replacement. The constriction had an hourglass type configuration. Homozygous type II hyperlipoproteinemia may be associated with severe atherosclerosis in the ascending aorta as well as with atherosclerotic type lesions in the aortic valve cusps themselves.[33] Recently, a patient with type II hyperlipoproteinemia was reported as having supravalvular aortic stenosis, but the obstruction was not documented hemodynamically.[34] Hudson[35] reported supravalvular aortic stenosis in a 61-year-old woman with syphilitic aortitis. The obstruction in the aorta, however, was not documented hemodynamically, and the patient's heart weighed only 370 gm.

References

1. Roberts, W. C., and Morrow, A. G.: *Congenital aortic stenosis produced by a unicommissural valve.* Br. Heart J. 27:505, 1965.
2. Falcone, M. W., Roberts, W. C., Morrow, A. G., and Perloff, J. K.: *Congenital aortic stenosis resulting from a unicommissural valve. Clinical and anatomic features in twenty-one adult patients.* Circulation 44:272, 1971.

3. ROBERTS, W. C., PERLOFF, J. K., AND COSTANTINO, T.: *Severe valvular aortic stenosis in patients over 65 years of age. A clinicopathologic study.* Am. J. Cardiol. 27:497, 1971.
4. MORROW, A G., FORT, L., III, ROBERTS, W. C., AND BRAUNWALD, E.: *Discrete subaortic stenosis complicated by aortic valvular regurgitation. Clinical, hemodynamic, and pathologic studies and the results of operative treatment.* Circulation 31:163, 1965.
5. MORROW, A. G., WALDHAUSEN, J. A., PETERS, R. L., BLOODWELL, R. D., AND BRAUNWALD, E.: *Supravalvular aortic stenosis. Clinical, hemodynamic and pathologic observations.* Circulation 20:1003, 1959.
6. LAMBERT, E. C., COLOMBI, M., WAGNER, H. R., AND VLAD, P.: *The clinical outlook of congenital aortic stenosis (valvar and discrete subvalvar) prior to surgery, in* Kidd, B. S. L., and Keith, J. D. (eds.): *The Natural History and Progress in Treatment of Congenital Heart Defects.* An International Symposium sponsored by the Ontario Heart Foundation in Cooperation with the Hospital for Sick Children and the University of Toronto. Charles C Thomas, Springfield, Ill., 1971, p. 205.
7. ROBERTS, W. B.: *The congenitally bicuspid aortic valve. A study of 85 autopsy cases.* Am. J. Cardiol. 26:72, 1970.
8. EDWARDS, J. E.: *Pathologic aspects of cardiac valvular insufficiencies.* Arch. Surg. 77:634, 1958.
9. ROBERTS, W. C.: *The structure of the aortic valve in clinically isolated aortic stenosis. An autopsy study of 162 patients over 15 years of age.* Circulation 42:91, 1970.
10. MCCOLL, I.: *Pericarditis due to a mycotic aneurysm in subacute bacterial endocarditis. Report of a case affecting congenitally stenosed quadricuspid aortic valve.* Guy's Hosp. Rep. 107:34, 1958.
11. HURWITZ, L. E., AND ROBERTS, W. C.: *The quadricuspid semilunar valve.* Am. J. Cardiol. (in press.)
12. MOLLER, J. H., NAKIB, A., ELIOT, R. S., AND EDWARDS, J. E.: *Symptomatic congenital aortic stenosis in the first year of life.* J. Pediatr. 69:728, 1966.
13. EDWARDS, J. E.: *The congenital bicuspid aortic valve.* Circulation 23:485, 1961.
14. ROBERTS, W. C.: *Anatomically isolated aortic valvular disease. The case against its being of rheumatic etiology.* Am. J. Med. 49:151, 1970.
15. MORROW, A. G., GOLDBLATT, A., AND BRAUNWALD, E.: *Congenital aortic stenosis. II. Surgical treatment and the results of operation.* Circulation 27:426, 1963.
15a. NEUFELD, H. N., WAGENVOORT, C. A., BURCHELL, H. B., AND EDWARDS, J. E.: *Idiopathic atrial fibrillation.* Am. J. Cardiol. 8:193, 1961.
16. BRAUNWALD, E., ROBERTS, W. C., GOLDBLATT, A., AYGEN, M. M., ROCKOFF, S. D., AND GILBERT, J. W.: *Aortic stenosis: Physiological, pathological, and clinical concepts.* Ann. Intern. Med. 58:494, 1963.
17. EWY, G. A., MARCUS, F. I., BOHAJALIAN, O., BURKE, H. L., AND ROBERTS, W. C.: *Muscular subaortic stenosis. Clinical and pathologic observations in an elderly patient.* Am. J. Cardiol. 22:126, 1968.
18. MORROW, A. G., ROBERTS, W. C., ROSS, J., JR., FISHER, R. D., BEHRENDT, D. M., MASON, D. T., AND BRAUNWALD, E.: *Obstruction to left ventricular outflow. Current concepts of management and operative treatment.* Ann. Intern. Med. 69:1255, 1968.
19. ROBERTS, W. C.: *Pathologic aspects of valvular and subvalvular (discrete and diffuse) aortic stenosis, in* Kidd, B. S. L., and Keith, I. D. (eds.): *The Natural History and Progress in Treatment of Congenital Heart Defects.* An International Symposium Sponsored by the Ontario Heart Foundation

in Cooperation with the Hospital for Sick Children and the University of Toronto. Charles C Thomas, Springfield, Ill., 1971, p. 221.

20. Ferrans, V. J., Morrow, A. G., and Roberts, W. C.: *Myocardial ultrastructure in idiopathic hypertrophic subaortic stenosis. A study of operatively excised left ventricular outflow tract muscle in 14 patients.* Circulation 45:769, 1972.
21. Simon, A. L., Ross, J., Jr., and Gault, J. H.: *Angiographic anatomy of the left ventricle and mitral valve in idiopathic hypertrophic subaortic stenosis.* Circulation 36:852, 1967.
22. Reis, R. L., Peterson, L. M., Mason, D. T., Simon, A. L., and Morrow, A. G.: *Congenital fixed subvalvular aortic stenosis. An anatomical classification and correlations with operative results.* Circulation 43 (Suppl. 1):11, 1971.
23. Edwards, J. E.: *Pathology of left ventricular outflow tract obstruction.* Circulation 31:586, 1965.
24. Braunwald, E., Ross, R. S., Morrow, A. G., and Roberts, W. C.: *Differential diagnosis of mitral regurgitation in childhood: Clinical pathological conference at the National Institutes of Health.* Ann. Intern. Med. 54:1223, 1961.
25. Shone, J. D., Sellers, R. D., Anderson, R. C., Adams, P., Jr., Lillehei, C. W., and Edwards, J. E.: *The developmental complex of "parachute mitral valve," supravalvular ring of left atrium, subaortic stenosis, and coarctation of aorta.* Am. J. Cardiol. 11:714, 1963.
26. Glancy, D. L., Chang, M. Y., Dorney, E. R., and Roberts, W. C.: *Parachute mitral valve. Further observations and associated lesions.* Am. J. Cardiol. 27:309, 1971.
27. Kahler, R. L., Braunwald, E., Plauth, W. H., Jr., and Morrow, A. G.: *Familial congenital heart disease. Familial occurrence of atrial septal defect with A-V conduction abnormalities, supravalvular aortic and pulmonic stenosis, and ventricular septal defect.* Am. J. Med. 40:384, 1966.
28. Garcia, R. E., Friedman, W. F., Kaback, M. M., and Rowe, R. D.: *Idiopathic hypercalcemia and supravalvular aortic stenosis. Documentation of a new syndrome.* New Eng. J. Med. 271:117, 1964.
29. Friedman, W. F., and Roberts, W. C.: *Vitamin D and the supravalvular aortic stenosis syndrome. The transplacental effects of vitamin D on the aorta of the rabbit.* Circulation 34:77, 1966.
30. Peterson, T. A., Todd, D. B., and Edwards, J. E.: *Supravalvular aortic stenosis.* J. Thorac. Cardiovasc. Surg. 50:734, 1965.
31. Neufeld, H. N., Wagenvoort, C. A., Ongley, P. A., and Edwards, J. E.: *Hypoplasia of ascending aorta: An unusual form of supravalvular aortic stenosis with special reference to localized coronary arterial hypertension.* Am. J. Cardiol. 10:746, 1962.
32. Page, H. L., Jr., Vogel, J. H. K., Pryor, R., and Blount, S. G., Jr.: *Supravalvular aortic stenosis. Unusual observations in three patients.* Am. J. Cardiol. 23:270, 1969.
33. Roberts, W. C., Levy, R. I., and Fredrickson, D. S.: *Hyperlipoproteinemia. A review of the five types with first report of necropsy findings in type III.* Arch. Pathol. 90:46, 1970.
34. Wennevold, A., and Jacobsen, J. G.: *Acquired supravalvular aortic stenosis in familial hypercholesterolemia. A hemodynamic and angiocardiographic study.* Am. J. Med. 50:823, 1971.
35. Hudson, R. E. B.: *Cardiovascular Pathology.* Williams & Wilkins Co., Baltimore, 1965, p. 1063.

Quadricuspid Semilunar Valve

LARRY E. HURWITZ, MD
WILLIAM C. ROBERTS, MD, FACC

Bethesda, Maryland

Clinical and necropsy findings are described in 10 patients with quadricuspid semilunar valves, and previous reports of 197 cases are reviewed. Quadricuspid semilunar valves occur infrequently, and usually the pulmonic valve is affected. The quadricuspid pulmonic valve typically functions normally. The quadricuspid aortic valve was functionally abnormal in 5 of 11 cases studied.

The most common major congenital anomaly involving the heart or great vessels is malformation of one or both semilunar valves.[1] Of the various congenital abnormalities affecting these valves, the most frequent by far is the bicuspid aortic valve (occurring in approximately 2 percent of the general population[1]); next in frequency is the unicuspid aortic valve.[2] Semilunar valves with 4 cusps are much less common than those with either 1 or 2 cusps. The bicuspid and unicuspid malformations of these valves have received considerable attention in recent years.[1,2] In contrast, the occurrence of 4 cusps in either the pulmonic or aortic valve has received relatively little attention. This report focuses on the quadricuspid semilunar valve. Clinical and necropsy observations in 10 patients studied by us are summarized, and observations previously recorded by others are reviewed.

Patients Studied

Pertinent information on the 10 patients is summarized in Table I. In 2 patients the aortic valve was quadricuspid (Fig. 1 and 2), and in the other 8 the pulmonic valve was quadricuspid (Fig. 3). Function of the quadricuspid valve appeared to have been normal in 8 patients and abnormal in 2. One of the latter, a 51 year old woman, had severe aortic regurgitation necessitating aortic valve replacement (Fig. 1). The other patient, a 3 day old boy, had a dysfunctioning quadricuspid valve with severe valvular pulmonic stenosis. He died shortly after operative alleviation of the right ventricular outflow obstruction. Other congenital cardiovascular anomalies—namely atrial septal defect of the fossa ovale type, partial atrioventricular canal and ventricular septal defect—were present in 3 of the 10 patients. Two other patients, each with a quadricuspid pulmonic valve, had rheumatic mitral and aortic valvular stenosis, but there was no evidence in either patient that the rheumatic process had involved the pulmonic valve.

Of the 2 patients with a quadricuspid aortic valve, 1 had a valve with 3 equal-sized cusps and 1 smaller cusp (Fig. 4), and the other had a valve with 2 equal larger and 2 unequal smaller cusps. In 5 cases, the pulmonic quadricuspid valve had 3 equal larger cusps and 1 smaller cusp; 1 valve had 4 equal-sized cusps, 1 had 2 equal larger and 2 equal smaller cusps, and 1 valve had 1 larger, 2 intermediate and 1 smaller cusp.

From the Section of Pathology, National Heart and Lung Institute, National Institutes of Health, Bethesda, Md. Manuscript received July 11, 1972, accepted September 14, 1972.

Address for reprints: William C. Roberts, MD, Section of Pathology, National Heart and Lung Institute, National Institutes of Health, Bethesda, Md. 20014.

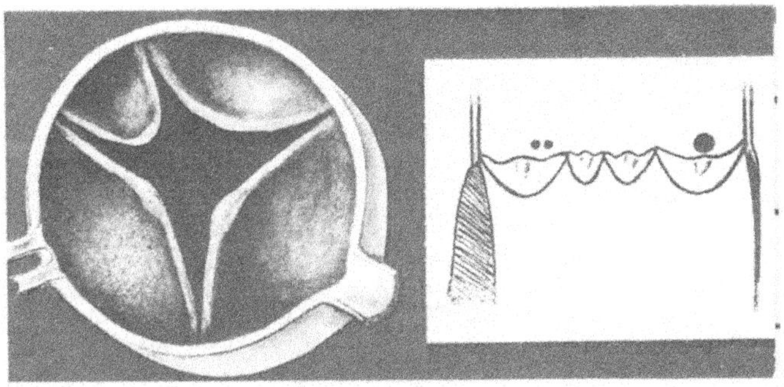

FIGURE 1. Case 1. Schematic diagram of the incompetent quadricuspid aortic valve in a 51 year old woman with angina pectoris and refractory congestive failure necessitating aortic valve replacement. At operation, the aortic valve was quadricuspid with 2 smaller and 2 larger cusps. A prosthesis was inserted. She died suddenly 17 days later. At necropsy, the heart weighed 520 g. Both ventricles were markedly dilated, and the left ventricular free wall measured up to 1.7 cm in thickness. Death was due to acute myocardial infarction secondary to an embolus to a coronary artery.

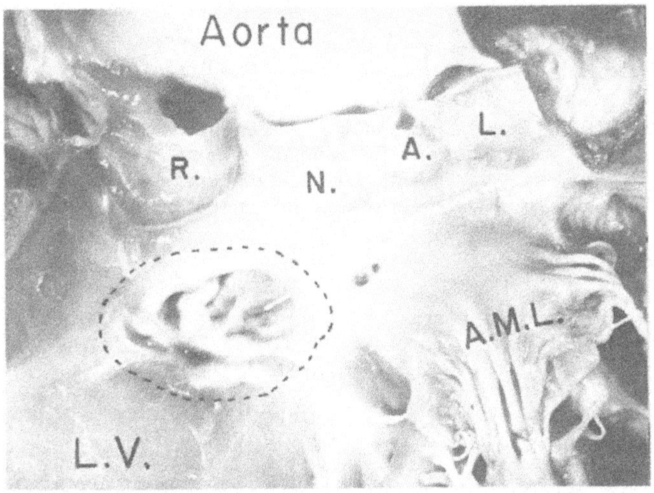

FIGURE 2. Case 2. A normally functioning quadricuspid aortic valve in an 11 year old girl with a known ventricular septal defect. Six months before death she was successfully treated for *alpha streptococcus* endocarditis; however, she died of progressive renal failure. At necropsy, the heart weighed 270 g. Both ventricles were dilated. The septal leaflet of the tricuspid valve was bound down to the ventricular septum by fibrous tissue, and a jet lesion (2 cm in diameter) was evident on the free wall of the right ventricle. There was no evidence of endocarditis on the quadricuspid aortic valve. The "closed" ventricular septal defect is outlined by the **dashed circle.** A = accessory valve cusp; A.M.L. = anterior mitral leaflet; L = left aortic valve cusp; L.V. = left ventricle; N = noncoronary valve cusp; R = right valve cusp.

TABLE I

Data on 10 Patients with Quadricuspid Semilunar Valves

Case no.	Age (yr) & Sex	Quadricuspid Valve	Functional Status	History RF	History IE*	Other Cardiac Abnormalities
1	51F	Aortic	Incompetent	0	0	0
2	11F	Aortic	Normal	0	+	VSD
3	40M	Pulmonic	Normal	0	0	0
4	3 daysM	Pulmonic	Stenotic	0	0	ASD
5	14M	Pulmonic	Normal	?	?	Partial A-V canal
6	57M	Pulmonic	Normal	+	+	Rheumatic MS, AS
7	46F	Pulmonic	Normal	0	0	0
8	81M	Pulmonic	Normal	0	0	0
9	41F	Pulmonic	Normal	0	0	HC
10	34M	Pulmonic	Normal	+	0	Rheumatic MS, AS

* Although 2 and possibly 3 patients had a positive history of infective endocarditis, none had vegetations involving the quadricuspid valve.

AS = aortic stenosis; ASD = atrial septal defect; A-V = atrioventricular; HC = hypertrophic cardiomyopathy without subaortic stenosis; IE = infective endocarditis; MS = mitral stenosis; RF = acute rheumatic fever; VSD = ventricular septal defect.

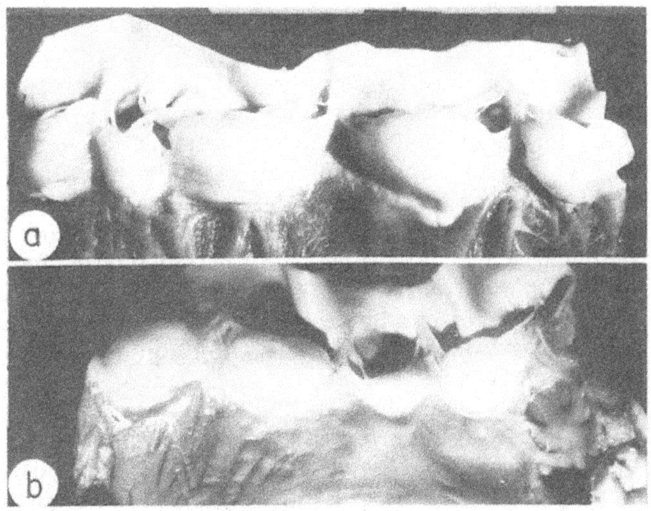

FIGURE 3. Quadricuspid pulmonic valves observed as incidental necropsy findings in 2 patients. *a*, Patient 3, who died of carcinoma of the pancreas. *b*, Patient 7, who died of acute leukemia. Neither patient had symptoms of cardiac dysfunction.

Comments

A quadricuspid semilunar valve is an uncommon condition. Review of previous reports yielded 197 cases: in 184 cases (93 percent) the affected valve was pulmonic[3-8] and in 13 cases (7 percent) was aortic.[5,7,9-14] It is unclear why the pulmonic valve is more commonly affected, since the aortic valve is more commonly bicuspid or unicuspid.[1,2] The quadricuspid pulmonic valve has been found in from 1 in 400[7] to 1 in 2,000 necropsies.[4] We found 8 quadricuspid pulmonic valves and 2 quadricuspid aortic valves during examination of 6,000 necropsies. Others have shown a similar smaller incidence of quadricuspid aortic valves. Neither Simonds[4] nor Simpson[8] found a quadricuspid aortic valve during examination of 6,252 necropsies; deVries[5] observed only 1 in 3,600 necropsies. These reports may underestimate the actual frequency of this anomaly since, unless they are specifically sought, minor abnormalities of the semilunar valves may be easily overlooked at necropsy examination.

Sex distribution: The quadricuspid pulmonic valve more commonly occurs in male subjects: of 79 affected patients whose sex was known, 52 (65 percent) were male and 27 (35 percent) were female. Unlike other malformations of the aortic valve that primarily affect male subjects,[1,2] the quadricuspid aortic valve appears to have an equal sex distribution. Of affected patients whose sex was known, 4 were male and 3 were female.

Valve function: The quadricuspid pulmonic valve nearly always appears to function normally. Consequently, most quadricuspid pulmonic valves represent incidental findings at necropsy. Why one quadricuspid valve functions normally and why another functions abnormally is uncertain. Of 158 quadricuspid pulmonic valves available for study or review, 6 (4 percent) functioned abnormally; of these, 2 were stenotic and 4 were purely incompetent. In contrast, the quadricuspid aortic valve frequently functions abnormally. Of 11 quadricuspid aortic valves, 1 was stenotic and 4 were incompetent. Valvular incompetence, the most common hemodynamic abnormality, was not observed in infants or young children, thus suggesting that the quadricuspid valve is not incompetent from birth. In no case was incompetence a result of infective endocarditis. The finding of a stenotic quadricuspid valve in a 3 day old infant (our Case 4) suggests that the quadricuspid valve, unlike the congenitally bicuspid valve,[1] may be stenotic from birth.

Other cardiac anomalies: The quadricuspid semilunar valve is rarely associated with other congenital cardiac anomalies. Seven patients (4 percent) with quadricuspid pulmonic valves had other abnormalities: 4 had atrial septal defect of the fossa ovale type, 1 had ventricular septal defect, 1 had partial atrioventricular canal and 1 had patent ductus arteriosus. One patient with a quadricuspid aortic valve had ventricular septal defect.

Endocarditis: The normally functioning quadricuspid valve does not appear to be more likely to have infective endocarditis than the normally formed valve. The only reported case of endocarditis involving a quadricuspid valve occurred on a previously stenotic valve.[13] Our Patient 2, who had a ventricular septal defect, had endocarditis of the right ventricular endocardium but no evidence of vegetation on the normally functioning quadricuspid aortic valve.

Although the rheumatic process has been demonstrated to involve the congenitally bicuspid aortic valve, it does not appear to involve quadricuspid semilunar or any other malformed valve with increased frequency. Although 2 of our patients had rheumatic disease of both mitral and aortic valves, the quadricuspid pulmonic valves were unaffected by the rheumatic process.

Anatomic variations: The anatomic variations of the quadricuspid valves are schematically presented in Figure 4. Of 121 quadricuspid pulmonic valves reviewed, 72 valves (60 percent) had 3 equal-sized cusps and 1 smaller cusp; 18 valves (15 percent) had

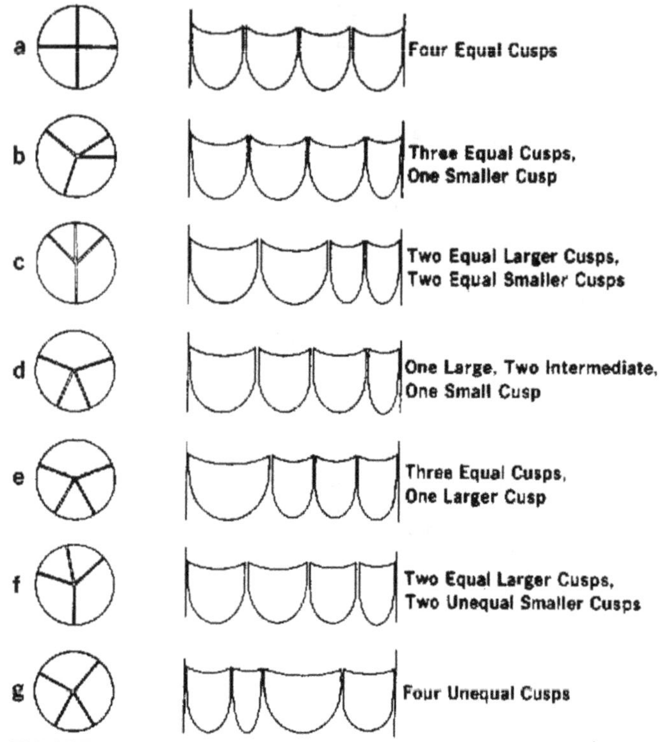

FIGURE 4. Seven described anatomic variations of quadricuspid valves. The most common variation in either aortic or pulmonic valve consisted of 3 equal-sized cusps and 1 smaller cusp (**b**). No correlation was found between anatomic variation and functional status.

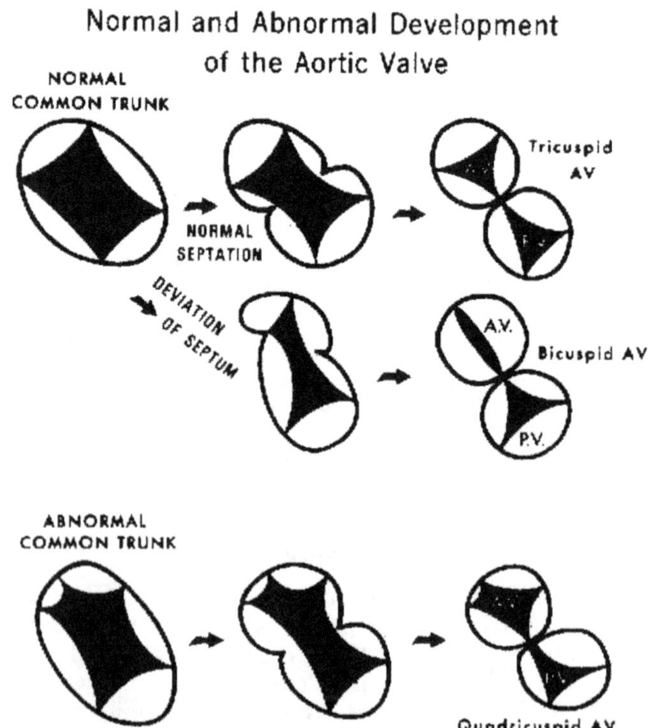

FIGURE 5. Diagrammatic portrayal of the probable mechanism of development of both normal and abnormal semilunar valves. Abnormalities may occur from either abnormal septal division or from abnormalities of mesenchymal proliferation in the common trunk. A.V. = aortic valve; P.V. = pulmonic valve.

2 equal larger and 2 equal smaller cusps; 15 valves (12 percent) had 4 equal cusps; 7 valves (6 percent) had 1 larger, 2 intermediate and 1 smaller cusp; 4 valves (3 percent) had 3 equal and 1 larger cusp; 3 valves (2 percent) had 2 equal and 2 smaller unequal cusps and 2 valves (2 percent) had 4 unequal-sized cusps. Of 7 quadricuspid aortic valves reviewed, 3 valves had 3 equal and 1 small cusp; 2 valves had 4 equal cusps; 1 valve had 3 equal and 1 larger cusp, and 1 valve had 4 unequal cusps.

Multiple small fenestrations were commonly observed in both quadricuspid aortic and pulmonic valves. In no patient were both aortic and pulmonic valves quadricuspid. In contrast, several patients with congenitally bicuspid pulmonic and aortic valves have been observed.

Embryology: Semilunar valve formation appears to occur as follows: By the fourth week of gestation, a pair of mesenchymal ridges have formed in the cephalad portion of the truncus arteriosus. With further growth these truncoconal ridges fuse and descend to the ventricles in a spiral fashion forming the aorticopulmonary septum and thus dividing the truncus into 2 distinct chambers. At the junction of the truncus and conus, the semilunar valves are formed by mesenchymal outgrowth from the development of 2 smaller mesenchymal proliferations, the intercolated valvular swellings, situated between the main truncoconal ridges.[15] Abnormal cusp formation, therefore, is due either to aberrant fusion of the aorticopulmonary septum or to abnormal proliferations in the common trunk (Fig. 5).

References

1. **Roberts WC:** The congenitally bicuspid aortic valve. A study of 85 autopsy cases. Amer J Cardiol 26:72–83, 1970
2. **Falcone WM, Roberts WC, Morrow AG, et al.:** Congenital aortic stenosis resulting from a unicommisural valve. Clinical and anatomic features in twenty-one adult patients. Circulation 44:272–280, 1971
3. **Kissin M:** Pulmonary insufficiency with a supernumerary cusp in the pulmonary valve. Report of a case with review of the literature. Amer Heart J 12:206–227, 1936
4. **Simonds JP:** Congenital malformations of the aortic and pulmonary valves. Amer J Med Sci 166:584–595, 1923
5. **DeVries WM:** Über Abweichungen in der Ishl der Semilunarklappen. Beitr Path Anat 64:39–54, 1918
6. **Dilg J:** Ein Beitrag zur Kenntniss seltener Herzanomalien im Anschluss an einen Fall von angeborner iinksseitiger Conusstenose. Virchow Arch Path Anat 91:193–259, 1883
7. **Ingham DW:** Congenital malformations of the pulmonic and aortic valves. Ann Int Med 12:609–613, 1938
8. **Simpson FO:** Congenital abnormalities of the heart in the insane. J Anat Physiol 32:678–686, 1898
9. **Hudson REB:** Cardiovascular Pathology, Vol 3. Baltimore, Williams & Wilkins, 1970, p S.1082
10. **Wyatt JP, Goldenberg H:** Supernumary aortic cusps with multiple fenestrations and with displacement of the left coronary orifice. Arch Path (Chicago) 45:784–786, 1948
11. **Robicsek F, Sanger PW, Daugherty HK, et al.:** Congenital quadricuspid aortic valve with displacement of the left coronary orifice. Amer J Cardiol 23:288–290, 1969
12. **Peretz DI, Chaugfoot GH, Goulay RH:** Four-cusped aortic valve with significant hemodynamic abnormality. Amer J Cardiol 23:291–293, 1969
13. **McColl I:** Pericarditis due to a mycotic aneurysm in subacute bacterial endocarditis. Report of a case affecting congenitally stenosed quadricuspid aortic valve. Guys Hosp Rep 107:34–47, 1958
14. **McRonald RE, Dean DC:** Congenital quadricuspid aortic valve. Amer J Cardiol 18:761–763, 1966
15. **Kramer TC:** The partitioning of the truncus and conus and the formation of the membranous portion of the interventricular septum in the human heart. Amer J Anat 71:343–370, 1942

Nonrheumatic Valvular Cardiac Disease: A Clinicopathologic Survey of 27 Different Conditions Causing Valvular Dysfunction

William C. Roberts, M.D.,
James C. Dangel, M.D., and
Bernadine H. Bulkley, M.D.

Until relatively recent years most valvular cardiac lesions in adults or older children were believed to be rheumatic in origin. During the past two decades, however, it has become increasingly apparent that rheumatic disease is only one of many causes of valvular dysfunction, and, indeed, not the most common. We have found it helpful to divide functionally significant valvular lesions into two groups: (1) those causing obstruction (with or without regurgitation) and (2) those causing pure regurgitation, i.e., without any element of obstruction (nonobstructive) (Table 1). Rheumatic disease continues to be a major cause of obstructive valve lesions but it plays a far less prominent role as a cause of nonobstructive lesions. Even in the obstructive group, however, the most common lesion is valvular aortic stenosis, which when isolated is rarely rheumatic in origin.[1-4] Mitral stenosis, on the other hand, is usually rheumatic in origin as are most combined valvular lesions.

We also have found it useful to divide the nonobstructive, i.e., purely incompetent, valvular lesions into two groups: (1) those associated with abnormalities of the ascending aorta and (2) those which do not affect the aorta (Table 1). Most lesions affecting the aorta cause aortic regurgitation, and most cases of

Table 1. A classification of nonrheumatic valvular cardiac disease

I. Obstructive lesions
  - A. Left-sided
    1. Obstruction to left ventricular outflow
       - a. Valvular aortic stenosis
       - b. Subvalvular
         - (1) Discrete
         - (2) Hypertrophic (asymmetric) cardiomyopathy
       - c. Supravalvular
    2. Obstruction to left ventricular inflow
  - B. Right-sided
    1. Obstruction to right ventricular outflow
    2. Obstruction to both right ventricular outflow and inflow
       - a. Carcinoid heart disease
  - C. Combined left-sided and right-sided

II. Nonobstructive lesions
  - A. With involvement of ascending aorta
    1. Syphilis
    2. Ankylosing spondylitis
    3. The Marfan syndrome including forme fruste variety
    4. The Hurler syndrome
    5. Osteogenesis imperfecta
    6. Pseudoxanthoma elasticum
    7. Ehlers-Danlos syndrome
    8. Takayasu's arteritis
  - B. Without involvement of ascending aorta
    1. Floppy atrioventricular valve
    2. Calcification of atrioventricular valve annuli
    3. Papillary muscle necrosis or fibrosis or both
    4. Infective endocarditis
    5. Congenital malformation
    6. Trauma
    7. Systemic lupus erythematosus
    8. Rheumatoid arthritis
    9. Endomyocardial fibrosis with and without eosinophilia
    10. Irradiation
    11. Idiopathic

pure aortic regurgitation result from abnormalities of the ascending aorta. Because pure aortic regurgitation most frequently results from conditions affecting the aorta rather than the aortic valve cusps, rheumatic disease is not a major cause of isolated aortic regurgitation. Pure mitral regurgitation, in contrast, is the major nonobstructive lesion not involving the aorta.

This report focuses on the nonrheumatic conditions causing valvular dysfunction. Patients with intracardiac or extracardiac shunts with a few exceptions have been excluded. The various entities will be discussed as outlined in Table 1. When possible, concrete data of patients studied at necropsy by the authors will be presented in place of or in addition to information derived from reports of others.

OBSTRUCTIVE LESIONS

Obstruction to Left Ventricular Outflow

Valvular Aortic Stenosis

It is now clear that isolated valvular aortic stenosis (with or without associated aortic regurgitation) is nearly always nonrheumatic in origin, and most commonly represents a congenital malformation of this valve.[1-4] Isolated valvular aortic stenosis is the most common cause of fatal valvular dysfunction in patients over 14 years of age. Of 543 patients with severe (functionally class III or IV [New York Heart Association Classification]) fatal valvular cardiac disease studied at necropsy by us, 182 patients or 34 per cent had isolated valvular aortic stenosis (with or without regurgitation) (Table 2). The second most common valvular

Table 2. Functional classification of valvular heart disease: data in 543 autopsy patients older than age 14 years

Functional Valve Lesion	No. Pts. (%)	Anatomic Classification				
		AV	MV	MV-AV	MV-TV	MV-AV-TV
1. Aortic Stenosis (AS)	182 (34)	158 (87)	0	23 (12.5)	0	1 (.5)
2. Mitral Stenosis (MS)	94 (17)	0	53 (57)	23 (24)	7 (7)	11 (12)
3. AS + MS	66 (12)	0	0	52 (79)	0	14 (21)
4. Aortic Regurgitation (AR)	60 (11)	50 (83)	0	9 (15)	0	1 (2)
5. Mitral Regurgitation (MR)	55 (10)	0	44 (80)	7 (13)	1 (2)	3 (5)
6. MS + AR	34 (6)	0	0	25 (74)	0	9 (26)
7. MR + AR	24 (5)	0	0	20 (83)	0	4 (17)
8. AS + MR	16 (3)	0	0	15 (94)	0	1 (6)
9. Tricuspid Stenosis + MS ± AS	12 (2)	0	0	0	1 (8)	11 (92)
TOTALS	543	208 (38)	97 (18)	174 (32)	9 (2)	55 (10)

lesion, namely mitral stenosis, is only half as frequent as aortic stenosis (Table 2). When aortic stenosis is the only functional valve lesion the remaining three cardiac valves are usually normal. As shown in Table 2, of the 182 patients with isolated valvular aortic stenosis, the other three cardiac valves were anatomically normal in 87 per cent of them. In contrast, of the 94 patients with isolated mitral stenosis (with or without regurgitation) only 57 per cent had anatomic involvement limited to the mitral valve.

We have found it useful to subdivide patients with valvular aortic stenosis into three groups according to ages[5]: (1) patients less than 15 years old; (2) patients 15 to 65 years old; and (3) patients older than 65 years.[4] Little anatomic data is available in the group less than 15 years of age. The data available tends to indicate that the aortic valves in these young individuals are either unicuspid or bicuspid and only occasionally tricuspid. In the group aged 15 to 65 years, the aortic valve is congenitally malformed in about 60 per cent of them (Table 3). Of the patients older than 65 years of age, the aortic valve is tricuspid in more than 90 per cent and congenitally malformed (biscuspid) in less than 10 per cent (Table 4).

Table 3. Aortic valve structure in clinically isolated aortic stenosis: ages 15–65 years

Valve Structure	No. Pts. (%)	Age Range (Avg.)	No. Males (%)	Hx ARF or chorea	LV-SA PSG (mm. Hg)
1. Unicommissural	18 (12)	16-62 (44)	14 (78)	1	10-158 (78)
2. Bicuspid	72 (46)	16-65 (49)	53 (73)	5	12-165 (91)
3. Tricuspid	57 (37)	21-64 (49)	49 (86)	15	20-155 (82)
MV Normal	36	28-64 (50;	29 (81)	1	20-155 (90)
MV Thickened	21	21-61 (48)	20 (95)	14	20-120 (74)
4. Uncertain	8 (5)	41-58 (52)	7 (87)	0	52-105 (81)
TOTALS	155	16-65 (46)	123 (79)	21 (13%)	10-165 (86)*

* 121 pts.

Table 4. Aortic valve structure in clinically isolated aortic stenosis: ages greater than 65 years

Valve Structure	No. Pts. (%)	Age Range (Avg.)	No. Males (%)	Hx ARF or chorea	LV-SA PSG (mm. Hg)
1. Unicommissural	0				
2. Bicuspid	2 (7)	75 + 79	1 (50)	0	–
3. Tricuspid	25 (93)	66-90 (77)	13 (52)		20-160 (88)
MV Normal	23	66-90 (77)	13 (56)	0	20-160 (92)
MV Thickened	2	74 + 76	0	0	70
4. Uncertain	0				
TOTALS	27	66-90 (78)	14 (52)	0	20-160 (88)

Although valvular aortic stenosis frequently involves a congenitally malformed aortic valve, the stenosis is usually not congenital but acquired, the result of fibrosis and calcification of the malformed cusps. Thus, acquired valvular aortic stenosis is fundamentally of two types: (1) that involving a previously congenitally malformed but initially normally functioning valve and (2) that involving a previously normally formed valve.

Several types of congenitally malformed aortic valves occur. Each type is determined by its number of cusps and commissures. At least two types of *unicuspid* aortic valves exist. In one, the orifice is centrally located and the cusp is devoid of lateral attachments to the wall of the aorta (simple dome or *acommissural* valve). This type valve also is usually the one underlying valvular pulmonic stenosis. Often three remnants of commissures are observed, and the undeveloped commissures have caused it to be confused with tricuspid semilunar valves. A second type of unicuspid valve is the *unicommissural* one.[6] This valve, described by Edwards,[7] is characterized by an eccentrically located orifice with only one lateral attachment to the aortic wall and that at the level of the orifice. From above, this valve has the appearance of an exclamation mark. Remnants of undeveloped commissures also are present in the unicommissural valve.[6] This is the most frequent malformation found in fatal valvular aortic stenosis in children less than one year of age.[8]

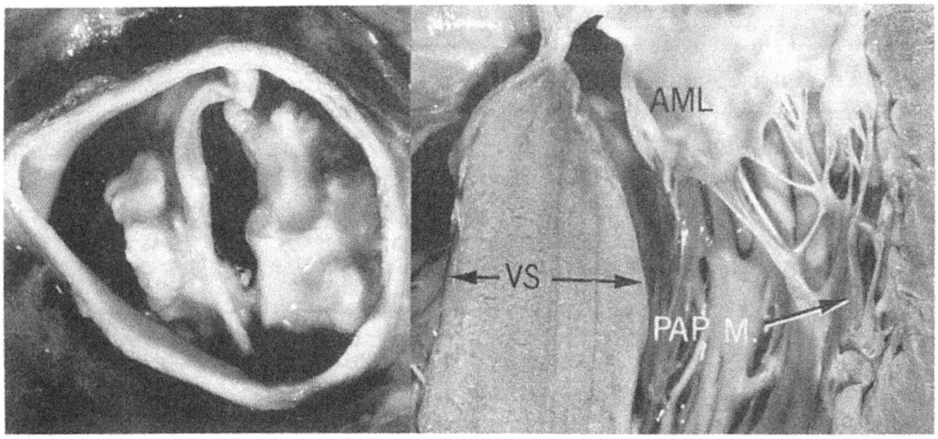

Figure 1. Stenotic congenitally bicuspid aortic valve and atrophied and scarred left ventricular papillary muscle (PAP M.) in a 52-year-old woman (A68–105). She had symptoms of cardiac dysfunction for three years and a murmur of mitral regurgitation as well as a murmur of aortic stenosis. The peak systolic pressure gradient across the aortic valve was 130 mm. Hg. She died of congestive cardiac failure. VS = ventricular septum. AML = anterior mitral leaflet.

The most frequent malformation of the aortic valve is the presence of only two cusps[3] (Fig. 1). The *bicuspid* valve is basically of two types: in one the cusps are located right and left, the commissures anteriorly and posteriorly, a raphe or false commissure, if present, is always in the right cusp, and a coronary artery arises from behind each cusp; in the second type, the cusps are located anteriorly and posteriorly, the commissures right and left, a raphe, if present, is always in the anterior cusp, and both coronary arteries arise in front of the anterior cusp. These two types are divided about equally among patients with congenitally bicuspid aortic valves.

Of 107 patients over 14 years of age with congenitally bicuspid aortic valves studied at necropsy by one of us (W.C.R.), 75 had aortic stenosis, 17 had pure aortic regurgitation, and 15 had functionally normal valves (Table 5). Why one patient with a congenitally bicuspid aortic valve develops stenosis, why another develops infection with subsequent regurgitation, why another (rarely) develops

Table 5. Congenitally bicuspid aortic valve: summary of 107 autopsied patients older than age 14 years

Group	No. Pts.	Age at Death Range (Avg.) Years	Sex M	Sex F	Infective Endocarditis	LV-SA PSG Range (Avg.) mm.Hg	AV Calcium Deposits
AS with or without AR	75	16 – 79 (48)	54	21	6	18 – 165 (94)	73
Pure AR	17	15 – 55 (34)	15	2	14	0 – 0 (0)	5
Functionally normal valve	15	23 – 59 (45)	9	6	0	–	4
TOTALS	107	15 – 79 (46)	78 (72%)	29 (28%)	2 (18%)		82 (77%)

pure regurgitation without infection, and why another never develops any of these complications during an entire lifetime is uncertain. The 15 patients with normally functioning congenitally bicuspid valves (Table 5) were found during routine examination of 1600 hearts at necropsy, none of which had dysfunctioning cardiac valves or shunts. How many patients with bicuspid aortic valves at birth develop complications (stenosis, regurgitation, infection) and how many never develop any of these complications is unknown. The biscuspid condition of the aortic valve appears to be the most common congenital malformation of the heart or great vessels; possibly as many as 2 per cent of births have this anomaly.[3] Stenosis, not infection, is by far the most common complication of the congenitally biscuspid aortic valve.

Occasionally a tricuspid aortic valve is malformed. When this occurs, the cusps are of unequal size. Minor differences in cuspal size are frequent but major differences appear to constitute a congenital malformation. There may be some basis for believing that contact of unequal sized cusps with one another can lead to focal cuspal fibrosis with eventual calcification and stenosis.[2] A quadricuspid aortic valve on rare occasion may be stenotic.[9] Most quadricuspid valves, however, function normally.[9] Although six-cuspid valves may occur (persistent truncus arteriosus), stenosis of these multi-cuspid valves is rare.

Function of the malformed aortic valves at birth is variable. The fewer the number of cusps and commissures the greater the likelihood that the valve is stenotic at birth. The acommissural and unicommissural unicuspid valves are stenotic from birth: the orifices of these valves are small and there is little opportunity for the valvular orifice to alter its size during either phase of the cardiac cycle. Most patients with unicuspid aortic valves have precordial murmurs from birth whereas this is probably not the case in most patients with congenitally bicuspid aortic valves.[6]

Whether or not the bicuspid aortic valve is ever stenotic at birth is unclear. Probably most often this valve becomes stenotic only as it thickens and calcifies. Of 30 patients, mostly children, with congenital valvular aortic stenosis operated upon by Morrow,[10] however, 18 were said to have bicuspid valves, 11 tricuspid, and one a unicommissural unicuspid valve. Unicommissural valves are most frequent in fatal congenital aortic valve stenosis in the first year of life.[8] Tricuspid aortic valves rarely appear to be stenotic at birth. If stenosis is present at birth and the aortic valve is three-cuspid, the stenosis is more usually the result of a very small aortic *annulus* rather than the result of fusion of the cusps. Acquired stenosis of a three-cuspid aortic valve, in contrast, is common. Of 155 patients aged 15 to 65 years with clinically isolated aortic stenosis (with or without regurgitation) studied at necropsy (Table 3), 57 (37 per cent) had tricuspid valves, and among the 27 patients older than age 65 years (Table 4), 25 (93 per cent) had tricuspid valves. In the 15 to 65 year age group, about half of the 57 patients with clinically isolated aortic stenosis had diffuse fibrous thickening of the mitral leaflets as well. The associated diffuse mitral leaflet thickening in them is strong evidence that the etiology of the stenosis in this group is rheumatic.[1] Also, about 70 per cent of this group had positive histories of acute rheumatic fever, whereas only 6 per cent of the other group, i.e., those with anatomically normal mitral valves, with valvular aortic stenosis had positive histories. The etiology of the aortic stenosis in the patients with anatomically normal mitral valves is unsolved. Possibly, as mentioned earlier, minor abnormalities in cuspal size from birth sets the stage for abnormal leaflet contact with resultant fibrosis and finally stenosis.[2]

Stenosis of the aortic valve in patients greater than age 65 years is usually characteristic.[4] The valves are tricuspid, nodular calcific deposits are rather uniformly distributed on the aortic aspects of each cusp, and the commissures are not fused. Obstruction results from the calcific deposits which prevent the cusps from retracting adequately during ventricular systole. Because the commissures are usually not fused, associated aortic regurgitation is infrequent.

Clinically, aortic stenosis in the elderly is characterized by several features which are either absent or more prominent than in younger subjects with this valvular lesion: the systemic arterial pulse pressure may be increased due to systolic hypertension; a harsh right basal systolic murmur may be relatively inconspicuous while a pure musical systolic murmur may be prominent at the apex; a coexisting apical systolic murmur of mitral regurgitation may be related to mitral annular calcification and not to left ventricular failure; and systemic systolic hypertension can result in a comparatively small pressure gradient despite severe left ventricular outflow obstruction.

The cause of the aortic stenosis in elderly patients is uncertain but simple wear-and-tear or degeneration appears to be the most reasonable explanation. The presence in the same hearts of other wear-and-tear lesions such as calcified mitral annuli, calcified coronary arteries, and focal thickening of other valve leaflets supports this contention.

Discrete Left Ventricular Outflow Obstruction (Discrete Subaortic Stenosis [DDS])

Although this congenital malformation does not primarily involve a cardiac valve, it may be confused with valvular aortic stenosis and it may cause secondary damage to the aortic valve cusps (Fig. 2).

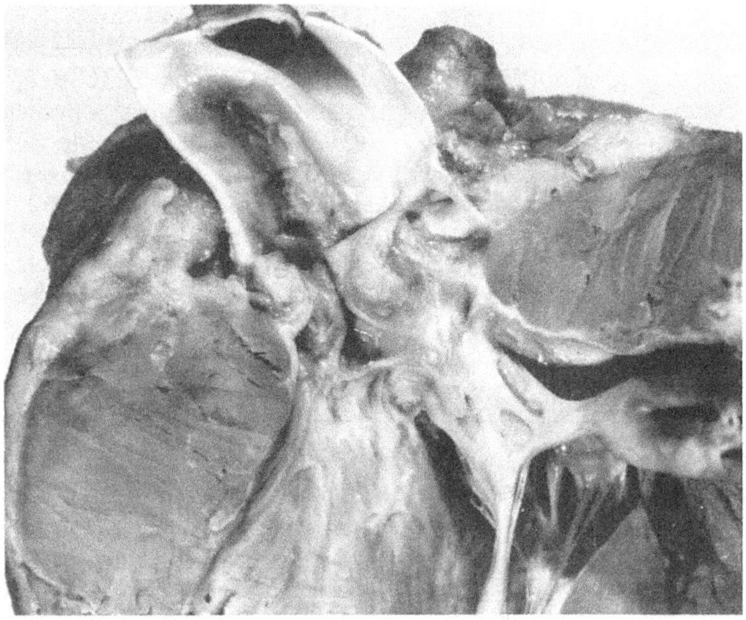

Figure 2. Discrete subaortic stenosis with scarring of the aortic valve. Opened aorta, aortic valve, and left ventricular outflow tract of a 13-year-old boy (A72–115) who died while swimming. Subaortic stenosis had been diagnosed by catheterization at age five. He had two operative procedures (ages five and seven) for removal of the subaortic membrane. Residual gradients of 132 mm. Hg and 60 mm. Hg, respectively, remained after these operations. At necropsy, a tough fibrous membrane was present. The aortic valve cusps were thickened and the aorta was smaller than normal.

We have studied at necropsy seven patients, aged 13 to 47 years (average 24), with DSS (Table 6). Five were male, and two were female. All seven had precordial diastolic murmurs (grade 1–3/6) typical of aortic regurgitation in addition to systolic thrills and loud murmurs (grade 3–5/6) typical of aortic stenosis. The one patient (#6, Table 6) with valvular stenosis also had an ejection click. Left ventricular peak systolic pressure gradients in 6 patients varied from 70 to 170 mm. Hg (avg. 115) and pressure tracings or left ventricular cineangiographic studies in each indicated discrete obstruction in the subvalvular region. The narrowed left ventricular outflow tract area ranged from 0.23 to 0.40 cm.^{2} (avg. 0.34) in the four patients in whom it was calculated. Two patients, at ages 28 and 41 years respectively, developed infective endocarditis of the aortic valve causing severe regurgitation in each. Five patients underwent operative resection of the subaortic membrane and one also had aortic valve replacement because of aortic regurgitation. Three died within a month of operation and one died suddenly seven years later because of residual obstruction. The patient in whom the aortic valve was replaced died six years postoperatively because of prosthetic dysfunction.

Two of the seven patients with DSS had other congenital cardiovascular malformations—one had a parachute mitral valve (which apparently functioned normally), a small aortic valve "ring," and a small coarctation of the aorta; the second had a large patent ductus arteriosus and mild coarctation of the aorta.

Subaortic "membrane" tissue was present at necropsy in all seven patients.

Table 6. Discrete subaortic stenosis: clinical and necropsy findings

Patient	Age	Sex	Murmurs AS	Murmurs AR	Pressures LV S/D	Pressures SA S/D	Pressures LV-SA PSG	Area of LVOT (cm.²)	Operative resection of subvalvular membrane	LV-SA PSG (mm.Hg) postoperative	Anatomic findings: Aortic valve	Anatomic findings: Associated malformations
1. A57–133	18	M	4/6	2/6	156/–	86/55	70	0.4	+	0	Thickened	0
2. A62–305	30	F	5/6	2/6	270/24	100/55	170	0.23	+	10	Thickened	0
3. A64–20	28	M	3/6	2/6	—	—	—	—	0	—	Infected	0
4. 05–23–07	47	F	3/6	3/6	260/55	100/60	160	—	+*	12	Infected	PDA, C of A
5. A60–164	17	M	4/6	1/6	200/8	122/65	78	—	+	—	Thickened	Parachute MV
6. GT71A–215	14	M	4/6	2/6	165/30	85/60	80	0.4	0	—	Bicuspid stenotic	C of A VSD (closed)
7. A72–115	13	M	5/6	1/6	240/9	108/64	132	0.32	+	65	Thickened	0

* Also, aortic valve replacement

AR = aortic regurgitation. AS = aortic stenosis. C of A = coarctation of aorta. LV = left ventricle. LVOT = left ventricular outflow tract. MV = mitral valve. PDA = patent ductus arteriosus. PSG = peak systolic gradient. SA = systemic artery. S/D = systolic/diastolic. VSD = ventricular septal defect.

The discrete membrane (fibrous tissue) was, or had been, located in circumferential fashion on a plane approximately 1 cm. below the base of the aortic cusps corresponding with the ventricular aspect of the basal attachment of the anterior mitral leaflet. The ventricular aspects of the aortic valve cusps in all seven patients were thickened by fibrous tissue. The focal fibrous thickening in each of the six with tricuspid valves caused them to be incompetent. The ascending aorta and aortic root was hypoplastic in two patients (#6 and #7). The ventricular papillary muscles were focally scarred in all patients.

These seven patients emphasize the frequency of acquired lesions of the aortic valve in DSS. The aortic valves may become thickened and incompetent, and resulting jet lesions infected.[11]

Hypertrophic (Asymmetric) Cardiomyopathy with or without Subaortic Stenosis (Idiopathic Hypertrophic Subaortic Stenosis [IHSS])

Like discrete subaortic stenosis, diffuse muscular left ventricular outflow tract obstruction (IHSS) does not primarily involve a cardiac valve but it also may be confused with valvular heart disease and it also secondarily affects a cardiac valve (mitral) to produce varying degrees of regurgitation.

We have studied at necropsy 34 patients with IHSS. Cardiac catheterization had been performed in 28: 17 had systolic pressure gradients (20 to 162 [avg. 93]) at rest between left ventricular body and a systemic artery, and 11 had no pressure gradients at rest. Patients with gradients at rest differed in one respect anatomically from those without gradients at rest: those with gradients had uniformly thickened left ventricular free walls whereas those without gradients at rest had free walls, at least that portion immediately behind posterior mitral leaflet, of normal thickness. The cardiac anatomic features in these 34 patients were: (1) disproportional hypertrophy of the ventricular septae, i.e., the ventricular septae were thicker than the left ventricular free walls (28 patients); (2) small or normal-sized left and right ventricular cavities (31 patients); (3) endocardial mural plaques, left ventricular outflow tract (25 patients); (4) thickened mitral valves (25 patients); (5) dilated left and right atria (32 patients); (6) hypertrophied free walls of all four cardiac chambers (34 patients); (7) normal or nearly normal aortic valve cusps (31 patients); and (8) normal sized aortae (34 patients).

In contrast to discrete subaortic stenosis, the aortic valve is not involved in IHSS. The reason appears to be related to the relatively long distance between the site of left ventricular outflow obstruction and the aortic valve. In IHSS the gradient appears to be located on a plane corresponding to the distal margin of the anterior mitral leaflet. The caudal margin of the endocardial mural plaque in the left ventricular outflow tract also corresponds to the distal margin of the anterior mitral leaflet. The caudal margin of the endocardial mural plaque in the left ventricular outflow tract also corresponds to the distal margin of the anterior mitral leaflet. The caudal extension of this plaque is about 3 to 4 cm. below the base of the aortic valve cusps, and thus any jet produced at the site of obstruction is diffused by the time blood contacts the aortic valve cusps. In discrete subaortic stenosis, in contrast, the obstruction occurs about 1 cm. below the base of the aortic valve cusps, the jet is unable to be diffused before contacting the aortic cusps, and the cusps become thickened and prone to infection.

The cardiac valve which is made abnormal in IHSS is the mitral one. The ventricular aspect of the anterior leaflet is usually thickened by contacting the mural endocardium in the left ventricular outflow tract during ventricular systole. The left ventricular cavity in IHSS is relatively small, and when the left ventricular walls contract, the posterior leaflet is squeezed abnormally so that portions of it contact other portions like an accordian causing focal fibrous thickening. Although it may be impressive in IHSS, the fibrous thickening of the mitral leaflets and chordae tendineae does not appear to be the explanation for mitral regurgitation, which occurs in the majority of patients with IHSS because the mitral regurgitation nearly always disappears following adequate left ventricular myotomy of myectomy.[12] Distortion of the anterior left ventricular papillary muscle during ventricular systole by the massively hypertrophied ventricular septum may better explain the mitral regurgitation in these patients.[13]

Although mitral regurgitation is to be expected in patients with IHSS, the

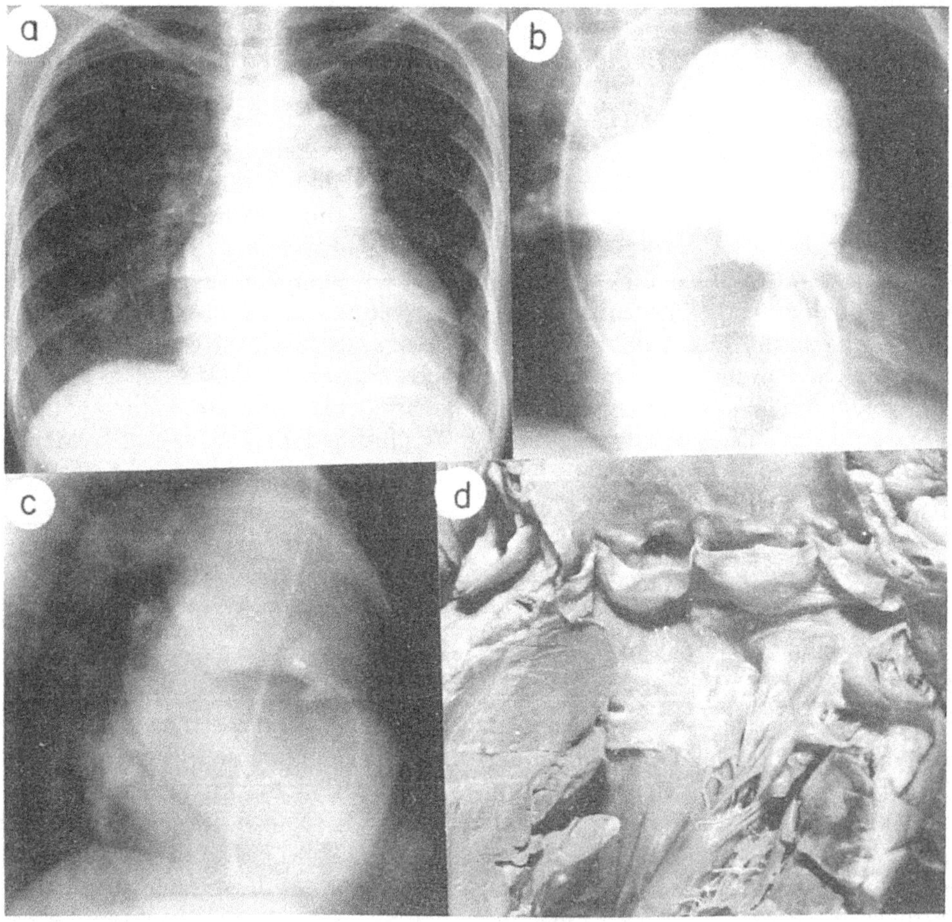

Figure 3. Hypertrophic (asymmetric) cardiomyopathy (idiopathic hypertrophic subaortic stenosis [IHSS]) presenting as pure mitral regurgitation. This 41-year-old woman (A63–77) was found to have a precordial murmur and cardiomegaly on insurance examination at age 33 and overt right-sided

and left-sided congestive cardiac failure, which progressed, appeared at age 38 years. When examined a month before death she was severely ill (functionally class IV). A grade 4/6 blowing pansystolic precordial murmur, loudest along the lower left sternal border, was audible. Electrocardiogram showed atrial fibrillation and a marked clockwise rotation. By x-ray (a, b, c), the heart was enlarged and the pulmonary trunk was aneurysmally dilated. The total serum protein was 5.3 with albumin 1.9 gm. per 100 ml., and 2.2 gm. of protein were measured in the urine in a 24-hour period. The total serum cholesterol was 318 mg. per 100 ml. At catheterization, the pressures (in mm. Hg) were: pulmonary artery, 34/7; right ventricle, 34/5; right atrial mean, 4; pulmonary arterial wedge, mean 11, v14; left ventricle, 112/11; and femoral artery, 122/65. The cardiac output (Fick method) was 1.6 L./min./m.^{2}. Left ventricular cineangiogram disclosed 4 /4 mitral regurgitation. (Retrospective examination of this angiogram was strongly suggestive of hypertrophic cardiomyopathy.) Aortic root injection of contrast material showed no aortic regurgitation. A day before death, cardiotomy was performed to replace the severely incompetent mitral valve. At operation, however, no systolic thrill was palpable over the left atrium which expanded hardly at all during ventricular systole. Examination of the mitral valve after cardiopulmonary bypass was instituted disclosed that the mitral leaflets and chordae were "normal" and that the left ventricular cavity was not dilated. Therefore, valve replacement was not carried out. The patient died the next day because of inadequate cardiac output. At necropsy, a large transmural acute myocardial infarct involved the posterior left ventricular free wall. Histologic study indicated that the infarct was about 14 days old. The mitral leaflets and chordae were focally thickened but the annulus was not dilated and the left ventricular cavity was of normal size. In the outflow tract of the left ventricle, a mural endocardial plaque, in direct apposition to the anterior mitral leaflet, was present (d). Since the aortic valve cusps were normal, it was clear that this endocardial plaque indicated that *hypertrophic cardiomyopathy* was the proper diagnosis. The ventricular septum was nearly twice as thick as was the left ventricular free wall. Thus, this patient demonstrates how IHSS may present as pure mitral regurgitation. The cause of the aneurysmal dilatation of the pulmonary trunk is uncertain. (At operation, a diastolic thrill had been palpated over this artery indicating the presence of pulmonic regurgitation.)

amount of regurgitation is usually minimal or mild. On rare occasions, however, mitral regurgitation is the dominant lesion (Fig. 3) and valve replacement, although hazardous in this condition, has been performed.

Supravalvular Aortic Stenosis (SAS)

Like subaortic stenosis, this condition does not primarily affect a cardiac valve but it too may be confused with valvular aortic stenosis and it also may

Figure 4. Valvular aortic stenosis from arteriosclerosis in homozygous type II hyperlipoproteinemia. a, Opened aortic valve and ascending aorta showing severe atherosclerosis of the aorta and severe fibrous thickening of the aortic valve cusps which are relatively rigid. b, Radiograph of heart at necropsy showing extensive calcific deposits in the ascending aorta and in the coronary arteries. c, Photograph of patient showing xanthomas on elbows, buttocks, and ankles. d, Photomicrograph (hematoxylin-eosin stain X 63) of portion of anterior mitral leaflet showing extensive collections of foam cells. Similar lesions were present in the aortic valve cusps. This 28-year-old man (A70–64), who died suddenly, had xanthomas noted at age two years. He ate low-fat foods most of his life. He was asymptomatic until age 17 years when angina pectoris appeared. At age 23, the first of several episodes of syncope occurred and at age 26 he had an episode of acute pulmonary edema without evidence of acute myocardial infarction. When studied a month later, he had mild exertional dyspnea and angina. He slept flat in bed. Several family members, including both parents, had type II hyperlipoproteinemia. In addition to large widespread tuberotendinous xanthomas, he had a sustained left ventricular lift and a grade 3/6 mid-systolic, ejection-type murmur over the left sternal border with radiation into the neck. He had no signs of congestive cardiac failure. The blood pressure was 115/65 mm. Hg. The heart was of normal size on chest roentgenogram. The initial serum total cholesterol was 588 with beta, alpha, and VLDL fractions 529, 31, and 28 mg. per 100 ml., respectively. The total serum triglyceride was 100 mg. per 100 ml. Protein electrophoresis showed a bifid peak in the beta region with a quantitation of 1.3 gm. per 100 ml. During his last two years he was treated with a low-cholesterol diet and high doses (48 gm. daily) of cholestyramine. The total serum cholesterol fell to 340 mg. per 100 ml., the xanthomas softened slightly and became less yellow. The immediate cause of death was not determined at necropsy.

be associated with fibrous thickening of the aortic valvular cusps. In this condition, the site of obstruction is the ascending aorta, most frequently (66 per cent) on a level corresponding to the most cephalad extension of the aortic valve cusps.[14] Maximal narrowing at this site produces an hourglass type obstruction. The narrowing results both from thickening of the aortic media and from superimposed fibrous intimal proliferation. Less frequently (21 per cent), the supravalvular obstruction results from diffuse hypoplasia of the entire ascending aorta or from a fibrous membrane just above the aortic sinuses associated with a central opening and a more normal-sized aorta (13 per cent).[14] Each of these three anatomic

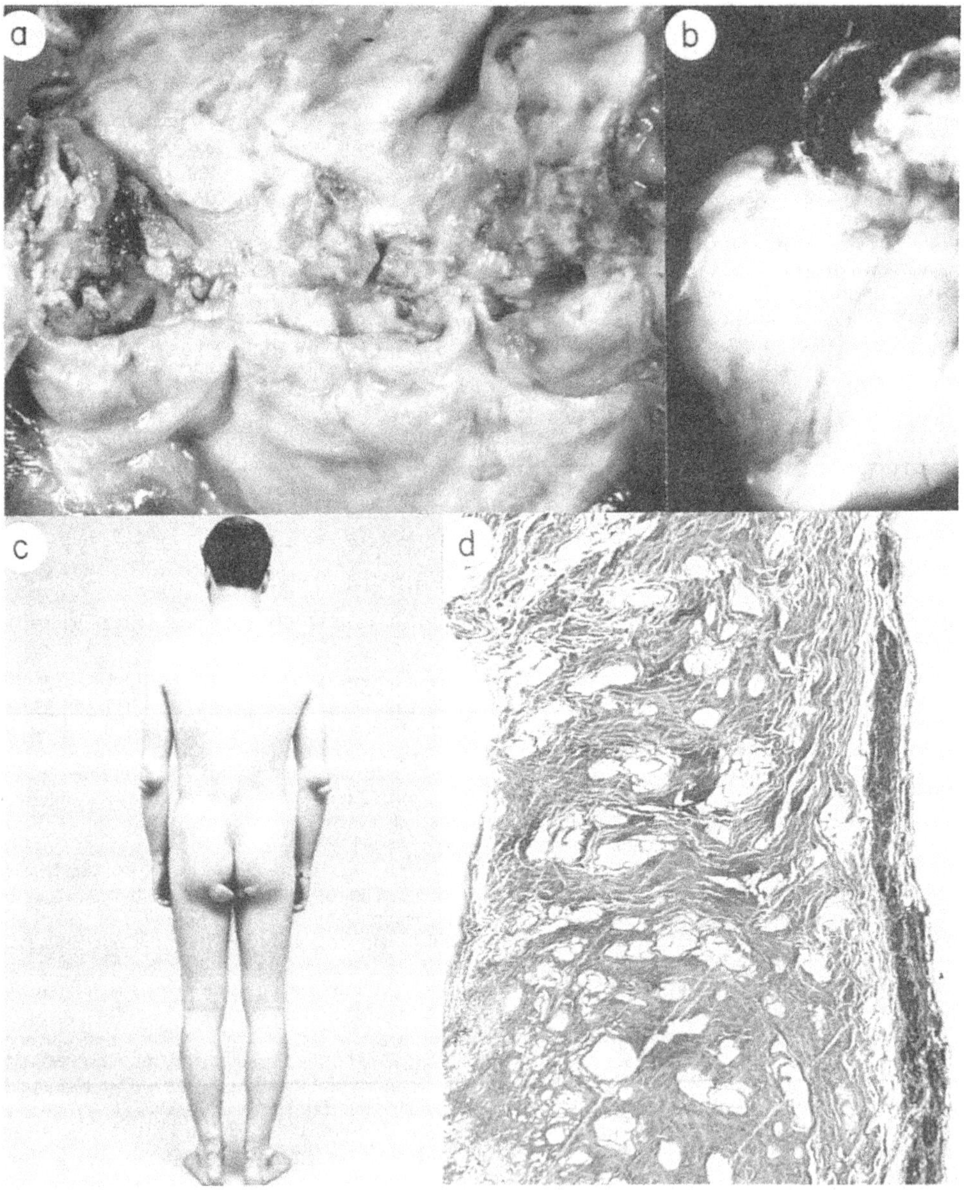

types may be associated with fibrous thickening of the aortic valve cusps, and may produce valvular aortic stenosis. Aortic valve cusps were thickened in 30 per cent of 68 necropsy cases of supravalvular aortic stenosis analyzed from the literature.[14] Occasionally, the margin of one or more cusps may be adherent to the aortic wall at the site of supravalvular obstruction and these deformities may produce aortic regurgitation. We have studied at necropsy two patients with supravalvular aortic stenosis.[15] Both had the hourglass type deformity: in one the aortic valve cusps were normal and in the second the cusps were diffusely thickened and adherent to the area of supravalvular stenosis probably causing valvular dysfunction.

Infection on the intima of the aorta above the aortic valve may complicate supravalvular aortic stenosis and the infection may extend retrogradely to involve the area of narrowing just above the aortic valve and the valve itself.

Although usually congenital in origin, SAS on rare occasion may be acquired. Healing of an aortotomy incision may constrict the aorta in an hourglass-type deformity. Homozygous type II hyperlipoproteinemia may be associated with severe atherosclerosis in the ascending aorta as well as in the aortic valve cusps themselves[16] (Fig. 4). Recently, a patient with type II hyperlipoproteinemia was reported as having supravalvular aortic "stenosis."[17]

Obstruction to Left Ventricular Inflow

Congenital Mitral Stenosis

Obstruction to left ventricular inflow at the level of the mitral valve may be congenital in origin or acquired. In the latter, the cause is usually filling defects

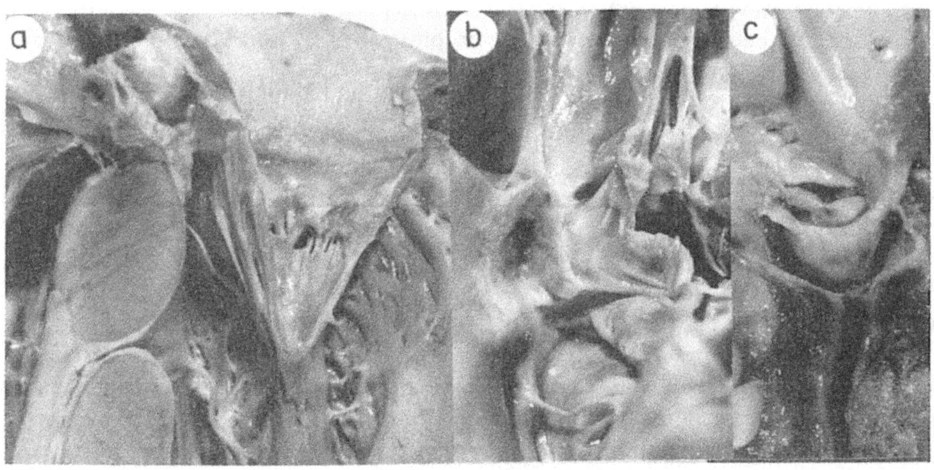

Figure 5. Single left ventricular papillary muscle (a) (Parachute mitral valve), discrete subaortic stenosis (b), and stenotic congenitally bicuspid aortic valve (c) in a 14 year-old boy (GT 71A–215) who had an 80 mm. Hg peak systolic pressure gradient between left ventricle and systemic artery. He had been asymptomatic until one year before death from pulmonary edema. No abnormality of the mitral valve had been appreciated clinically. a, Longitudinal section across mitral and aortic valves and ventricular septum demonstrating the parachute mitral deformity. A defect in the muscular portion of the ventricular septum had closed spontaneously by fibrous-tissue proliferation. b, View of discrete subaortic stenosis from left ventricle. c, View of bicuspid, stenotic aortic valve from above.

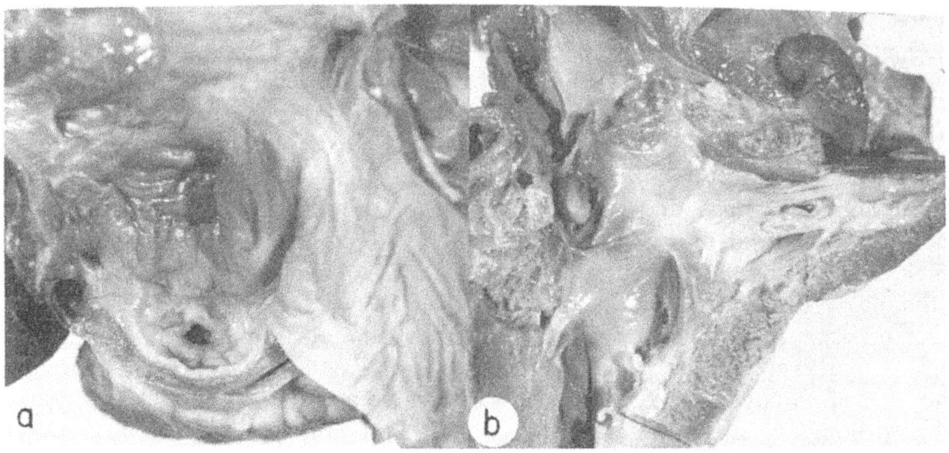

Figure 6. Congenital mitral stenosis with parachute mitral valve and supravalvular left atrial ring in a young child (A69–264). a, Mitral valve area viewed from left atrium. A fibrous diaphragm with a narrowed central orifice is present at the level of the annulus. The endocardium of the dilated left atrium is severely thickened. b, Opened left ventricle, aortic valve, and aorta. The thickened chordae tendineae insert into a single papillary muscle which is located in an anterolateral position. The valve orifice is stenotic. In addition, this child had a defect in the membranous portion of the ventricular septum (it nearly was closed by septal tricuspid leaflet), a persistent patent ductus arteriosus, and a coarctation of the aorta.

in the left atrium which protrude into the mitral orifice during ventricular diastole. These filling defects include left atrial myxomas,[18] fungal masses[19] and malignant neoplasms.[20] The latter two generally originate in the lung and extend into the left atrium via pulmonary veins.

Nonrheumatic valvular obstruction involving mitral leaflets is virtually limited to congenital anomalies. In one type of congenital mitral stenosis (MS) the leaflets are thickened and fibrosed with rudimentary or fused commissures and short and fused chordae.[21] Anatomically, the valve is funnel-shaped and resembles a rheumatically diseased valve. Another variety is the parachute deformity[22-23] (Figs. 5 and 6), in which the chordae are shortened and converge to insert on a single papillary muscle thus restricting the motion of the leaflets. Left ventricular inflow is limited primarily to openings between chordae. Both anomalies often are complicated by discrete supravalvular fibrous diaphragms arising from the atrial aspect of the valve annuli (Fig. 6). Either the valvular deformity or the annular diaphragm or both may cause obstruction. Parachute mitral valves are usually associated with other developmental anomalies including coarctation of the aorta (often with a bicuspid aortic valve), discrete subvalvular left ventricular outflow obstruction, and supravalvular mitral ring, which may or may not be stenotic. Congenital MS also may result from an arcade type deformity of the valve[24] (Fig. 7).

The hemodymanic consequences of congenital MS are similar to those caused by acquired (rheumatic) MS. Auscultation, however, may differ. Many patients with congenital MS do not have detectable diastolic murmurs, and opening snaps

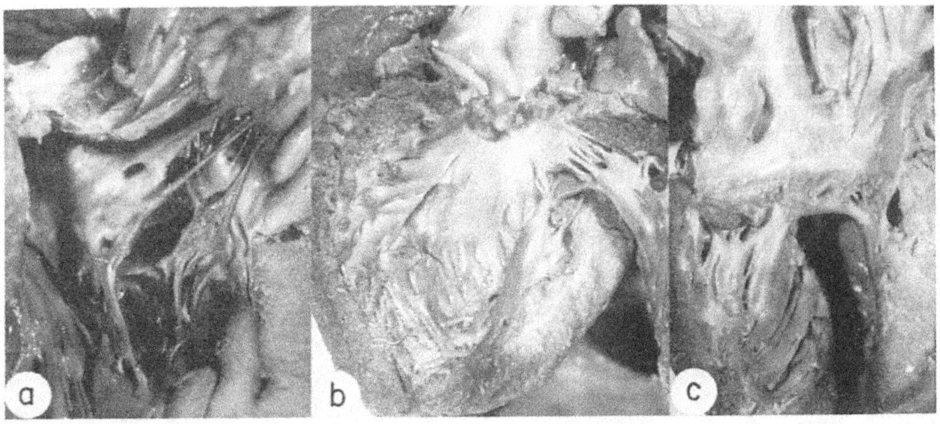

Figure 7. Congenital mitral stenosis due to "arcade" type deformity of the valve. This 3-day-old boy (A67–212), who died during catheterization, was diagnosed clinically as having "hypoplastic left heart." At necropsy, the mitral valve appeared stenotic. a, View of mitral valve from left ventricle. b, Opened left ventricle, aortic valve, and aorta. The endocardium is thickened, and the aortic valve consisted of rudimentary cusps. c, Opened mitral valve showing short chordae tendineae and thickened cuspal margins. The patient also had a large patent ductus arteriosus.

are rare. These auscultatory differences may be explained by their rapid heart rates, by the increased tendency of the right ventricle to occupy the apex and obscure the murmur, and by the severly reduced mobility of the leaflets.[25]

Congenital MS, even when associated with other anomalies, is rare, but when isolated is extremely rare.[26] We have not observed congenital MS as an isolated defect. The heart of a child with a stenotic supravalvular ring and a parachute deformity of the mitral valve is illustrated in Figure 6.

Obstruction to Right Ventricular Outflow

Isolated Valvular Pulmonic Stenosis

Congenital valvular pulmonic stenosis (PS) with intact ventricular septum is the most common form of isolated right ventricular outflow obstruction and comprises about 10 per cent of all major congenital cardiovascular anomalies in patients surviving beyond infancy.[27] The stenotic valve usually has a

Table 7. Isolated congenital pulmonic stenosis: clinical and necropsy findings

Patient	*Age (yrs.)*	*Sex*	*Duration (yrs.) symptoms*	*Cyanosis*	*Right-sided CHF*	*RV-PA PSG (mm. Hg)*	*Heart weight (gm.)*	*Pulmonic valve*	*VC-PFO*
1. A55–59	4	F	2	+	+	124	270*	Dome	+
2. A64–135	43	F	35	+	+	161	400	Dome	+
3. NNMC# A71–24	38	F	—	0	+	88	450	Bicuspid	0

* Expected weight = 75 gm.
CHF = congestive heart failure. PA = pulmonary artery. PSG = peak systolic gradient. RV= right ventricle. VC-PFO = valvular competent patent foramen ovale.

domed shape or funnel shape with a small (less than 5 mm.) opening at the apex. Three raphes extend from the valve to the pulmonary trunk and these probably represent vestigial commissures. Rarely, three separate cusps are identifiable but when this occurs additional developmental defects usually are present.[28] The mean age of death in unoperated patients with isolated PS is 25 years.[29] Older patients with this malformation may develop calcific deposits in the valve.[30,31]

We have studied at necropsy three patients with isolated congenital valvular PS (Table 7, Figs. 8–11). All three died within two months of pulmonic val-

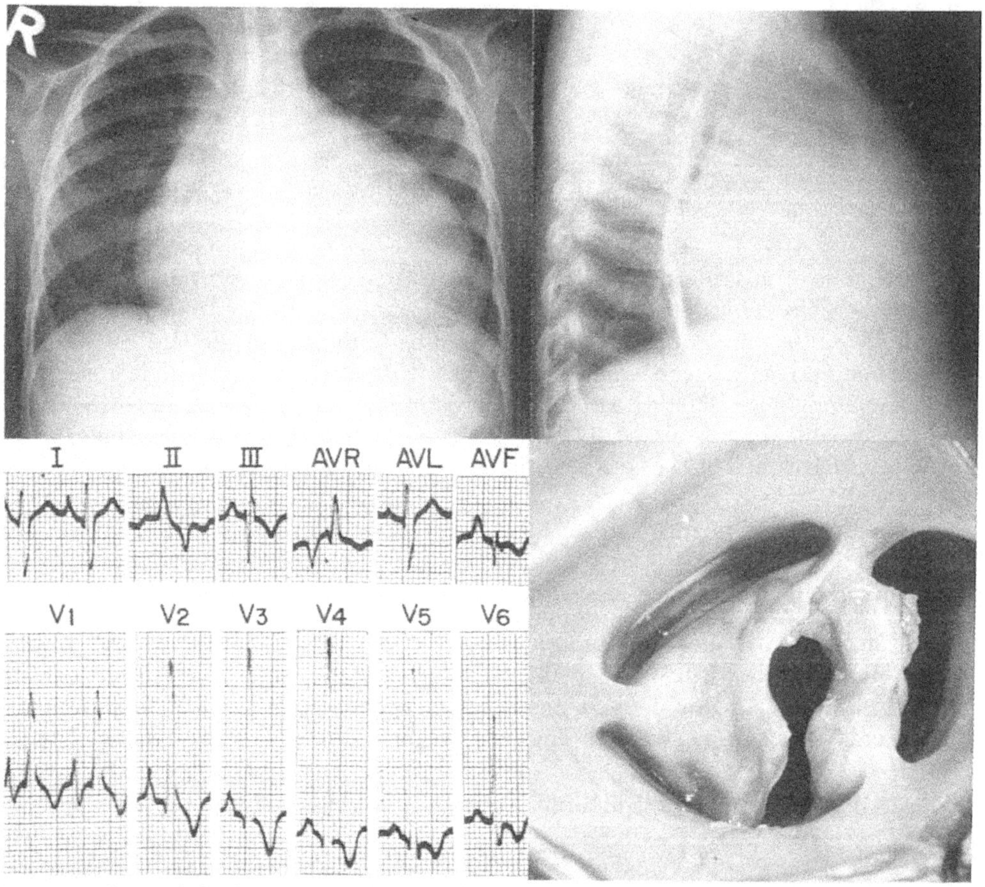

Figure 8. Congenital valvular pulmonic stenosis. Posteroanterior and lateral chest roentgenograms, electrocardiogram, and pulmonary valve from a four-year-old girl (A55–59) who died just after pulmonic valvulotomy. A precordial murmur had been heard at six months of age and by two years cyanosis was present. By age three she was in right-sided cardiac failure and had episodes of precordial pain. Chest roentgenogram reveals severe cardiomegaly with marked right ventricular enlargement and decreased pulmonary vascular markings. Electrocardiogram shows right atrial enlargement and right ventricular hypertrophy. The cardiac size and monophasic R waves in V_1 through V_6 contrast sharply with those of the adult patient in Figure 9. A single incision had been made in the valve at operation but the domed structure, small central orifice, and fused commissures with raphes attached to the wall of the pulmonary trunk are well preserved.

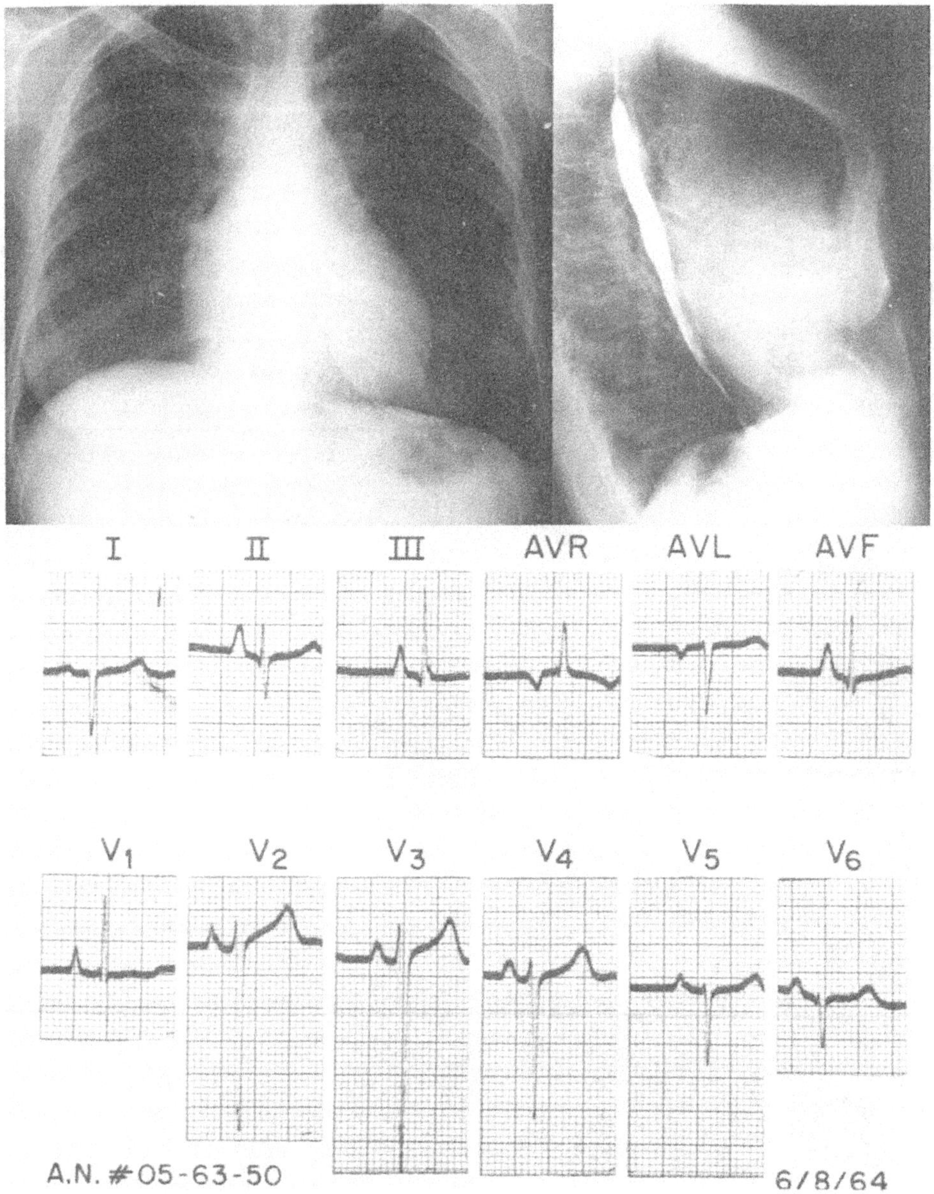

Figure 9. Congenital valvular pulmonic stenosis. Posteroanterior and lateral chest roentgenograms and electrocardiogram of a 43-year-old woman (A64–135) who died during pulmonic valvulotomy. She had symptoms of cardiac dysfunction since age five years. For several years before death she had episodes of severe precordial pressure and dyspnea associated with mild exertion. Despite these symptoms she underwent two normal pregnancies and worked on a factory assembly line until hospitalization. On examination, she was cyanotic with clubbed fingers and toes. Chest roentgenogram revealed right atrial and right ventricular enlargement, a prominent pulmonary segment, normal to decreased pulmonary vascular markings, and pectus carinatum. Electrocardiogram showed right axis deviation (120 degrees) and right atrial and right ventricular hypertrophy.

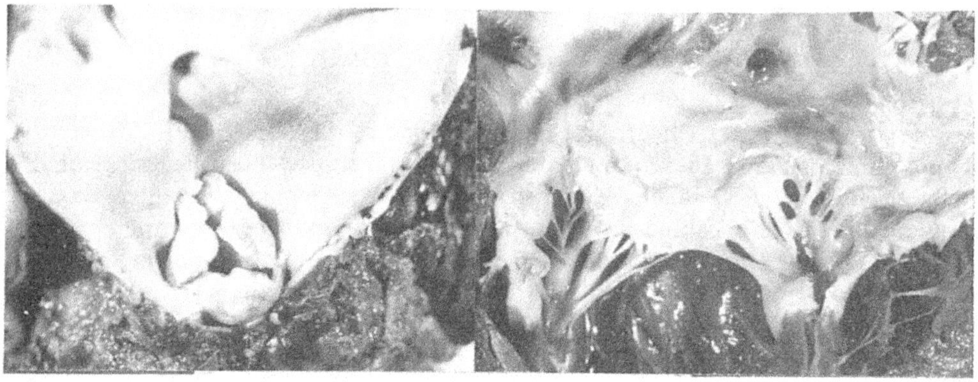

Figure 10. Congenital valvular pulmonic stenosis. Anatomic findings from woman whose electrocardiogram and roentgenogram are depicted in Figure 9. *Left,* Opened pulmonary trunk showing stenotic three-cuspid pulmonic valve after commissurotomy. *Right,* Although there was no clinical evidence of mitral valve dysfunction, the mitral leaflets and chordae were thickened.

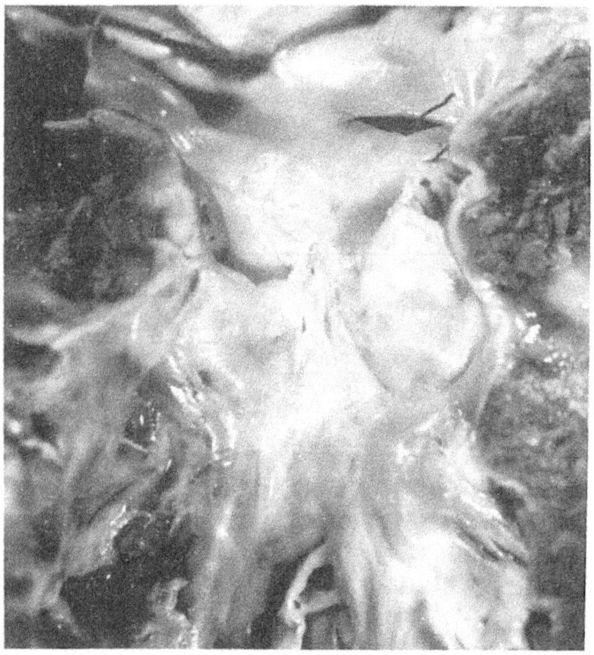

Figure 11. Pulmonic valve stenosis with bicuspid valve. Opened pulmonic valve and pulmonary trunk of a 34-year-old woman (NNMC# A71-24) who died of sepsis from an infected hematoma several months after pulmonic valvulotomy. The cusps are thickened and stiff.

vulotomy. Two had dome-shaped valves and one had a congenitally bicuspid valve. The valves in each were thickened, scarred, and stiff.

Congenitally bucuspid pulmonic valves are rare in comparison with the frequency of congenitally bicuspid aortic valves. Although they are commonly associated with other congenital cardiovascular malformations, particularly tetralogy of Fallot, congenitally bicuspid pulmonic valves appear to be extremely rare in patients with isolated pulmonic stenosis.[32] Indeed, we have found no reports describing isolated pulmonic stenosis complicating the congenitally bicuspid valve.

Obstruction to Both Right Ventricular Outflow and Inflow

The Carcinoid Syndrome

First recognized as a distinct entity in 1954,[33] this syndrome is caused by a metastasizing carcinoid tumor located usually in the small intestine, occasionally in the bronchus[34] or stomach,[35] and rarely elsewhere. The tumor produces several biologically active substances, including serotonin (5-hydroxytryptamine), histamine, and kinin peptides (bradykinin).[36] Diagnosis is established on the basis of increased urinary excretion of 5-hydroxyindole acetic acid (HIAA), a breakdown product of serotonin.[37] Dermal flushing and diarrhea occur in almost all patients with the syndrome; wheezing occurs in approximately a third, and a peculiar but specific cardiac disease is present in over one half.[38,39] Of 32 necropsy patients with the carcinoid syndrome studied by us, 18 had carcinoid heart disease and 14 did not (Table 8).

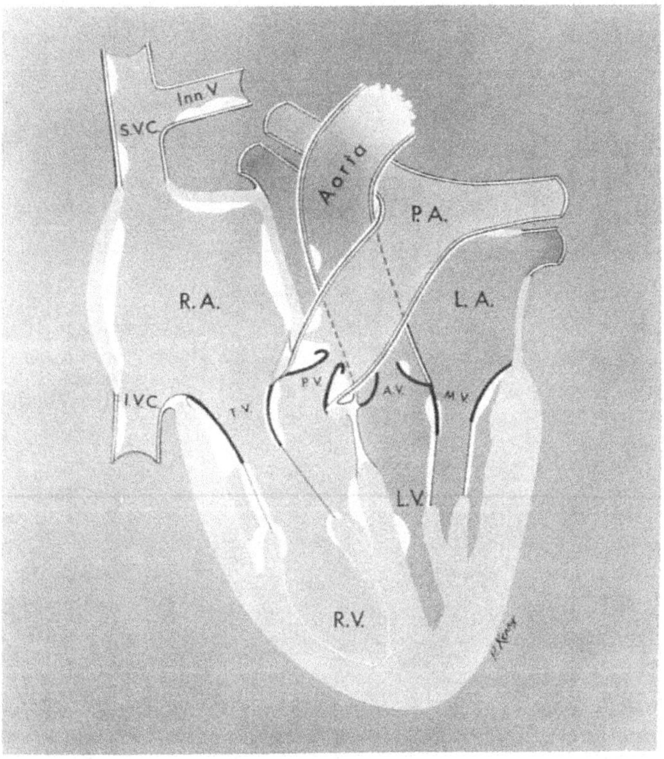

Figure 12. Carcinoid heart disease. Summary diagram demonstrating (in white) the sites where fibrous plaques occur in patients with the carcinoid syndrome. In patients with abdominal carcinoid tumors the lesions are always more numerous and more extensive on the right side of the heart. The white plaques often are extensive in right atrium (R.A.) and tricuspid (T.V.) and pulmonic (P.V.) valves. The lesions have not been observed in the pulmonary arteries (P.A.) except in the immediate vicinity of the valve or in the left atrium (L.A.). Inn. V. = innominate vein. S.V.C. = superior vena cava. I.V.C. = inferior vena cava. R.V. = right ventricle. M.V. = mitral valve. L.V. = left ventricle. A.V. = aortic valve.

Table 8. The carcinoid syndrome: clinical and necropsy data

	No. pts.	Ages range (avg.) (years)	F	M	Length of illness (mo.) (avg.)	Diarrhea	Flushing	Asthma	Precordial murmur	Urinary 5-HIAA excretion (mg./24 hrs.)	Small intestinal primary	Hepatic metastases	Organ weights (gm.) Liver	Heart	Spleen
With heart disease	18*	32–69 (53)	8	10	10–156 (58)	18	17	8	18	120–1270 (418)	18	18	1600–7400 (2723)	200–475 (283)	40–475 (159)
Without heart disease	14†	28–75 (56)	4	10	12–108 (45)	13	14	4	8‡	14–900 (284)	10 ¶	13	500–6100 (3015)	150–450 (284)	30–730 (247)
TOTALS	32	28–75 (55)	12	20	10–156 (53)	31	31	12	26	14-1270 § (357)§	28 ¶	31	1600–7400 (2847)	150–475# (285)	30–730** (200)

* 3 black; 15 white
† All white
‡ One had a large atrial septal defect; another had a large left atrial myxoma; another had severe valvular aortic stenosis.
§ The range and average are of the highest values for each patient.
¶ Bronchus in three; stomach in one.
\# Only four (two from each group) of 32 hearts weighed more than 400 gm. and each patient had a history of systemic hypertension.
** Weight more than 300 gm. in five patients, two with and three without carcinoid heart disease.

The cardiovascular lesions associated with the carcinoid syndrome are pathognomonic and bear little resemblance to those in other cardiac diseases.[38] The involvement consists of focal or diffuse collections of a peculiar type of fibrous tissue which is deposited on the endocardium of the valvular cusps and cardiac chambers and on the intima of the great veins, coronary sinus, and occasionally great arteries (Figs. 12–14). The valvular cusps per se and mural endocardium are normal, and are clearly separated from the fibrosing process by the endocardial elastic membrane. The deposits, which are often referred to as fibrous, white, or carcinoid plaques, are most frequent and extensive in the right side of the

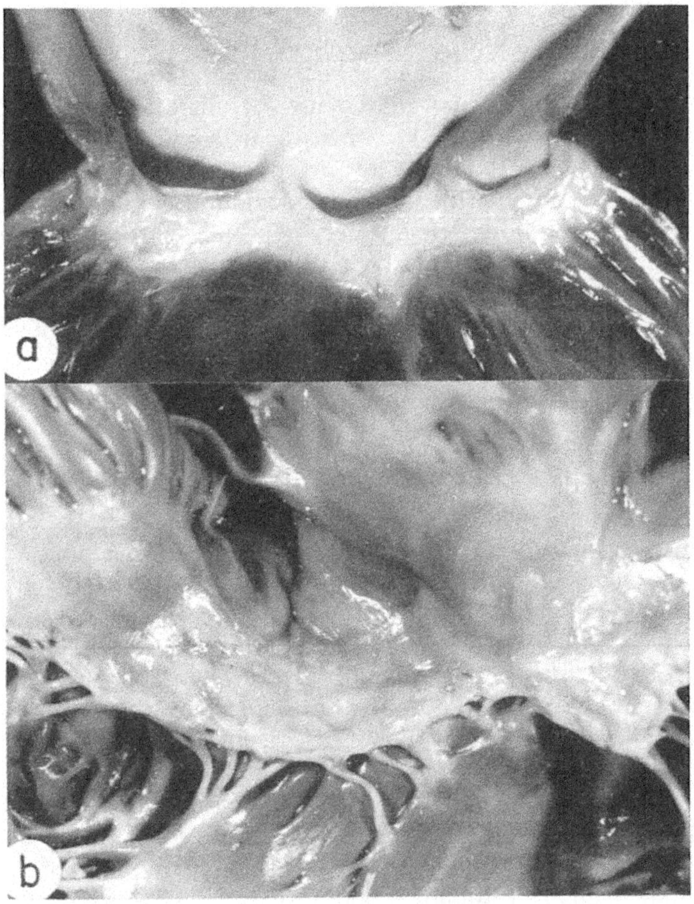

Figure 13. Carcinoid heart disease. Opened pulmonic (a) and tricuspid (b) valves in a 61-year-old woman (A72–96) who had had diarrhea and dermal flushing for 12 months. She had evidence clinically of tricuspid regurgitation and pulmonic stenosis. She developed severe ascites and subcutaneous edema and died of massive gastrointestinal hemorrhage. A carcinoid tumor was present in the ileum and carcinoid metastases were present in abdominal lymph nodes and in liver. The heart was small (240 gm.) but she was cachectic. Carcinoid plaques were present on tricuspid and pulmonic valves, right atrial endocardium, and coronary sinus. The pulmonic valve ring was constricted and the cusps were retracted (a). The tricuspid valve cusps and chordae also were thickened and contracted (b).

heart. Of our 18 patients with carcinoid heart disease, plaques were present on the tricuspid and pulmonic valves in all: on right atrium in 17, right ventricle in 11, vena cava in 7, coronary sinus and veins in 8, and pulmonary trunk in 4. In every patient the tricuspid and pulmonic valves were contracted, relatively rigid, and both stenotic and incompetent. The predominant hemodynamic lesion of the tricuspid valve, however, was regurgitation, and that of the pulmonic valve, stenosis. The diffuse deposition of fibrous tissue on the endocardium of the right atrium causes its wall to be relatively noncompliant.[39] The deposits on the right ventricle, in contrast, are always small and functionally insignificant.

Left-sided cardiac lesions in the carcinoid syndrome are more common than initially believed and occurred in seven patients: mitral valve lesion in all seven, left ventricle in three, aortic valve in one, and ascending aorta in one. Although two patients had diffuse mitral valvular deposits, the valvular orifices did not appear stenotic or incompetent. The aortic valve carcinoid plaque occurred in only one of the three cusps and caused no valvular dysfunction. No patients with left-sided lesions had intracardiac or extracardiac shunts nor carcinoid tumor in the lungs. The right-sided cardiac lesions in these seven patients were always more extensive than the left-sided ones. Carcinoid plaquing limited entirely to the left side of the heart, however, has been reported with bronchial carcinoid.[40]

With the exception of the anterior tricuspid and anterior mitral leaflets, the fibrous plaques were located on the ventricular surfaces of the atrioventricular cusps. The deposits on the posterior and septal tricuspid leaflets adhered these cusps to the underlying right ventricular wall, and the semilunar valvular deposits were located entirely within the sinuses.

The right ventricle and right atrium were mildly hypertrophied and dilated in each of the 18 patients with carcinoid heart disease, but, overall, the hearts of the 18 patients with carcinoid heart disease were identical in weight to those of the 14 patients without cardiac involvement (Table 8). Four patients had hearts weighing more than 400 gm. and each had histories of systemic hypertension. Interstitial and replacement myocardial fibrosis is not part of carcinoid heart disease and if present can be attributed to another condition.

Carcinoid plaques are composed of layers of collagen and acid mucopolysaccharide; the cellular elements are narrow, elongated, arranged parallel to the surface of the plaque, and stain intensely with phosphotungstic acid hematoxylin. The distinctive histologic feature of carcinoid plaques, however, is the absence of elastic tissue. The underlying internal elastic lamina of the endocardium is intact. Electron-microscopic examination shows that the carcinoid plaque consists of smooth muscle cells, fibrils of young and developing collagen, layered material similar to that of basement membranes of smooth muscle cells, and small spicules of unknown composition.[41]

The most useful clinical finding for distinguishing patients with carcinoid heart disease from those without is the presence of a precordial murmur suggestive of tricuspid regurgitation or pulmonic stenosis. The most frequent murmur in the 18 patients with cardiac involvement was fairly harsh in quality, grade 1 to 3/6 in intensity, systolic in time, and located along the upper left sternal border. Less frequently, a systolic blowing murmur which increased with inspira-

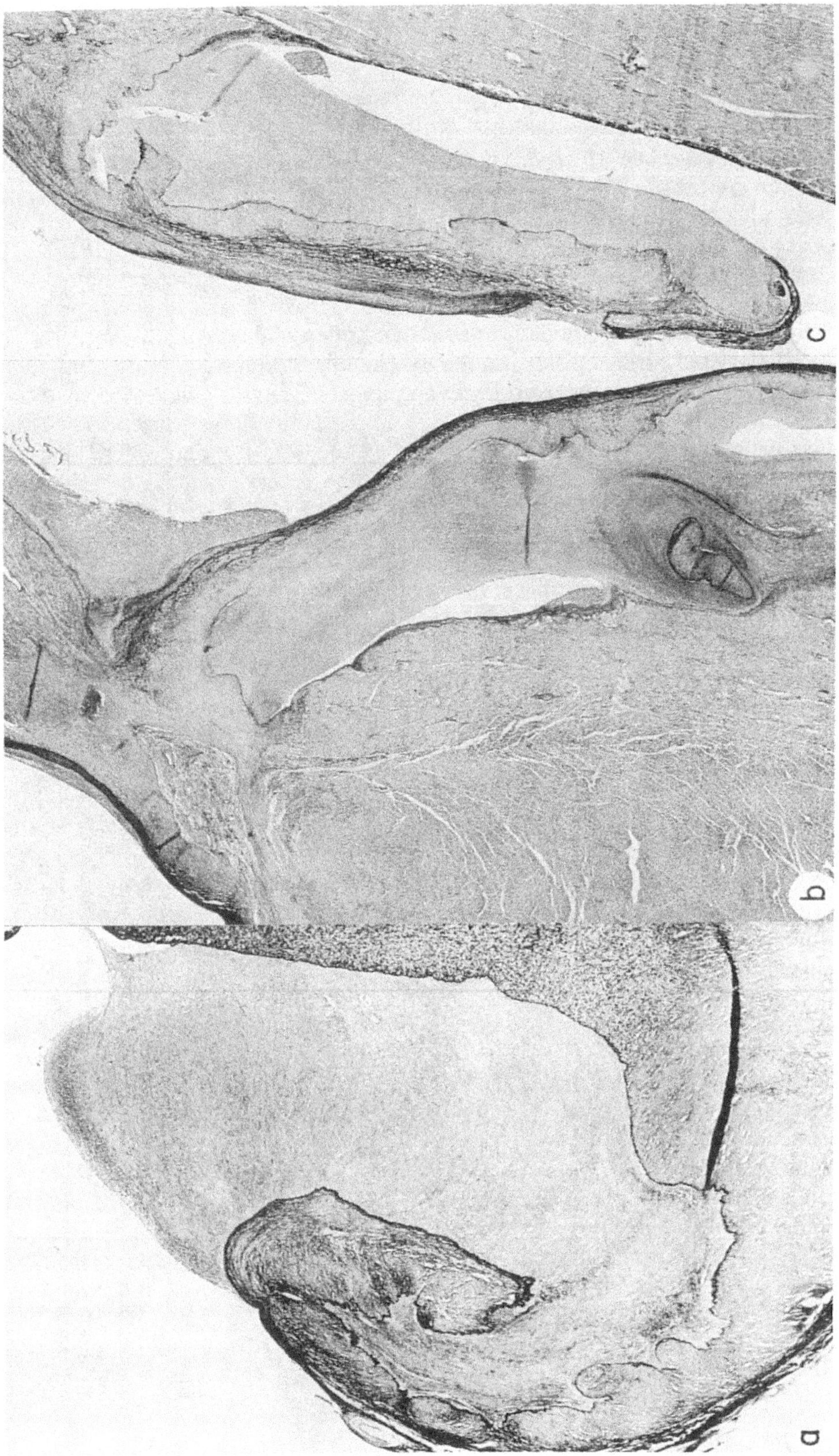

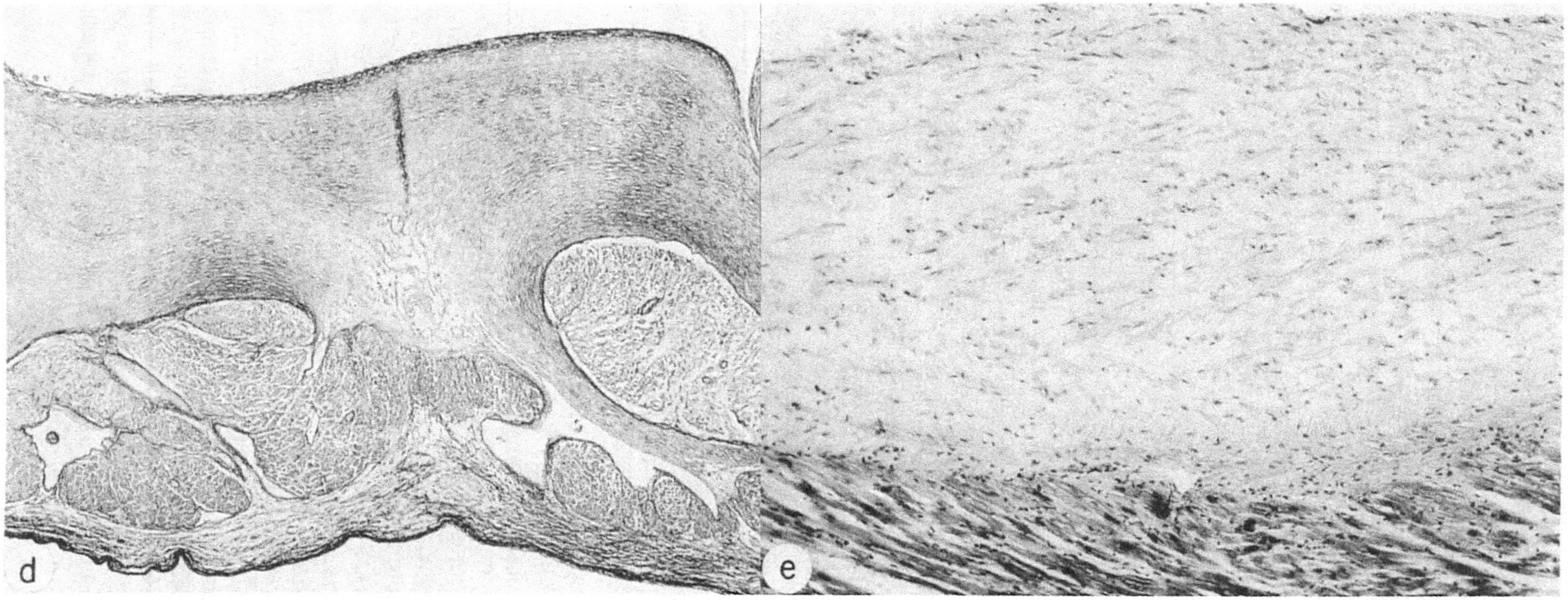

Figure 14. Carcinoid heart disease. Photomicrographs of carcinoid plaques in pulmonic valve (a), tricuspid valve (b), mitral valve (c), and right atrium (d and e). a, The carcinoid plaque which consists of an unusual type of elastic fiber, is located entirely on the sinus side of the cusp, i.e., the side which does not have the initial contact with the blood stream. The normal valve cusp is clearly separated from the superimposed fibrous tissue by a black staining elastic membrane (A61–68). b, Tricuspid valve showing extensive carcinoid plaquing on the ventricular aspect of the cusp. The plaque adheres the valve leaflet to the underlying mural endocardium. The penetrating portion of the atrioventricular bundle also is visible on this section (A61–193). c, Posterior mitral leaflet. The carcinoid plaque is on the undersurface of the cusp, which remains normal (A61–193). d, Right atrial wall showing a large carcinoid plaque superimposed on normal right atrial endocardium (A59–223). e, Close-up of carcinoid atrial plaque showing that it consists of strap cells, arranged parallel to its surface, separated by an amorphous ground substance (A61–193). a-d, Elastic van Gieson stains. e, Hematoxylin-eosin stain. [Reduced 15 per cent from × 39(a), × 14(b), × 18(c), × 40(d), and × 108 (e).]

tion was heard along the lower left sternal border. In none of the seven patients with mitral carcinoid disease was the diagnosis apparent clinically. Prominent v waves often were detectable in the superficial jugular veins; a waves were occasionally prominent also. The liver was sometimes pulsatile.

The chest roentgenogram and electrocardiogram are of little value in determining the presence or absence of carcinoid heart disease. Although the lateral chest roentgenogram sometimes discloses enlargement of the right ventricle, the overall size of the heart on posteroanterior projection is usually normal. Low voltage, the most frequent electrocardiographic abnormality in patients with this syndrome, occurred in 9 of 18 patients with carcinoid heart disease and in 3 of the 14 patients without it. Electrocardiographic evidence of right ventricular hypertrophy occurred in only 2 patients, and evidence of right atrial enlargement (peaked P waves) occurred in 4 of 18 patients with carcinoid heart disease.

Cardiac catheterization in patients with carcinoid heart disease has disclosed tricuspid regurgitation and pulmonic stenosis to be the most frequent valvular lesions. The right atrial pressures are commonly very elevated, and probably higher than would be expected with rheumatic tricuspid regurgitation of similar severity.[39] Although the cardiac output has been reported to be elevated in patients with the carcinoid syndrome without carcinoid heart disease, it is generally normal or low in patients who have carcinoid heart disease.

One of the best means of producing severe right-sided failure in animals is by making the pulmonary trunk stenotic and the tricuspid valve incompetent. These are the two principal valvular lesions which occur in patients with carcinoid heart disease. This cardiac disease, however, does not appear to decrease longevity. The length of illness from onset of symptoms to death in the 18 patients with carcinoid heart disease averaged 58 months, and in the 14 without it, 45 months. Peripheral edema and ascites appear to be worse in patients with carcinoid cardiac disease, but these signs appear to result more commonly from associated hepatic dysfunction (due to metastases) and hypoalbuminemia.

The pathogenesis of the carcinoid plaque is uncertain. An intriguing feature of the carcinoid plaque is the lack of varying stages of development. No "early" lesions have been observed. All plaques are similar whether on valvular or mural endocardium. Initially, serotonin was believed to cause the endocardial fibrosis, but there is no evidence to substantiate this belief. It has not been possible to produce the cardiac lesions in animals by giving serotonin or other substances, and urinary levels of the breakdown product of serotonin (5-hydroxyindole acetic acid) and blood serotonin levels have been similar in patients with the carcinoid syndrome with and without cardiac involvement.[42] Serotonin initially also was believed to be responsible for the dermal flush in this syndrome, but this hypothesis has been discounted.[43] A kinin peptide, such as bradykinin, appears the more likely cause of the flush,[43] and it may also cause the carcinoid endocardial lesions, but this has not been demonstrated. Our identification of the cells in carcinoid plaques as smooth muscle cells is of interest in this respect since the clinical features of the carcinoid syndrome, i.e., flushing, wheezing, and diarrhea, are mediated through effects on smooth muscle. The same circulating factor responsible for the aforementioned clinical manifestations may stimulate smooth muscle cells in endocardium to proliferate and to synthesize collagen and basement membrane-like material. The importance of other unknown factors in the formation of carcinoid endocardial plaques is shown by the selective localization of the plaques and by their lack of elastic tissue.

Combined Stenosis of Right and Left-Sided Cardiac Valves

Stenosis of multiple valves usually indicates rheumatic heart disease. Rarely, however, one valve on both right and left sides of the heart may be stenotic when the etiology is congenital rather than rheumatic. The usual combination is congenital pulmonic and aortic stenosis,[44-45] and rarely tricuspid stenosis with aortic or mitral stenosis or both.[46] The occurrence of combined congenital pulmonic and mitral stenosis also is rare,[47] but we have studied two such patients at necropsy. Mitral stenosis was diagnosed only at catheterization in one, and never clinically in the second.[48] The latter patient underwent pulmonic valvulotomy, and died shortly thereafter of pulmonary edema, the consequence of the undiagnosed and untreated mitral stenosis.[48] Both patients had dome-shaped pulmonic valves. The mitral valve leaflets and chordae in one were thickened, stiff, and shortened; the other had a parachute mitral valve.

Stenotic right-sided lesions regardless of etiology protect to varying degrees against pulmonary vascular congestion resulting from associated mitral stenosis. When both right and left-sided stenotic lesions are present the left-sided stenosis should be relieved first. Unfortunately, the same conditions which delay the onset of incapacitating symptoms may obscure the clinical diagnosis of mitral stenosis as was true in both our patients.

NONOBSTRUCTIVE LESIONS

With Involvement of Ascending Aorta

Syphilis

Syphilis remains an important cause of severe aortic regurgitation. We have studied at necropsy nine patients with aortic regurgitation secondary to syphilitic aortitis (Table 9). Six were men, three were women, and their ages ranged from 19 to 80 years. Serological tests for syphilis were positive in six of the eight patients in whom the tests were performed. No patient had received penicillin at the time of the primary infection. In seven of nine patients, symptoms of congestive cardiac failure developed within three years of detection of a precordial murmur. In each, aortic regurgitation was severe, caused congestive failure, and was responsible for death in all but one. The latter patient died of a stroke.

At necropsy, the hearts weighed 600 to 850 gm. (avg. 695), and in each the left ventricular cavities were dilated and their walls, hypertrophied. The ascending aorta was diffusely dilated in all patients. In seven, the entire ascending aorta was involved by the luetic process and in the other two, the process was limited to that portion behind the sinuses of Valsalva (Figs. 15–17). The luetic process caused the aortic wall to be up to four times thicker than normal. The thickening

Table 9. Aortic regurgitation secondary to syphilis: clinical and necropsy observations

Patient	Age	Sex	STS	Age (yrs.) onset		Conduction disturbances by ECG	Pressures (mm./Hg)		Heart weight (gm.)	Saccular AA aneurysm
				Murmur	CHF		LV	SA		
1. A58–280	19	M	+	17	17	0	105/33	148/33	800	0
2. A61–192	37	M	0	34	32	0	160/20	170/50	600	+
3. A4344	44	M		43	43	1°HB	175/5	175/85	850	+
4. 70A–369	50	M	+	50	50	0	—	160/50	720	+
5. A65–31	53	M	+	53	48	0	143/18	152/40	600	+
6. A64–223	56	F	0	52	55	0	106/25	108/27	800	0
7. A67–43	69	M	+	63	63	1°HB	—	170/50*	640	0
8. A69–226	69	F	+	56	54	0	—	200/90*	650	+
9. A72–137	80	F	+	44	60	0	—	210/70*	600	0

AA = ascending aorta. CHF = congestive heart failure. LV = left ventricle. SA = systemic artery. STS = serologic test for syphilis. 1°HB = prolonged P–R interval (P–R greater than 0.20 sec.).
* Arm cuff pressure.

was due to both intimal proliferation and to dense adventitial scarring (Fig. 16). The aortic media, in contrast, was not thickened, and many of its elastic fibers had been replaced by scar tissue. The walls of the vasa vasorum were thickened and their lumens were narrowed. Collections of lymphocytes and plasma cells surrounded many vasa vasorum. Arteriosclerotic plaques were superimposed on the diseased aorta in all patients, including the 19-year-old. No spirochetes were found on special stains of aorta. The aortic "annuli" were dilated in all nine patients, preventing coaptation of the aortic valve cusps. The distal margins of the cusps were thickened in all patients, but the valves remained mobile and

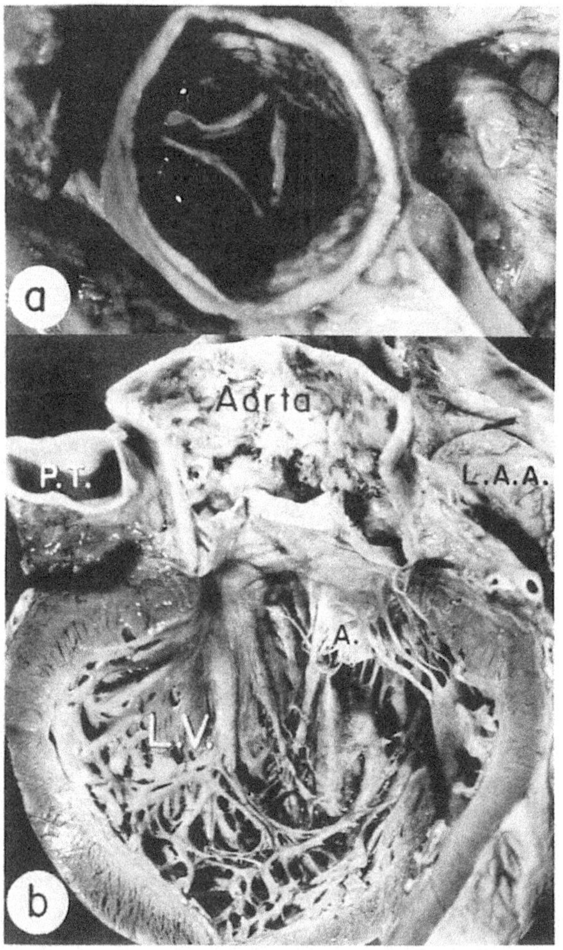

Figure 15. Cardiovascular syphilis with severe aortic regurgitation. Shown here is the aortic valve from above (a) and the opened aorta, aortic valve, and left ventricle (b) in a 69-year-old man (A67–43) who died of congestive cardiac failure. His blood pressure was 170/50 mm. Hg. The regurgitation resulted from inability of the cusps to coapt during ventricular diastole (a). Dilatation of the aortic root stretched the cusps between any two commissures but no one commissure was widened. The wall of the entire ascending aorta is involved by the syphilitic process. The left ventricle (L.V.) is very dilated. P.T. = pulmonary trunk. A. = anterior mitral leaflet. L.A.A. = left atrial appendage.

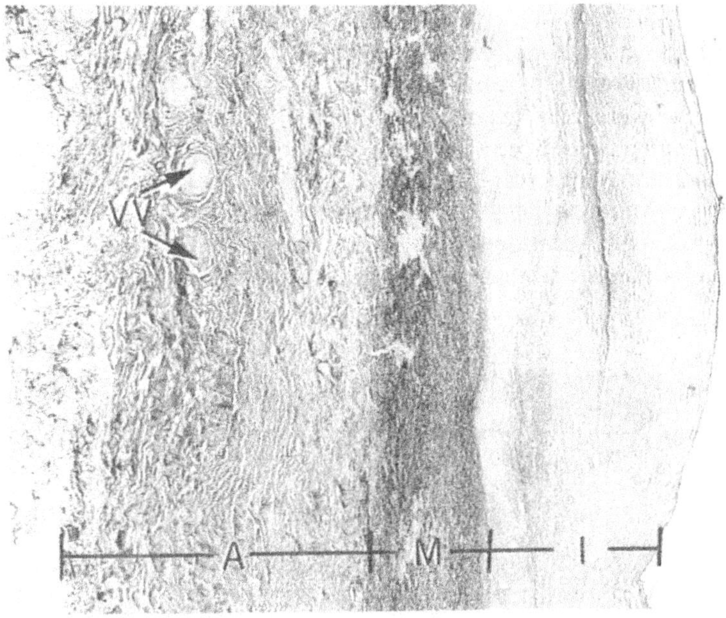

Figure 16. Syphilis of the aorta. Photomicrograph of a cross section of aortic wall from a 55-year-old man (DCGH #72A–115) with luetic aortitis. The intima (I) is thickened by fibrous tissue. The media (M) is thinned due to elastic fiber degeneration. The stellate scars resulted from focal disruption of the darkly staining elastic fibers. The adventitia (A) also is thickened by a dense scarring process and the vasa vasorum (VV) are severely thickened by the obliterative endocarditis. Infiltrate of lymphocytes, not evident at this magnification, are present in the adventitia. Elastic tissue stain; × 21.

otherwise grossly and histologically normal. In only two patients were the commissures widened.

Aortic regurgitation occurs in about 30 per cent[49-51] of patients with cardiovascular syphilis. The regurgitation is due primarily to aortic root dilatation, the result of destructive aortitis. Stretched across a dilated aortic annulus, the cusps are unable to meet in diastole and a central regurgitant stream results. The fibrosis of the rolled free margins of the aortic valve cusps appears to be secondary to regurgitation and not due to a valvulitis per se. The sparing of the valvular cusps might result from their being relatively avascular.

Syphilitic aortitis is a focal disease of the ascending aorta with skip areas that are grossly and histologically normal. The site of disease in the aorta is the major determinant of valvular dysfunction. All our patients with aortic regurgitation had severe aortic root involvement and variable involvement of other portions of ascending aorta. Extensive destruction of ascending aorta, even with formation of aneurysms, may occur in the absence of aortic regurgitation if the aortic wall immediately behind the sinuses is spared (Fig. 17). Thus, the aortic root is the important determinant of aortic valve function and alteration in its structure may prevent normal valve closure.

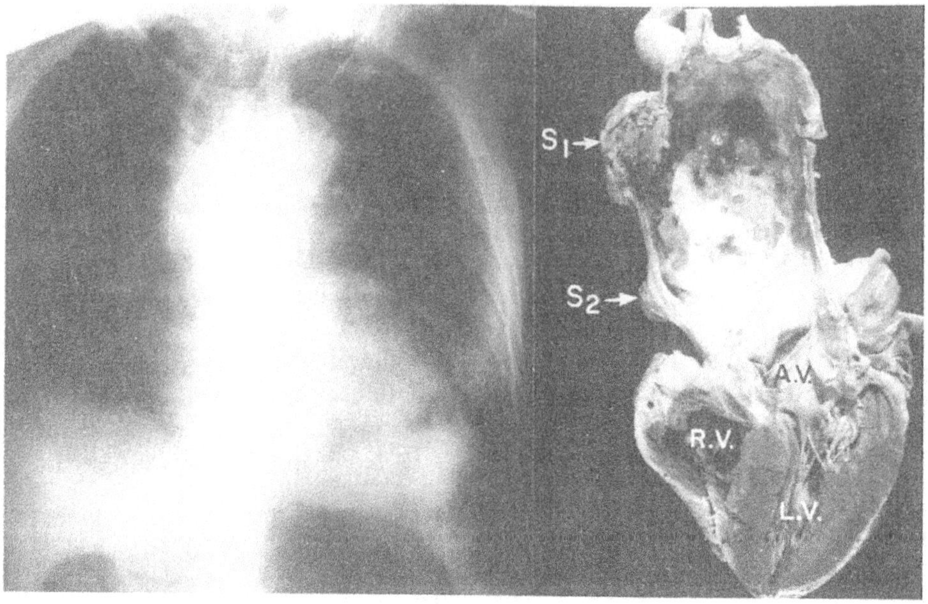

Figure 17. Cardiovascular syphilis without aortic regurgitation. Incidental finding in an 81-year-old man (A67–177) who died of pneumonia but never had evidence of cardiac dysfunction. Syphilitic aortitis led to severe destruction and aneurysmal dilatation of aorta, and formation of two smaller saccular aneurysms (S and S_2). Chest roentgenogram demonstrates a diffusely dilated aorta with a calcified wall. In contrast to the patient illustrated in Figure 15, aortic regurgitation did not occur in this patient since the walls of the sinuses of Valsalva were not involved by the syphilitic process. Neither aortic root nor left ventricle (L.V.) was dilated. R.V. = right ventricle. A.V. = aortic valve.

Ankylosing Spondylitis

We have studied eight patients with combined ankylosing spondylitis and aortic regurgitation (Table 10). All were men, aged 34 to 57 years. All had severe (functionally class III or IV) congestive cardiac failure and signs and symptoms of joint involvement consistent with ankylosing spondylitis. In all eight patients, the joint symptoms antedated those of congestive cardiac failure, in seven of them by 10 to 20 years. In five of the eight patients, however, precordial murmurs of aortic regurgitation were noted at the same time, or within one year of onset of joint symptoms. Serologic test (VDRL) for syphilis was negative in all patients. Conduction disturbances were present in six of eight patients: five had prolonged (greater than 0.20 sec.) P–R intervals, one associated with right bundle branch block and another with left bundle branch block; and one had complete heart block. At catheterization, the left ventricular and systemic arterial diastolic pressures were equal in five of seven patients studied. Aortic valve replacement was carried out in five patients. Death in seven patients was directly related to the aortic valvular disease and occurred at an average of six years from the onset of congestive cardiac failure; the eighth patient died of lung carcinoma.

At necropsy, the hearts weighed 520 to 1100 gm. (avg. 756). The aortic valve cusps were shortened and thickened, particularly at their attachments. Focal calcific deposits were present along the bases of the cusps in four patients, and in one the deposit extended to the anterior mitral leaflet and membranous septum. The ascending aorta was diffusely dilated. The thickening was limited to the

Table 10. Ankylosing spondylitis: clinical and necropsy observations

Patient	Age (years) at death	Sex	Age (years) onset arthritis	Age (years) onset cardiac disease		Duration (years) of arthritis	Duration (years) of cardiac disease		Conduction disturbances by ECG	Pressures (mm. Hg)		AR	Heart weight (gm.)	AV cusps		Sub AV ridge	Thickening of aorta of sinuses
				Murmur	CHF		Murmur	CHP		LV	SA			thick	short		
1. A61–99	52	M	24	37	43	28	15	9	1°HB RBBB	160/18	168/30	+	850	+	+	+	+
2. A61–262	55	M	45	45	53	15	15	2	1°HB	114/40	124/40	+	680	+	+	+	+
3. A61–274	34	M	18	31	31	16	3	3	1°HB	100/22	120/25	+	700	+	+	+	+
4. A64–17	35	M	6	6	29	29	29	6	0	170/12	170/50	+	840	+	+	+	+
5. A66–127	57	M	42	41	55	16	17	2	0	—	180/40	+	520	+	+	+	+
6. A68–142	38	M	13	14	32	25	24	6	1°HB	170/16	190/20	+	1100	+	+	+	+
7. A68–300	54	M	40	40	48	14	14	6	CHB	170/52	170/50	+	750	+	+	+	+
8. A68–350	46	M	18	38	38	28	8	8	LBBB	128/32	128/32	+	610	+	+	+	+
Averages	46		26	32	41	21	16	6									

AR = aortic regurgitation. AV = aortic valve. CHB = complete heart block. CHF = congestive cardiac failure. 1°HB = first degree heart block (P–R interval greater than 0.20 sec.). LBBB = left bundle branch block. LV = left ventricle. RBBB = right bundle branch block. SA = systemic artery.

most proximal 3 to 4 cm. of ascending aorta, and the wall behind the sinuses of Valsalva was always involved. The thickening resulted from dense connective tissue in the adventitia of the aorta. The adventitial scarring continued downward in the groove between the anterior mitral leaflet and the aortic valve cusps, producing a fibrous ridge between the base of the aortic valve cusps and the anterior mitral leaflet (Fig. 18). In four patients the fibrous tissue involved the membranous ventricular septum as well. A few mononuclear cells were present in the adventitia of the aorta, and the lumens of the vasa vasorum were narrowed by extensive intimal fibrous proliferation and medial hypertrophy. The media of the aorta behind the sinuses showed evidence of severe degeneration, and the overlying intima was thickened by proliferated fibrous tissue.

Although aortic regurgitation has been described previously in ankylosing spondylitis,[52-57] the distinctive morphologic features of the cardiovascular lesion have not been clearly defined. The aortic valve cusps, particularly near their aortic attachments, are shortened and diffusely thickened by fibrous tissue. The extension of the dense adventitial fibrosis below the attachments of the aortic valve cusps to anterior mitral leaflet and membranous ventricular septum distinguished these patients morphologically from those with aortic regurgitation of other etiologies. The extension of the scarring process below the aortic valve also explains the frequency of conduction disturbances in ankylosing spondylitis.

Although the aortic valve cusps are abnormal in as high as 20 per cent,[56] aortic regurgitation is said to occur clinically in only about 3 per cent of patients with ankylosing spondylitis.[56,58,59] Symptoms of arthritis usually antedate the cardiac disease by 10 to 20 years. In five of our patients and in patients described by others,[54,59-62] precordial murmurs were noted within two years of the onset of joint symptoms. Symptoms of cardiac dysfunction, however, developed much later. This observation suggests that the joints and the aortic root area may be attacked at the same time, but that it takes many years for the sclerosing process to produce aortic regurgitation.

Ankylosing spondylitis has been described as a benign disease.[62-64] Seven of our eight patients, however, died of consequences of aortic regurgitation at a mean age of 46 years with death occurring within six years of the first symptoms of heart disease. The age at death in the 16 patients with ankylosing spondylitis and aortic regurgitation reported by Clark et al.[54] was 45 years, and the interval from the onset of symptomatic heart disease to death was six years. In contrast, the overall mortality of patients with ankylosing spondylitis has been reported to be similar to that of the general population.[64] Thus, the presence of aortic regurgitation appears to be a prime determinant of whether or not ankylosing spondylitis shortens life.

The Marfan Syndrome

This heritable disorder involves the bones, joints, eye, heart, and blood vessels.[65] The extremities are long and thin (dolichostenomelia), the ligaments and joint capsules are redundant, the lenses are dislocated (ectopia lentis), the ascending aorta is dilated, and one or both left-sided cardiac valves usually are incompetent.

We have studied at necropsy 11 patients with the classic features of the

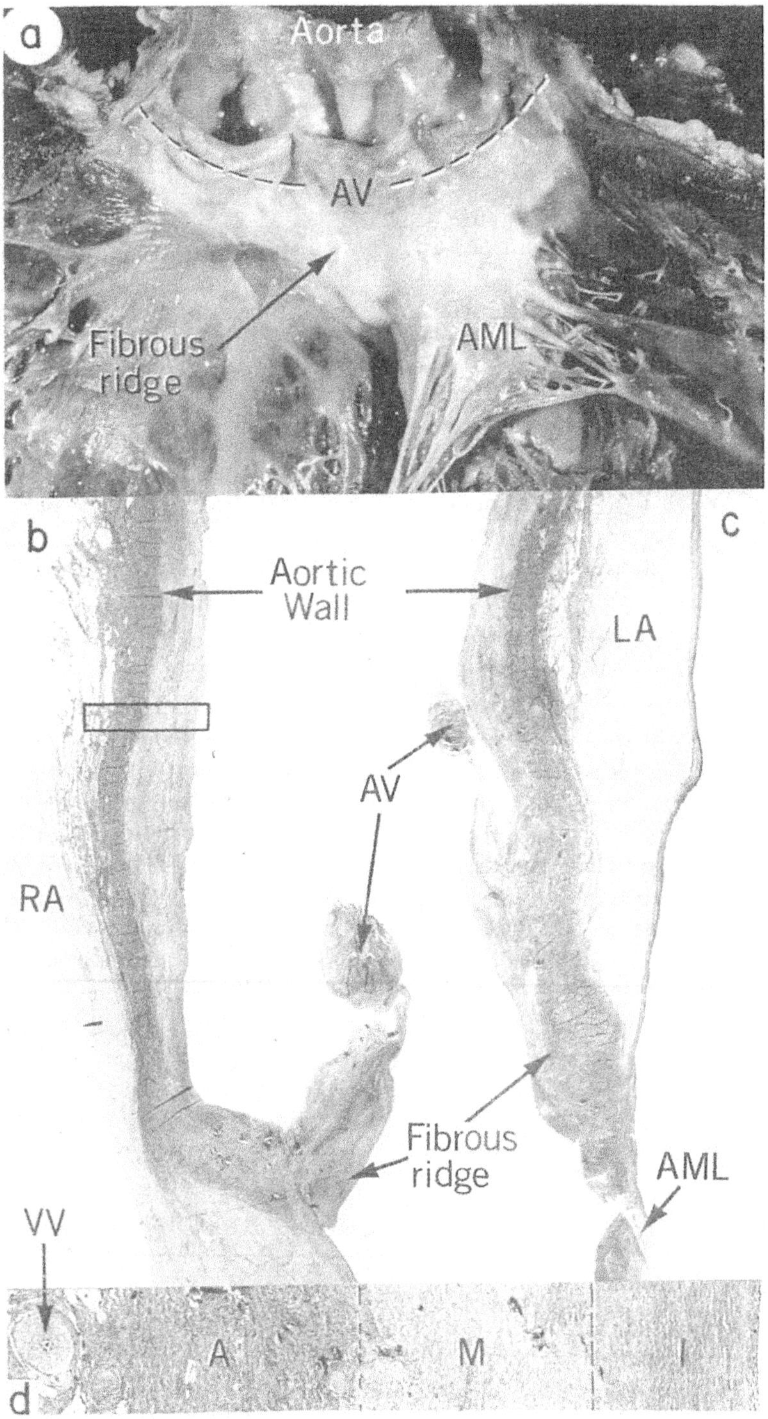
a
Aorta
AV
Fibrous ridge
AML
b
c
Aortic Wall
LA
AV
RA
Fibrous ridge
AML
VV
A
M
I
d

Marfan syndrome and four other patients without the bone, joint, or eye features of the syndrome but with similar lesions in the ascending aorta (Table 11) (Figs. 19–22). The youngest died of congestive cardiac failure from mitral regurgitation at two days of age and the oldest, at age 59 years of congestive failure from aortic regurgitation. Thirteen were males, two were females; 12 were white and three, black. Fourteen had congestive cardiac failure, and the fifteenth died suddenly of rupture of the ascending aorta before congestive failure had appeared. All 15 had precordial murmurs consistent with mitral regurgitation, and 12 had murmurs of aortic regurgitation. Operations to alleviate valvular regurgitation were performed in eight patients, and in another, an aortic coarctation was resected.

At necropsy (or operation), the ascending aorta was dilated in 13 patients, all but one of whom had had clear evidence of aortic regurgitation. The sinuses of Valsalva were especially dilated and their walls, thinner than normal. In addition, focal outpouching was present in the ascending aorta in these 13 patients. Their walls were markedly thinned and contained few if any elastic fibers. The intima of these thinned areas had an orange-peel appearance whereas the other areas of intima usually were grossly normal. Elastic fibers in the grossly normal portions of aorta, however, also were severly decreased in number and the amount of acid mucopolysaccharide material, focally increased. Few medial scars were present in any portion of ascending aorta. Neither adventitia nor intima was thickened and the vasa vasorum were not narrowed.

Other than mild focal thickening of their margins, the aortic valve cusps were grossly normal (Fig. 22). On histologic study, however, the aortic cusps, as well as the mitral ones, contained increased quantities of acid mucopolysaccharide material. The mitral valve leaflets and chordae were elongated, both transversely and longitudinally, in most patients, and in several the leaflets and chordae were focally thickened. In four patients calcific deposits were present in the mitral annuli behind the posterior mitral leaflets. All four valve annuli in all 15 patients were dilated.

The two major functional valve lesions in the Marfan and Marfan-like (forme fruste) syndromes are mitral regurgitation[65-71] and aortic regurgitation.[65,71] All 15 of our patients had clinical evidence of mitral regurgitation and 13 of them had aortic regurgitation. The aortic regurgitation appears to result from dilatation of the aortic root, the result of massive degeneration of elastic fibers (and probably

Figure 18. Ankylosing spondylitis associated with aortic regurgitation and complete heart block. This 54-year-old man (A68–300) had crippling ankylosing spondylitis which progressed over a 14-year period. Coincident with his initial skeletal symptoms was the development of a murmur of aortic regurgitation. He subsequently developed congestive cardic failure and complete heart block. a, The aortic valve cusps are shortened and thickened and a dense fibrous band or ridge extends along the base of the cusps to the anterior mitral leaflet. b, Photomicrograph of longitudinal section through right coronary cusp, right atrium (RA), and adjacent aortic wall. The latter is thickened by intimal proliferation and by dense adventitial scar which extends below the base of the valve forming the fibrous ridge. c, Photomicrograph of a longitudinal section through left coronary cusp, left atrium (LA), and anterior mitral leaflet (AML). Dense scar extends from adventitia of aorta below the aortic valve to the AML. d, Close-up of full thickness of aortic wall showing dense fibrosis of adventitia (A) with narrowing of lumen of vasa vasorum (VV), degeneration of medial (M) elastic tissue, and thickening of intima (I) by fibrous tissue proliferation. These changes are virtually indistinguishable from the changes seen in syphilitic aortitis. b and c, Elastic tissue stains. d, Hematoxylin-eosin stain. [$\times$ 3.5 (b), $\times$ 2.5 (c), and $\times$ 24 (d).]

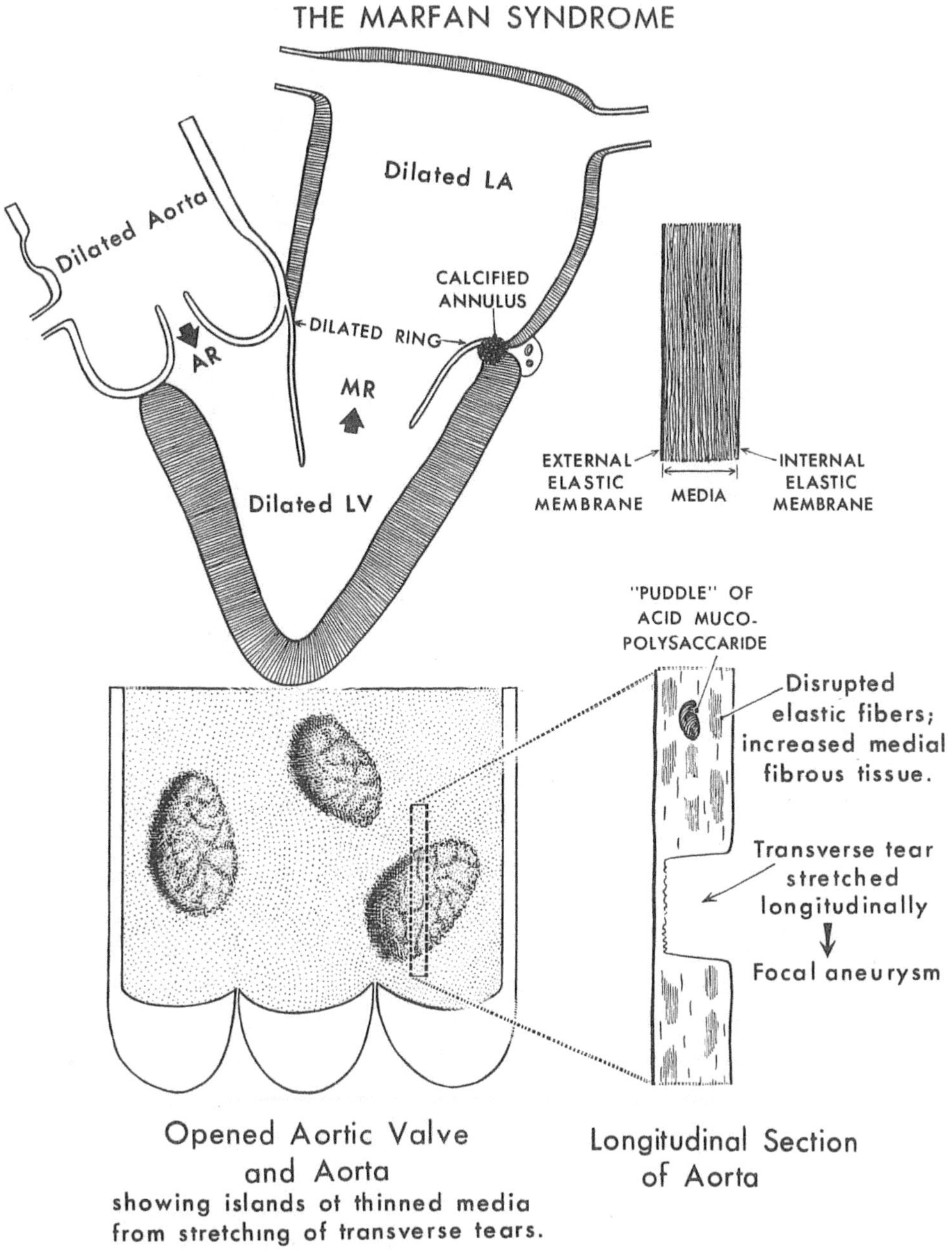

Figure 19. Diagram demonstrating the various cardiovascular abnormalities found in the Marfan syndrome. The aortic regurgitation appears to be related primarily to dilatation of the aorta. The mitral regurgitation probably results from a combination of factors: dilatation of the left ventricular cavity altering the papillary muscle–mitral leaflet angle; dilatation of the mitral annulus; calcification of the mitral annulus; and elongation of the mitral leaflets and chordae allowing prolapse of the leaflets into left atrium during ventricular systole. Shown on top right is a longitudinal section of normal aorta. At bottom right is a longitudinal section in a patient with the Marfan syndrome. There is severe loss of elastic fibers, deposition of abnormal amounts of acid mucopolysaccharide material, and tears in the wall. These tears expand to cause islands of thinning noted in the view of the opened aortic valve and aorta.

Table 11. The Marfan syndrome and its forme fruste variety

Patient	Age (yrs.)	Sex	CHF	Murmurs AR	Murmurs MR	SA press. (mm. Hg)	Operation AVR	Operation AAR	Ascending aorta: Medial degen.	Ascending aorta: Diffuse aneurysm	Ascending aorta: Complete rupture	Heart weight (gm.)	Ca^{++} MV annulus	Other lesions
The Marfan syndrome														
1. A56-132	31	M	+	2/6	4/6	135/40¶	O*	O	+	+	O	700	+	Hx IE
2. A58-150	15	M	+	3/6	3/6	150/0	O	O	+	+	O	750	O	Hx IE
3. A58-206	36	F	+	4/6	2/6	—	O	O	+	+	O	750	O	O
4. A59-134	20	M	+	3/6	3/6	160/60¶	O	O†	O	+	O	850	+	C of A† bicuspid AV
5. A63-25	28	M	+	0	5/6	130/80¶	O	O	O	O	O	850	+	O
6. A64-224	21	M	+	4/6	2/6	158/62¶	+‡	+	+	+	O	700	+	O
7. A65-64	41	M	+	5/6	1/6	105/35¶	+	+	+	+	O	750	O	An., desc. thoracic aorta
8. A67-120	21	M	O	O§	2/6	130/80§	O	O	+	+	+	460	O	O
9. A69-278	48	F	+	4/6	2/6	150/40¶	+	+	+	+	O	520	O	O
10. A67-236	2 days	M	+	O	4/6	—	O	O	+	O	O	—	O	O
11. 37468	47	M	+	4/6	2/6	108/39¶	+	+	+	+	O	—	O	O
The forme fruste variety														
12. A68-197	52	M	+	3/6	2/6	160/60¶	+	+	+	+	O	850	O	O
13. A70-102	32	M	+	4/6	2/6	110/45¶	+	+	+	+	O	650	O	C of A bicuspid AV
14. A59-169	59	M	+	3/6	2/6	190/80¶	O	O	+	+	O	820	O	O
15. 37429	48	M	+	3/6	2/6	135/54¶	+	+	+	+	O	900	O	Bicuspid AV

* This patient underwent insertion of a Hufnagel ball-value prosthesis in his descending thoracic aorta in 1956 and died from rupture of the proximal aortic suture line a month later.

† This patient died in the operating room from bleeding after insertion of a conduit proximal and distal to the coarctation of the aorta.

‡ Replacement of the ascending aorta and aortic valve was performed nine months before death and mitral valve replacement (for mitral regurgitation) was carried out 15 days before death.

§ This recording was at age 12 (nine years before sudden death). Since his ascending aorta was quite dilated at necropsy, it is highly likely that aortic regurgitation was present and the systemic arterial diastolic pressure was low for some time before death.

¶ Direct pressure recording during catheterization.

AAR = ascending aorta replacement. An. = aneurysm. AR = aortic regurgitation. AV = aortic valve. AVR = aortic valve replacement. Ca^{++} = calcium. CHF = congestive cardiac failure. C of A = coarctation of aorta. degen. = degeneration. desc. = descending. Hx = history of. IE = infective endocarditis. MR = mitral regurgitation. MV = mitral valve. SA systemic artery.

also of some smooth muscle cells) of the media. The especially severe dilatation of the sinuses of Valsalva appears to cause peripheral migration of the aortic valve cusps which tilt or prolapse toward left ventricle. The focal thickening of the cuspal margins appears to be secondary to the aortic regurgitation and not a factor in causing it.

At least four factors are important in causing mitral regurgitation in this syndrome: (1) Papillary muscle dysfunction resulting from the tremendous left ventricular dilatation.[72,73] The dilatation appears to alter the angle of pull of these structures making it more difficult for the leaflets to coapt during ventricular systole. (2) Dilatation of the mitral annulus. This annulus is probably more dilatated in patients with the Marfan or Marfan-like syndromes than in any other condition. (3) Calcification of the mitral annulus.[74] It is well known that calcific deposits in the annulus of the posterior leaflet can inhibit the sphincter-like action of this ring, an action which occurs normally during ventricular systole. (4) Floppiness of the mitral leaflets. Not only are the leaflets stretched transversely as the annulus dilates, but they also are stretched longitudinally by the dilating left ventricular cavity. It is possible that the increased quantities of acid-mucopolysaccharide material in the mitral leaflets allow this abnormal stretching. The chordae tendineae also are stretched and this in turn allows abnormal prolapsing of the leaflets toward left atrium during ventricular systole. Possibly none of the four factors alone could account for severe regurgitation, but in combination severe regurgitation may result. Tricuspid regurgitation and floppy tricuspid valve leaflets and chordae tendineae also may occur in this condition as illustrated by our patient #11 and as described by others.[68]

Although floppiness of the atrioventricular valves is a prominent feature of the Marfan and Marfan-like syndromes, the major cause of cardiovascular dysfunction results from involvement of ascending aorta. The major lesion here appears to be degeneration of elastic fibers and not the presence of increased quantities of acid-mucopolysaccharide material. In our view, the latter deposits have been too strongly emphasized and therefore the name *medial cystic necrosis* is probably not the most appropriate one. Dissection of the aorta did not occur in any of our 15 patients. What has been called "dissection" may represent tears beginning in the intima and extending for varying distances into the media or through the media to be enclosed by adventitia.

The occurrence of congenitally bicuspid aortic valves in three of our 15 patients is a frequency too high to be attributed to chance alone. Bicuspid aortic valves were present in one of the 11 patients with the Marfan syndrome and in two of the four without the syndrome but with similar lesions in the ascending aorta. Two of the three also had aortic coarctation. It is possible that the ascending aorta is structurally congenitally weak in patients with congenitally malformed aortic valves. If this postulate is correct, it might be reasoned that congenitally weak elastic fibers in the ascending aorta are more likely to degenerate than are structurally normal elastic fibers. If coarctation also is present the increased pressure in the ascending aorta might accelerate the elastic-fiber-degeneration process. When aortic elastic fibers degenerate, the spaces may be filled with acid-mucopolysaccharide material to produce a lesion which is typical of that

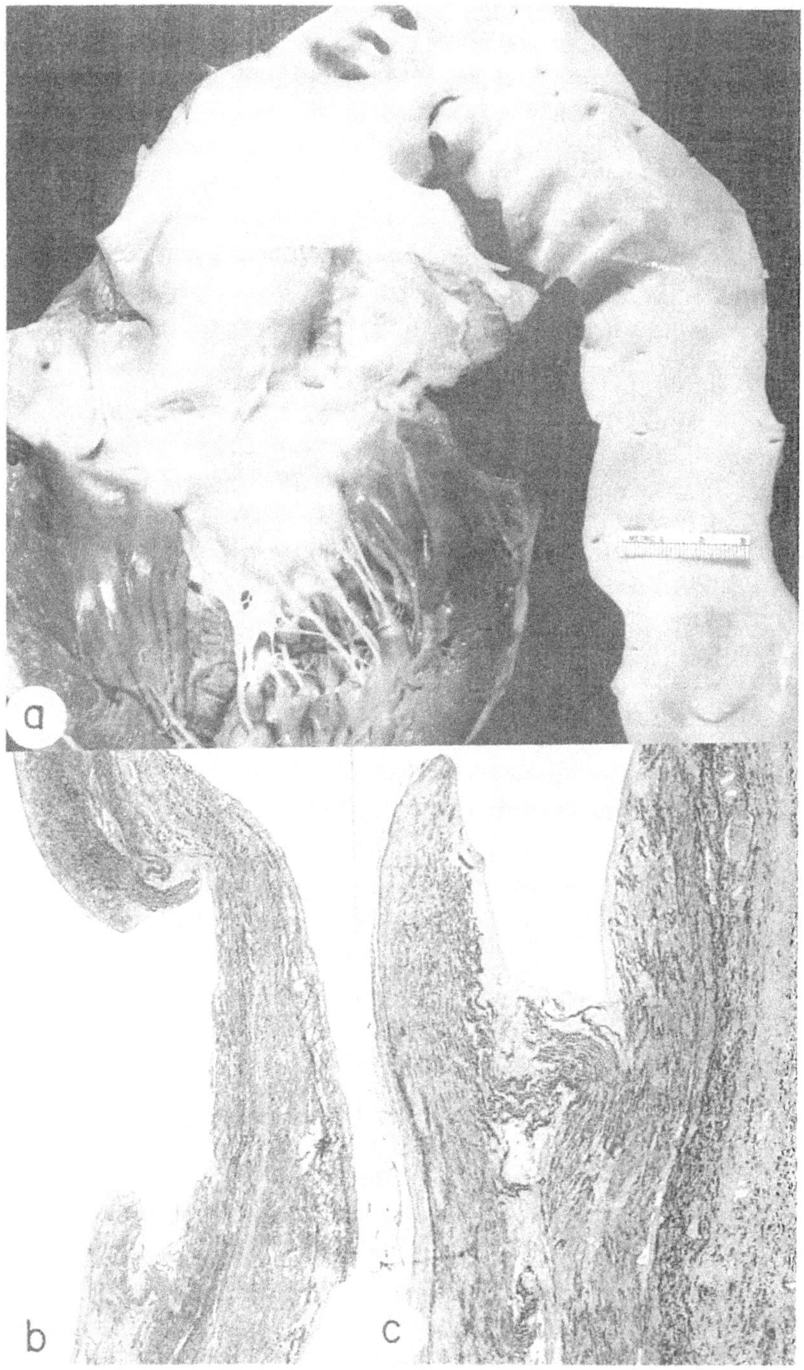

Figure 20. The Marfan syndrome. This 21-year-old man (A67–120) with typical skeletal and optic features of this syndrome had always been asymptomatic. He was found dead in his parked car after playing in a band during the several previous hours. At necropsy, the precordial sac was filled with blood. A through-and-through rupture had occurred in the ascending aorta (a) just above the aortic valve. In addition, several partial ruptures or tears also were present in ascending aorta. A histologic section of one tear is shown in b. A close-up of an adjacent section of b is shown in c. There is severe degeneration of elastic fibers of the media. b and c, Elastic tissue stains. [× 7 (b) and × 18 (c).]

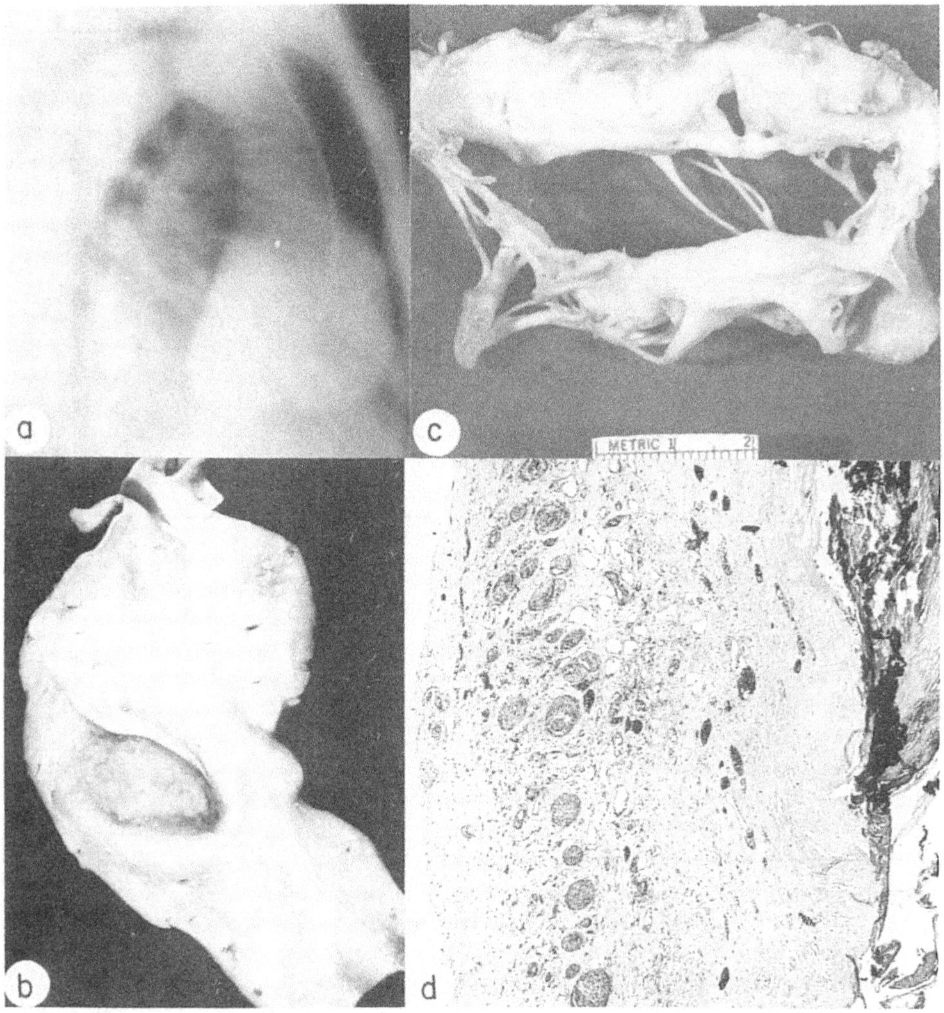

Figure 21. The Marfan syndrome with both aortic and mitral regurgitation in a 21-year-old man (A64–224). This patient had a precordial murmur at birth. Four siblings also had the Marfan syndrome. He was asymptomatic until about one year before death when episodes of rapid atrial fibrillation appeared. He had one episode of sudden heavy retrosternal chest pain 10 months before death. He died after replacement of both aortic and mitral valves with prostheses. The ascending aorta had been resected at operation. a, Lateral aortogram showing dilatation of the aortic sinuses, a typical cardiovascular feature of the Marfan syndrome. b, Excised ascending aorta showing two punched out aortic tears or splits. The nontorn portion of aorta grossly appears normal but histologically the aorta showed extensive loss of elastic fibers and focal collections of acid mucopolysaccharide material. c, Excised mitral valve. The leaflets are thickened, the annulus is dilated, and focal deposits of calcium are present at the line of excision (annulus). d, Histologic section of portion of mitral leaflet, which is thickened by vascularized fibrous tissue. Vascularization of valvular leaflet at one time was considered typical of rheumatic heart disease but this is not so as demonstrated here. Also, a deposit of calcium (near the annulus) is present. Hematoxylin-eosin stain. (Reduced 25 per cent from × 56.)

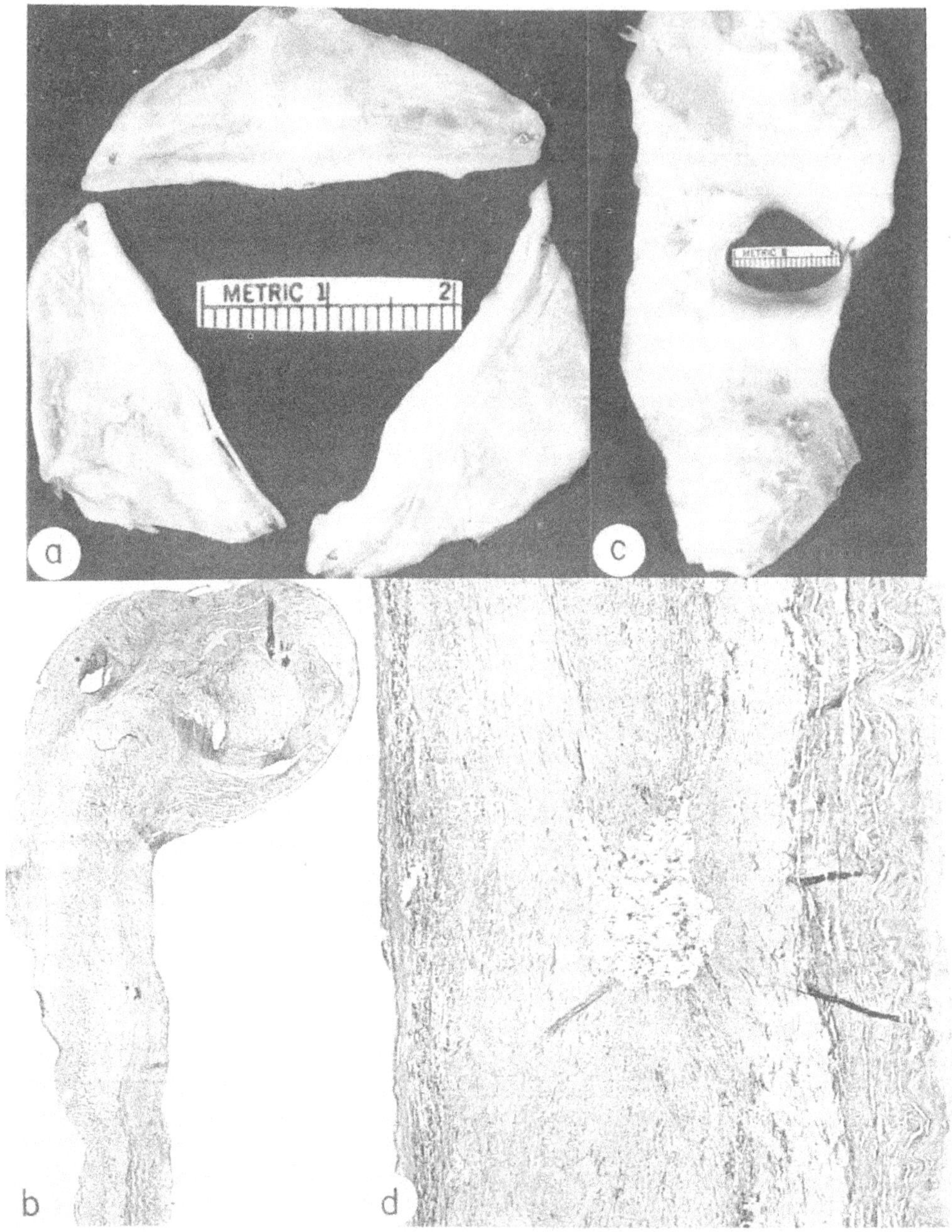

Figure 22. The Marfan syndrome with severe aortic regurgitation in a 41-year-old man (A65–64). This patient underwent replacement of his aortic valve and ascending aorta two months before death from complications of the nephrotic syndrome. At necropsy, he was found to have a large aneurysm filled with organized thrombus in the descending thoracic aorta. a, Excised aortic valve showing mild thickening of the margins of each of the three cusps. Otherwise, the aortic valve grossly appears normal. This is the typical appearance of the aortic valve in a patient with the Marfan syndrome. b, Photomicrograph of portion of one aortic valve cusp showing increased spongiosa and therefore increased acid-mucopolysaccharide material. c, Excised ascending aorta. d, Photomicrograph of portion of ascending aorta showing virtual total disappearance of elastic fibers and a puddle of acid-mucopolysaccharide material. b, Hematoxylin-eosin stain. d, Elastic van Gieson stain. [Reduced 15 per cent from × 24 (b) and × 58 (d).]

Table 12. The Hurler syndrome: data in three necropsy patients

Patient	Age-race-sex	Cardiac symptoms	Murmur	CE by x-ray	ECG	Cardiac involvement: Heart weight (gm.)	All four valves	Mural endocardium of four chambers	Cor. art.	Myocardium	MV annulus Ca^{++}
1. A65-89	6 WF	0	+	Slight	Normal*	95(101)†	+	+	+	+	0
2. A66-199	9 WM	0	0	0	LAE	110(138)†	+	+	+	+	+
3. A70-236	12 WM	0	+	Slight	RAE, RAD, VPCs	150(169)†	+	+	+	+	+

* Recorded eight years before death.
† Expected weight for age and sex.

Ca^{++} = calcium. CE = cardiac enlargement. Cor. art. = coronary artery. LAE = left atrial enlargement. MV = mitral valve. RAD = right axis deviation. VPCs = ventricular premature contractions. RAE = right atrial enlargement.

which occurs in the Marfan syndrome in subjects with three-cuspid aortic valves. Furthermore, aortic medial degeneration with cystic necrosis also has been observed in patients with valvular aortic stenosis.[75,76] The stenosis in most of the latter patients probably is superimposed on a congenitally malformed aortic valve.

The Hurler Syndrome (Mucopolysaccharidosis I)

Virtually all patients with this syndrome have anatomically abnormal cardiac valves. Three children (one girl, two brothers) with typical clinical, chemical, and morphologic features of this syndrome were studied (Table 12). Each had moderate dwarfism, grotesque facial appearances, protuberant abdomens, joint contractures, and mental retardation. Acid mucopolysaccharides, mainly chondroitin sulfate B and heparitin sulfate, in increased amounts were found in the urine of each patient. Although none had symptoms of cardiac dysfunction, two had precordial systolic murmurs (grade 2/6 intensity), loudest at the apices, two had slight cardiomegaly by chest roentgenograms, and two had abnormal electrocardiograms.

At necropsy, each heart was smaller than normal, the ventricular walls were

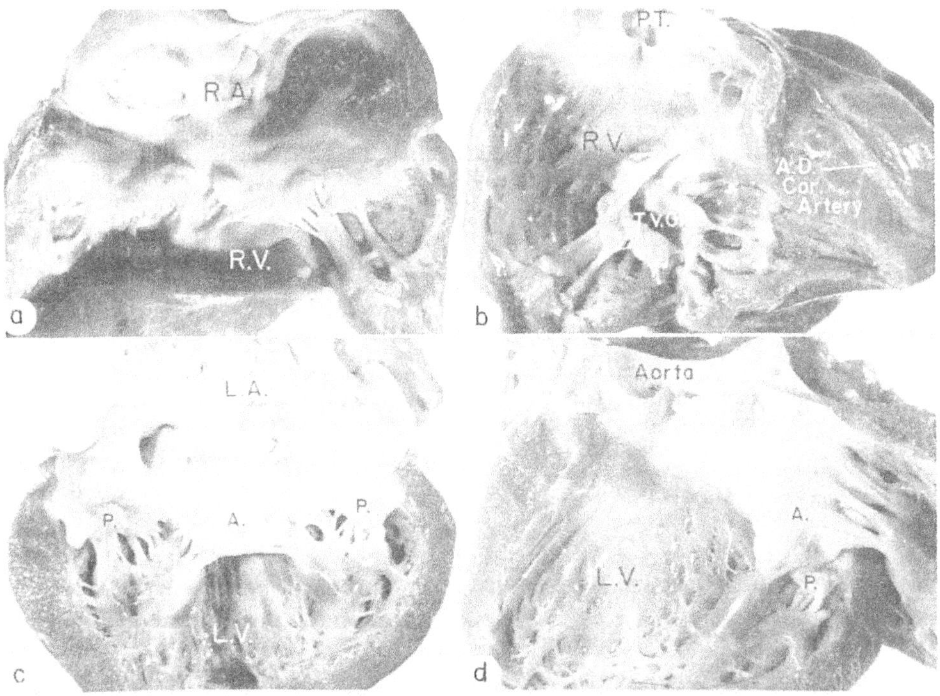

Figure 23. The Hurler syndrome. Opened right (a and b) and left (c and d) sides of the heart in a six-year-old girl (A65–89) with typical features of the Hurler syndrome. She had a precordial murmur but no evidence of cardiac dysfunction. All four cardiac valves and the mural endocardium of all four chambers were thickened. a, Opened right atrium (R.A.), tricuspid valve, and right ventricle (R.V.). b, Opened pulmonary trunk (P.T.) and right ventricle (R.V.) showing the thickened valves and the tricuspid valve orifice (T.V.O.). The anterior descending (A.D.) coronary (Cor.) artery is thickened. c, Opened left atrium (L.A.), mitral valve, and left ventricle (L.V.). A. = anterior mitral leaflet. P. = posterior mitral leaflet. d, Opened left ventricle (L.V.) and aorta showing thickening of both valves and the mural endocardium.

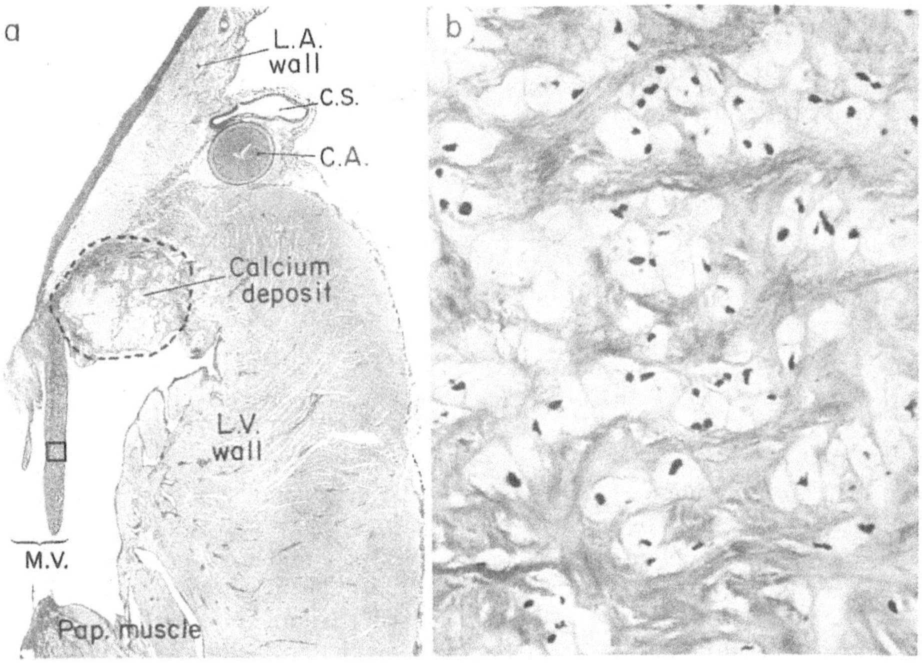

Figure 24. The Hurler syndrome. a, Photomicrograph of section of left atrium (L.A.), posterior mitral valve (M.V.) leaflet, and left ventricular (L.V.) wall showing a heavy deposit of calcium in the mitral annular region and an extremely narrowed coronary artery (C.A.). A close-up of calcium deposit area seen in (a) from a portion of a chorda tendinea is shown in (b). These are typical Hurler cells with vacouloted cytoplasm. These cells were present in valve leaflets, mural endocardium, and in coronary arteries. This patient was a 9-year-old boy (A65–89) without evidence of cardiac dysfunction. a, Elastic tissue stain. b, Hematoxylin-eosin stain. [Reduced 25 per cent from × 4.5 (a) and × 290 (b).]

firmer than normal in consistency, and the mural endocardium of all four chambers of all three patients was diffusely thickened, more on the left than right. The leaflets of all four cardiac valves and many chordae tendineae of all three patients were diffusely thickened (Fig. 23). The mitral and aortic valves were thickened the most, followed by the tricuspid and pulmonic valves. In two patients, calcific deposits were present in mitral annuli (Fig. 24), and smaller calcific deposits were present on the anterior mitral leaflets and on the aortic aspects of one or more aortic valvular cusps. In no patient did the anatomic abnormalities appear to produce clinically significant valvular dysfunction. The lumens of the major coronary arteries were narrowed at some sites more than 75 per cent. Despite the narrowing, however, no myocardial necrosis was observed and fibrosis was limited to the left ventricular papillary muscles (in the two brothers only). Many yellow and fibrous atherosclerotic plaques were present in the aorta of each patient.

Histologic studies disclosed that the valvular thickening and the coronary luminal narrowing were due mainly to the presence of large cells with clear cytoplasm (gargoyle, Hurler, clear or balloon cells) and to bundles of fibrous tissue between the cells. The membranous ventricular septa and atrioventricular valve annuli were thickened by similar clear cells and by collagenous and calcific deposits. The thickening of the mural endocardium resulted primarily from proliferation of elastic fibrils (endocardial fibroelastosis), but a few clear cells also were observed.

Electron microscopic study[77,78] of valvular endocardium and of proliferated tissue within the lumens of the coronary arteries disclosed large clear vacuolated cells and lipid deposits. Although they appeared normal by light microscopic examination, the cardiac muscle cells were found to contain organized lipid and amorphous material by electron microscopy.

Virtually all patients with the Hurler syndrome have been found at necropsy to have anatomically abnormal hearts. Furthermore, all portions of the heart have been shown to be involved, including valvular and mural endocardium, coronary arteries, myocardial fibers, cardiac fibrous skelton, and epicardium. The involvement consists of proliferation of fibrous tissue within which is enmeshed varying numbers of gargoyle cells and ground substance containing acid-mucopolysaccharide material. The result of this involvement is thickening of the valvular leaflets and chordae tendineae, thickening of mural endocardium, and narrowing of the lumens of the coronary arteries.

Of the four cardiac valves, the one most frequently involved in the Hurler syndrome is the mitral. Of 40 necropsy patients with the Hurler syndrome gathered from the literature by Okada et al.,[79] the mitral was involved in 90 per cent, the pulmonic in 20 per cent, and the aortic and tricuspid, each in about 40 per cent. In each of our three patients all four cardiac valves were thickened and contained numerous gargoyle cells.

Another valvular abnormality in this syndrome, one rarely commented on in previous publications, is the occurrence of mitral annular calcification. The Hurler syndrome is probably the most common cause of annular calcification in childhood. Small calcific deposits also may occur on the ventricular aspect of the anterior mitral leaflet and on the aortic aspects of the aortic valvular cusps.

Although there may be no functional consequence of the valvular involvement in the Hurler syndrome, valvular regurgitation of some degree probably occurs eventually in most patients. Because leaflet and chordal thickening is more severe on the left than on the right side of the heart, the mitral valve is the one involved by annular calcification, and the left-sided pressures are higher, regurgitation is usually limited to the mitral or aortic valve or both. Although precordial murmurs have been described in many patients with the Hurler-Hunter syndrome, including one of Hunter's original two patients,[80] hemodynamic and angiographic observations were not reported until 1965 when Krovetz et al.[81] demonstrated mitral regurgitation in six and aortic regurgitation in one of 15 children. Only one of the seven had auscultatory evidence of valvular dysfunction. Although regurgitation is the usual valvular lesion of the Hurler syndrome, mitral stenosis was described at necropsy in a five-year-old child with atypical gargoylism.[82]

Although it is a striking anatomic finding, valvular involvement does not explain the sudden cardiovascular collapse or progressive congestive cardiac failure which causes about 50 per cent of the deaths in this syndrome. Systemic hypertension, coronary arterial luminal narrowing, and lipid deposits in myocardial fibers are probably more important factors.

Other Heritable Disorders of Connective Tissues Associated with Cardiac Valvular Regurgitation

Occurrence of cardiac valvular lesions in pseudoxanthoma elasticum (PXE) and in the Ehlers-Danlos (E-D) syndrome is not well known. About 10 patients with either PXE or E-D and valvular lesions have been described.[65,83-90] Elongated mitral and tricuspid valve leaflets and chordae (floppy valves) have been observed in both conditions, and aortic regurgitation, the result of severe degeneration of elastic fibers of the aorta with or without dissecting aneurysm, has been seen in the E-D syndrome. Dilated aortic roots with severe aortic regurgitation were observed in three men with *osteogenesis imperfecta* (OI) studied by Criscitiello et al.[91] One had had probable infective endocarditis as well. Other patients with aortic and mitral valvular incompetence associated with OI also have been reported.[92] Although not proved, it appears reasonable to believe that the valvular lesions accompanying OI, PXE and E-D syndrome are the result of an underlying disorder of connective tissue.

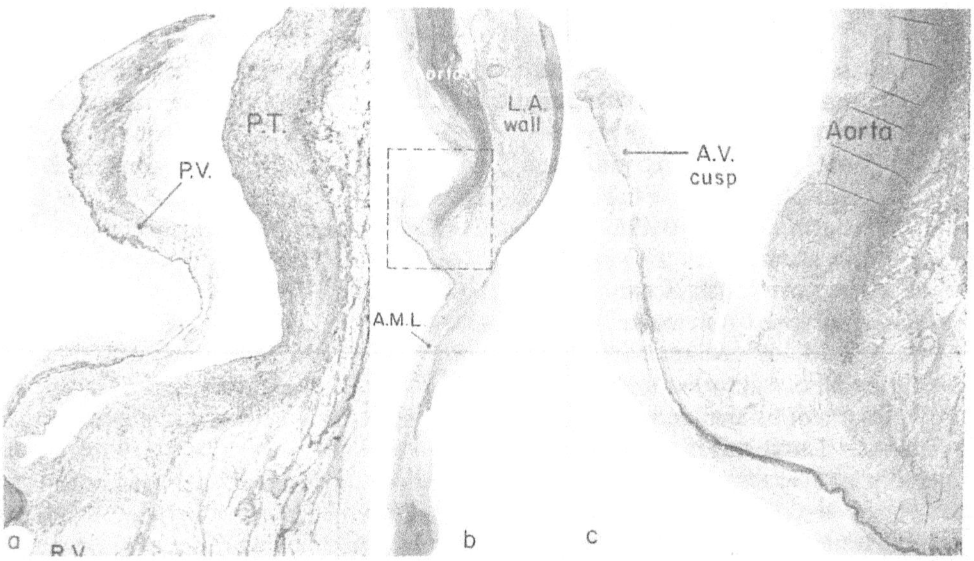

Figure 25. Valvular lesions in Takayasu's arteritis. This 46-year-old woman (A66–237) had panarteritis involving aorta and all vessels arising from it. She presented with fever of unknown origin and changing precordial murmurs. All four cardiac valves were thickened and both atrioventricular valves were mildly incompetent. Histologic sections of three cardiac valves are shown here. a, Pulmonic valve (P.V.) cusp is delineated by the black-staining elastic membrane. Superimposed on this membrane is fibrous tissue which contains few elastic fibers. P.T. = pulmonary trunk. R.V. = right ventricle. b, Section includes anterior mitral leaflet (A.M.L), aortic valve cusp, and walls of the aorta and left atrium (L.A.). Both mitral and aortic leaflets are diffusely thickened as is the wall of the aorta. c, Close-up of aortic valve (A.V.) shown in b. The cusp per se is normal but fibrous tissue, devoid of elastic fibers, is superimposed on it. a-c, Elastic tissue stains. [Reduced 40 per cent from × 15 (a), × 3 (b), and × 11 (c).]

Takayasu's Arteritis

Takayasu's disease is a panarteritis of the aorta and its major branches leading to progressive vascular occlusion. This rare syndrome occurs predominantly in women and is characterized by fever, elevation of erythrocyte sedimentation rate, and diminished or absent peripheral pulses. Vascular compromise most frequently causes neurologic dysfunction. Since any branch of aorta may be affected, however, its clinical manifestations are protean and may include angina pectoris, myocardial infarction, and sudden death.[93-97]

Although considered a disease of arteries, Takayasu's syndrome may cause valvular dysfunction before or after peripheral pulses disappear.[98] One such patient studied by us at necropsy had both tricuspid and mitral regurgitation.[98] The aorta and all four cardiac valves were involved by an unusual fibrosing process (Fig. 25) which may be unique for this condition. The fibrous tissue contained mononuclear cells, mainly lymphocytes, and vascular channels and no elastic fibers. The fibrous tissue was superimposed on both surfaces of the valvular leaflets, which appeared intact. The mural endocardium was focally involved by a similar process. Although aortic, mitral, and tricuspid regurgitation have been described clinically in at least 20 patients with Takayasu's arteritis, few gross and no other histologic descriptions of these valves have appeared. The cause of the diffuse valvular and focal endocardial fibrosis in these patients is uncertain, but it is reasonable to believe that its etiology is the same as that causing the panarteritis and aortitis.

NONOBSTRUCTIVE LESIONS

Without Involvement of Ascending Aorta

The Floppy Valve

The floppy valve as a cause of mitral valvular dysfunction is a relatively new concept. The innocence of apical systolic clicks and late systolic murmurs was refuted by Barlow[99] in 1963 when he demonstrated by left ventricular cineangiocardiography mild mitral regurgitation in these patients. He also suggested that the mid-late systolic clicks were not extracardiac in origin, but resulted from "snapping of fibrosed chordae." Subsequent reports confirmed his observations, and demonstrated prolapse of the posterior mitral leaflet into left atrium coincident with the regurgitant murmur.[101-103] Using intracardiac phonocardiograms, Criley et al.[100] showed that the systolic click coincided with maximum prolapse of the valve leaflet into left atrium. Hence, a syndrome of "mid-late systolic click and late systolic murmur" became synonymous with the "billowing or ballooning mitral leaflet syndrome" or "floppy valve syndrome." Although by cineangiocardiography the valve lesions appeared similar, the clinical syndrome was described in many conditions, including the Marfan syndrome, trauma, atrial septal defect, hypertrophic (asymmetric) cardiomyopathy, and even ischemic and rheumatic heart disease.[66, 104-110] The syndrome was described in all ages, newborn to elderly. In most patients valve dysfunction was asymptomatic. Electrocardiographic abnormalities, namely T wave and ST segment changes suggestive of posterior

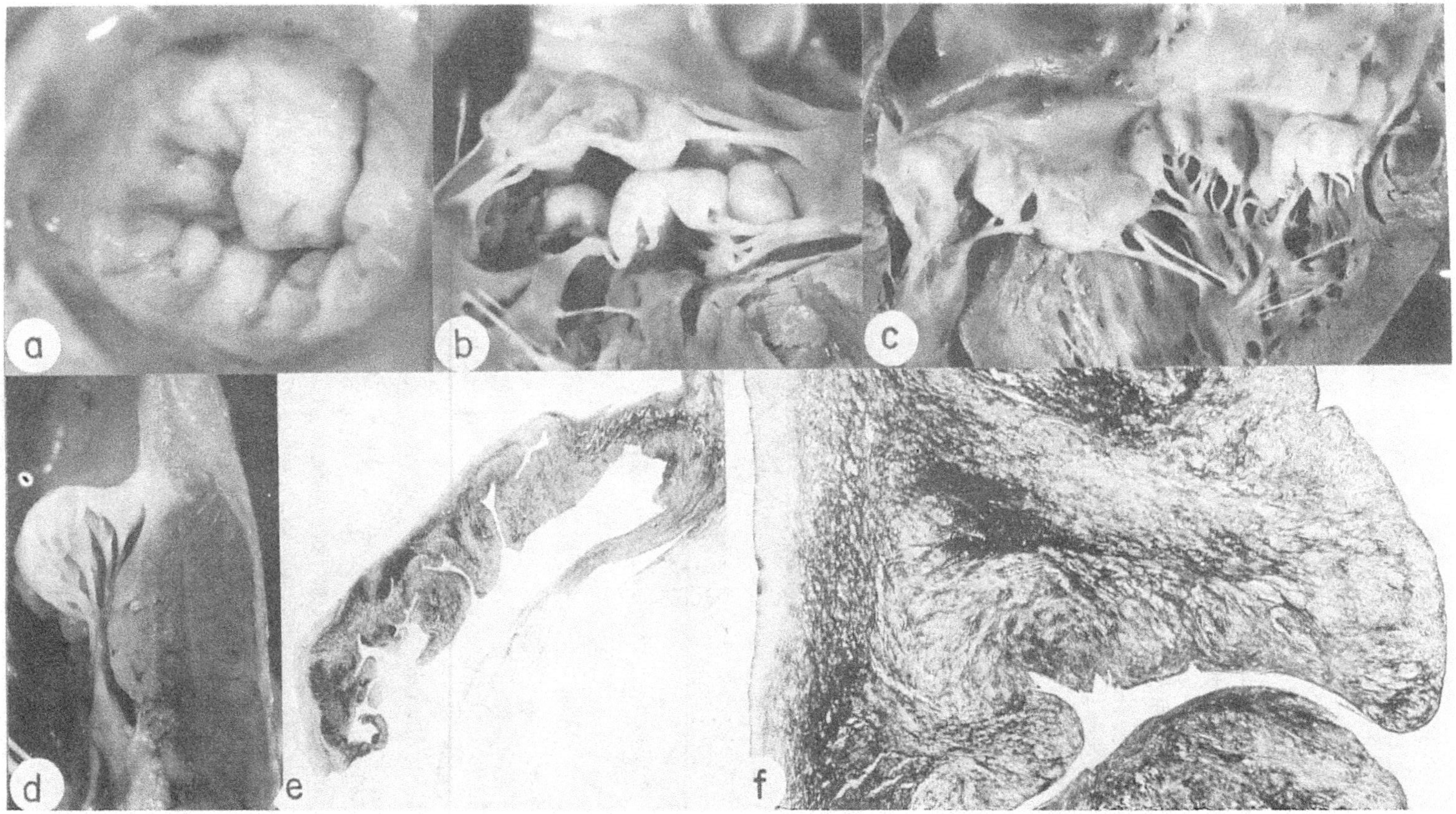

Figure 26. Floppy mitral valve, an incidental necropsy finding. This 18-year-old girl (A71–172), who died of Ewing's sarcoma, never had symptoms of cardiac dysfunction despite an active life. She had a mid-systolic click and a grade 3/6 ejection type systolic murmur over the precordium, left axilla, and back, loudest over the apex. At necropsy, she had an Ebstein's malformation of the tricuspid valve in addition to the floppy mitral valve. The mitral valve leaflets are elongated, but in contrast to those seen in Figure 27 the chordae are not elongated. a, Prolapsed mitral valve leaflets as viewed from left atrium. b, View of floppy leaflets from left ventricle. c, Opened mitral valve showing elongated and focally thickened anterior and posterior leaflets. d, Longitudinal section through left atrium, posterior mitral leaflet, and left ventricle showing the billowed posterior leaflet. e, Photomicrograph of the leaflet demonstrates focal thickening and increased acid-mucopolysaccharide (AMP) deposits. f, Higher power magnification showing AMP deposits (dark-staining). e and f, Acid-mucopolysaccharide stains (Rinehart). [Reduced 10 per cent from × 5(e) and × 36 (f).]

wall ischemia, were frequent, prompting still another name, "the auscultatory-electrocardiographic syndrome."

Necropsy observations[109-113] (Figs. 26–29) on patients with clear-cut clinical evidence of the floppy mitral valve syndrome have been sparse. A major reason for the sparcity of morphologic data is the good prognosis of most patients with this clinical complex. The term "floppy valve syndrome," however, also has been used to describe patients with morphologic evidence of a floppy leaflet whether or not clinically detectable valvular dysfunction is present and therefore includes a wide spectrum of patients. Floppy valve has become synonymous with *myxomatous degeneration,* a histologic description which needs further clarification.

In most valvular heart diseases, the spongiosa component of leaflets is either partially or completely replaced by the fibrous component. In the condition under consideration, the spongiosa is the component which proliferates. Because the spongiosa is the portion of the valve which contains acid-mucopolysaccharide

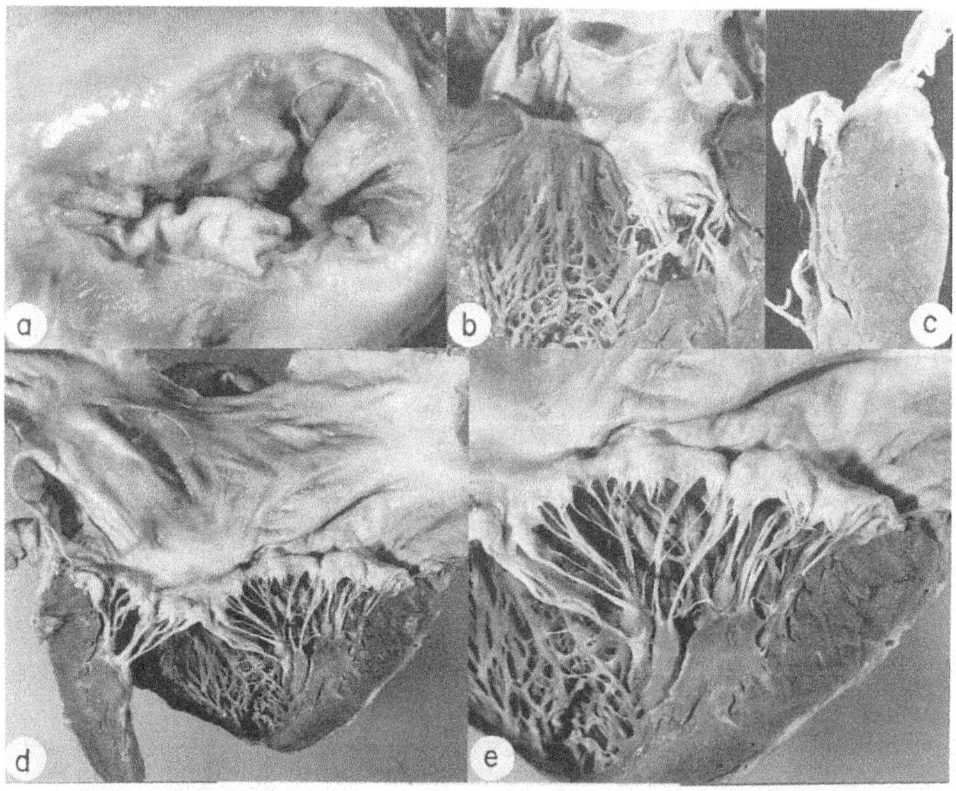

Figure 27. Floppy mitral valve. This 70-year-old man (A71–152), who died of gastric carcinoma, had had a grade 3/6 pansystolic blowing murmur. He never had symptoms of cardiac dysfunction. a, Mitral valve as viewed from left atrium. The leaflets protrude toward the atrium because the chordae tendineae are too long. Photographs of opened mitral valve and left ventricle (b, d, e) show elongated chordae and voluminous anterior and posterior mitral leaflets. A longitudinal section (c) through the left atrium, posterior mitral leaflet, and left ventricle shows the billowed leaflet and small calcific deposits in the annulus.

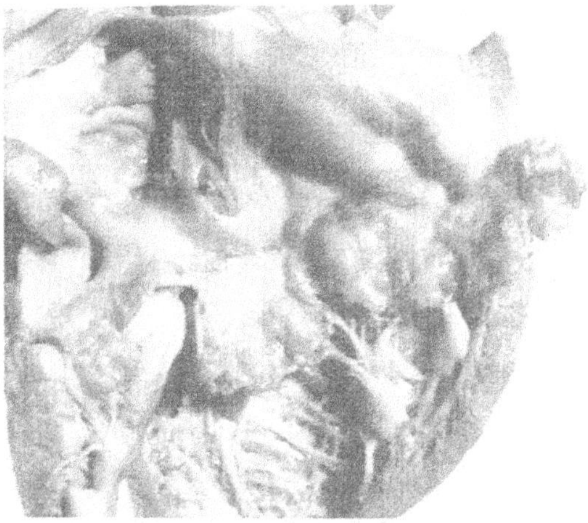

Figure 28. Floppy mitral valve. This two-day-old boy (A67–236), with long toes and fingers and a high-arched palate, had a grade 3/6 precordial systolic murmur typical of mitral regurgitation. Shown here is the opened left atrium, mitral valve, and left ventricle. The mitral leaflets are considerably elongated in both longitudinal and transverse dimensions. The left atrium is dilated. This case is important because it shows that the floppy valve may be present from birth.

(AMP) material, there is an increased amount of AMP in floppy leaflets. In the floppy valve the spongiosa has been described as being disorganized, giving rise to what has been called mucoid or myxomatous degeneration, but little information regarding normal organization of the spongiosa is available for comparison.

Because spongiosa (and therefore AMP material) is part of the normal valve, it is not surprising that it also is part of the diseased valve. Most cardiac valves, excised for either stenosis or incompetency or both, contain myxoid stroma.[110] Stenotic valves, however, appear to contain a much smaller percentage of myxoid material than do purely incompetent valves.

A wide spectrum of leaflet abnormalities may be associated with an isolated increase in valvular myxoid stroma. In some patients the change is evident only by histologic examination, and grossly the leaflet appears normal. We have called this change grade 1 on a scale of 1 to 4. When myxoid stroma is increased enough to cause valve leaflet to be grossly abnormal, the leaflet may prolapse without causing valvular incompetence (grade 2), the valve may prolapse and be mildly incompetent (grade 3), or the valve may be moderately to severely incompetent with or without congestive cardiac failure (grade 4). Similar myxomatous changes also have been described in tricuspid, aortic, and pulmonic valves, most frequently in the Marfan and Marfan-like syndromes, and they also may be incompetent.[68,114,115]

The common denominator of the floppy valve syndrome is an abnormal prolapse of one or both mitral valve leaflets toward left atrium during ventricular systole. Whether or not mitral regurgitation (MR) is a consequence of leaflet prolapse is determined by the extent of the prolapse. Abnormal prolapse without MR generally results in a systolic click without an accompanying murmur (stage I) (Table 13). Additional prolapse generally produces mild MR as manifested by a late systolic murmur with retention of the systolic click (stage II) (Barlow syndrome). Severe prolapse produces moderate to severe MR as manifested by prolongation of the murmur throughout systole (pansystolic) and disappearance of the systolic click (stage III). Thus, MR represents a consequence of the prolapsing (floppy) mitral valve. Other complications, namely infective endocarditis,

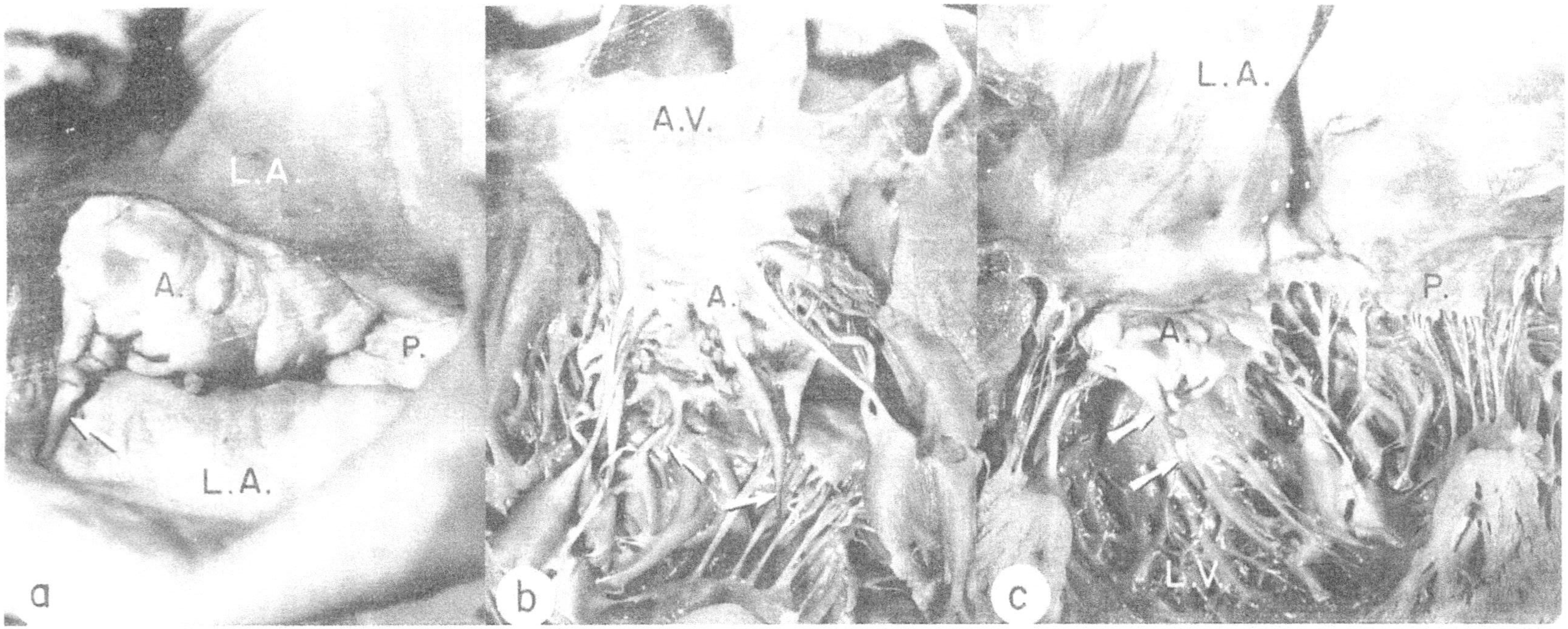

Figure 29. Prolapsed anterior mitral leaflet with chordae, probably involving an initially focally floppy valve. This 71-year-old man (A67–66) had a precordial murmur first noted at age 20 and it suddenly increased from grade 2/6 to 4/6 two years before death when heart failure appeared. At necropsy, the mitral regurgitation was explained by rupture of the chordae attached to the anterior mitral leaflet. There was no clinical or necropsy evidence of active endocarditis or of myocardial infarction. a, Left atrial (L.A.) view showing prolapsed anterior (A.) mitral leaflet. P. = posterior mitral leaflet. b, Opened aortic valve (A.V.) and left ventricle showing aortic aspect of anterior mitral leaflet (A.). The leaflet is thickened and two chordae are ruptured (arrows). c, Opened left atrium, mitral valve and left ventricle (L.V.). Arrows point to a ruptured chorda. The posterior mitral leaflet (P.) is normal. The case may represent spontaneous rupture of chordae tendineae in association with floppy mitral valve.

Table 13.

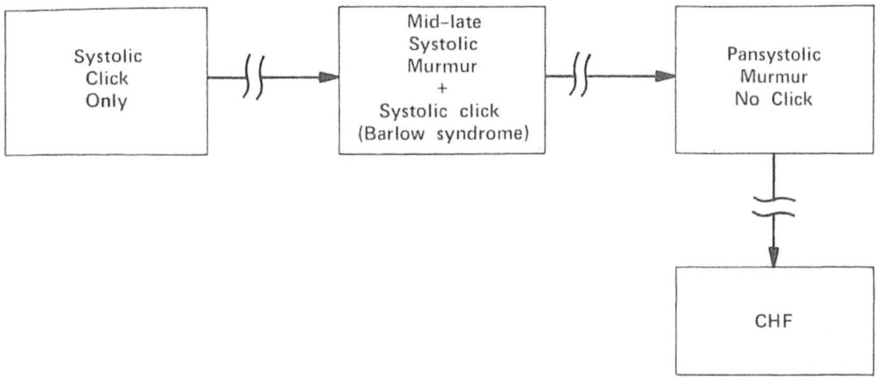

rupture of chordae tendineae without infection, rupture of valvular leaflet, calcification of the mitral annulus, arrhythmias, chest pain, and sudden death may occur at any of the three stages. Although probably most patients enter the scene at stage I, initial entrance may be at stage II or III. Although little information is available regarding progression from stage I to stage III, it appears reasonable to believe that progression is in this order even though one may remain only briefly at one stage or skip stage II entirely.

The actual frequency with which mitral regurgitation complicates myxomatous degeneration of the mitral valve is uncertain. A recent necropsy study of 35 patients with these valves disclosed that less than 25 per cent had mitral regurgitation and more than 50 per cent had symptoms of cardiac dysfunction.[111] It is well established that floppy mitral valves have a predisposition to develop infective endocarditis, and therefore antibiotics before operative procedures are warranted. It is less well appreciated that spontaneous rupture of chordae tendineae may be a complication of floppiness,[111] and even less well recognized that myxomatous degeneration may result in aneurysmal dilatation and rupture of a mitral leaflet. Whether or not calcification of the mitral annulus is a complica-

Table 14. Cause of prolapse (overshooting) of mitral valve leaflet(s) into left atrium during ventricular systole

I. Abnormal leaflets only
    A. Elongation
        1. Focal
        2. Diffuse
II. Abnormal chordae tendineae only
    A. Elongation
    B. Rupture
III. Abnormal leaflets and chordae
IV. Normal leaflets and chordae
    A. Shortened left ventricular cavity (old age)
    B. Necrosis, fibrosis, or ischemia of papillary muscle(s)
    C. Rupture of papillary muscle
        1. Whole trunk
        2. One or more heads

tion of floppiness is uncertain. It is frequently seen in the elderly, and appears to be accelerated by conditions which elevate left ventricular pressure and cause increased wear and tear on the valve. The snapping back of the mitral leaflet in systole may cause added stress on the mitral annulus and also accelerate or increase the likelihood of calcification of the annulus. Calcification of the annulus in the Marfan syndrome may be an expression of this complication of floppiness.

The causes of abnormal prolapse of mitral valve leaflets into left atrium during ventricular systole may be divided anatomically into four categories (Table 14). The mitral leaflets themselves may be enlarged (redundant) leading to billowing of the valve. This had been described most frequently in association with histologic changes of myxomatous degeneration of leaflet and marked increase in acid-mucopolysaccharide material. These histologic changes may not be unique to this syndrome, however, since the aging process may lead to anatomic and functional floppy mitral valves which show little or no evidence of mucoid degeneration microscopically.[116-118] Chordae tendineae which are ruptured or elongated may cause the leaflets to prolapse. The resulting laxity of the valve may lead secondarily to stretching and elongation of the leaflets. In the Marfan syndrome, abnormality in both mitral chordae and leaflets may result in billowing of the valve. An inborn defect of connective tissue of leaflet and chorda appears responsible. Intrinsically normal valves may become floppy because of left ventricular wall abnormalities. The shrunken left ventricular cavity of old age may cause the mitral valve to be redundant. A dysfunctioning or ruptured left ventricular papillary muscle may lead to slackening of the mitral valve in systole with prolapse into left atrium. A left ventricular contraction ridge has been seen by cineangiocardiography in some patients with the billowing mitral leaflet syndrome. This ridge may represent an abnormality of papillary muscle or of adjacent left ventricular wall, that is either cause or consequence of the valvular lesion.[104,119]

Thus, floppiness of the mitral valve is an anatomic and functional abnormality of diverse etiology and it is an important cause of nonrheumatic valvular regurgitation.

Calcification of the Mitral Annulus

Calcification of the mitral annulus is one of the most frequent abnormalities of the heart. Mitral annular calcification is generally considered to be a disease of elderly women. Indeed, of 14 patients with massive mitral annular calcification reported by Korn et al.[120] in 1962, all were women and all were over 65 years of age. It is incorrect, however, to believe that this entity is reserved entirely for a particular sex at a particular time in life. During the past four years one of us (W.C.R.) has examined at necropsy the hearts of 95 patients in whom varying amounts of calcium involved the mitral annulus. Of the 95 patients, 46 were male and 49 were female. Sixty-five patients (27 male, 38 female) were greater than 65 years of age and 30 patients (19 male, 11 female) were less than 66 years of age. Of the latter 30 patients, 8 were less than 40 years of age: three of them had the Marfan syndrome; two had the Hurler syndrome; and three had metabolic disturbances with hypercalcemia.

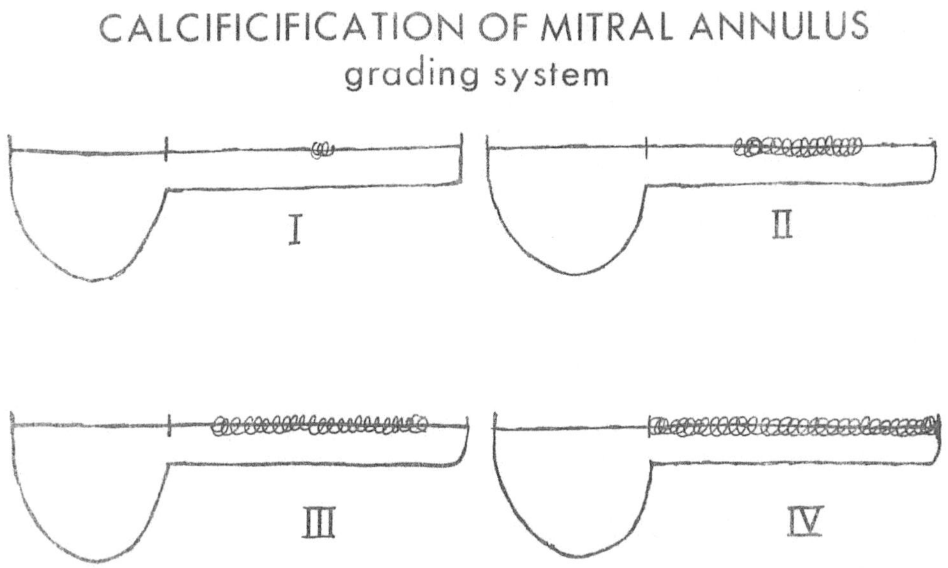

Figure 30. Method of grading mitral annular calcification. Grade I indicates only a single small deposit, grade II a large single or more than one small deposit. Grades III and IV represent extensive deposits. The entire annulus behind the posterior leaflet is involved in grade IV and, on rare occasion, calcific deposits also may extend across the anterior leaflet.

The extent of mitral annular calcification was graded 1+ to 4+ (Fig. 30): 49 patients (30 male, 19 female) had 1+ or 2+ deposits, and 46 (16 male, 30 female) had 3+ or 4+ deposits. Thus, this condition is as frequent in both sexes, but the larger deposits (those likely to be seen on chest roentgenogram) are more frequent in women. The smaller deposits (grade 1+ and 2+) have no functional importance. The larger deposits (grade 3+ and 4+) (Fig. 31), in contrast, may produce mitral regurgitation. Although stenosis has been mentioned as a possible complication of massive mitral annular calcification, obstruction has never been confirmed hemodynamically. Wide-open severe mitral regurgitation, likewise, is probably never due to mitral annular calcification.

Among patients with calcific deposits in the mitral annulus, similar calcific deposits often also are observed in the aortic valve cusps and in the extramural or epicardial coronary arteries. Of the 95 patients with mitral annular calcification,

Figure 31. Calcification of the mitral valve annulus. This 71-year-old woman (PH# A72-68) had had second degree heart block with ventricular rates as low as 40 beats per minute for two years. Bundle of His studies by Dr. Ross Fletcher had showed normal conduction through the atrioventricular node with block distal to the atrioventricular bundle. A pacemaker had been inserted 23 months before death. She died suddenly after climbing a flight of stairs at home. Necropsy disclosed acute myocardial infarction with rupture of the left ventricular apex and a blood-filled tense pericardial sac. Necropsy disclosed a large calcific deposit in the area behind the posterior mitral leaflet (a, b, c). Calcium had extended from this area into the ventricular septum in the area of the atrioventricular bundle. a, Radiograph at necropsy of the heart with pacing catheter in the right ventricle. Electrocardiogram at necropsy disclosed that the pacemaker was functioning normally, firing at 70 beats per minute. Calcific deposits also are present in the walls of the coronary arteries and aorta. b, Longitudinal section showing calcific deposit beneath the posterior mitral leaflet. c, Radiograph of heart specimen from above showing circumferential extent of the mitral annular calcific deposits.

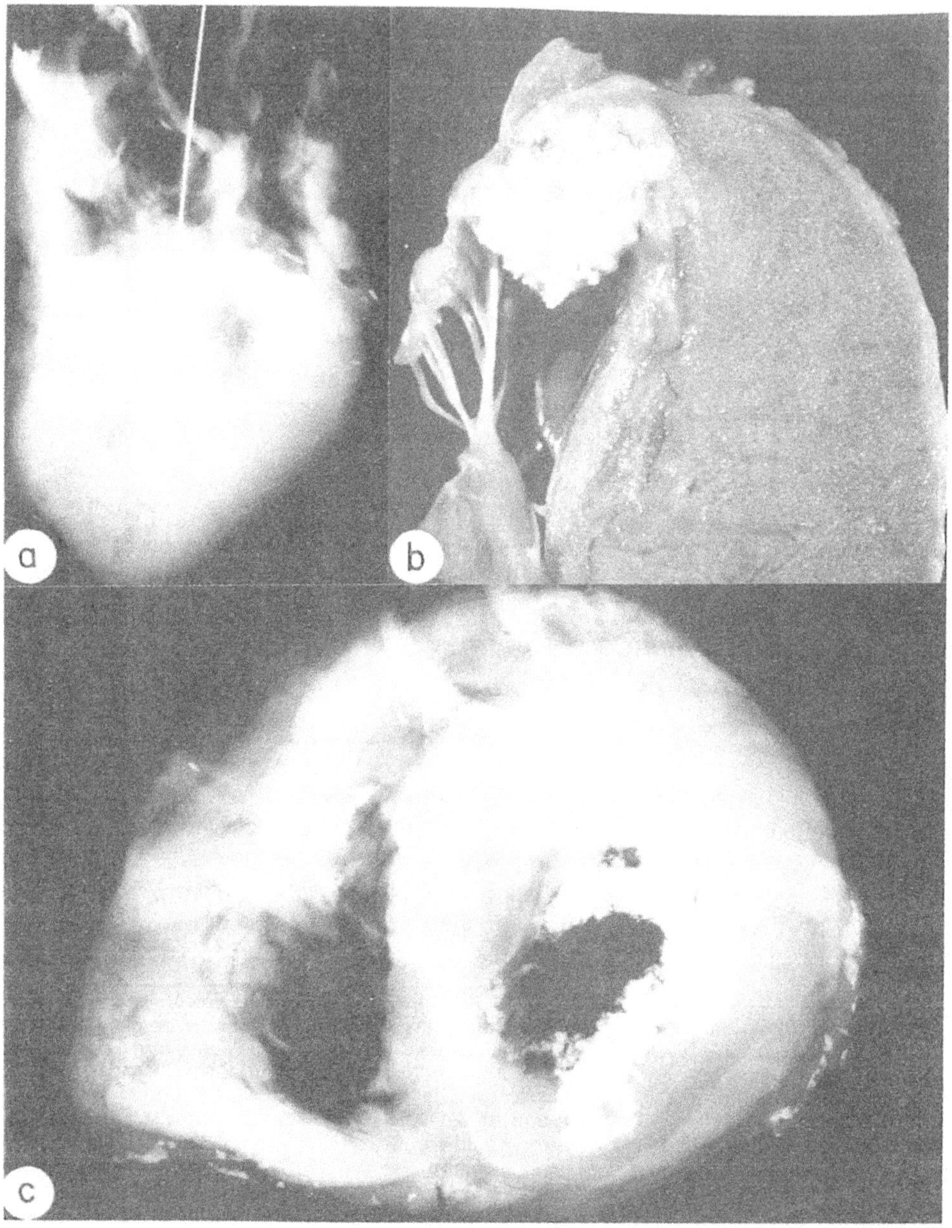
a
b
c

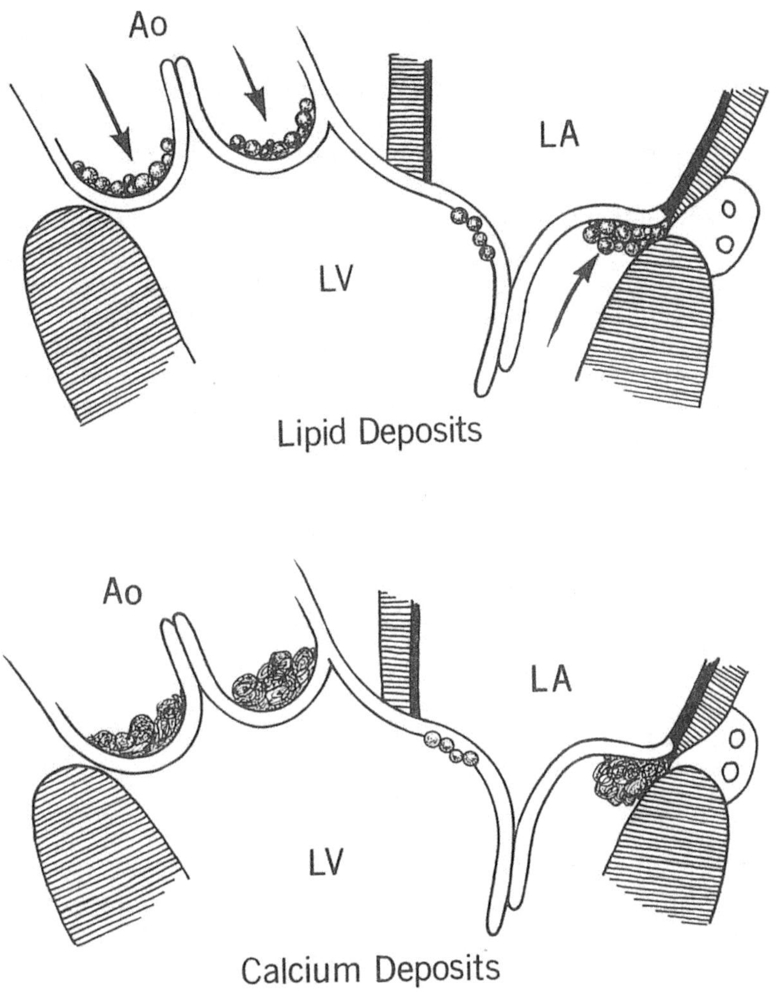

Figure 32. The cause of calcification of the mitral annulus is uncertain. Since most patients with mitral annular calcific deposits also have calcific deposits in the aortic valve cusps and coronary arteries, it seems reasonable to believe that the cause of the calcification in each of these sites is similar. In young adults, yellow deposits are nearly always seen on the ventricular surface of both mitral leaflets and on the aortic surfaces of the aortic valve cusps. The lipid may be both intracellular and extracellular. Degeneration of the lipid probably leads to the calcification. The latter occurs behind the posterior mitral leaflet and on the aortic aspects of the cusps because these are the sites of high pressure and there is nowhere else for the blood to go, so, in effect, it is pushed into the valve leaflets. In contrast, the high pressure on the anterior leaflet is reflected off into the aorta. In other words, the impact of pressure contacts the posterior mitral leaflet and aortic valve cusps at right angles to the cusps, whereas the angle of contact with the anterior leaflet approaches a 180 degree angle.

68 (72 per cent) also had calcific deposits in the aortic valve and in 35 of them the deposits were so extensive that the aortic valve orifice appeared stenotic. Large peak systolic pressure gradients were recorded across the aortic valve in several.[4] The aortic valve in this situation usually contains calcific deposits only on its aortic surfaces, the commissures are not fused, and there is no associated incompetence.[4] Calcific deposits were observed grossly in the coronary arteries in 83 (87 per cent) of the 95 patients. Nine of 12 patients *without* coronary arterial calcific deposits were less than 53 years of age. Of the 65 patients greater than 65 years of age with mitral annular calcification, 62 (95 per cent) had calcific deposits in the coronary arteries and 51 (78 per cent) had calcific deposits in the aortic valve cusps. Thus, deposits of calcium in these three locations—mitral annulus, aortic valve, and coronary artery—are seen most frequently in the elderly and suggest a common etiology. The deposits occur on the undersurface, i.e., ventricular surface of the posterior mitral leaflet at or below the annulus and on the aortic surfaces of the aortic valve cusps. Foam (lipid-containing) cells are common in these locations in younger adults. Probably, breakdown of these lipid deposits is responsible for the calcification at these sites (Fig. 32).

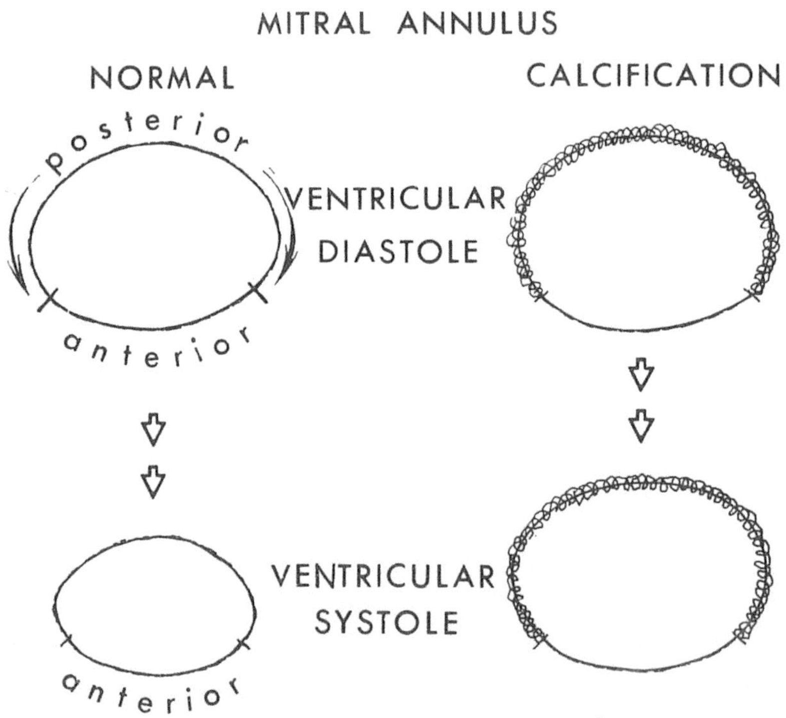

Figure 33. The mechanism of mitral regurgitation in patients with calcification of the mitral annulus is depicted here. During ventricular systole the base of the left ventricle contracts like a sphincter. Included in the base of the left ventricle is the annulus behind the posterior mitral leaflet. Thus, this circumference decreases during systole. If, however, the annulus behind the posterior mitral leaflet is calcified, the sphincter-like contraction of the left ventricular base no longer takes place. Thus, the area of the mitral orifice is not decreased and mild degrees of mitral regurgitation may be the result.

Calcification in the mitral annular area appears to be accelerated by conditions which elevate left ventricular pressure, namely systemic hypertension, aortic valvular stenosis, and hypertrophic cardiomyopathy,[121] and by conditions which accelerate atherosclerosis, for example, diabetes mellitus. The former conditions increase the mitral closing pressure and the latter appear to increase the supply of lipids. An intrinsic defect of the fibrous skeleton of the heart appears to be the explanation for early mitral annular calcification in the Marfan and Hurler syndromes. The mechanism by which mitral regurgitation is produced in patients with calcified mitral annuli is discussed in Figure 33.

In contrast to calcification of the mitral annulus, calcification of the tricuspid valve annulus is rare and the deposits are always focal and usually small. Tricuspid annular calcification may occur in two circumstances: (1) In patients with heritable connective tissue defects. We have observed tricuspid annular calcification in a patient with the Marfan syndrome and in another with the Hurler syndrome. (2) In patients with right ventricular hypertension from any cause. This is by far the most common underlying abnormality in these patients. We have observed tricuspid annular calcific deposits in patients with so-called pure pulmonic stenosis, primary pulmonary hypertension, and tetralogy of Fallot. Others have made similar observations.[122-124]

Papillary Muscle Dysfunction

A significant advance in clinical cardiology during the decade of the 1960s was the appreciation of the important contribution of the left ventricular papillary muscles to maintenance of mitral valve competence during ventricular systole. It is now well recognized that hypoxia, necrosis, or fibrosis of the left ventricular papillary muscles may be associated with varying degrees of mitral regurgitation. Discrepancies exist, however, in correlating papillary muscle structure with function. Although it most commonly results from coronary atherosclerosis, papillary muscle necrosis or fibrosis may occur when the coronary arteries are normal. Patients without clinical evidence of mitral valve dysfunction at necropsy have had severe necrosis or fibrosis or both, of one or both left ventricular papillary muscles; severe mitral regurgitation during or after acute myocardial infarction has been found at necropsy to be associated with normal papillary muscles, normal mitral leaflets and chordae tendineae, and normal-sized mitral annuli. This section seeks to clarify these discrepancies. Types and causes of papillary muscle damage are outlined in Table 15.[72]

Transient ischemia of papillary muscles is believed to be common and probably results in varying degrees of mitral regurgitation.[73] A murmur of mitral regurgitation may occur during an attack of angina pectoris and be absent during pain-free periods. Transient systolic murmurs during and after myocardial infarction probably result from papillary muscle ischemia. Arterial perfusion of the left ventricular papillary muscles even may be influenced by body position.[125] Possibly, transient ischemia of papillary muscles occurs during emotional stress in individuals with normal or nearly normal coronary arteries in a manner similar to that which leads to constriction of the peripheral vascular beds during anxiety or during cigarette smoking.

Table 15. Spectrum of left ventricular papillary muscle disease

- I. Anatomically normal papillary muscles but papillary muscle dysfunction
  - A. Transient ischemia
  - B. Left ventricular dilatation from any cause
    - 1. Generalized
    - 2. Localized
  - C. Necrosis or fibrosis in adjacent left ventricular free wall
    - 1. With coronary arterial narrowing
    - 2. Without coronary arterial narrowing
  - D. "Small" left ventricular cavity (hypertrophic cardiomyopathy)
- II. Necrosis or fibrosis of papillary muscle(s) without rupture
  - A. With coronary arterial narrowing
    - 1. Acute myocardial infarction
    - 2. Healed myocardial infarction
  - B. Without coronary arterial narrowing
    - 1. Acute
      - a. Shock
      - b. Acute valvular regurgitation (infective endocarditis)
    - 2. Chronic
      - a. Anemia
      - b. Left ventricular outflow obstruction
        - (1) Valvular aortic stenosis
        - (2) Discrete and diffuse subaortic stenosis
        - (3) Supravalvular aortic stenosis
      - c. Systemic hypertension
      - d. Origin of left coronary artery or of both coronary arteries from pulmonary trunk
      - e. Primary endocardial fibroelastosis of left ventricle
      - f. Endomyocardial disease and eosinophilia
        - (1) Löffler's fibroplastic parietal endocarditis
        - (2) Endomyocardial fibrosis of Davies
      - g. Idiopathic cardiomegaly (primary or diffuse myocardial disease)
      - h. Focal myocardial disease
        - (1) Idiopathic
        - (2) "Neurogenic" heart disease
          - (a) Progressive muscular dystrophy
          - (b) Friedreich's ataxia
          - (c) Myotonic muscular dystrophy
- III. Necrosis or fibrosis of papillary muscle(s) with rupture
  - A. Acute myocardial infarction from coronary heart disease
  - B. Trauma
  - C. Miscellaneous
- IV. Infiltrative diseases of papillary muscles
  - A. Pyogenic abscess
  - B. Granulomas
    - 1. Aschoff bodies
    - 2. Sarcoid
  - C. Amyloid
  - D. Neoplasm
  - E. Calcium
  - F. Iron
  - G. Other
- V. Congenital malformations of papillary muscle(s)
  - A. Single papillary muscle (parachute mitral valve syndrome)
  - B. Accessory papillary muscle
  - C. Abnormally large and malpositioned papillary muscles
  - D. Abnormally small and malpositioned papillary muscle
  - E. Insertion of papillary muscle directly into mitral leaflet
- VI. Miscellaneous afflictions of papillary muscle(s)
  - A. Excision, partial or complete, during mitral valve replacement
    - 1. Atrophy of nonexcised portion of papillary muscle after valve replacement
    - 2. Left ventricular aneurysm at site of papillary muscle excision
  - B. Disuse atrophy after excision of mitral leaflets and chordae without excision of papillary muscle(s)

Left ventricular dilatation is a frequent cause of papillary muscle dysfunction.[126] Although the papillary muscles may contract normally under such circumstances, the spatial relationships between them, chordae tendineae, and orifices are altered by the caudal and lateral migration of the left ventricular walls away from the mitral annuli. The valve leaflets thus are pulled downward toward the left ventricle and consequently the mitral orifice becomes incompetent.

Although it may accompany left ventricular dilatation, mitral annular dilatation is probably an infrequent cause of mitral regurgitation, and most cases of mitral regurgitation attributed to annular dilatation probably result from papillary muscle dysfunction. Mitral annular dilatation must be massive to cause regurgitation for at least two reasons: (1) normally the surface area of the mitral leaflets is about two times the area of the mitral orifice and (2) the mitral ring has a sphincter-like action which causes the annulus to contract during ventricular systole.[127] Furthermore, a fibrous skeleton at the base of the heart inhibits mitral annular dilatation. Indeed, in the dilated heart the widest diameter occurs not at the left ventricular base, the area which includes the mitral annulus, but in the midportion of the chamber between apex and base.

It is now well appreciated that dilated left ventricles, per se, with or without fibrosis or necrosis of ventricular walls, may be associated with mitral regurgitation. It is less well recognized that mitral regurgitation may be associated with necrosis or fibrosis of the left ventricular free wall without accompanying left ventricular dilatation or papillary muscle or mitral valve lesions. Necrotic or scarred myocardium adjacent to papillary muscles, which fail to move or move paradoxically during ventricular systole, and the abnormal ventricular contraction may lead to abnormal papillary-muscle anchoring with resulting mitral regurgitation. Anatomic left ventricular aneurysms unassociated with papillary muscle necrosis or fibrosis also may cause mitral regurgitation by a similar mechanism. In hypertrophic cardiomyopathy the septal hypertrophy bends or distorts the papillary muscles causing mitral regurgitation.[72,73]

Necrosis or fibrosis of one or both left ventricular papillary muscles is extremely common. It may be focal or diffuse, involve only one papillary muscle or both, and auscultatory mitral regurgitation may or may not be present. Experimental studies show[128] that mitral regurgitation is not a consequence of fibrosis of papillary muscles alone. The free wall beneath the papillary muscle must also be fibrotic for mitral regurgitation to occur. We have observed at necropsy many patients who had no audible precordial murmurs in life but had extensive fibrosis or necrosis of one or both left ventricular papillary muscles. Papillary muscle fibrosis or necrosis causing mitral regurgitation, however, does not necessarily assure the appearance of a precordial murmur. Several patients without a regurgitant murmur have been shown to have mitral regurgitation by cineangiocardiography, and at necropsy to have extensive necrosis or fibrosis of papillary muscle and of left ventricular free wall.[129] Silent mitral regurgitation during acute myocardial infarction has been attributed to a diminished flow velocity across the mitral valve secondary to diminished myocardial contractility.

The most common cause of papillary muscle necrosis or fibrosis is narrowing of the coronary arterial lumen by atherosclerosis. The posteromedial papillary

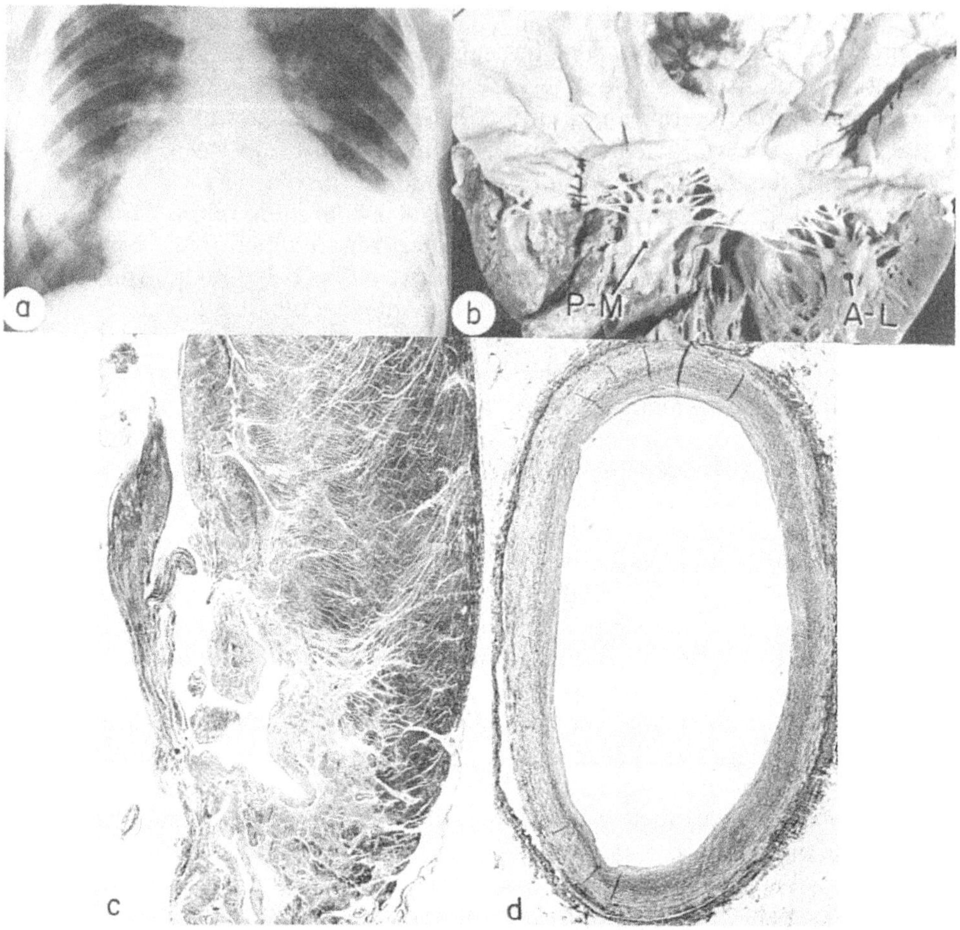

Figure 34. Possible focal myocarditis with subsequent fibrosis causing severe mitral regurgitation in an 84-year-old man (A66–213). A precordial murmur had been known to be present for 44 years. During his last 20 years he had periodic overt congestive cardiac failure and a grade 4/6 pansystolic blowing murmur typical of mitral regurgitation. He never had chest pain, systemic hypertension, rheumatic fever, or infective endocarditis. The heart was enlarged (a). The mitral leaflets and chordae tendineae were virtually normal. The posteromedial (P-M) papillary muscle was diffusely fibrotic as was the adjacent left ventricular free wall beneath it (b). No other myocardial scars were present and the coronary arteries were wide open. c, Longitudinal section of posteromedial papillary muscle and adjacent left ventricular free wall. Both are severely scarred and thinned. d, Section of right coronary artery which is wide open. All his coronary arteries were widely patent. c, Masson stain. d, Elastic van Gieson stain. [Reduced 30 per cent from × 4 (c) and × 21 (d).]

muscle is usually involved in posterior wall infarction, but in anterior wall infarction the anterolateral papillary muscle may be spared. Necrosis or fibrosis of one or both left ventricular papillary muscles may be unassociated with luminal narrowing of the extramural coronary arteries (Fig. 34). Inadequate oxygenation of the papillary muscles may occur if the amount of oxygen in the blood is low (i.e., anemia) or if the cardiac output for any reason is below a critical level. To perfuse the apices of the papillary muscles the coronary arteries must extend

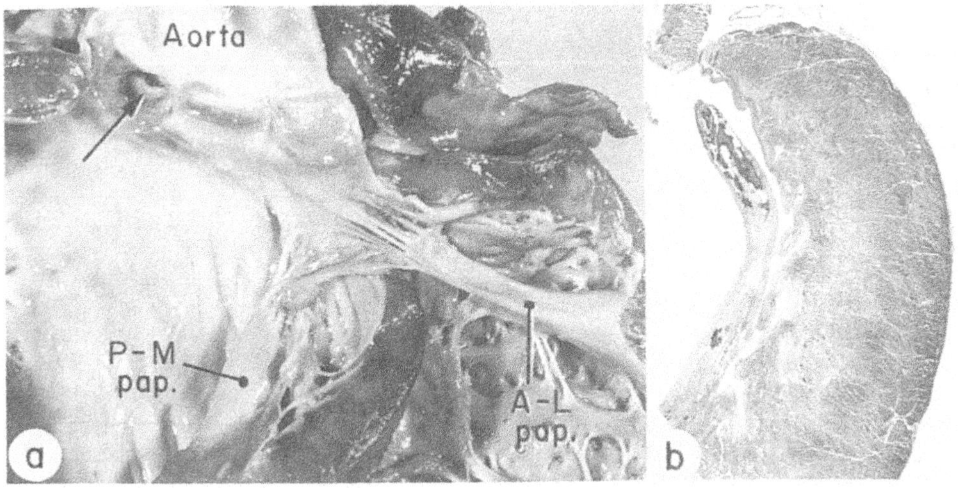

Figure 35. Mitral regurgitation due to origin of left coronary artery from the pulmonary trunk. Severe fibrosis and calcification in the anterolateral left ventricular papillary muscle in a nine-month-old girl (A56–14) in whom the left coronary artery arose from the pulmonary trunk. She had had evidence of congestive cardiac failure since age three weeks. Examination at age eight months disclosed a grade 3/6 systolic precordial murmur consistent with mitral regurgitation. The heart was huge, and electrocardiogram showed evidence of left ventricular hypertrophy and ischemia. She died during cardiac operation. At necropsy, the left ventricle was considerably dilated and its endocardium showed diffuse fibroelastosis (a). The anterolateral papillary muscle was severely thinned, scarred and calcified (b). b, Hematoxylin-eosin stain. [Reduced 15 percent from × 4 (b).]

through the entire thicknesses of the myocardial free walls, turn up hill, and ascend distances of at least one and often two thicknesses of the free wall. Hence, the papillary muscles (particularly the posteromedial one) are the most sensitive markers of inadequate myocardial oxygenation. Foci of necrosis also are common in patients with fatal severe valvular regurgitation of recent onset. Among 47 patients dying of active valvular infective endocarditis, 34 (72 per cent) had necrotic lesions in one or both left ventricular papillary muscles and none had significant narrowing of the extramural coronary arteries.[130-132] Severely diminished cardiac output with resultant poor myocardial perfusion appeared to cause the papillary muscle necrosis in them.

Fibrosis with atrophy of the papillary muscles is seen in patients with primary

Figure 36. Diagrammatic representation of the types of, and possible consequences of, papillary muscle rupture during acute myocardial infarction. It is likely that rupture of the entire trunk (*left*) is incompatible with survival in any patient since a major portion of the support to both valve leaflets is destroyed. With rupture of an apical head (*right*), survival would appear to depend on the extent to which the function of the left ventricle has been impaired by the infarct. With severely impaired ventricular function, the additional burden of even modest mitral regurgitation may be intolerable, and death will ensue. If the left ventricle is less severely compromised, survival is possible for weeks or months, but congestive cardiac failure will almost invariably develop. *Lower,* Rupture of a portion of one papillary muscle during acute myocardial infarction in a 51-year-old man (S67–813) who underwent mitral valve replacement three months after the onset of infarction. Preoperatively, the pulmonary arterial pressure was 60/28 (mean 40); pulmonary arterial wedge pressure, mean 28, v42; left ventricular pressure 74/17; and cardiac index, 1.7 L./min./m^2. Shown here is the excised mitral valve (by Dr. Andrew G. Morrow). The leaflets are normal but the posteromedial papillary muscle is necrotic and fibrotic and a portion of it is entwined in chordae tendineae at the margin of the anterior mitral leaflet. This is a view of the ventricular aspects of the leaflets.

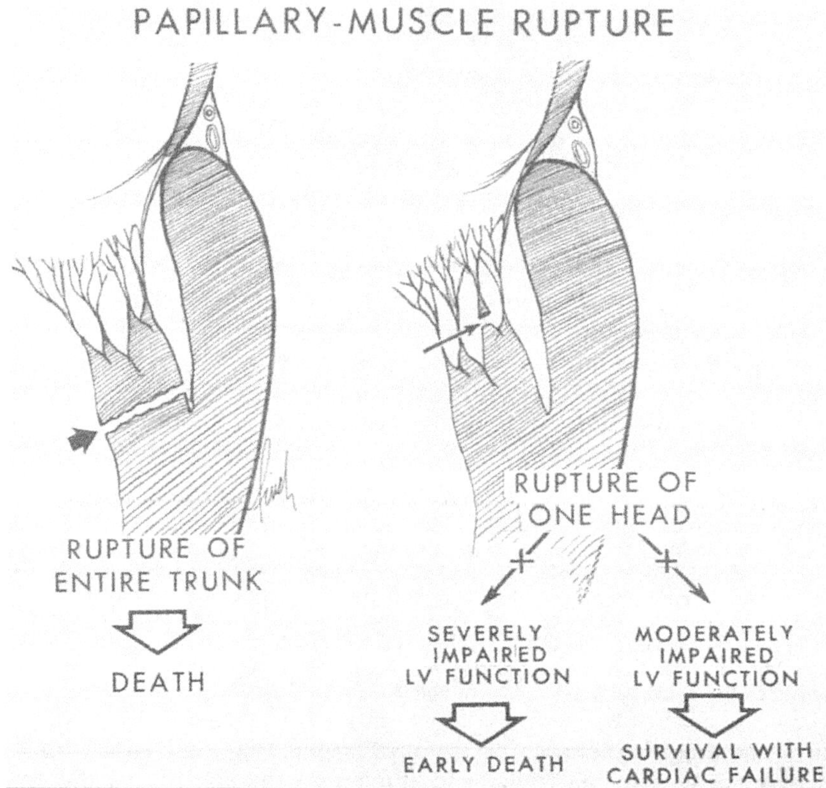
PAPILLARY-MUSCLE RUPTURE
RUPTURE OF
ENTIRE TRUNK
DEATH
RUPTURE OF
ONE HEAD
SEVERELY
IMPAIRED
LV FUNCTION
EARLY DEATH
MODERATELY
IMPAIRED
LV FUNCTION
SURVIVAL WITH
CARDIAC FAILURE

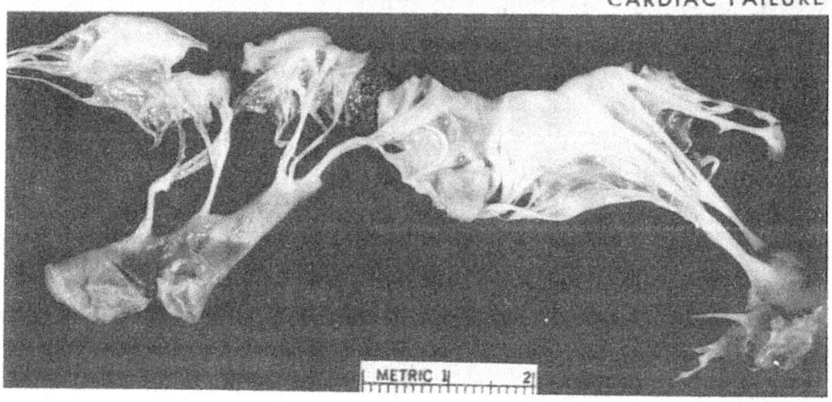
METRIC 1 2

endocardial fibroelastosis of the left ventricle.[133] The endocardial scarring as well as the papillary muscle fibrosis may be an anatomic expression of chronically inadequate coronary arterial perfusion of the left ventricle. In the congenital condition, origin of the left[134] or both[135] coronary arteries from the pulmonary trunk, diffuse endocardial fibroelastosis of the left ventricle, and fibrosis and atrophy of the left ventricular papillary muscles are associated lesions. These patients may present clinically with features of pure mitral regurgitation[136] (Fig. 35). Similarly, the African conditions, endomyocardial fibrosis and Löffler's fibroplastic parietal endocarditis may be associated with scarring of one or both papillary muscles, and rarely, patients with primary or secondary forms of cardiomyopathy may have scarred and dysfunctioning papillary muscles.[137-140]

In contrast to necrosis of a papillary muscle which occurs in over 50 per cent of patients with fatal acute myocardial infarction, rupture of a papillary muscle is rare, occurring in less than 1 per cent of patients with fatal acute myocardial infarction. The rupture may be of two types (Fig. 36).[141] One involves

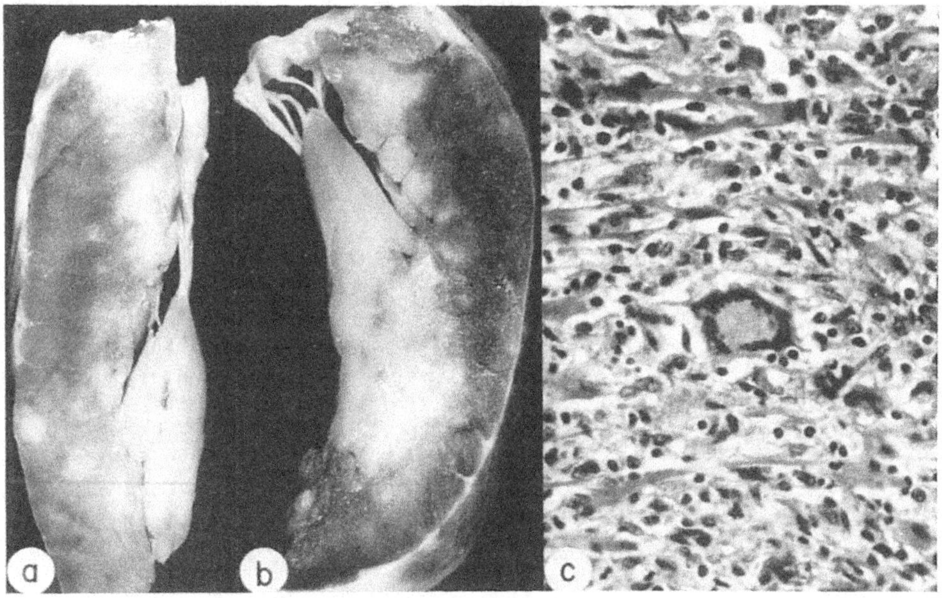

Figure 37. Sarcoidosis of papillary muscles causing mitral regurgitation. Anterolateral (a) and posteromedial (b) left ventricular papillary muscles in a 26-year-old woman (PGGH A-70-541) who was asymptomatic until 10 days before death when dyspnea appeared. The dyspnea rapidly worsened, and when hospitalized on the day of death she was in acute pulmonary edema. The blood pressure was 80/70 mm. Hg, heart rate 160 beats/minute, and a grade 3–4/6 pansystolic blowing apical murmur, which radiated into the axilla, was audible. Chest roentgenogram showed congested lungs, cardiomegaly, and prominent hilar adenopathy. Electrocardiogram showed nonspecific ST–T wave changes and atrial hypertrophy. Several hours after admission ventricular fibrillation occurred; she was resuscitated, but complete heart block appeared. A transvenous pacemaker was inserted, but asystole occurred shortly thereafter. At necropsy, large firm white deposits were present in the walls of all four cardiac chambers and completely replaced both left ventricular papillary muscles (a and b). On histologic section, the firm white areas represented hard granulomas typical of sarcoidosis (c). Similar hard granulomas were present in lymph nodes, liver, spleen, and lung. Stains for acid-fast organisms, other bacteria, and fungi were negative. (Specimen was kindly provided by Dr. James Hutchinson.) c, Hematoxylin-eosin stain. [Reduced 25 per cent from × 400 (c).]

the entire central muscle belly of the papillary muscle, and this type rupture is incompatible with survival since half the support of each valve leaflet is destroyed and mitral regurgitation of overwhelming severity results. The second type of rupture involves only one or two apical heads of a papillary muscle. The resulting mitral regurgitation is of lesser magnitude and immediate survival is then dependent upon the degree to which the function of the left ventricle has been impaired by the infarct. In patients who survive after papillary muscle rupture, the functional capacity of the left ventricle also governs the extent of clinical and hemodynamic improvement after mitral valve replacement.

The papillary muscles are subject to various infiltrative processes just like any other portion of myocardium.[72,142] Pyogenic abscesses, Aschoff bodies, granulomas,[142] neoplasms,[143-145] amyloid,[146] and iron[147] have all been observed in these structures. Congestive heart failure from severe mitral regurgitation may be the initial symptom of sarcoidosis[72] (Fig. 37).

Infective Endocarditis

Infective endocarditis (IE) continues to be a major cause of fatal valvular heart disease. Clinical and necropsy observations in 57 necropsy patients with IE have recently been reported[130,131] from this laboratory and major findings from these studies are summarized in Table 16. Although IE may involve both right-sided and left-sided cardiac valves, or mural endocardium only,[148] it is useful to separate cases with right-sided vegetations (with or without associated left-sided vegetations) from those with isolated left-sided vegetations (Table 16).

The frequency with which infection attacks previously normal as opposed to previously abnormal valves is somewhat uncertain. It has long been stated

Table 16. Infective endocarditis: data in 57 necropsy patients

	Isolated Left-sided Vegetations	Isolated Right-sided Vegetations	Right and Left-sided Vegetations	Totals
Patients	45	6	6	57
Ages (years): Range (avg)	17-70(38)	25-65(40)	1-62(40)	1-70(39)
Males	32(71%)	3	5	40(70%)
Females	13(29%)	3	1	17(30%)
Alcoholics	7(15%)	1	4	12(21%)
Heroin addicts	6(13%)	4	0	10(18%)
Acute meningitis	6(13%)	2	3	11(19%)
Acute pneumonia	4(9%)	5	5	14(25%)
Antemortum diagnosis	36(80%)	3	2	41(72%)
Previous symptomatic H.D.	12(27%)	0	1	13(23%)
Rheumatic H.D.	10(22%)	0	0	10(18%)
Congenital H.D.	8(18%)	0	1	9(16%)
Anatomically normal valve	24(53%)	6	5	35(61%)
Anatomically abnormal valve	21(47%)	0	1	22(39%)
Functionally normal	10(22%)	—	1	11(19%)
Functionally abnormal	11(24%)	—	0	11(19%)
Stenosis	7(15%)	—	0	7(12%)
Incompetent	4(9%)	—	0	4(7%)
Staphylococcus	12(27%)	5	1	18(32%)
Streptococcus	9(20%)	0	1	10(18%)
Pneumococcus	4(9%)	1	3	8(14%)
Acute myocarditis	23(51%)	1	2	26(46%)
Papillary muscle necrosis	22/39(56%)	0	3	25/50(50%)

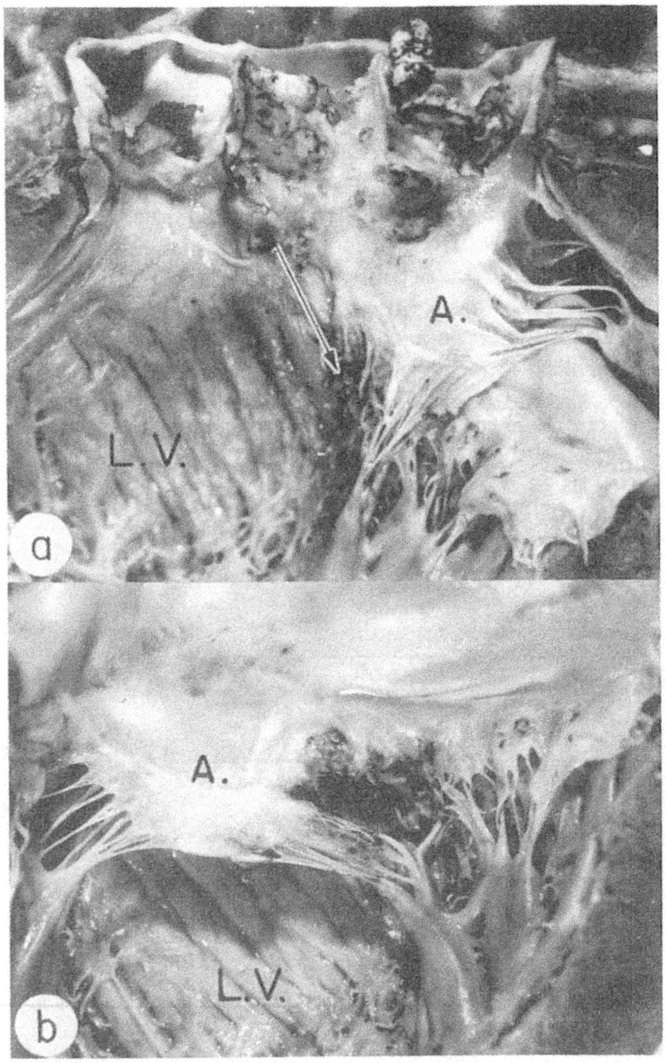

Figure 38. Streptococcus faecalis endocarditis involving both aortic and mitral valves in a 61-year-old man (DCGH# 71A-120). Symptoms and signs of active infective endocarditis appeared three weeks after catheterization of his urinary bladder. Both valves probably were normal before they became sites of infection. a, Opened left ventricle (L.V.) and aortic valve. The vegetations have partially destroyed each cusp causing severe aortic regurgitation. Vegetation on the left ventricular outflow endocardium, mitral leaflet, and chordae tendineae almost certainly resulted from retrograde spread of the aortic vegetations by the aortic regurgitant stream (arrow). A. = anterior mitral leaflet. b, Opened mitral valve showing vegetations at the posteromedial commissure area. Many chordae have ruptured.

that IE tends to affect persons with known valvular heart disease, but that the cardiac condition is compensated, i.e., the patient is usually asymptomatic before infection appears. This view indicates, therefore, that infection tends to involve valves which are anatomically abnormal but functionally normal. From a necropsy standpoint, however, fatal active IE more frequently involves previously anatomically normal valves (Figs. 38–41). Of our 45 necropsy patients with left-sided IE, the affected valve was previously anatomically normal in 24 (53 per cent), and of the 21 (47 per cent) affecting previously anatomically abnormal valves, only 11 of them had been functionally abnormal (valve stenosis in seven, pure incompetency in four). Of our 12 patients with right-sided vegetations, the involved valve had been anatomically normal before IE in 11, and functionally normal in all 12. Because infection of previously anatomically normal valves is nearly always by virulent organisms, and because the infective process can more easily destroy a thin, delicate (normal) valve as opposed to a thick, tough (abnormal) valve, the frequency of involvement by IE of previously anatomically normal

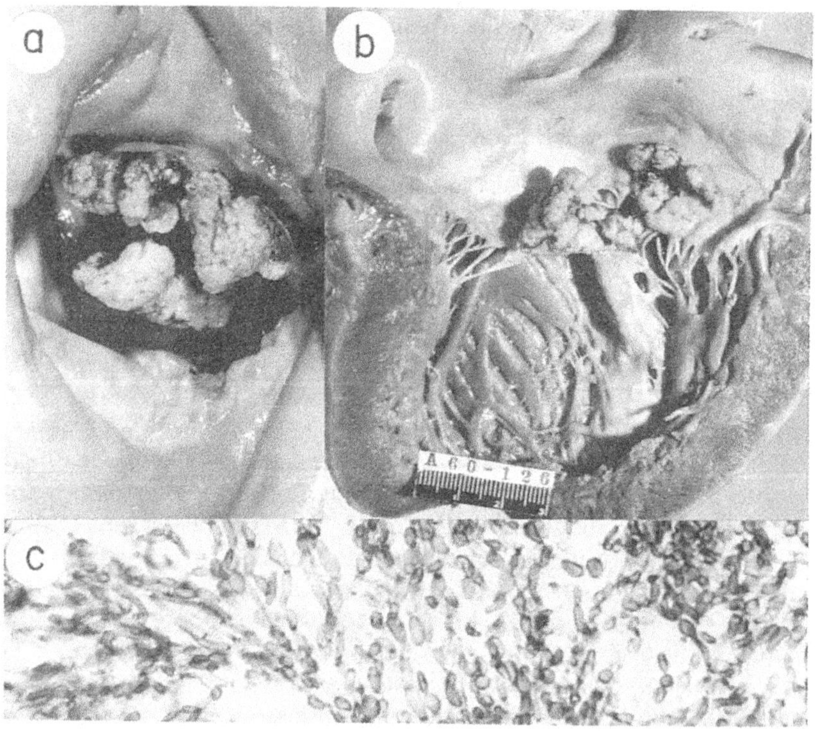

Figure 39. Candida parapsilosis endocarditis on a previously normal mitral valve of a 68-year-old man (A60–126) with chronic lung disease and coronary heart disease. Five months before death he had fever, and 45 days later he was hospitalized. A grade 2/6 apical systolic murmur was present. Despite amphotericin B therapy, blood cultures remained positive, and he died of congestive heart failure. A large embolus to the left common iliac artery occurred during hospitalization. a, Mitral valve viewed from left atrium showing huge vegetations on both leaflets. b, Opened left heart showing large vegetations on both mitral leaflets. Although they were large, the vegetations did not destroy the valvular leaflets or rupture chordae tendineae. c, Photomicrograph of portion of vegetation showing spores and pseudomycelia of Candida species. Methenamine silver stain × 500.

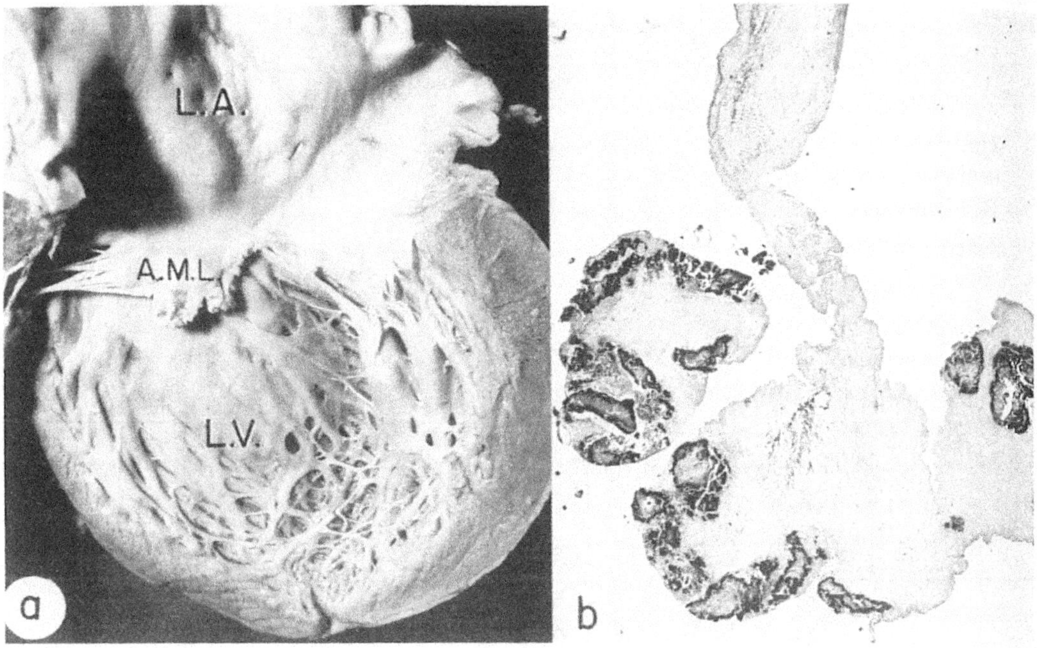

Figure 40. Acute mitral regurgitation from rupture of chordae tendineae secondary to Streptococcus faecalis endocarditis in a 24-year-old woman (A62–19) who had been well until five months earlier when symptoms of infective endocarditis appeared shortly after an abortion. Despite antibiotic therapy, severe congestive cardiac failure and pulmonary hypertension developed. The vegetation healed but she died of results of rupture of many mitral chordae tendineae. a, Opened left atrium (L.A.), mitral valve, and left ventricle (L.V.) showing severence of all chordae on the posterior half of the anterior mitral leaflet (A.M.L.). The valve before infection was normal. b, Histologic section of portion of anterior mitral leaflet showing calcific deposits, almost certainly a consequence of healing of the vegetation. Hematoxylin-eosin stain × 16.

valves in a necropsy study might be abnormally high. The incidence of IE, however, is clearly greater among persons with underlying valvular heart disease as opposed to the incidence of IE among persons with previously normal hearts. But, because there are many more persons with four normal valves compared to persons with one or more abnormal ones, this numerical difference alone may explain the greater frequency with which normal valves are involved by IE. The frequency of certain predisposing factors (malignancy, heroin addiction, alcoholism, long-term intravenous catheters, etc.) allowing entrance of virulent or unusual organisms or alterations in host defense mechanisms also is important in explaining the frequency of IE on normal valves.

Valvular dysfunction is by no means an inevitable consequence of active IE. It was unequivocally a consequence of IE in 59 per cent, and possibly as high as 74 per cent, of our 45 patients with left-sided IE but in none of our six patients with isolated right-sided vegetations. Congestive cardiac failure is common in fatal IE. It occurred in 74 per cent of our patients with left-sided IE, and in each was the result of valvular dysfunction, not the result of associated myocardial lesions. Although the latter occurred in 87 per cent of the patients

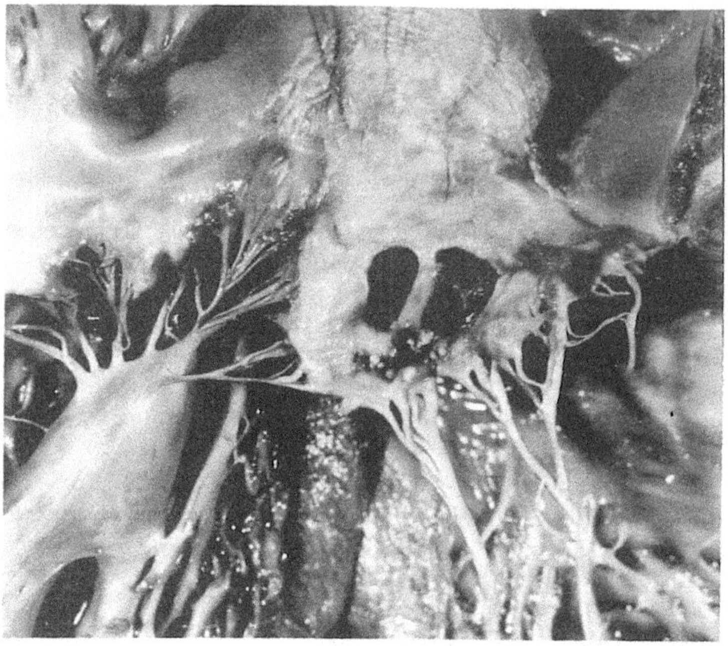

Figure 41. Infective endocarditis with perforation of mitral leaflet and severe regurgitation. This young woman (A69–154) had been well until the appearance of infective endocarditis about one year before death. The infection was "cured" by antibiotics but mitral regurgitation was a consequence. She died of progressive congestive cardiac failure from mitral regurgitation. Perforation of a mitral valve cusp by infection, as shown here, is infrequent. Mitral regurgitation in infective endocarditis far more commonly results from rupture of chordae tendineae. It appears that the valve shown here was anatomically normal before infection appeared.

with isolated left-sided vegetations, in none did they appear large or diffuse enough to account by themselves for congestive cardiac failure. Papillary muscle necrosis was present in 58 per cent, but in none did it appear to cause mitral regurgitation. Valve ring abscesses occurred in 12 or 31 per cent of patients with aortic valve vegetations and in none of 26 with mitral valve vegetations. Ring abscesses indicate severe destruction of valvular cusps and severe valvular dysfunction, and they also usually indicate that the infection is the result of a highly virulent organism. Aortic regurgitation, when it occurred, was the result of destruction (tears or perforations) of the cusps by the infective process. Mitral regurgitation resulted from rupture of chordae tendineae by the infective process, and only 2 of 26 patients with mitral vegetations had cuspal perforations.

Of the 12 patients with right-sided cardiac valvular vegetations, six also had vegetations on left-sided cardiac valves (Table 16). In only one of the latter, however, was the IE definitely primary on the left side of the heart. The tricuspid valve was the site of IE in 11 patients and the pulmonic valve in one. The organisms responsible for the IE were Staphylococcus aureus in six patients, Diplococcus pneumoniae in four, Alpha streptococcus in one and Aspergillus flavus in one.

Five patients were alcoholics, four were heroin addicts, two had blood dyscrasias, and one had congenital cardiac disease (ventricular septal defect). The IE in each of the nine patients with alcoholism or heroin addiction and in the one with congenital heart disease was primary in the heart; in the remaining two patients, it was secondary to generalized infection affecting many body organs. Acute pneumonia was a dominant clinical feature in 10 of the 12 patients and appeared to be secondary to dislodgment of material from the right-sided cardiac vegetations. Six patients also had acute meningitis. Although the vegetations caused considerable damage to the right-sided cardiac valves, evidence of cardiac dysfunction was either absent or attributable to acute *cor pulmonale* secondary to the acute pneumonia. The tetrad of chronic alcoholism, acute pneumonia, acute meningitis, and infective endocarditis is common.[149] In 9 of the 12 patients the right-sided vegetations did not extend to involve the basal attachments of the leaflets to the annuli. Thus, in these nine patients total excision of the valve leaflets would have eradicated their valvular endocarditis.

The two major causes of acute valvular regurgitation are acute myocardial infarction and IE. Among 55 patients with fatal pure mitral regurgitation studied by one of us (W.C.R.), rupture of mitral chordae tendineae was the second most frequent etiology and IE was the most common cause of rupture.[150] Since infection most commonly involves previously normal valves, valvular destruction may be rapid and lead to severe regurgitation and decompensation. Rupture of previously normal mitral chordae leads to sudden severe elevation of left atrial pressures and the left atrial v waves may be similar in magnitude to the left ventricular systolic pressure (ventricularization of left atrial pressure) (Fig. 42). This circumstance occurs because the left atrium does not dilate initially, and as a consequence the high left atrial pressure is reflected to the pulmonary circuit with resulting severe pulmonary and right ventricular hypertension. When the left atrium finally dilates in pure mitral regurgitation from this mechanism, its pressure, along with that in the pulmonary vessels and right ventricle, also decreases.[150]

Although many reports have appeared on active IE, few reports have appeared on the morphologic aspects of *healed* IE. Recently, a study from this laboratory[151] examined cardiac valves in 59 patients with positive histories of IE searching for anatomic evidence of healed IE. Of the 59 patients, healed cuspal perforations were present in 16, healed ruptured chordae tendineae in 15, and healed ring abscesses in 5. A total of 30 of the 59 patients had one or more of these anatomic findings. Thus, about half of the patients with positive histories of IE had clear-cut anatomic evidences of IE. The relationship of healed valvular perforations and

Figure 42. Diagram depicting the two extremes of the spectrum of pure mitral regurgitation. When severe mitral regurgitation appears suddenly in individuals with previously normal or near-normal hearts, the left atrium (LA) is relatively small and the high pressure within it is reflected back into the pulmonary vessels and right ventricle (RV). The anatomic indicator of this latter physiologic event is severe hypertrophy of the left atrial and right ventricular walls and marked intimal proliferation and medial hypertrophy of the pulmonary arteries (PA), arterioles, and veins (PV). In the other extreme, the left atrial cavity is of giant size and its wall is thin. It is thus able to "absorb" the left ventricular (LV) pressure without reflecting it back into the pulmonary vessels or right ventricle. As a consequence, the pulmonary vessels remain normal and the right ventricular wall does not thicken. PT = pulmonary trunk. RA = right atrium.

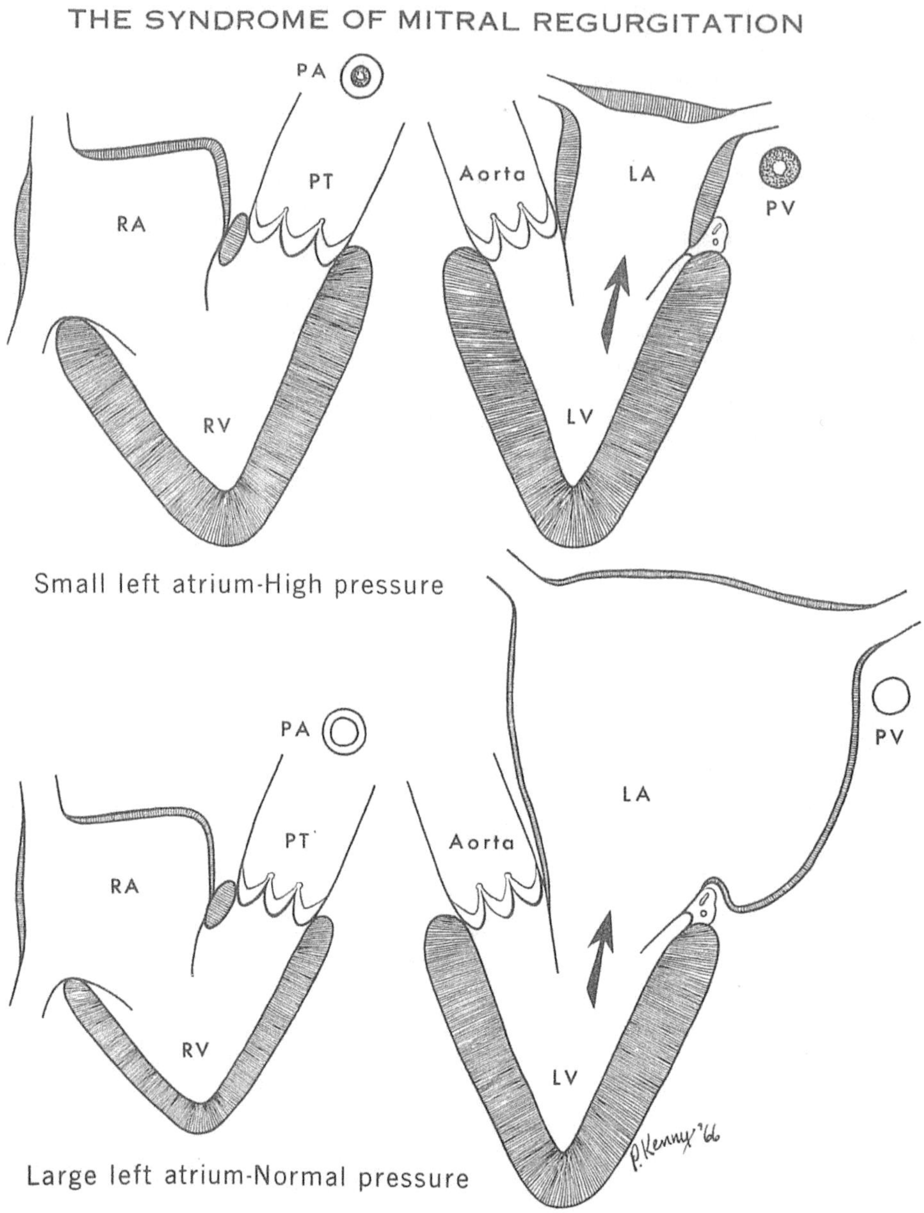
THE SYNDROME OF MITRAL REGURGITATION
PA
PT
RA
RV
Aorta
LA
PV
LV
Small left atrium-High pressure
PA
PT
RA
RV
Aorta
LA
PV
LV
P. Kenny '66
Large left atrium-Normal pressure

Table 17. Ebstein's anomaly: clinical and necropsy fiindings

Patient	Age	Sex	Age (yrs.) onset of symptoms	Cyanosis	Precordial murmurs: Systolic	Precordial murmurs: Diastolic	CE by x-ray	Electrocardiogram: SVA	Electrocardiogram: P Pulmonale	Electrocardiogram: RBBB	Cause of death	Necropsy findings: DDDTV (0-4+)	Necropsy findings: Associated lesions
1. A57-55	20	M	14	+	+	0	+	+	+	+	Operation*	4+	VI-PFO
2. A58-122	31	F	8	+	+	0	0	0	+	+	Operation†	3+	ASD,anomalous left SVC
3. A66-217	26	M	24‡	0	+‡	0	0	+	0	+	Sudden§	2+	Stenotic bicuspid AV
4. A68-2	18	F	15	0	+	0	0	+	0	0¶	SVA, VA	1+	0
5. A71-172	18	F	—#	0	+	0	0	0	0	0	Ewing's sarcoma	4+	Floppy MV
6. NNMC A72-97	37	F	33	+	+	0	+	+	0**	+	CHF heart block	4+	ASD

* Closure of valvular incompetent patent foramen ovale (VI-PFO) shortly before death.
† Closure of fossa ovale type atrial septal defect shortly before death.
‡ Symptoms and murmur consistent with aortic stenosis.
§ Ventricular fibrillation 18 days after aortic valve repair.
¶ Wolff-Parkinson-White pattern.
\# Asymptomatic.
** Atrial fibrillation.

ASD = atrial septal defect, fossa ovale type. AV = aortic valve. CE = cardiac enlargement. CHF = congestive heart failure. DDDTV = degree of downward displacement of tricuspid valve. MV = mitral valve. RBBB = right bundle branch block. SVA = supraventricular arrhythmias. SVC = superior vena cava. VA = ventricular arrhythmias.

ruptured chordae tendineae to antecedent positive histories of active IE also was examined. Of 18 patients with valve perforations, all 18 had had positive histories of active IE. Of 43 patients with healed ruptured chordae tendineae, only 15 (35 per cent) had had positive histories of active IE.

Congenital Tricuspid Regurgitation

Congenital tricuspid regurgitation most commonly is the result of displacement of the basal attachment of one or more tricuspid valve leaflets into right ventricle. This downward displacement is the characteristic feature of the malformation first described in 1866 by Ebstein.[152] Now over 300 patients have been reported with *Ebstein's anomaly* including one series of 108 patients.[153]

We have studied at necropsy six patients, aged 18 to 37 years, with Ebstein's anomaly (Table 17) (Figs. 43–46). Four were women. Three had been cyanotic, and they were the only ones with atrial septal defects. All six had systolic murmurs, but in two (#2 and #4) they appeared to be caused by associated mitral and aortic lesions and not by tricuspid regurgitation. None had diastolic murmurs. Four had ventricular diastolic gallops. Four had supraventricular arrhythmias. Roentgenograms revealed globular-shaped hearts (Fig. 43) in only two. The degree of caudal displacement of the tricuspid valve leaflets varied. Two (#1 and #5) of the three patients with the most marked downward displacement (Figs. 43–45) had classic clinical features of the anomaly and both had severe congestive failure

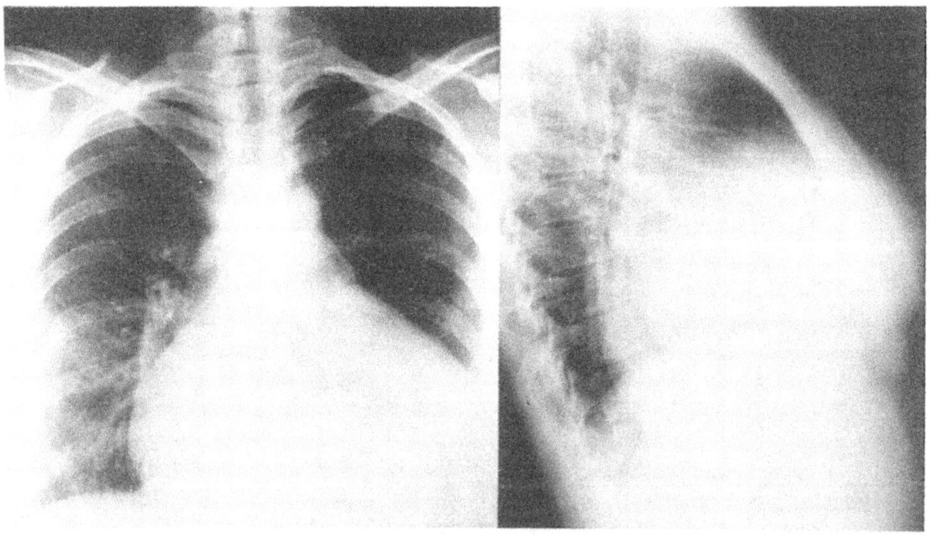

Figure 43. Ebstein's anomaly. Posteroanterior and lateral chest roentgenograms of a 37-year-old woman (NNMC A72–97) who died of severe cardiac failure and heart block. She had had profound cyanosis, chest pain, and episodes of syncope. At necropsy, severe downward displacement of the septal and posterior leaflets of the tricuspid valve and parchment-like thinning of the atrialized portion of right ventricle were found. In addition, a fossa-ovale type atrial septal defect was present. The radiograph reveals globular-shaped cardiomegaly in contrast to the patient in Figures 44 and 45 whose anatomic findings were similar in type and severity.

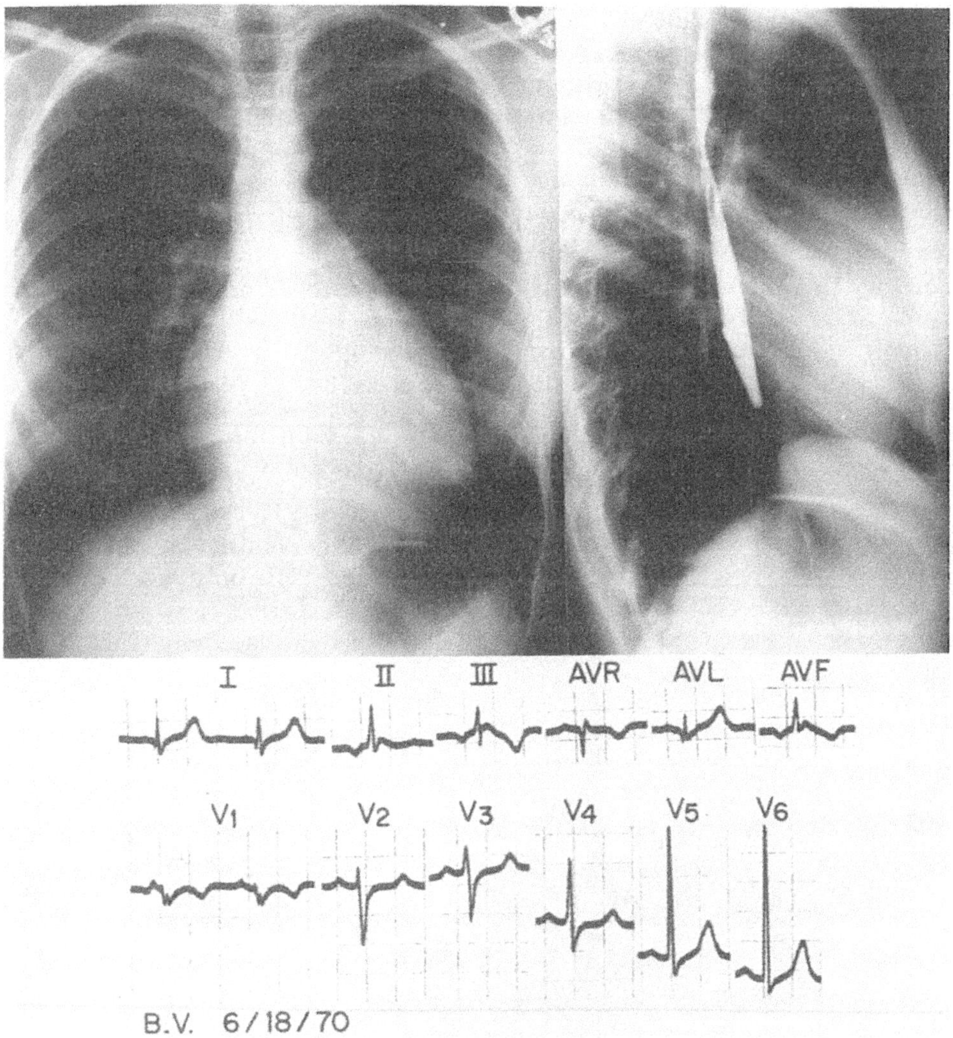

Figure 44. Severe Ebstein's anomaly of tricuspid valve, an incidental necropsy finding. Posteroanterior and lateral chest roentgenogram and electrocardiogram from the patient (A71–172) whose anatomic findings are demonstrated in Figure 45. The roentgenogram suggests right atrial enlargement and borderline cardiomegaly. The anteroposterior thoracic width, however, is narrow. The electrocardiogram reveals an atrioventricular junctional rhythm without tachycardia and an abnormally superior T wave vector. The P amplitude is normal and there are no clearcut defects in atrioventricular or intraventricular conduction.

before death or operation. In contrast, the patients with less caudal displacement did not die of congestive cardiac failure (Fig. 46). The displacement involved primarily the septal and posterior tricuspid valve leaflets, the basal attachments of these leaflets were displaced caudally from 2 to 8 cm. below the normal tricuspid valve annuli. In two patients (#5 and #6) functioning right ventricle was limited to outflow tract. In all patients one or more leaflets adhered to the ventricular walls by short chordae. An accessory tricuspid valve orifice was present in two patients. The tricuspid valve "annuli" were dilated in five patients. Right atrial and right ventricular dilatation was present in all and varied from mild to severe. In two patients the atrialized portion of the right ventricle was parchment-like.

The tricuspid valve in Ebstein's malformation is usually incompetent. Decompensation in these patients, however, appears to result primarily from inadequate pumping of the right ventricle and not from tricuspid regurgitation.[154,155] The portion of right ventricle cephalad to the displaced tricuspid leaflets is atrialized, i.e., the muscle is thin and contracts poorly, if at all. The functioning mass of right ventricular muscle may be reduced to outflow portion. As a result, pulmonary blood flow may decrease and the right atrial and systemic venous pressures may rise. Prognosis in patients with Ebstein's anomaly depends, in general, on the degree of caudal displacement of the tricuspid leaflets and the magnitude of associated valvular incompetency.[156] The average life expectancy is 37 years.[27,157] In its most severe form Ebstein's anomaly has been the presumed cause of intrauterine and perinatal death,[158,159] but survival into the seventh and eight

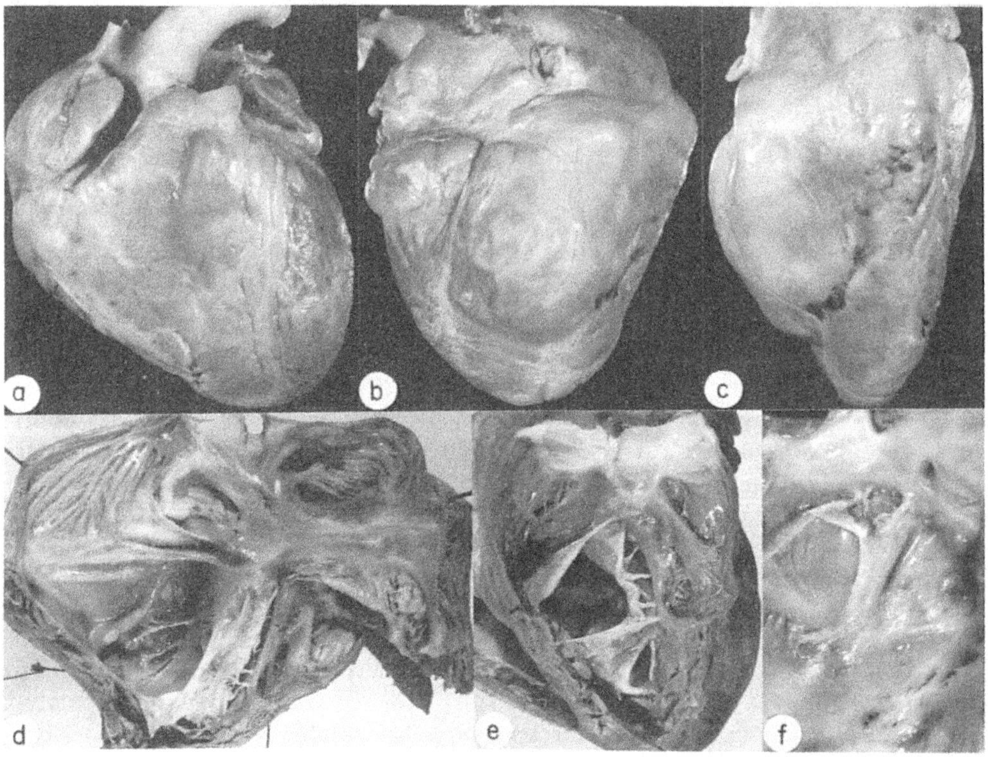

Figure 45. Severe Ebstein's anomaly of the tricuspid valve, an incidental necropsy finding. This 18-year-old girl (A71–172), who died of Ewing's sarcoma, had no symptoms of cardiac dysfunction despite an active life. a, b, and c, Anterior, posterior, and lateral views, respectively, of the external aspect of the heart demonstrating a thinned, parchment-like (atrialized) right ventricular wall bulging posteriorly above the attachment of the tricuspid leaflets. d, Opened right atrium and ventricle showing marked downward displacement of the posterior and septal tricuspid leaflets. The atrialized portion of right ventricle behind the posterior leaflet is the part that bulges (b and c). e, Tricuspid valve from above displaced deep into right ventricular cavity. Two valvular orifices are present. f, Intact atrial septum from left atrium with valvular-competent foramen ovale. The patient was never cyanotic.

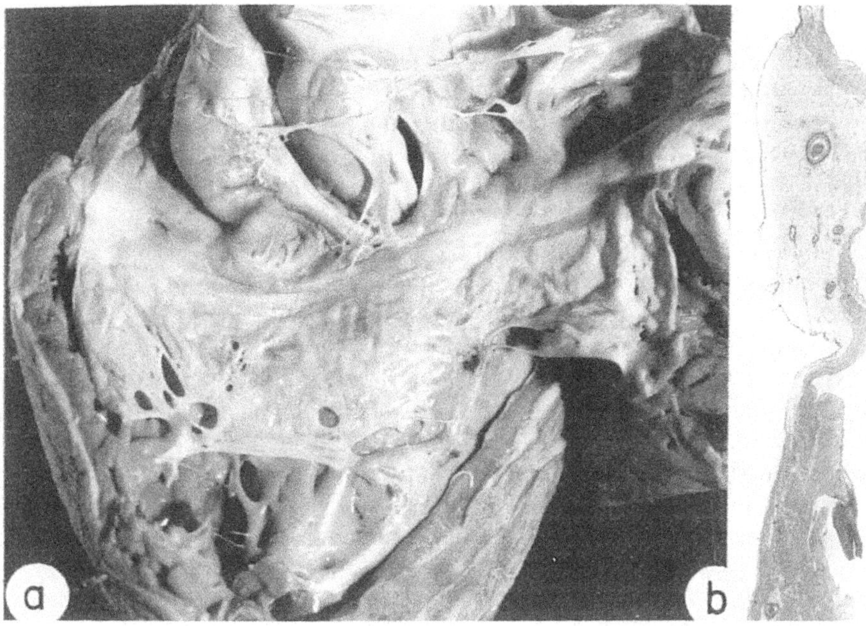

Figure 46. Mild Ebstein's anomaly in two patients. a, Opened tricuspid valve of a 25-year-old man (A66–217) who died 20 days after operation for severe valvular aortic stenosis. Tricuspid valvular dysfunction was not suspected clinically. At necropsy, it was seen that the tricuspid leaflets inserted into the right ventricular wall just below the annulus fibrosis. The tricuspid leaflets were bound down to the ventricular endocardium. b, Photomicrograph of a longitudinal section through right atrioventricular sulcus including a portion of right atrium and right ventricle. The basal attachment of the leaflet of the tricuspid valve is to the ventricular wall 1.8 cm. below the annulus. Hematoxylin-eosin stain × 2. This 18-year-old girl (A68–2) had a systolic precordial murmur of unknown cause and type B Wolff-Parkinson-White syndrome. She died of ventricular tachycardia and fibrillation during treatment of one of many episodes of supraventricular tachycardia. At necropsy, the right atrium, right ventricle, and tricuspid annulus were dilated.

decades may occur.[27,157,158,160,161] Death most frequently (about 40 per cent) results from congestive cardiac failure, another 20 per cent from supraventricular arrhythmias, and the remainder from miscellaneous causes.[158] About 75 per cent of these patients have an atrial septal defect with some right-to-left shunting. Most defects are valvular-incompetent patent foramina ovale.[153,160]

The clinical features of Ebstein's anomaly were first well described in 1950 by Engle et al.[162] The typical patient is fatigued, dyspneic, often cyanotic, and has a large, "quiet" globular heart, gallop rhythm, systolic and scratchy diastolic murmurs, right bundle branch block, and occasionally atrioventricular conduction delay (Wolff-Parkinson-White [type B] in 10 per cent). Diagnosis of this anomaly, however, may be difficult. Of our six patients, three (#2, #3, and #4) were not diagnosed correctly despite repeated clinical examinations. Some patients may be acyanotic, asymptomatic, and devoid of diagnostically useful physical findings.[163] In this situation, the electrocardiogram may be helpful.[164] Diagnosis in patients surviving past the fourth decade may be confused with more common forms of acquired heart disease, as was true of our patient #5 in whom the initial diagnosis was coronary heart disease. Unless strongly suspected, diagnosis of Ebstein's anomaly may be easily missed at catheterization.[165]

Pure Congenital Pulmonic Regurgitation

Isolated pure congenital pulmonary regurgitation (PR) is rare. It may complicate idiopathic dilatation of the pulmonary trunk,[166] hypoplasia or aplasia[167-170] of the pulmonic cusps, congenitally bicuspid[171,172] or quadricuspid[9] valves or malformed tricuspid valves. The congenitally aplastic or bicuspid pulmonic valve is usually associated with other congenital cardiac malformation, notably tetralogy of Fallot.[173] Of 158 patients reported with congenitally quadricuspid pulmonic valves, only four appeared incompetent.[9]

The natural history of congenital PR is unclear. When secondary to an aplastic valve, severe congestive heart failure and death have occurred in infancy.[167,168] Death in adults with pure congenital PR may be sudden[171] or after periods of progressive right-heart failure.[172] Evidence of right ventricular dysfunction without symptoms of congestive cardiac failure also may occur in adults.[174] Most reported patients, however, are young and asymptomatic. Although they may have abnormal right ventricular and pulmonary arterial pulsations and enlarged pulmonary trunks, the right ventricular and pulmonary arterial pressures are usually normal. The presumed benign nature of congenital PR is derived from reports of older adults with little or no evidence of cardiac decompensation.[170,175,176]

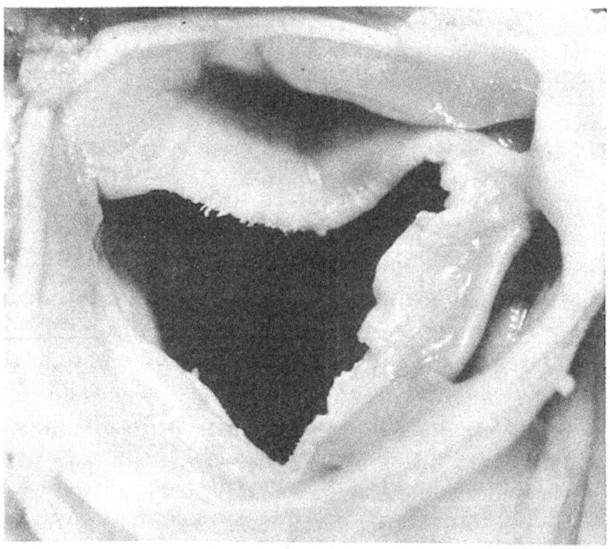

Figure 47. Congenital pulmonic valvular regurgitation in a 67-year-old man (36451) who died suddenly of a myocardial infarction. He had been told that he had "heart disease" at age 35, and cardiomegaly was known to be present at age 40. At age 49 he was found to be in congestive cardiac failure with cardiomegaly and a prominent pulmonary arterial segment on roentgenogram. Systolic and diastolic precordial murmurs were present and the electrocardiogram disclosed complete right bundle branch block. The clinical diagnosis at this time was valvular aortic stenosis and regurgitation. At age 58, pulmonic stenosis and regurgitation were diagnosed after catheterization. Right ventricular systolic pressure was 44 mm. Hg and a 10 mm. Hg peak systolic pressure gradient between right ventricle and pulmonary trunk was recorded on pullback. At necropsy all three pulmonic valve cusps were hypoplastic, thickened, and retracted. The valve did not appear stenotic. The right ventricle was severely dilated.

We have studied a 67-year-old man with isolated congenital PR who died of consequences of systemic atherosclerosis. Cardiac disease had been diagnosed when he was about 35 years of age and his heart was enlarged by age 40. At necropsy, the pulmonic valve was tricuspid but congenitally malformed and severely incompetent (Fig. 47).

Congenital Mitral Regurgitation

Congenital abnormalities of the mitral valve resulting in regurgitation are most often associated with other congenital cardiovascular anomalies. We have studied at necropsy, however, nine patients with fatal congenital mitral regurgitation (MR) presenting with this valve lesion (Table 18). Six were females, three were males, and they ranged in age from 9 months to 44 years. The MR in four patients was associated with and possibly caused by *diffuse endocardial fibroelastosis* of the left ventricle.[133, 177, 178] Two patients had *congeni-*

Table 18. Congenital mitral regurgitation: clinical and necropsy data

Autopsy number	*Age (yrs.)*	*Sex*	*Age (yrs.) murmur first heard*	*ECG*	*Pressures (mm. Hg)* *PA (s/d)*	*LA (V/mean)*	*LV (s/d)*	*SA (s/d)*	*LV angio (MR = 1+-4+)*
Diffuse endocardial fibroelastosis									
1. A61-133	9	F	7	AF LAH, LVH	30/12	14/8	—	—	—
2. A62-120	8	M	3	AF LVH, RVH	66/36	32/21	102/12	116/72	—
3. A63-33	14	F	7	↑PR LAE, LVH RVH	65/26	23/19	120/20	120/70	+++
4. A66-54	14	F	5	LAE, RVH	58/5*	19/11	95/10	111/63	++++
Corrected transposition of the great arteries									
5. A63-142	44	F	26	$S_{1,2,3}$ QSV_1	98/41	50/34	139/24	—	—
6. UKMC A158-71	22	F	Birth	—	—	—	—	—	—
Partial atrioventricular canal									
7. A59-253	13	M	6	AF LAD, LVH	55/15	27/15	—	—	++++
Origin of left coronary artery from pulmonary trunk									
8. A56-14	9 mo.	F	8 mo.	ALMI	50/—	—	—	—	—
Parachute mitral valve									
9. A66-189	22	M	19	LBBB, LAE	54/28	30/30	96/29	96/67	++++

* Right ventricular pressure. Pulmonary artery not entered.

AF = atrial fibrillation. ALMI = anterolateral myocardial infarction. ECG = electrocardiogram. LA = left atrium. LAD = left axis deviation. LAE = left atrial enlargement. LBBB = left bundle branch block. LV = left ventricle. LVH = left ventricular hypertrophy. MR = mitral regurgitation. PA = pulmonary artery. ↑PR = interval >0.20 sec. QSV_1 = Q and S wave in lead V_1. RVH = right ventricular hypertrophy. $S_{1,2,3}$ = S wave standard leads 1, 2, and 3. SA = systemic artery. s/d = systolic/diastolic.

tally corrected transposition (CCT).[179] During life, one was believed to have rheumatic MR[180] and the second underwent mitral valve replacement shortly before death. Anamalies of the left-sided or systemic atrioventricular valves (anatomic tricuspid valve) in CCT are extremely common (about 80 per cent).[179,181] Although the usual cause of MR in these patients is an Ebstein-type malformation of the so-called mitral valve, neither of our patients with CCT had this anomaly. The mitral leaflets and chordae, however, in each were malformed. Another patient also was considered before cardiac catherization to have severe rheumatic MR, but at operation the severe MR was found to be the result of a complete cleft in the anterior mitral leaflet. Thus, this patient's condition is an example of *partial persistent atrioventricular canal* presenting as MR.[182-184] A small defect (1 cm. size) was found in the lowermost portion of the atrial septum in this patient but the amount of shunting through the defect was small. *Parachute mitral valve* (single papillary muscle) may cause massive MR (patient #8).[185,186] This anomaly most commonly, however, produces stenosis.[187] *Origin of the left coronary artery from the pulmonary trunk* may cause severe fibrosis and atrophy of one or both left ventricular papillary muscles with resulting MR. Indeed, MR may be the presenting or major clinical feature of this condition.[134,136] Another cause of congenital MR is the *arcade type deformity of the mitral valve*.[188] We have studied at necropsy one patient with this anomaly. The patient also had a patent ductus arteriosus and therefore is not included herein. Arcade mitral valve may occur, however, without associated shunts.[188,189] It is well to keep in mind that severe anatomic malformations of the mitral valve may occur without any functional consequence. An example is the double orifice mitral valve.[190]

Isolated Congenital Pure Aortic Regurgitation

Aortic regurgitation (AR) commonly occurs in patients with congenitally malformed aortic valves, particularly the bicuspid one.[3] The degree of AR, however, is usually mild unless the valve has previously been the site of infection. Of 17 necropsy patients with fatal pure AR complicating a congenitally bicuspid aortic valve, infective endocarditis was the cause of the fatal AR in 15 of them.[3,15] The congenitally unicuspid aortic valve appears never to be a cause of pure AR.[6] A quadricuspid aortic valve, an extremely rare malformation, on occasion may lead to pure AR. At least four patients with quadricuspid aortic valves and pure AR have been reported.[9] Although a unicuspid, bicuspid or quadricuspid aortic valve represents a congenital malformation, the aortic valve may be tricuspid and still congenitally malformed. In this situation, one cusp is probably smaller than the other two (see below). Usually, however, pure AR complicating a tricuspid aortic valve represents an acquired lesion.

We have studied at necropsy four patinets with fatal pure AR unassociated with infective endocarditis or shunts (Table 19). The murmur of AR was recognized in all before the age of 18 years and none had clinical or necropsy evidence of acute rheumatic fever. Two patients had bicuspid aortic valves: in one (#1), a fibrous band, extending from the margin of one cusp to the wall of ascending

Table 19. Congenital aortic regurgitation: clinical and necropsy findings

Patient	Age	Sex	Age (yrs.) murmur first heard	Murmurs "AS"	Murmurs AR	Murmurs AF	ECG	Pressures (mm. Hg) BA (s/d)	Pressures (mm. Hg) LV (s/d)	Valve replacement	No. AV cusps	AV calcium	Heart weight (gm.)
1. A66-6	27	M	17	2/6	3/6	2/6	↑PR, LVH, LAD	126/54	125/25	+	2	0	800
2. A66-233	18	M	5	3/6	3/6	2/6	LVH, LVS, LAD	122/40†	—	+*	3	0	570
3. A66-234	23	M	8	5/6	4/6	3/6	LVH	120/45	120/11	+	2	0	600
4. A68-325	51	F	17	3/6	3/6	3/6	↑PR LVH	210/80†	—	+	4	0	520

* Replacement of right coronary cusp only.
† Indirect.

AF = Austin Flint. AR = aortic regurgitation. AS = "aortic stenosis." AV = aortic valve. BA = brachial artery. ECG = electrocardiogram. LV = left ventricular. LVH = left ventricular hypertrophy. LVS = left ventricular strain. ↑PR = interval >0.20 sec. LAD = left axis deviation. s/d = systolic/diastolic.

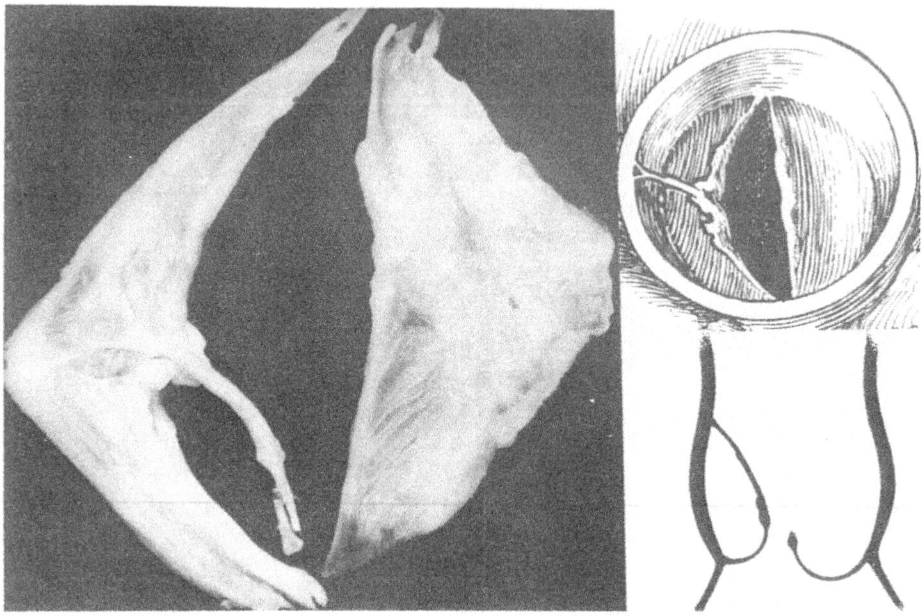

Figure 48. Congenital aortic regurgitation with bicuspid aortic valve. Surgical specimen and diagrams of the aortic valve in situ of a 27-year-old man (A66–6) who was found to have aortic regurgitation at age 17. At age 25 years, evaluation confirmed free aortic regurgitation and he underwent successful prosthetic aortic valve replacement by Dr. Andrew G. Morrow. Thirteen months postoperatively he died suddenly while playing football. Attached to the free margin in the mid-portion of one cusp is a fibrous band which inserts onto the wall of the aorta. This structure prevented closure of the valve during ventricular diastole with resultant severe aortic regurgitation.

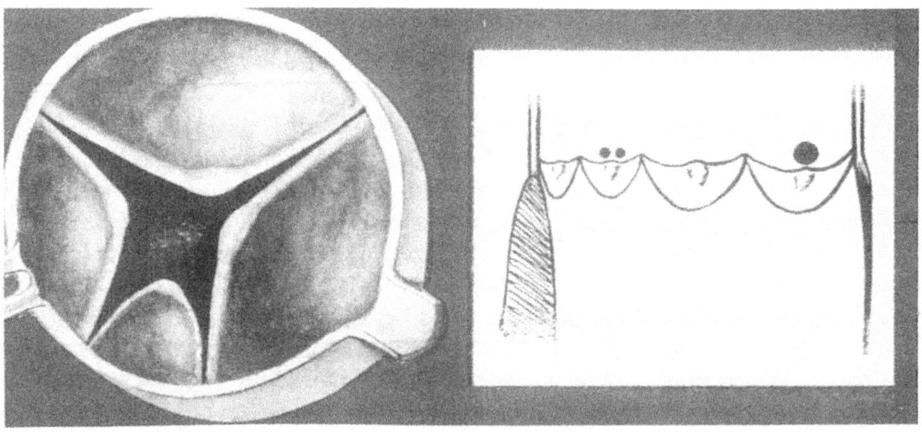

Figure 49. Congenital aortic regurgitation with quadricuspid aortic valve. Diagrams of aortic valve from above (left) and opened (right) of a 51-year-old woman (A68–325) who died shortly after aortic valve replacement. A precordial murmur had been heard at age 17 years. At age 45, she developed congestive cardiac failure and signs of free aortic regurgitation. The aortic valve had four cusps, two hypoplastic ones and two normal ones.

aorta, pulled the cusp cephalad preventing coaptation during ventricular diastole (Fig. 48); in the second (#3), the mechanism of AR is uncertain. Likewise, the mechanism of AR in the patient with a tricuspid aortic valve is uncertain. A murmur of AR had been heard in him at age five years, and a valvular operation was carried out when he was 13 years old. The patient with a quadricuspid aortic valve had two hypoplastic cusps which prevented cuspal coaptation during ventricular diastole[9] (Fig. 49).

Trauma

The heart and vessels may be injured by either blunt or penetrating trauma, and both may lead to valvular regurgitation.

Penetrating trauma results from the passage of projectiles into or through the cardiovascular structures. The speed of entry, the type of projectile, and the structures penetrated determine the kind of injury which results and the length of survival. Laceration or avulsion or both of myocardium or great vessel usually leads to rapid death from hemorrhage into the pericardial sac (cardiac tamponade) or elsewhere. Damage to the cardiac valves from penetrating trauma is rare. Of 456 fatalities from penetrating wounds of the heart and aorta compiled in 1958,[191] the valves were damaged in only a few patients and none survived longer than several days. During the past 14 years, other studies of penetrating cardiac trauma have revealed isolated patients with valvular damage and most of them died quickly.[192-195] Significant valvular regurgitation from penetrating trauma to the aortic,[196-201] mitral,[202,203] or tricuspid[203] valves has been described and recognized clinically in about 10 patients. Valve replacement or repair is necessary.

Blunt or compressive trauma, in contrast to the penetrating variety, is a more common cause of clinically apparent valvular dysfunction (Fig. 50). Since injury to the intracardiac structures may occur without damage to the myocardium or vessels, the patient is more likely to survive until signs of valvular dysfunction appear. Excessive physical effort or strain, a form of blunt trauma, commonly damages only valvular or supporting structures. Like other forms of blunt trauma, the diagnosis of valvular damage may be masked initially by cardiac contusion, pericardial effusion, or myocardial rupture.

Aortic regurgitation (AR) is the most common clinically recognized valvular lesion resulting from blunt trauma.[204] Nevertheless, it is an infrequent consequence and limited almost exclusively to men. Only two of 64 reported patients with AR from nonpenetrating trauma were women.[205,206] The AR may result from muscular strain or from some type of thoracic compression. Of 44 necropsy patients reviewed by Howard in 1928,[205] 30 had AR secondary to muscular strain. Since his review, however, only two additional patients have been described in the English literature as having AR from this mechanism.[207,208] Compressive thoracic trauma, mainly from automotive steering wheel injuries, today is by far the most common cause of valvular regurgitation from nonpenetrating trauma.[206] Although it appears to be an immediate consequence of blunt chest trauma, AR is not always clinically evident or diagnosed in the early post-trauma period, apparently because it is masked by other consequences of the trauma

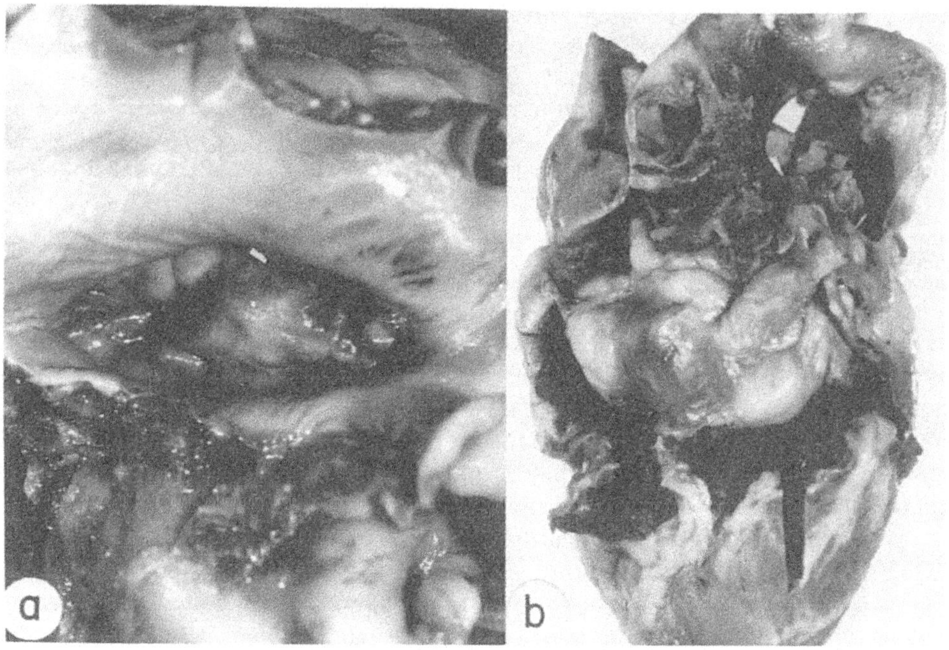

Figure 50. Mitral regurgitation from blunt trauma in a 23-year-old man (NNMC #A71–72) who died instantaneously in an airplane crash. a, Mitral valve viewed from left atrium. The anterior leaflet is flail due to rupture of papillary muscles. b, External aspect of the heart viewed anteriorly. In most cases when blunt trauma results in severe mitral regurgitation, extensive injury to myocardium and great vessels also occurs. This patient sustained an 80 per cent circumferential transmural laceration of both ventricles as well as a large tear in the ascending aorta. Thus, the prolapse of the mitral leaflet was of no consequence.

or because medical attention has not been sought. The murmur of AR may not be detected until weeks or months after the event when symptoms of cardiac dysfunction appear.[209] It has been described as cooing, whistling, buzzing, humming, or whining in character. The AR results from detachment of one or more cusps with prolapse or from tearing or fenestration of one or more cusps without detachment, or from both. Cuspal detachment, similar to that produced by trauma, however, may occur without a clear history of trauma (Fig. 51). The left anterior cusp appears to be the one most commonly involved. Valvular reconstruction or replacement is frequently required for survival.[206]

Atrioventricular valvular regurgitation from blunt trauma is even less common than AR. Of 546 patients described by Parmley et al.,[204] 39 had anatomic evidence of mitral (MR) or tricuspid regurgitation and all but one of them had associated myocardial rupture with rapid death (Fig. 50). By 1964, 18 patients with mitral valve damage due to blunt trauma had been reported in the English literature.[210] Leaflet damage appears to be the least common cause of MR and was responsible in only one patient, described by McLaughlin et al.,[210] and in one patient described subsequently.[211] Rupture of chordae tendineae due to trauma or exertion has long been implicated as a couse of MR, but it too appears to be an infrequent cause of the hemodynamic lesion. Rupture of a papillary muscle by trauma is rare. Sanders et al. in 1957 collected six cases[212] and at least two more have

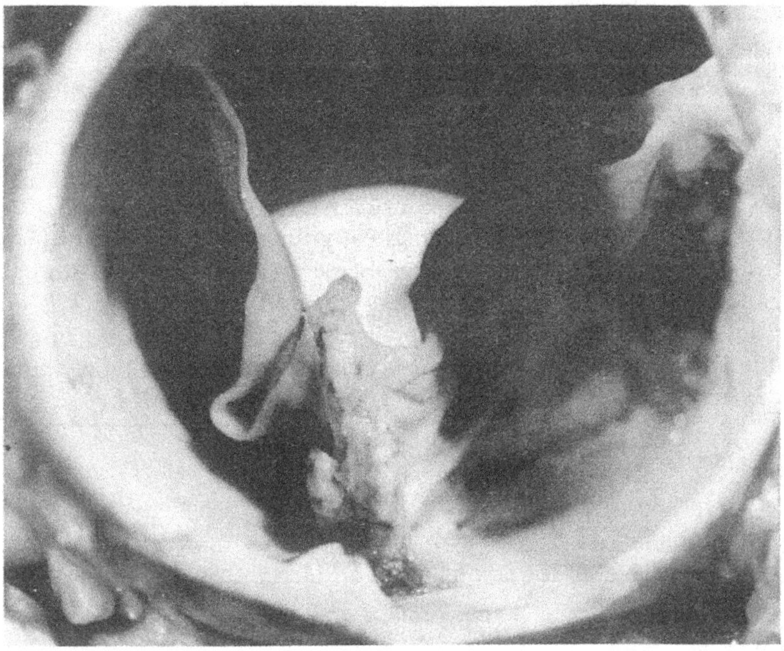

Figure 51. Possible traumatic aortic regurgitation without history of trauma in a 47-year-old man (37266) with no symptoms of cardiac dysfunction until two weeks before death when he suddenly developed fulminant congestive heart failure. Clinical signs of free aortic regurgitation were present and he was treated for infective endocarditis (despite no supporting clinical features and negative blood cultures). At necropsy, the commissure between two of the aortic cusps was torn loose from the aorta causing prolapse of these cusps into left ventricle. The tricuspid aortic valve and aorta were otherwise normal. There was no evidence of infective endocarditis.

been described subsequently.[213,214] All patients had severely compressed thoraces with fulminant pulmonary edema, shock, and rapid death.

Tricuspid regurgitation due to blunt trauma is less common than MR but better tolerated. Several patients have survived over 20 years.[215-218] Parmley et al.[204] described a five-month survivor among their 39 patients with traumatic atrioventricular valve incompetence, and he had a ruptured right ventricular papillary muscle. Associated myocardial rupture is infrequent in trauma-indiced tricus-

Table 20. Systemic lupus erythematosus (SLE): clinical and necropsy data in 26 patients

	No. pts.	*Ages (years) Range (avg.)*	*F*	*M*	*Age onset symptoms SLE range (avg.) (years)*	*Duration (yrs.) of symptoms range (avg.)*	*CHF*	*Renal failure*	*HT*
1. With L-E endocarditis	12	17-61 (30)	11	1	14-61 (26)	1-9 (4)	6	8	10
2. Without L-E endocarditis	14	8-55 (31)	13	1	7-55 (29)	0.5-7 (2)	2	10	9
TOTALS	26	8-61 (31)	24	2	7-61 (28)	0.5-9 (3)	8	18	19

* Purulent in one and granulomatous in one.
AV = aortic valve. CHF = congestive heart failure. HT = hypertension. L-E = lupus-erythematosus. MV = mitral valve.

pid regurgitation and was present in only one of 26 patients previously reported.[219] Symptoms often appeared within days of violent chest trauma but were usually mild. When evaluated weeks to years later because of progressive clinical decompensation, signs of florid tricuspid regurgitation were invariably present. The proper clinical diagnosis was occasionally confused by associated lesions such as traumatic ventricular septal defect, traumatic constrictive pericarditis (secondary to longstanding hemopericardium), and congenital atrial septal defect.[219,220] One patient was followed clinically for many years with the diagnosis of Ebstein's anomaly.[216] The incompetence in 21 patients in whom anatomic data was available resulted primarily from ruptured chordae tendineae and papillary muscles, but six of them also sustained a laceration or avulsion of one or more valve leaflets. Of the 26 patients, 15 underwent tricuspid valvular repair or replacement.[215-221]

Systemic Lupus Erythematosus

Congestive heart failure and systemic hypertension (usually of renal origin) are the predominant cardiovascular consequences of systemic lupus erythematosus (SLE). Valvular lesions also are frequent and often unique but rarely of functional significance.

We have studied at necropsy 26 patients with SLE, and 12 (46 per cent) had valvular lesions consistent with atypical verrucous endocarditis (Table 20). There were no significant differences in age, sex, duration of illness, presence of precordial murmurs, or presence of systemic hypertension between patients with and without SLE endocarditis. All but two had received steroid therapy. Seven of 12 Libman-Sacks (L-S) endocarditis had diffuse fibrinous pericarditis, and only two of 14 without L-S endocarditis had pericarditis and in them it was due to infection. Mitral valvular lesions were present in 12 patients (Figs. 52, 53), one of whom also had aortic valvular verrucae. Only one of the 12 patients had clinical evidence of valvular dysfunction. The pulmonic and tricuspid valves were normal in all 12 patients. The involved leaflets were thickened to some degree by vascularized fibrous tissue in all 12 patients. The mural endocardium beneath the involved leaflets was similarly involved in most patients. In addition, seven patients had valvular lesions variously described in the past as "raised or flat, dry or wet, granular or smooth, single or conglomerate, yellow or gray, tawny or pink, pinhead to 4 mm. in size, shaped like beads or pyramids,

Table 20. (Continued)

Precordial murmur	*Steroid therapy*	*Heart weight (gm.) range (avg.)*	*Valvular involvement MV*	*AV*	*Diffuse pericarditis*	*Hematoxylin bodies in heart*	*Valve leaflet fibrin and/or necrosis*	*Leaflet or mural endocardial fibrous thickening*
6	11	270-600 (385)	12	1	7	7	10	12
7	13	180-400 (306)	0	0	2*	0	0	0
13	24	180-600 (343)	12	1	9	7	10	12

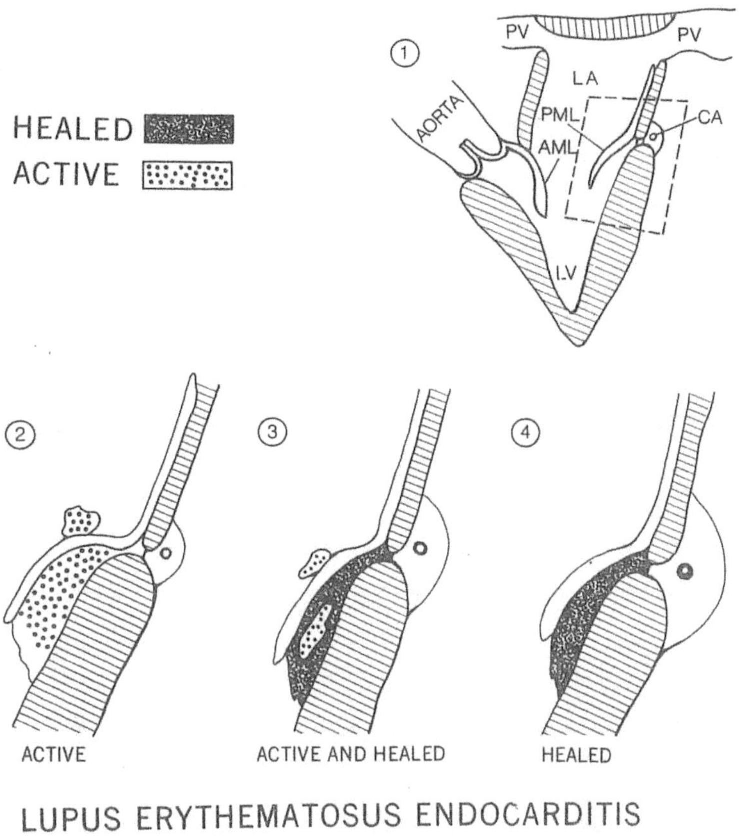

Figure 52. Lupus erythematosus (LE) endocarditis. 2, Active lesions of LE endocarditis, or verrucae, are accumulations of fibrin and cellular debris and project from either surface of the valve leaflet. When located on the atrial surface they usually appear like polyps or vegetations, but when located on the under surface of the leaflet they become adherent to leaflet and mural endocardium and may go unnoticed. 3, As the process heals fibrous tissue appears and it may lead to shortening and thickening of leaflet and chordae. 4, Healed LE endocarditis with fibrous scarring of valve and no evidence of the earlier active process. This complete healing may be a consequence of steroid therapy. The amount of adipose tissue in the atrioventricular sulcus progressively increases, and the lumens of the coronary arteries may become narrowed by atherosclerosis. PV = pulmonic veins. LA = left atrium. LV = left ventricle. CA = coronary artery. AML = anterior mitral leaflet. PML = posterior mitral leaflet.

arranged in mulberry-like clusters or in trails.''[222-224] These lesions considered active and represent the verrucae of classic L-S endocarditis. They may be located on either side of a valvular cusp but most frequently are found on the under or ventricular surface of the posterior mitral leaflet or in the valve ring and they infrequently involve the anterior mitral leaflet.

Histologically, the verrucae consist of fibrin partially surrounded by varying quantities of cellular and vascularized fibrous tissue. In seven patients, hematoxylin bodies were present. The fibrin usually appeared to be organizing into fibrous tissue which was continuous with the involved leaflet and usually with the mural endocardium. As the process "heals," fibrous scarring of the undersurface of the posterior mitral leaflet and of the chordae may shorten and thicken these

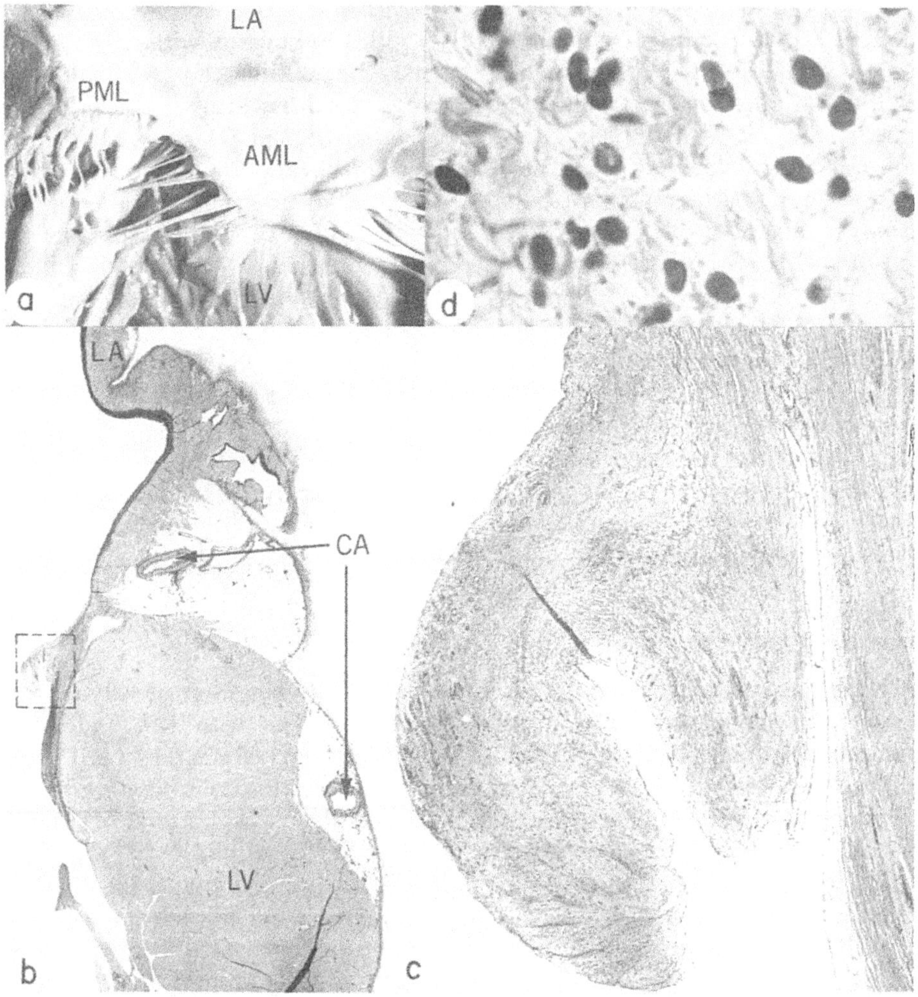

Figure 53. Active and healed lupus erythematosus (LE) endocarditis. This 22-year-old woman (A61–294), who had systemic LE for four years, died of renal failure. She had received steroids for three years. At necropsy, she had a diffuse fibrous pericarditis. a, Her mitral valve was thickened and the under surface of the posterior mitral leaflet (PML) was adherent to left ventricular (LV) mural endocardium. AML = anterior mitral leaflet. LA = left atrium. b, Longitudinal section through left atrium (LA), posterior mitral leaflet, and left ventricle (LV) demonstrating a thickened, contracted leaflet and thickening of the mural endocardium beneath it. c, Photomicrograph of the posterior mitral leaflet shown (----) in b. There is proliferation of vascularized fibrous tissue. Here "active" inflammatory changes are present in the leaflet. d, Numerous hematoxylin bodies were present within the loose posterior mitral leaflet. These bodies are pathognomonic of SLE. b, Elastic tissue stain. c and d, Hematoxylin-eosin stains. [Reduced 25 per cent from × 3.2 (b), × 37 (c), and × 690 (d).]

structures and in one patient this process was severe enough to cause clinically apparent mitral regurgitation. In addition, this same patient had active lesions, including verrucae on two valves and extensive necrosis of the base of the posterior mitral leaflet.

Although Libman-Sacks (L-S) endocarditis, probably better termed lupus erythematosus (LE) endocarditis, is a frequent anatomic finding in SLE, clinically detectable valvular dysfunction in these patients is rare. Moreover, precordial murmurs are detected as frequently (50 per cent) in patients without as in those with endocarditis.[225-227] Steroid therapy may be altering the morphology and location and possibly the frequency of LE endocarditis. Early reports described endocarditis in 33 to 65 per cent of patients with SLE.[228,229] More recent studies[230,231] involving steroid-treated lupus patients reported endocarditis in 13 to 50 per cent; 46 per cent of our 26 patients had endocarditis and only two had not received steroids. An equal frequency of involvement of valves on both sides of the heart in patients with SLE was stressed in early writings.[222-224] In contrast, none of our patients had right-sided valvular lesions and of the 12 with valvular lesions, the mitral valve was involved in each. Others have found a similar preponderance of mitral involvement by LE endocarditis.[230-232] The valvular lesions of SLE also appear to be smaller and fewer in number in the steroid-treated compared to nonsteroid-treated patients. Gross[223] described extensive multivalvular involvement and frequent necrosis of valvular tissue in many of his 23 necropsy patients. In contrast to his findings, the endocarditis in our patients was more limited, and healed lesions were more frequent than active ones.

Rheumatoid Arthritis

Rheumatoid arthritis (RS) is associated with a unique form of valvular heart disease. We have studied at necropsy three patients with RA and cardiac rheumatoid nodules (Table 21). Each had had symptoms of RA for over 15 years. Each had had pansystolic precordial murmurs and one, a diastolic blowing murmur. One patient had left a bundle branch block and another, a prolonged P–R interval. Only one patient had congestive heart failure, and it was mild.

At necropsy, their hearts weighed 260, 350, and 550 gm. respectively. In each, the pericardial space was diffusely obliterated by fibrous adhesions. In two patients, numerous rheumatoid nodules were present in all four cardiac valves (Fig. 54), in membranous ventricular septum, in myocardium of both ventricles, in endocardium of both atria, and in pericardium. In the third patient, rheumatoid nodules were present only in mitral valve and in left ventricular myocardium immediately beneath the posterior leaflet (Fig. 55). The rheumatoid nodules were histologically similar to those classically seen in subcutaneous tissue.

In all three patients the mitral valves were thickened, and the normal cuspal tissue was replaced by rheumatoid nodules. With one exception, the rheumatoid nodules were located *within* the valve leaflets and were enclosed by a border of fibrous tissue. In one patient, however, the nodule had erupted with extrusion of its central necrotic material. The involved aortic valves (two patients) were

Table 21. Rheumatoid arthritis: clinical and necropsy findings

	Age (yrs.)	*Sex*	*Age (yrs.) at onset of arthritis*	*Duration (yrs.) of arthritis*	*CHF*	*Precordial murmur*		*Heart weight (gm.)*	*Location, rheumatoid nodules*		
						Systolic	*Diastolic*		*Pericardium*	*Myocardium*	*Valves*
1. A66-100	65	F	50	15	+	+	+	550	+	+	MV, AV, TV, PV
2. A67-1	72	M	36	36	0	+	0	350	+	+	MV, AV TV, PV
3. A69-19	67	F	27	40	0	+	0	260	0	+	MV

AV = aortic valve. CHF = congestive heart failure. MV = mitral valve. PV = pulmonic valve. TV = tricuspid valve.

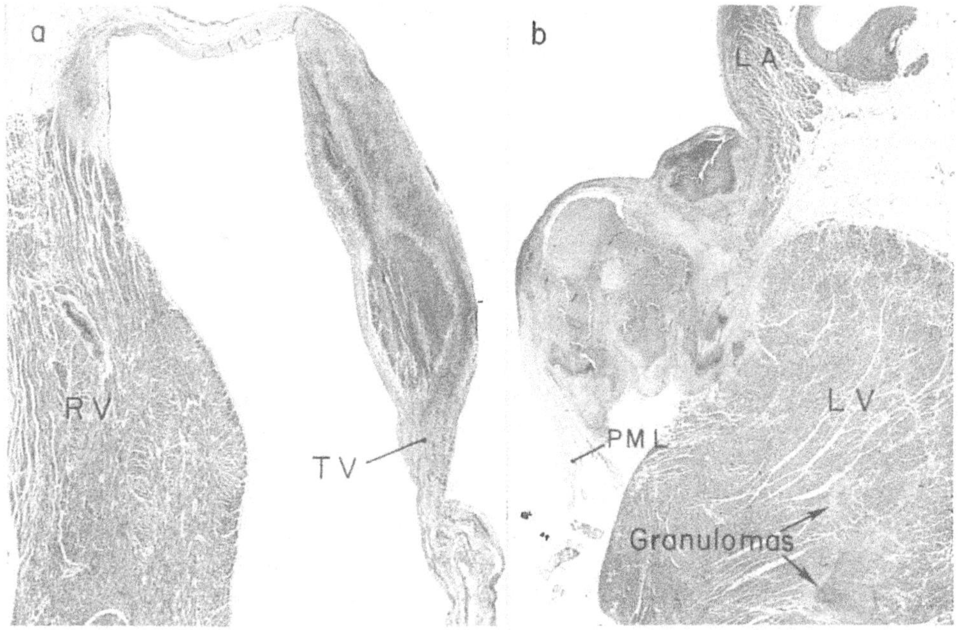

Figure 54. Valvular lesions of rheumatoid arthritis. This 72-year-old man (A67–1) had rheumatoid arthritis for 36 years. He had a grade 1/6 systolic precordial murmur for several years but no signs of cardiac dysfunction, despite extensive involvement of pericardium, myocardium, and endocardium by rheumatoid nodules. a, Tricuspid valve (TV) leaflet showing a typical rheumatoid granuloma within the substance of the leaflet. RV = right ventricle. b, A large rheumatoid granuloma within posterior mitral leaflet (PML). A smaller nodule involves endocardium of left atrium (LA) as well. Arrows indicate rheumatoid granulomas within left ventricular (LV) wall. a and b, Hematoxylin-eosin stain. [Reduced 30 per cent from × 12 (a) and × 6.5 (b).]

similarly thickened by numerous rheumatoid nodules. In the two patients with right-sided valvular lesions, the nodules were localized to the basal attachments of tricuspid and pulmonic valve cusps with little disruption of the normal valve structure.

Although nonspecific forms of pericarditis, myocarditis, and coronary arthritis have been observed at necropsy in patients with rheumatoid arthritis (RA),[233-236] rheumatoid nodules (granulomas) similar to subcutaneous nodules are pathognomonic and occur in the heart in 1 to 3 per cent of necropsied patients with this condition.[237] At least 24 patients with rheumatoid granulomas involving cardiac valves or valvular rings have been reported[235] (Table 22). Nine of the 24 patients had auscultatory evidence of mitral or aortic regurgitation or both, and 11 had hearts weighing more than 300 gm. Most frequently, the valvular lesions were focal. In two of our three patients the mitral and aortic valvular lesions were diffuse and the valves incompetent. Although coronary arterial narrowing is frequent, cardiac dysfunction in RA often can be explained on the basis of valvular cardiac disease.

Although rheumatoid nodules in hearts of patients with RA have been well described, little attention has been given to the exact location of these lesions

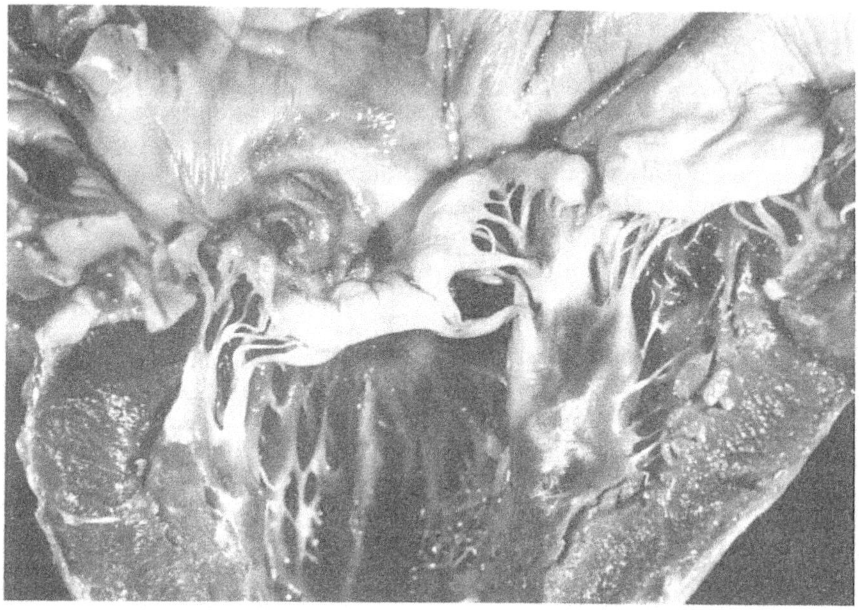

Figure 55. Erupted rheumatoid nodule of mitral valve. This 67-year-old woman (A69–19) had rheumatoid arthritis for 47 years. She had a grade 2/6 systolic murmur but no symptoms of cardiac dysfunction. Shown here is the opened mitral valve. A large rheumatoid nodule, which has erupted, is present in the anterior leaflet. The valve is probably mildly incompetent.

Table 22. Rheumatoid nodules in cardiac valves

Mitral	19	
Aortic	11	
Tricuspid	5	
Pulmonic	4	
	39	of possible 96 valves involved in 24 necropsy patients

in the valve leaflets and rings. The location and size of the cardiac rheumatoid nodules were similar in two of our three patients. The lesions grossly were yellow, firm, smooth, and focal or diffuse. On the tricuspid valve the lesions were focal and located at the basal attachment of the septal and anterior leaflets. The posterior tricuspid leaflets were uninvolved. A single nodule was present at the basal attachment of a pulmonic valvular cusp in both patients with extensive lesions. These right-sided cardiac lesions did not interfere with valvular function because most of the valvular tissue was uninvolved. In contrast to the right-sided lesions in the two patients, those on left-sided cardiac valves were diffuse; nearly all areas of both mitral and aortic leaflets were thickened.

Histologically, the lesions were located within the valve leaflets leaving a border of fibrous tissue to enclose the necrotic material. This fibrous capsule probably represents the original and uninvolved valve tissue. Thus, the process appears to begin as a reaction within the core or central portion of the valve leaflet preserving peripheral portions. The valvular involvement in rheumatoid heart disease is in direct contrast to that of carcinoid heart disease, in which the valve itself remains normal and atypical fibrous tissue is deposited on the surface of the valvular cusp. Also, it differs from rheumatic valvular disease in which the entire leaflet, both its central and peripheral portions, is involved, often leaving no residual normal or near-normal valvular tissue. Cardiovascular differences between rheumatoid arthritis, syphilis, ankylosing spondylitis, and the Marfan syndrome are summarized in Table 23.

Table 23. Cardiovascular manifestations of conditions causing aortic regurgitation

	Syphilis	*Ankylosing Spondylitis*	*Rheumatoid arthritis*	*Marfan*
Avg. age	50	45	70	30
Sex	Men	Men	Women	Men
Aortic regurgitation	++++	++++	+	++++
Mitral regurgitation	0	++	+	+++
Conduction disturbances	+	++++	++	+
Serology (STS)	+	0	0	0
Morphology of aorta				
Thickened adventitia	++++	++++	+	+
Degenerated media	+++	+++	0	++++
Intimal proliferation	+++	+++	0	+
Vasa vasora abnormal	++++	++++	0	0
Calcium	++	+	0	0
Aneurysms	+++	0	0	+++
Rupture	+	0	0	+
Dissection	0	0	0	+
Limited to sinuses	0	+	0	0
Morphology of aortic valve				
Cuspal thickening				
Diffuse	0	+	0	0
Focal	+	0	+	+
Cuspal calcification	0	0	0	0
↑AMP	0	0	0	+
Shortening	0	+	0	0
Commissural abnormality	+	+	0	0

The reason the cardiac valves are involved at all in RA is unclear. If vasculitis is considered to be an intrinsic part of the development of the subcutaneous nodules, as proposed by Sokoloff et al.,[238] then involvement of valvular blood vessels must occur. The cardiac valves, however, contain few blood vessels. Certainly, if vasculitis predisposes to the development of rheumatoid granulomas, these lesions might be expected to be much more frequent in the myocardium than in the endocardium (valves), although this is not the situation.

Endomyocardial Disease with and without Eosinophilia

In 1936 Löffler described two patients with "fibroplastic parietal endocarditis with blood eosinophilia."[239] Since then about 100 patients with this condition have been reported, some under the heading "eosinophilic leukemia."[139,140,142] These conditions are characterized by endocardial fibrosis of one or both ventricles, blood eosinophilia, and usually mitral regurgitation. Death characteristically results from congestive cardiac failure.

The endocardial thickening is located primarily in the inflow tracts of the ventricles. It appears to begin in the apices and progresses retrogradely to involve the endocardium beneath the posterior mitral leaflet and occasionally to involve that behind the posterior or septal tricuspid valve leaflet. Superimposed on the fibrotic mural endocardium is fibrin thrombus. The posterior mitral leaflet may adhere to the underlying mural endocardium and lead to mitral regurgitation. A similar process may cause tricuspid regurgitation. The left ventricular cavity may be prevented from expanding adequately during ventricular diastole by the thickened mural endocardium and the cavity may be considerably decreased in size by thrombus.

We have studied at necropsy six patients, all men, aged 25 to 52 years, with endomyocardial disease and eosinophilia.[139,140,142] Each had symptoms from 11 to 42 months (avg. 24). The highest leukocyte counts ranged from 79,000

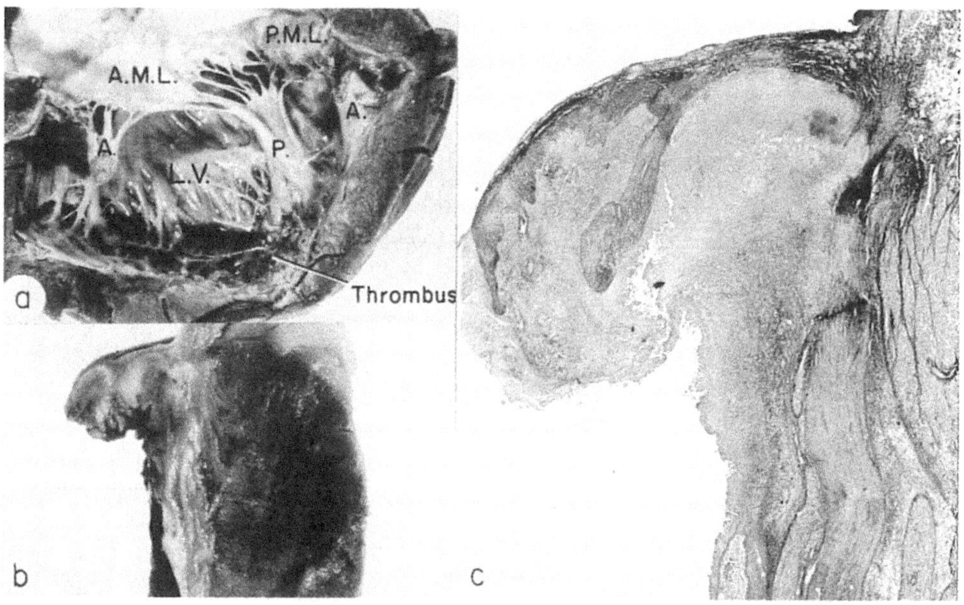

Figure 56. Löffler's fibroplastic parietal endocarditis with thickening of the mitral valve and papillary muscle fibrosis. This 35-year-old man (A65–211) had been well until 12 months before death when recurring headaches, weakness, weight loss, and anorexia appeared and he sought his physician. He was found to have leukocytosis with 70 per cent eosinophils on differential smear. Precordial examination showed no murmur. He died of congestive cardiac failure with chronic eosinophilia and hepatosplenomegaly. At necropsy, the heart weighed 430 gm. and the coronary arteries were clean. Both left ventricular papillary muscles were extensively scarred and mural thrombi were present at the apices of both ventricles. a, Opened left ventricle (L.V.) and mitral valve. Both posteromedial (P.) and anterolateral (A.) papillary muscles are severely scarred and the endocardium covering them is thckened. Much organizing fibrous tissue is present behind the posterior mitral leaflet (P.M.L.). A.M.L. = anterior mitral leaflet. b, Longitudinal section including posterior mitral leaflet and left ventricular well. c, Photomicrograph of posterior mitral leaflet seen in b. The thickening is due to vascularized fibrous tissue located entirely on the ventricular aspect of the cusp and on the mural endocardium. The leaflet is made immobile by its adherence to the underlying mural endocardium.

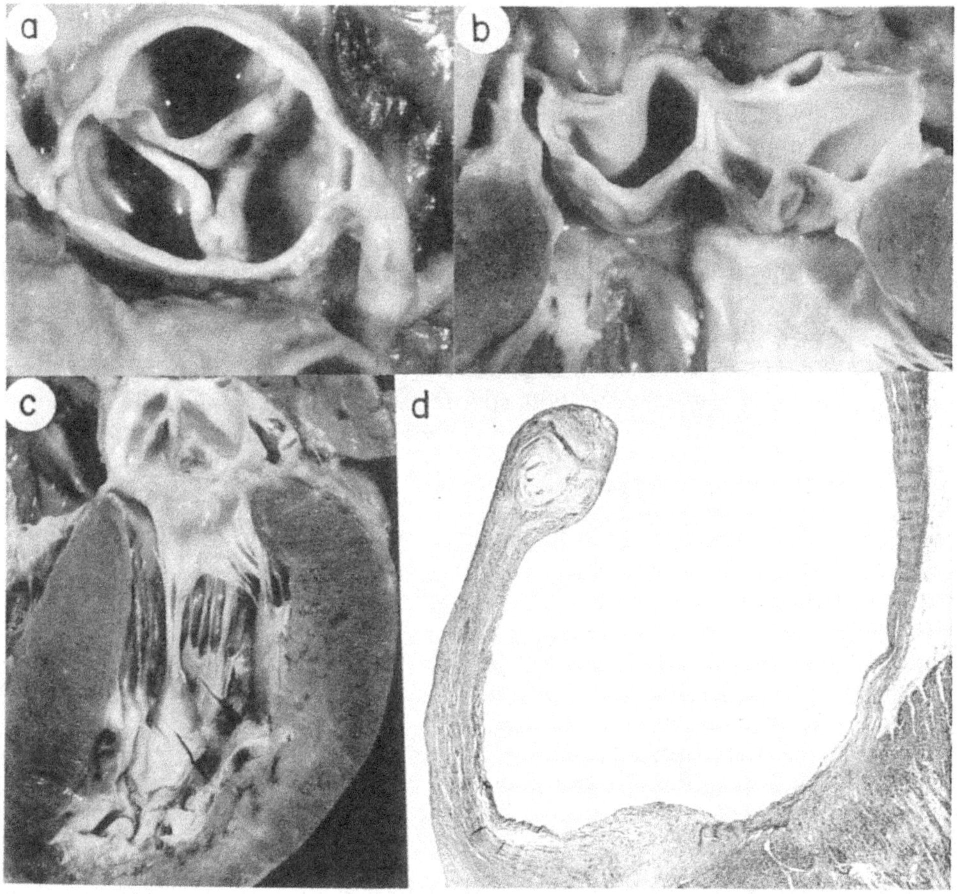

Figure 57. Löffler's fibroplastic parietal endocarditis (LFPE) associated with valvular aortic stenosis. It is well known that patients with LFPE may have mitral regurgitation secondary to extensive thickening of mural endocardium with superimposed thrombosis in the left ventricular inflow tract. That aortic valvular disease can be a part of LFPE is uncertain but highly suggestive from the case shown here. This 46-year-old man (A71–250) had been well until 42 months before death when fatigue and headache were noted and he was found to have eosinophilia (70 per cent). During the next 40 months his white count ranged from 40,000 to 60,000 per cu. mm. and the per cent of eosinophils from 70 to 90. When examined initially no precordial murmur was audible but when examined 22 months before death a grade 2/6 systolic ejection murmur and a grade 1/6 diastolic blowing murmur were audible over the cardiac base and along the left sternal border. Electrocardiogram showed left ventricular hypertrophy and strain and left atrial abnormality. By seven months before death, the precordial systolic murmur had increased to grade 4/6 intensity and the diastolic murmur, to grade 3/6 intensity. He died of progressive congestive cardiac failure. At necropsy, the heart weighed 520 gm. Each of the three valve cusps were thickened and two of the commissures were fused. a, Aortic valve from above. b, Opened aortic valve showing one fused commissure. The adherence of the commissures was produced by thrombus formation on the ventricular aspects of the cusps adjacent to the commissures. d, Photomicrograph of a portion of one aortic valve cusp. The cuspal thickening resulted from fibrous proliferation. Close-up disclosed that the underlying cusp was normal and that the thickening resulted from superimposition of vascularized fibrous tissue on the ventricular aspects of the cusps. c, Left ventricle and aortic valve showing severe endocardial thickening in apical one third of the chamber. The mitral valve is normal. d, Hematoxylin-eosin stain. [Reduced 15 per cent from × 7 (d).]

to 108,000 per cu. mm. and the highest percentage of eosinophils on differential smear of peripheral blood, from 35 to 90 per cent. Although greatly increased in number, the eosinophils appeared structurally normal in each patient. All six patients had overt right-sided and left-sided congestive cardiac failure, which was the dominant clinical feature in each patient, and the major cause of death. Four had precordial murmurs; in three they were consistent with mitral regurgitation and in one, murmurs of aortic stenosis and regurgitation were present. At necropsy, the hearts weighed 420 to 530 gm. (avg. 472). All four cardiac chambers were mildly dilated and the walls of all four chambers were mildly thickened. In each patient, the endocardium in left ventricular inflow tract and apex was thickened by dense fibrous tissue, devoid of elastic fibrils, and overlain by fibrin-platelet-leukocyte-erythrocyte thrombi. Right ventricular apical endocardial scars were present in every patient, with superimposed mural thrombi in two. Left ventricular subendocardial scarring occurred in all six patients. Eosinophilic leukocytes, usually few in number, were found in sections of heart. The mitral regurgitation in three patients appeared to result from the adherence of the posterior mitral leaflets to the underlying mural endocardium (Fig. 56). The aortic valve cusps in the patient with clinical evidence of aortic stenosis and regurgitation were thickened by vascularized fibrous tissue which was superimposed on the ventricular aspects of each of the three cusps (Fig. 57) in a manner directly opposite that causing leaflet thickening in patients with carcinoid heart disease. In addition, two of the three commissures were fused by a fibrin-platelet process similar to that of the mural thrombosis in the left ventricular cavity.

Endomycardial fibrosis (EMF) without eosinophilia (less than 15 per cent) has been observed in the African and their hearts are similar in many respects to those observed in Löffler's fibroplastic parietal endocarditis. One of us (W.C.R.) has examined the hearts of 16 patients with fatal EMF and cardiac dysfunction. Their ages ranged from 3 to 50 years (avg. 27); 11 were males and 5 females. Cardiac symptoms were present from 2 weeks to 24 months (avg. 7 months).

At necropsy, the hearts weighed 370 to 500 gm. Endocardial fibrous tissue devoid of elastic fibers was present in the left ventricle in all patients, and in 14 it was severe. Right ventricular endocardial fibrosis was present in 13. The endocardial fibrosis was located almost exclusively in the ventricular inflow tracts, and frequently beneath the posterior mitral or posterior and septal tricuspid valve leaflets. When the endocardial scars were small, they were usually limited to the ventricular apices. The configuration of the heart, i.e., the size of the various cardiac chambers and of the pulmonary trunk, depend primarily on which ventricle contained the largest deposits of endocardial scar tissue or superimposed thrombi or both. When the amount of endocardial plaquing was severe in the left ventricle and absent, mild, or moderate in the right ventricle, the heart usually had the appearance of a mitral stenotic heart, i.e., the left atrium, pulmonary trunk, right ventricle, and right atrium were dilated; the left ventricular cavity was small, being constricted by the extensive endocardial scarring. The left ventricle in this situation appears to be noncompliant and acts to some extent as an impediment to flow. The mitral lesion in this circumstance, however, is not stenotic unless another disease, i.e., rheumatic, coexists, but the mitral orifice in EMF is frequently made incompetent by the mural endocardial fibrosis which adheres to the undersurface of the posterior mitral leaflet causing the latter to be immobile. When the right ventricular endocardial scarring is more severe than that in the left ventricle, the right ventricle acts as an impediment to flow. The right atrium dilates, at times even to giant proportions (as it did in one of the 16 patients), the right ventricle is usually constricted, and the left atrium and left ventricle remain more or less normal in size. This type of heart may be viewed as the tricuspid incompetent one. When the amount of endocardial plaquing is similar in both ventricles, each atrium becomes quite dilated and the ventricular cavities usually remain small or at least not dilated.

Although it is usually confined to the inflow tract, the ventricular endocardial fibrosis in EMF on rare occasion may extend into the left ventricular outflow tract as it did in one of the 16 patients, and it also may be present in the atria. Also, in one patient both atria contained large endocardial plaques. Infective endocarditis may complicate EMF; three of the 16 patients had superimposed bacterial endocarditis of the mitral valve causing rupture of several chordae tendineae in each patient.

Radiation

Irradiation may produce several morphologic changes in the heart; the most frequent is thickening of parietal and visceral paricardia with or without development of pericardial effusion or tamponade. The second most frequent change reported has been interstital and perivascular myocardial fibrosis of varying degrees. Although mural endocardial thickening has been described from irradiation, cardiac valvular lesions produced by this means have not been described. We have studied 11 necropsy patients who received large doses of radiation to the chest and at necropsy each had lesions involving one or more cardiac valves. All 11 had lymphomas. Only two had clinical evidence of cardiac dysfunction and each had constrictive pericarditis.[145] No patient had evidence of cardiac dysfunction from valvular lesions. Precordial murmurs were recorded in five patients; one had right ventricular outflow tract obstruction secondary to tumor;[145] in the other four patients the cause of the precordial murmurs (grade 1/6 to 2/6) is uncertain. Four had pericardial friction rubs. The number of rads received to mediastinum in the 11 patients ranged from 3,000 to 6,000 (average 4,400). The time interval from completion of irradiation to death ranged from one to eight years (avg. three).

Abnormally large collections of serous fluid were present in the body cavities of all patients. Five had pericardial effusions (100 to 375 ml.) and four had obliterated pericardial sacs from fibrous adhesions. Seven patients had focal or diffuse fibrinous or fibrofibrinous pericarditis. The hearts in the 11 patients weighed 170 to 290 gm. (avg. 220). The right ventricular mural endocardium was focally thickened in all 11 patients. The tricuspid and mitral valve leaflets and chordae tendineae were focally thickened in all 11 patients, the aortic valve in eight, and the pulmonic valve in one (Fig. 58). The extramural coronary arteries in all 11 patients were normal.

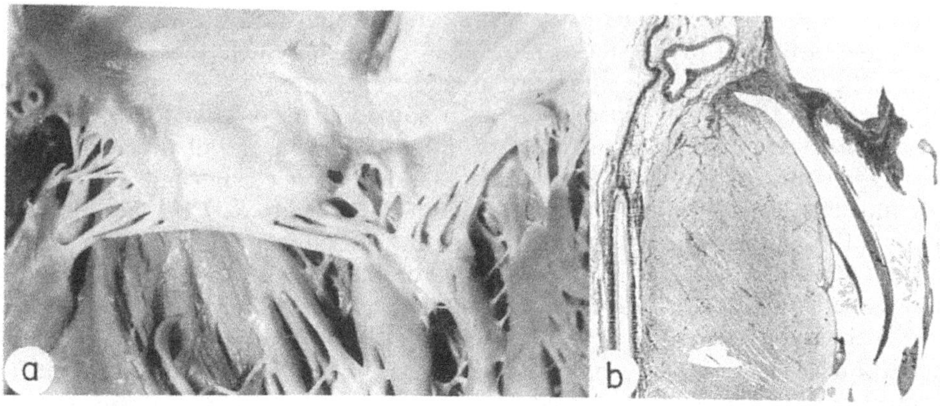

Figure 58. Radiation-induced valvular heart disease. This 29-year-old woman (A71–141) with Hodgkin's disease for four years received total body irradiation including 5335 rads to the anterior chest. A grade 1/6 systolic precordial murmur consistent with mitral regurgitation was audible. At necropsy, the pericardial sac was obliterated by fibrous adhesions. The tricuspid, mitral, and aortic valvular cusps were focally scarred and the mural endocardium of both ventricles was thickened. The myocardium appeared normal. a, Opened mitral valve showing fibrous thickening of the anterior leaflet and of its attached chordae. b, Longitudinal section of thickened posterior mitral leaflet with adjacent left atrial and left ventricular walls. b, Elastic van Gieson stain. [Reduced 20 per cent from × 3.5 (b).]

The valvular lesions in the 11 patients described almost certainly were the consequence of irradiation. All patients were relatively young, none had histories of acute rheumatic fever or infective endocarditis or other types of known valvular disease. The distribution of the lesions also was peculiar in that they involved mainly the tricuspid and mitral valves and the lesions were about as severe on the tricuspid as on the mitral valve. The valvular thickenings were focal: the anterior tricuspid leaflet and anterior mitral leaflet always were more involved than the posteriorly-located leaflets. In no patient were the valvular lesions extensive enough to cause dysfunction of the valve.

Idiopathic

Although a reasonable explanation for valvular dysfunction can usually be provided by necropsy examination of the heart and great arteries, the latter examination on occasion may fail to be enlightening in patients known to have varying degrees of valvular dysfunction during life. Such was the case in the patient described in Figure 59.[240] Mild degrees of aortic regurgitation in the elderly occasionally may be difficult at times to attribute to aortic root dilatation alone. Patients with systemic hypertension may have whiffs of aortic regurgitation, and at necropsy the aortic valve and aorta may be normal. An anatomic explanation of tricuspid regurgitation is often lacking.

SUMMARY

This review has focused on nonrheumatic causes of valvular cardiac disease. A quick survey of the structural alterations observed in a few of these conditions is shown in Figure 60. It appears clear that there are relatively few causes of

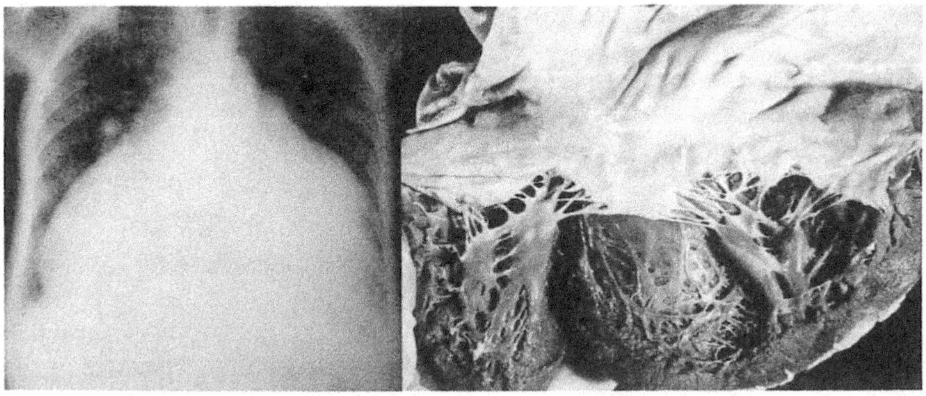

Figure 59. Mitral regurgitation of unknown etiology. This 60-year-old woman (A66–95) had been known to have congestive cardiac failure since age 34. She never had an illness consistent with or diagnostic of acute rheumatic fever or of infective endocarditis. A precordial murmur consistent with mitral regurgitation was heard when she was 43 years old, and her heart was shown enlarged by chest roentgenogram at this time. Thyrotoxicosis was diagnosed and treated at age 50. Although elevated blood pressures (180/105 mm. Hg) had been recorded during her 40s, the pressures were normal during her 50s. The congestive heart failure became severe during her last five years and the pansystolic murmur increased in intensity (to grade 4/6) and a murmur of tricuspid regurgitation also appeared. She was in atrial fibrillation for 26 years. The chest roentgenogram shown here was taken when she was 60 years old. At necropsy, the cause of the mitral regurgitation was not determined. The opened mitral valve (right) shows very pliable, only minimally thickened leaflets and the chordae are not thickened. The left atrium was enormously dilated. The papillary muscles and free wall myocardium are free of foci of fibrosis or necrosis. The mitral annulus is dilated but this in itself does not appear adequate to explain the severe mitral regurgitation. Thus, mitral regurgitation may be present clinically for years and necropsy may fail to provide an explanation for the valvular dysfunction.

valvular stenosis. When a rheumatic etiology is eliminated, most valvular stenotic lesions are congenital in origin, or, in the case of the aortic valve, the result of wear and tear of aging. In contrast to the relatively few causes of valvular stenosis, there are numerous causes and conditions associated with pure valvular regurgitation. Therefore, it is useful to separate valve dysfunction not into predominately stenotic or predominately incompetent lesions, but into purely incompetent lesions and those with elements of stenosis. Purely incompetent valvular lesions may be further divided into those which affect the ascending aorta and into those in which the aorta is normal. The latter primarily are the conditions causing pure mitral regurgitation and the former, the conditions causing aortic regurgitation.

The puzzle of valvular heart disease is beginning to be put together from a morphologic standpoint, but the end of the road is a long way from the beginning and there are many roadblocks and detours along the way.

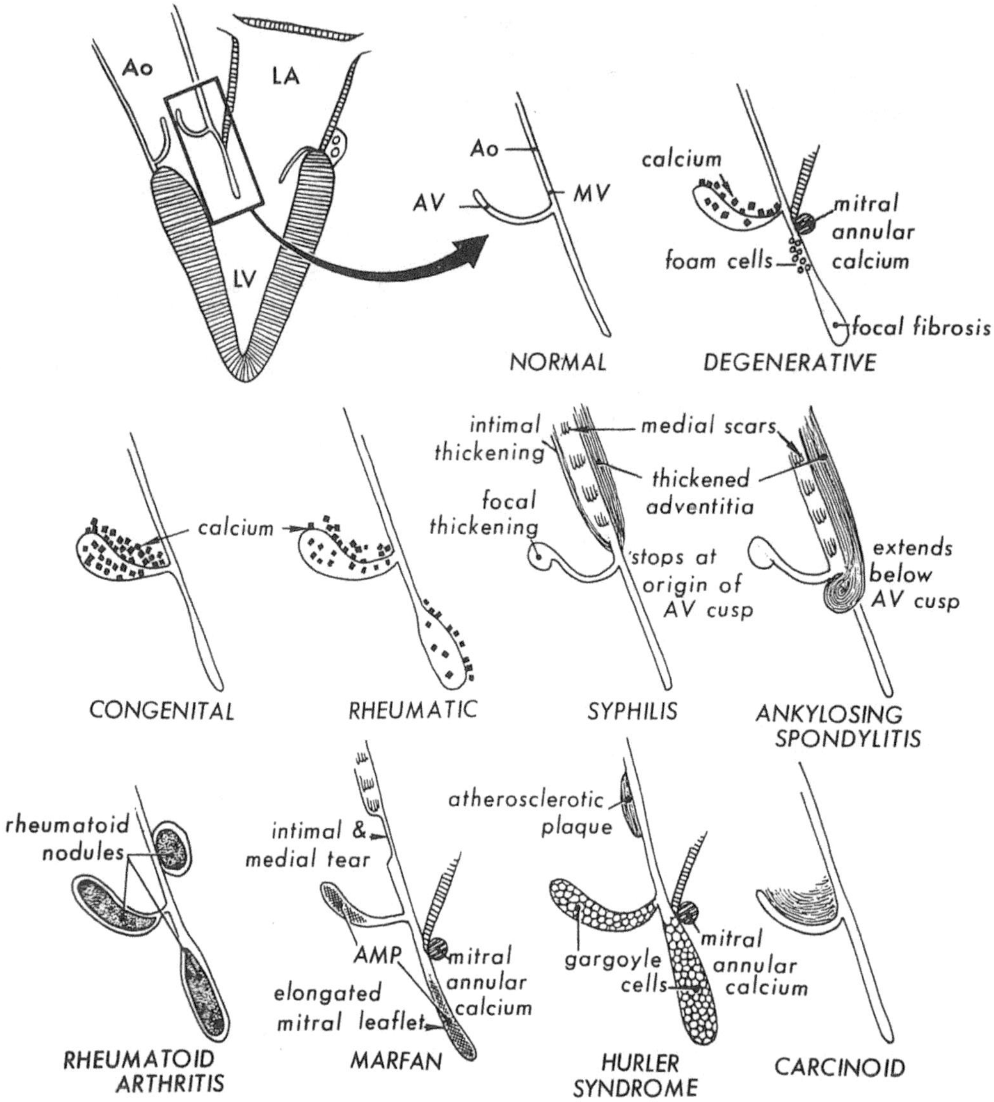

Figure 60. Diagrammatic portrayal of some of the conditions affecting the mitral and aortic valve leaflets. Degenerative, congenital, and rheumatic conditions frequently are associated with some degree of valvular stenosis. Syphilis never affects the mitral leaflets but ankylosing spondylitis extends below the aortic valve and may even lead to some mitral regurgitation. Rheumatoid arthritis, floppy valves with or without the Marfan syndrome, and the Hurler syndrome produce purely incompetent lesions. Carcinoid usually affects, or more severely affects, the right-sided cardiac valves but carcinoid plaques also have been observed on the mitral and aortic leaflets. Ao = aorta. LV = left ventricle. LA = left atrium. AV = aortic valve. MV = mitral valve. AMP = acid-mucopolysaccharide material.

REFERENCES

1. ROBERTS, W. C.: *Anatomically isolated aortic valvular disease. The case against its being of rheumatic origin.* Am. J. Med. 49:151, 1970.

2. ROBERTS, W. C.: *The structure of the aortic valve in clinically isolated aortic stenosis. An autopsy study of 162 patients over 15 years of age.* Circulation 42:91, 1970.

3. ROBERTS, W. C.: *The congenitally bicuspid aortic valve. A study of 85 autopsy cases.* Am. J. Cardiol. 26:72, 1970.

4. ROBERTS, W. C., PERLOFF, J. K., AND CONSTANTINO, T.: *Severe valvular aortic stenosis in patients over 65 years of age. A clinicopathologic study.* Am. J. Cardiol. 27:497, 1971.

5. ROBERTS, W. C.: *Valvular, subvalvular and supravalvular aortic stenosis. Morphologic features.* Cardiovasc. Clin. 5 (1):97, 1973.

6. FALCONE, M. W., ROBERTS, W. C., MORROW, A. G., AND PERLOFF, J. K.: *Congenital aortic stenosis resulting from a unicommissural valve. Clinical and anatomic features in twenty-one adult patients.* Circulation 44:272, 1971.

7. EDWARDS, J. E.: *Pathologic aspects of cardiac valvular insufficiencies.* Arch. Surg. 77:634, 1958.

8. MOLLER, J. H., NAKIB, A., ELIOT, R. S., AND EDWARDS, J. E.: *Symptomatic congenital aortic stenosis in the first year of life.* J. Pediatr. 67:728, 1966.

9. HURWITZ, L. E., AND ROBERTS, W. C.: *The quadricuspid semilunar valve.* Am. J. Cardiol. (in press).

10. MORROW, A. G., GOLDBLATT, A., AND BRAUNWALD, E.: *Congenital aortic stenosis. II. Surgical treatment and the results of operation.* Circulation 27:426, 1963

11. MORROW, A. G., FORT, L., III, ROBERTS, W. C., AND BRAUNWALD, E.: *Discrete subaortic stenosis complicated by aortic valvular regurgitation. Clinical, hemodynamic, and pathologic studies and the results of operative treatment.* Circulation 20:1003, 1959.

12. MORROW, A. G.: *Hypertrophic subaortic stenosis. Some physiologic concepts and the role of operative treatment.* Arch. Surg. 99:677, 1969.

13. ADELMAN, A. G., MCLOUGHLIN, M. J., MARQUIS, Y., AUGER, P., AND WIGLE, E. D.: *Left ventricular cineangiographic observations in muscular subaortic stenosis.* Am. J. Cardiol. 24:689, 1969.

14. PETERSON, T. A., TODD, D. B., AND EDWARDS, J. E.: *Supravalvular aortic stenosis.* J. Thorac. Cardiovasc. Surg. 50:734, 1965.

15. ROBERTS, W. C.: *Pathologic aspects of valvular and subvalvular (discrete and diffuse) aortic stenosis, in* Kidd, B. S. L., and Keith, I. D. (eds.): *The Natural History and Progress in Treatment of Congenital Heart Defects. An International Symposium Sponsored by the Ontario Heart Foundation in Co-operation with the Hospital for Sick Children and the University of Toronto.* Charles C Thomas, Springfield, 1971, p. 221.

16. ROBERTS, W. C., FERRANS, V. J., LEVY, R. I., AND FREDRICKSON, D. S.: *Cardiovascular pathology in hyperlipoproteinemia. Anatomic observa-*

tions in 41 necropsy patients with normal or abnormal serum lipoprotein patterns. Am. J. Cardiol. (in press).

17. Wennevold, A., and Jacobsen, J. G.: *Acquired supravalvular aortic stenosis in familial hypercholesterolemia. A hemodynamic and angiographic study*. Am. J. Med. 50:823, 1971.

18. Ferrans, V. J., and Roberts, W. C.: *Structural features of cardiac myxomas. Histology, histochemistry and electron microscopy*. Hum. Pathol. 4:111, 1973.

19. Buchbinder, N. A., and Roberts, W. C.: *Active infective endocarditis confined to mural endocardium. A study of six necropsy patients*. Arch. Pathol. 93:435, 1972.

20. MacLowery, J. D., and Roberts, W. C.: *Metastatic choriocarcinoma of the lung. Invasion of pulmonary veins with extension into left atrium and mitral orifice*. Am. J. Cardiol. 18:938, 1966.

21. Ferencz, C., Johnson, A. L., and Wiglesworth, F. W.: *Congenital mitral stenosis*. Circulation 9:161, 1954.

22. Shone, J. D., Sellers, R. D., Anderson, R. C., Adams, P., Jr., Lillehei, C. W., and Edwards, J. E.: *The developmental complex of "parachute mitral valve," supravalvular ring of left atrium, subaortic stenosis, and coarctation of aorta*. Am. J. Cardiol. 11:714, 1963.

23. Glancy, D. L., Chang, M. Y., Dorney, E. R., and Roberts, W. C.: *Parachute mitral valve. Further observations and associated lesions*. Am. J. Cardiol. 27:309, 1971.

24. Castaneda, A. R., Anderson, R. C., and Ewards, J. E.: *Congenital mitral stenosis resulting from anomalous arcade and obstructing papillary muscles. Report of correction by use of ball valve prosthesis*. Am. J. Cardiol. 24:237, 1969.

25. Van Den Horst, R. L., and Hastreiter, A. R.: *Congenital mitral stenosis*. Am. J. Cardiol. 20:773, 1967.

26. Shem-Tov, A., Yahini, J. H., Deutsch, V., Katznelson, D., and Neufeld, H. N.: *Congenital mitral stenosis*. Cardiologica 54:65, 1969.

27. Fontana, R. S., and Edwards, J. E.: *Congenital Cardiac Disease: A Review of 357 Cases Studied Pathologically*. W. B. Saunders Co., Philadelphia, 1962.

28. Koretzky, B. S., Moller, J. H., Korns, M. E., Schwartz, C. J., and Edwards, J. E.: *Congenital pulmonary stenosis resulting from dysplasia of the valve*. Circulation 40:43, 1969.

29. Campbell, M.: *Natural history of congenital pulmonary stenosis*. Br. Heart J. 31:394, 1969.

30. Roberts, W. C., Mason, D. T., Morrow, A. G., and Braunwald, E.: *Calcific pulmonic stenosis*. Circulation 37:973, 1968.

31. Rodriguez, G. R., Bennette, K. R., and Lehan, P. H.: *Calcification of the pulmonic valve*. Chest 59:160, 1971.

32. Hudson, R. E. B.: *Cardiovascular Pathology*. Edward Arnold Ltd., London, 1965, p. 1953.

33. Thörson, A., Biörck, G., Björkman, G., and Waldenström, J.: *Malignant carcinoid of the small intestine with metastases to the liver, valvular disease of the heart (pulmonic stenosis and tricuspid regurgitation without septal defects), peripheral vasomotor symptoms, bronchoconstriction, and an unusual type of cyanosis. A clinical and pathologic syndrome.* Am. Heart J. 47:795, 1954.

34. Melmon, K. L., Sjoerdsma, A., and Mason, D. T.: *Distinctive clinical and therapeutic aspects of the syndrome associated with bronchial carcinoid tumors.* Am. J. Med. 39:568, 1965.

35. Oates, J. A., and Sjoerdsma, A.: *A unique syndrome associated with secretion of 5-hydroxytryptophan by metastatic gastric carcinoids.* Am. J. Med. 32:333, 1962.

36. Oates, J. A., Melmon, K., Sjoerdsma, A., Gillespie, L., and Mason, D. T.: *Release of kinin peptide in the carcinoid syndrome.* Lancet 1:514, 1964.

37. Sjoerdsma, A., Weissbach, H., and Udenfriend, S.: *A clinical, physiologic and biochemical study of patients with malignant carcinoid (argentaffinoma).* Am. J. Med. 20:520, 1956.

38. Roberts, W. C., and Sjoerdsma, A.: *The cardiac disease associated with the carcinoid syndrome (carcinoid heart disease).* Am. J. Med. 36:5, 1964.

39. Roberts, W. C., Mason, D. T., and Wright, L. D., Jr.: *The nondistensible right atrium of carcinoid disease of the heart.* Am. J. Clin. Pathol. 44:627, 1965.

40. Von Bernheimer, H., Ehringer, H., Heistracher, P., Kraupp, O., Lachnit, V., Obiditsch-Mayer, I., and Wenzl, M.: *Biologisch aktives, nicht metastasierendes Bronchuscarcinoid mit Linksherz-syndrom.* Wien. Klin. Wochenschr. 72:867, 1960.

41. Ferrans, V. F., and Roberts, W. C.: *Ultrastructural features of the carcinoid cardiac plaque.* (In preparation).

42. Sjoerdsma, A., Weissbach, H., Terry, L. L., and Udenfriend, S.: *Further observations on patients with malignant carcinoid.* Am. J. Med. 23:5, 1957.

43. Levine, R. J., and Sjoerdsma, A.: *Pressor amines and the carcinoid flush.* Ann. Intern. Med. 58:818, 1963.

44. Brock, R.: *The surgical treatment of pulmonary stenosis.* Br. Heart J. 23:337, 1961.

45. Horlick, L., and Merriman, J. E.: *Congenital valvular stenosis of pulmonary and aortic valves with atrial septal defect.* Am. Heart J. 54:615, 1957.

46. Salazar, E., Benavides, P., Contreras, R., and Espino-Vela, J.: *Congenital mitral and tricuspid stenosis.* Am. J. Cardiol. 16:358, 1965.

47. Van Den Horst, R. L., and Hastreiter, A. R.: *Congenital mitral stenosis.* Am. J. Cardiol. 20:773, 1967.

48. Roberts, W. C., Goldblatt, A., Mason, D. T., and Morrow, A. G.: *Combined congenital pulmonic and mitral stenosis.* N. Engl. J. Med. 267:1298, 1962.

49. Martland, H. S.: *Syphilis of the aorta and heart.* Am. Heart J. 6:1, 1930.

50. Carr, J. G.: *The gross pathology of the heart in cardiovascular syphilis.* Am. Heart J. 6:30, 1930.

51. Heggtveit, H. A.: *Syphilitic aortitis. A clinicopathologic autopsy study of 100 cases.* Circulation 29:346, 1964.

52. Clark, W. S., and Bauer, W.: *Cardiac changes in rheumatoid arthritis.* Ann. Rheum. Dis. 7:39, 1948.

53. Schilder, D. P., Harvey, W. P., and Hufnagel, C. A.: *Rheumatoid spondylitis and aortic insufficiency.* N. Engl. J. Med. 255:11, 1956.

54. Clark, W. S., Kulka, J. P., and Bauer, W.: *Rheumatoid aortitis with aortic regurgitation.* Am. J. Med. 22:580, 1957.

55. Graham, D. C., and Smythe, H. A.: *The carditis and aortitis of ankylosing spondylitis.* Bull. Rheum. Dis. 9:171, 1958.

56. Davidson, P., Baggenstross, A. H., Slocumb, C. H., and Daugherty, G. W.: *Cardiac and aortic lesions in rheumatoid spondylitis.* Proc. Mayo Clin. 36:427, 1963.

57. Liu, S. M., and Alexander, C. S.: *Complete heart block and aortic insufficiency in rheumatoid spondylitis.* Am. J. Cardiol. 23:888, 1969.

58. Bernstein, L.: *Cardiac complications in spondyl-arthritis ankylopoietica.* Rheumatism 7:18, 1951.

59. Toone, E. C., Pierce, E. L., and Hennigar, G. R.: *Aortitis and aortic regurgitation associated with rheumatoid spondylitis.* Am. J. Med. 26:255, 1959.

60. Valaitis, J., Pilz, C. G., and Montgomery, M. M.: *Aortitis with aortic valve insufficiency in rheumatoid arthritis.* Arch. Pathol. 63:207, 1957.

61. Malette, W. G., Eisman, B., Danielson, G. K., Mazzoleni, A., and Rams, J. J.: *Rheumatoid spondylitis and aortic insufficiency.* J. Thorac. Cardiovasc. Surg. 57:471, 1969.

62. Gleckler, W. J.: *Rheumatoid spondylitis with carditis.* Am. J. Med. 16:284, 1954.

63. Bernstein, C., and Broch, O. J.: *Cardiac complications in spondyl-arthritis ankylopoietica.* Acta Med. Scand. 135:185, 1949.

64. Blumberg, B., and Ragan, C.: *Natural history of rheumatoid spondylitis.* Medicine 35:1, 1956.

65. McKusick, V. A.: *Heritable Disorders of Connective Tissue,* ed. 3. C. V. Mosby Co., St. Louis, 1966.

66. Read, R. C., Thal, A. P., and Wendt, V. E.: *Symptomatic valvular myxomatous transformation (the floppy valve syndrome). A possible forme fruste of the Marfan syndrome.* Circulation 32:897, 1965.

67. Ragib, G., Jue, K. L., Anderson, R. C., and Edwards, J. E.: *Marfan's syndrome with mitral insufficiency.* Am. J. Cardiol. 16:127, 1965.

68. Shankar, K. R., Hultgren, M. K., Laver, R. M., and Diehl, A. M.: *Lethal tricuspid and mitral regurgitation in Marfan's syndrome.* Am. J. Cardiol. 20:122, 1967.

69. Dietzman, R. H., Peter, E. T., Wang, Y., and Lillehei, R. C.: *Mitral insufficiency in Marfan's syndrome. A case report of surgical correction.* Dis. Chest 51:650, 1967.

70. Crocker, D. W.: *Marfan's syndrome confined to the mitral valve region: two cases in siblings.* Am. Heart J. 76:538, 1968.

71. Jortner, R., Shahin, W., Eshkol, D., Gueron, M., and Levy, M. J.: *Cardiovascular manifestations and surgery for Marfan's syndrome.* Dis. Chest 56:24, 1969.

72. Roberts, W. C., and Cohen, L. S.: *Left ventricular papillary muscles. Description of the normal and a survey of conditions causing them to be abnormal.* Circulation 46:138, 1972.

73. Perloff, J. K., and Roberts, W. C.: *The mitral apparatus. Functional anatomy of mitral regurgitation.* Circulation 46:227, 1972.

74. Grossman, M., Knott, A. P., Jr., and Jacoby, W. J., Jr.: *Calcified annulus fibrosis with mitral insufficiency with Marfan's syndrome.* Arch. Intern. Med. 121:561, 1968.

75. McKusick, V. A., Logue, R. B., and Bahnson, H. T.: *Association of aortic valvular disease and cystic medial necrosis of the ascending aorta. Report of four instances.* Circulation 16:188, 1957.

76. Heath, D., Edwards, J. E., and Smith, L. A.: *The rheologic significance of medial necrosis and dissecting aneurysm of the ascending aorta in association with calcific aortic stenosis.* Proc. Mayo Clin. 33:228, 1958.

77. Lagunoff, D., Ross, R., and Benditt, E. P.: *Histochemical and electron microscopic study of a case of Hurler's disease.* Am. J. Pathol. 41:273, 1962.

78. Ferrans, V. F., and Roberts, W. C.: *Ultrastructural features of cardiac lesions of the Hurler syndrome.* In preparation.

79. Okada, R., Rosenthal, I. M., Scaravelli, G., and Lev, M.: *A histopathologic study of the heart in gargoylism.* Arch. Pathol. 84:20, 1967.

80. Hunter, C.: *A rare disease in two brothers.* Proc. R. Soc. Med. 10:104, 1917.

81. Krovetz, L. J., Lorincz, A. E., and Schiebler, G. L.: *Cardiovascular manifestations of the Hurler syndrome. Hemodynamic and angiographic observations in 15 patients.* Circulation 31:132, 1965.

82. Vanace, P. W., Friedman, S., and Wagner, B. M.: *Mitral stenosis in an atypical case of gargoylism: a case report with pathologic and histochemical studies of the cardiac tissues.* Circulation 21:80, 1960.

83. Frieden, J., Hurwitt, E. S., and Leader, E.: *Ruptured aortic cusp with an heritable disorder of connective tissue.* Am. J. Med. 33:615, 1962.

84. Tucker, D. H., Miller, D. E., and Jacoby, W. J.: *Ehlers-Danlos syndrome with a sinus of Valsalva aneurysm and aortic insufficiency simulating rheumatic heart disease.* Am. J. Med. 35:715, 1963.

85. Madison, W. R., Jr., Bradley, E. J., and Castillo, A. J.: *Ehlers-Danlos syndrome with cardiac involvement.* Am. J. Cardiol. 11:689, 1963.

86. Browell, J. M., Jr., and Dreke, E. H.: *Aortic valve lesions associated with osteogenesis imperfecta.* Henry Ford Hosp. Med. Bull. 14:245, 1966.

87. Green, G. J., Schuman, B., and Barron, J.: *Ehlers-Danlos syndrome complicated by acute hemorrhagic diverticulitis with an unusual mitral valve abnormality.* Am. J. Med. 41:622, 1966.

88. Huang, S., Ganraj, K., Steele, H., and Park, J. O.: *Cardiac involvement in pseudoxanthoma elasticum.* Am. Heart J. 74:680, 1967.

89. Heckman, B. A., and Steinberg, I.: *Congenital heart disease (mitral regurgitation) in osteogenesis imperfecta.* Am. J. Roentgenol. Radium Ther. Nucl. Med. 103:601, 1968.

90. Goodman, R. W., Baba, M., and Wooley, C. F.: *Observations on the heart in a case of combined Ehlers-Danlos and Marfan syndromes.* Am. J. Cardiol. 24:134, 1969.

91. Criscitiello, M. G., Ronan, J. A., Besterman, E. M. M., and Schoenwetter, W.: *Cardiovascular abnormalities in osteogenesis imperfecta.* Circulation 31:255, 1965.

92. Jorriod, J., Rothlin, M., and Uehlinger, E.: *Anomalies cardiovasculaires de la Maladie de Lobstein.* Schweiz. Med. Wochenschr. 98:795, 1968.

93. Allen, E. V.: *Primary arteritis of the aortic arch.* Circulation 11:486, 1955.

94. Kalmansohn, R. B., and Kalmansohn, R. W.: *Thrombotic obliteration of the branches of the aortic arch.* Circulation 15:237, 1957.

95. Nasu, T.: *Pathology of pulseless disease.* Angiology 14:225, 1963.

96. Strachan, R. W.: *The natural history of Takayasu's arteriopathy.* J. Med. 33:57, 1964.

97. Roberts, W. C., and Wibin, E. A.: *Idiopathic panaortitis, supraaortic arteritis, granulomatous myocarditis and pericarditis.* Am. J. Med. 41:453, 1966.

98. Roberts, W. C., MacGregor, R. R., DeBlanc, H. J., Beiser, G. B., and Wolff, S. M.: *The prepulseless phase of pulseless disease, or pulseless disease with pulses. A newly recognized cause of cardiac disease, monoclonal gammopathy and fever of unknown origin.* Am. J. Med. 46:313, 1969.

99. Barlow, J. B., Pocock, W. A., Marchand, P., and Denny, M.: *The significance of late systolic murmurs.* Am. Heart J. 66:443, 1963.

100. Criley, J. M., Lewis, K. B., Humphries, J. O., and Ross, R. S.: *Prolapse of the mitral valve: Clinical and cine-angiocardiographic findings.* Br. Heart J. 28:488, 1966.

101. Stannard, M., Sloman, J. G., Hare, W. S., and Goble, A. J.: *Prolapse of the posterior leaflet of the mitral valve. A clinical, familial and cineangiographic study.* Br. Med. J. 3:71, 1967.

102. Barlow, J. B., Bosman, C. K., Pocock, W. A., and Marchand, P.: *Late systolic murmurs and non-ejection ('mid-late') systolic clicks; An analysis of 90 patients.* Br. Heart J. 30:203, 1968.

103. Jeresaty, R. M.: *Ballooning of the mitral valve leaflets. Angiographic study of 24 patients.* Radiology 100:45, 1971.

104. Ehlers, K. H., Engle, M. A., Levin, A. R., Grossman, H., and Fleming, R. J.: *Left ventricular abnormality with late mitral insufficiency and abnormal electrocardiogram.* Am. J. Cardiol. 26:333, 1970.

105. Edynak, G. M., and Rawson, A. J.: *Ruptured aneurysm of the mitral valve in a Marfan-like syndrome.* Am. J. Cardiol. 11:674, 1963.

106. Pocock, W. A., and Barlow, J. B.: *Etiology and electrocardiographic features of the billowing posterior mitral leaflet syndrome.* Am. J. Med. 51:731, 1971.

107. McDonald, A., Harris, H., Jefferson, K., Marshall, J., and McDonald, L.: *Association of prolapse of posterior cusp of mitral valve and atrial septal defect.* Br. Heart J. 33:383, 1971.

108. Pocock, W. A., and Barlow, J. B.: *An association between billowing posterior mitral leaflet syndrome and congenital heart disease, particularly atrial septal defect.* Am. Heart J. 81:720, 1971.

109. Davis, R. H., Schuster, B., Knoebel, S. B., and Fisch, C.: *Myxomatous degeneration of the mitral valve.* Am. J. Cardiol. 28:449, 1971.

110. Kern, W. H., and Tucker, B. L.: *Myxoid changes in cardiac valves: pathologic, clinical and ultrastructural studies.* Am. Heart J. 84:294, 1972.

111. Pomerance, A.: *Ballooning deformity (mucoid degeneration) of atrioventricular valves.* Br. Heart J. 31:343, 1969.

112. Sherman, E. B., Char, F., Dungan, W. T., and Campbell, G. S.: *Myxomatous transformation of the mitral valve producing mitral insufficiency. Floppy valve syndrome.* Am. J. Dis. Child. 119:171, 1970.

113. Edwards, J. E.: *Mitral insufficiency resulting from 'overshooting' of leaflets.* Circulation 43:606, 1971.

114. Bowers, D.: *An electrocardiographic pattern associated with mitral valve deformity in Marfan's syndrome.* Circulation 23:30, 1961.

115. Frable, W. J.: *Mucinous degeneration of the cardiac valves: the floppy valve syndrome.* J. Thorac. Cardiovasc. Surg. 58:62, 1969.

116. Pomerance, A.: *Cardiac pathology and systolic murmurs in the elderly.* Br. Heart J. 30:687, 1968.

117. Pomerance, A.: *Ageing changes in human heart valves.* Br. Heart J. 29:222, 1967.

118. Sell, S., and Scully, R. E.: *Aging changes in the aortic and mitral valves.* Am. J. Pathol. 46:345, 1965.

119. Kittredge, R. D., Shimomura, S., Cameron, A., and Bell, A. L.: *Prolapsing mitral valve leaflets; cineangiographic demonstrations.* Am. J. Roentgenol. Radium Ther. Nucl. Med. 109:84, 1970.

120. Korn, D., De Sanctis, R. W., and Sell, S.: *Massive calcification of the mitral annulus.* N. Engl. J. Med. 267:900, 1962.

121. Ewy, G. A., Marcus, F. I., Bohajalian, O., Burke, H. L., and Roberts, W. C.: *Muscular subaortic stenosis. Clinical and pathologic observations in an elderly patient.* Am. J. Cardiol. 22:126, 1968.

122. ROGERS, J. B., CHANDLER, N. W., AND FRANCH, R. H.: *Calcification of the tricuspid annulus*. Am. J. Roentgenol. Radium Ther. Nucl. Med. 106:550, 1969.

123. COOKSEY, J. D., PARKER, B. M., AND WELDON, C. S.: *Atrial septal defect and calcification of the tricuspid valve*. Br. Heart J. 32:409, 1970.

124. ARNOLD, J. R., GHAHRAMANI, A. R., HERNANDEZ, F. A., AND SOMMER, L. S.: *Calcification of annulus of tricuspid valve (observation in two patients with congenital pulmonary stenosis)*. Chest 60:229, 1971.

125. BRODY, W., AND CRILEY, J. M.: *Intermittent severe mitral regurgitation: hemodynamic studies in a patient with recurrent acute left-sided heart failure*. N. Engl. J. Med. 283:673, 1970.

126. BURCH, G. E., DE PASQUALE, N. P., AND PHILLIPS, J. H.: *The syndrome of papillary muscle dysfunction*. Am. Heart J. 75:399, 1968.

127. BROCK, R. C.: *The surgical and pathological anatomy of the mitral valve*. Br. Heart J. 14:489, 1952.

128. MITTAL, A. K., LANGSTON, M., JR., COHN, K. E., SELZER, A., AND KERTH, W. J.: *Combined papillary muscle and left ventricular wall dysfunction as a cause of mitral regurgitation: An experimental study*. Circulation 44:174, 1971.

129. FALCONE, M. W., RONAN, J. A., JR., AND ROBERTS, W. C.: *Silent mitral regurgitation complicating silent myocardial infarction: hemodynamic and morphologic decumentation*. Chest 62:226, 1972.

130. ROBERTS, W. C., AND BUCHBINDER, N. A.: *Right-sided valvular infective endocarditis. A clinicopathologic study of twelve necropsy patients*. Am. J. Med. 53:7, 1972.

131. BUCHBINDER, N. A., AND ROBERTS, W. C.: *Left-sided valvular active infective endocarditis. A study of forty-five necropsy patients*. Am. J. Med. 53:20, 1972.

132. ROBERTS, W. C., AND BUCHBINDER, N. A.: *Papillary muscle necrosis in active valvular infective endocarditis*. Am. J. Cardiol. 29:287, 1972.

133. MOLLER, J. H., LUCAS, R. B., JR., ADAMS, P., JR., ANDERSON, R. C., JORGENS, J., AND EDWARDS, J. E.: *Endocardial fibroelastosis. A clinical and anatomic study of 47 patients with emphasis on its relationship to mitral insufficiency*. Circulation 30:759, 1964.

134. NOREN, G. R., RAGHIB, G., MOLLER, J. H., AMPLANTZ, K., ADAMS, P., JR., AND EDWARDS, J. E.: *Anomalous origin of the left coronary artery from the pulmonary trunk with special reference to the occurrence of mitral insufficiency*. Circulation 30:171, 1964.

135. ROBERTS, W. C.: *Anomalous origin of both coronary arteries from the pulmonary artery*. Am. J. Cardiol. 10:595, 1962.

136. BURCHELL, H. B., AND BROWN, A. L., JR.: *Anomalous origin of coronary artery from pulmonary artery masquerading as mitral insufficiency*. Am. Heart J. 63:388, 1962.

137. MARCUS, F. I., GOMEZ, L., GLANCY, D. L., EWY, G. A., AND ROBERTS, W. C.: *Papillary muscle fibrosis in primary myocardial disease.* Am. Heart J. 77:681, 1969.

138. PERLOFF, J. K., ROBERTS, W. C., DE LEON, A. C., AND O'DOHERTY, D.: *The distinctive electrocardiogram of Duchenne's progressive muscular dystrophy. An electrocardiographic-pathologic correlative study.* Am. J. Med. 42:179, 1967.

139. ROBERTS, W. C., BUJA, L. M., AND FERRANS, V. J.: *Löffler's fibroplastic parietal endocarditis, eosinophilic leukemia, and Davis' endomyocardial fibrosis: The same disease at different stages?* Pathol. Microbiol. 35:90, 1970.

140. ROBERTS, W. C., LIEGLER, D. G., AND CARBONE, P. P.: *Endomycardial disease and eosinophilia: A clinical and pathologic spectrum.* Am. J. Med. 46:28, 1969.

141. MORROW, A. G., COHEN, L. S., ROBERTS, W. C., BRAUNWALD, N. S., AND BRAUNWALD, E.: *Severe mitral regurgitation following acute myocardial infarction and ruptured papillary muscle: Hemodynamic findings and results of operative treatment in four patients.* Circulation 38 (Suppl.): II-124, 1968.

142. ROBERTS, W. C., AND FERRANS, V. J.: *Morphologic observations in the cardiomyopathies, in* Fowler, N. O. (ed.): *The Cardiomyopathies.* Grune & Stratton, New York, 1973, (in press).

143. ROBERTS, W. C., BODEY, G. P., AND WERTLAKE, P. T.: *The heart in acute leukemia. A study of 420 autopsy cases.* Am. J. Cardiol. 21:388, 1968.

144. GLANCY, D. L., AND ROBERTS, W. C.: *The heart in malignant malanoma. A study of 70 autopsy cases.* Am. J. Cardiol. 21:555, 1968.

145. ROBERTS, W. C., GLANCY, D. L., AND DEVITA, V. T., JR.: *Heart in malignant lymphoma (Hodgkin's disease, lymphosarcoma, reticulum cell sarcoma and mycosis fungoides). A study of 196 autopsy cases.* Am. J. Cardiol. 22:85, 1968.

146. BUJA, L. M., KHOI, N. B., AND ROBERTS, W. C.: *Clinically significant cardiac amyloidosis. Clinicopathologic findings in 15 patients.* Am. J. Cardiol. 26:394, 1970.

147. BUJA, L. M., AND ROBERTS, W. C.: *Iron in the heart. Etiology and clinical significance.* Am. J. Med. 51:209, 1971.

148. BUCHBINDER, N. A., AND ROBERTS, W. C.: *Active infective endocarditis confined to mural endocardium. A study of six necropsy patients.* Arch. Pathol. 93:435, 1972.

149. BUCHBINDER, N. A., AND ROBERTS, W. C.: *Alcoholism—An important but unemphasized factor predisposing to infective endocarditis with reemphasis on the syndrome of pneumococcal endocarditis, meningitis and pneumonitis in alcholics.* Arch. Intern. Med. (in press).

150. ROBERTS, W. C., AND PERLOFF, J. K.: *Mitral valvular disease. A combined clinical and pathologic survey of the conditions causing the mitral valve to function abnormally.* Ann. Intern. Med. 77:939, 1972.

151. ROBERTS, W. C., BUCHBINDER, N. A., AND MORROW, A. G.: *Healed infective endocarditis: An anatomic study of patients with histories of active*

infective endocarditis and a clinical analysis of anatomically confirmed cases of healed rupture of mitral chordae tendineae or of perforation of mitral or aortic valve cusps. (in preparation).

152. Schiebler, G. L., Gravenstein, J. S., and Van Mierop, L. H. S.: *Ebstein's anomaly of the tricuspid valve. Translation of the original description with comments.* Am. J. Cardiol. 22:867, 1968.

153. Vacca, J. B., Bussmann, D. W., and Mudd, J. G.: *Ebstein's anomaly, complete review of 108 cases.* Am. J. Cardiol. 2:210, 1958.

154. Kezdi, P., and Wennemark, J.: *Ebstein's malformation: Clinical findings and hemodynamic alterations.* Am. J. Cardiol. 2:200, 1958.

155. Spencer, F. C.: *Surgery of the tricuspid valve.* Cardiovasc. Clin. 3(2):301, 1971.

156. Becker, A. E., Becker, M. J., and Edwards, J. E.: *Pathologic spectrum of dysplasia of the tricuspid valve. Features in common with Ebstein's malformation.* Arch. Pathol. 91:169, 1971.

157. Markous, N., and Vander Veer, J. B.: *Ebstein's anamaly and life expectancy. Report of a survival to over age 79.* Am. J. Cardiol. 18:100, 1966.

158. Genton , E., and Blount, S. G.: *The spectrum of Ebstein's anomaly.* Am. Heart J. 73:395, 1967.

159. Newfeld, E. A., Cole, R. B., and Paul, M. H.: *Ebstein's malformation of the tricuspid valve in the neonate. Functional and anatomic pulmonary outflow tract obstruction.* Am. J. Cardiol. 19:727, 1967.

160. Mayer, F. E., Nadas, A. S., and Ongley, P. A.: *Ebstein's anomaly. Presentation of 10 cases.* Circulation 16:1057, 1957.

161. Harris, R. H. D.: *Ebstein's anomaly: Discovered in a 75 year old subject in the dissecting laboratory.* Canad. Med. Assoc. J. 83:653, 1960.

162. Engle, M. A., Payne, T. P. B., Bruins, C., and Taussig, H. B.: *Ebstein's anomaly of the tricuspid valve. Report of three cases and analysis of the clinical syndrome.* Circulation 1:1246, 1950.

163. Pocock, W. A., Tucker, R. B. K., and Barlow, J. B.: *Mild Ebstein's anomaly.* Br. Heart J. 31:327, 1969.

164. Lowe, K. G., and Emslie-Smith, D.: *Scalar, vector and intracardiac electrocardiograms in Ebstein's anomaly.* Br. Heart J. 30:617, 1968.

165. Moles, S. S., Jacoby, W. J., Jr., and McIntosh, H. D.: *Ebstein's malformation. Discordant intracavitary electrocardiographic and pressure relationship.* Am. J. Cardiol. 14:720, 1964.

166. Brayshaw, J. R., and Perloff, J. K.: *Congenital pulmonary insufficiency complicating idiopathic dilatation of the pulmonary artery.* Am. J. Cardiol. 10:282, 1962.

167. Smith, R. D., Dushane, J. W., and Edwards, J. A.: *Congenital insufficiency of the pulmonary valve. Including a case of fetal cardiac failure.* Circulation 20:554, 1959.

168. Ito, T., Engle, M. A., and Holswade, G. R.: *Congenital insufficiency of the pulmonic valve. A rare cause of neonatal heart failure.* Pediatrics 28:712, 1961.

169. D'Cruz, I. A., Leudrum, B. L., and Novak, G.: *Congenital absence of the pulmonary valve*. Am. Heart J. 68:728, 1964.

170. Pouget, J. M., Kelly, C. E., and Pilz, C. G.: *Congenital absence of the pulmonic valve. Report of case in a 73 year old man*. Am. J. Cardiol. 19:732, 1967.

171. Ford, A. B., Hellerstein, H. K., Wood, C., and Kelley, H. B.: *Isolated congenital bicuspid pulmonary valve: Clinical and pathologic study*. Am. J. Med. 20:474, 1956.

172. Dickens, J., Raber, G. T., and Goldberg, H.: *Dynamic pulmonary regurgitation associated with a bicuspid valve*. Ann. Intern. Med. 48:851, 1958.

173. Miller, R. A., Leu, M., and Paul, M. H.: *Congenital absence of the pulmonary valve. The clinical syndrome of tetralogy of Fallot with pulmonary regurgitation*. Circulation 26:266, 1962.

174. Nemickas, R., Roberts, J., Gunnar, R., and Tobin, J. R., Jr.: *Isolated congenital pulmonic insufficiency*. Am. J. Cardiol. 14:456, 1964.

175. Holmes, J. C., Fowler, N. O., and Kaplan, S.: *Pulmonary valvular insufficiency*. Am. J. Med. 44:851, 1968.

176. Rokseth, R.: *Isolated pulmonic valvular regurgitation*. Acta Med. Scand. 185:489, 1969.

177. Carney, E. K., Braunwald, E., Roberts, W. C., Aygen, M., and Morrow, A. G.: *Congenital mitral regurgitation. Clinical, hemodynamic and angiographic findings in nine patients*. Am. J. Med. 33:223, 1962.

178. Ainger, L. E.: *Mitral and aortic valve incompetence in endocardial fibroelastosis. Diagnostic and hemodynamic significance*. Am. J. Cardiol. 28:309, 1971.

179. Berry, W. B., Roberts, W. C., Morrow, A. G., and Braunwald, E.: *Corrected transposition of the aorta and pulmonary trunk. Clinical, hemocynamic and pathologic findings*. Am. J. Med. 36:35, 1964.

180. Roberts, W. C., Ross, R. S., and Davis, F. W., Jr.: *Congenital corrected transportation of the great vessels in adulthood simulating rheumatic valvular disease*. Bul. Johns Hopkins Hosp. 144:157, 1964.

181. Schiebler, G. L., Edwards, J. C., Burchell, H. B., DuShane, J. W., Ongley, P. A., and Wood, E. H.: *Congenital corrected transposition of the great vessels. A study of 33 cases*. Pediatrics 27:851, 1961.

182. Braunwald, E., Ross, R. S., Morrow, A. G., and Roberts, W. C.: *Differential diagnosis of mitral regurgitation in childhood: clinical pathological conference at the National Institutes of Health*. Ann. Intern. Med. 54:1223, 1961.

183. Brockenbrough, E. C., Braunwald, E., Roberts, W. C., and Morrow, A. G.: *Partial persistent atrioventricular canal simulating pure mitral regurgitation*. Am. Heart J. 63:9, 1962.

184. MacLeod, C. A.: *Endocardial cushion defects with severe mitral insufficiency and small atrial septal defect*. Circulation 26:755, 1962.

185. Glancy, D. L., Chang, M. Y., Dorney, E. R., and Roberts, W. C.: *Parachute mitral valve. Further observations and associated lesions*. Am. J. Cardiol. 27:309, 1971.

186. Scheiken, R. M., Freidman, S., Waldhausen, J., and Johnson, J.: *Isolated congenital mitral insufficiency: Pathologic and surgical variations in five children*. J. Pediatr. Surg. 6:49, 1971.

187. Shone, J. D., Sellers, R. D., Anderson, R. C., Adams, P., Jr., Lillehei, C. W., and Edwards, J. E.: *The developmental complex of "parachute mitral valve," supravalvular ring of left atrium, subaortic stenosis and coarctation of the aorta*. Am. J. Cardiol. 11:714, 1963.

188. Layman, T. E., Edwards, J. E.: *Anomalous mitral arcade. A type of congenital mitral insufficiency*. Circulation 35:389, 1967.

189. Davachi, F., Moller, J. H., and Edwards, J. E.: *Diseases of the mitral valve in infancy. An anatomic review of 55 cases*. Circulation 43:565, 1971.

190. Rosenberg, J., and Roberts, W. C.: *Double orifice mitral valve. Study of the anomaly in two calves and a summary of the literature in humans*. Arch. Pathol. 86:77, 1968.

191. Parmley, L. F., Mattingly, T. W., and Manion, W. C.: *Penetrating wounds of the heart and aorta*. Circulation 17:953, 1958.

192. Yao, S. T., Vanecko, R. M., Printen, K, and Shoemaker, W. C.: *Penetrating wounds of the heart. A review of 80 cases*. Ann. Surg. 168:67, 1968.

193. Jones, E. W., and Helmsworth, J.: *Penetrating wounds of the heart: Thirty years' experience*. Arch. Surg. 96:671, 1968.

194. Sugg, W. L., Rea, W. J., Ecker, R. R., Webb, W. R., Rose, E. F., and Shaw, R. R.: *Penetrating wounds of the heart: An analysis of 459 cases*. J. Thorac. Cardiovasc. Surg. 56:531, 1968.

195. Wilson, R. F., and Bassett, J. S.: *Penetrating wounds of the pericardium and its contents*. J.A.M.A. 195:513, 1966.

196. Mulder, D. G.: *Stab wound of the heart*. Ann. Surg. 160:287, 1964.

197. Bland, E. F., and Beebe, G. W.: *Missiles in the heart. A twenty year follow-up report of World War II cases*. N. Engl. J. Med. 274:1039, 1965.

198. Riemer, R.: Indiscussion of paper by Sugg, W. L., et al.: *Penetrating wounds of the heart*. J. Thorac. Cardiovasc. Surg. 56:545, 1968.

199. Berger, R. L., Gibson, H., Reimer, R. W., and Ramaswamy, K.: *Traumatic aortic regurgitation, ventricular septal defect and fistula of the sinus of Valsalva*. N. Engl. J. Med. 281:887, 1969.

200. Hutchinson, J. E., Beach, P. M., Kaplan, S., and Garvey, J. W.: *Management of penetrating cardiac trauma*. N. Y. State J. Med. 71:1932, 1971.

201. Cleveland, R. J., Kemp, E. V., and Lower, R. R.: *Acute aortic valve insufficiency as a result of a bullet wound. Report of a case of successful treatment*. J. Thorac. Cardiovasc. Surg. 55:123, 1968.

202. Hardy, J. O., and Timmis, H. H.: *Repair of intracardiac gunshot wounds. Report of three cases*. Ann. Surg. 169:906, 1969.

203. Pate, J. W., and Richardson, R. L.: *Penetrating wounds of the cardiac valves*. J.A.M.A. 207:309, 1969.

204. PARMLEY, L. F., MANION, W. C., AND MATTINGLY, T. W.: *Nonpenetrating traumatic injury of the heart.* Circulation 18:371, 1958.

205. HOWARD, C. P.: *Aortic insufficiency due to rupture by strain of a normal aortic valve.* Can. Med. Assoc. J. 19:12, 1928.

206. LOOP, F. D., HOFMEIR, G., AND GROVES, L. K.: *Traumatic disruption of the aortic valve.* Cleve. Clin. Q. 38:187, 1971.

207. NAJAFI, H., DYE, W. S., JAVID, H., HUNTER, J. A., AND JULIAN, O. C.: *Rupture of an otherwise normal aortic valve: Report of two cases and review of the literature.* J. Thorac. Cardiovasc. Surg. 56:57, 1968.

208. SPURNY, O. M., AND HARA, M.: *Rupture of the aortic valve due to strain.* Am. J. Cardiol. 8:125, 1961.

209. LEVINE, R. J., ROBERTS, W. C., AND MORROW, A. G.: *Traumatic aortic regurgitation.* Am. J. Cardiol. 10:1962.

210. MCLAUGHLIN, J. S., COWELY, R. A., SMITH, G., AND MATHESON, M. A.: *Mitral valve disease from blunt trauma.* J. Thorac. Cardiovasc. Surg. 48:261, 1964.

211. GOGGIN, M. J., THOMPSON, F. D., AND JACKSON, J. W.: *Deceleration trauma to the heart and great vessels after road traffic accidents.* Br. J. Med. 2:767, 1970.

212. SANDERS, R. J., NEUBUERGER, K. T., AND RAVIN, A.: *Rupture of papillary muscles: Occurrence of rupture of the posterior muscle in posterior myocardial infarction.* Dis. Chest 31:316, 1957.

213. GOMEZ, A. R., AND JACKSON, H. A.: *Traumatic rupture of a papillary muscle in a child.* Am. Heart J. 7:522, 1966.

214. FRY, W. A., AND BASINGER, C. E.: *Traumatic rupture of a papillary muscle of the heart.* Dis. Chest 51:100, 1967.

215. BRANDENBURG, R. O., MCGOON, D. C., CAMPEAU, L., AND GUILLIANI, E.: *Traumatic rupture of the chordae tendineae of the tricuspid valve. Successful repair 24 years later.* Am. J. Cardiol. 18:911, 1966.

216. TACHOVSKY, T. H., GIULIANI, E. R., AND ELLIS, F. H.: *Prosthetic valve replacement for traumatic tricuspid insufficiency. Report of a case originally diagnosed as Ebstein's malformation.* Am. J. Cardiol. 26:200, 1970.

217. MORGAN, J. R., AND FORKER, A. D.: *Isolated tricuspid regurgitation.* Circulation 43:559, 1971.

218. CROXSON, M. S., O'BRIEN, K. P., AND LOWE, J. B.: *Traumatic tricuspid regurgitation. Long term survival.* Br. Heart J. 33:750, 1971.

219. KREMER, R., CHALANT, C. H., HEKSTER, C., TIMMERMANS, A., GIELAN, A., AND LAVENNE, F.: *Insuffisance Tricuspidienne it communication Interventriculaire dues a un Traumatisme Ferme du Thorax, Correction Surgicale.* Acta Cardiol. (Brux.) 22:381, 1967.

220. SHABETAI, R., VADAKEPAT, A., DANIELSON, G., AND BRYANT, L.: *Traumatic hemopericardium with tricuspid incompetence.* J. Thorac. Cardiovasc. Surg. 57:294, 1969.

221. YAMADA, J, NAGAOKA, H., KONDO, N., TANIGUCHI, K., AND SHINTOMI, Y.: *Surgical treatment of teaumatic tricuspid insufficiency.* Bull. Tokyo Med. Dent. Univ. 17:319, 1970.

222. LIBMAN, E., AND SACKS, B.: *A hitherto undescribed form of valvular and mural endocarditis*. Arch. Intern. Med. 33:701, 1924.

223. GROSS, L.: *The cardiac lesions in Libman-Sacks disease; with a consideration of its relationship to acute diffuse lupus erythematosus*. Am. J. Pathol. 16:375, 1940.

224. KLEMPERER, P., POLLACK, A. D., AND BAEHR, G.: *Pathology of disseminated lupus erythematosus*. Arch. Pathol. 32:569, 1941.

225. GRIFFITH, G. C., AND VURAL, I. L.: *Acute and subacute disseminated lupus erythematosus: A correlation of clinical and post mortem findings in eighteen cases*. Circulation 3:492, 1951.

226. BENNET, J. C., CLAYBROOK, J., KINSEY, H., AND HOLLEY, H. L.: *The clinical manifestations of systemic lupus erythematosus*. J. Chronic Dis. 13:411, 1961.

227. KONG, T. Q., KELLUM, R. E., AND HASERICK, J. R.: *Clinical diagnosis of cardiac involvement in systemic lupus erythematosus*. Circulation 26:7, 1962.

228. BAEHR, G., KLEMPERER, P., AND SCHIFRIN, A.: *A diffuse disease of the peripheral circulation (usually associated with lupus erythematosus and endocarditis)*. Trans. Assoc. Am. Physicians 50:139, 1935.

229. HUMPRIES, E. M.: *The cardiac lesions of acute disseminated lupus erythematosus*. Ann. Intern. Med. 28:12, 1948.

230. SHEARN, M. A.: *The heart in systemic lupus erythematosus*. Am. Heart J. 58:452, 1959.

231. HEJTMANCIK, M. R., WRIGHT, J. C., QUINT, R., AND JENNINGS, I. L.: *The cardiovascular manifestations of systemic lupus erythematosus*. Am. Heart J. 68:119, 1964.

232. HARVEY, A. M., SCHULMAN, L. E., TUMULTY, P. A., CONLEY, C. L., AND SCHOENRICH, E. H.: *Systemic lupus erythematosus: Review of the literature and clinical analysis of 138 cases*. Medicine 33:291, 1954.

233. BAGGENSTOSS, A. H., AND ROSENBERG, E. F.: *Cardiac lesions associated with chronic fectious arthritis*. Arch. Intern. Med. 67:241–258, 1941.

234. LIEBOWITZ, W. B.: *The heart in rheumatoid arthritis (rheumatoid disease)*. Ann. Intern. Med. 58:102, 1963.

235. ROBERTS, W. C., KEHOE, J. A., CARPENTER, D. F., AND GOLDEN, A.: *Cardiac valvular lesions in rheumatoid arthritis*. Arch. Intern. Med. 122: 141, 1968.

236. CARPENTER, D. F., GOLDEN, A., AND ROBERTS, W. C.: *Quadrivalvular rheumatoid heart disease associated with left bundle branch block*. Am. J. Med. 43:922, 1967.

237. SOKOLOFF, L.: *The heart in rheumatoid arthritis*. Am. Heart J. 45:635, 1953.

238. SOKOLOFF, L., MCCLUSKEY, R. T., AND BUNIM, J. J.: *Vascularity of the early subcutaneous nodule of rheumatoid arthritis*. Arch. Pathol. 55:475, 1953.

239. LÖFFLER, W.: *Endocarditis parietalis fibroplastica mit Bluteosinophilie*. Schweiz. Med. Wochenschr. 66:817, 1936.

240. ROBERTS, W. C., ROSS, R. S., EGGLESTON, J. C., AND MASSUMI, R. A.: *Chronic mitral regurgitation of unresolved etiology in the elderly. A clinicopathologic study of two patients*. Johns Hopkins Med. J. 122:26, 1968.

Combined Acute Rheumatic Fever and Congenitally Bicuspid Aortic Valve

A Hitherto Unconfirmed Combination*

*Richard A. McReynolds, M.D.;*** *Nayab Ali, M.D.;*†
Michael Cuadra, M.D.;‡ *and*
William C. Roberts, M.D., F.C.C.P.§

An 18-year-old man is described in whom rheumatic heart disease, as evidenced by the presence of classic Aschoff bodies, occurred in combination with a congenitally bicuspid (purely incompetent) aortic valve. To our knowledge, this is the first report documenting the presence of rheumatic heart disease and congenitally bicuspid aortic valve in the same patient.

Although fusion of two of three aortic valve cusps (one of three commissures) causing "acquired" bicuspid valve is common in rheumatic heart disease, the occurrence of a congenitally bicuspid aortic valve in a patient with unequivocal rheumatic disease, *ie,* with Aschoff bodies present, has not been reported. The report which follows describes this association in the same patient.

*From the Section of Pathology, National Heart and Lung Institute, National Institutes of Health, Bethesda, Maryland and the Cardiac Laboratory, Howard University Medical Service, and the Department of Pathology, D.C. General Hospital, Washington, D.C.
**Presently Assistant Professor of Pathology, University of Alabama School of Medicine, Birmingham.
†Assistant Professor of Medicine, Howard University School of Medicine; Cardiologist, D.C. General Hospital.
‡Chief, Autopsy Service, D.C. General Hospital, Washington, D.C.
§Chief, Section of Pathology, National Heart and Lung Institute, National Institutes of Health, Bethesda.
Reprint requests: Dr. Roberts, NIH Bldg 10A, Room 3E20, Bethesda, 20014

Case Report

An 18-year-old black man was well until two years before death when he developed flank pain for which he was hospitalized. Examination at that time disclosed blood pressure of 140/80 mm Hg, collapsing peripheral pulses, and grade 3/6 basal systolic and diastolic precordial murmurs consistent with aortic "stenosis" and regurgitation. Electrocardiogram (Fig 1) and chest roentgenogram (Fig 2) showed cardiomegaly. After several days, the flank pain subsided; its etiology was never determined. Infective endocarditis was ruled out by repeatedly negative blood cultures. After discharge, he remained well and active until he suddenly collapsed and died while at work.

At necropsy the heart weighed 800 gm. Both ventricular cavities were dilated and their walls hypertrophied (Fig 3). Neither atrial cavity was dilated. No foci of myocardial fibrosis or necrosis were noted grossly. The aortic valve was congenitally bicuspid. Each cusp was diffusely fibrotic and retracted but mobile, and devoid of calcium (Fig 3). The valve orifice was not stenotic, but it was incompetent. Both coronary arteries arose in front of the anterior cusp, which contained a raphe. The mitral leaflets were mildly but diffusely thickened by fibrous tissue, but the chordae tendineae were normal. The tricuspid and pulmonic valves were normal. The left ventricular endocardium was diffusely opaque, and the right ventricular endocardium was focally opaque. Histologic examination disclosed multiple typical Aschoff bodies in the endocardium of both atria and in the endocardium and interstitium of both ventricles (Fig 4).

Comments

Although each is a fairly common condition, a congenitally bicuspid aortic valve and rheumatic heart disease have not previously been clearly demonstrated to be present simultaneously in the same patient. Previous studies[1-3] from this laboratory have shown that congenitally bicuspid aortic valves may occur in as high as 2 percent of the population, and the incidence of rheumatic heart disease clinically has been reported to be as high as 6 percent of the population.[4] Thus, it is surprising that the two conditions have not been described previously in the same patient. One of the reasons for this discrepancy may be different criteria utilized for defining the congenitally bicuspid condition of the aortic valve and for designating valvular disease as rheumatic in type. Our criteria for designating an aortic valve as congenitally bicuspid have been delineated elsewhere.[1] In essence, there are only two aortic valve cusps, only two true commissures, and, in about half of the cases, a false commissure or raphe also is present. The cusps are oriented either anteriorly and posteriorly (and if a raphe is present it is always in the anterior cusp) or right and left (and if a raphe is present it is always in the right cusp). The distance circumferentially between any two true commissures is always greater than between a true and a false commissure. The raphe rarely extends as far cephalad in the aorta as do the true commissures.

The only unequivocal criterion of rheumatic heart disease is the presence of Aschoff bodies. Although a number of different stages of Aschoff bodies have been described,[5] only in the granulomatous stage can an Aschoff body be unequivocally identified.[6] In our labo-

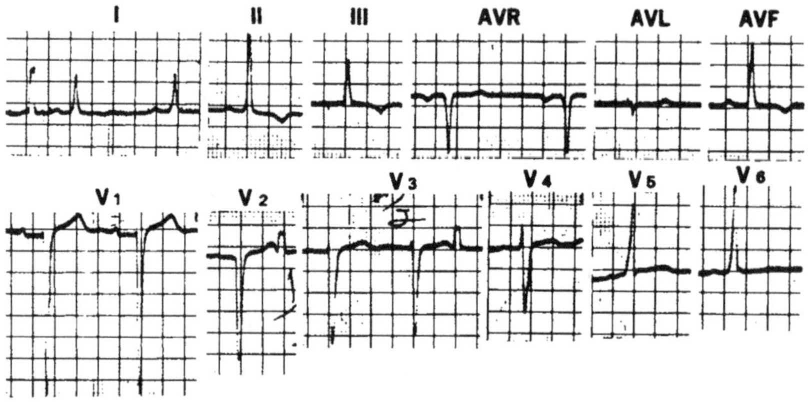

FIGURE 1. Electrocardiogram showing left ventricular hypertrophy and sinus rhythm.

ratory, we have found Aschoff bodies at necropsy or in biopsies of atrial appendages[7] or papillary muscles obtained at operation only in patients with diffuse disease, nearly always stenosis, of the mitral valve. About 5 percent of our patients with fatal mitral valve disease studied at necropsy had Aschoff bodies.[8] We have never observed an Aschoff body in the heart of a patient with anatomically isolated aortic valve disease, *ie*, an anatomically normal mitral valve, and indeed we have been unable to find any report demonstrating an Aschoff body in the heart of a patient with isolated aortic valve disease, irrespective of the number of aortic valve cusps present. Among approximately 200 adult patients with congenitally biscuspid aortic valves studied by us at necropsy, only the patient described herein had an Aschoff body in his heart.

At least two previous authors, however, have mentioned the occurrence of Aschoff bodies in patients with bicuspid aortic valves. Gross[9] described Aschoff bodies in 5 of 16 hearts with "so-called congenital bicuspid aortic valve." It is clear from study of his paper, however, that his criteria for Aschoff bodies were extremely loose, indeed unacceptable, and furthermore that several of his patients almost surely had acquired bicuspid aortic valves rather than congenital malformations. Hall and Ichioka[10] found Aschoff bodies in five of eight patients with "bicuspid aortic valves." Three of these five patients were over 65 years of age and a fourth was 53. Thus,

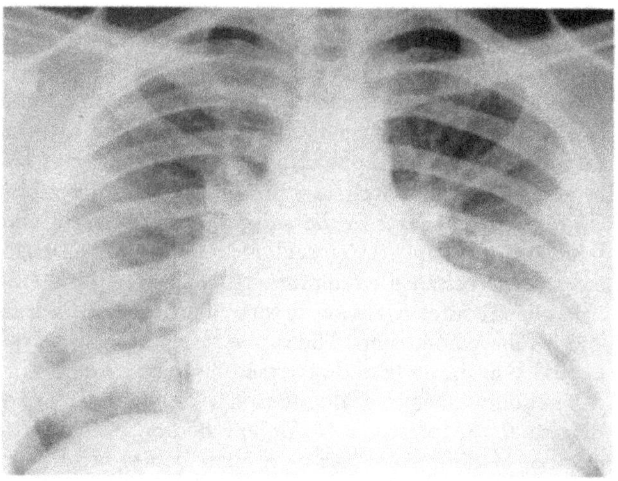

FIGURE 2. Chest roentgenogram showing considerable cardiomegaly of the left ventricular type.

three of their patients may have had aortic valve disease of the elderly, probably degenerative in origin,[3] rather than congenital malformations. These authors also used the loose, nonspecific criteria of Gross and Ehrlich[5] for identification of Aschoff bodies. In addition, none of their five patients had anatomic disease of the mitral valve. To reemphasize, we have never observed an Aschoff body, using the criteria defined by Saphir,[6] in a patient without anatomic disease of the mitral valve. Almost surely in years past there has been an "over-

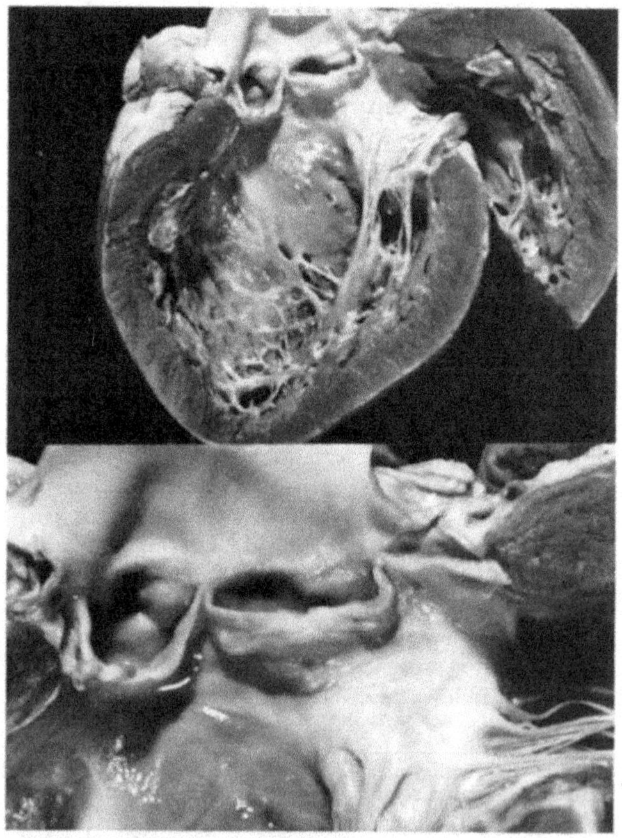

FIGURE 3. Heart. *Upper*: Opened aorta, aortic valve, and left ventricle. The left ventricular cavity is quite dilated, its endocardium mildly thickened, and its wall, very thick. *Lower*: Close-up view of the opened aortic valve. The anterior cusp, the one containing the raphe, has been severed during the opening of the valve. The posterior cusp, from which no coronary arteries arose, is intact. The anterior leaflet of the mitral valve (shown here) also is thickened by fibrous tissue. No inflammatory cells were found in histologic sections of any of the four cardiac valves.

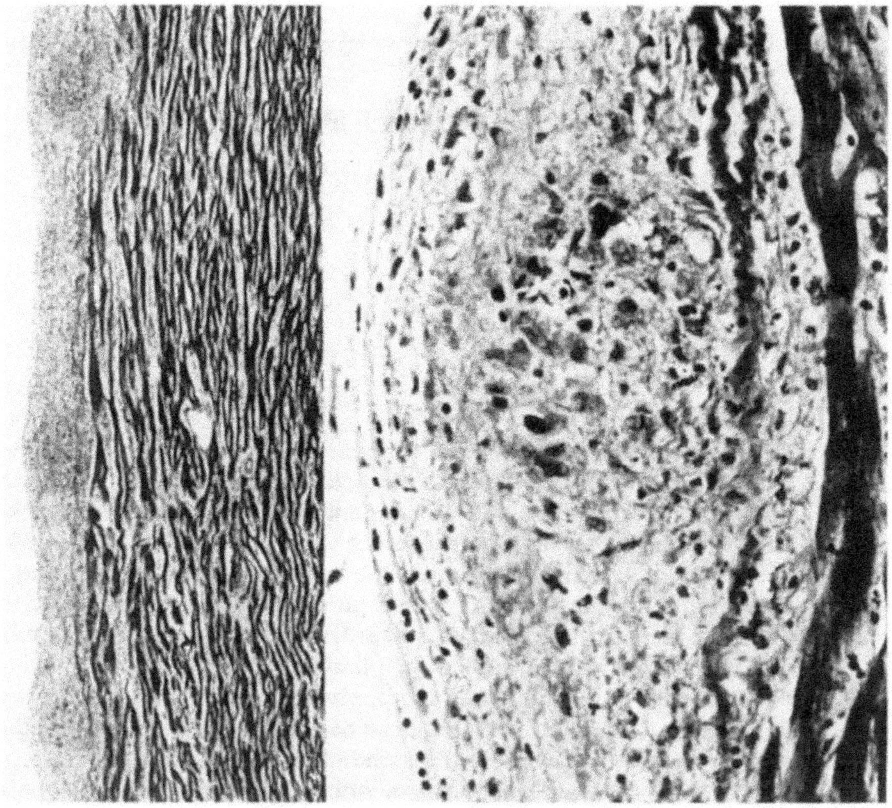

FIGURE 4. Left ventricular endocardium with multiple typical Aschoff bodies. *Left*: Low-power (x55) view showing three discrete Aschoff bodies in the thickened endocardium. *Right*: Close-up (x350) view of one of the Aschoff bodies (hematoxylin and eosin stains).

diagnosis" of Aschoff bodies at necropsy, using loose criteria which may include nonspecific inflammatory lesions of the heart.

Our patient had a classic congenitally bicuspid aortic valve and numerous classic Aschoff bodies in the heart at necropsy. To our knowledge, this combination has neither been clearly documented nor illustrated previously.

References

1 Roberts WC: The congenitally bicuspid aortic valve. A study of 85 autopsy cases. Am J Cardiol 26:72-83, 1970

2 Roberts WC: The structure of the aortic valve in clinically-isolated aortic stenosis. An autopsy study of 162 patients over 15 years of age. Circulation 42:91-97, 1970

3 Roberts WC, Perloff JK, Constantino T: Severe valvular aortic stenosis in patients over 65 years of age. A clinicopathologic study. Am J Cardiol 27:497-506, 1971

4 Marienfield CJ, Robins M, Sandidge RP, et al: Rheumatic fever and rheumatic heart disease among U.S. college freshmen, 1956-60. Pub Health Rep 79:789-811, 1964

5 Gross L, Ehrlich JC: Studies on the myocardial Aschoff body: descriptive classification of lesions. Am J Pathol 10:467-488, 1934

6 Saphir O: The Aschoff nodule (editorial). Am J Clin Pathol 31:534-539, 1959

7 Vermani R, Roberts WC: Incidence and significance of Aschoff bodies in atrial appendages removed at operation: an analysis of 800 patients. (In preparation)

8 Roberts WC: Anatomically isolated aortic valvular disease. The case against its being of rheumatic etiology. Am J Med 49:151-159, 1970

9 Gross L: So-called congenital bicuspid aortic valve. Arch Pathol 23:350-362, 1937

10 Hall EM, Ichioka T: Etiology of calcified nodular aortic stenosis. Am J Pathol 16:761-785, 1940

Congenitally Bicuspid Aortic Valve Causing Severe, Pure Aortic Regurgitation Without Superimposed Infective Endocarditis

Analysis of 13 Patients Requiring Aortic Valve Replacement

WILLIAM C. ROBERTS, MD, FACC
ANDREW G. MORROW, MD, FACC
CHARLES L. McINTOSH, MD
MICHAEL JONES, MD
STEPHEN E. EPSTEIN, MD, FACC

Bethesda, Maryland

Although stenosis and infective endocarditis are commonly appreciated complications of the congenitally bicuspid aortic valve, pure *severe* aortic regurgitation complicating this congenital malformation, unassociated with either stenosis or infection, is not well recognized. Among 189 patients who had aortic valve replacement at the National Heart, Lung, and Blood Institute because of isolated pure aortic regurgitation, the congenitally bicuspid aortic valve, never the site of infective endocarditis, was responsible for the aortic regurgitation in 13 (7 percent). This report describes certain clinical and morphologic findings in 13 men, aged 26 to 65 years (mean 43), who required aortic valve replacement because of severe aortic regurgitation secondary to a noninfected, nonstenotic congenitally bicuspid aortic valve. Although not generally recognized, the noninfected congenitally bicuspid aortic valve is an important cause of pure aortic regurgitation severe enough to warrant aortic valve replacement.

The congenitally bicuspid aortic valve frequently becomes stenotic, and because most stenotic valves are also regurgitant, the most frequent circumstance in which aortic regurgitation is found with this congenital anomaly is in association with aortic valve stenosis.[1] In this situation the aortic regurgitation is usually of only mild or moderate degree. Also, the congenitally bicuspid aortic valve is often the site of infective endocarditis.[1] Although it may be superimposed on a stenotic congenitally bicuspid aortic valve, infective endocarditis far more commonly involves the previously normally functioning bicuspid valve or the one previously only slightly regurgitant.[1,2] The usual consequence of the infection in this circumstance is severe pure aortic regurgitation. Mild degrees of pure aortic regurgitation also are commonly observed in patients with a congenitally bicuspid aortic valve and elevated pressure in the ascending aorta from associated aortic isthmic coarctation. However, *severe* aortic regurgitation due to a nonstenotic and noninfected congenitally bicuspid aortic valve is believed to be decidedly infrequent and, indeed, no reports, to our knowledge, have focused specifically on this complication of the bicuspid valve condition. In this report, we describe observations in 13 men who underwent aortic valve replacement because of severe pure aortic regurgitation unassociated with aortic valve stenosis or infective endocarditis.

From the Pathology, Surgery and Cardiology Branches, National Heart, Lung, and Blood Institute, National Institutes of Health, Bethesda, Maryland. Manuscript received August 4, 1980; revised manuscript received September 16, 1980; accepted September 18, 1980.
Address for reprints: William C. Roberts, MD, Building 10A, Room 3E-30, National Institutes of Health, Bethesda, Maryland 20205.

Clinical Features of Patients

Clinical findings (Table I): At the time of aortic valve replacement, the ages of the 13 men studied ranged from 26 to 65 years (mean 43). Preoperatively, one patient had been in functional class I (New York Heart Association classification[3]), three patients in class II, eight in class III and one in class IV. The one patient who was asymptomatic preop-

TABLE I

Clinical and Operative Observations in 13 Men With Aortic Valve Replacement for Pure Severe Aortic Regurgitation and Noninfected Congenitally Bicuspid Aortic Valve

Case	Age (yr) at AVR	Age (yr) M First Heard	Age (yr) Onset of Cardiac Symptoms	Pressures (s/d) (mm Hg) LV	SA	Site of AV Cusps	AV Raphe	AV Ca^{++}	AV Wt (g)
1	26	17	20	125/25	125/54	R-L	+	0	
2	26	13	21	150/24	150/60	A-P	+	0	1.2
3	28	6	27	200/32	235/70	?		0	1.0
4	30	16	29	135/11	160/55	A-P	0	0	0.9
5	30	27	27	118/6	118/52	R-L	+	0	0.7
6	40	11	35	200/32	200/80	A-P	+	+	2.9
7	46	20	44	125/7	130/50	A-P	+	0	?
8	48	13	40	170/12	170/60	?	+	+	2.2
9	49	20	?	118/5	120/58	R-L	0	0	1.5
10	56	27	27	165/17	165/72	A-P	+	0	1.4
11	57	22	44	160/14	170/75	R-L	+	+	1.8
12	63	45	60	155/7	155/55	?	+	+	2.3
13	65	60	65	138/36	160/53	R-L	+	+	1.7

A = anterior; AV = aortic valve; AVR = aortic valve replacement; Ca^{++} = calcium; L = left; LV = left ventricle; M = murmur; P = posterior; R = right; SA = systemic artery; s/d = peak systole/end-diastole; Wt = weight; ? = not known; + = present or positive; 0 = absent or negative.

eratively underwent aortic valve replacement because of severe aortic regurgitation associated with a dilated left ventricular cavity[4] (left ventricular end-systolic cavity dimension on echocardiogram = 56 mm). None of the 13 patients at any time had had clinical evidence of either active infective endocarditis or acute rheumatic fever.

A precordial murmur had been heard for the first time initially as early as age 6 years to as late as age 60 years (mean 23). By auscultation, all 13 patients had grade 3-5/6 murmurs typical of aortic regurgitation, and by aortic root angiograms the degree of aortic regurgitation was graded in each as either 3+/4+ or 4+/4+. The direct aortic diastolic pressures preoperatively ranged from 45 to 80 mm Hg (mean 61). All 13 patients also had basal precordial systolic murmurs, but at catheterization none had a peak systolic pressure gradient between the left ventricle and a major systemic artery or on pullback from the left ventricle to the aorta. Precordial ejection sounds were absent in all 13 patients. Aortic root angiograms were obtained in all patients, but the bicuspid condition of the aortic valve could not be established by this method. Also, the bicuspid nature of the valve was not recognized in any of the seven patients who had echocardiograms.

Three patients (Cases 3, 4 and 6) had aortic isthmic coarctation, with a peak systolic pressure gradient across the coarctation of 70, 50 and 70 mm Hg, respectively. One (Patient 1) had a right aortic arch. No patient had evidence of mitral regurgitation. The father of Patient 2 had had aortic valve replacement because of a stenotic (60 mm Hg peak systolic pressure gradient) congenitally bicuspid aortic valve.

Surgical and morphologic findings: At aortic valve replacement, only two aortic valve cusps were identified in each of the 13 patients (Fig. 1 to 4). In 10 valves, a

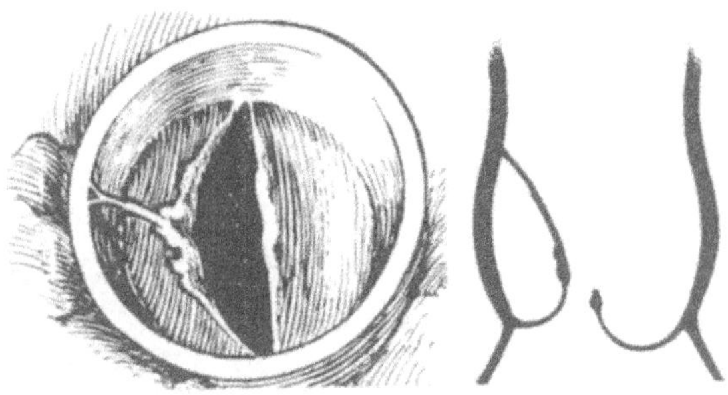

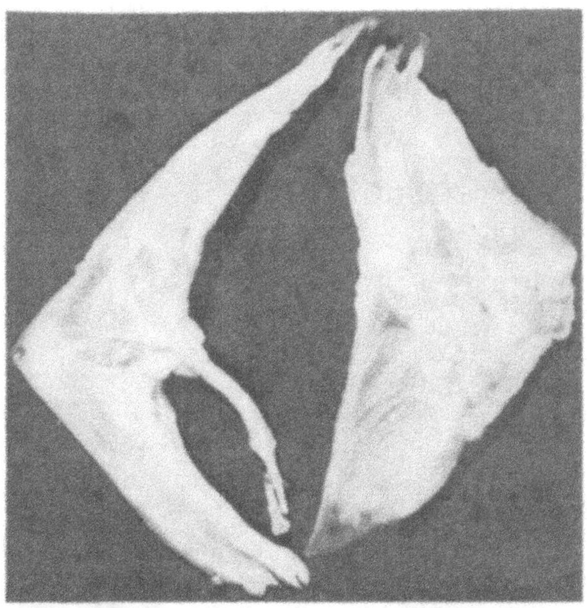

FIGURE 1. Aortic valve in Case 1. The fibrous band on the right cusp (**below**) was attached to the wall of the ascending aorta as shown in the diagram (**above**).

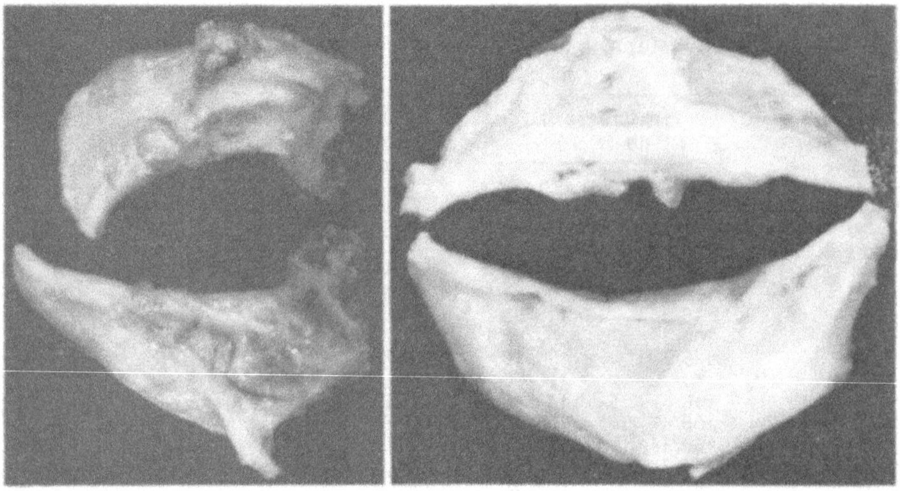

FIGURE 2. Aortic valve in Case 6 (**left**) and Case 7 (**right**). In each valve, the larger cusp is the anterior one. Calcium deposits are present in the valve on the **left**, but not in the one on the **right**.

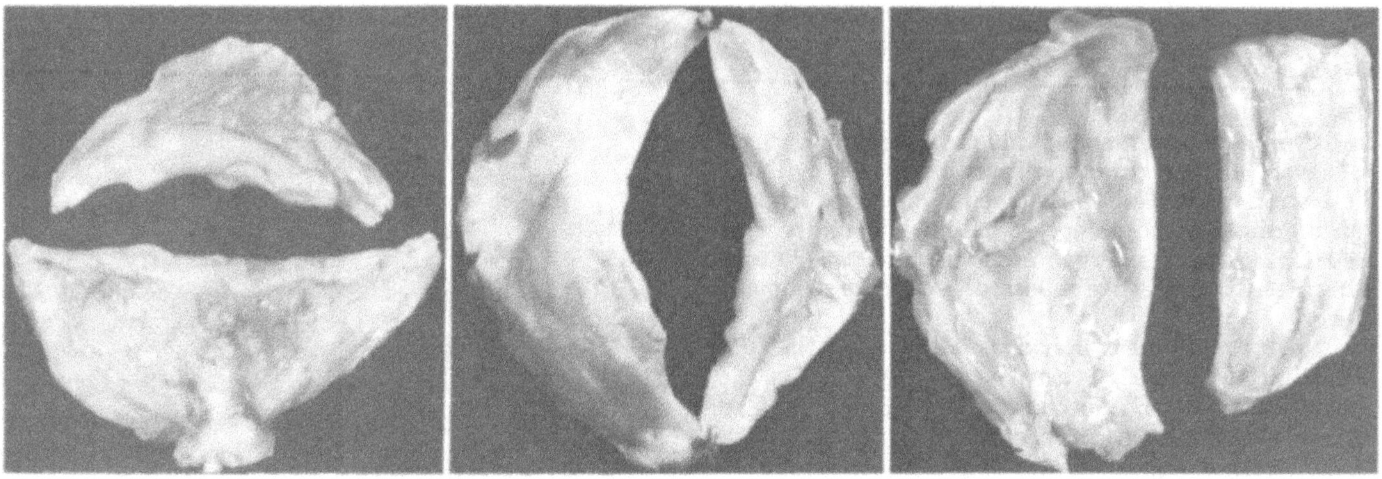

FIGURE 3. Aortic valve in Case 8 (**left**), Case 9 (**middle**) and Case 13 (**right**). The orientation of the cusps is uncertain in Case 8; calcium is present in the raphe in the larger cusp. In both Case 9 and Case 13, the larger cusp is the right one, and the smaller cusp, the left one.

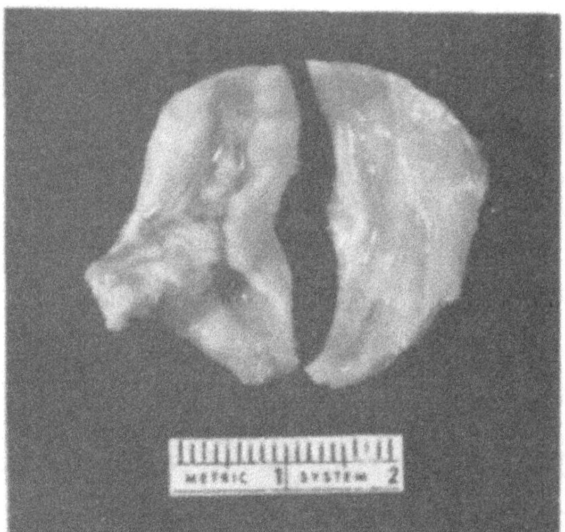

FIGURE 4. Aortic valve in Case 12. The orientation of the two cusps in this patient is not known. The raphe is calcified.

congenital raphe (false commissure) was identified. Each cusp of all 13 aortic valves was thickened by fibrous tissue; no cusp contained vegetations or perforations, indentations, or other evidences of healed infective endocarditis.[5] Calcific deposits, all small, were present in 5 of the 13 excised aortic valves; the deposits in 3 were limited to the raphes.

Comments

Frequency at necropsy of pure regurgitation in bicuspid aortic valve: Each of the 13 patients had aortic regurgitation severe enough to require aortic valve replacement, and at operation each was found to have a congenitally bicuspid aortic valve that neither was stenotic nor had evidence of past infective endocarditis. Furthermore, no patient had had a past clinical illness compatible with active infective endocarditis. Among the complications of a congenitally bicuspid aortic valve, pure severe aortic regurgitation unrelated to infective endocarditis is the least common. Among 200 patients over age 15 years with a congenitally bicuspid aortic valve studied by one of us (W.C.R.) at *necropsy*, only 3 had pure severe aortic regurgitation unassociated with infective endocarditis.[1] Of the 200 necropsy patients, however, 179 had some degree of aortic regurgitation, but it was associated with aortic valve stenosis in 157 and was the result of infective endocarditis in 19; in the remaining 21 patients the bicuspid valve functioned normally. Of 152 necropsy patients with a congenitally bicuspid aortic valve reported on by Fenoglio et al.,[6] 4 apparently had pure aortic regurgitation without evidence of infective endocarditis; however, the severity of the aortic regurgitation in their patients was not stated.

Frequency of congenitally bicuspid valve in pure aortic regurgitation (operative experience): Although the two studies cited provide some information on the frequency of pure aortic regurgitation unassociated with infective endocarditis among *necropsy* patients with a congenitally bicuspid aortic valve, no information is available concerning the frequency of the congenitally bicuspid aortic valve unassociated with infective endocarditis among patients with pure *severe* aortic regurgitation. Accordingly, we reviewed the clinical and operative records and the excised aortic valves in 189 patients aged 18 to 70 years who had aortic valve replacement at the National Heart, Lung, and Blood Institute from 1963 to 1979 because of *isolated* (unassociated with dysfunction of another cardiac valve) *pure* (no element of valve stenosis) aortic regurgitation (Table II). In 13 (7 percent) of the 189 patients the aortic regurgitation was the result of a congenitally bicuspid aortic valve that was not and had not been the site of infective endocarditis. In contrast to the 13 patients that form the basis of this report, only 7 patients (among the 189) had pure aortic regurgitation because of infective endocarditis involving a congenitally bicuspid aortic valve. Thus, the congenitally bicuspid aortic valve unaffected by infective endocarditis is an important cause of pure aortic regurgitation severe enough to warrant aortic valve replacement.

TABLE II

Etiology of Isolated Pure Aortic Regurgitation in 189 Patients Aged 18 to 70 Years Having Aortic Valve Replacement

Cause	Patients n	Patients %
1.* Rheumatic	94	49
2.* Infective endocarditis	41	22
Bicuspid (n = 7)		
Tricuspid (n = 34)		
3. Marfan and Marfan-type	15	8
4.* Congenital (bicuspid valve)	13	7
5.* Prolapse from ventricular septal defect	10	5
6. Syphilis	9	5
7. Aortic dissection	2	7 (7–10)
8. Ankylosing spondylitis	2	
9.* With subaortic stenosis	2	4 (7–10)
Discrete subaortic stenosis (n = 1)		
Hypertrophic cardiomyopathy (n = 1)		
10. Trauma	1	
Total	189	100

* Aortic regurgitation resulted from abnormality of the aortic valve only and not from abnormality of the aorta.

References

1. **Roberts WC.** The congenitally bicuspid aortic valve. A study of 85 autopsy cases. Am J Cardiol 1960;23:72–83.
2. **Roberts WC.** Characteristics and consequences of infective endocarditis (active or healed or both) learned from morphologic studies. In: Rahimtoola SH, ed. Infective Endocarditis. New York; Grune & Stratton, 1978;55–123.
3. Criteria Committee of the New York Heart Association. Nomenclature and Criteria for Diseases of the Heart and Great Vessels. 8th ed. Boston; Little, Brown, 1979:349.
4. **Henry WL, Bonow RO, Rosing DR, Epstein SE.** Observations on the optimum time for operative intervention for aortic regurgitation. II. Serial echocardiographic evaluation of asymptomatic patients. Circulation 1980;61:484–92.
5. **Roberts WC, Buchbinder NA.** Healed left-sided infective endocarditis: a clinicopathologic study of 59 patients. Am J Cardiol 1977; 40:876–88.
6. **Fenoglio JJ, McAllister HA, DeCastro CM.** The congenital bicuspid aortic valve after age 20. Am J Cardiol 1977;39:164–9.

Electrocardiographic observations in severe aortic valve stenosis: Correlative necropsy study to clinical, hemodynamic, and ECG variables demonstrating relation of 12-lead QRS amplitude to peak systolic transaortic pressure gradient

Most ECG studies in patients with aortic valve stenosis (AS) have involved living patients in whom the status of the left ventricular (LV) myocardium, epicardial coronary arteries, and mitral valve was not precisely known. We examined the 12-lead ECG recorded within 2 months of death in 50 patients aged 16 to 65 years (mean 48) with peak systolic pressure gradients (PSPG) across the aortic valve ranging from 52 to 180 mm Hg (mean 98) and anatomically normal mitral valves. Excluding four patients with complete left bundle branch block (LBBB), 44 (96%) of the other 46 patients had the usual voltage criteria for LV hypertrophy (LVH). Measurement of the total 12-lead QRS amplitude, which ranged from 144 to 417 mm (10 mm = 1 mV), (mean 257) proved useful for it correlated directly with PSPG across the aortic valve and, when the four LBBB patients were excluded, with the peak LV systolic pressure. The total 12-lead QRS amplitude (mm) was similar in most patients to the LV systolic pressure (mm Hg). Thus, subtraction of the indirect systemic arterial systolic pressure (mm Hg) from the total 12-lead QRS amplitude (mm) provides a reasonable noninvasive prediction of the PSPG across the aortic valve in patients with moderate to severe AS. Additionally, the mean of the total 12-lead QRS amplitude was significantly ($p < 0.05$) greater in the 11 younger (≤ 40 years) than in the 39 older patients (278 mm vs 257 mm), in the 14 women than in the 36 men (277 mm vs 249 mm), in the 22 patients with heavier (> 600 gm) hearts (274 mm vs 244 mm), in the 34 patients without compared to the 16 with significant coronary arterial narrowing (270 mm vs 238 mm), and in the 22 patients without compared to the 24 with ECG myocardial damage patterns (269 mm vs 236 mm). (Am Heart J 103:210, 1982.)

Robert J. Siegel, M.D., and William C. Roberts, M.D. *Bethesda, Md.*

The usual ECG findings in patients with aortic valve stenosis (AS) are well recognized, the most characteristic one being excessive voltage indicative of left ventricular hypertrophy (LVH). Among adults with AS and ECG criteria of LVH, the latter correlate poorly with the presence of symptoms of cardiac dysfunction, the amount of obstruction across the aortic valve, or prognosis in the absence of symptoms. Adults with AS frequently also have associated atherosclerotic coronary disease (CAD) which also may alter the ECG. In most ECG studies in adults with AS, the status of the coronary arteries, LV myocardium and mitral valve (MV), and the weight of the heart have not been known. In studies before 1950, the pressure gradient across the aortic valve was not available.

In an attempt to determine the ECG finding attributable only to AS, with or without aortic regurgitation (AR), we analyzed the ECG in 50 necropsy patients aged 16 to 65 years with severe or moderately severe AS, all of whom had ECG and cardiac catheterization performed within 2 months of death, and thorough examination of the major coronary arteries, LV myocardium and MV at necropsy. The total amplitude of the QRS complexes in all 12 leads was measured in each patient

From the Pathology Branch, National Heart, Lung and Blood Institute, National Institutes of Health.

Received for publication Sept. 4, 1981; accepted Sept. 28, 1981.

Reprint requests: William C. Roberts, M.D., Pathology Branch, NHLBI-NIH, Bldg. 10A, Room 3E-30, Bethesda, MD 20205.

Table I. Clinical and necropsy finding in severe isolated aortic valve stenosis

Parameter	*Number*
1. Age (years)	16-65 (mean 48)
2. Male: female (pts)	36:14
3. Angina pectoris (pts)	34
4. Pressures (mm Hg)	
Left ventricle (LV) peak systolic	149-270 (avg 210)
Systemic artery (SA) systolic	63-180 (avg 112)
LV-SA peak systolic gradient	52-180 (avg 98)
LV end-diastolic	4-45 (avg 18)
SA end-diastolic	34*-88 (avg 62)
Cardiac index (L/min/m²)	1.3-4.5 (mean 2.7)
Aortic valve area (cm²)	0.16-0.89 (mean 0.53)
Aortic valve area index (cm²/BSA)	0.16-0.44 (mean 0.29)
5. Aortic regurgitation murmur (pts)	24
6. Heart weight (Gm)	380-880 (mean 606)
7. Narrowed (> 75%) coronary artery (pts)	16
8. Gross LV scar (pts)	7

*LVSP only 63 mm in this patient.
pts = patients.

and correlated with the age, sex, pressure gradient across the aortic valve, LV peak systolic pressure, heart weight, and the presence of angina pectoris, CAD, LV scarring, and ECG myocardial damage pattern.

METHODS

Patient criteria. Criteria for patient inclusion in this study included the following: (1) peak systolic pressure gradient across the aortic valve of > 50 mm Hg demonstrated at catheterization within 2 months of death; (2) age of death > 15 years and < 66 years; (3) ECG recorded within 2 months of death and available for reexamination, and recorded before an operation was performed on the aortic valve; and (4) anatomically normal MV, tricuspid, and pulmonic valves at necropsy. The first 50 patients in the files of the Pathology Branch, NHLBI, fulfilling these above four criteria form the basis of this study.

ECG criteria. ECG criteria utilized for LVH were the point-score system of Romhilt and Estes.[1] Four or more points were considered evidence of LVH. A LV strain pattern was diagnosed when the ST segment was displaced and the T wave was directed 180 degrees away from the major QRS axis at least in leads V_5 and V_6. Left atrial (LA) abnormality was diagnosed when the P wave in lead V_1 was diphasic with the negative component reaching at least 1 mm in amplitude and at least 120 msec in width, and when the P wave in leads I, II, or aV_L was notched and at least 120 msec in width. Right atrial (RA) abnormality was diagnosed when the P wave amplitude in leads II, III, of aV_F was 3 mm or greater. Left axis deviation (LAD) was diagnosed when the QRS axis in the frontal plane was −30 degrees or less and right axis deviation (RAD) when it was 110 degrees or greater. Left bundle branch block (LBBB) was defined by: (1) QRS duration > 12 seconds in the extremity leads; (2) presence of broad monophasic R wave in leads I, V_5 and V_6, and (3) displacement of the ST segment and T wave 180 degrees away from the major QRS defection. Two myocardial damage patterns were diagnosed: type A, when the R wave in V_1 was absent and < 5 mm in amplitude in lead V_3; type B, when Q waves > 30 msec were present in two or more leads posteriorly (leads II, III, aV_F) or laterally (leads I, aV_L, V_4 to V_6).

Table II. ECG observations in severe isolated aortic valve stenosis

Finding	*Number*
1. Rhythm (pts)	
Sinus	45
Atrial fibrillation	5
2. Atrial abnormality (pts)	
Left only	16
Right only	0
Both	1
3. Ventricular premature complexes (pts)	7
4. PR interval > 0.20 sec (pts)	7
5. Left axis deviation (pts)	12
6. Left ventricular hypertrophy and strain without BBB (pts)	44
7. Left bundle branch block (BBB) (pts)	4
8. QRS amplitude (mm)	
All 12 leads	144-417 (mean 257)
Leads I-III only	12-78 (mean 39)
9. Myocardial damage pattern (without BBB) (pts)	24
A. Poor precordial R-wave progression	18
B. Q waves > 30 ms in ≥ 2 leads	2
1. II, III, AVF = 2	
2. I, AVL, V_{4-6} = 0	
C. A + B1	2
D. A + B2	2

Clinical observations. The 50 patients ranged in age from 16 to 65 years (mean 48); 36 (72%) were male and 14 (28%) were female (Table I). The peak systolic pressure gradient between LV and systemic artery ranged from 52 to 180 mm Hg (mean 98), the aortic valve area (AVA) from 0.16 to 0.89 cm² (mean 0.53), the AVA indices from 0.16 to 0.44 cm²/m² (mean 0.29) and the cardiac index (CI) from 1.3 to 4.7 L/min/m² (mean 2.7). Precordial murmurs of AR were recorded in 24 patients (48%) and AR was observed by angiography in 4 of the 13 patients in whom contrast material was injected into the proximal portion of ascending aorta. Of the 50 patients, 34 (68%) had angina pectoris; none had had a clinical event compatible with acute myocardial infarction. An operation on the aortic valve was performed in 38 (76%) patients: 20 died within 24 hours of operation, 11 others within 2 weeks, and seven

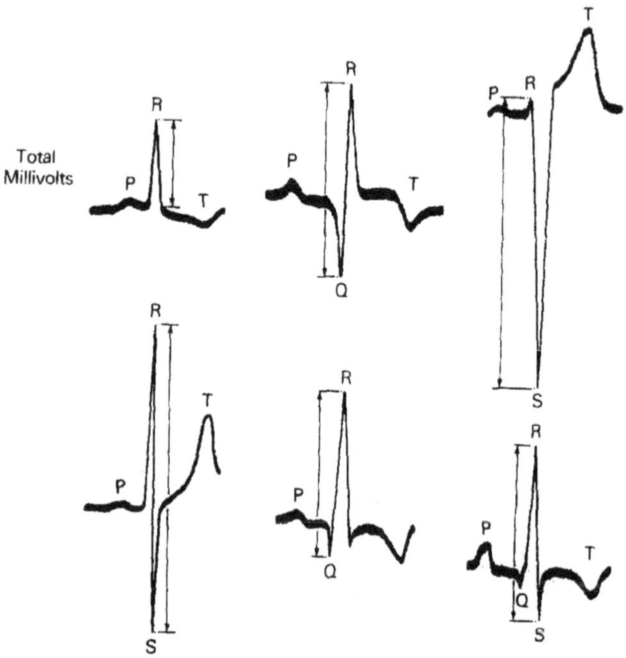

Fig. 1. Various QRS complexes showing how each was measured.

others from 2 to 6 weeks postoperatively. Two other patients died during induction of anesthesia or during the skin incision for planned aortic valve operation. All 50 patients were in functional classes III or IV (New York Heart Association classification). In the 10 unoperated patients, aortic valve operations had been planned or recommended in each, but death occurred, usually suddenly, before they were performed.

Necropsy observations. The hearts ranged in weight from 380 to 880 gm (mean 606). All were examined by one of us (WCR) and most by RJS as well (Table I). The number of cusps in the aortic valve (identified at operation by the surgeon, by examination of the excised valve by one of us [WCR] or from examination of the heart at necropsy) were the following: one cusp (unicuspid unicommissural) = five patients (10%); two cusps (bicuspid) = 29 patients (58%); three cusps (tricuspid) = 15 patients (30%); and uncertain structure =one patient. One or more of the four major epicardial coronary arteries was narrowed > 75% in cross-sectional area by atherosclerotic plaques in 16 patients (32%). LV scars were present at necropsy in seven patients (14%) and in each they were relatively small: subendocardial (inner one half of wall) only in two patients and transmural (> the inner one half of the wall) in five patients. Only one patient had gross evidence of LV necrosis and this patient died 33 days after the ring of a caged-ball prosthesis had severely narrowed the ostium of his right coronary artery.

RESULTS

General ECG observations. These are summarized in Table II. Sinus rhythm was present in 45 patients and chronic atrial fibrillation in five. None had atrial premature contractions or supraventricular tachycardia recorded; seven patients had ventricular premature complexes recorded. Abnormal configuration of the P wave was recorded in 16 patients, of the LA type in 15. The PR interval was greater than 0.20 second in seven patients. LAD was present in 12 patients and none had RAD. Four patients had LBBB and none had right bundle branch block or complete heart block. Excluding the four patients with LBBB, 44 (99%) of the remaining 46 patients had ECG evidence of LVH, with a LV strain pattern in 43. Although all 50 patients at necropsy had right ventricular hypertrophy (RVH), none had ECG evidence of RVH.[1] Myocardial damage patterns were present in 24 patients: poor precordial R-wave progression only in 18 patients, Q waves > 30 msec in width in two or more leads only in two patients, and combinations of the two in four patients. In each of the 12 leads in all 50 patients, the amplitude of the QRS complexes were measured from the peak of the R wave to the maximal dip of the S or Q wave, whichever was greatest (Fig. 1). The sum of the amplitude of the QRS complexes in all 12 leads in the 50 patients ranged from 144 to 417 mm (mean 257) (10 mm = 1 mV) and the sum of the amplitude of the QRS complexes in leads I, II, and III in all patients ranged from 12 to 78 mm (mean 39).

Correlation of age and gender to clinical, hemodynamic, ECG, and necropsy findings. Compared to the 11 patients aged 40 years and under, the 39 patients over age 40 had a higher frequency of angina pectoris (30 of 39 [77%] vs 4 of 11) ($p < 0.005$), lower average peak systolic pressure gradients across the aortic valve (94 mm Hg vs 113 mm Hg) ($p < 0.025$), more frequent significant CAD (16 of 39 [41%] vs 0 of 11) and LV scarring (7 of 39 [18%] vs 0 of 12) ($p < 0.025$), and lower average total QRS amplitude in the 12 leads (257 mm vs 278 mm) ($p < 0.05$). (Table III). Compared to the 14 women, the 36 men had lower average peak systolic pressure gradients between LV and a systemic artery (91 mm Hg vs 144 mm Hg) ($p < 0.01$), higher mean heart weights (639 gm vs 521 gm) ($p < 0.01$), and lower total QRS amplitude in the 12 leads (249 mm vs 277 mm) ($p < 0.05$) (Table IV).

Correlation of transaortic pressure gradient, LV systolic pressure and heart weight to clinical, hemodynamic, ECG, and necropsy findings. The total amplitude of the QRS complexes in the 12 leads in the 33 patients with LV to systemic arterial peak systolic pressure gradients ≤ 100 mm Hg (mean 82) averaged 244 mm and in the 17 patients with higher gradients, 281 mm ($p < 0.05$) (Table V). The average LV peak systolic pressure in the patients with

Table III. Comparison of 12 patients aged 16 to 40 years to 38 patients aged 41 to 65 years with isolated severe aortic valve stenosis

Age (years)	*16-40 (n = 11)*	*41-65 (n = 39)*	*p value*
Mean age (years)	31	53	< 0.0005
Male:Female (pts)	6:5	30:9	ns
Angina pectoris (pts)	4	30 (77%)	< 0.005
LV-SA psg (mm Hg)	70-180 (113)	52-145 (94)	< 0.025
LVSP (mm Hg)	175-270 (220)	149-260 (208)	ns
Aortic valve area (cm²)	0.40-0.58 (.44)	0.16-0.89 (0.54)	ns
CI (L/min/m²)	2.0-4.3 (2.9)	1.6-4.8 (2.5)	ns
Heart weight (gm)	380-880 (593)	400-880 (614)	ns
CA narrowing > 75% (pts)	0	16 (41%)	< 0.025
LV scar (pts)	0	7 (18%)	ns
Electrocardiogram			
VPC (pts)	1 (9%)	6 (15%)	ns
LAD (pts)	1 (9%)	11 (28%)	ns
MDP (pts)	6 (55%)	18 (46%)	ns
QRS amplitude (mm)			
12 leads	193-395 (278)	144-417 (257)	< 0.05
I-III	26-58 (40)	12-78 (38)	ns

Abbreviations: CA = coronary artery; LAD = left axis deviation; LV = left ventricular; LVSP = left ventricular systolic pressure; MDP = myocardial damage pattern; psg = peak systolic pressure gradient; SA = systemic artery, VPC = ventricular premature complex; ns = $p > 0.05$.

Table IV. Comparison of 35 men to 15 women with severe isolated aortic valve stenosis

Sex	*Men (n = 36)*	*Women (n = 14)*	*p value*
Age (years)	16-64 (48)	16-65 (47)	ns
Angina pectoris (pts)	23 (64%)	11 (79%)	ns
LV-SA psg (mm Hg)	52-160 (91)	70-180 (107)	< 0.01
LVSP (mm Hg)	149-260 (203)	192-270 (228)	< 0.01
Aortic valve areas (cm²)	0.16-0.89 (0.59)	0.28-0.54 (0.42)	< 0.0025
CI (L/min/m²)	1.2-4.8 (2.7)	2.0-4.2 (2.7)	ns
Heart weight (gm)	440-880 (639)	380-700 (521)	< 0.01
CA narrowing > 75% (pts)	11 (31%)	5 (36%)	ns
LV scar (pts)	6 (17%)	1 (7%)	ns
Electrocardiogram			
VPC (pts)	5 (14%)	2 (14%)	ns
LAD (pts)	10 (28%)	2 (14%)	ns
MDP (pts)	19 (53%)	5 (40%)	ns
QRS amplitude (mm)			
12 leads	144-417 (249)	193-376 (277)	< 0.05
I-III	12-78 (36)	27-72 (47)	< 0.002

Abbreviations as in Table III.

gradients ≤ 100 mm Hg was 198 mm Hg and in those with higher gradients, 234 mm Hg ($p < 0.0005$).

The 22 patients with peak LV systolic pressure ≤ 200 mm Hg had smaller peak systolic pressure gradients across the aortic valve (80 mm Hg vs 122 mm Hg) ($p < 0.0005$) and lower total QRS amplitudes (247 mm vs 265 mm) ($p < 0.05$) than did those with higher pressures (Table VI). Compared to the 28 patients with smaller hearts, the 22 patients with hearts weighing over 600 gm were more often men (20 of 22 [91%] vs 16 of 28 [57%]) ($p < 0.025$), had lower average LV peak systolic pressures (205 mm Hg vs 214 mm Hg) ($p < 0.05$), more commonly had LAD (39% vs 7%) ($p < 0.01$), and higher average total QRS amplitude (274 mm vs 244 mm) ($p < 0.025$) (Table VII).

Correlation of angina, CAD, and LV scarring to clinical, hemodynamic, ECG, and necropsy findings. The 34 patients with angina had smaller mean heart

Table V. Comparison of 33 patients with transaortic peak systolic pressure gradients (psg) of 51 to 100 mm Hg to 17 patients with gradients >100 mm Hg in isolated severe aortic valve stenosis

LV-SA psg (mm Hg)	*51-100 (n = 33)*	*>100 (n = 17)*	*p value*
Age (years)	16-65 (50)	18-63 (46)	ns
Male:female (pts)	28:5	8:9	< 0.005
Angina pectoris (pts)	24 (73%)	10 (59%)	ns
LV-SA psg (mm Hg)	52-100 (82)	105-180 (135)	< 0.0005
LVSP (mm Hg)	149-255 (198)	192-270 (234)	< 0.0005
Aortic valve areas (cm^2)	0.30-0.67 (0.54)	0.28-0.89 (0.50)	ns
CI ($L/min/m^2$)	1.3-4.3 (2.49)	2.0-4.5 (2.79)	ns
Heart weight (gm)	380-880 (583)	400-770 (612)	ns
CA narrowing > 75% (pts)	12 (36%)	4 (23%)	ns
LV scar (pts)	6 (18%)	1 (6%)	ns
Electrocardiogram			
VPC (pts)	6 (18%)	1 (6%)	ns
LAD (pts)	9 (27%)	3 (3%)	ns
MDP (pts)	15 (45%)	9 (53%)	ns
QRS amplitude (mm)			
12 leads	144-417 (244)	216-370 (281)	< 0.05
I-III	12-78 (37)	25-58 (41)	ns

Abbreviations as in Table III.

Table VI. Comparison of 22 patients with peak left ventricular systolic pressure (LVSP) ≤ 200 mm Hg to 28 patients with LVSP > 200 mm Hg in isolated severe aortic valve stenosis

LVSP (mm Hg)	*≤200 (n = 22)*	*>200 (n = 28)*	*p value*
Age (years)	18-65 (49)	16-64 (48)	ns
Male:female (pts)	19:3	17:11	ns
Angina pectoris (pts)	14 (64%)	20 (71%)	ns
LV-SA psg (mm Hg)	52-129 (80)	60-180 (112)	< 0.0005
LVSP (mm Hg)	149-200 (185)	202-270 (230)	< 0.0005
Aortic valve areas (cm^2)	0.3-0.7 (0.54)	0.2-0.9 (0.51)	ns
CI ($L/min/m^2$)	1.3-3.7 (2.49)	1.8-4.5 (2.68)	ns
Heart weight (gm)	410-880 (613)	380-880 (600)	ns
CA narrowing > 75% (pts)	8 (36%)	8 (29%)	ns
LV scar (pts)	4 (18%)	3 (11%)	ns
Electrocardiogram	3 (14%)	4 (14%)	ns
VPC (pts)			
LAD (pts)	7 (32%)	5 (18%)	ns
MDP (pts)	11 (50%)	13 (46%)	ns
QRS amplitude (mm)			
12 leads	144-417 (247)	193-395 (265)	< 0.05
I-III	12-78 (38)	20-58 (39)	ns

Abbreviations as in Table III.

weights than the 16 patients without (580 gm vs 661 gm) ($p < 0.025$), more frequent ventricular premature complexes recorded (7 of 34 vs 0 of 16) ($p < 0.05$), less frequent occurrence of LAD (3 of 34 vs 9 of 16) ($p < 0.0005$), and higher QRS amplitude in leads I to III (42 mm vs 32 mm) ($p < 0.005$) (Table VIII). Compared to the 34 patients with lesser degrees of coronary narrowing, the 16 patients with > 75% cross-sectional area coronary narrowing by atherosclerotic plaques of one or more of the four major (right, left main, left anterior descending, left circumflex) epicardial coronary arteries were older (54 years vs 46 years) ($p < 0.01$), had higher frequency of LV scars at necropsy (31% vs 6%) ($p < 0.01$), ECG myocardial damage patterns (81% vs 32%) ($p < 0.025$), and lower total 12-lead QRS amplitude (238 mm vs 270 mm) ($p < 0.05$) (Table IX). No significant differences occurred in the amount of ST segment depression or the depth of T wave inversion between patients with and without significant coronary narrowing. Compared to the 43 patients without, the seven patients with grossly visible LV scars were older (53 years vs 47 years) ($p < 0.05$), had lower average peak systolic gradients across the

Table VII. Comparison of 28 patients with heart weight ≤600 gm to 22 patients with larger hearts in isolated severe aortic valve stenosis

Heart weight (gm)	*≤600 (n = 28)*	*>600 (n = 22)*	*p value*
Age (years)	16-65 (49)	31-64 (48)	ns
Male:female (pts)	16:12	20:2	< 0.025
Angina pectoris (pts)	21 (75%)	13 (59%)	ns
LV-SA psg (mm Hg)	52-180 (97)	52-160 (99)	ns
LVSP (mm Hg)	149-270 (214)	155-255 (250)	< 0.05
Aortic valve areas (cm^2)	0.28-0.89 (0.28)	0.4-0.68 (0.32)	ns
CI ($L/min/m^2$)	1.28-4.5 (2.74)	1.8-3.2 (2.46)	ns
Heart weight (gm)	380-600 (517)	610-880 (719)	< 0.0005
CA narrowing > 75% (pts)	10 (36%)	6 (27%)	ns
LV scar (pts)	3 (11%)	4 (18%)	ns
Electrocardiogram			
VPC (pts)	3 (11%)	4 (18%)	ns
LAD (pts)	3 (11%)	9 (41%)	< 0.01
MDP (pts)	16 (57%)	8 (36%)	ns
QRS amplitude (mm)			
12 leads	144-376 (244)	200-417 (274)	< 0.025
I-III	12-72 (39)	21-78 (39)	ns

Abbreviations as in Table III.

Table VIII. Comparison of 34 angina patients to 16 patients without angina in isolated severe aortic valve stenosis

Angina pectoris	*Present (n = 34)*	*Absent (n = 16)*	*p value*
Age (years)	18-65 (50)	16-63 (45)	ns
Male:female (pts)	27:7	9:7	ns
LV-SA psg (mm Hg)	52-180 (97)	70-153 (99)	ns
LVSP (mm Hg)	149-270 (212)	175-255 (203)	ns
Aortic valve areas (cm^2)	0.16-0.89 (0.54)	0.30-0.77 (0.05)	ns
CI ($L/min/m^2$)	1.8-4.7 (2.7)	1.2-4.3 (2.5)	ns
Heart weight (gm)	380-840 (580)	410-880 (661)	< 0.025
CA narrowing > 75% (pts)	12 (35%)	4 (25%)	ns
LV scar (pts)	6 (18%)	1 (6%)	ns
Electrocardiogram			
VPC (pts)	7 (21%)	0	< 0.05
LAD (pts)	3 (9%)	9 (56%)	< 0.0005
MDP (pts)	14 (41%)	10 (62%)	ns
QRS amplitude (mm)			
12 leads	144-417 (265)	162-395 (242)	ns
I-III	19-78 (42)	12-50 (32)	< 0.005

Abbreviations as in Table III.

aortic valve (77 mm Hg vs 101 mm Hg) ($p < 0.025$), and more frequent CAD (6 of 7 vs 9 of 43) ($p < 0.001$) (Table X).

Correlation of ECG myocardial damage pattern, QRS amplitude, AF and LBBB to clinical, hemodynamic, ECG, and necropsy findings. Excluding the four patients with LBBB, the mean total 12-lead QRS amplitude was lower in the 24 patients with ECG myocardial damage patterns than in the 24 patients without (243 mm vs 269 mm) ($p < 0.05$) (Table XI). Compared to the 26 patients with total 12-lead QRS amplitude ≤ 250 mm, the 24 patients in whom this amplitude was > 250 mm had a higher frequency of angina pectoris (79% vs 58%) ($p < 0.001$) and a lower frequency of ECG myocardial damage patterns (33% vs 58%) ($p < 0.01$) (Table XII).

The five patients (four men) with *atrial fibrillation* (AF) ranged in age from 45 to 63 years (mean 53) and the peak systolic pressure gradients across their aortic valves, from 52 to 140 mm Hg (average 75). Three had LAD, three had ventricular premature complexes, and three had ECG myocardial damage patterns (poor R wave progression in precordial leads). The total 12-lead QRS amplitude ranged from 199 to 306 mm (mean 245), and in the other 33 patients over age 40 years with sinus rhythm it averaged 259 mm. The QRS amplitude in leads I to III ranged from 21 to 51 mm (mean 31).

Table IX. Comparison of 15 patients with severe coronary narrowing to 35 patients without CAD in isolated severe aortic valve stenosis

Coronary narrowing	*≤75%* *(n = 16)*	*>75%* *(n = 34)*	*p value*
Age (years)	16-65 (46)	41-64 (54)	< 0.01
Male:female (pts)	24:10	12:4	ns
Angina pectoris (pts)	23 (68%)	11 (69%)	ns
LV-SA psg (mm Hg)	52-180 (99)	60-145 (95)	ns
LVSP (mm Hg)	145-270 (209)	149-260 (208)	ns
Aortic valve areas (cm^2)	0.28-0.89 (0.47)	0.33-0.77 (0.44)	ns
CI ($L/min/m^2$)	1.28-4.5 (2.7)	1.8-3.2 (2.5)	ns
Heart weight (gm)	380-880 (602)	450-840 (615)	ns
LV scar (pts)	2 (6%)	5 (31%)	< 0.01
Electrocardiogram			
VPC (pts)	6 (18%)	1 (6%)	ns
LAD (pts)	9 (26%)	3 (19%)	ns
MDP (pts)	11 (32%)	13 (81%)	< 0.025
QRS amplitude (mm)			
12 leads	144-329 (270)	162-417 (238)	< 0.05
I-III	12-78 (35)	19-57 (41)	ns
ST segment depression*	0-0.4 (0.17)	0-0.2 (0.13)	ns
T wave inversion depth*	0-13 (4.9)	0-6 (3.8)	ns

*Excludes patients with complete bundle branch block.
Abbreviations as in Table III.

Table X. Comparison of seven patients with grossly visible left ventricular scars to 43 patients without scar in isolated severe aortic valve stenosis

LV scar	*Present* *(n = 7)*	*Absent* *(n = 43)*	*p value*
Age (years)	16-65 (47)	41-64 (53)	< 0.05
Male:female (pts)	6:1	30:13	ns
Angina pectoris (pts)	6	28 (65%)	ns
LV-SA psg (mm Hg)	52-111 (77)	52-180 (101)	< 0.025
LVSP (mm Hg)	149-240 (196)	175-270 (212)	ns
Aortic valve areas (cm^2)	0.52-0.68 (0.60)	0.16-0.89 (0.50)	ns
CI ($L/min/m^2$)	1.8-2.6 (2.2)	1.3-4.5 (2.3)	ns
Heart weight (gm)	450-840 (646)	380-880 (599)	ns
CA narrowing >75% (pts)	6	9 (21%)	< 0.001
Electrocardiogram			
VPC (pts)	2	5 (12%)	ns
LAD (pts)	2	13 (30%)	ns
MDP (pts)	5	19 (44%)	ns
QRS amplitude (mm)			
12 leads	144-417 (259)	162-395 (257)	ns
I-III	19-78 (37)	12-72 (39)	ns

Abbreviations as in Table III.

The hearts ranged in weight from 520 to 750 gm (mean 645). The aortic valves were tricuspid in four and bicuspid in one. Two of the five patients had one or more major coronary arteries narrowed > 75% in cross-sectional area by atherosclerotic plaques and one of them had a small transmural LV scar. Four patients had no grossly visible LV scarring.

The four patients with *complete LBBB* were aged 19 to 56 years (mean 42); three were over age 40 years. Two were women and two were men. All four had sinus rhythm, three had LAD, one had prolonged PR interval, and two had LA abnormality. The peak systolic pressure gradients were 75, 75, 102, and 145 mm Hg (average 100) and the total 12-lead QRS amplitude was 256, 417, 376, and 216 mm (mean 316), respectively. In the other 46

Table XI. Comparison of 24 patients with myocardial damage pattern (in absence of bundle branch block) to 22 patients without in isolated severe aortic valve stenosis

Myocardial damage pattern	*Present (n = 24)*	*Absent (n = 22)*	*p value*
Age (years)	16-63 (48)	31-65 (50)	ns
Male:female (pts)	19:5	15:7	ns
Angina pectoris (pts)	14 (58%)	15 (68%)	ns
LV-SA psg (mm Hg)	52-180 (102)	52-160 (94)	ns
LVSP (mm Hg)	149-270 (213)	175-255 (209)	ns
Aortic valve areas (cm^2)	0.16-0.89 (0.58)	0.23-0.66 (0.52)	ns
CI ($L/min/m^2$)	1.28-4.5 (2.64)	2.8-3.6 (2.58)	ns
Heart weight (gm)	380-880 (590)	410-780 (621)	ns
CA narrowing >75% (pts)	12 (50%)	13 (59%)	ns
LV scar (pts)	5 (21%)	1 (4%)	ns
Electrocardiogram			
VPC (pts)	2 (8%)	4 (18%)	ns
LAD (pts)	6 (25%)	4 (18%)	ns
QRS amplitude (mm)			
12 leads	144-353 (236)	199-395 (269)	< 0.05
I-III	12-72 (37)	20-72 (39)	ns

Abbreviations as in Table III.

Table XII. Comparison of 26 patients with total (12-lead) QRS amplitude ≤250 to 24 patients with amplitude >250 mm in isolated severe aortic valve stenosis

Total QRS amplitude (mm)	*≤250 (n = 26)*	*>250 (n = 24)*	*p value*
Age (years)	32-63 (50)	16-65 (46)	ns
Male:female (pts)	20:6	16:8	ns
Angina pectoris (pts)	15 (58%)	19 (79%)	< 0.001
LV-SA psg (mm Hg)	52-158 (93)	52-180 (105)	ns
LVSP (mm Hg)	149-260 (205)	155-270 (215)	ns
Aortic valve areas (cm^2)	0.28-0.89 (0.54)	0.39-0.66 (0.51)	ns
CI ($L/min/m^2$)	1.3-4.5 (2.6)	1.8-4.2 (2.7)	ns
Heart weight (gm)	380-880 (595)	400-880 (614)	ns
CA narrowing >75% (pts)	10 (38%)	6 (25%)	ns
LV scar (pts)	3 (12%)	4 (17%)	ns
Electrocardiogram			
VPC (pts)	3 (12%)	4 (17%)	ns
LAD (pts)	7 (27%)	5 (21%)	ns
MDP (pts)	15 (58%)	8 (33%)	< 0.01
QRS amplitude (mm)			
12 leads	144-250 (207)	252-417 (305)	< 0.001
I-III	12-55 (42)	28-78 (46)	< 0.01

Abbreviations as in Table III.

patients in whom the QRS width was < 0.12 seconds, the 12-lead amplitude averaged 252 mm. The sum of the QRS amplitude in leads I to III in the four patients ranged from 36 to 51 mm (mean 42). The hearts ranged in weight from 400 to 880 gm (mean 615). The aortic valves were congenitally malformed in each. None had significant narrowing of any of the major epicardial coronary arteries, and only one had a LV scar which was small and subendocardial.

DISCUSSION

Initial substantive necropsy study of abnormal ECG correlations in hemodynamically documented isolated severe AS. Although there are many reports on ECG observations in patients with pressure overloaded left ventricles (systemic hypertension,[2-6] aortic valve stenosis,[4, 7-29] hypertrophic cardiomyopathy,[30, 31] and discrete subaortic stenosis[14]), virtually none have focused on necropsy patients in whom direct hemodynamic data were obtained shortly before death.

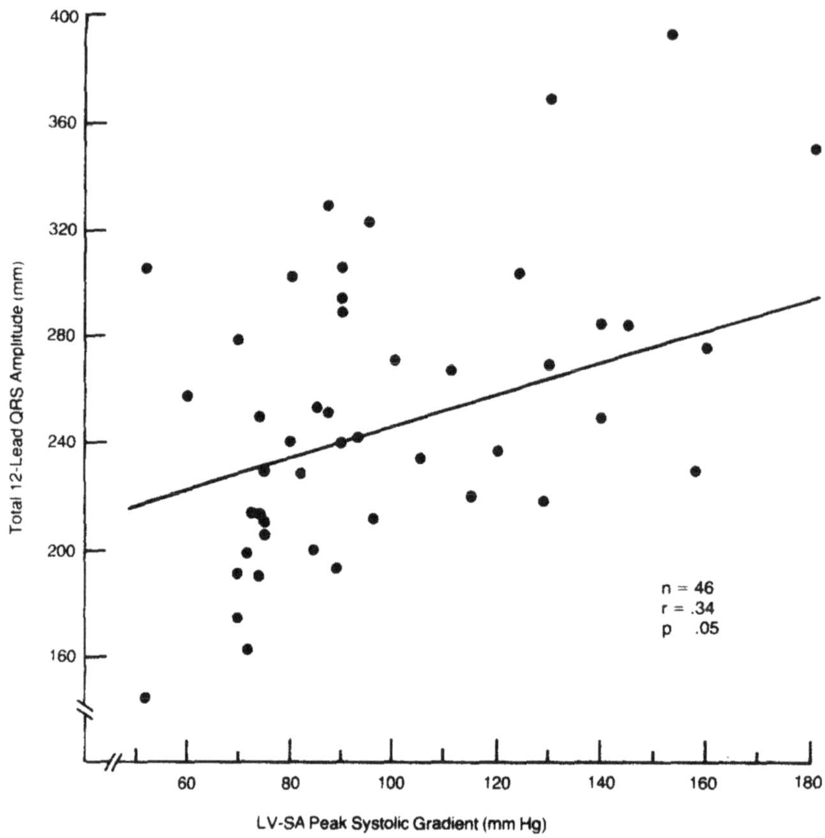

Fig. 2. Relation between the total 12-lead QRS amplitude (in mm) and the peak left ventricular *(LV)* systemic arterial *(SA)* pressure gradient in 46 necropsy patients with aortic valve stenosis without bundle branch block.

All 50 patients included herein had isolated AS, i.e., anatomically normal tricuspid, pulmonic, and mitral valves, with peak systolic pressure gradients between LV and a systemic artery of > 50 mm Hg (average = 98) and all had necropsy examination of the heart. Of the 15 parameters analyzed in each patient (Tables III to XII), 10 were further analyzed to compare patients with to those without, or those with greater than to those with less than a certain figure. Of these 10 categories in which the 15 parameters were compared, excluding the factor analysed, 33 (22%) of the 150 were significantly ($p < 0.05$) different between the two groups.

Total 12-lead QRS amplitude best single predictor of most marked AS without CAD in young adult males in severe AS patients. Of the 15 parameters analyzed, the one most often showing significant differences between the 10 groups compared was total 12-lead QRS amplitude. The mean of the total 12-lead QRS amplitude was significantly greater in the younger (≤ 40 years) than in the older patients (278 mm vs 257 mm); in the women than in the men (277 mm vs 249 mm), in the patients with higher (> 100 mm Hg) peak systolic pressure gradients across the aortic valve (281 mm vs 244 mm); in the patients with heavier (> 600 gm) hearts (274 mm vs 244 mm); in the patients without versus those with significant CAD (270 mm vs 238 mm), and in those without compared to those with ECG myocardial damage patterns (269 mm vs 236 mm). Although the mean values of the total QRS amplitude were significantly different between these six groups, comparison of patients with total 12-lead QRS amplitude of ≤ 250 mm to those with higher amplitude disclosed the frequency of angina pectoris and of ECG myocardial damage patterns to be the only factors significantly different. Although the mean values of the total 12-lead QRS amplitude was not significantly different in the groups of patients with and without angina pectoris, the sum of the QRS amplitude in leads I, II, and III was significantly greater in the patients with compared to those without angina (42 mm vs 32 mm). In contrast to the significant mean differences between total 12-lead QRS amplitude in 6 of the 10 groups compared and in QRS amplitude in leads I to III in 2 of the 10 groups compared, the frequency of the usual ECG criteria of LVH was similar in all 10 groups compared because all but 2 of

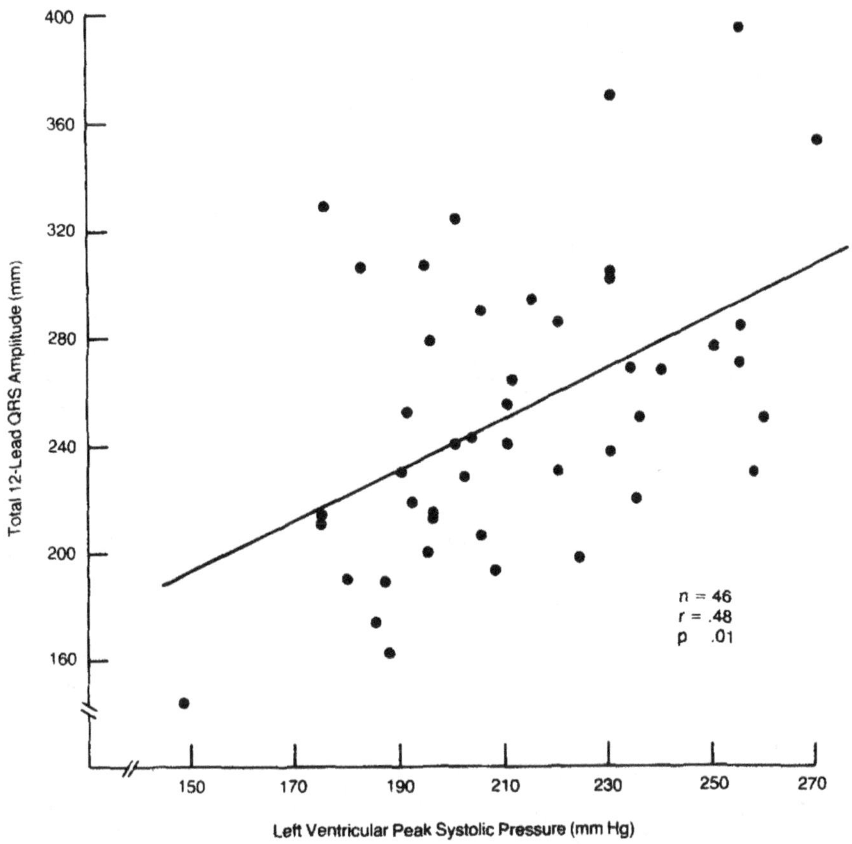

Fig. 3. Relation between the total 12-lead QRS amplitude (in mm) and the left ventricular peak systolic pressure (in mm Hg) in 46 necropsy patients with aortic valve stenosis without bundle branch block.

the 46 patients without LBBB had LVH by ECG utilizing common criteria.[1]

Total QRS amplitude (peak LV systolic pressure) minus peak systolic systemic arterial pressure implies peak systolic transaortic pressure gradient in severe AS patients. Using regression analysis, the total 12-lead QRS amplitude correlated directly with the peak systolic pressure gradient across the aortic valve ($p < 0.05$, $r = 0.31$) and when the four patients with LBBB were excluded, this correlation improved ($r = 0.34$) (Fig. 2). When the four patients with LBBB were excluded, the total 12-lead QRS amplitude correlated directly with the LV peak systolic pressure ($p < 0.01$, $r = 0.48$) (Fig. 3). Indeed, the LV systolic pressure (in mm Hg) was generally similar to the total 12-lead QRS amplitude (in mm) (Fig. 4). Thus measurement of the total 12-lead amplitude (in mm) appears to allow a reasonable prediction of LV systolic pressure and subtraction of the systemic arterial systolic pressure from the total 12-lead amplitude (in mm) appears to provide a reasonable noninvasive means of predicting the peak systolic pressure gradient across the aortic valve among patients with moderate to severe AS and without LBBB (Fig. 4).

We found no previous reports describing amplitude of the QRS complexes in all 12 precordial leads in patients with AS. Simonson,[32] however, has provided data on the upper and lower limits of amplitude of the QRS complexes in each of the 12 leads in normal men and women aged 20 to 59 years. (The mean for the normals is not available.) The upper and lower limits of normal for men aged 50 to 59 years was 277 and 36 mm, and for the women 248 and 27 mm, respectively. The upper and lower limits of amplitude in all 12 leads in our 50 patients with AS was 417 and 144 mm, respectively, and averaged 260 mm. For the 36 men in our study, the total QRS voltage (all 12 leads) averaged 249 mm and for the 14 women, 277 mm.

Only three other ECG findings differed significantly between any of the 10 groups analyzed. LAD occurred in 3 (11%) of the 28 patients with hearts weighing < 600 gm and in 9 (41%) of the 22 patients with larger hearts ($p < 0.01$). Additionally, LAD occurred in 9 (56%) of the 16 patients without angina pectoris and in only 3 (9%) of the 34 patients with angina ($p < 0.0005$). Ventricular premature complexes were recorded on routine ECG in 7 (20%) of the 34 patients with angina and in none of the 16

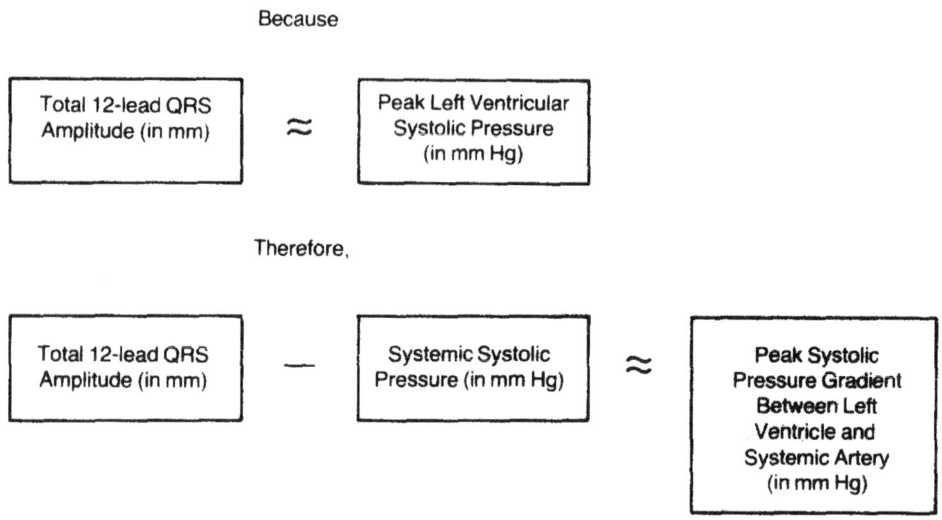

Fig. 4. Usefulness of measuring the total 12-lead QRS amplitude in predicting left ventricular–systemic arterial pressure gradient in valvular aortic stenosis unassociated with bundle branch block.

patients without angina ($p > 0.05$). Finally, ECG myocardial damage patterns were significantly more frequent in the 16 patients with CAD at necropsy compared to the 34 patients without (81% vs 32%) ($p < 0.025$). The frequency of myocardial ischemic changes (ST segment depression and depth of T wave inversion) was not significantly different in the patients with and without coronary narrowing.

Concomitant CAD suggested by ECG myocardial damage patterns and less increased QRS amplitude in older adults, but not by angina. Certain factors did suggest the presence of significant (> 75% in cross-sectional area) CAD. All 16 patients with narrowing of one or more major coronary arteries were over 40 years of age (mean 54); it occurred in 16 (41%) of the 39 patients over age 40 years and in none of the 11 aged 40 years or under. ECG myocardial damage patterns occurred in 13 (81%) of the 16 patients with CAD and in 11 (32%) of the 34 patients without significant narrowing. The patients with CAD also had lower total amplitude of QRS complexes in the 12 leads compared to those without coronary narrowing (238 mm vs 270 mm) and also a much higher frequency of grossly visible myocardial scarring: in 5 (31%) of the 16 patients with CAD and in 2 (6%) of the 34 patients without CAD ($p < 0.001$). As demonstrated by others,[33-37] the frequency of angina pectoris was similar in the patients with and without significant CAD (69% and 68%).

The presence of grossly visible LV scars did not alter the ECG finding in our patients with AS. All seven with scars, however, were among the 39 patients over age 40 years (mean 53), six of the seven had significantly (> 75%) narrowed coronary arteries ($p < 0.001$) and the average peak transaortic gradient in the seven patients with compared to the 43 patients without scars was smaller (77 mm Hg vs 101 mm Hg) ($p < 0.025$).

REFERENCES

1. Romhilt DW, Estes EH: A point-score system for the ECG diagnosis of left ventricular hypertrophy. Am Heart J **75**:752, 1968.
2. Sokolow M, Lyon TP: The ventricular complex in left ventricular hypertrophy as obtained by unipolar precordial and limb leads. Am Heart J **37**:161, 1949.
3. Sannersdedt R, Bjure J, Varnauskas E: Correlation between electrocardiographic changes and systemic hemodynamics in human arterial hypertension. Am J Cardiol **26**:117, 1970.
4. Kini PM, Eddelman EE, Pipberger HV: Electrocardiographic differentiation between left ventricular hypertrophy and anterior myocardial infarction. Circulation **42**:875, 1970.
5. McCaughan D, Littmann D, Pipberger HV: Computer analysis of the orthogonal electrocardiogram and vectorcardiogram in 939 cases with hypertensive cardiovascular disease. Am Heart J **85**:467, 1973.
6. Toshima H, Koga Y, Kimura N: Correlations between electrocardiographic, vectorcardiographic, and echocardiographic findings in patients with left ventricular overload. Am Heart J **94**:547, 1977.
7. Mitchell AM, Sackett CH, Hunzicker WJ, Levine SA: The clinical features of aortic stenosis. Am Heart J **48**:684, 1954.
8. Bergeron J, Abelmann WH, Vazquez-Milan H, Ellis LB: Aortic stenosis—clinical manifestations and course of the disease. Review of one hundred proved cases. Arch Intern Med **94**:911, 1954.
9. Wood P: Aortic stenosis. Am J Cardiol **1**:553, 1958.
10. Hancock EW, Fleming PR: Aortic stenosis. Q J Med **29**:209, 1960.
11. Reynolds JL, Nadas AS, Rudolph AM, Gross RE: Critical congenital aortic stenosis with minimal electrocardiographic changes. N Engl J Med **262**:276, 1960.
12. Björk VO, Cullhed I, Lodin H: Aortic stenosis. Correlations between pressure gradient and left ventricular angiography. Circulation **23**:509, 1961.
13. Hugenholtz PG, Lee MM, Nadas AS: The scalar electrocardiogram, vectorcardiogram, and exercise electrocardiogram in the assessment of congenital aortic stenosis. Circulation **26**:79, 1962.

14. Braunwald E, Goldblatt A, Aygen MM, Rockoff SD, Morrow AG: Congenital aortic stenosis. I. Clinical and hemodynamic findings in 100 patients. Circulation **27**:426, 1963.
15. Morris JJ Jr, Estes WH Jr, Whalen RE, Thompson HK Jr, McIntosh HD: P-wave analysis in valvular heart disease. Circulation **27**:242, 1964.
16. Cullhed I: Aortic stenosis. A clinical study of aortic stenosis, isolated or combined with aortic insufficiency, with special reference to hemodynamic and angiographic observations. Stockholm, 1964, Alxqvist & Wiksell, pp 154.
17. Gamboa R, Hugenholtz PG, Nadas AS: Comparison of electrocardiograms and vectorcardiograms in congenital aortic stenosis. Br Heart J **27**:344, 1965.
18. Fowler RS: Ventricular repolarization in congenital aortic stenosis. AM HEART J **70**:603, 1965.
19. Gooch AS, Calatayud JB, Rogers JB, Corman PA: Analysis of the P wave in severe aortic stenosis. Dis Chest **49**:459, 1966.
20. Myler RK, Sanders CA: Aortic valve disease and atrial fibrillation. Report of 122 patients with electrographic, radiographic, and hemodynamic observations. Arch Intern Med **121**:530, 1968.
21. Postell WN, Rainey RL, Witham, AC, Edmonds JH Jr: Vectorcardiographic and electrocardiographic manifestations of increasing left ventricular pressure overload. AM HEART J **77**:33, 1969.
22. Holt JH Jr, Barnard ACL, Lynn MS: A study of the human heart as a multiple dipole electrical source. II. Diagnosis and quantitation of left ventricular hypertrophy. Circulation **40**:697, 1969.
23. Hilsenrath J, Hamby RI, Glassman E, Hollman I: Pitfalls in prediction of coronary arterial obstruction from patterns of anterior infarction on electrocardiogram and vectorcardiogram. Am J Cardiol **29**:164, 1972.
24. Kornreich F, Brismee D: II. Diagnosis of left ventricular hypertrophy and myocardial infarction from "total" surface waveform information. Circulation **48**:996, 1973.
25. Bennett DH, Evans DW: Correlation of left ventricular mass determined by echocardiography with vectorcardiographic and electrocardiographic voltage measurements. Br Heart J **36**:981, 1974.
26. Dhingra RC, Amat-y-Leon F, Pietras RJ, Wyndham C, Deedwania PC, Wu D, Denes P, Rosen KM: Sites of conduction disease in aortic stenosis. Significance of valve gradient and calcification. Ann Intern Med **87**:275, 1977.
27. Yankopoulos NA, Haisty W, Pipberger HV: Computer analysis of the orthogonal electrocardiogram and vectorcardiogram in 257 patients with aortic valve disease. Am J Cardiol **40**:707, 1977.
28. Friedman HS, Zaman Q, Haft JI, Melendez S: Assessment of atrioventricular conduction in aortic valve disease. Br Heart J **40**:911, 1978.
29. Thompson R, Mitchell A, Ahmed M, Towers M, Yacoub M: Conduction defects in aortic valve disease. AM HEART J **98**:3, 1979.
30. Estes EH Jr, Whalen RE, Roberts SR Jr, McIntosh HD: The electrocardiographic and vectorcardiographic findings in idiopathic hypertrophic subaortic stenosis. AM HEART J **65**:155, 1963.
31. Savage DD, Seides SF, Clark CE, Henry WL, Maron BJ, Robinson FC, Epstein SE: Electrocardiographic findings in patients with obstructive and nonobstructive hypertrophic cardiomyopathy. Circulation **58**:402, 1978.
32. Simonson F: Differentiation between normal and abnormal in electrocardiography. St. Louis, Mo, 1961, The CV Mosby Co, p 328.
33. Moraski RE, Russell RO Jr, Mantle JA, Rackley CE: Aortic stenosis, angina pectoris, coronary artery disease. Cathet Cardiovasc Diagn **2**:157, 1976.
34. Paquay PA, Anderson G, Diefenthal H, Nordstrom L, Richman HG, Gobel FL: Chest pain as a predictor of coronary artery disease in patients with obstructive aortic valve disease. Am J Cardiol **38**:863, 1976.
35. Graboys TB, Cohn PF: The prevalence of angina pectoris and abnormal coronary arteriograms in severe aortic valvular disease. AM HEART J **93**:683, 1977.
36. Miller DC, Stinson EB, Oyer PE, Rossiter SJ, Reitz BA, Shumway NE: Surgical implications and results of combined aortic valve replacement and myocardial revascularization. Am J Cardiol **43**:494, 1979.
37. Storstein O, Enge I: Angina pectoris in aortic valvular disease and its relation to coronary pathology. Acta Med Scand **205**:275, 1979.

No cardiac catheterization before cardiac valve replacement—a mistake

William C. Roberts, M.D. *Bethesda, Md.*

In the November 21, 1981, issue of the *New England Journal of Medicine,* St. John Sutton et al.[1] described results of an investigation carried out in the Brompton Hospital, London, in 1978, to determine the usefulness of *routine* cardiac catheterization before operative replacement of one or both left-sided cardiac valves. The authors concluded that routine cardiac catheterization is unnecessary before valve replacement and this view was supported in an accompanying editorial by Brandenburg[2] from the Mayo Clinic. Before accepting the conclusion of the Brompton Hospital study, another look at the data collected is warranted.

During a single year, 243 patients with valvular heart disease and without previous cardiac catheterization were referred to physicians at the Brompton Hospital. In each patient, a decision to perform cardiac catheterization was delayed until an analysis was made of the history and physical signs, ECG and chest roentgenograms, and, in those in whom it was obtained, M-mode echocardiograms. After these data were collected, the diagnosis appeared "unequivocal" in 184 patients (76%) and catheterization in them was not performed. In the remaining 59 patients (24%), cardiac catheterization was performed because of "... persistent doubt about the severity of the valve lesions, clinical evidence of aortic root disease, evidence of substantial coronary artery disease, or discordance between clinical and echocardiographic data."[1] The decision regarding the usefulness of preoperative cardiac catheterization was evaluated postoperatively by comparison of *operative mortality, 2-year mortality, extent of symptom relief,* and *frequency of "... subsequent valve replacement for untreated aortic valve or mitral valve regurgitation"* between the groups having and not having this invasive procedure preoperatively. Additionally, 62 other patients with valvular heart disease and previous cardiac catheterization were referred to the Brompton Hospital during the same year and they too were included in their analysis.

The operative and 2-year mortality and extent of symptom relief were similar in the groups of patients having and not having preoperative cardiac catheterization, and no uncorrected valvular lesions became apparent in the 2-year follow-up period in the uncatheterized patients. Thus the authors concluded that *routine* cardiac catheterization was unnecessary before valve replacement. But is their conclusion applicable to patients with valvular heart disease being evaluated for valve replacement operations at other medical centers? The Brompton Hospital patients were *younger, less symptomatic,* and had a *much higher frequency of mitral valve disease* than patients having cardiac valve replacement at most Western World medical centers.

Of their 305 patients, 42% were less than 50 years of age, and of course significant associated coronary narrowing is relatively infrequent in this younger age group, especially in persons from Third World countries, the source of a significant percentage of their patients. Of their 177 patients (58%) aged 50 years and older, 57 (32%) had coronary angiograms of which 15 (36%) were abnormal and five patients received aortocoronary bypass conduits. Thus only five (1.6%) of their 305 patient having valve replacement also had aortocoronary bypass, a much lower percent than observed in the USA.

Nearly one half (48%) of their patients were in New York Heart Association functional class I (asymptomatic) or II, a sharp contrast to that of most patients having valve replacement in the major medical centers in the USA. Did all those class I and II patients really need a cardiac operation, especially a valve replacement compared to a valve commissurotomy (mitral group)?

In comparison to the higher frequency of aortic valve replacement in the USA, mitral valve replace-

From the Pathology Branch, National Heart, Lung and Blood Institute, National Institutes of Health.

Received for publication Feb. 8, 1982; accepted Feb. 9, 1982.

Reprint requests: William C. Roberts, M.D., Pathology Branch, NHLBI-NIH, Bldg. 10A, Room 3E-30, Bethesda, MD 20205.

ment was more frequent than aortic valve replacement among the Brompton Hospital patients. Of their 305 patients, 209 (69%) had mitral valve replacement (with or without aortic valve replacement) and 166 (54%) had aortic valve replacement (with or without mitral valve replacement). Of their 235 patients having isolated valve replacement, 59% involved the mitral, and 41% the aortic valve. Although the specific types of hemodynamic valve lesions present in their patients were not provided, it can be inferred that mitral stenosis was the most common type of valvular dysfunction, because rheumatic heart disease was stated to be the etiology of the valvular heart disease in 164 (67%) of the 305 patients. This is a much higher percentage than observed in most major medical centers in the USA today where aortic valve stenosis is the most frequent type of valvular dysfunction necessitating valve replacement. The reason that rheumatic heart disease was so frequent in their patients appears to be related to the fact that many were from abroad, particularly from Third World Countries, where the frequency of rheumatic heart disease is quite high.

Assuming ideal follow-up (which was not the case with the Brompton study), can comparison of operative and 2-year postoperative mortality and evaluation of symptoms and new valve lesions between one group having and another group not having preoperative catheterization really provide sufficient data to answer the question, Is *routine* cardiac catheterization necessary before cardiac valve replacement? The method of follow-up of their patients apparently was primarily by correspondence and not by reexamination by a physician or repeat M-mode echocardiographic or hemodynamic study. Meaningful comparisons using one type of prosthetic cardiac valve versus another cannot be obtained simply by analysis of the operative and 2-year postoperative mortality and evaluation of symptoms at 2 years postoperatively, and it is unlikely that these parameters are sensitive enough to provide meaningful information on the usefulness of routine cardiac catheterization as a preliminary to cardiac valve replacement. If the usefulness of a procedure, namely cardiac catheterization, is to be evaluated, it seems unlikely that the necessary information can be obtained simply by avoiding the performance of the procedure being evaluated.

Although the authors stated that only 62 of the 305 patients with valvular heart disease referred to them in 1978 had had cardiac catheterization previously, it is likely that most or all of their 50 patients who underwent reoperation without cardiac catheterization did indeed have this invasive procedure performed before the initial cardiac operation. If these 50 patients were added to their 50 (of 243 evaluated) who underwent cardiac catheterization before their first cardiac operation, the number of patients (excluding those who had catheterization before referral to Brompton) having catheterization before valve replacement would increase from 24% to 45%.

The paper by St. John Sutton et al.[1] and previous investigations by others[3] do indeed indicate that valve replacement can be performed successfully without prior cardiac catheterization, but they do not indicate whether or not valve replacement was necessary in the first place, because the severity of the valve lesions(s) most often was not determined. Nearly half of the patients studied by St. John Sutton et al. were asymptomatic or had only mild symptoms and it is of course difficult to improve on an asymptomatic state when relief of or diminution of symptoms and lack of death are the only bases for the judgment of improvement or success. That valve surgery can be performed "successfully" without preoperative catheterization is of course not new. In the 1950's many patients having mitral valve commissurotomy had no previous cardiac catheterization, or if they had it was usually limited to the right side of the heart and the operation, nevertheless, usually was quite beneficial.

In the 1950's, echocardiography was not available. Has the additional information provided by the M-mode and 2-dimensional (2DE) echocardiogram supplanted *routine* cardiac catheterization before cardiac valve replacement today? The answer is "No." Although the echocardiogram does record certain aspects of the functional *anatomy* of the cardiac valves and hemodynamic parameters record the functional *effects* of valvular dysfunction, the echocardiogram has not proved as useful as originally hoped in diagnosing and quantitating valvular dysfunction. The M-mode echocardiogram, for example, has proved to be highly useful in diagnosing mitral stenosis, but it has not proven useful in indicating the severity of the obstruction[4] and *it is the severity of the valve lesion not the presence of it which is the major determinant of whether or not valve replacement or commissurotomy is indicated.*

2DE has proved to be more useful in predicting the severity of mitral stenosis, but many pitfalls confront the estimator of mitral valve area by this means alone and therefore considerable caution must be exerted in using it quantitatively.[4] Just as the ECG is poor in predicting the severity of aortic valve stenosis,[5] both the M-mode echogram and 2DE are poor, not only in predicting its severity but also are frequently not helpful in diagnosis of aortic valve stenosis. Likewise, echocardiography has proved highly useful in diagnosing or confirming mitral valve prolapse, but it is not very helpful in indicating the presence of or degree of mitral valve regurgitation irrespective of the cause. Additionally, the echocardiogram has been extremely useful in determining the presence of aortic root dilatation (anuloaortic ectasia), but it is not very good in determining the degree of, and at times even the presence of, aortic regurgitation. Of course, the echocardiogram has been extremely helpful in evaluating the size of the left ventricle in both phases of the cardiac cycle, but with the exception of pure aortic regurgitation, left ventricular size *per se* does not determine whether valve replacement is indicated or will predictably be successful,[6,7] And finally, the standard M-mode echogram and 2DE are not reliable in delineating associated tricuspid valve disease, especially tricuspid regurgitation.[4] Contrast echocardiography, however, has been useful in this regard.[8] (It is surprising, incidentally, that associated tricuspid valve stenosis or regurgitation was not mentioned in any of the 305 patients reported by St. John Sutton et al.) Thus the echocardiogram is helpful in diagnosing some valve lesions, but it is not reliable in predicting the severity of most valvular lesions.

In patients with valvular heart disease, *cardiac catheterization is the only presently available procedure which provides accurate information on the severity of the valvular lesion(s).* Symptoms of cardiac dysfunction are not necessarily proportional to the degree of valvular stenosis or regurgitation. In patients with valvular heart disease, symptoms of cardiac dysfunction cannot be attributed to valvular dysfunction unless the degree of valvular dysfunction is considerable. Some patients with large gradients or severe degrees of regurgitation involving either the mitral or aortic valves or both have minimal symptoms, and some patients with small gradients or mild degrees of regurgitation involving one or both of these valves have severe symptoms. Improvement may occur postoperatively in some patients irrespective of the amount of reduction in valvular gradient or degree of regurgitation. Thus when nearly one half of the patients having valve replacement reported by St. John Sutton et al. were functionally class I or II preoperatively, it is impossible to know whether the operation was indicated in the first place or whether it was beneficial in the second place, without knowing the degree of valvular obstruction or regurgitation present preoperatively. The only way to obtain that information at the present time is by preoperative cardiac catheterization. Judging degrees of valvular obstruction by visual inspection at operation is fraught with enormous error, as is determining the degree of valvular regurgitation by manual palpation within the downstream chamber.

When a patient enters the operating room for a cardiac valve operation, be it commissurotomy, anuloplasty or replacement, the surgeon should have as much precise information as possible available to him (her) regarding which valve(s) functions abnormally and the extent of the dysfunction. It is expecting too much for surgeons uniformly to make proper decisions on which valve to excise or incise by visual inspection or palpation alone at operation. The most stenotic orifice of the mitral valve, for example, is at a level corresponding to the distal margins of the leaflets, and this portion of the valve is not necessarily seen well from the left atrium. The gold standard for the degree of obstruction across a valve is that obtained by measurement of pressures on either side of a valve, not by anatomic inspection or palpation. I have seen calcified aortic valves of diminished mobilty which by visual inspection appeared stenotic but by catheterization a short time earlier had shown no or minimal peak systolic pressure differences across the valve. The least errors are produced when most decisions regarding replacement of cardiac valves are made before the patient and surgeon enter the operating room on the basis of hemodynamic and angiographic data.[9] Echocardiographic data should be viewed mainly as supplemental and primarily diagnostic because it provides limited information on the severity of valve lesions.

Information regarding the level of the pulmonary arterial pressure of course is useful in following patients with mitral valve disease, and this pressure cannot be obtained accurately without cardiac catheterization. Pressures obtained at operation of course are not nearly as reliable as those obtained while the patient is awake. The right ventricular systolic pressure is most useful in evaluating the anatomic status of the tricuspid valve in patients with tricuspid regurgitation. Patients having tricuspid regurgitation associated with high right ventricular systolic pressure usually have anatomically normal tricuspid leaflets and chordae tendineae and dilated tricuspid valve anuli; patients with tricuspid regurgitation and normal or only mildly elevated right ventricular systolic pressures usually have anatomically abnormal tricuspid valve leaflets and chordae, and these valves in contrast to the former more likely require replacement.

To determine the status of the epicardial coronary arteries, there is no substitute for coronary angiography. If the patient population is mainly less than 50 years of age from Third World countries where the frequency of associated coronary disease is small, and the majority have mitral rather than aortic valve disease, the likelihood of associated significant coronary narrowing is relatively small. But patients in most Western World medical centers being considered for valve replacement are over 50 years of age, have a high frequency of associated coronary narrowing, and more commonly have aortic rather than mitral valve disease. The presence of associated significant coronary arterial narrowing in patients with aortic valve stenosis and angina pectoris, for example, cannot be determined reliably without cardiac catheterization (coronary angiography). Some patients with valve disease and symptoms of severe myocardial ischemia have insignificant coronary narrowing by coronary angiogram and vice versa. Knowing the status of the epicardial coronary arteries in patients over age 50 years, or possibly over age 40 years, being considered for cardiac valve replacement appears to be a fundamental preoperative requirement in 1982. Even when aortocoronary bypass grafting is not planned, if the patient has trouble being weaned from cardiopulmonary bypass after valve replacement, this additional procedure nevertheless might be warranted. No one can reliably determine the degree of narrowing of the epicardial coronary arteries by visual inspection or palpation, either in the operating room or in the necropsy room. This information needs to be obtained by selective coronary angiography preoperatively.

When the decision regarding the necessity of cardiac valve replacement arises, no procedure provides the information required as objectively as that obtained from preoperative cardiac catheterization. Cardiac catheterization today, including measurements of pressures in all four cardiac chambers and in both great arteries, and both selective coronary and left ventricular and aortic root angiography, is a procedure, which in skilled and experienced hands, takes only about 1 hour to perform. It is minimally traumatic to the patient. It not only provides the only conclusive data available regarding the severity of the valvular lesions, but it also provides objective baseline data to which postoperative studies can be compared. Its expense is relatively small compared to the expense of the cardiac operation and it may even prevent at times the latter from being performed. Cardiac catheterization can be performed many times in a lifetime, but the number of times that thoractomy and cardiotomy can be performed in a lifetime is limited. Therefore, the indications for the latter must be as precise as possible to achieve the maximal benefit when performed and to prevent the operation's being performed if the valve lesion(s) is not of sufficient severity to expect considerable improvement.

In some *emergency* situations in patients with valvular heart disease of course, it may be more advantageous to omit preoperative cardiac catheterization and proceed directly to the operating room. These circumstances might include extremely low cardiac output states from a stenosed or detached prosthetic or bioprosthetic cardiac valve, sudden severe valvular regurgitation (mainly aortic valve) from active infective endocarditis, and papillary muscle dysfunction in the setting of acute myocardial infarction. But, *for elective valve replacement in a stable patient, preoperative cardiac catheterization will increase the diagnostic accuracy, determine accurately the severity of the valvular dysfunction, provide information on the status of the epicardial coronary arteries, prevent surprises at operation, and provide a baseline of information to which postoperative data can be compared,* and this information cannot be obtained reliably today from any procedure other than cardiac catherization.

REFERENCES

1. St John Sutton MG, St John Sutton M, Oldershaw P, Sacchetti R, Paneth M, Lennox SC, Gibson RV, Gibson DG: Valve replacement without preoperative cardiac catheterization. N Engl J Med **305**:1233, 1981.
2. Brandenburg RO: No more routine catheterization for valvular heart disease. N Engl J Med **305**:1277, 1981.
3. Brandenburg RO, Fuster V, Giuliani ER: Indications for cardiac catheterization and coronary arteriography in the adult. *In* Brandenburg RO, editor: Office cardiology, Philadelphia 1980, FA Davis, Co p 83.
4. Feigenbaum H: Echocardiography. 3rd ed. Philadelphia, 1981, Lea & Febiger, p 239.
5. Braunwald E, Goldblatt A, Aygen MM, Rockoff SD, Morrow AG: Congenital aortic stenosis. I. Clinical and hemodynamic findings in 100 patients. Circulation **27**:426, 1963.
6. Henry WL, Bonow RO, Borer JS, Ware JH, Kent KM, Redwood DR, McIntosh CL, Morrow AG, Epstein SE: Observations on the optimum time for operative intervention for aortic regurgitation. I. Evaluation of the results of aortic valve replacement in symptomatic patients. Circulation **61**:471, 1980.
7. Henry WL, Bonow RO, Rosing DR, Epstein SE: Observations on the optimum time for operative intervention for aortic regurgitation. II. Serial echocardiographic evaluation of asymptomatic patients. Circulation **61**:484, 1980.
8. Lieppe W, Behar VS, Scallion R, Kisslo JA: Detection of tricuspid regurgitation with two-dimensional echocardiography and peripheral vein injections. Circulation **57**:128, 1978.
9. Roberts WC: Choosing a substitute cardiac valve: Type, size, surgeon. Am J Cardiol **38**:633, 1976.

REASONS FOR CARDIAC CATHETERIZATION BEFORE CARDIAC-VALVE REPLACEMENT

In a recent article in the *Journal,* St. John Sutton and his associates[1] described a study conducted in the Brompton Hospital, London, to determine the usefulness of routine cardiac catheterization before operative replacement of one or both left-sided cardiac valves. Of 243 patients analyzed, 184 (76 per cent) had cardiac catheterization and 59 (24 per cent) did not. The operative and two-year mortality and the relief of symptoms were similar in the patients who did and did not have preoperative cardiac catheterization, and no uncorrected valvular lesions became apparent in the two-year follow-up period in the uncatheterized patients. Thus, the authors concluded that routine cardiac catheterization was unnecessary before valve replacement. But is their conclusion applicable to patients with valvular heart disease who are being evaluated for valve replacement at other medical centers? The Brompton patients were younger and less symptomatic than patients who have cardiac valve replacement at most medical centers in the western world; they had a higher frequency of mitral-valve disease and had less coronary narrowing.

Assuming ideal follow-up (which was not the case), can comparison of operative and two-year postoperative mortality and evaluation of symptoms and new valve lesions between one group having preoperative catheterization and another group not having it really provide sufficient data to determine whether cardiac catheterization is necessary before cardiac-valve replacement? Meaningful comparison of one type of prosthetic cardiac valve with another cannot be obtained by analysis of the operative and two-year postoperative mortality and by evaluation of symptoms two years after the operation, and it is unlikely that these data are sensitive enough to provide meaningful information on the usefulness of routine cardiac catheterization as a preliminary to cardiac-valve replacement. If the usefulness of a procedure is to be evaluated, it seems unlikely that one can obtain the necessary information simply by avoiding the performance of the procedure being evaluated.

The paper by St. John Sutton and his associates[1] and the observations of others[2] indicate that valve replacement can be performed successfully without prior cardiac catheterization, but they do not indicate whether replacement was necessary in the first place, because the severity of the valve lesion or lesions most often was not determined. Nearly half the Brompton patients (48 per cent) were asymptomatic or had only mild symptoms, and it is of course difficult to improve on an asymptomatic state when relief or diminution of symptoms and lack of death are the only bases for the judgment of improvement or success.

In the 1950s, when cardiac operations were commonly performed without previous cardiac catheterization, echocardiography was not available. Has this technique supplanted routine cardiac catheterization before cardiac-valve replacement today? Of course not. The echo is not as useful in diagnosing and quantitating valvular dysfunction as many originally hoped. The M-mode echocardiogram is useful in diagnosing mitral-valve stenosis but not useful in indicating its severity,[3] and it is the severity of a valve lesion, not its presence, that is the major determinant of whether valve replacement or another valve operation is indicated. The two-dimensional echo is more useful in predicting the severity of mitral stenosis, but estimating mitral-valve area by this means alone is hazardous.[3] Just as the electrocardiogram is poor in predicting the severity of aortic-valve stenosis,[4] both the M-mode and two-dimensional echo techniques are poor in predicting its severity and even in diagnosing its presence. Although useful in diagnosing or confirming mitral-valve prolapse, echo is rarely helpful in indicating the presence or degree of mitral regurgitation, regardless of its cause. In addition, the echo is useful in determining the presence of aortic-root dilatation, but it is not good in determining the degree of aortic regurgitation, or at times even its presence. The echo is helpful in determining left ventricular size, but only with pure aortic regurgitation is left ventricular size helpful in determining whether valve replacement is indicated or will be successful.[5,6] Standard M-mode and two-dimensional echocardiograms are not reliable in delineating associated tricuspid-valve disease, especially tricuspid regurgitation.[3] Thus, the echo is helpful in the diagnosis of some valvular lesions, but it is not reliable in determining the severity of most of them.

Cardiac catheterization is the only available means of acquiring accurate information on the severity of a valvular lesion. Symptoms of cardiac dysfunction are not necessarily proportional to the degree of valvular stenosis or regurgitation. Some patients with large gradients or severe degrees of regurgitation involving the mitral or aortic valves or both have minimal symptoms, and some patients with small gradients or mild regurgitation have severe symptoms. Improvement may occur after surgery, regardless of the amount of reduction in the valvular gradient or the degree of regurgitation. Thus, since nearly half the Brompton patients were in Functional Class I or II before the operation, it is impossible to know whether the operation was indicated, or whether it was beneficial, without knowing the degree of preoperative valvular obstruction or regurgitation.

When a patient enters the operating room for a cardiac-valve operation, the surgeon should have as much precise information as possible about which valve or valves function abnormally and about the extent of the dysfunction. It is expecting too much to think that surgeons can uniformly make proper decisions on which valve to excise or incise by visual inspection or palpation alone at operation. Judging degrees of valvular obstruction by visual inspection at operation is fraught with error, as is determining the degree of valvular regurgitation by manual palpation within the downstream chamber. The gold standard for the degree of valvular obstruction is the difference in pressures on either side of a valve. The least errors are produced when most decisions regarding cardiac-valve operations are made before the patient and the surgeon enter the operating room, on the basis of hemodynamic and angiographic data.[7]

The level of the pulmonary arterial or right ventricular pressure is useful in evaluating the anatomic status of the tricuspid valve in patients with tricuspid regurgitation. Patients who have tricuspid regurgitation associated with high right ventricular systolic pressure usually have anatomically normal tricuspid leaflets and chordae tendineae and dilated tricuspid-valve anuli; patients with tricuspid regurgitation and normal or only mildly elevated right ventricular systolic pressure usually have anatomically abnormal tricuspid-valve leaflets and chordae, and these valves are more likely to require replacement.

Coronary angiography is the only certain means of determining the status of the epicardial coronary arteries during life. If patients are under 50 years old and from countries where coronary disease is infrequent, and if they have mitral-valve disease rather than aortic-valve disease, the likelihood of associated coronary narrowing is small. But patients undergoing valve replacement in most western medical centers are over 50, have a high frequency of associated coronary narrowing, and more commonly have aortic-valve disease than mitral-valve disease. The presence of associated coronary-arterial narrowing in patients with aortic-valve stenosis and angina pectoris cannot be determined reliably without coronary angiography. Knowing the status of the epicardial coronary arteries before surgery in patients over 50 (or even over 40) who are undergoing cardiac-valve replacement is fundamental. Even when aortocoronary-bypass grafting is not planned, if trouble arises during the discontinuation of cardiopulmonary bypass after valve replacement this additional procedure may be warranted. No one can reliably determine the degree of narrowing of the epicardial coronary arteries by visual inspection or palpation, either in the operating room or at autopsy.

No procedure provides information about the necessity of cardiac-valve replacement as objectively as preoperative cardiac catheterization. Measurement of pressures in all four cardiac chambers and in both great arteries and selective coronary, left ventricular, and aortic-root angiography are procedures that in skilled and experienced hands take only about one hour to perform. Such study is minimally traumatic to the patient. It not only provides the only conclusive data available about the severity of valvular lesions, but it also provides objective base-line data with which postoperative measurements can be compared. Its expense is relatively small as compared with that of the cardiac operation, and it may prevent that operation from being performed. Cardiac catheterization can be performed many times in a lifetime, but thoracotomy and cardiotomy can be performed only a few times. Therefore, the indications for the operation must be as precise as possible to achieve maximal benefit and to prevent its performance when the valve lesion is not of sufficient severity to require surgery.

In some emergency situations in patients with valvular heart disease, it may be more advantageous to omit preoperative cardiac catheterization and proceed directly to the operating room. These circumstances include extremely low cardiac-output states from a stenosed or detached prosthetic or bioprosthetic cardiac valve, sudden and severe valvular regurgitation from active infective endocarditis, and papillary-muscle dysfunction from acute myocardial infarction. But for elective valve replacement in a stable patient, preoperative cardiac catheterization will increase the diagnostic accuracy, determine accurately the severity of the valvular dysfunction, provide information on the status of the epicardial coronary arteries, prevent surprises and the need for subjective judgments at operation, and provide base-line information with which postoperative data can be compared. This information cannot be obtained reliably today from any means other than cardiac catheterization.

National Heart, Lung,
and Blood Institute
Bethesda, MD 20205

WILLIAM C. ROBERTS, M.D.

1. St. John Sutton MG, St. John Sutton M, Oldershaw P, et al. Valve replacement without preoperative cardiac catheterization. N Engl J Med. 1981; 305:1233-8.
2. Brandenburg RO. No more routine catheterization for valvular heart disease? N Engl J Med. 1981; 305:1277-8.
3. Feigenbaum H. Echocardiography. 3d ed. Philadelphia: Lea & Febiger, 1981:239-327.
4. Braunwald E, Goldblatt A, Aygen MM, Rockoff SD, Morrow AG. Congenital aortic stenosis. I. Clinical and hemodynamic findings in 100 patients. Circulation. 1963; 27:426-62.
5. Henry WL, Bonow RO, Borer JS, et al. Observations on the optimum time for operative intervention for aortic regurgitation. I. Evaluation of the results of aortic valve replacement in symptomatic patients. Circulation. 1980; 61:471-83.
6. Henry WL, Bonow RO, Rosing DR, Epstein SE. Observations on the optimum time for operative intervention for aortic regurgitation. II. Serial echocardiographic evaluation of asymptomatic patients. Circulation. 1980; 61:484-92.
7. Roberts WC. Choosing a substitute cardiac valve: type, size, surgeon. Am J Cardiol. 1976; 38:633-44.

Aortic valve stenosis and left ventricular apical aneurysm and/or rupture: Real or potential complications of persistent left ventricular systolic hypertension after acute myocardial infarction

William C. Roberts, M.D., Ernest N. Arnett, M.D., Seena C. Aisner, M.D., and Paul Techlenberg, M.D.
Bethesda and Baltimore, Md.

When acute myocardial infarction (MI) occurs in patients with systemic hypertension, the systemic arterial and left ventricular (LV) pressure generally returns to or toward normal if the MI was fairly large. When acute MI occurs in patients with significant aortic valve stenosis (AS), however, the LV systolic pressure remains elevated and the continuation of this pressure elevation increases the likelihood of LV rupture or aneurysmal formation, particularly when the MI involves the LV apical wall which normally is several times thinner than the LV basal wall.[1,2] Such was the case in a 67-year-old man, who died of progressive congestive heart failure after healing of more than one (by history) acute MI in the previous 5 years. At necropsy he had a severely stenotic congenitally bicuspid aortic valve and a large apical aneurysm at the site of a healed LV MI (Fig. 1). The heart weighed 630 gm. Both the left anterior descending and left circumflex coronary arteries were narrowed 76% to 100% in cross-sectional area by atherosclerotic plaques. The occurrence of LV free wall rupture and/or aneurysmal formation has not been reported previously in a patient with severe AS. This fact is surprising in view of the elderly age of many patients with AS.

From the Pathology Branch, National Heart, Lung and Blood Institute, National Institutes of Health; and the Departments of Cardiology and Pathology, Franklin Square Hospital.

Received for publication July 8, 1982; accepted July 27, 1982.

Reprint requests: William C. Roberts, M.D., National Institutes of Health, Bldg. 10A, Room 3E-30, Bethesda, MD 20205.

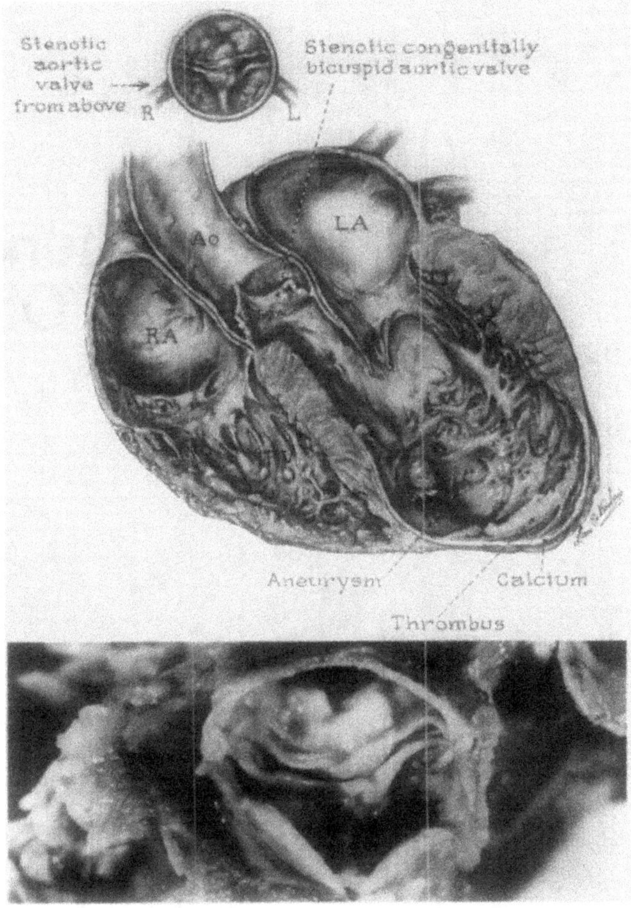

Fig. 1. Drawing of heart *(upper panel)* showing the healed left ventricular apical aneurysm and the congenitally bicuspid, stenotic aortic valve; and a photograph of the valve *(lower panel)*.

REFERENCES

1. Roberts WC, Ronan JA Jr, Harvey WP: Rupture of the left ventricular free wall (LVFW) or the ventricular septum (VS) secondary to acute myocardial infarction (AMI): An occurrence virtually limited to the first transmural AMI in the hypertensive individual (abstr). Am J Cardiol **35:**166, 1975.
2. Cabin HS, Roberts WC: True left ventricular aneurysm and healed myocardial infarction. Clinical and necropsy observations including quantification of degrees of coronary arterial narrowing. Am J Cardiol **46:**754, 1980.

Aortic Valve Stenosis: Estimating the Severity of Obstruction

William C. Roberts, M.D.

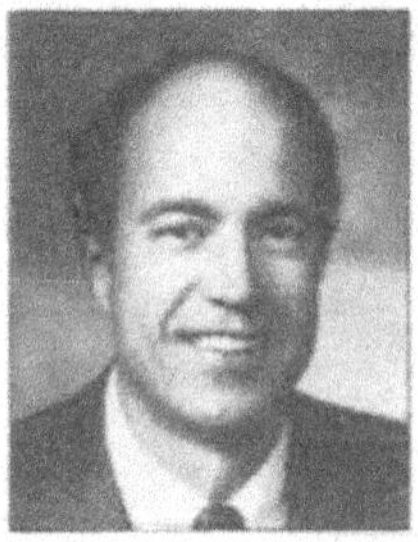

Pathology Branch
National Heart, Lung, and Blood Institute
National Institutes of Health
Bethesda, Maryland

Robert J. Siegel, M.D.

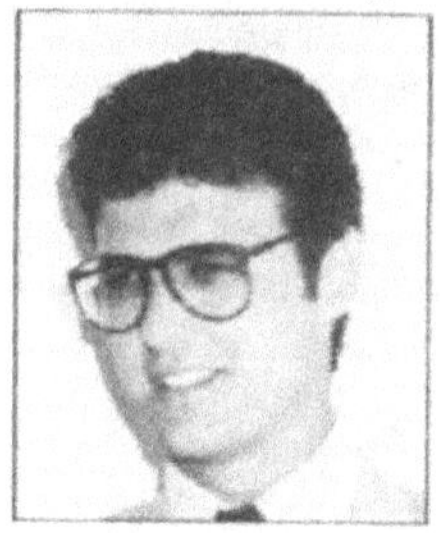

Cedars Sinai Medical Center
Los Angeles, California

Subtraction of the indirect systemic arterial systolic pressure, (in mmHg) from the total 12-lead QRS amplitude (in mm) may provide a reasonable noninvasive prediction of the peak systolic pressure gradient across the aortic valve in patients with moderate to severe aortic valve stenosis (AS). Most studies of the electrocardiogram (ECG) in patients with AS have involved living patients in whom the status of the left ventricular myocardium, epicardial coronary arteries, and mitral valve was not precisely known. We examined the 12-lead ECG recorded within 2 months of death in 50 patients aged 16–65 years (mean age: 48) with peak systolic pressure gradients across the aortic valve in the range of 52–180 mmHg (mean: 98) and anatomically normal mitral valves. Excluding 4 patients with complete left bundle branch block (LBBB), 44 (96 per cent) of the other 46 patients had the usual voltage criteria for left ventricular hypertrophy. Measurement of the total 12-lead QRS amplitude, which ranged from 144 to 417 mm (10 mm = 1 mV; mean: 257) correlated directly with the peak systolic pressure gradient across the aortic valve and, when the 4 patients with complete LBBB were excluded, with the peak left ventricular systolic pressure. The total 12-lead QRS amplitude (in mm) was similar in most patients to the left ventricular systolic pressure (in mmHg). The mean of the total 12-lead QRS amplitude was significantly ($P<0.05$) greater in the 11 younger (<40 years) than in the 39 older patients (278 mm vs 257 mm), in the 14 women than in the 36 men (277 mm vs 249 mm), in the 22 patients with heavier (>600 g) hearts (274 mm vs 244 mm), in the 34 patients without, compared to the 16 with, significant coronary arterial narrowing (270 mm vs 238 mm), and in the 22 patients without, compared to the 24 with, myocardial damage patterns on ECG: 269 mm vs 236 mm.

The most characteristic electrocardiographic finding in patients with aortic valve stenosis (AS) is excessive voltage, indicating left ventricular hypertrophy. Among adults with AS, the electrocardiographic criteria of left ventricular hypertrophy correlate poorly with symptoms of cardiac dysfunction, the amount of obstruction across the aortic valve, or prognosis in the absence of symptoms. Frequently, adults with AS have atherosclerotic coronary heart disease as well, which may also alter the electrocardiogram (ECG).

In most ECG studies in adults with AS, the status of the coronary arteries, left ventricular myocardium and mitral valve, and the weight of the heart have not been known, and before 1950 the pressure gradient across the aortic valve could not be ascertained. To determine which electrocardiographic finding could be attributed only to AS, with or without aortic regurgitation, we analyzed ECGs from 50 necropsy patients ages 16–65 years with severe or moderately severe AS. All of these patients had had ECGs and cardiac catheterization performed within 2 months of death. At necropsy the major coronary arteries, left ventricular myocardium, and mitral valve were thoroughly examined. In each patient, the total amplitude of the QRS complexes in all 12 leads was measured and correlated with the patient's age and sex, the pressure gradient across the aortic valve, left ventricular peak systolic pressure, heart weight, and whether or not angina pectoris, coronary arterial narrowing or left ventricular scarring were present and myocardial damage pattern appeared on the ECG.

Criteria for Patient Inclusion

Included in this study were only patients over the age of 16 and under 66, who had a peak systolic pressure gradient across the aortic valve of > 50 mmHg, demonstrated at catheterization within 2 months of death; an ECG recorded within 2 months of death and available for reexamination, and recorded before an operation was performed on the aortic valve; and who had anatomically normal mitral, tricuspid, and pulmonic valves at necropsy. The first 50 patients in the files of the Pathology Branch, NHLBI, who fulfilled these criteria were studied.

FAST TAKE

Necropsy studies of patients who had ECG and underwent cardiac catheterization no more than 2 months before death brought to light clinically useful correlations concerning the status of the coronary arteries, the left ventricular myocardium, the mitral valve, and heart weight.

ECG Criteria

Four or more points in the point-score system of Romhilt and Estes[1] were considered evidence of left ventricular hypertrophy.

A **strain pattern** was diagnosed when the ST segment was displaced and the T wave was directed 180° away from the major QRS axis, at least in leads V_5 and V_6.

Left atrial abnormality was diagnosed when the P wave in lead V_1 was diphasic with the negative component reaching at least 1 mm in amplitude and at least 120 milliseconds (msec) in width, and when the P wave in leads I, II, or aVL was notched and at least 120 msec in width.

Right atrial abnormality was diagnosed when the P-wave amplitude in leads II, III, or aVF was 3 mm or greater.

Left-axis deviation was diagnosed when the QRS axis in the frontal plane was −30° or less, and **right-axis deviation** when it was 110° or greater.

Table 1
Electrocardiographic Observations in 50 Patients Aged 16–65 Years with Isolated Aortic Valve Stenosis (pressure gradients >50 mmHg)

Finding	Number
1. Rhythm	
Sinus	45
Atrial fibrillation	5
2. Atrial abnormality	
Left only	16
Right only	0
Both	1
3. Premature ventricular complexes	7
4. PR Interval >0.20 sec	7
5. Left-axis deviation	12
6. Left ventricular hypertrophy without BBB (with strain = 43)	44
7. Left bundle branch block (LBBB)	4
8. QRS amplitude	
All 12 leads	144–417 (mean: 257)
Leads I-III only	12–78 (mean: 39)
9. Myocardial damage pattern (without LBBB)	24
A. Poor precordial R-wave progression	18
B. Q waves >30 msec in >2 leads	2
1. II, III, aVF = 2	
2. I, aVl, V_{4-6} = 0	
C. A + B1	2
D. A + B2	2

Left bundle branch block was defined by: QRS duration > 12 seconds in the extremity leads; the presence of broad monophasic R waves in leads I, V_5, and V_6, and displacement of the ST segment and T wave 180° away from the major QRS defection.

Two **myocardial damage patterns** were diagnosed: In type A, the R wave in V_1 was absent and <5 mm in amplitude in lead V_2; in type B, Q waves >30 ms were present in 2 or more leads posteriorly (leads II, III, aVF) or laterally (leads I, aVL, V_5, V_6).

Clinical Observations

The 50 patients had a mean age of 48; 36, or 72 per cent were male and 14 (28 per cent) female. The peak systolic pressure gradient between left ventricle and systemic artery range was 52–180 mmHg with a mean of 98; the aortic valve areas were 0.16–0.89 cm^2 (mean: 0.53); the aortic valve area indices range was 0.16–0.44 $cm^2/M2$ (mean: 0.29), and the cardiac indices were 1.3–4.7 liters/minute/M^2 (mean: 2.7).

Precordial murmurs of aortic regurgitation were recorded in 24 patients (48 per cent) and aortic regurgitation observed on angiography in 4 of the 13 patients in whom contrast material was injected into the proximal portion of ascending aorta. Of the 50 patients studied, 34 (68 per cent) had angina pectoris; none had experienced a clinical event compatible with acute myocardial infarction.

An operation on the aortic valve was performed in 38 (76 per cent) patients: 20 died within 24 hours of surgery, 11 others within 2 weeks, and 7 others from 2 to 6 weeks postoperatively. Two other patients died during anesthesia induction or skin incision for planned aortic valve operations. All 50 patients were in functional classes III or IV of the New York Heart Association Classification. Aortic valve operations had been planned or recommended in each of the 10 unoperated patients.

Necropsy Observations

The hearts ranged in weight from 380 to 880 g, with a mean of 606 g. The number of cusps in the aortic valve, which was identified either by the surgeon at operation, by our own examination of the excised valve, or at necropsy examination of the heart, were: 1 cusp (unicuspid, unicommissural) was found in 5 patients (10 per cent); 2 cusps (biscuspid) in 29 patients (58 per cent); 3 cusps (tricuspid) in 15 patients (30 per cent), and uncertain structure found in 1 patient. The cross-sectional area of one or more of the 4 major epicardial coronary arteries was narrowed more than 75 per cent by atherosclerotic plaques in 16 patients (32 per cent). Left ventricular scars were present at necropsy in 7 patients (14 per cent), and in each they were relatively small: subendocardial (inner half of wall) in only 2 patients and transmural (more than the inner half of the wall) in 5 patients. Only 1 patient had gross evidence of left ventricular necrosis and died 33 days after the ring of a caged-ball prosthesis had severely narrowed the ostium of his right coronary artery.

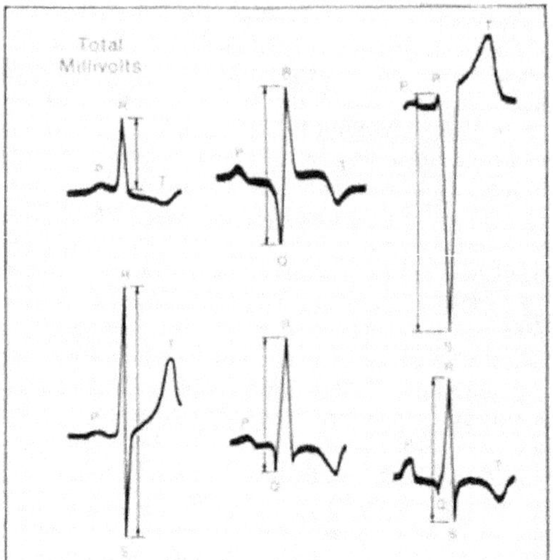

Fig. 1. Various QRS complexes showing how each was measured.

ECG Observations

We measured the amplitude of the QRS complexes from the peak of the R wave to the maximal dip of the S or Q wave, whichever was greatest, in each of the 12 leads in all 50 patients. The sum of the amplitude of the QRS complexes in all 12 leads in the 50 patients ranged from 144 to 417 mm for a mean of 257 (10 mm = 1 m V). The sum of the amplitude of the QRS complexes in leads I, II, and III in all patients ranged from 12 to 78 mm; mean: 39.

FAST TAKE

Operation on the aortic valve was performed in more than three-quarters of the study group. All 50 of the patients investigated were in functional classes III or IV of the N.Y. Heart Association classification. More than two-thirds had angina pectoris, but none had had a clinical event compatible with acute MI.

Age

Compared to the 11 patients aged 40 years and under, the 39 patients over age 40 had a higher frequency of angina pectoris (30 of 39, or 77 per cent vs 4 of 11;

P<0.005). They also had lower average peak systolic pressure gradients across the aortic valve (94 mmHg vs 113 mmHg; P<0.025), more frequent significant coronary narrowing (16 of 39 or 41 per cent vs 0 of 11) and left ventricular scarring (7 of 39, or 18 per cent vs 0 of 12; P<0.025), and lower average total QRS amplitude in the 12 leads (257 mm vs 278 mm P<0.05).

Sex

The 36 men had lower average peak systolic pressure gradients between the left ventricle and a systemic artery (91 mmHg vs 114 mmHg; P<0.01): higher mean heart weights (639 g vs 521 g; P< 0.01); and lower total QRS amplitude in the 12 leads (249 mm vs 277 mm; P<0.05) than the 14 women.

Aortic Pressure Gradient

The total amplitude of the QRS complexes in the 12 leads in the 33 patients with left ventricular to systemic arterial peak systolic pressure gradients of 100 mmHg or less (mean: 82) averaged 244 mm. In the 17 patients with higher gradients, it averaged 281 mm (P<0.05). The average left ventricular peak systolic pressure in the patients with gradients of 100 mmHg or less was 198 mmHg, and in those with higher gradients, it was 234 mmHg (P<0.0005).

Left Ventricular Systolic Pressure

The 22 patients with peak left ventricular systolic pressures of 200 mmHg or less had smaller peak systolic pressure gradients across the aortic valve (80 mmHg vs 122 mmHg; P<0.0005) and lower total QRS amplitudes (247 mm vs 265 mm; P<0.05) than did those with higher pressures.

Heart Weight

Compared to the 28 patients with smaller hearts, the 22 patients with hearts weighing over 600 g were more often men (20 of 22, or 91 per cent vs 16 of 28, or 57 per cent; P<0.25); had lower average left ventricular peak systolic pressures (205 mmHg vs 214 mmHg; P<0.05), more commonly had left-axis deviation (39 per cent vs 7 per cent; P<0.01) and higher average total QRS amplitude (274 mm vs 244 mm; P<0.025).

Angina Pectoris

The 34 patients with angina had smaller mean heart weights than the 16 patients without angina (580 g vs 661 g; P<0.025), more frequent premature ventricular complexes recorded (7 of 34 vs 0 of 16; P<0.05), less frequent occurrence of left-axis deviation (3 of 34 vs 9 of 16; P<0.0005) and higher QRS amplitude in leads I-III (42 mm vs 32 mm).

Coronary Narrowing

Compared to the 34 patients with less degrees of narrowing, the 16 patients with a greater than 75 per cent cross-sectional area narrowing of 1 or more of the 4 major epicardial coronary arteries by atherosclerotic plaques were older (54 years vs 46 years; P<0.01), had a higher frequency of left ventricular scars at necropsy (31 per cent vs 6 per cent; P<0.01), a higher frequency of myocardial damage patterns by ECG (81 per cent vs 32 per cent; P<0.025) and lower total 12-lead QRS amplitude (238 mm vs 270 mm; P<0.05). There was no significant difference in the amount of ST-segment depression or the depth of T-wave inversion between the patients with and without significant coronary narrowing.

Left Ventricular Scarring

Compared to the 43 patients without them, the 7 patients with grossly visible left ventricular scars were older (53 years vs 47 years; P<0.05), had lower average peak systolic gradients across the aortic valve (77 mmHg vs 101 mmHg; P<0.025), and more frequent coronary narrowing (6 of 7 vs 9 of 43; P<0.001).

Myocardial Damage Pattern

Excluding the 4 patients with LBBB, the mean total 12-lead QRS amplitude was lower in the 24 patients with myocardial damage patterns on ECG than in the 24 patients without such damage (243 mm vs 269 mm; P<0.05).

12-Lead QRS Amplitude

Compared to the 26 patients with total 12-lead QRS amplitude of 250 mm or less, the 24 patients in whom this amplitude was greater than 250 mm had a higher frequency of angina pectoris (79 per cent vs 58 per cent; P<0.001) and a lower frequency of myocardial damage patterns on ECG (33 per cent vs 58 per cent; P<0.01).

Atrial Fibrillation

The 5 patients with atrial fibrillation, 4 of them men, ranged in age from 45 to 63 years with a mean of 53. The peak systolic pressure gradients across their aortic valves ranged from 52 to 140 mmHg (average: 75 mmHg). Three had left-axis deviation, 3 had premature ventricular complexes, and 3 had myocardial damage patterns: poor R-wave progression in precordial leads. The total 12-lead QRS amplitude range was 199-306 mm (mean: 245 mm), and in the other 33 patients over age 40 with sinus rhythm it averaged 259 mm. The range of QRS amplitude in leads I-III was 21-51 mm (mean: 31 mm).

The heart weight range was 520-750 g (mean: 645 g).

The aortic valves were tricuspid in 4 and bicuspid in 1. Two of the 5 patients had 1 or more major coronary arteries narrowed more than 75 per cent in cross section by atherosclerotic plaques and 1 of them had a small, transmural left ventricular scar. Four patients had no grossly visible left ventricular scarring.

FAST TAKE

Coronary artery narrowing by more than 75 per cent due to atherosclerotic plaques was found in only 16 patients, who were, on average, older than the 34 with lesser degrees of stenosis, had a higher frequency of left ventricular scarring, greater myocardial damage pattern on ECG, and a lower total 12-lead QRS amplitude.

Left Bundle Branch Block

The 4 patients (2 women and 2 men) with complete LBBB ranged in age from 19 to 56, with a mean of 42. Three were over age 40. All 4 had sinus rhythm, 3 had left-axis deviation, 1 had a prolonged P-R interval, and 2 had left atrial abnormality. The peak systolic pressure gradients were 75, 75, 102, and 145 mmHg (average: 100 mmHg) and the total 12-lead QRS amplitude was 256, 417, 376, and 216 mm (mean: 316 mm), respectively. In the other 46 patients, in whom the QRS width was <0.12 seconds, the 12-lead amplitude averaged 252mm.

The sum of the QRS amplitude in leads I-III in the 4 patients ranged from 36–51 mm (mean: 42 mm). The hearts ranged in weight from 400–800 g (mean: 615 g). The aortic valves were congenitally malformed in each. None had significant narrowing of any of the major epicardial coronary arteries, and only 1 had a left ventricular scar, which was small and subendocardial.

Although there are many reports on electrocardiographic observations in patients with pressure overloaded left ventricles as in systemic hypertension,[2-6] aortic valve stenosis(AS)[4,7-9] hypertrophic cardiomyopathy,[10,11] and discrete subaortic stenosis,[14] virtually none have focused on necropsy patients in whom direct hemodynamic data was obtained shortly before death.

All 50 patients whom we studied had isolated AS, that is, anatomically normal tricuspid, pulmonic, and mitral valves, with peak systolic pressure gradients between the left ventricle and a systemic artery of more than 50 mmHg and all had necropsy examination of the heart. Of the 15 parameters analyzed in each patient, 10 were analyzed further to compare patients with the feature in question to those without it, or to compare those with more to those with less than a certain value. Of these 10 categories in which the 15 parameters were compared, excluding the factor analyzed, 33 (22 per cent) of the 150 showed significant ($P<0.05$) differences between the 2 groups.

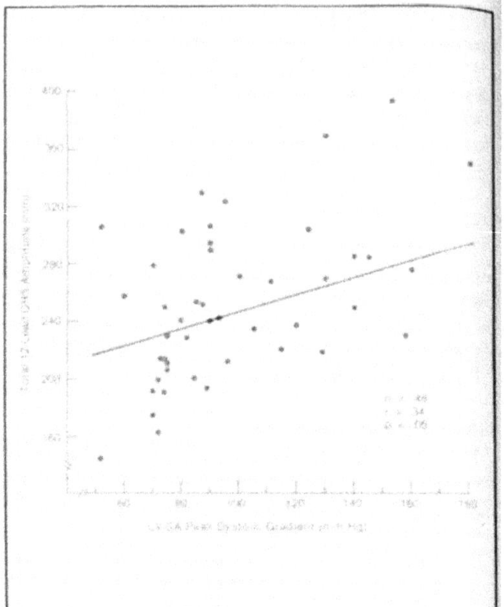

Fig. 2. Relation between the total 12-lead QRS amplitude and the peak left ventricular systemic arterial pressure gradient in 46 necropsy patients with aortic valve stenosis without bundle branch block.

Of the 15 parameters analyzed, the one that showed significant differences most often was total 12-lead QRS amplitude. Its mean was significantly greater in the patients under age 40 than in the older patients (278 mm vs 257 mm); in the women than in the men (277 mm vs 249 mm), in the patients with higher (>100 mmHg) peak systolic pressure across the aortic valve (281 mm vs 244 mm); in the patients with heavier (>600 g) hearts (274 mm vs 244 mm); in the patients without significant coronary narrowing: 270 mm vs 238 mm in those with significant narrowing, and in those without myocardial damage patterns compared to those with them on ECG: 269 mm vs 236 mm.

Although the mean values of the total QRS amplitude were significantly different among these 6 groups, comparing patients with total 12-lead QRS amplitude of 250 mm or less, with those who had higher amplitudes disclosed that the frequency of angina pectoris and myocardial damage patterns on ECG were the only factors differing significantly. The mean values of the total 12-lead QRS amplitude were not significantly different in the groups of patients with and without angina pectoris, but the sum of the QRS amplitude in leads I,

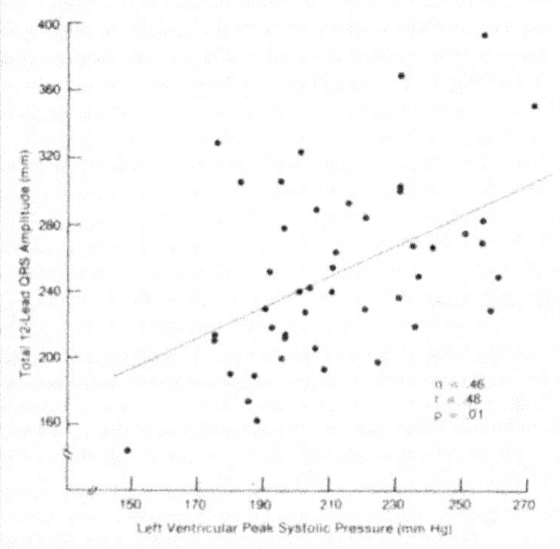

Fig. 3. Relation between the total 12-lead QRS amplitude and the left ventricular peak systolic pressure in 46 necropsy patients with aortic valve stenosis without bundle branch block.

II, and III was significantly greater in the patients with angina: 42 mm vs 32 mm.

In contrast to the significant mean differences between total 12-lead QRS amplitude in 6 of the 10 groups compared and in QRS amplitude in leads I-III in 2 groups, the frequency of electrocardiographic criteria for left ventricular hypertrophy was similar in all 10 groups, because on ECG utilizing common criteria, all but 2 of the 46 patients without LBBB had left ventricular hypertrophy.

Using regression analysis, the total 12-lead QRS amplitude correlated directly with the peak systolic pressure gradient across the aortic valve ($P<0.05$, $r=0.31$) and when the 4 LBBB patients were excluded, this correlation improved ($r=0.34$). When these 4 patients were excluded, the total 12-lead QRS amplitude correlated directly with the left ventricular peak systolic pressure ($P<10.01$, $r=0.48$). Indeed, the left ventricular systolic pressure (in mmHg) was roughly similar to the total 12-lead amplitude (in mm).

Thus, measurement of the total 12-lead amplitude appears to allow a reasonable prediction of left ventricular systolic pressure, and subtraction of the systemic arterial systolic pressure from the total 12-lead amplitude appears to provide a reasonable noninvasive means of predicting the peak systolic pressure gradient across the aortic valve among patients with moderate to severe AS and without LBBB.

We found no previous reports describing amplitude of the QRS complexes in all 12 precordial leads in AS patients. Simonson,[12] however, has provided data on the upper and lower limits of amplitude of the QRS complexes in each of the 12 leads among normal men and women ages 20–59 years. The mean for the normals is not available. The upper and lower limits of normal for men 40–59 years old were 277 and 36 mm, and for the women, 248 and 27 mm. The upper and lower limits of amplitude in all 12 leads in our 50 AS patients were 417 and 144 mm, and averaged 249 mm; for the 14 women the average was 277 mm.

FAST TAKE

LV systolic pressure in mmHg was roughly similar to the total 12-lead QRS amplitude in mm. Measuring the latter appears to provide a reasonable noninvasive means for predicting the peak systolic pressure gradient across the aortic valve among patients with moderate to severe AS without LBBB.

Only 3 other electrocardiographic findings differed significantly between any of the 10 groups analyzed. Left-axis deviation occurred in 3 (11 per cent) of the 28 patients with hearts weighing less than 600 g and in 9, or 41 per cent, of the 22 patients with larger hearts ($P<0.01$). Additionally, left-axis deviation occurred in 9 (56 per cent) of the 16 patients without angina pectoris and only 3 (9 per cent) of the 34 patients with angina ($P<0.0005$). Premature ventricular complexes were recorded on routine ECG in 7 (20 per cent) of the 34 patients with angina and in none of the 16 patients without angina ($P>0.05$). Finally, myocardial damage patterns on the ECG were significantly more frequent in the 16 patients with significantly narrowed coronary arteries at necropsy than among the 34 patients without them: 81 per cent vs 32 per cent; $P<0.025$. The frequency of myocardial ischemic changes, ST-segment depression and depth of T-wave inversion, did not differ significantly in the patients with and without coronary narrowing.

Practice Procedures

Predicting Peak LV-Systemic Arterial Pressure Gradient in Aortic Stenosis

Because:
Total 12-lead QRS amplitude in mm is similar to peak LV systolic pressure in mmHg;

Therefore:
Total 12-lead QRS amplitude in mm minus systolic pressure in mmHg;

Is similar to:
Peak systolic pressure gradient between left ventricle and systemic artery, in mmHg.

Certain factors suggested the presence of significant coronary stenosis. All 16 patients with narrowing of one or more major coronary arteries were over age 40 (mean age: 54); it occurred in 16 (41 per cent) of the 39 patients over 40 and in none of the 11 aged 40 or under. Myocardial damage patterns on ECG occurred in 13 (81 per cent) of the 16 patients with narrowed coronary arteries and in 11 (32 per cent) of the 34 patients without significant narrowing. The patients with stenosed coronary arteries also had lower total amplitude of the QRS complexes in the 12 leads compared with those without narrowing (238 mm vs 270 mm) and a much higher incidence of grossly visible myocardial scarring in 5 (31 per cent) of the 16 patients with narrowed arteries and in 2 (6 per cent) of the 34 patients without narrowing ($P<0.001$). As demonstrated by others,[11, 12] the frequency of angina pectoris was similar in the patients with and those without significantly stenosed coronary arteries (69 and 68 per cent).

The presence of grossly visible left ventricular scars did not alter the electrocardiographic findings in our patients with AS. All 7 with scars, however, were among the 39 patients over age 40 (mean age: 53); 6 of the 7 had significantly narrowed coronary arteries ($P<0.001$) and the average peak gradient in the 7 patients with scars compared to the 43 patients without scars was smaller (77 mmHg vs 101 mmHg; $P<0.025$). □

References

1. Romhilt DW and Estes EH: A point-score system for the ECG diagnosis of left ventricular hypertrophy. Am. Heart J. *75*:752, 1968.
2. Sokolow M and Lyon TP: The ventricular complex in left ventricular hypertrophy as obtained by unipolar precordial and limb leads. Am. Heart J. *37*:161, 1949.
3. Sannersdedt R, Bjure J, and Varnauskas E: Correlation between electrocardiographic changes and systemic hemodynamics in human arterial hypertension. Am. J. Cardiol. *26*:117, 1970.
4. Kini PM, Eddelman EE, and Pipberger HV: Electrocardiographic differentiation between left ventricular hypertrophy and anterior myocardial infarction. Circulation *42*:875, 1970.
5. McCaughan D, Littmann D, and Pipberger HV: Computer analysis of the orthogonal electrocardiogram and vectorcardiogram in 939 cases with hypertensive cardiovascular disease. Am. Heart J. *85*:467, 1973.
6. Toshima H, Koga Y, and Kimura N: Correlations between electrocardiographic, vectorcardiographic, and echocardiographic findings in patients with left ventricular overload. Am. Heart J. *94*:547, 1977.
7. Mitchell AM, Sackett CH, Hunzicker WJ, et al: The clinical features of aortic stenosis. Am. Heart J. *48*:684, 1954.
8. Bergeron J, Abelmann WH, Vazquez-Milan H, et al: Aortic stenosis—clinical manifestations and course of the disease. Review of one hundred proved cases. Arch. Int. Med. *94*:911, 1954.
9. Wood P: Aortic stenosis. Am. J. Cardiol. *1*:553, 1958.
10. Hancock EW and Fleming PR: Aortic stenosis. Quart. J. Med. *29*:209, 1960.
11. Reynolds JL, Nadas AS, Rudolph AM, et al: Critical congenital aortic stenosis with minimal electrocardiographic changes. New Engl. J. Med. *262*:276, 1960.
12. Bjork VO, Cullhed I, and lodin H: Aortic stenosis. Correlations between pressure gradient and left ventricular angiography. Circulation *23*:509, 1961.
13. Hugenholz PG, Lee MM, and Nadas AS: The scalar electrocardiogram, vectorcardiogram, and exercise electrocardiogram in the assessment of congenital aortic stenosis. Circulation *26*:79, 1962.
14. Braunwald E, Goldblatt A, Aygen MM, et al: Congenital aortic stenosis. I. Clinical and hemodynamic findings in 100 patients. Circulation *27*:426, 1963.
15. Morris JJ Jr, Estes WH Jr, Whalen RE, et al: P-wave analysis in valvular heart disease. Circulation *27*:242, 1964.
16. Cullhed I: Aortic stenosis. *In* A Clinical Study of Aortic Stenosis, Isolated or Combined with Aortic Insufficiency, with Special Reference to Hemodynamic and Angiographic Observations, Stockholm, Almqvist & Wiksell, 1964, p 154.

17. Gamboa R, Hugenholtz PG, and Nadas AS: Comparison of electrocardiograms and vectorcardiograms in congenital aortic stenosis. Br. Heart J. *27*:344, 1965.
18. Fowler RS: Ventricular repolarization in congenital aortic stenosis. Am. Heart J. *70*:603, 1965.
19. Gooch AS, Calatayud JB, Rogers JB, et al: Analysis of the P wave in severe aortic stenosis. Dis. Chest *49*:459, 1966.
20. Myler RK and Sanders CA: Aortic valve disease and atrial fibrillation. Report of 122 patients with electrographic, radiographic, and hemodynamic observations. Arch. Int. Med. *121*:530, 1968.
21. Postell WN, Rainey RL, Witham AC, et al: Vectorcardiographic and electrocardiographic manifestations of increasing left ventricular pressure overload. Am. Heart J. *77*:33, 1969.
22. Holt JH Jr, Barnard ACL, and Lynn MS: A study of the human heart as a multiple dipole electrical source. II. Diagnosis and quantification of left ventricular hypertrophy. Circulation *40*:697, 1969.
23. Hilsenrath J, Hamby RI, Glassman E, et al: Pitfalls in prediction of coronary arterial obstruction from patterns of anterior infarction on electrocardiogram and vectorcardiogram. Am. J. Cardiol. *29*:164, 1972.
24. Kornreich F and Brismee D: II. Diagnosis of left ventricular hypertrophy and myocardial infarction from "total" surface waveform information. Circulation *48*:996, 1973.
25. Bennett DH and Evans DW: Correlation of left ventricular mass determined by echocardiography with vectocardiographic and electrocardiographic voltage measurements. Br. Heart J. *36*:981, 1974.
26. Dhingra RC, Amat-y-Leon F, Pietras RJ, et al: Sites of conduction disease in aortic stenosis. Significance of valve gradient and calcification. Ann. Int. Med. *87*:275, 1977.
27. Yankopoulos NA, Haisty W, and Pipberger HV: Computer analysis of the orthogonal electrocardiogram and vectorcardiogram in 257 patients with aortic valve disease. Am. J. Cardiol. *40*:707, 1977.
28. Friedman HS, Zaman Q, Haft JI, et al: Assessment of atrioventricular conduction in aortic valve disease. Br. Heart J. *40*:911, 1978.
29. Thompson R, Mitchell A, Ahmed M, et al: Conduction defects in aortic valve disease. Am. Heart J. *98*:3, 1979.
30. Estes EH Jr, Whalen RE, Roberts SR Jr, et al: The electrocardiographic and vectorcardiographic findings in idiopathic hypertrophic subaortic stenosis. Am. Heart J. *65*:155, 1963.
31. Savage DD, Seides SF, Clark CE, et al: Electrocardiographic findings in patients with chronic obstructive and nonobstructive hypertrophic cardiomyopathy. Circulation *58*:402, 1978.
32. Simonson E: Differentiation between normal and abnormal in electrocardiography. St. Louis, CV Mosby, 1961, p 328.
33. Moraski RE, Russell RO Jr, Mantle JA, et al: Aortic stenosis, angina pectoris, coronary artery disease. Catheter. Cardiovasc. Diagn. *2*:157, 1976.
34. Paquay PA, Anderson G, Diefenthal H, et al: Chest pain as a predictor of coronary artery disease in patients with obstructive aortic valve disease. Am. J. Cardiol. *38*:863, 1976.
35. Graboys TB and Cohn PF: The prevalence of angina pectoris and abnormal coronary arteriograms in severe aortic valvular disease. Am. Heart. J. *93*:683, 1977.
36. Miller DC, Stinson EB, Oyer PE, et al: Surgical implications and results of combined aortic valve replacement and myocardial revascularization. Am. J. Cardiol. *43*:494, 1979.
37. Storstein O and Enge I: Angina pectoris in aortic valvular disease and its relation to coronary pathology. Acta Med. Scand. *205*, 275, 1979.

Detailed Anatomy of the Normally Functioning Aortic Valve in Hearts of Normal and Increased Weight

MARC A. SILVER, MD, and WILLIAM C. ROBERTS, MD

The area, weight and 4 linear variables were measured in each aortic valve cusp in 100 necropsy patients with normally functioning aortic valves, and the volume of each sinus of Valsalva and the aortic area at the sinotubular junction were determined in the same patients. The sums of the aortic valve cuspal areas, cuspal weights and sinus of Valsalva volumes increased with age ($p < 0.001$) and with heart weight ($p < 0.001$). All 3 variables (cuspal area, cuspal weight and sinus of Valsalva volume) also increased with age and heart weight relative to each other. The luminal area of aorta at the sinotubular junction also increased with age and heart weight and it also increased as the sum of the aortic valve cuspal areas and weights and sinus of Valsalva volumes increased. In only 16% of the 100 patients were the 3 aortic valve cusps of similar size (less than 5% difference in area between cusps); in 51%, 1 cusp was of different size than the other 2, and in 33% of patients all 3 cusps were of different sizes.

(Am J Cardiol 1985;55:454–461)

Although various features of dysfunctioning human aortic valves have been described, few reports are available describing results of detailed measurements of normally functioning human aortic valves. This report describes results of measuring at necropsy various dimensions of each aortic valve cusp, the volume of each sinus of Valsalva, and the luminal area of aorta at the sinotubular junction in 100 patients with normally functioning aortic valves.

Definitions

A *normal valve* may be defined as a thin, mobile layer of tissue located in a canal or passage, and this tissue allows free flow through the passageway and prevents reflux of the contents passing by it. When this definition of "valve" is applied to the normal aortic valve, it is applicable only to the 3 cusps (or leaflets). If the 3 aortic valve cusps are excised, an aortic valve is no longer present. Thus, the aortic valve is a structure located between left ventricular outflow tract and the tubular portion of aorta and within the sinus portion of aorta, and it consists of 3 freely mobile cusps. Although they affect both structure and function of the 3 aortic valve cusps, the structures contacted by the aortic valve cusps are not considered part of the aortic valve. The 3 aortic valve cusps are designated right, left and posterior. The term "non-coronary cusp" is best avoided because a coronary artery may originate from the wall of aorta behind the posterior cusp or a coronary ostium may be absent from 1 or both anteriorly located cusps.

A *sinus of Valsalva* is a space that exists between the aortic surface of an aortic valve cusp and the wall of aorta behind that cusp (Fig. 1). It is bounded caudally by the basal attachment of the aortic cusp (to wall of aorta, membraneous or muscular ventricular septum or anterior mitral leaflet) and above by the sinotubular junction. The space serves as a reservoir of blood during ventricular diastole. The *tubular portion of ascending aorta* is that portion beginning at the most cephalad extension of the sinuses of Valsalva and extending to the origin of the innominate artery (Fig. 1).

Methods

During an 18-month period, the measurements described herein were carried out in 100 hearts, which had been fixed in 10% buffered formalin. Death in all 100 patients was either the result of a noncardiac condition or to consequences of atherosclerotic coronary heart disease, a condition that does not affect the aortic valve. Patients with valvular, congenital, pericardial and primary myocardial diseases, patients in whom a cardiac operation had been performed, and patients younger than 18 years of age at death were excluded. If the heart was increased in mass the cause of the cardiomegaly was attributable only to systemic hypertension. Of the 100 patients, 2 were aged 18 to 20 years, 7 aged 21 to 30, 9 aged 31 to 40, 9 aged 41 to 50, 19 aged 51 to 60, 31 aged 61 to 70, 16 aged 71 to 80, 2 aged 81 to 90 and 5 aged 91 to 100 years. The heart weighed less than 400 g in 54 patients and more than 400 g in 46 patients. Of the 61 men, 28 (46%) had hearts less than 400 g and 33 (54%) had hearts more than 400 g; of the 39 women, 26 (67%) had hearts less than 400 g and 13 (33%) had hearts more than 400 g.

From the Pathology Branch, National Heart, Lung, and Blood Institute, National Institutes of Health, Bethesda, Maryland. Dr. Silver's present address: Section of Cardiology, Rush-Presbyterian-St. Luke's Medical Center, 1753 West Congress Parkway, Chicago, Illinois 60612. Manuscript received September 12, 1984, accepted October 8, 1984.

Address for reprints: William C. Roberts, MD, Building 10A, Room 3E30, National Institutes of Health, Bethesda, Maryland 20205.

One or more measurements were made in each patient on 6 structures or spaces. Of the 6, one measurement per patient was made in 2: heart weight and area of aortic lumen at the sinotubular junction. Of the other 4 structures or spaces, 3 measurements per patient were made because each patient had 3 aortic valve cusps and 3 sinuses of Valsalva. These 4 structures or spaces were: volume capacity of each sinus of Valsalva; weight of each aortic valve cusp; area of each aortic valve cusp; length of free margin of each cusp (measurement 1 [Fig. 2]); length of attachment margin of each cusp (measurement 2 [Fig. 2]); length from midportion of free margin to midportion of attachment margin (cuspal height) in each cusp (measurement 3 [Fig. 2]); and the straight-line distance between 2 junctions where free margins meet attachment margins of each cusp (cuspal width) (measurement 4 [Fig. 2]). Thus, in the 100 patients, 2,300 measurements of the 6 structures or spaces were possible; of these, 2,146 (93%) were carried out. The heart weight was determined in all 100 patients. The area of the aortic lumen at the level of the sinotubular junction was determined in 75 patients. The capacity of all 3 sinuses of Valsalva was determined in 68 patients or in 204 (68%) of the 300 sinuses. The weight of all 3 cusps individually was determined in 89 patients or in 267 of the 300 separate aortic valve cusps. The area of all 3 cusps was determined in all 100 patients or in all 300 of the possible 300 cusps. All 4 linear measurements (Fig. 2) were performed on each of the 3 aortic valve cusps in all 100 patients, yielding a total of 1,200 measurements of a possible 1,200 measurements.

The heart was weighed after cleaning all 4 cavities of postmortem clot and after excising both the ascending aorta and the pulmonary trunk about 2 cm above the cephalad extension of the semilunar valve cusps.

The volume capacity of each sinus of Valsalva was determined via a 2-ml pipette calibrated into 0.1-ml units. The pipette was filled to its capacity with water. While holding the heart with the sinuses of Valsalva roughly perpendicular to the long axis of the pipette, each sinus was filled to its capacity with water and the amount delivered by the pipette was recorded to the nearest 0.1 ml.

The luminal area of the aorta at the sinotubular junction was determined by incising circumferentially the aorta exteriorly while observing the blade of the knife within the aortic lumen. The thickness of the aortic wall circumferentially at the sinotubular junction was then blackened by a felt-tipped marking pen. The blackened aortic wall was then imprinted on white paper. Tracing paper was then superimposed over the black ring and the inner circumference was traced onto tracing paper. The cross-sectional area (in mm^2) of the aortic lumen then was determined directly by planimetry (KE-compensatory polar planimeter) using a video method described elsewhere.[1] The system was calibrated to 1-cm-square grid (100 mm^2). Each tracing then was placed under a focused camera and the resultant video signal was passed through an electronic integrator and displayed on a television monitor, which ensured that the area being measured was accurate. The analog output voltages of the video planimeters provided on-line measurements of the cross-sectional areas by a digital readout.

The aorta at the level of the aortic valve usually was opened between 2 cusps so that each cusp remained intact. Each of the 3 aortic valve cusps was excised intact along their curved line of attachment (just inside line 2 in Figure 2). Each cusp was then weighed using a Mettler P1210 scale, which has an accuracy to 0.01 g. Then each cusp was flattened (usually simply by applying water) on a sheet of white paper and the attachment margin (measurement 2 [Fig. 2]) and the free margin (measurement 1 [Fig. 2]) was traced onto the paper. The area enclosed by the tracing was measured by videoplanimetry as described above. Measurements 1 to 4 (Fig. 2) were made from the tracing by a flexible plastic metric ruler calibrated in 1-mm units.

Statistical methods: The comparison of means was done using an uncorrelated Student *t* test, and the correlation coefficients were calculated using a Pearson's product moment test. Significance was judged if the test yielded a p value <0.05.

Results

The findings are summarized in Tables I and II and in Figures 3 to 16.

The *sum of the areas of the 3 aortic valve cusps* increased with age (Fig. 3) ($r = 0.40$, $p < 0.001$), with heart weight (Fig. 4) ($r = 0.62$, $p < 0.001$); with total volume of the 3 sinuses of Valsalva (Fig. 5) ($r = 0.61$, $p < 0.001$); with the sum of the weight of the 3 aortic valve cusps (Fig. 6) ($r = 0.77$, $p < 0.001$), and with the aortic area at the sinotubular junction (Fig. 7) ($r = 0.75$, $p < 0.001$).

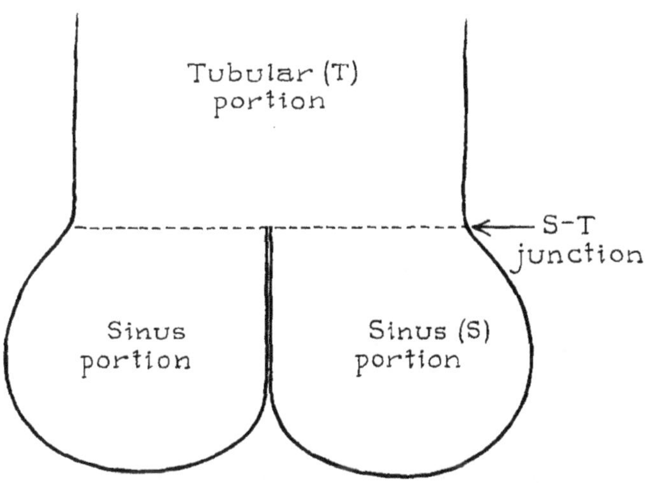

FIGURE 1. Diagram of the sinus and tubular portions of ascending aorta.

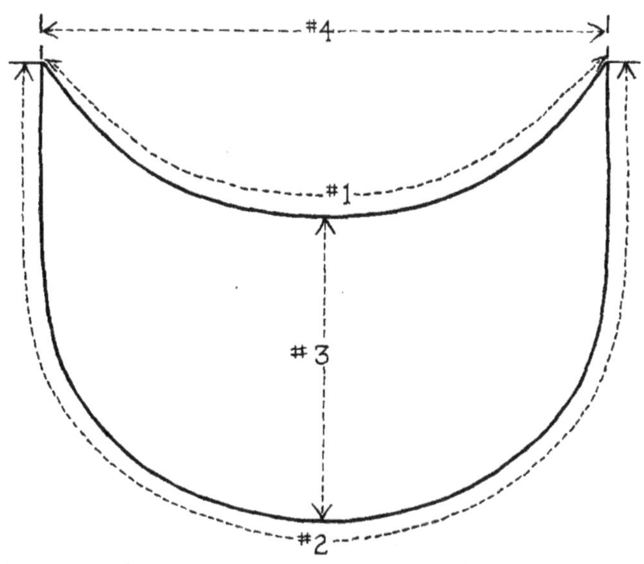

FIGURE 2. Diagram of a single aortic valve cusp illustrating the 4 linear measurements.

TABLE I Summary of Aortic Valve Cuspal and Sinus of Valsalva Measurements in 54 Patients with Normal Sized and in 46 Patients with Enlarged Hearts*

Structure or Space Measured	Cusp or Sinus of Valsalva					
	Right		Left		Posterior	
Heart weight (g)	≤400 (n = 54)	>400 (n = 46)	≤400 (n = 54)	>400 (n = 46)	≤400 (n = 54)	>400 (n = 46)
Area (mm^2)	127–480 (302 ± 77)	266–629 (384 ± 74)	161–456 (300 ± 74)	227–562 (376 ± 70)	162–473 (320 ± 70)	267–614 (381 ± 75)
Sinus volume (ml)	0.4–2.0 (1.0 ± 0.4)	0.8–3.0 (1.4 ± 0.4)	0.4–1.8 (0.9 ± 0.3)	0.6–2.0 (1.2 ± 0.3)	0.4–2.0 (1.1 ± 0.4)	0.6–2.8 (1.4 ± 0.4)
Weight (g)	0.06–0.32 (0.15 ± 0.06)	0.11–0.42 (0.20 ± 0.06)	0.07–0.28 (0.14 ± 0.05)	0.09–0.47 (0.21 ± 0.06)	0.07–0.32 (0.18 ± 0.06)	0.10–0.46 (0.22 ± 0.06)
Free margin (mm) (#1)	21–40 (31 ± 4)	27–46 (34 ± 4)	20–36 (29 ± 4)	25–49 (33 ± 5)	21–35 (30 ± 4)	25–45 (34 ± 4)
Attachment margin (mm) (#2)	32–60 (46 ± 6)	41–71 (51 ± 6)	33–60 (46 ± 7)	40–71 (50 ± 6)	35–60 (47 ± 6)	42–67 (50 ± 5)
Height (mm) (#3)	9–18 (13 ± 2)	11–20 (15 ± 2)	11–18 (14 ± 2)	11–20 (15 ± 2)	10–19 (14 ± 2)	12–18 (15 ± 2)
Width (mm) (#4)	19–40 (30 ± 5)	23–43 (34 ± 4)	18–35 (28 ± 4)	24–46 (32 ± 5)	20–35 (30 ± 4)	25– 43 (33 ± 5)

* The differences in all 8 measurements within each of the 3 cusps or sinuses between hearts that weighed 400 g or less and those that weighed more than 400 g were highly significant (p <0.01).

The *sum of the volumes of the 3 sinuses of Valsalva* increased with age (Fig. 8) (r = 0.52, p <0.001); with heart weight (Fig. 9) (r = 0.58, p <0.001); with the sum of the aortic valve cuspal area (Fig. 5) (r = 0.61, p <0.001); with the sum of the weight of each of the 3 aortic valve cusps (Fig. 10) (r = 0.58, p <0.001); and with the aortic area at the sinotubular junction (Fig. 11) (r = 0.63, p <0.001).

The *sum of the weights of the 3 aortic valve cusps* increased with age (Fig. 12) (r = 0.40, p <0.001); with heart weight (Fig. 13) (r = 0.57, p <0.001); with the sum of the area of the 3 aortic valve cusps (Fig. 6) (r = 0.77, p <0.001); with the sum of the volume of the 3 sinuses of Valsalva (Fig. 8) (r = 0.52, p <0.001, and with the aortic area at the sino-tubular junction (Fig. 14) (r = 0.62, p <0.001).

The *aortic area at the sinotubular junction* increased with age (Fig. 15) (r = 0.69, p <0.001); with heart weight (Fig. 16) (r = 0.55, p <0.001); with the sum of the area of the 3 aortic valve cusps (Fig. 7) (r = 0.75, p <0.001); with the sum of the volume of the 3 sinuses of Valsalva (Fig. 11) (r = 0.63, p <0.001); and with the sum of the weight of the 3 aortic valve cusps (Fig. 14) (r = 0.62, p <0.001).

The ranges and means of the aortic valve cuspal and sinus measurements of each of the 3 aortic valve cusps and sinuses of Valsalva in the patients with hearts that weighed 400 g or less in those with hearts that weighed more than 400 g are summarized in Table I. The mean

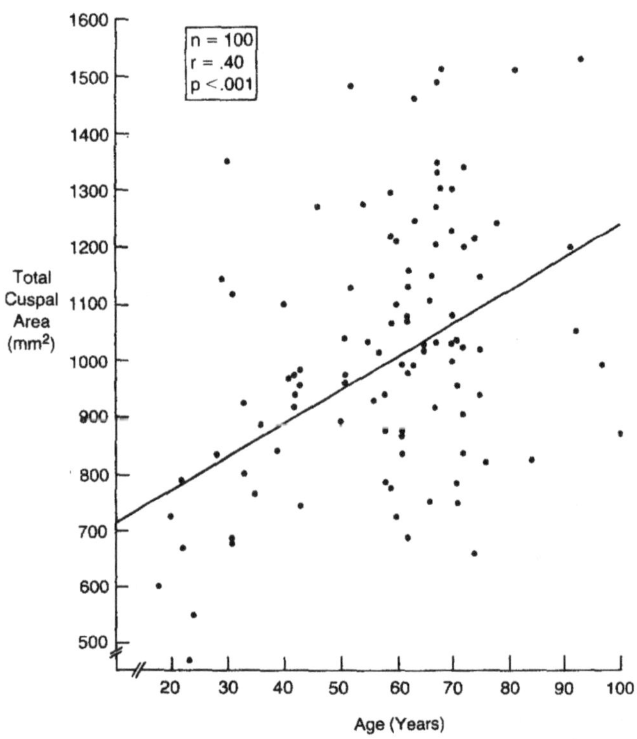

FIGURE 3. Relation of total aortic valve cuspal area to age.

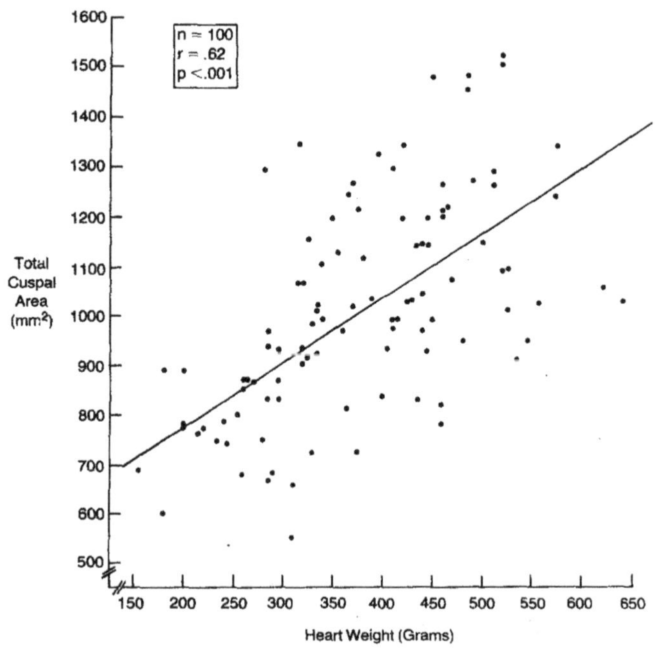

FIGURE 4. Relation of total aortic valve cuspal area to heart weight.

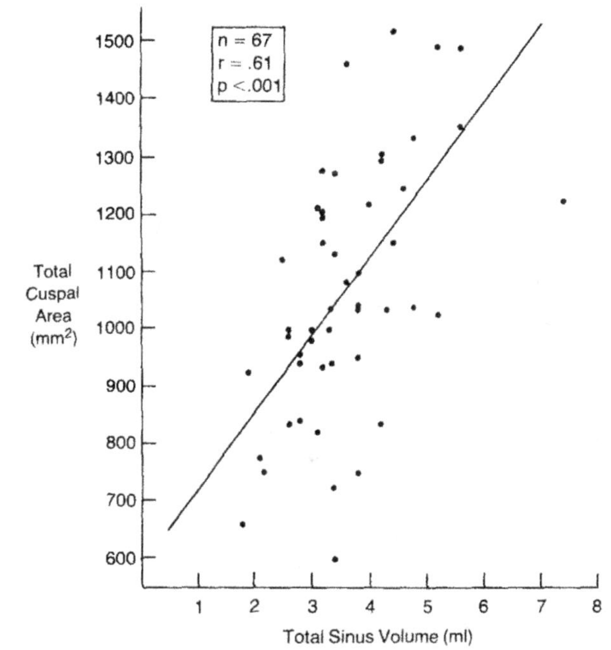

FIGURE 5. Relation of the sum of the 3 aortic valve cusps to the sum of the volumes of the 3 sinuses of Valsalva.

TABLE II Cuspal Differences* in Normally Functioning Aortic Valves in 54 Hearts of Normal Weight and in 46 Hearts of Increased Weight

	Heart Weight (g)		
Cusp Size	≤400	>400	Totals
0 equal-sized cusps (all 3 different)	23 (42.5%)	10 (22%)	33 (33%)
Largest cusp			
Right (R)	4	2	6 (18%)
Left (L)	5	2	7 (21%)
Posterior (P)	14	6	20 (61%)
Smallest cusps			
Right (R)	12	4	16 (49%)
Left (L)	8	4	12 (36%)
Posterior (P)	3	2	5 (15%)
2 equal-sized cusps (1 cusp different)	23 (42.5%)	28 (61%)	51 (51%)
The different cusp			
Right (R)	7	7	14 (28%)
Left (L)	8	9	17 (33%)
Posterior (P)	8	12	20 (39%)
Smaller	13	12	25 (49%)
Larger	10	16	26 (51%)
3 equal-sized cusps (no cusp different)	8 (15%)	8 (17%)	16 (16%)
Total	54 (100%)	46 (100%)	100 (100%)

* Difference more than 5% from the average cuspal area for the 3 cusps of an aortic valve (measured in mm²).

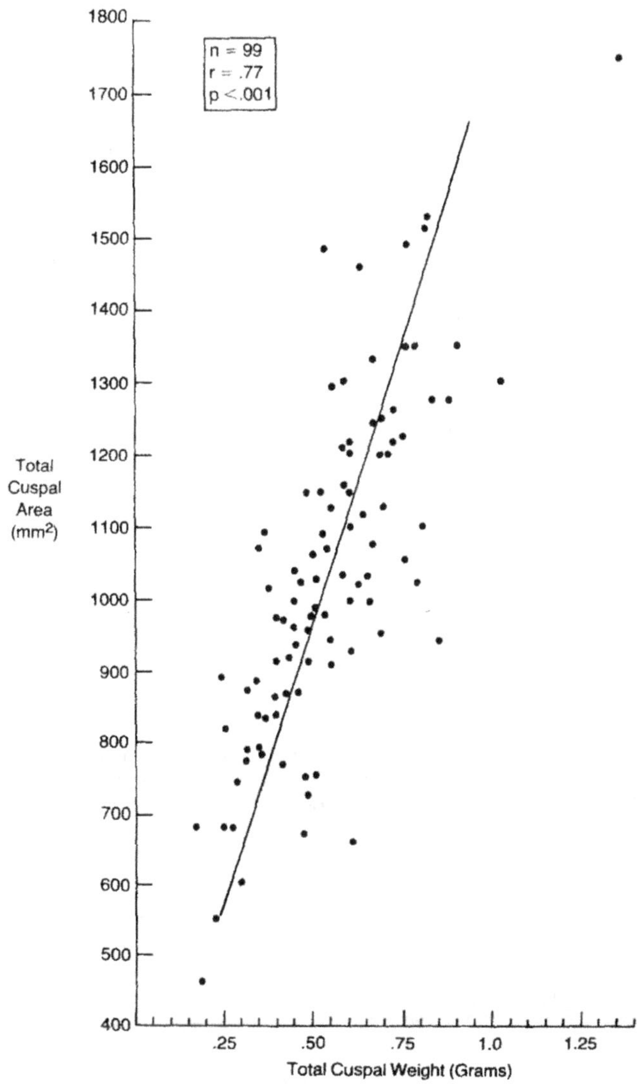

FIGURE 6. Relation of sum of areas of the 3 aortic valve cusps to sum of weights of the 3 aortic valve cusps.

cuspal area, mean cuspal weight, mean sinus of Valsalva volume, and the means of the 4 cuspal linear measurements (numbers 1 to 4 [Fig. 2]) were highly ($p < 0.01$) significantly different for each cusp or sinus in patients with normal sized hearts (≤400 g) compared with the patients with hearts of increased mass (>400 g).

Smaller, insignificant differences occurred in mean sinus of Valsalva volume, and the means of the 4 cuspal

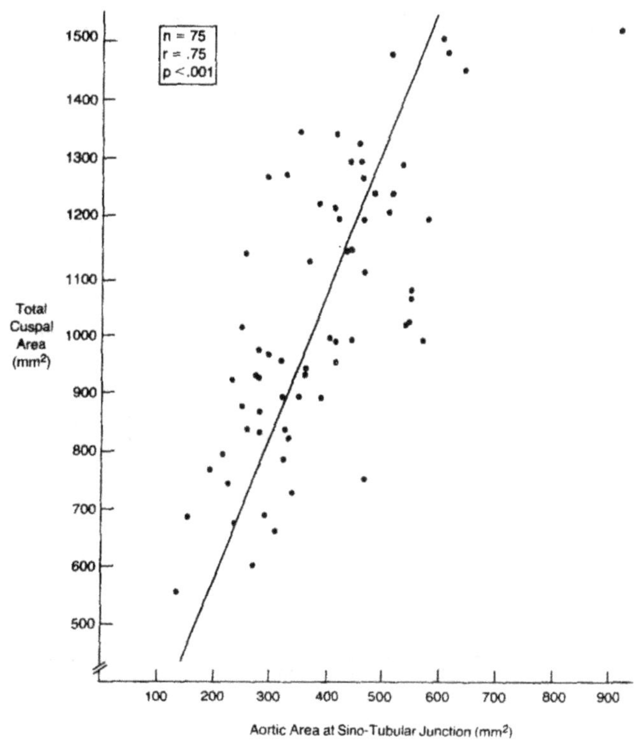

FIGURE 7. Relation of sum of the areas of the 3 aortic valve cusps to aortic area at the sinotubular junction.

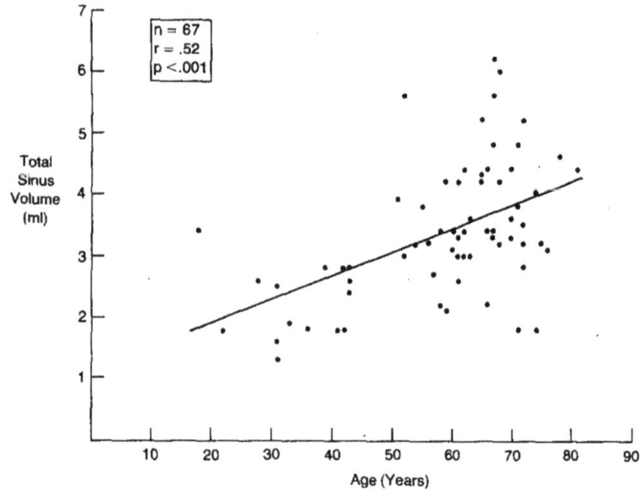

FIGURE 8. Relation of sum of volumes of the 3 sinuses of Valsalva to age.

linear measurements among the 3 cusps or sinuses between the 54 patients with normal-sized hearts (≤400 g) and those with hearts of increased mass (>400 g) (Table I). The posterior cusp, compared to both right and left ones, however, had a larger mean area and mean weight (Table I).

As summarized in Table II, only 16 patients had 3 equal-sized aortic valve cusps; 51 patients had 2 equal-sized cusps (1 different cusp), and 33 patients had no equal-sized cusps (all 3 cusps different). Among the 51 patients with 2 equal-sized cusps, the different-sized cusp was smaller than the other 2 in 25 patients and larger in 26 patients. The different-sized cusp was nearly equally split between the right, left and posterior locations. Of the 33 patients in whom none of the 3 cusps was of equal size, the posterior cusp was the largest in 20, the left in 7 and the right in 6; the posterior

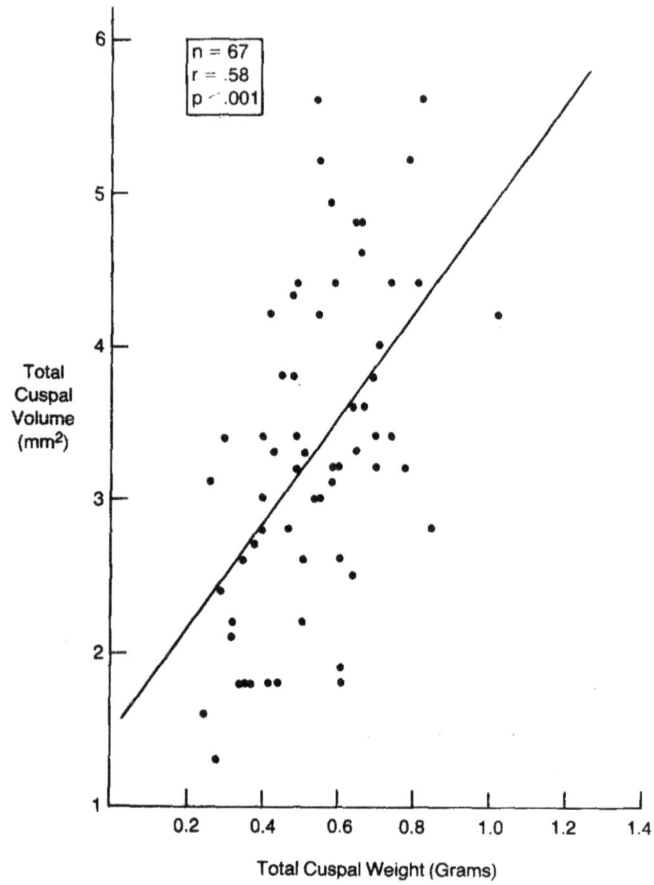

FIGURE 10. Relation of sum of volumes of all 3 sinuses of Valsalva to sum of weights of the 3 aortic valve cusps.

cusp was the smallest in 5, the left in 12 and the right in 16 (Table II).

The luminal area of aorta at the sinotubular junction (measured in 75 patients) ranged from 139 to 915 mm^2 (mean 392 ± 108); the range in the 40 patients with

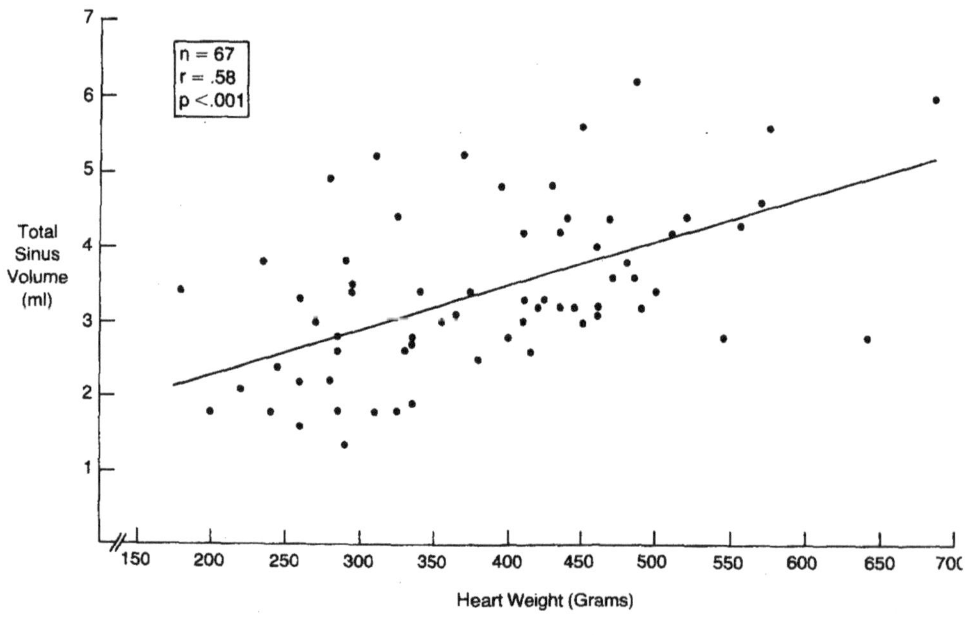

FIGURE 9. Relation of sum of volumes of the 3 sinuses of Valsalva to heart weight.

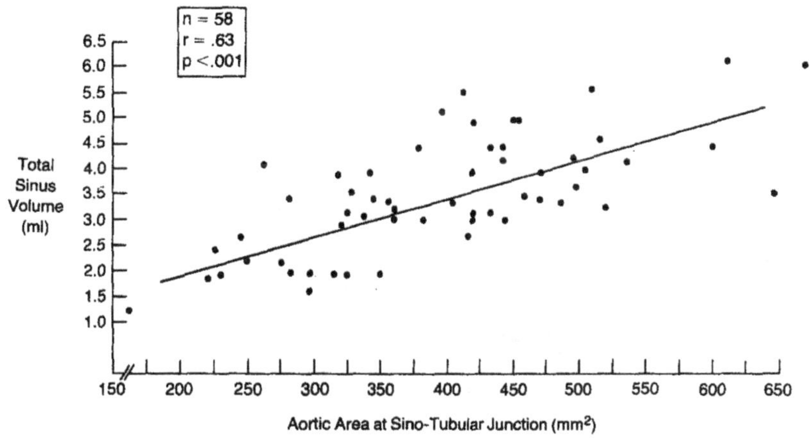

FIGURE 11. Relation of sum of volumes of all 3 sinuses of Valsalva to aortic area at sinotubular junction.

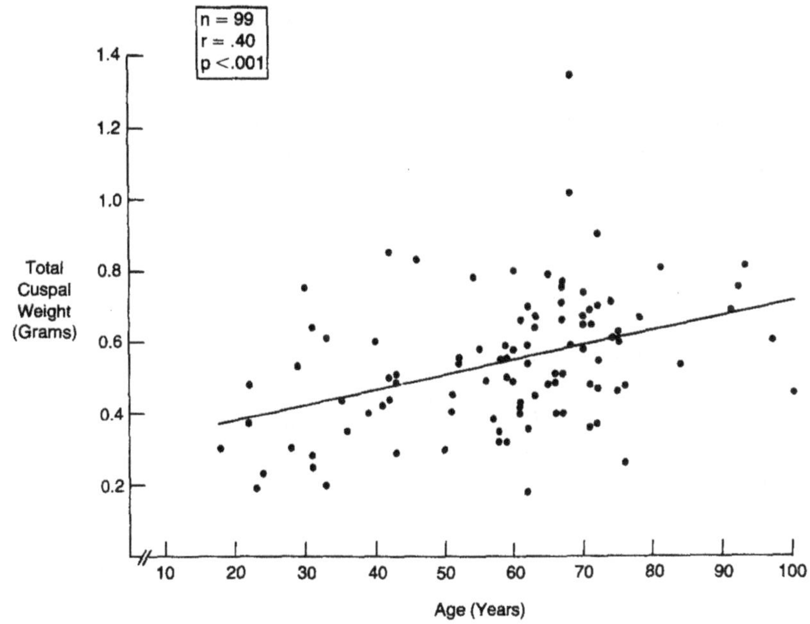

FIGURE 12. Relation of sum of weights of the 3 aortic valve cusps to age.

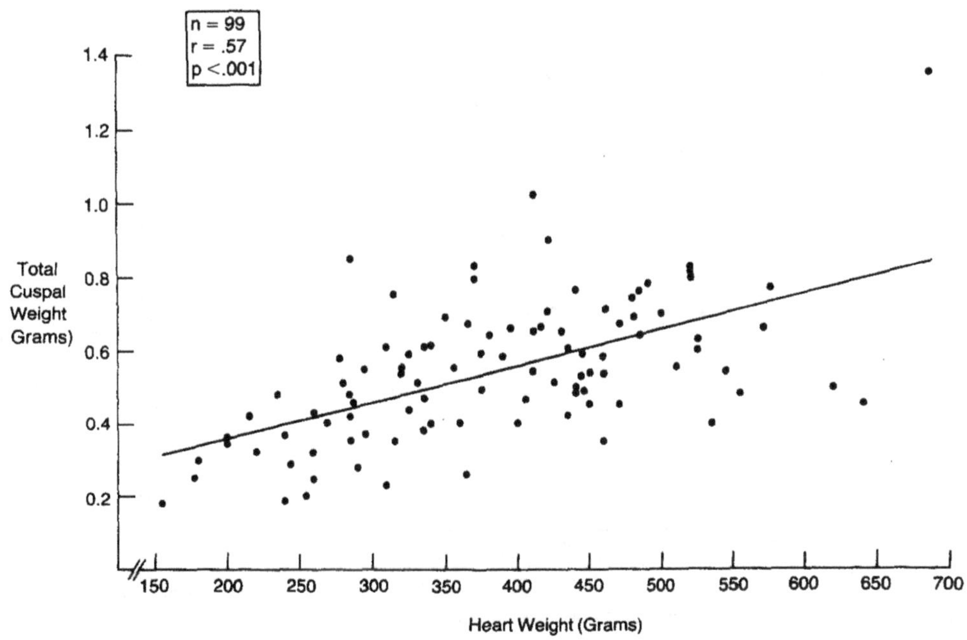

FIGURE 13. Relation of sum of weights of the 3 aortic valve cusps to heart weight.

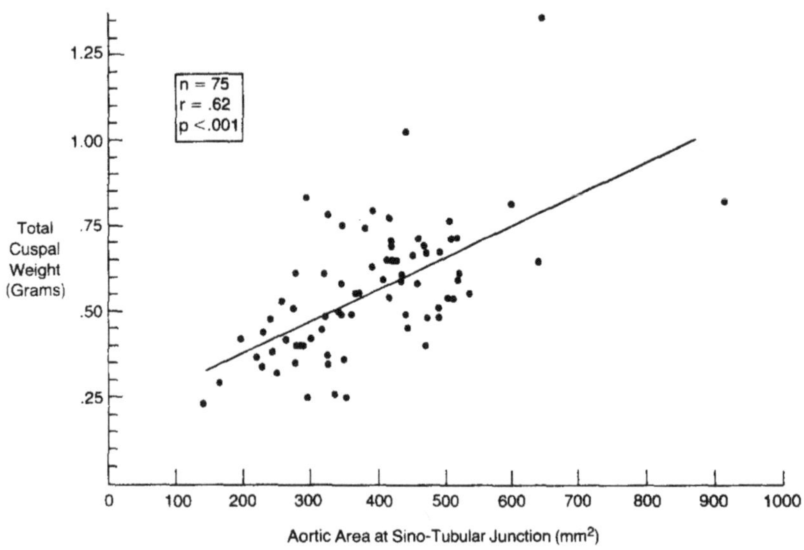

FIGURE 14. Relation of sum of weights of the 3 aortic valve cusps to aortic area at sinotubular junction.

hearts ≤400 g was 139 to 520 mm^2 (mean 333 ± 94); and in the 35 patients with hearts >400 g it was 256 to 915 mm^2 (mean 459 ± 124).

Discussion

The present observations provide detailed data on the area, weight and certain linear measurements on each of the aortic valve cusps and on the volumes of the sinuses of Valsalva in necropsied persons with normally functioning aortic valves. The sums of the aortic valve cuspal areas, cuspal weights and sinus of Valsalva volumes increased with age (p <0.001) and with heart weight (p <0.001). All 3 variables (cuspal area, cuspal weight and sinus of Valsalva volume) also increased with age and heart weight relative to each other. Additionally, the luminal area at the sinotubular junction also increased with age and heart weight, and it also increased as the sum of the aortic valve cuspal areas and weights and sinus of Valsalva volumes increased.

Detailed measurements of the aortic valve cusps disclosed that in only 16% of the patients were the 3 aortic valve cusps of similar sizes (<5% difference in area between cusps); in 51% of patients 1 cusp was of different size from the other 2, and in 33% of patients all 3 cusps were of different sizes. That aortic valve cusps are often of different size was pointed out by Roberts[2] in 1970, but actual measurements on each cusp were not performed. Vollebergh and Becker[3] in 1977 measured the "width," a measurement corresponding to our measurement 4 (Fig. 2), and "height," a mea-

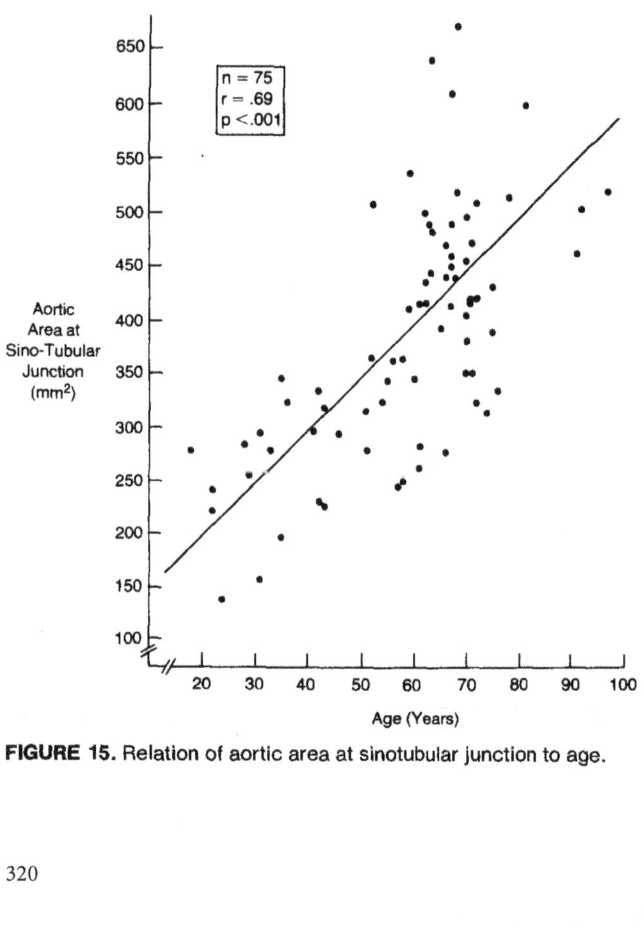

FIGURE 15. Relation of aortic area at sinotubular junction to age.

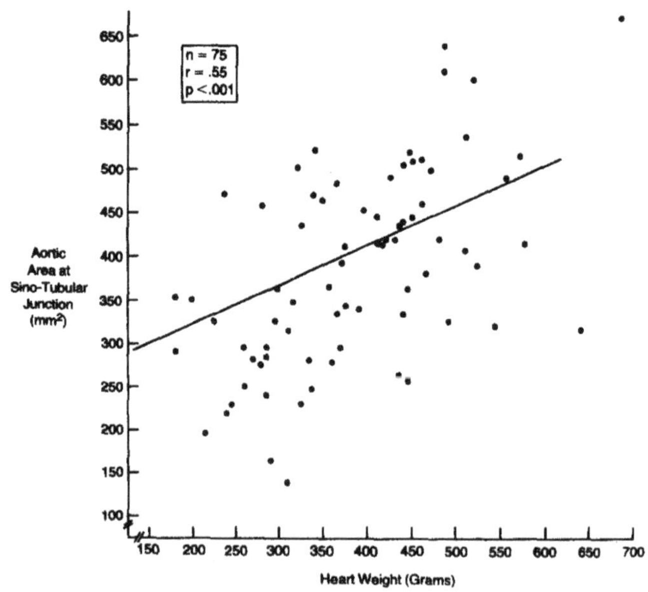

FIGURE 16. Relation of aortic area at sinotubular junction to heart weight.

surement corresponding to our measurement 3 (Fig. 2), in 200 necropsy patients "... who had no clinical signs of aortic stenosis and no other cardiac abnormality that could have affected the aortic valve." Both height and width of each cusp were usually different in each patient. The actual heights of the 3 cusps were not provided, however; the results of these measurements were expressed as a percentage of the width of the same cusp. The average width of the right cusp was 25.9 mm; that of the posterior cusp 25.5 mm and that of the left cusp 25.0 mm. Whether or not these differences are significant was not stated. These investigators also calculated the area of each cusp by applying the formula $\pi/4$ (width $\times$ height). Using this formula, they found that only 5 of the 200 hearts had cusps of equal areas and that 53 of the 54 hearts of patients younger than 40 years of age had cusps of unequal areas.

In contrast to the few studies describing measurements on the aortic valve in human beings,[3,4] several reports have described results of measurements on the ascending aorta. Krovetz[5] recalculated data gathered initially by Sutter[6] in 1897 and by Kani[7] in 1910 and demonstrated that the size of the aorta, at the level of the sinuses of Valsalva and 1 cm above the sinotubular junction and expressed as cross-sectional area per square meter of body surface area, decreases during the first 20 years of life and increases thereafter (r = 0.77). Several groups of investigators have described results of measuring the circumference of the aorta, presumably at the sinotubular junction, at necropsy. De La Cruz et al,[8] Rowlatt et al,[9] and Eckner et al[10] measured aortic circumference in children and found that it related to body surface area, weight and age. Hutchins and Anaya,[11] Davies[12] and Westaby et al[13] found wide variation in the circumference or diameter of the proximal aorta in adults and it was not importantly related to the size of the patient but it did increase with age.

Acknowledgment: We thank Robert Fatula and Sandra York for their assistance with the videoplanimetry measurements.

References

1. **Dvorak JA, Schutte WH, Whitehouse WC.** A simple video method for the quantification of microscopic objects. J Microscopy 1974;102:71–76.
2. **Roberts WC.** The structure of the aortic valve in clinically isolated aortic stenosis. An autopsy study of 162 patients over 15 years of age. Circulation 1970;42:91–97.
3. **Vollebergh FEMG, Becker AE.** Minor congenital variations of cusp size in tricuspid aortic valves. Possible link with isolated aortic stenosis. Br Heart J 1977;39:1006–1011.
4. **Swanson WM, Clark RE.** Dimensions and geometric relationships of the human aortic valve as a function of pressure. Circ Res 1974;35:871–882.
5. **Krovetz LJ.** Age-related changes in size of the aortic valve annulus in man. Am Heart J 1975;90:569–574.
6. **Suter F.** Über das Verhalten des aortenumfanges unter physiologischen und pathologischen Bedingungen. Arch Exp Pathol Pharmacol 1887;39: 289–299.
7. **Kani I.** Systematische Lichtungs und Dickenmessungen des grossen Arterien und ihre Bedeutung für die Pathologie des Getässe. Virchows Arch Pathol Anat 1910;201:45–59.
8. **De La Cruz MV, Anselmi G, Romero A, Monroy G.** A qualitative and quantitative study of the ventricles and great vessels of normal children. Am Heart J 1960;60:675–690.
9. **Rowlatt UF, Rimoldi HJA, Lev M.** The quantitative anatomy of the normal child's heart. Pediatr Clin North Am 1963;10:499–588.
10. **Eckner FAO, Brown BW, Davidson DL, Glagov S.** Dimensions of normal human hearts after standard fixation by controlled pressure coronary perfusion. Arch Pathol 1969;88:497–507.
11. **Hutchins AM, Anaya OA.** Measurements of cardiac size, chamber volumes and valve orifices at autopsy. Johns Hopkins Med J 1973;133:96–106.
12. **Davies MJ.** The aortic valve. *In* Crawford T, ed. Pathology of Cardiac Valves. London: Butterworths, 1980:1–61.
13. **Westaby S, Karp RB, Blackstone EH, Bishop SP.** Adult human valve dimensions and their surgical significance. Am J Cardiol 1984;53:552–556.

Aortic Valve Perforation With Calcific Aortic Valve Stenosis and Without Infective Endocarditis or Significant Aortic Regurgitation

WILLIAM C. ROBERTS, MD
CHARLES L. McINTOSH, MD
ROBERT B. WALLACE, MD

Small lucunae adjacent to commissures are often observed in the aortic valve cusps of older persons, and they have no functional consequences. Larger perforations in the more central portions of 1 or more aortic valve cusps, in contrast, are uncommon, nearly always the consequence of infective endocarditis; they usually produce severe aortic regurgitation, and rarely involve valves that are either calcified or stenotic.[1,2] Recently, we encountered 3 patients with large perforations in an aortic valve cusp associated with cuspal calcific deposits, large enough in 2 patients to cause aortic valve stenosis and warrant valve replacement; only 1 had associated aortic regurgitation, and none had a clinical event compatible with infective endocarditis. Such cases have not been reported previously.

From the Pathology and Surgery Branches, National Heart, Lung, and Blood Institute, National Institutes of Health, Bethesda, Maryland, and the Department of Surgery, Georgetown University Medical Center, Washington, D.C. Manuscript received and accepted August 21, 1986.

Pertinent findings in the 3 patients are summarized in Table I and illustrated in Figures 1 through 4. Both men had congenitally bicuspid aortic valves that were stenotic, and each was excised and replaced (Fig. 1 to 3). Patient 3, an 85-year-old woman, died from a noncardiac condition. In each of the 3 patients, a protruding calcific nodule on the ventricular aspect of 1 cusp closed the perforation in the apposing cusp. The portion of the cusp in the vicinity of the perforation was devoid of calcific deposits, whereas the cusp in apposition to the perforation contained prominent calcific deposits.

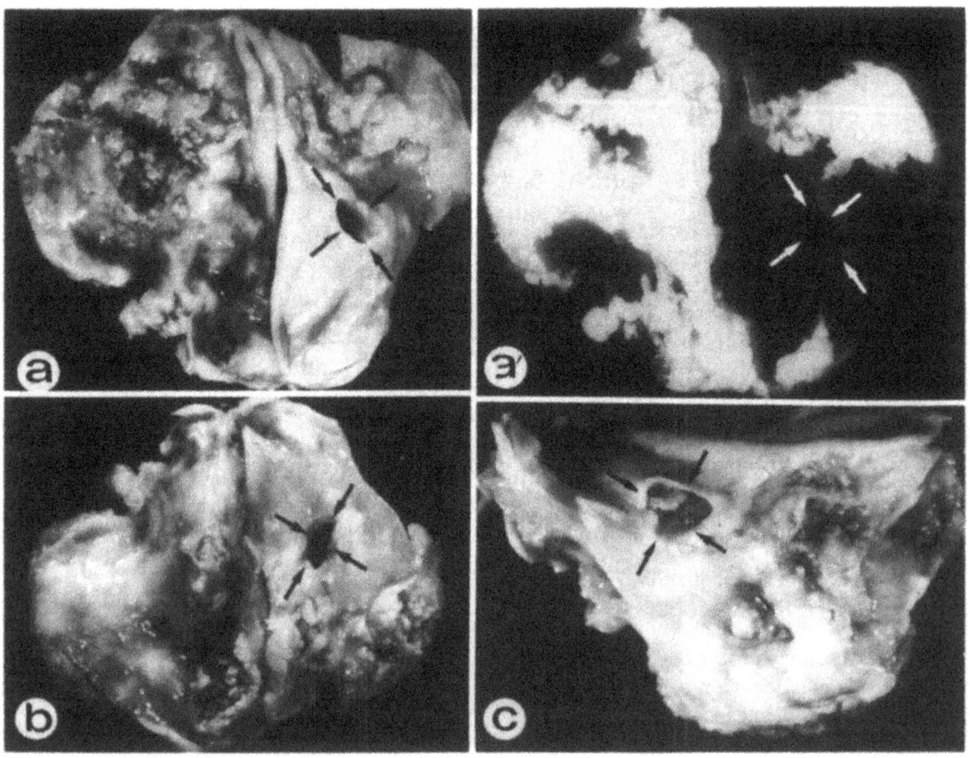

FIGURE 1. Patient 1. Operatively excised congenitally bicuspid aortic valve from the aortic aspect (*a*) and radiograph (*a'*), from the ventricular aspect (*b*), and a view of the aortic aspect of the cusp with calcium protruding into the cusp (*c*). The perforation is designated by the *arrow*.

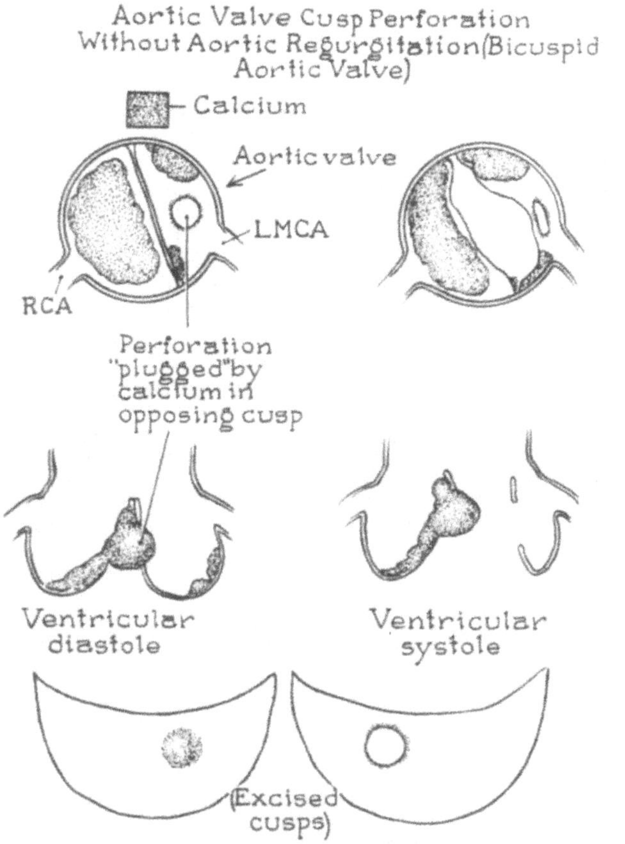

FIGURE 2. Patient 1. Drawing of the aortic valve illustrating the mechanism of the cuspal perforation. LMCA = left main coronary artery; RCA = right coronary artery.

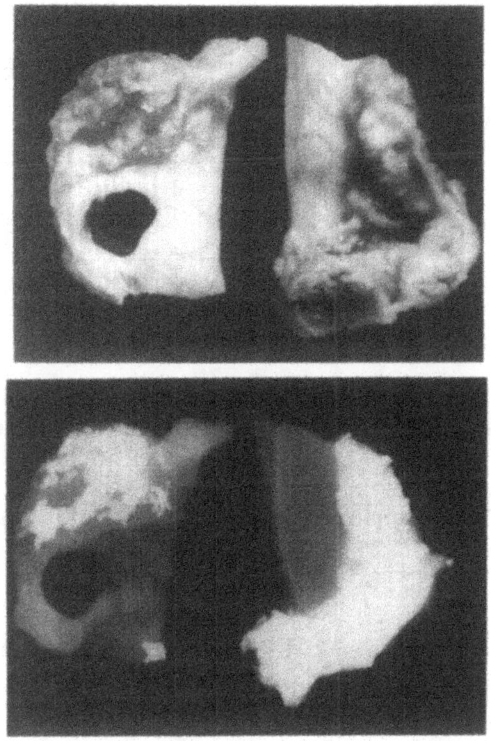

FIGURE 3. Patient 2. Operatively excised congenitally bicuspid aortic valve with radiograph. The perforation is located in the noncalcified portions of the cusp in apposition to heavy calcific deposits in the other cusp.

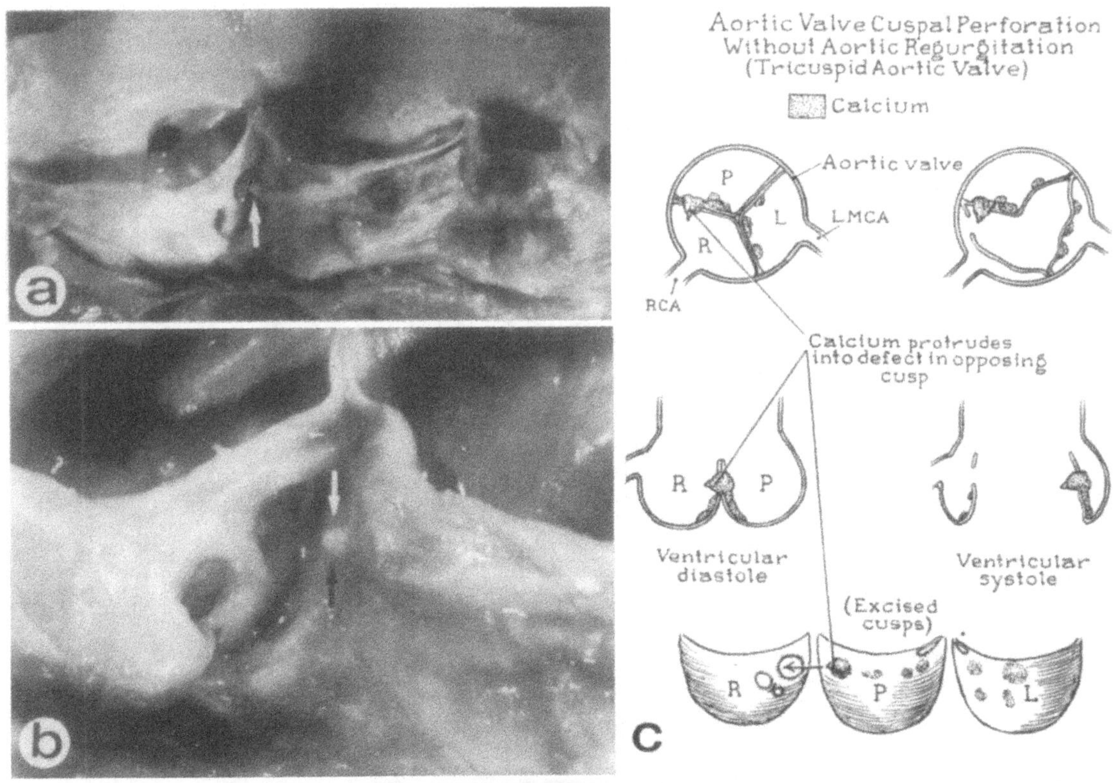

FIGURE 4. Patient 3. *a* and *b*, 2 views of the opened 3-cuspid aortic valve showing 2 large and 1 small perforation in the right cusp and a calcific spur from the posterior cusp protruding into 1 of the perforations in the right cusp. *c*, diagram illustrating the mechanism of cuspal perforation. L = left; LMCA = left main coronary artery; P = posterior; R = right; RCA = right coronary artery.

TABLE I Pertinent Observations in the Three Patients

Case	Age (year) at AVR or Death	Sex	Pressures (mm Hg) LV (s/d)	SA (s/d)	LV-SA psg	AR by AA Cine (0-3+)	Murmur of AR	No. AV Cusps	HW (g)
1	62	M	240/20	185/85	55	0	0	2	...
2	64	M	220/9	155/90	65	1+	2/6	2	620
3	85	F	...	160/100	...	...	0	3	440

AA = ascending aorta; AR = aortic regurgitation; AV = aortic valve; AVR = aortic valve replacement; HW = heart weight; LV = left ventricle; psg = peak systolic gradient; SA = systemic artery; s/d = peak systole/end diastole.

Thus, perforation of 1 aortic valve cusp in each of the 3 patients resulted from the trauma engendered by a calcific nodule in 1 cusp, protruding into and finally perforating a noncalcified portion of the apposing cusp. This mechanism of cuspal perforation has not been described previously and neither has aortic valve cuspal perforation without aortic regurgitation.

1. Roberts WC, Buchbinder NA. *Healed left-sided infective endocarditis: a clinicopathologic study of 59 patients. Am J Cardiol 1977;40:876–888.*

2. Roberts WC. *Characteristics and consequences of infective endocarditis (active or healed or both) learned from morphologic studies. In: Rahimtoola SH, ed. Infective Endocarditis. New York: Grune & Stratton, 1978: 55–123.*

FROM THE EDITOR

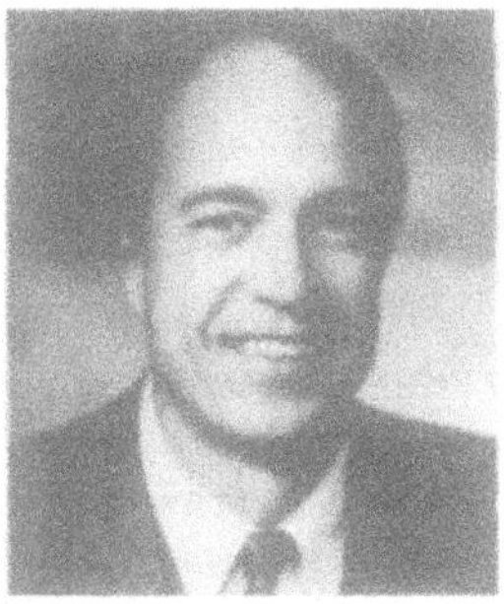

Examining Operatively Excised Cardiac Valves

Recently, I received a letter from a cardiovascular surgeon (Henry E. Martinez, MD, Amarillo, Texas) describing how operatively excised cardiac valves are handled by the pathologist at his hospital and inquiring whether or not I agreed with the method of handling. His letter stated ". . .we have rules in our hospital that require that all cardiac valves excised be sent to the pathologists for processing. There they are fixed and slide preparations are made. The pathologist then looks at the slides, sends a detailed report and accompanying bill to the patient. It has been my opinion for a long time that these reports are of no

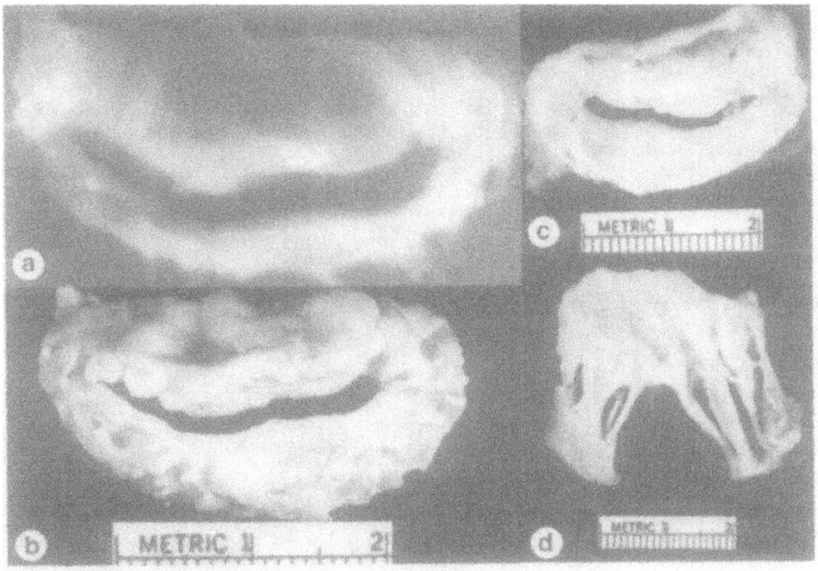

FIGURE 1. Operatively excised severely stenotic mitral valve in a 63-year-old woman (S67-815) who several years earlier had undergone mitral commissurotomy. *a*, radiograph showing 2 minute-sized calcific deposits. *b*, view of ventricular aspect after excision of chordae tendineae and papillary muscles. *c*, view of atrial aspect. *d*, view of anterior mitral leaflet and its attached chordae tendineae. This would have been a good valve for repeat commissurotomy either by finger, instrument or balloon. There was no mitral regurgitation.

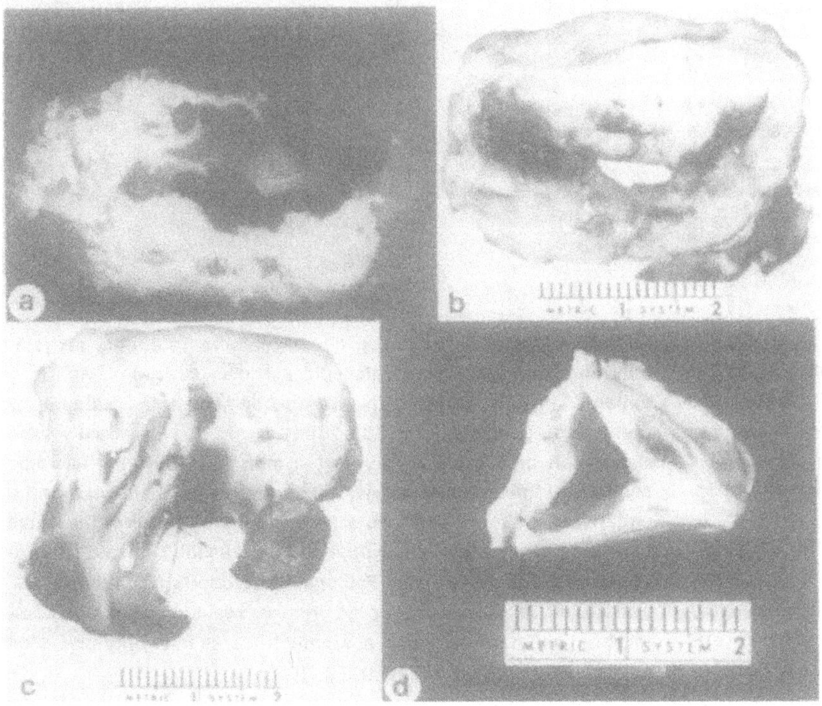

FIGURE 2. Operatively excised severely stenotic mitral valve (*a*, *b* and *c*) and stenotic and regurgitant aortic valve (*d*) in a 30-year-old woman (S74-5035). *a*, radiograph of mitral valve showing heavy calcific deposit. *b*, mitral valve from left atrial aspect. *c*, mitral valve showing ventricular aspect of the anterior mitral leaflet and its attached chordae tendineae and papillary muscle. *d*, aortic aspect of a 3-cuspid aortic valve with fusion of 1 of the 3 commissures. A suture was placed at the sites of the nonfused commissures so that the photograph could show how the valve appeared when intact.

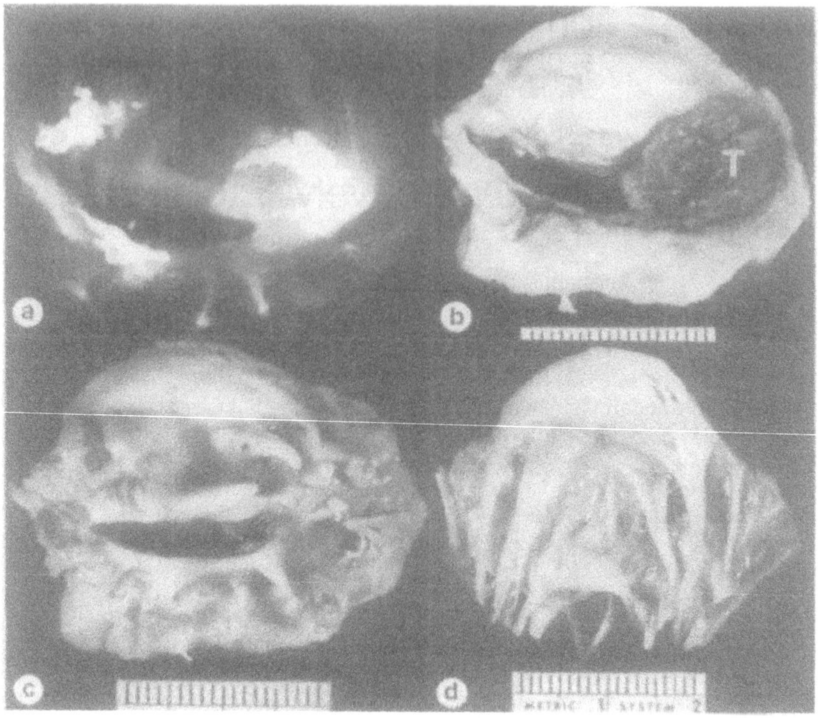

FIGURE 3. Operatively excised severely stenotic mitral valve in a 72-year-old woman (S76-76). ***a*****, radiograph showing 3 calcific deposits.** ***b*****, view from atrial aspect showing a thrombus (T) at the anterolateral commissure.** ***c*****, view from ventricular aspect.** ***d*****, view of ventricular aspect of anterior mitral leaflet. Neither papillary muscle had been excised. Balloon valvulotomy would be undesirable in the presence of thrombus adjacent to the valve orifice, but fortunately, thrombus at this location is rare.**

value. . .in the patient's subsequent course or in educating the medical personnel associated with the patient."

I agree completely with Dr. Martinez and discussed this subject in an article in 1966.[1] In my laboratory, the only operatively excised cardiac valves that are divided into smaller pieces for histologic examination are those with obvious vegetations or those suspected of containing vegetative material, and these type valves are relatively infrequently seen. The final anatomic diagnosis of all other operatively excised cardiac valves is based entirely on gross inspection, and no histologic sections are prepared.

In my view, the surgeon should make every attempt to excise the cardiac valve intact. During the past 25 years, I have examined hundreds of cardiac valves excised by a number of different surgeons. Usually, it is possible to identify the operating surgeon by examining the operatively excised valve. Some surgeons virtually routinely excise the valve intact; others virtually never excise the valve intact. It is likely that the chance of dislodgment of fragments of the valve is less when the valve is removed intact than when it is removed in multiple pieces. In the 1960s most operatively excised mitral valves received in my laboratory contained portions of both papillary muscles. Today, papillary muscles are less often excised, and therefore, accuracy in detecting ruptured chordae tendineae is less than in the early period of valve replacement. Also today, portions of the posterior mitral leaflet are often not excised when valve replacement is performed for pure mitral regurgitation.

The most important procedure to be performed on the operatively excised valve is a good photograph of it (Fig. 1 to 5). Ideally, the photograph should be a part of the official report describing gross anatomic features of the excised valve. In my laboratory, all stenotic and most purely regurgitant operatively excised valves are x-rayed, and these radiographs provide precise records of the presence and the amount of calcific depos-

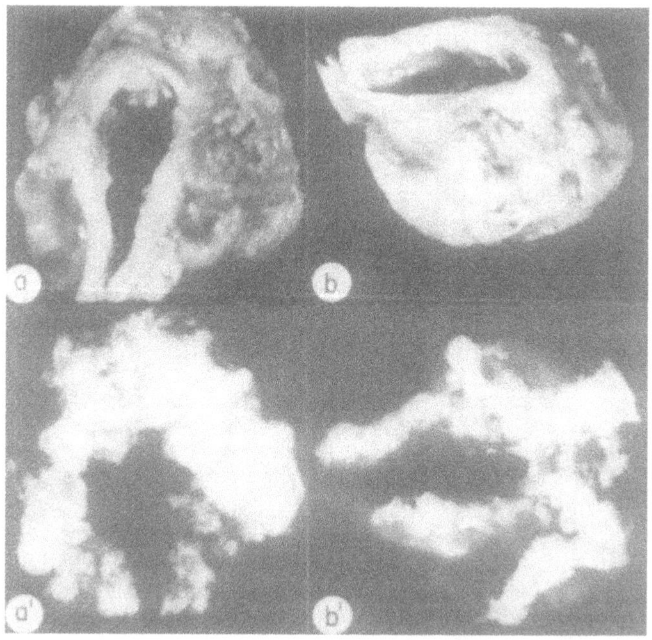

FIGURE 4. Operatively excised, heavily calcified, stenotic, congenitally unicommissural and unicuspid aortic valves from each of 2 patients. ***a*** **and** ***a'*****, view of valve from aortic aspect and radiography of it in a 53-year-old man (S69-2699).** ***b*** **and** ***b'*****, view of valve and radiograph of it from a 41-year-old man (S70-3087). Histologic sections of these valves would, of course, not have shown that the underlying malformation was a congenital one and that the valve consisted of a single cusp rather than the usual 3 cusps. (Reproduced with permission from Falcone MW, Roberts WC, Morrow AG, and Perloff JK. Congenital aortic stenosis resulting from a unicommissural valve. Clinical and anatomic features in twenty-one adult patients. Circulation 1971;44:272–280).**

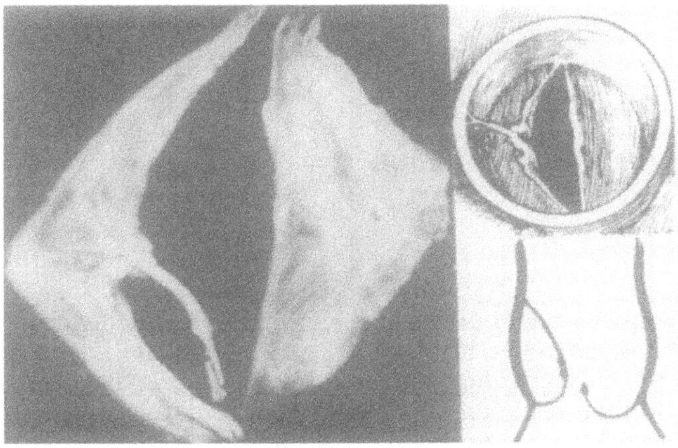

FIGURE 5. Operatively excised, purely regurgitant, congenitally bicuspid aortic valve in a 26-year-old man (A66-6). One of the cusps was attached to the wall of aorta cephalad to the sinotubular junction as shown in the drawing. (The photograph of the noncalcified valve is reproduced with permission from reference 6.)

its. Finally, all operatively excised valves are retained. This retention and storage of all valves allows studies of the causes of the various types of valvular dysfunction during different periods and other clinicomorphologic studies.[2–19]

In summary, the operatively excised cardic valve should not be processed as a "routine surgical specimen." The most precise morphologic diagnosis results from careful gross inspection of the valve and not from histologic examination of sections of it. Photographs of the valve provide the most effective record of the pathologic findings, and permit correlations between the anatomic abnormalities and clinical, hemodynamic and operative findings.

William C. Roberts, MD
Editor in Chief

1. Roberts WC, Morrow AG. *Cardiac valves and the surgical pathologist.* Arch Pathol 1966;82:309–313.
2. Roberts WC, Buchbinder NA. *Healed left-sided infective endocarditis: a clinicopathologic study of 59 patients.* Am J Cardiol 1977;40:876–888.
3. Lachman AS, Roberts WC. *Calcific deposits in stenotic mitral valves. Extent and relation to age, sex, degree of stenosis, cardiac rhythm, previous commissurotomy and left atrial body thrombus from study of 164 operatively-excised valves.* Circulation 1978;57:808–815.
4. Covarrubias EA, Sheikh MU, Isner J, Gomes M, Hufnagel CA, Roberts WC. *Calcific pulmonic stenosis in adulthood. Treatment by valve replacement (porcine xenograft) with postoperative hemodynamic evaluation.* Chest 1979;75:399–402.
5. Roberts WC, Lachman AS. *Mitral valve commissurotomy versus replacement. Considerations based on examination of operatively excised stenotic mitral valves.* Am Heart J 1979;98:56–62.
6. Roberts WC, Morrow AG, McIntosh CL, Jones M, Epstein SE. *Congenitally bicuspid aortic valve causing severe, pure aortic regurgitation without superimposed infective endocarditis. Analysis of 13 patients requiring aortic valve replacement.* Am J Cardiol 1981;47:206–209.
7. Waller BJ, Morrow AG, Maron BJ, Del Negro AA, Kent DM, McGrath FJ, Wallace RB, McIntosh CL, Roberts WC. *Etiology of clinically isolated, severe, chronic, pure mitral regurgitation: analysis of 97 patients over 30 years of age having mitral valve replacement.* Am Heart J 1982;104:276–288.
8. Waller BF, Kishel JC, Roberts WC. *Severe aortic regurgitation from systemic hypertension.* Chest 1982;82:365–368.
9. Waller BF, McManus BM, Roberts WC. *Mitral valve stenosis produced by or worsened by active bacterial endocarditis.* Chest 1982;82:498–500.
10. Byram MT, Roberts WC. *Frequency and extent of calcific deposits in purely regurgitant mitral valves: analysis of 108 operatively excised valves.* Am J Cardiol 1983;52:1059–1061.
11. Waller BF, Maron BJ, Del Negro AA, Gottdiener JS, Roberts WC. *Frequency and significance of M-mode echocardiographic evidence of mitral prolapse in clinically isolated pure mitral regurgitation: analysis of 65 patients having mitral valve replacement.* Am J Cardiol 1984;53:139–147.
12. Day PJ, Roberts WC. *Relation of level of total serum cholesterol to amount of calcific deposits in operatively excised stenotic mitral valves: analysis of 155 cases.* Am J Cardiol 1984;53:157–159.
13. Subramanian R, Olson LJ, Edwards WD. *Surgical pathology of pure aortic stenosis: a study of 374 cases.* Mayo Clin Proc 1984;59:683–690.
14. Olson LJ, Subramanian R, Edwards WD. *Surgical pathology of pure aortic insufficiency: a study of 225 cases.* Mayo Clin Proc 1984;59:835–841.
15. Jeresaty RM, Edwards JE, Chawla SK. *Mitral valve prolapse and ruptured chordae tendineae.* Am J Cardiol 1985;55:138–142.
16. Subramanian R, Olson LJ, Edwards WD. *Surgical pathology of combined aortic stenosis and insufficiency: a study of 213 cases.* Mayo Clin Proc 1985;60:247–254.
17. Hanson TP, Edwards BS, Edwards JE. *Pathology of surgically excised mitral valves: one hundred consecutive cases.* Arch Pathol Lab Med 1985;109:823–828.
18. Peterson MD, Roach RM, Edwards JE. *Types of aortic stenosis in surgically removed valves.* Arch Pathol Lab Med 1985;109:829–832.
19. Roberts WC, McIntosh CL, Wallace RB. *Mechanisms of severe mitral regurgitation in mitral valve prolapse determined from analysis of operatively excised valves.* Am Heart J 1987;113:1316–1323.

Cardiac Valve Replacement for Stenotic Bicuspid Aortic Valve in Husband and for Purely Regurgitant Prolapsed Mitral Valve in Wife

JESSICA M. MANN, MD
CHARLES L. McINTOSH, MD
NEVIN M. KATZ, MD
WILLIAM C. ROBERTS, MD

Congenital heart disease is recognized to occur in families, i.e., in a parent or grandparent and in 1 or more siblings. The occurrence of congenital heart disease in both husband and wife must indeed be rare, and even more so is the occurrence of cardiac valve replacement in both husband and wife. Such was the case, however, in 2 recently studied patients. Each had the most common congenital heart disease that occurs in their sex, namely, mitral valve prolapse in women and bicuspid aortic valve in men.[1]

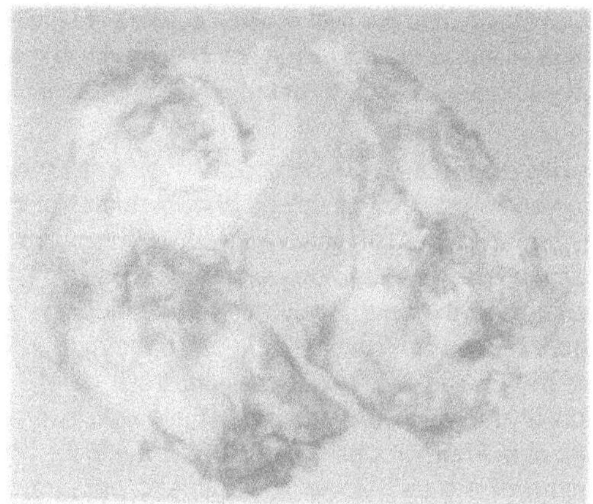

FIGURE 1. View of the operatively excised stenotic bicuspid aortic valve.

From the Pathology and Surgery Branches, National Heart, Lung, Blood Institute, National Institutes of Health, Bethesda, Maryland 20892, and the Department of Surgery, Georgetown University, Washington, D.C. Manuscript received and accepted 18 March 1987.

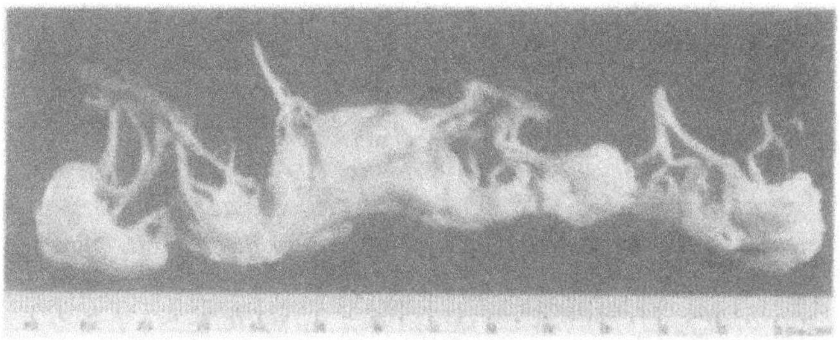

FIGURE 2. View of the operatively excised purely regurgitant and prolapsed mitral valve.

The husband was 63 years old at the time of aortic valve replacement for a congenitally bicuspid stenotic aortic valve (Fig. 1). The wife was 69 years old at the time of mitral valve replacement for mitral regurgitation secondary to a severely prolapsed valve (Fig. 2). The husband's aortic valve was replaced with a Björk-Shiley prosthesis (no. 23). The wife's mitral valve was initially replaced with a porcine aortic valve, which degenerated rapidly because of her oral consumption of calcium supplements.[2] The degenerated porcine bioprosthesis was replaced 18 months after the initial operation by a Medtronic-Hall prosthesis (no. 31). Both husband and wife are on daily warfarin therapy and both are asymptomatic.

The occurrence of cardiac valve replacement in both husband and wife has not been described previously.

1. Roberts WC. *The 2 most common congenital heart diseases. From the editor. Am J Cardiol 1984;53:1198.*

2. Moront M, Katz NM. *Early degeneration of a porcine aortic valve bioprosthesis in the mitral valve position in an elderly woman and its association with long-term calcium carbonate therapy. Am J Cardiol 1987;59:1006–1007.*

Morphologic Findings in Stenotic Aortic Valves That Have Had "Successful" Percutaneous Balloon Valvuloplasty

Jay M. Kalan, MD, Jessica M. Mann, MD, Martin B. Leon, MD, Augusto Pichard, MD, Kenneth M. Kent, MD, and William C. Roberts, MD

Percutaneous transluminal aortic valvuloplasty in adults was first reported in 1986 and since then multiple reports have described successful and unsuccessful consequences of this procedure. Despite these multiple reports surprisingly few morphologic descriptions have been reported of stenotic aortic valves that have been subjected to this procedure. Such is the purpose of this report.

From the Pathology and Cardiology Branches, National Heart, Lung, and Blood Institute, National Institutes of Health, Bethesda, Maryland, the Division of Cardiology, Department of Medicine, Washington Hospital Center, Washington, DC, and the Division of Cardiology, Department of Medicine, Georgetown University Hospital, Washington, DC.
Manuscript received March 3, 1988; revised manuscript received and accepted April 5, 1988.

Clinical and necropsy findings in our 3 patients are summarized in Table I. All 3 had symptoms of congestive heart failure before valvuloplasty and patient no. 1 also had angina pectoris and syncope. The 3 patients tolerated the procedure well and no complications were apparent while they were in the cardiac catheterization laboratory. Hypotension developed in patient no. 1 two

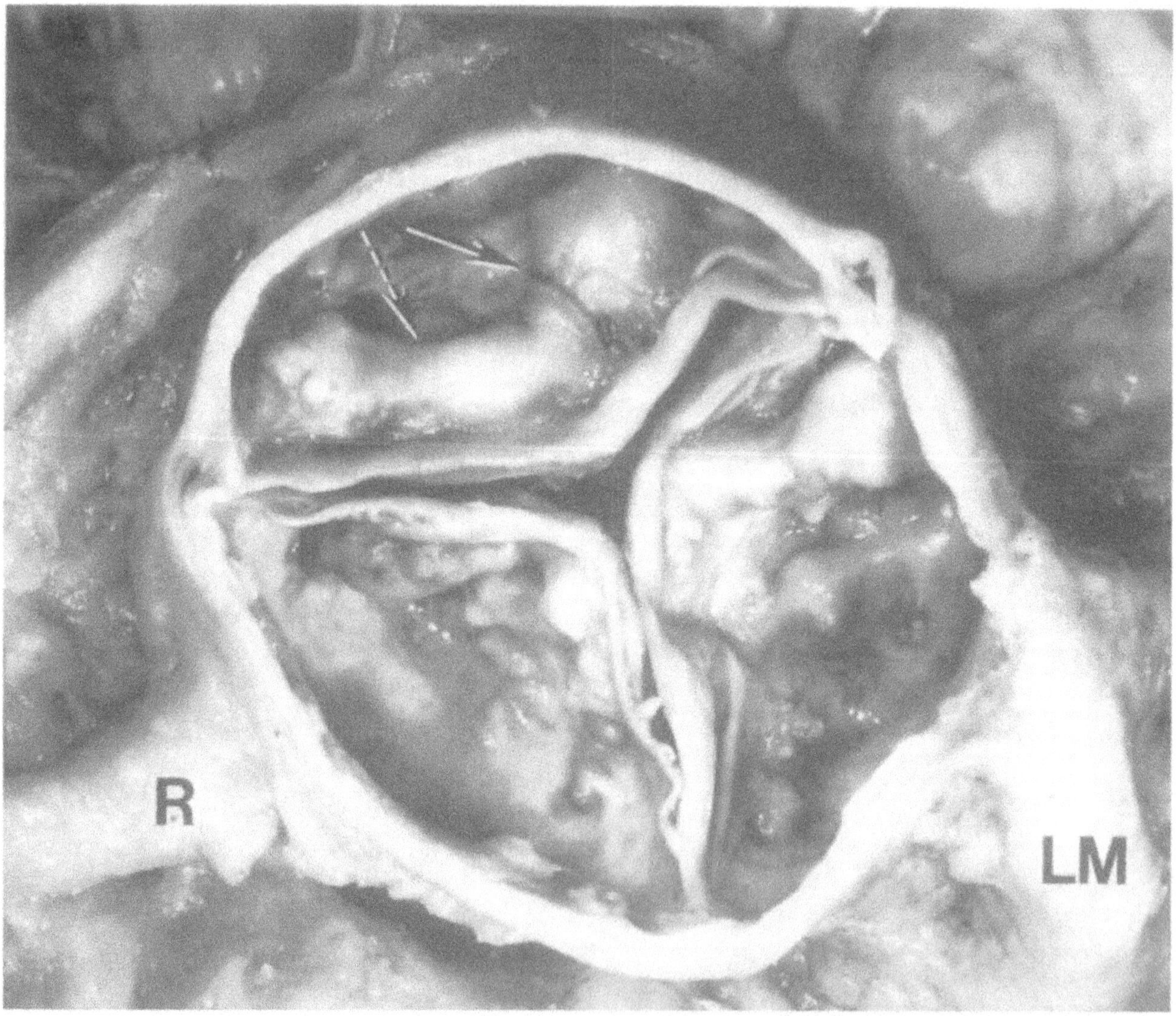

no commissural fusion. A crack is visible through the calcific bar in the posterior cusp (*solid arrow*). A partial crack was seen on a roentgenogram of the aortic valve, but it is not seen in this view (*dashed arrow*). A third crack was present through the calcific bar in the left cusp (not shown). No crack was present in the calcific deposits in the right cusp. LM = left main coronary artery; R = right coronary artery.

TABLE I Clinical and Morphologic Features of Three Patients Studied at Necropy After Percutaneous Aortic Valvuloplasty

Pt	Age (yrs), Sex	Pressures (mm hg): Immediately Before Valvuloplasty				Immediately After Valvuloplasty				Interval Valvuloplasty to Death	HW (g)	No. Fractured Calcium Deposits	AR (0–3+)		Balloon Size (mm)				Balloon Rupture
		LV	Aorta	PSG	AVA	LV	Aorta	PSG	AVA				Pre	Post	15	18	20†	23	
1	89, M	220/22	150/45	70	0.5	160/20	120/42	40	0.9	3 hrs	445	2	+	+	0	0	+	0	+ (20 mm)
2	81, F	210/10	130/60	80	0.4	180/12	140/160	40	0.7	36 hrs	560	3	+	+	+	+	+	+	+ (15 mm)
3	72, M	155/8	105/50	50	0.3	120/5	90/45	30	0.7	194 days	490	3	++	++	0	0	+	0	0
						140/2*	105/40*	35*	0.55*										

* Values obtained 184 days after valvuloplasty, 10 days before death.
† Only 1 balloon used at a time.
AR = aortic regurgitation; AVA = aortic valve area in cm^2; HW = heart weight; LV = left ventricle; PGS = peak systolic gradient; + = present; 0 = absent.

hours afterwards, and it was followed quickly by fatal electromechanical dissociation. Patient 2 had a thrombectomy and evacuation of a large hematoma of her thigh the day after valvuloplasty, and she became bradycardic and hypotensive the next day; these findings were followed by fatal electromechanical dissociation. Patient 3 was asymptomatic for 2 months and then dyspnea reappeared and progressed. Six months after valvuloplasty repeat cardiac catheterization was performed (Table I). Cardiac arrest occurred the following day: he never regained consciousness and died 5 days later. At necropsy, all 3 aortic valves were 3-cuspid (Figures 1 through 3). All had heavy calcific deposits in each cusp. In 2 patients none of the 3 commissures was fused; in patient 3, one of 3 commissures was fused, and the fusion was unaffected by the valvuloplasty. Deposits of calcium were fractured in 2 of the 3 cusps in each patient (Figures 1 through 3). None of the cusps in any patient was torn or perforated.

Percutaneous balloon dilatation of a stenotic aortic valve in adults was first described by Cribier et al[1] in 1986. Later that year McKay et al[2] described consequences of balloon angioplasty of 5 stenotic aortic valves dilated at necropsy and of 5 other stenotic aortic valves dilated intraoperatively before valve replacement: in 2 necropsy valves calcific deposits were fractured and in the 3 valves with fused commissures there was partial or complete separation of the fused cusps. In 1987, McKay et al[3] described necropsy findings (without illustrations) in 3 patients who had undergone percutaneous balloon valvuloplasty of stenotic aortic valves: each had fracture of at least 1 calcific deposit. Safian et al[4] reported consequences of balloon valvuloplasty of stenotic aortic valves in 33 patients at necropsy and in 6 patients at operation: calcific cuspal deposits were fractured in 16 patients, 5 had separation of fused cusps and 6 had both cuspal fracture and cuspal separation. Drobinski et al[5] reported morphologic data in 2 necropsy and 3 surgical patients who had had percutaneous aortic balloon valvuloplasty: calcific deposits were fractured in 1 cusp of a congenitally bicuspid valve; no specific findings were noted in 2 other bicuspid valves or in two 3-cuspid valves with fused commissures. Robicsek and Harbold[6] measured orifice size and cuspal mobility before and after valvuloplasty at operation immediately before valve replacement in 16 patients: of the 10 patients with bicuspid aortic valves the only anatomic consequence was separation of fused cusps in 2 of the 4 patients who had fused commissures; in 2 patients with unicuspid valves, no change was noted; and in the 4 patients with 3-cuspid aortic valves, fractures in calcific deposits occurred in 3 patients. Isner et al[7] described morphologic features of "successful" percutaneous aortic valvuloplasty in 3 patients studied at necropsy; grossly visible fractures of the calcific deposits in 1 or more cusps were seen in all 3 patients. Of the 16 patients described by Robicsek and Harbold, 7 were younger than 65 years of age. In contrast, of the total of 60 patients described by McKay,[2] Safian,[4] Drobinski[5] and their coworkers, all but a few were over 65 years of age.

All of our 3 patients were over 65 years of age, all had 3-cuspid aortic valves and all had a significant reduction in valve gradient by the procedure without development of, or worsening of, aortic regurgitation and without dislodgement of calcific debris. Two died suddenly shortly after the procedure and 1 died 6 months after the procedure. Distinct fractures occurred in the calcific aortic valve cuspal deposits in 2 or 3 of the cusps in each patient.

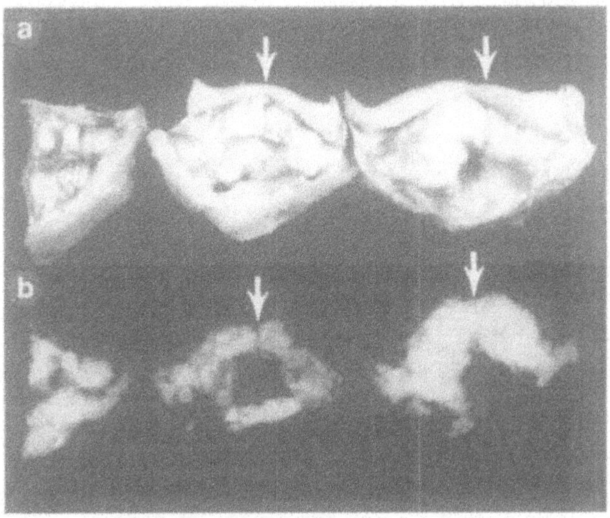

FIGURE 2. Patient no. 2. Photograph and roentgenogram of the excised 3-cuspid aortic valve. *a* shows a single crack in each of the calcific deposits in the right and left aortic valve cusps (*arrows*). *b* the roentgenogram confirms the presence of the crack in the calcific deposits (*arrows*). A crack was present on the posterior cusp at necropsy (not shown).

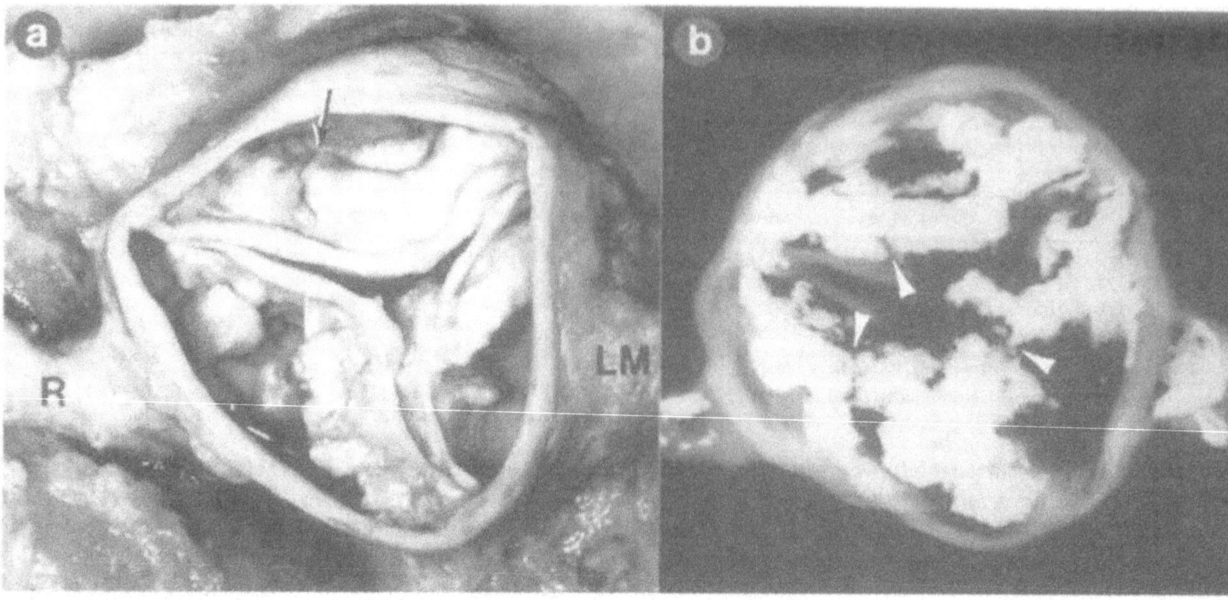

FIGURE 3. Patient no. 3. Photograph and roentgenogram of the 3-cuspid aortic valve. *a*, all 3 aortic valve cusps have extensive calcific deposits and the right and left cusps are completely fused. A crack is visible in the posterior cusp (*arrow*). The calcific bar in the left cusp also was cracked, but this crack is not seen in this view. The right and left cusps remain fused. *b*, the roentgenogram of the excised aortic valve shows a single crack in each of the 3 cusps (*arrows*). LM = left main coronary artery; R = right coronary artery.

The fractures in the cusps 6 months after the procedure in 1 patient were indistinguishable from those occurring within hours of the procedure in the other 2 patients.

Although the initial enthusiasm for aortic valvuloplasty in elderly patients has waned, this procedure nevertheless appears to produce clean anatomic effects, which may benefit elderly persons with stenotic 3-cuspid aortic valves.

1. Cribier A, Savin T, Saoudi N, Rocha P, Berland J, Letac B. *Percutaneous transluminal valvuloplasty of acquired aortic stenosis in elderly patients: an alternative to valve replacement? Lancet 1986;1:63–67.*

2. McKay RG, Safian RD, Lock JE, Mandell VS, Thurer RL, Schnitt SJ, Grossman W. *Balloon dilatation of calcific aortic stenosis in elderly patients: postmortem, intraoperative, and percutaneous valvuloplasty studies. Circulation 1986;74:119–125.*

3. McKay RG, Safian RD, Lock JE, Diver DJ, Berman AD, Warren SE, Come PC, Baim DS, Mandell VE, Royal HD, Grossman W. *Assessment of left ventricular and aortic valve function after aortic balloon valvuloplasty in adult patients with critical aortic stenosis. Circulation 1987;75:192–203.*

4. Safian RD, Mandell VS, Thurer RE, Hutchins GM, Schnitt SJ, Grossman W, McKay RG. *Postmortem and intraoperative balloon valvuloplasty of calcific aortic stenosis in elderly patients: mechanisms of successful dilation. JACC 1987;9:655–660.*

5. Drobinski G, Lechat P, Metzger JP, Lepailleur C, Vacheron A, Grosgogeat Y. *Results of percutaneous catheter valvuloplasty for calcified aortic stenosis in the elderly. Eur Heart J 1987;8:322–328.*

6. Robicsek F, Harbold NB, Jr. *Limited value of balloon dilatation in calcified aortic stenosis in adults: direct observations during open heart surgery. Am J Cardiol 1987;60:857–864.*

7. Isner JM, Samuels DA, Slovenkai GA, Halaburka KR, Hougen TJ, Desnoyers MR, Fields CD, Salem DN. *Mechanism of aortic balloon valvuloplasty: fracture of valvular calcific deposits. Ann Intern Med 1988;108:377–380.*

Development of Severe Stenosis in a Previously Purely Regurgitant, Congenitally Bicuspid Aortic Valve

Jay M. Kalan, MD, Charles L. McIntosh, MD, PhD, Robert O. Bonow, MD, and William C. Roberts, MD

A congenitally bicuspid aortic valve may function normally, it may be stenotic with or without associated regurgitation or it may be purely regurgitant (no associated stenosis).[1,2] Such a valve may function normally for many years and then it may become stenotic (as calcific deposits build up) or it may become purely regurgitant (because of superimposed infective endocarditis or because of reasons unclear). Once a bicuspid valve develops some degree of stenosis, its course thereafter is one of gradually worsening stenosis; once a bicuspid valve develops some degree of pure regurgitation (without associated stenosis), its course thereafter is one of gradually worsening regurgitation. Recently, we encountered a man who 8 years earlier had evidence of severe pure aortic regurgitation (no element of stenosis) and thereafter he went on to develop severe aortic valve stenosis with virtual loss of the regurgitation. To our knowledge, conversion from pure aortic regurgitation to severe aortic stenosis has not been reported. This report records such an occurrence.

A.H., a 70-year-old white man, had a precordial murmur when inducted into the armed forces at about age 25. At age 60, two transient episodes of paroxysmal nocturnal dyspnea occurred and digoxin therapy was started. He remained without symptoms of cardiac dysfunction, able to swim and play tennis, until age 70, when aortic valve replacement was done. At age 62 (1979) his blood pressure was 160/70 mm Hg. Peripheral signs of aortic regurgitation were present, including a rapid carotid artery upstroke, water-hammer pulse and Quincke's sign. A grade 3/6 precordial systolic ejection murmur radiated to the neck, and a grade 3/6 diastolic blow was present and loudest at the left sternal border. Echocardiographic and catheterization data are shown in Table I and Figure 1. Ejection fraction by radionuclide angiography was 63% at rest and 52% with exercise. Exercise capacity by exercise stress test was good. He remained asymptomatic but gradually

From the Pathology, Surgery and Cardiology Branches, National Heart, Lung, and Blood Institute, National Institutes of Health, Bethesda, Maryland 20892. Manuscript received May 19, 1988; revised manuscript received and accepted June 19, 1988.

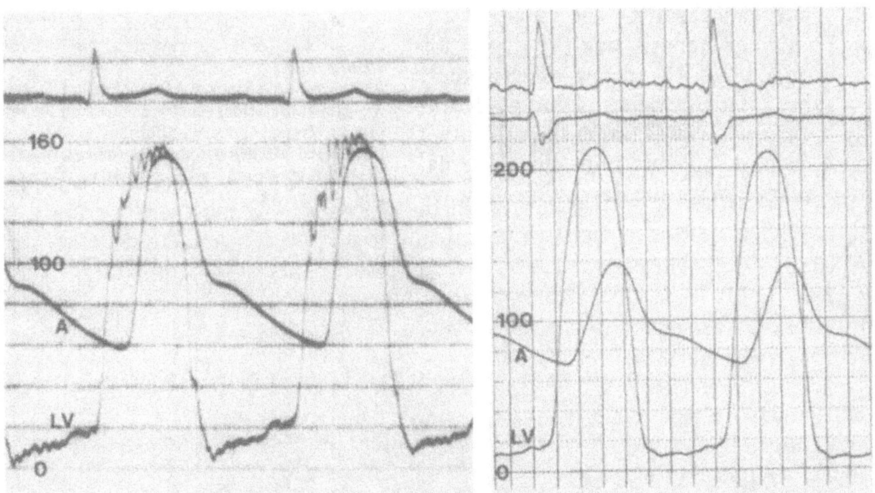

FIGURE 1. Simultaneous pressure tracings from the aorta (A) and left ventricle (LV) at catheterization at age 62 (*left*) and at age 70 (*right*). The left tracing shows no pressure gradient at peak systole across the aortic valve and the right tracing shows a 75-mm Hg peak systolic pressure gradient across the aortic valve.

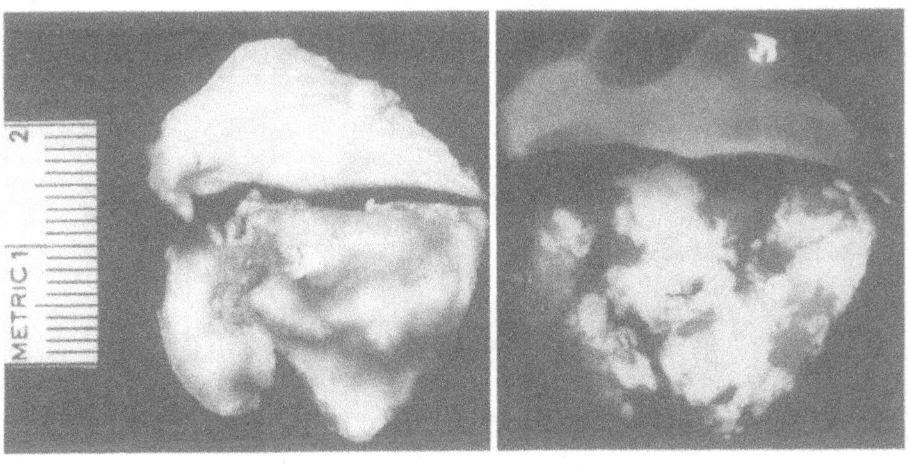

FIGURE 2. Photograph and roentgenogram of the excised aortic valve showing heavy calcific deposits in the anterior cusp and a single small deposit in the posterior cusp.

developed left ventricular hypertrophy without dilatation (Table I). At age 70, transient second-degree heart block was seen on electrocardiogram. The systemic blood pressure was 130/90 mm Hg and the carotid upstroke was delayed. A harsh, grade 4/6 systolic precordial murmur that radiated to the neck was present. No precordial diastolic murmur was heard. Cardiac catheterization (Table I) now showed a 75-mm Hg peak systolic pressure gradient across the aortic valve (Figure 1). The aortic valve was replaced (August 1987) with a 23-mm Hancock porcine bioprosthesis. Seven months postoperatively, he is asymptomatic and active, with an ejection fraction by radionuclide angiography of 70% at rest.

The excised native aortic valve consisted of 2 cusps weighing together 5.9 g (Figure 2). The posterior cusp was mobile but thickened by fibrous tissue; it contained a single small deposit of calcium. The anterior cusp, in contrast, was immobile and contained heavy calcific deposits.

TABLE I Echocardiographic and Catheterization Data

	Age 62	Age 70
Dimensions		
Left ventricular wall (mm)	12	18
Left ventricular cavity (ed/ps) (mm)	60/35	53/35
Fractional shortening (%)	42	34
Pressures (mm Hg)		
Right atrium (mean)	7	7
Right ventricle (ps/ed)	30/10	32/8
Pulmonary artery (ps/ed)	28/12	28/15
Pulmonary artery wedge (mean)	12	10
Left atrium (mean)	12	10
Left ventricle (ps/ed)	155/13	210/17
Aorta (ps/ed)	155/60	135/70
Aorta to left ventricle peak systolic gradient	0	75
Cineangiogram		
Aortic regurgitation	3+/4	trace
Aortic valve calcium	0	3+/4+
Cardiac output (liter/min)	5.7	6.5
Cardiac index (liter/min/m^2)	2.8	3.1

Ed/ps = end-diastole/peak systole.

When calcium is deposited on a congenitally bicuspid valve, it usually is distributed relatively evenly on each of the 2 cusps.[1] In the aforementioned patient, 1 cusp contained heavy deposits and the second was nearly devoid of calcific deposits. The reason for this uneven distribution of the calcific deposits is unclear. There was never clinical evidence of infective endocarditis. The cause of the valvular stenosis was the deposition on one of the cusps of extremely heavy calcific deposits that made this cusp, which was larger than the other cusp, completely immobile. The explanation for the deposition of heavy deposits of calcium on a previously purely regurgitant aortic valve is unclear, but such a documentation has not been recorded previously.

1. Roberts WC. The congenitally bicuspid aortic valve. A study of 85 autopsy cases. *Am J Cardiol 1970;26:72–83.*

2. Roberts WC, Morrow AG, McIntosh CL, Jones M, Epstein SE. Congenitally bicuspid aortic valve causing severe, pure aortic regurgitation without superimposed infective endocarditis. Analysis of 13 patients requiring aortic valve replacement. *Am J Cardiol 1981;47:206–209.*

Congenitally Quadricuspid Aortic Valve: Analysis of Six Necropsy Patients

Daniel J. Fernicola, MD, Jessica M. Mann, MD, and William C. Roberts, MD

Congenitally quadricuspid aortic valves are rare and usually cause no valvular dysfunction. Herein we describe clinical and anatomic findings in 6 patients with quadricuspid aortic valves.

From the Pathology Branch, National Heart, Lung, and Blood Institute, National Institutes of Health, Bethesda, Maryland 20892. Manuscript received July 14, 1988; revised manuscript received and accepted September 15, 1988.

Dr. Fernicola's present address: Department of Medicine, Thomas Jefferson Hospital, Philadelphia, Pennsylvania.

Pertinent findings in the 6 patients are listed in Table I. One quadricuspid aortic valve was severely regurgitant, necessitating surgical replacement. The 5 remaining valves (Figures 1 through 5) functioned normally and each of these 5 patients died from a noncardiac condition. Other congenital cardiac abnormalities were present in 2 of the 6 patients: case 1 had a "ventricular septal defect" that had closed spontaneously (Figure 1),[1] and case 2 had a congenitally deficient posterior half of the anterior mitral leaflet and no attached chordae ten-

TABLE I Clinical and Necropsy Findings in Six Patients with Quadricuspid Aortic Valve

Case No.	Figure No.	Age (yrs), Sex	AR	CAD	HW (g)	Location of Accessory Cusp
1	1	11, F	0	0	270	L-P
2	2	45, M	0	+	425	R-L
3	—	51, F	+	0	520	R-P
4	3	54, M	0	+	395	R-P
5	4	74, M	0	+	765	R-P
6	5	76, F	0	+	410	R-P

AR = aortic regurgitation; CAD = coronary artery disease; HW = heart weight; L = left; P = posterior; R = right; + = present; 0 = absent; — = no information available.

dineae. The accessory cusp in all 6 patients was smaller than any of the other 3 cusps, which were similar in size. The accessory cusp was between the right and posterior cusps in 4 patients (cases 3, 4, 5 and 6), between the left and posterior cusps in case 1 and between the right and left cusps in case 2. The right coronary artery was dominant in the 5 patients in whom coronary dominance was known.

Some findings at necropsy have been reported in at least 18 patients with quadricuspid aortic valves.[1-7] In the 13 patients with detailed information, 11 were male,[2-7] the aortic valve was regurgitant in 5,[1,4,6] infective endo-

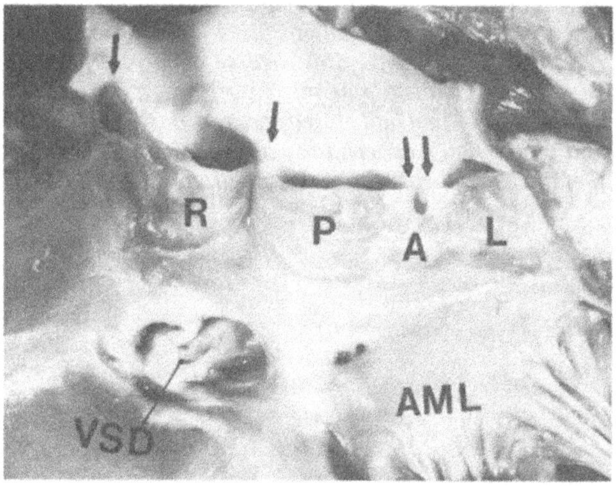

FIGURE 1. Case 1. View of opened ascending aorta, aortic valve and left ventricular outflow tract showing the accessory (A) cusp between the left (L) and posterior (P) cusps. The 4 commissures are designated by *arrows*. A spontaneously closed congenital "ventricular septal defect" (VSD) is present. AML = anterior mitral leaflet; R = right.

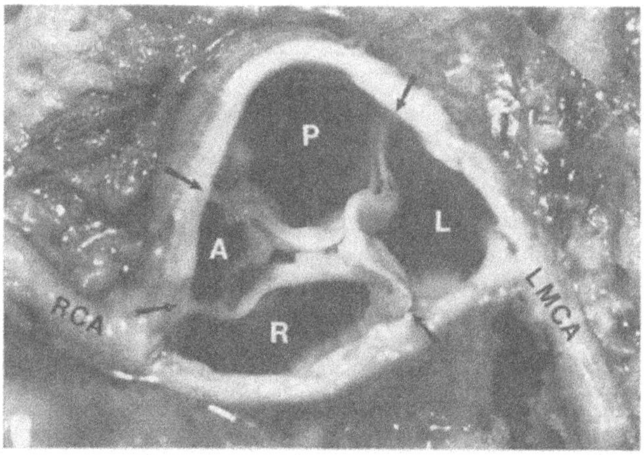

FIGURE 3. Case 4. View of the aortic valve from above showing the accessory (A) cusp located between the right (R) and posterior (P) cusps. The 4 commissures are designated by *arrows*. L = left; LMCA = left main coronary artery; RCA = right coronary artery.

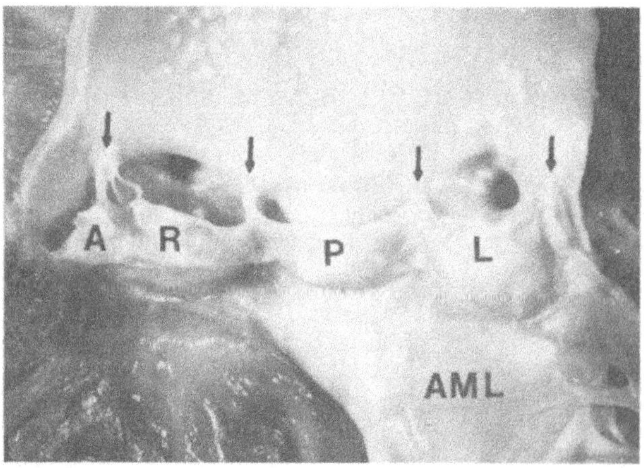

FIGURE 2. Case 2. View of opened ascending aorta, aortic valve and left ventricular outflow tract showing the accessory (A) cusp located between the right (R) and left (L) cusps. The 4 commissures are designated by *arrows*. Other abbreviations as in Figure 1.

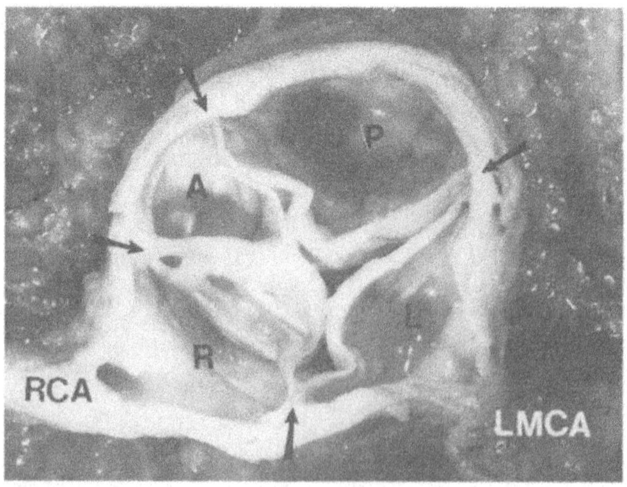

FIGURE 4. Case 5. View of the aortic valve from above showing the accessory (A) cusp between the right (R) and the posterior (P) cusps. The 4 commissures are designated by *arrows*. Other abbreviations as in Figure 3.

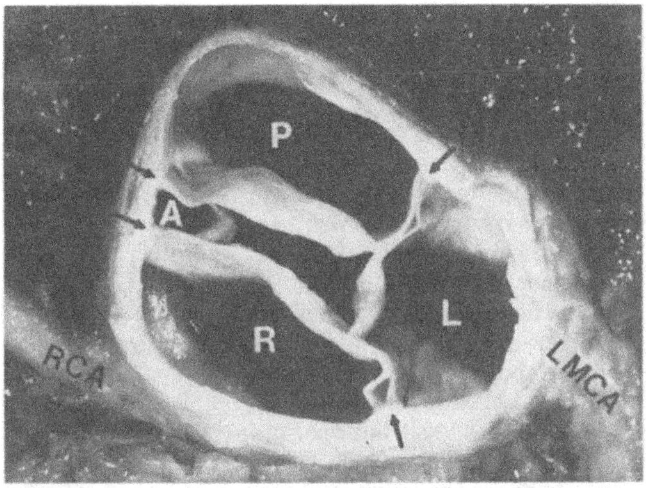

FIGURE 5. Case 6. View of the aortic valve from above showing the accessory (A) cusp between the right (R) and posterior (P) cusps. The 4 commissures are designated by *arrows*. Other abbreviations as in Figure 3.

carditis involving the aortic valve occurred in 2[2,4] and other congenital cardiac anomalies were present in 2 patients: a patent ductus arteriosus in 1[2] and a ventricular septal defect in 1.[1]

The first report describing aortic valve replacement in a patient with a quadricuspid aortic valve appeared in 1969,[8] and since then, at least 10 more cases have been reported.[9–17] Of the 11 cases, 8 were men; the aortic valve was purely regurgitant in 10, both stenotic and regurgitant in 1 and subaortic stenosis was present in 1.[12]

Diagnosis of quadricuspid aortic valve has been made by echocardiogram.[18] Whether or not prophylactic antibiotics are necessary in patients with this condition has not been determined. None of our 6 necropsy patients had infective endocarditis; 2 of 18 reported necropsy patients and none of 11 reported surgical patients with quadricuspid aortic valves had clinical or anatomic evidence of infective endocarditis.

1. Hurwitz LE, Roberts WC. Quadricuspid semilunar valve. *Am J Cardiol 1973;31:623–626.*
2. Simonds JP. Congenital malformations of the aortic and pulmonary valves. *Am J Med Sci 1923;166:584–595.*
3. Wyatt JP, Goldenberg H. Supernumerary aortic cusps with multiple fenestrations and with displacement of the left coronary orifice. *Arch Pathol 1948; 45:784–786.*
4. McColl I. Pericarditis due to a mycotic aneurysm in subacute bacterial endocarditis. *Guys Hosp Rep 1958;107:34–47.*
5. McRonald RE, Dean DC. Congenital quadricuspid aortic valve. *Am J Cardiol 1966;18:761–763.*
6. Davia JE, Fenoglio JJ, DeCastro CM, McAllister HA Jr, Cheitlin MD. Quadricuspid semilunar valves. *Chest 1977;72:186–189.*
7. Kurosawa H, Wagenaar SS, Becker AE. Sudden death in a youth—a case of quadricuspid aortic valve with isolation of origin of left coronary artery. *Br Heart J 1981;46:211–215.*
8. Peretz DI, Changfoot GH, Gourlay RH. Four-cuspid aortic valve with significant hemodynamic abnormality. *Am J Cardiol 1969;23:291–293.*
9. Robicsek F, Sanger PW, Daugherty HK, Montgomery CC. Congenital quadricuspid aortic valve with displacement of the left coronary orifice. *Am J Cardiol 1969;23:288–290.*
10. Nalbantgil I, Cagatay G. Quadricuspid aortic valve. *Chest 1975;67:623–624.*
11. Salvatore L, Mincione G, Baldelli P. Valvola aortica quadricuspide con insufficienza aortica. *G Ital Cardiol 1976;6:323–326.*
12. Iglesias A, Oliver J, Munoz JE, Nunez L. Quadricuspid aortic valve associated with fibromuscular subaortic stenosis and aortic regurgitation treated by conservative surgery. *Chest 1981;80:327–328.*
13. Sievers HH, Regensburger D, Bernhard A. Quadricuspid aortic valve with significant insufficiency. *Thorac Cardiovasc Surg 1982;30:44–45.*
14. Olson LJ, Subramanian R, Edwards WD. Surgical pathology of pure aortic insufficiency: a study of 225 cases. *Mayo Clin Proc 1984;59:835–841.*
15. Luisi VS, Pasque A, Verunelli F, Aliboni M, Urbano U, Reginato E. Quadricuspid aortic valve. *J Cardiovasc Surg 1984;25:252–254.*
16. Subramanian R, Olson LJ, Edwards WD. Surgical pathology of combined aortic stenosis and insufficiency: a study of 213 cases. *Mayo Clin Proc 1985;60:247–254.*
17. Matsumoto M, Miki S, Kusuhara K, Ueda Y, Ohkita Y, Tahata T, Komeda M. Quadricuspid aortic valve associated with severe aortic regurgitation. *Jpn Circ J 1985;49:190–191.*
18. Coeurderoy A, Biron Y, Laurent M, Almange C. Quadricuspidie aortique congenitale. *Arch Mal Coeur 1986;79:745–748.*

Living with a Congenitally Bicuspid Aortic Valve

A healthy, weight-lifting, athletic, 32-year-old former fellow of mine while spending time recently in an echocardiography laboratory had an esophageal echocardiogram "to see what it was like". To his surprise, the echocardiogram disclosed that he had a bicuspid aortic valve, which was noncalcified and competent. He called to relay this news and we discussed how he might prevent complications from developing on the congenitally malformed valve. I recommended the following:

Avoid infection. Prophylactic antibiotics obviously are required during dental and other operative procedures. Sir William Osler was the one who pointed out in 1885 the extreme propensity of the bicuspid aortic valve to be the site of infective endocarditis.[1–3] Certainly one with a bicuspid aortic valve should not use illicit drugs intravenously. Opiate addicts with bicuspid aortic valves do not live long.[4,5]

Discontinue lifting weights. This type of exercise puts undue stress, i.e., pressure, although for short periods, on the aortic valve.

Maintain a normal systemic blood pressure. Although the bicuspid aortic valve probably is not affected adversely by the left ventricular systolic pressure irrespective of its level, the level of the valve's closing pressure, i.e., the aortic diastolic pressure, probably plays a prominent role in determining whether the bicuspid valve becomes stenotic, or purely regurgitant (without superimposed infective endocarditis) or functions normally throughout life.

Keep the heart rate relatively slow. It is reasonable to believe that if the aortic valve closes only 55 times a minute rather than 75 times a minute (a 27% heart rate reduction) that the wear and tear received by the aortic valve from the aorta's closing pressure would be reduced. The best way to produce a relatively slow heart rate is by various aerobic exercises. Although the heart rate increases during the exercise, the total 24-hour heart beats probably would be reduced substantially. Beta-blocker therapy could be useful to achieve this objective.

Keep the serum total cholesterol level relatively low. The major reason a bicuspid aortic valve becomes stenotic is because large calcific deposits develop on the aortic aspects of the cusps and the large deposits impart an immobility to the cusps which prevent their opening adequately during ventricular systole.[1–3] Thus, prevention of calcific deposits is essential for prevention of stenosis. In older persons in the Western world it is common to develop calcific deposits on the aortic aspects of the aortic valve cusps, on the ventricular aspects of the posterior mitral leaflet (mitral "anular" calcium), and in atherosclerotic plaques in the coronary arteries (as well as in plaques in other arteries).[6] The development of calcific deposits on the aortic valve, mitral anulus and coronary arteries with age occurs only in those populations with serum total cholesterol levels >150 mg/dl and usually in those persons with levels >200 mg/dl. Thus, maintaining a low serum total cholesterol level prevents calcific deposits on a normally formed aortic valve, and therefore it is reasonable to believe that maintaining a low level would have similar effect on a bicuspid aortic valve. Calcific deposits are never present on the aortic valve at birth; they are always acquired. Calcific deposits are less common on stenotic mitral valves (rheumatic origin) in persons residing in the undeveloped nations of the world (where the serum total cholesterol levels often are <150 mg/dl) than in persons in the Western World where these levels are usually >150 mg/dl. Thus, maintaining a relatively low serum total cholesterol level might deter calcific deposition on a bicuspid aortic valve, and if no calcium, no stenosis. Preventing calcific deposits, however, would not prevent the development of pure aortic regurgitation or infective endocarditis.[7,8]

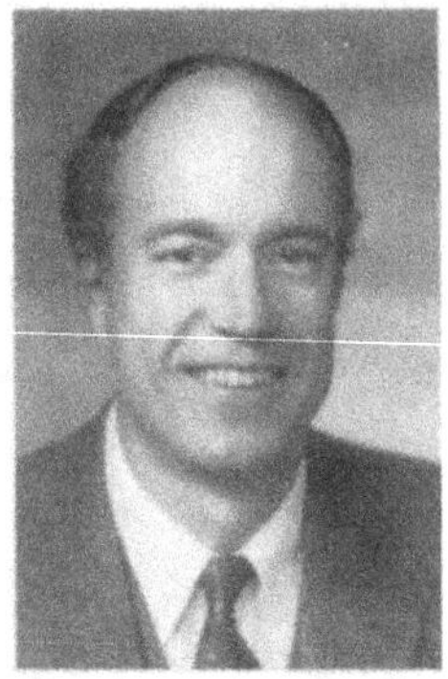

Try to forget that the aortic valve is bicuspid. As long as the bicuspid valve functions normally there is nothing to worry about, and no one can predict which bicuspid aortic valve will function normally for a full lifetime and which one will become stenotic, purely regurgitant (without superimposed infective endocarditis) or infected. In other words, the natural history of a congenitally bicuspid aortic valve is unknown. It appears that about 1% of live births have a congenitally bicuspid valve. If that be the case about 50 million (of 5 billion) persons on planet earth have a congenitally bicuspid aortic valve, and about 2.5 million persons in the USA have a bicuspid aortic valve. What percentage of them in a lifetime will develop stenosis, pure regurgitation, infection, or no complications is unknown. Thus, life must continue and the focus must be on things other than the bicuspid aortic valve. Even with the worst scenario, aortic valve replacement is usually highly successful.

The echocardiogram will continue to detect abnormalities in the heart that at the time cause no trouble. As a consequence, this instrument at times will produce worry and concern in both patient and physician. It also can provide superb information on the natural history of many cardiac abnormalities.

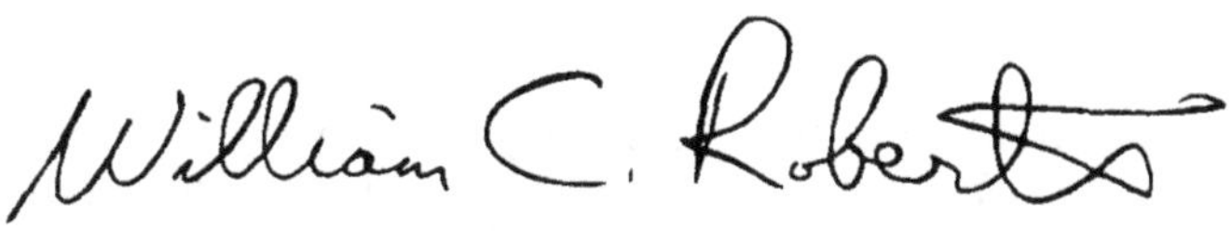

William Clifford Roberts, MD
Editor in Chief

1. Roberts WC. The congenitally bicuspid aortic valve. A study of 85 autopsy cases. *Am J Cardiol 1970;26:72–83.*
2. Roberts WC. Anatomically isolated aortic valvular disease. The case against its being of rheumatic etiology. *Am J Med 1970;49:151–159.*
3. Roberts WC. The structure of the aortic valve in clinically-isolated aortic stenosis. An autopsy study of 162 patients over 15 years of age. *Circulation 1970;42:91–97.*
4. Dressler FA, Roberts WC. Infective endocarditis in opiate addicts: analysis of 80 cases studied at necropsy. *Am J Cardiol 1989;63:1240–1257.*
5. Dressler FA, Roberts WC. Modes of death and types of cardiac diseases in opiate addicts: analysis of 168 necropsy cases. *Am J Cardiol 1989;64:909–920.*
6. Roberts WC. The senile cardiac calcification syndrome. *Am J Cardiol 1986;58:572–574.*
7. Roberts WC, Morrow AG, McIntosh CL, Jones M, Epstein SE. Congenitally bicuspid aortic valve causing severe, pure aortic regurgitation without superimposed infective endocarditis. Analysis of 13 patients requiring aortic valve replacement. *Am J Cardiol 1981;47:206–209.*
8. Arnett EW, Roberts WC. Pathology of active infective endocarditis: a necropsy analysis of 192 patients. *Thorac Cardiovasc Surg 1982;30:327–335.*

Combined Obstructive Hypertrophic Cardiomyopathy and Stenotic Congenitally Bicuspid Aortic Valve

Paul S. Brown, Jr., MD, Charles Stewart Roberts, MD, Charles L. McIntosh, MD, PhD, William C. Roberts, MD, and Richard E. Clark, MD

Hypertrophic cardiomyopathy (HC) is a congenital heart disease. Persons with 1 type of congenital heart disease are more prone to a second congenital heart condition than are persons without any congenital cardiac condition. The frequency of the congenitally bicuspid aortic valve in the general population is believed to be about 1%.[1] Therefore, it might be expected to be present in an occasional patient with a more uncommon condition, such as HC. The present report describes findings in 4 patients with coexisting HC and a congenitally bicuspid aortic valve.

The records of the Surgery Branch, National Heart, Lung, and Blood Institute, were searched for all patients who had a cardiac operation for HC and who had coexisting aortic valve disease. From 1960 to 1990 a total of 525 patients with HC underwent ventricular septotomy and partial septectomy (hereafter referred to as myotomy and myectomy) and 29 (5%) of them had coexisting aortic valve disease: pure aortic regurgitation in 20 patients and aortic valve stenosis with or without regurgitation in 9 patients. Of the latter 9 patients, 5 had tricuspid aortic valves, and 4 had bicuspid aortic valves. This report focuses on the 4 patients with combined HC and stenotic congenitally bicuspid aortic valves.

Pertinent findings in the 4 patients are summarized in Table I. All 4 patients were in New York Heart Association Functional class III or IV. Patients 1 and 2 had other family members with HC. Grade 3/6 systolic precordial murmurs, loudest along the left sternal border, were audible in all 4 patients, and the murmur was made louder by standing or by the Valsalva maneuver. Patients 1, 3 and 4 had a second systolic murmur that radiated to the neck, suggestive of valvular aortic stenosis. By echocardiogram the thickness of the ventricular septum was considerably greater (ratio >1.6) than that of the left ventricular free wall, and systolic anterior motion of the anterior mitral leaflet was present in all 4 patients. The peak systolic pressure gradient between the left ventricle and ascending aorta was >70 mm Hg in all 4 patients (Figure 1). At operation, all 4 patients had calcified, stenotic, congenitally bicuspid aortic valves (Figure 2). A typical mural endocardial plaque in apposition to the anterior mitral leaflet was present in all 4 patients. The ventricular septum by palpation was severely thickened and typical of that found in HC associated with a normal aortic valve. The portions of excised ventricular septum histologically had myofibril disorganization consistent with HC. All 4 patients had a lessening of their symptoms of cardiac dysfunction late postoperatively.

Coexisting HC and valvular aortic stenosis have been reported in at least 30 patients since 1960,[2-4] but usually the only evidence of HC was a ventricular septum thicker than the left ventricular free wall. Although asymmetric septal hypertrophy is usually present in HC, it also occurs in about 10% of patients with valvular aortic stenosis, and in about 10% of patients with systemic hypertension.[5,6] Thus, to diagnose HC in the presence of valvular aortic stenosis, findings other than a disproportionately thickened ventricular septum are necessary, and such was the case in the 4 patients described here.

The congenitally bicuspid aortic valve appears to occur with the same frequency in patients with obstructive HC as in the general population (each about 1%). At least 2 patients with HC and a congenitally bicuspid stenotic aortic valve have been reported by others. One,[3] a 52-year-old man, had a 73-mm Hg peak systolic left ventricular outflow pressure gradient, a ventricular septum con-

From the Surgery and Pathology Branches, National Heart, Lung, and Blood Institute, National Institutes of Health, Room 2N244, Building 10, Bethesda, Maryland 20892. Manuscript received June 7, 1990; revised manuscript received and accepted July 5, 1990.

TABLE I Findings in Four Patients with Combined Hypertrophic Cardiomyopathy and Congenitally Bicuspid Stenotic Aortic Valves

		Preoperative Catheterization								Echo Data				Morphologic Data				AV Prosthesis		Six Months Postoperative Catheterization					Follow-Up After MM+AVR		
				LVP	AAP	LV–AA															LVP	AAP	LV–AA psg§				
Pt. No.	Age (Yr)/ & Sex	FH of HC	FC (1–4)	s/d (mm Hg)	s/d (mm Hg)	psg (mm Hg)	CI	AR (0–4)	+VPC Response	VS (mm)	LVFW (mm)	LA (mm)	SAM	Amount VS Excised (g)	LVOT Mural Plaque	AV Ca (0–4)	AV Weight (g)	Type	(Size)	FC (1–4)	s/d (mm Hg)	s/d (mm Hg)	Rest (mm Hg)	Provoked (mm Hg)	CI	(yrs)	FC
1	57/F	+	4	235/12	93/56	142*	2.4	2+	+	22	12	45	+	4.7	+	4+	4.7	BS	(21)	1	150/5	140/72	10	50	2.2	16.5	1
2	57/M	+	3	238/10	123/62	115*	2.3	0	+	21	13	46	+	1.1	+	2+	1.4	BS‡	(19)	2	160/10	142/80	22	50	2.8	7.2	2
3	58/M	0	3	195/5	110/65	95*,†	2.6	1+	+	21	12	45	+	1.4	+	4+	7.2	SJM‡	(27)	1	150/10	125/80	25	30	2.5	2.6	1
4	64/M	0	4	220/9	145/60	75	1.8	2+	+	25	10	48	+	1.0	+	3+	—	H	(27)	2	—	130/80	—	—	—	7.3	2

* Left ventricle to ascending aorta pullback pressure measurements demonstrated <25 mm Hg aortic valvular component to the gradient; † provokable gradient to 125 mm Hg with isoproterenol; ‡ concomitant coronary artery bypass grafting; § highest provokable gradient measured during Valsalva maneuver, inhalation of amyl nitrite or infusion of isoproterenol; ‖ all patients were alive at 4/1/90.

AA = ascending aorta; AAP = ascending aortic pressure; AR = aortic regurgitation; AV = aortic valve; AVR = aortic valve replacement; BS = Bjork Shiley; Ca = calcification; CI = cardiac index (liters/min/m^2); F = female; FC = functional class (New York Heart Association); FH = family history; H = Hancock bioprosthesis; HC = hypertrophic cardiomyopathy; LA = left atrium; LV = left ventricular; LVFW = left ventricular free wall; LVP = left ventricle pressure; M = male; MM = myotomy and myectomy; psg = peak systolic gradient; SAM = systolic anterior motion of the anterior mitral leaflet; s/d = peak systolic/end-diastolic pressure; SJM = St. Jude Medical; VPC = ventricular premature complex; VS = ventricular septum; + = present; 0 = absent; — = unknown.

siderably thicker than the left ventricular free wall, and systolic anterior motion of the anterior mitral leaflet; he underwent both aortic valve replacement and myotomy and myectomy. The second,[4] a 48-year-old woman with a family history of HC, had a 120-mm Hg peak systolic pressure gradient between the left ventricle and aorta, and a ventricular septum considerably thicker than the left ventricular free wall; she underwent aortic valve replacement only.

The operatively excised valves in our 4 patients actually appeared considerably more stenotic than was the degree of valvular stenosis found at preoperative cardiac catheterization. In our 4 patients, however, valvular aortic stenosis was anticipated because of the presence of an additional precordial murmur, calcific deposits in the aortic valve on chest x-ray, and aortic regurgitation.

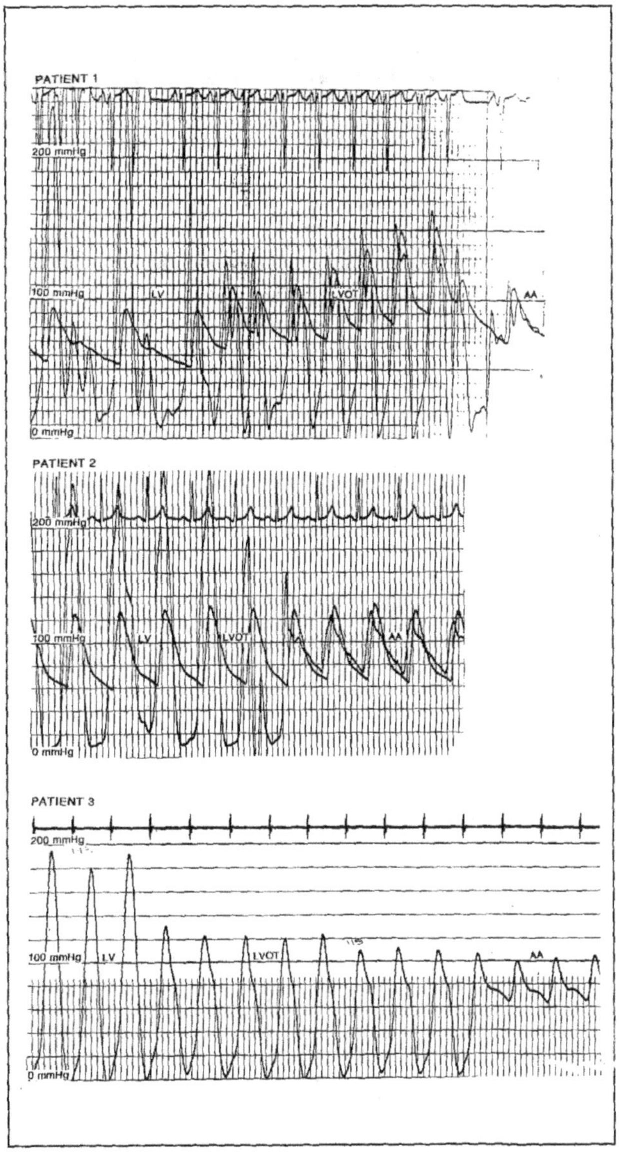

FIGURE 1. Left ventricle to ascending aorta pullback pressure tracings. The pressure gradient was primarily subvalvular with a <25 mm Hg valvular component in patients 1 to 3. AA = ascending aorta; LV = left ventricle; LVOT = left ventricular outflow tract.

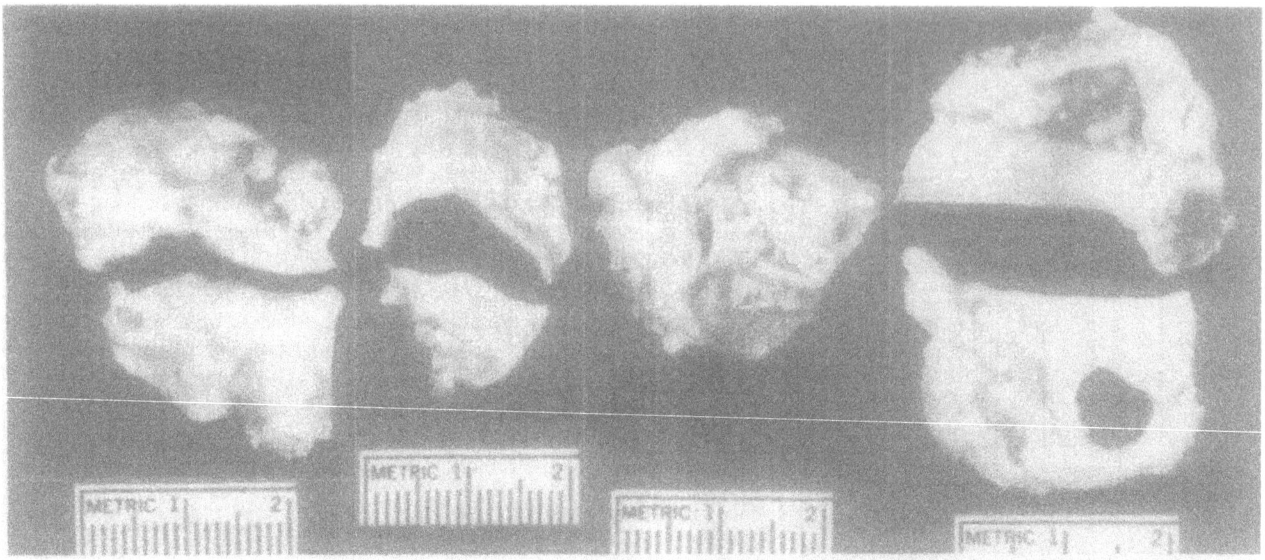

FIGURE 2. Excised stenotic bicuspid aortic valves from the 4 patients are shown from left to right. Valve no. 4 had a large perforation that was blocked by an area of calcium from the opposite leaflet.

1. Roberts WC. The congenitally bicuspid aortic valve. A study of 85 autopsy cases. *Am J Cardiol* 1970;26:72–83.

2. Nanda NC, Gramiak R, Shaw PM, Stewart S, DeWeese JA. Echocardiography in the diagnosis of idiopathic hypertrophic subaortic stenosis co-existing with aortic valve disease. *Circulation* 1974;50:752–757.

3. Stewart S, Nanda N, DeWeese J. Simultaneous operative correction of aortic valve stenosis and idiopathic hypertrophic subaortic stenosis. *Circulation* 1975; 51/52(suppl 1):I-34–I-39.

4. Feize O, Farrer-Brown G, Emanuel R. Familial study of hypertrophic cardiomyopathy and congenital aortic valve disease. *Am J Cardiol* 1978;41:956–964.

5. Parker D, Kaplan MA, Connolly JE. Coexistent aortic valvular and functional hypertrophic subaortic stenosis. *Am J Cardiol* 1969;24:307–317.

6. Panza JA, Maron BJ. Valvular aortic stenosis and asymmetric septal hypertrophy; diagnostic consideration and clinical and therapeutic implication. *Eur Heart J* 1988;9(suppl E):71–76.

Cardiovascular findings in alkaptonuric ochronosis

Amy H. Kragel, MD, Joyce A. Lapa, MD, and
William C. Roberts, MD. *Bethesda, Md.*

Hereditary alkaptonuric ochronosis is an autosomal recessive metabolic disorder that affects about one in one million persons and has been shown to exist for over 3500

From the Pathology Branch, National Heart, Lung, and Blood Institute, National Institutes of Health, and the Department of Laboratory Medicine, National Naval Medical Center.

Reprint requests: William C. Roberts, MD, NHLBI-NIH, Building 10, Room 2N258, 9000 Rockville Pike, Bethesda, MD 20892.

4/4/24306

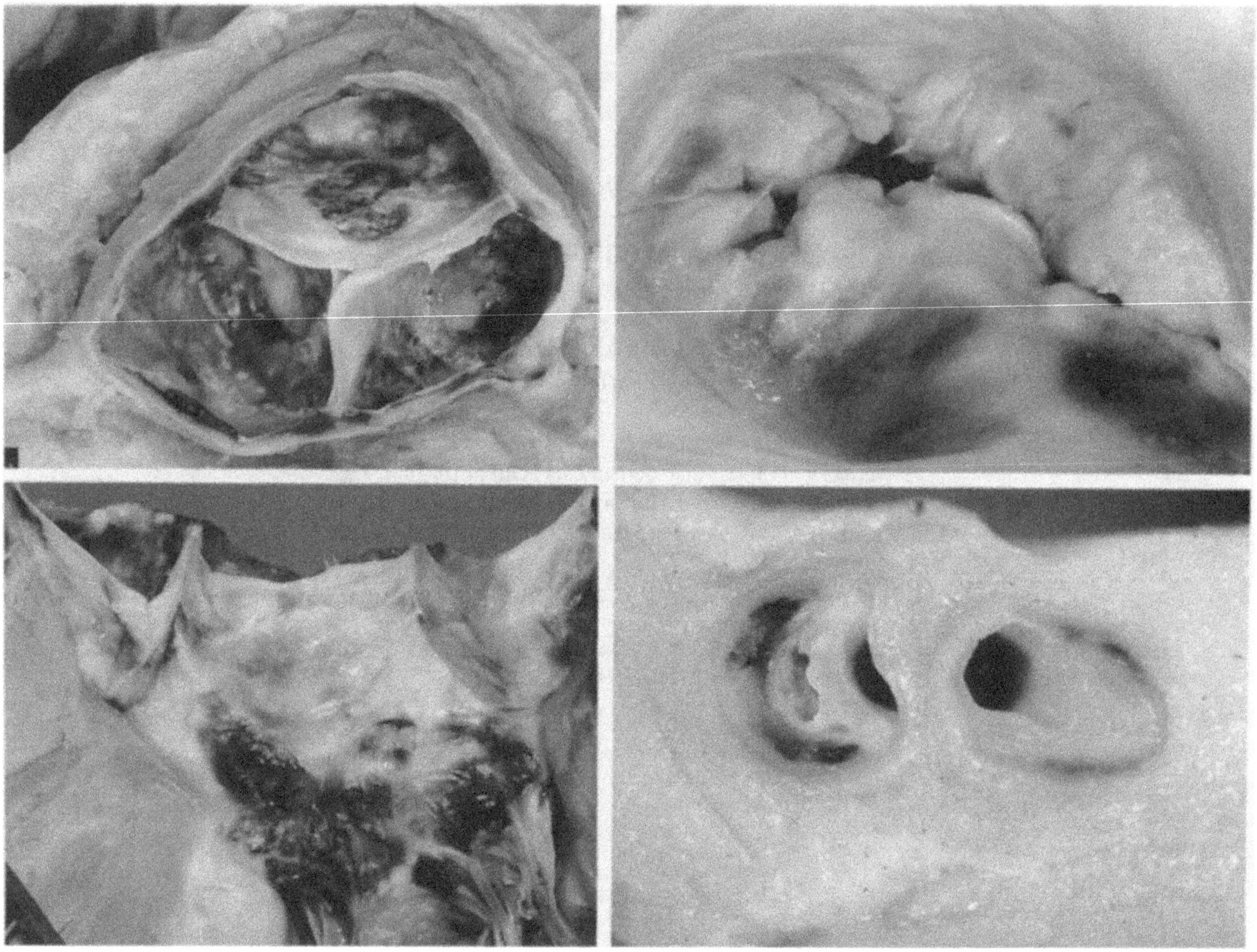

Fig. 1. Pigmented heart. **Top left,** Aortic valve viewed from above. **Top right,** Mitral valve from left atrium. **Bottom right,** Cross-sections of the proximal left anterior descending and first diagonal coronary arteries. The blue-black pigment represents ochronotic deposits. Pigment deposition is heaviest in areas associated with calcific deposits, that is, the aortic aspect of the aortic valve, the ventricular aspect of the mitral valve, and calcified atherosclerotic plaque in epicardial coronary arteries.

years.[1,2] The disorder is due to a deficiency of the enzyme homogentisic acid oxidase and the deficiency leads to elevation of body levels of homogentistic acid. The homogentisic acid is either excreted in the urine, where it oxidizes in an alkaline pH causing darkening of the urine, or (after polymerization) deposits in the connective tissues of the body causing characteristic pigmentation.[1,2] While the most debilitating complication of alkaptonuria is ochronotic arthropathy, a variety of cardiovascular abnormalities have been described in ochronosis. In this report we describe typical cardiovascular findings in alkaptonuric ochronosis.

R.B., a 72-year-old man, developed severe degenerative arthritis during his 30s and was diagnosed then as having alkaptonuria. His arthritis was progressive and severely limited his activity. At age 54, angina pectoris appeared and at age 55 he had an uncomplicated acute myocardial infarction. Subsequently, he had angina pectoris with moderate exertion, but his activity was limited primarily by the arthritis. Other medical problems included systemic hypertension, Raynaud's phenomenon, severe chronic obstructive pulmonary disease, chronic urinary obstruction with a nonfunctioning right kidney, orchiectomy for a benign teratoma, and an abdominal aortic aneurysm. He was admitted to the hospital 19 days before death because of severe respiratory distress. The blood pressure was 160/80 mm Hg; the pulse was 109 beats/min and irregular, and the respiratory rate was 28 breaths/min. He had diffuse pulmonary wheezes. He had a grade 2/6 systolic ejection murmur over both base and apex and a third heart sound. The electrocardiogram showed multifocal atrial tachycardia and Q waves were present in leads II, III, AVF, V_5 and V_6. Shortly before death, he developed electrocardiographic changes consistent with an anterior wall acute myocardial infarction. He died of severe respiratory failure.

Necropsy (NNMC No. A88-41) findings included severe degenerative bone disease with extensive black pigmentation of his skeleton, emphysema, generalized atherosclerosis, obstruction of the right ureter with a black pigmented stone, and an adjacent papillary transitional cell carcinoma

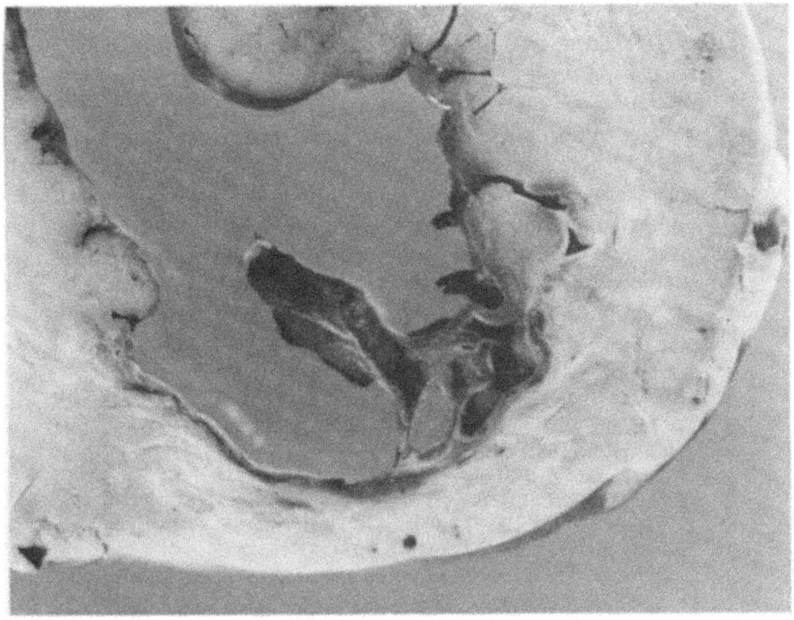

Fig. 2. Transverse section of posterolateral left ventricular free wall showing a healed transmural infarct. The posterior free wall and adjacent papillary muscle are thin and fibrotic. Ochronotic pigment is present within some of the scarred tissues.

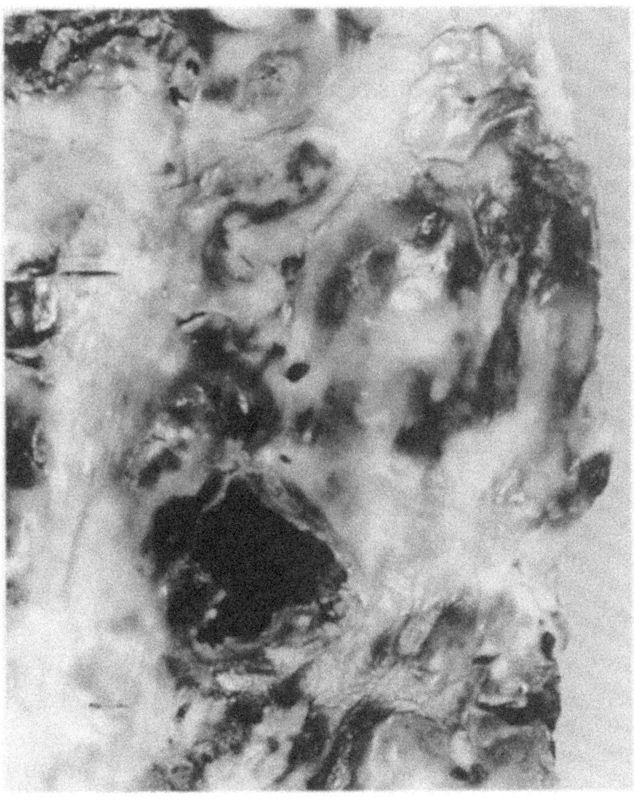

Fig. 3. Portion of opened descending thoracic aorta showing pigmented, calcified, and ulcerated atherosclerotic plaques.

of the ureter. Multiple pigmented stones also were present in the prostate gland. The heart weighed 645 gm. Large deposits of dark pigment were present on the aortic and mitral valve cusps and in atherosclerotic plaques of the coronary arteries (Fig. 1). Calcific deposits were present in the mitral valve anulus and on the aortic aspects of the aortic valve cusps. Neither the mitral nor aortic valves were stenotic. The lumens of the left anterior descending, left circumflex, and right coronary arteries were narrowed >75% in cross-sectional area by calcified, pigmented plaque. A healed, focally pigmented, transmural infarct was present in the posterior left ventricular wall (Fig. 2). The posteromedial papillary muscle was atrophied, focally pigmented, and focally calcified. The aorta was extensively calcified, ulcerated, and pigmented (Fig. 3). The abdominal aorta was aneurysmal (4 cm wide). Hematoxylin and eosin stained sections of the transmural left ventricular scar showed black pigment within areas of fibrosis. Similar pigment was seen within plaque in the epicardial coronary arteries. This pigment stained with the Nile blue stain.

Alkaptonuric ochronosis has been associated with pigmentation of various cardiovascular structures including the aortic, pulmonic, and mitral valves, mitral anulus, mural endocardium, areas of replacement myocardial fibrosis, and in atherosclerotic plaques of aorta and epicardial coronary arteries.[3-12] Pigment is deposited both intracellularly and extracellularly. It may be seen within macrophages and fibrocytes of endocardial and valvular tissue.[12] Pigment may be seen in all three layers (intima, media, and adventitia) of the arterial wall, in atherosclerotic plaque, and in the smooth muscle cells of media.[11, 12]

Both fatal and symptomatic atherosclerotic coronary artery disease and aortic stenosis have been described in association with alkaptonuric ochronosis.[4, 6-11] O'Brien et al.[1] found no increase in the frequency of either aortic stenosis or coronary artery disease in a large series of patients. Others, however, have suggested that the frequency of aortic stenosis may be increased[8, 11] and that ochronotic pigment in the aortic valve may lead to acceleration of degenerative changes in that structure.[11] Although the aortic valve in our patient was focally thickened by fibrous tissue, calcium, and ochronotic pigment, it was not stenotic.

REFERENCES

1. O'Brien WM, LaDu BN, Bunim JJ. Biochemical, pathologic and clinical aspects of alcaptonuria, ochronosis and ochronotic arthropathy. Review of world literature (1584-1962). Am J Med 1963;34:813-38.
2. Lee SL, Stenn FF. Characterization of mummy bone ochronotic pigment. JAMA 1978;240:136-8.
3. Skinsnes OK. Generalized ochronosis. Report of an instance in which it was misdiagnosed as melanosarcoma, with resultant enucleation of an eye. JAMA 1942;120:552-8.
4. Lichtenstein L, Kaplan L. Hereditary ochronosis. Pathologic changes observed in two necropsied cases. Am J Pathol 1954;30:99-119.
5. Nishimori I, Itoh J, Hakuno T. An autopsy case of alkaptonuria with ochronosis. Acta Pathol Jpn 1970;20:505-12.
6. Reginato A, Riera M, Martinez V, et al. Alcaptonuria, artropatia ochronotica y estenosis aortica. Rev Med Chil 1972;100:529-33.
7. Gould L, Reddy CVR, DePalma D, et al. Cardiac manifestations of ochronosis. J Thorac Cardiovasc Surg 1976;72:788-91.
8. Levine HD, Parisi AF, Holdsworth DE, et al. Aortic valve replacement for ochronosis of the aortic valve. Chest 1978;74:466-7.
9. Ptacin M, Sebastian J, Bamrah VS. Ochronotic cardiovascular disease. Clin Cardiol 1985;8:441-5.
10. Vlay SC, Hartman AR, Culliford AT. Alkaptonuria and aortic stenosis [Abstract]. Ann Intern Med 1986;104:446.
11. Gaines JJ, Pai GM. Cardiovascular ochronosis. Arch Pathol Lab Med 1987;111:991-4.
12. Gaines JJ. The pathology of alkaptonuric ochronosis. Hum Pathol 1989;20:40-6.

Dissection of the Aorta Associated With Congenital Malformation of The Aortic Valve

CHARLES S. ROBERTS, MD, WILLIAM C. ROBERTS, MD, FACC

Bethesda, Maryland

The association of congenital aortic valve malformation and aortic dissection is analyzed. Over a 30 year period, 186 patients with noniatrogenic aortic dissection were studied at necropsy. The aortic valve was tricuspid in 170 (91.4%), bicuspid in 14 (7.5%) and unicuspid in 2 (1.1%). Among the 16 patients with aortic dissection and a congenitally malformed valve, the age at death ranged from 17 to 82 years (mean 52) and 13 (81%) were men.

The entrance tear of the aortic dissection was located in the ascending aorta in all 16 patients with a malformed valve but in only 68% of those with a tricuspid aortic valve. The aortic valve was stenotic in 6 of the 16 patients with a congenitally malformed valve. Fatal rupture of the false channel occurred after acute ascending aortic dissection in each of the 11 patients (none with healed dissection) who did not have operative therapy for the dissection. Two of the 16 patients with a malformed valve compared with no patient with a tricuspid aortic valve had aortic isthmic coarctation. Histologic sections of aorta from 10 patients disclosed severe degeneration of the elastic fibers of the media in 9 patients.

Thus, a congenitally malformed aortic valve appears to be present at least 5 times more frequently in adults with than in those without aortic dissection, and in our patients the entrance tear was always in the ascending aorta, which usually had severe loss of elastic fibers in its media.

(J Am Coll Cardiol 1991;17:712–6)

Previous studies (1–4) have reported the association of aortic dissection with congenital abnormality of the aortic valve. During the past 30 years, we have studied at necropsy 186 patients with spontaneous aortic dissection. The aortic valve was normal (tricuspid) in 170 patients (91%) and abnormal (bicuspid or unicuspid) in 16 (9%). This report describes certain findings in the aortic valve and ascending aorta in the latter 16 patients and compares these findings with those in the 170 patients with tricuspid aortic valve.

Methods

Sources of patients. The necropsy records of the Pathology Branch, National Heart, Lung, and Blood Institute from 1959 to June 1990 were searched for cases coded as "aortic dissection." Nearly all of the cases came from 1 of 12 Washington, D.C. area medical centers. A total of 199 cases were so coded. Thirteen were excluded from this analysis because of an iatrogenic origin of the aortic dissection; that is, the entrance tear was adjacent to an aortotomy or resulted from insertion of an aortic balloon. The records of each of the remaining 186 necropsy patients were reviewed. The heart and aorta of all 186 patients were originally examined and classified by W.C.R., and most were reexamined later by C.S.R.

Of the 16 patients with a malformed aortic valve, 2 were studied at necropsy from 1959 to 1970, 4 from 1971 to 1980 and 10 from 1981 to 1990. The 16 cases were submitted from nine hospitals, eight local and one nonlocal. The study was approved by the director of intramural research of the National Heart, Lung, and Blood Institute.

Examination of ascending aorta. In 10 of the 16 cases in which the heart was available for reexamination, two or more segments of ascending aorta were excised for histologic study. Each segment was taken approximately 2 cm cephalad to the sinotubular junction perpendicular to the longitudinal axis of the aorta. Each segment was fixed in formalin, processed in alcohols and xylene, dehydrated and embedded in paraffin; a histologic section was prepared from each segment and stained by the Movat method.

Results

Clinical findings. Pertinent clinical and necropsy findings in each of the 16 patients with a congenitally malformed aortic valve are summarized in Table 1, and the appearance of the aortic valve and ascending aorta in two patients are shown in Figures 1 and 2. The age at death in the 16 patients ranged from 17 to 81 years (mean 52); 13 were men (81%). In 6 (38%) of the 16 patients the diagnosis of aortic dissection had been established during life. No patient had skeletal or known ocular features of the Marfan syndrome.

From the Surgery and Pathology Branches, National Heart, Lung, and Blood Institute, National Institutes of Health, Bethesda, Maryland.

Manuscript received June 19, 1990; revised manuscript received August 22, 1990, accepted September 10, 1990.

Address for reprints: William C. Roberts, MD, Pathology Branch, National Heart, Lung, and Blood Institute, National Institutes of Health, Building 10, Room 2N258, Bethesda, Maryland 20892.

Table 1. Clinical and Morphologic Characteristics of 16 Patients Who Had Fatal Acquired Dissection of the Aorta Associated With Congenital Malformation of the Aortic Valve

Case No.	Age (yr)/ Gender	SH	Angiogram LV	Angiogram Aorta	AD Dx in Life	Operation AA	Operation AVR	Operation CABG	Interval From Op to Death	Rupture AA	Portion of Aorta Dissected AA	Portion of Aorta Dissected T	Portion of Aorta Dissected DT	Portion of Aorta Dissected Abd	Aortic Reentry Tear	PAH	Healed AD	AIC	Number AV Cusps	AS	Location AV Cusps A-P	Location AV Cusps L-R	EFD (0-3) AA	HW (g)
1	17/M	0	+	+	–	0	+*	0	6 yr	+	+	+	0	0	0	0	0	+*	2	+	A	P	–	500
2	30/M	0	0	0	0	0	0	0	–	+	+	+	0	0	0	+	0	+	2	0	L	R	3	390
3	32/M	0	0	0	0	0	0	0	–	+	+	+	0	0	0	+	+	0	2	0	R	L	3	470
4	46/M	+	0	+	+	0	0	0	–	+	+	+	0	+	0	0	0	0	2	0	A	P	–	440
5	48/M	+	+	+	+	+	0	0	21 days	†	+	+	+	+	+	0	+	0	2	0	A	P	3	–
6	52/M	0	0	0	0	0	0	0	–	0	+	0	+	0	0	0	0	0	2	0	A	P	3	510
7	55/M	–	+	+	+	+	+	+	0	†	+	0	0	0	0	0	0	0	2	0	A	P	3	530
8	57/M	+	0	+	+	+	0	0	0	†	+	+	0	+	0	0	0	0	2	0	A	P	0	–
9	62/M	+	+	+	0	+‡	+	0	–	†	+	+	+	+	0	0	0	0	2	+	L	R	3	620
10	67/M	+	0	0	0	0	0	0	–	+	+	0	+	0	0	0	0	0	2	0	A	P	–	–
11	69/F	0	0	0	0	0	0	0	–	+	+	0	0	0	0	+	0	0	2	0	A	P	–	–
12	69/F	–	0	0	0	0	0	0	–	+	+	+	0	0	0	+	0	0	2	+	A	P	3	400
13	71/F	0	0	0	0	0	0	0	–	+	+	+	0	0	+	+	0	0	2	0	A	P	3	430
14	82/M	+	0	0	+	0	0	0	–	+	+	0	0	0	+	+	0	0	2	+	A	P	3	585
15	26/M	0	0	0	0	0	0	0	–	+	+	+	0	0	0	+	0	0	1	+	–	–	–	610
16	45/M	0	0	+	+	+	+	+	0	‡	+	+	0	0	–	+	0	0	1	+	–	–	–	–

*Coarctation of aorta resected at age 27 months, and aortic valve commissurotomy at age 11 years. †Underwent operative therapy for aortic dissection. ‡Aortic dissection diagnosed for first time at operation.
A = anterior; AA = ascending aorta; Abd = abdominal; AD = aortic dissection; AIC = aortic isthmic coarctation; AS = aortic stenosis with or without regurgitation; AV = aortic valve; AVR = aortic valve replacement; CABG = coronary artery bypass grafting; DT = descending thoracic; Dx = diagnosis; EFD = elastic fiber degeneration; HW = heart weight; L = left; LV = left ventricle; Op = operation; P = posterior; PAH = pulmonary adventitial hemorrhage; R = right; SH = systemic hypertension; T = transverse; – = no information available; + = present or positive; 0 = absent or negative.

Aortic valve function. The aortic valve was functionally abnormal in 6 of the 16 patients: in 4 of the 5 who had operative therapy for the dissection and in 2 of the 11 who did not. Valvular aortic stenosis developed early in life in one patient (Case 1), who underwent aortic valve commissurotomy at age 11 years; aortic dissection at age 17 years caused sudden death. None of the other five patients with an abnormally functioning aortic valve had an operative procedure on the aortic valve. Anatomic examination indicated that 10 of the 14 congenitally bicuspid aortic valves had functioned normally before the dissection and that 4 were stenotic (2 severely calcified). Of the 10 functionally normal valves before the dissection, 2 had aortic regurgitation as a consequence of the dissection. Each of the 2 congenitally unicuspid aortic valves was severely stenotic.

Location of aortic valve cusps. Of the 14 patients with a congenitally bicuspid aortic valve, the location of each cusp was noted in 13: in 10 patients, one cusp was anterior and the other posterior and both coronary arteries arose from the anterior sinus; in the other three patients, the cusps were right and left and a coronary artery arose from each aortic sinus. A raphe, present in 10 of the 14 cases, was always located in either the anterior or the right cusp.

Survival after aortic dissection. The interval from aortic dissection to death was ≤21 days in 15 patients and about 6 months in 1 patient (Case 5). Thus, the dissection healed in only 1 of the 16 patients. All 11 patients who had no operative intervention for aortic dissection died within 24 hours of onset of the dissection. Rupture of the false channel causing hemopericardium led to death in all 11 unoperated patients.

Extent of the dissection. In all 16 patients the aortic entrance tear was located in the ascending aorta (proximal to the innominate artery). The dissection also involved the transverse portion of aorta in six patients, and the descending thoracic and abdominal aorta in four other patients. Hemorrhage into the adventitia of the pulmonary trunk occurred in seven patients (5–7).

Aortic isthmic coarctation. One (Case 1) of the 16 patients had aortic isthmic coarctation that was resected when he was 27 months of age. The dissection terminated at the proximal suture line of the coarctation repair.

Aortic media. Histologic sections of ascending aorta, obtained in 10 cases, revealed severe degeneration or loss of elastic fibers in the media in 9 cases, and a normal aortic media in 1 case (Case 8). Some areas of media in the nine abnormal cases had no elastic fibers, and nearly all areas were deficient in elastic fibers.

Comparison of cases of congenitally malformed aortic valves with cases of tricuspid aortic valves. Pertinent findings in the 14 patients with a bicuspid aortic valve, the 2 patients with a unicuspid aortic valve and the 170 patients with a tricuspid aortic valve are listed in Table 2. None of the 16 patients with a congenitally malformed aortic valve but 54 (32%) of the 170 patients with a tricuspid aortic valve had a tear distal to the ascending aorta. Two (14%) of the 14 patients with a bicuspid aortic valve had aortic isthmic

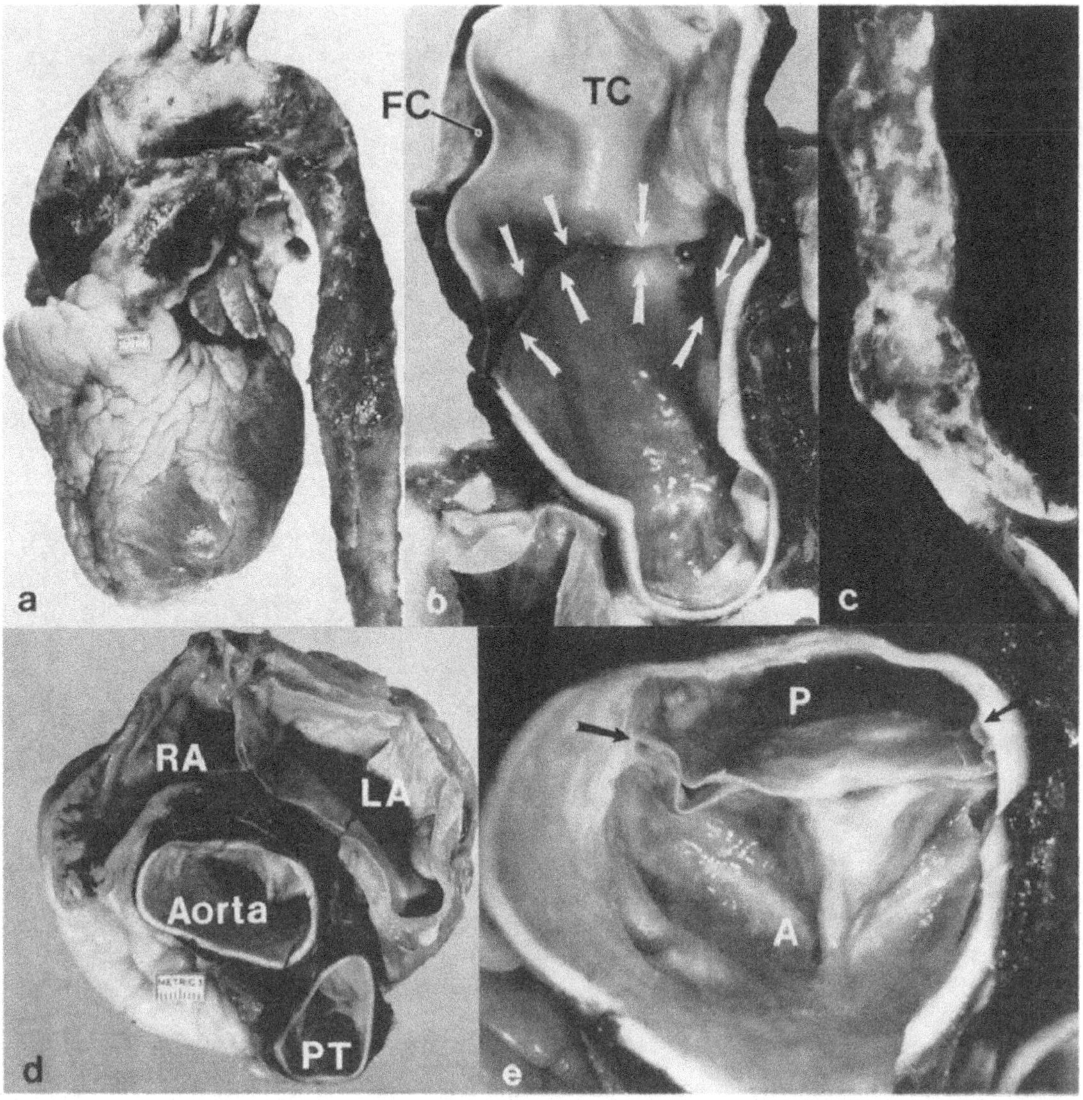

Figure 1. Case 11. Photographs and a radiograph of heart and aorta in a 69 year old woman who died suddenly from rupture of the false channel after ascending aortic dissection. **a**, View of the heart and aorta showing adventitial hemorrhage in the aortic root and pulmonary trunk. **b**, View of the lumen of the ascending aorta. **Arrows** point to the transverse linear entrance tear. The true channel (TC) and false channel (FC) are separated by the inner two-thirds of media. **c**, Postmortem radiograph of abdominal aorta showing extensive calcific deposits. Aortic dissection, which often terminates at the site of extensive atherosclerosis or calcific deposits, did not extend beyond the ascending aorta in this patient. **d**, Cephalad view of the heart showing the right atrium (RA), left atrium (LA) and the origin of the aorta and pulmonary trunk (PT). **e**, View of the bicuspid aortic valve from above showing the anterior (A) and posterior (P) cusps. A raphe is present in the anterior cusp. **Arrows** point to the two true commissures.

coarctation, compared with none of the 170 patients with a tricuspid aortic valve. None of the 16 patients with a malformed aortic valve had the Marfan syndrome, compared with 3 (2%) of the 170 patients with a tricuspid valve.

Discussion

Frequency of bicuspid aortic valve in aortic dissection. The frequency of a congenitally bicuspid aortic valve among persons >15 years of age appears to be 1% to 2%, closer to 1% (8). The finding of a congenitally bicuspid aortic valve in 14 (7.5%) of 186 necropsy patients with spontaneous aortic dissection indicates that the bicuspid aortic valve is at least 5 times more common in persons with aortic dissection than in the general adult population with a tricuspid aortic valve. A bicuspid aortic valve was present in 11 (13%) of 85 patients with aortic dissection reported by Gore and Seiwert (1), in 11 (9%) of 119 cases reported by Edwards et al. (2), in none of 204 cases reported by Wilson and Hutchins (3) and in 18 (11%) of 161 cases reported by Larson and Edwards (4). Wilson and Hutchins (3) reviewed autopsy protocols rather than actual heart specimens and their study covered a 92 year period. It is therefore likely that the presence of a bicuspid aortic valve was overlooked.

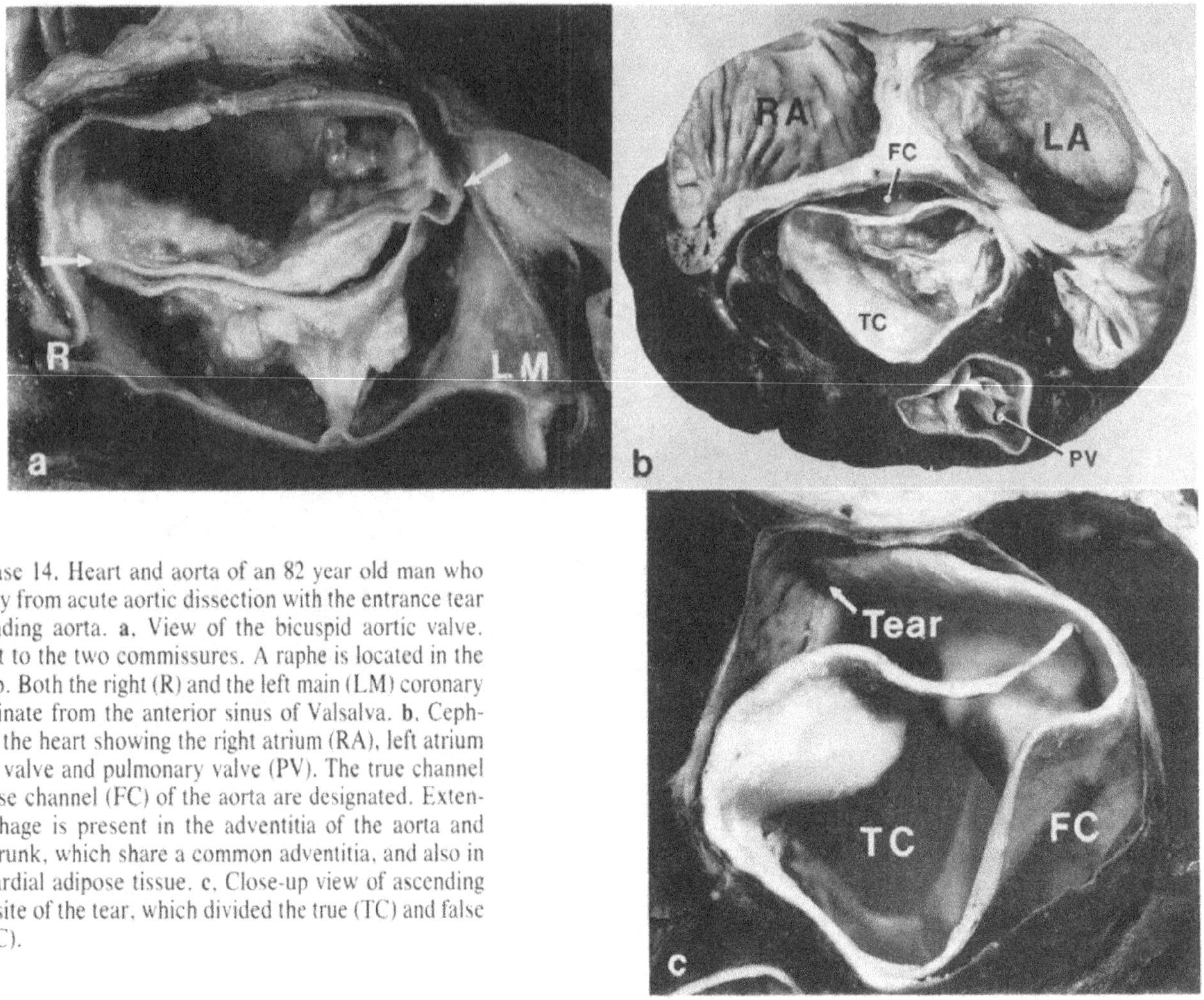

Figure 2. Case 14. Heart and aorta of an 82 year old man who died suddenly from acute aortic dissection with the entrance tear in the ascending aorta. **a.** View of the bicuspid aortic valve. **Arrows** point to the two commissures. A raphe is located in the anterior cusp. Both the right (R) and the left main (LM) coronary arteries originate from the anterior sinus of Valsalva. **b.** Cephalad view of the heart showing the right atrium (RA), left atrium (LA), aortic valve and pulmonary valve (PV). The true channel (TC) and false channel (FC) of the aorta are designated. Extensive hemorrhage is present in the adventitia of the aorta and pulmonary trunk, which share a common adventitia, and also in the subepicardial adipose tissue. **c.** Close-up view of ascending aorta at the site of the tear, which divided the true (TC) and false channels (FC).

Frequency of aortic dissection in persons with a bicuspid aortic valve. Fenoglio et al. (9) found aortic dissection in 8 (5%) of 152 necropsy patients ≥20 years of age with a bicuspid aortic valve. In the study by Larson and Edwards (4), 18 (6%) of 293 persons with a bicuspid aortic valve and 141 (0.67%) of 21,105 persons with a tricuspid aortic valve had aortic dissection, a ninefold difference. Their study included persons of all ages, not just those >15 or 20 years old. At the Pathology Branch, National Heart, Lung, and Blood Institute, of 328 patients >15 years of age with a congenitally bicuspid aortic valve studied (to June 1990) at necropsy, 14 (4%) had aortic dissection.

Frequency of aortic dissection in persons with a unicuspid aortic valve and vice versa. The frequency of aortic dissection among persons with a unicuspid aortic valve also appears to be higher than in patients with a tricuspid aortic valve. Among our 186 necropsy patients with aortic dissection, 2 (1.1%) had a unicuspid aortic valve. Larson and Edwards (4) found a unicuspid aortic valve in 2 (1.2%) of 161 patients with aortic dissection; of their 16 patients with a unicuspid aortic valve, 2 (12.5%) had aortic dissection. During the past 30 years, 29 patients with a congenitally unicuspid aortic valve have been studied at necropsy in the Pathology Branch of the National Heart, Lung, and Blood Institute, and 2 (7%) had aortic dissection. Thus, although the unicuspid aortic valve is far less frequent than a bicuspid valve, the frequency of associated aortic dissection may be similar to that observed with the bicuspid aortic valve.

Functional status of bicuspid aortic valve in aortic dissection. The bicuspid aortic valve in patients with aortic dissection can function either normally or abnormally. Among our 14 patients with a congenitally bicuspid aortic valve and aortic dissection, the valve had functioned normally before the dissection in 10 and was stenotic in the other 4. Among 18 patients with a bicuspid aortic valve and aortic dissection reported by Larson and Edwards (4), the valve had functioned normally in 9, was stenotic in 6 and was purely regurgitant in 3. The unicuspid aortic valve was severely stenotic in each of our two patients.

Frequency of aortic coarctation in aortic dissection with a bicuspid aortic valve. It is well established that aortic isthmic coarctation occurs more frequently in persons with a bicuspid (or unicuspid) aortic valve than in persons with a tricuspid aortic valve (8,9) and that aortic dissection occurs more frequently in persons with than in those without aortic coarctation (10,11). Abbott (10) found aortic dissection in 38 (19%) of 200 necropsy cases of unoperated aortic isthmic coarctation. The status of the aortic valve was known in 183

Table 2. Clinical and Morphologic Characteristics of 186 Necropsy Patients With Aortic Dissection and Either a Unicuspid, Bicuspid or Tricuspid Aortic Valve

	Number of Aortic Valve Cusps			
	1	2	3	Totals
No. of patients	2	14	170	186
Mean age (yr) at death (range)	36 (26–45)	54 (17–82)	62 (21–91)	60 (17–91)
Men	2	11 (79%)	103 (61%)	116 (62%)
Systemic hypertension	0/2	6/11 (55%)	103/136 (76%)	109/149 (73%)
Cardiomegaly	1/1	9/10	107/131 (82%)	117/142 (82%)
Location of aortic tear				
Ascending	2	14 (100%)	116 (68%)	132 (71%)
Transverse	0	0	12	12 (6%)
Descending	0	0	42	42 (22%)
Operation for AD	1	4 (29%)	33 (19%)	38 (20%)
Unoperated AD	1	10	137	148 (80%)
Interval from AD to death				
Acute	1*/1	10*/10	110*/137	121*/148 (82%)
Healed	0/1	0/10	27*/137	27*/148 (18%)
False channel rupture	1*/1	9*/10	105*/137	115*/148 (78%)
Aortic isthmic coarctation	0	2	0	2
The Marfan syndrome	0	0	3	3

*Excludes patients who had an operation for aortic dissection. Abbreviation as in Table 1.

of the 200 coarctation cases: in 46 of the 183 cases, the aortic valve was bicuspid and aortic dissection occurred in 17 (37%) of the 46. Among our 14 patients with a bicuspid aortic valve associated with aortic dissection, 1 patient had severe aortic isthmic coarctation (that had been operatively excised years earlier), and 1 had aortic pseudocoarctation, that is, an anatomic indentation at the aortic isthmus but not enough indentation to cause functional obstruction. Of the 18 cases with bicuspid aortic valve and aortic dissection reported by Larson and Edwards (4), two (11%) had aortic coarctation.

Aortic media in aortic dissection with bicuspid aortic valve: clinical implications. As has been recognized for some time (2), the media of the ascending aorta is usually, but not always (4), abnormal among patients with a congenitally bicuspid aortic valve with or without associated aortic isthmic coarctation (12,13). The aortic media was abnormal in 9 of 10 cases examined in the present study. The abnormal configuration of the elastic fibers, mainly a severe loss of these fibers, of the media is probably the cause of the increased frequency of aortic dissection among persons with a congenitally bicuspid aortic valve. Often the aortic media in the cases examined was so abnormal that it was similar to that observed in patients with the Marfan syndrome (14). The abnormality of the ascending aorta should be kept in mind when performing aortic valve replacement in patients with a congenitally bicuspid stenotic or purely regurgitant aortic valve, for these persons probably have a greater propensity for dissection (particularly originating at an aortotomy site after the valve replacement) than have persons undergoing a similar procedure for a tricuspid aortic valve.

References

1. Gore I, Seiwert VJ. Dissecting aneurysm of the aorta: pathologic aspects: an analysis of eighty-five fatal cases. Arch Pathol 1952;53:121–41.
2. Edwards WD, Leaf DS, Edwards JE. Dissecting aortic aneurysm associated with congenital bicuspid aortic valve. Circulation 1978;57:1022–5.
3. Wilson SK, Hutchins GM. Aortic dissecting aneurysms: causative factors in 204 subjects. Arch Pathol Lab Med 1982;106:175–80.
4. Larson EW, Edwards WD. Risk factors for aortic dissection: a necropsy study of 161 cases. Am J Cardiol 1984;53:849–55.
5. Buja LM, Ali N, Fletcher RD, Roberts WC. Stenosis of the right pulmonary artery: a complication of acute dissecting aneurysm of the ascending aorta. Am Heart J 1972;83:89–92.
6. Roberts WC. Aortic dissection: anatomy, consequences, and causes. Am Heart J 1981;101:195–214.
7. Roberts WC, Satler LF, Wallace RB. Hemodynamic confirmation of peripheral pulmonary stenosis caused by aortic dissection. Am J Cardiol 1989;63:1418–20.
8. Roberts WC. The congenitally bicuspid aortic valve: a study of 85 autopsy cases. Am J Cardiol 1970;26:72–83.
9. Fenoglio JJ Jr, McAllister HA Jr, DeCastro CM, Davia JE, Cheitlin MD. Congenital bicuspid aortic valve after age 20. Am J Cardiol 1977;39:164–9.
10. Abbott ME. Coarctation of the aorta of the adult type. II. A statistical study and historical retrospect of 200 recorded cases, with autopsy, of stenosis or obliteration of the descending arch in subjects above the age of two years. Am Heart J 1928;3:574–618.
11. Reifenstein GH, Levine SA, Gross RE. Coarctation of the aorta: a review of 104 autopsied cases of "adult type," 2 years of age or older. Am Heart J 1947;33:146–68.
12. McKusick VA, Logue RB, Bahnson HT. Association of aortic valvular disease and cystic medial necrosis of the ascending aorta: report of four instances. Circulation 1957;16:188–94.
13. McKusick VA. Association of congenital bicuspid aortic valve and Erdheim's cystic medial necrosis. Lancet 1972;1:1026–7.
14. Roberts WC, Honig HC. The spectrum of cardiovascular disease in the Marfan syndrome: a clinico-morphologic study of 18 patients and comparison to 151 previously reported necropsy patients. Am Heart J 1982;104:115–35.

Severe Mitral or Aortic Valve Regurgitation, or Both, Requiring Valve Replacement for Infective Endocarditis Complicating Hypertrophic Cardiomyopathy

WILLIAM C. ROBERTS, MD, FACC, JOAN C. KISHEL, MD, CHARLES L. McINTOSH, MD, FACC, RICHARD O. CANNON III, MD, FACC, BARRY J. MARON, MD

Bethesda, Maryland

Certain clinical and morphologic findings are described in 11 patients with hypertrophic cardiomyopathy complicated by infective endocarditis that produced severe mitral or aortic valve regurgitation, or both, necessitating valve replacement. All 11 patients had changes in the operatively excised valve or valves characteristic of healed infective endocarditis. The infection involved only the mitral valve in seven patients, only the aortic valve in three patients and both valves in one patient.

Study of the operatively excised mitral valves indicated that the healed vegetations were located most commonly on the left ventricular aspects of the anterior mitral leaflet, indicating that vegetation had formed at contact points of this leaflet with mural endocardium of the left ventricular outflow tract. In all 11 patients, the infective endocarditis either worsened preexisting valve regurgitation or initiated valve regurgitation and led to worsened signs and symptoms of cardiac dysfunction, necessitating valve replacement. Functional class improved in the nine patients who survived 7 to 101 months after valve replacement.

Hypertrophic cardiomyopathy appears to be a factor predisposing to infective endocarditis. Patients with hypertrophic cardiomyopathy should receive prophylactic antibiotic therapy during procedures that predispose to infective endocarditis.

(J Am Coll Cardiol 1992;19:365–71)

From 1961 through October 1989, 626 patients with hypertrophic cardiomyopathy underwent a cardiac operation at the Surgery Branch of the National Heart, Lung, and Blood Institute: partial septotomy/septectomy alone in 539 patients (86%); septotomy/septectomy followed later by mitral valve replacement in 19 patients (3%) and mitral valve replacement alone in 68 patients (11%). Of the 87 patients undergoing mitral valve replacement with or without septotomy/septectomy, mitral valve replacement was performed because of severe left ventricular outflow obstruction unassociated with severe thickening of the ventricular septum in 65 patients; damage to either the mitral or aortic valve at the time of earlier septotomy/septectomy in 5 patients; inability to wean the patient from cardiopulmonary bypass after septotomy/septectomy in 3 patients; severe regurgitation of uncertain etiology in 3 patients; and valvular regurgitation caused by or worsened by infective endocarditis in 11 patients. This report describes certain clinical and morphologic cardiac findings in the 11 patients with hypertrophic cardiomyopathy with severe mitral or aortic valvular regurgitation, or both, from infective endocarditis.

From the Pathology, Cardiology and Surgery Branches, National Heart, Lung, and Blood Institute, National Institutes of Health, Bethesda, Maryland.

Manuscript received May 8, 1991; revised manuscript received July 15, 1991, accepted July 29, 1991.

Address for reprints: William C. Roberts, MD, Building 10, Room 2N258, NHLBI-NIH, Bethesda, Maryland 20892.

Methods

Clinical characteristics (Tables 1 to 3). All 11 patients had clear clinical evidence of hypertrophic cardiomyopathy: 1) each had evidence of left ventricular hypertrophy on both the electrocardiogram (ECG) and the M-mode echocardiogram; 2) immediately before cardiac valve replacement, only 1 patient had a dilated left ventricular cavity as determined by left ventricular angiography and the dilation was of mild degree; 3) none had a history of systemic hypertension and, with one exception, all had systemic arterial indirect pressure recordings ≤140 mm Hg systolic and ≤90 mm Hg diastolic (Patient 3 had a systemic arterial direct pressure of 160/90 mm Hg recorded immediately before valve replacement, but other pressures recorded were normal); 4) although cardiac index was normal in only four of nine patients in whom it was recorded, the other five had evidence of severe valvular regurgitation (worsened by infective endocarditis) at the time of the recording; 5) the maximal thickness of the ventricular septum was greater than that of the left ventricular free wall in all patients before either valve replacement or partial ventricular septotomy/septectomy; and 6) all patients had hemodynamic documentation of subaortic obstruction at some time.

Characteristics of infective endocarditis. All 11 patients had evidence of active infective endocarditis at some time (Fig. 1 to 7). Ten patients had a typical clinical illness of active infective endocarditis. Of the nine patients with one

Table 1. Clinical and Morphologic Features in 11 Patients Having Valve Replacement for Valvular Regurgitation Due to or Worsened by Infective Endocarditis Complicating Hypertrophic Cardiomyopathy

Pt No.	Age (yr) at VR/ Gender	Diagnosis of HCM		NYHA Functional Class (I–IV)			Septotomy/Septectomy (7 patients)				Follow-Up After Valve Replacement (mo)	NYHA Class at Latest Follow-Up	Interval IE to VR (mo)	Type Valve Prosthesis		Morphology of Operatively Excised Valve				
		Before IE	After IE	Just Before IE	After IE	Just Before VR	Before IE	After IE	Before VR	With VR				MV (size)	AV (size)	MV Calcium	MV P	MV RCT	AV Calcium	AV P
1	12/M	+	0	II	IV	IV	0	0	0	0	7	I	17	SE	–	+	+	+	–	–
2	25/M	+	0	II	III	III	+	+	0	+	21	I	10	H (27 mm)	–	+	+	+	–	–
3	43/M	+	0	II	III	III	0	0	0	0	10	II	19	H (25 mm)	–	+	+	+	–	–
4	46/M	–	–	–	–	III	0	+	0	+	101	III	–	H (25 mm)	–	0	+	+	–	–
5	63/M	+	0	III	IV	IV	0	0	0	0	90	II	8	H (31 mm)	–	+	+	+	–	–
6	64/M	0	+	II	II	III	0	0	0	0	18	I	156	H (31 mm)	–	+	+	+	–	–
7	71/M	+	0	II	III	IV	0	–	+	0	30 days	Dead	204	H (31 mm)	–	+	+	+	–	–
8	51/M	0	+	I	IV	IV	0	–	0	+	72	I	3	–	SE (9A)	–	–	–	+	+
9	52/F	+	0	II	III	III	0	–	0	+	33	II	7	–	SE (9A)	–	–	–	+	+
10	64/F	0	+	I	III	IV	0	+	0	+	12	I	60	–	H (21 mm)	–	–	–	0	+
11	58/M	+	0	III	IV	IV	0	+	+	0	3 days	Dead	168	H (29 mm)	H (23 mm)	+	+	+	0	+

AV = aortic valve; F = female; H = Hancock; HCM = hypertrophic cardiomyopathy; IE = infective endocarditis; M = male; MV = mitral valve; NYHA = New York Heart Association; P = perforation or indentation (deficiency of leaflet tissue); Pt = patient; RCT = ruptured chordae tendineae; SE = Starr-Edwards; VR = valve replacement; 0 = absent or negative; + = present or positive; – = no information available or not applicable.

clinical episode of active infective endocarditis, the interval between active infective endocarditis and valve replacement ranged from 3 to 204 months (mean 54, median 17). This interval was <1 year in four patients. Patient 11 (Table 1) had two episodes of active infective endocarditis that occurred 168 and 27 months, respectively, before valve replacement (Fig. 7). Only the second episode caused clinical worsening of this patient's cardiac status. Patient 4 apparently never had a clinical illness diagnosed as active infective endocarditis, but examination of the operatively excised mitral valve disclosed a large deficit in the anterior mitral leaflet adjacent to several ruptured chordae tendineae, anatomic findings diagnostic of healed infective endocarditis (1). Of the 11 patients, 9 had active infective endocarditis before they were admitted to the National Institutes of Health; 1 had active infective endocarditis treated at another hospital, but hypertrophic cardiomyopathy had previously been diagnosed at the National Institutes of Health; and 1 patient had active infective endocarditis while hospitalized at the National Institutes of Health. Diagnosis of hypertrophic cardiomyopathy had been established previously in 7 of the 10 patients with a clinical illness diagnosed as active infective endocarditis; it was made in the other 3 patients after active infective endocarditis had healed. In five patients, a factor other than hypertrophic cardiomyopathy predisposing to infective endocarditis was apparent: dental procedures in Patients 4 and 5, cardiac catheterization in Patients 6 and 10 and opiate addiction in Patient 11.

During active infective endocarditis, information regarding the results of blood cultures were known in eight patients: in two, the blood cultures were negative and in six a bacterium was identified (alpha streptococcus in Patients 7, 10 and 11; group D streptococcus in two patients [nonenterococcal in Patient 2 and enterococcus in Patient 6]; and *Cardiobacterium hominis* in Patient 4). All 11 patients, however, had anatomic deficiencies of mitral or aortic valve cusps, and in those with infective endocarditis involving the mitral valve, there were associated ruptured chordae tendineae. The 10 patients with clear clinical evidence of active infective endocarditis received appropriate antibiotic treatment, and by the time of valve replacement, the infection had healed in all 10 patients. The M-mode echocardiogram immediately before valve replacement showed "echo densities" compatible with healed vegetations in four of seven patients in whom healed infective endocarditis involved the mitral valve and two of four in whom it involved the aortic valve.

Valvular regurgitation caused by infective endocarditis. Active infective endocarditis worsened the symptomatic status in nine patients by at least one New York Heart Association functional class. It also increased the intensity of the precordial systolic murmur (mitral regurgitation) in three of three patients in whom this information was known and caused the appearance of a basal diastolic murmur in all four patients with aortic regurgitation. Despite the appearance or worsening of valvular regurgitation, the left ventric-

Table 2. M-Mode Echocardiographic Data Before and After Operation in the 11 Patients With Infective Endocarditis Complicating Hypertrophic Cardiomyopathy and Requiring Valve Replacement

Pt No.	Interval Echo to VR (days)	Wall Thickness (mm) VSd	Wall Thickness (mm) LVd	Cavity (mm) LVd	Cavity (mm) LVs	Cavity (mm) LA	FS (%)	Echo Density MV	Echo Density AV	Flail MV	Flail AV	SAM
1	9 (MVR)	20	13	41	18	45	56	+	0	+	0	+
	PO	16	10	37	18	35	51	–	0	–	0	–
2												
3	78 (MVR)	17	14	36	16	56	55	0	0	+	0	+
	PO	—	—	—	—	—	—	–	–	–	–	–
4	12 (MVR)	19	15	40	18	40	55	0	0	0	0	–
	PO	15	—*	—*	—*	57	—	–	0	–	0	–
5	65 (MVR)	32	14	46	28	55	39	±	0	0	0	+
	PO	14	—	—	—	57	—	–	0	–	0	–
6	16 (MVR)	26	13	56	38	68	32	+	0	0	0	+
	PO	—	—	—	—	—	—	–	–	–	–	–
7	33 (MVR)	—	—	—	—	72	—	0	0	±	0	–
	PO	—	—	—	—	63	—	–	0	–	0	–
8	8 (AVR)	20	13	40	22	43	45	0	+	0	–	0
	PO	10	10	—*	—*	40	—	0	–	0	–	0
9	37 (AVR)	26	14	44	22	49	50	0	+	0	+	0
	PO†		11	51	29	45	43	0	–	0	–	0
10	41 (AVR)	24	13	53	41	60	23	0	0	0	0	–
	PO	11	11	—*	—*	52	—	0	–	0	–	0
11	10 (MVR, AVR)	—	—	—	—	54	—	0	0	0	0	0
	PO	—	—	—	—	—	—	–	–	–	–	–

*Paradoxical movement; †ventricular septal defect created at operation. AV = aortic valve; AVR = aortic valve replacement; d = end-diastole; Echo = echocardiography; FS = fractional shortening; LA = left atrium; LV = left ventricle; MV = mitral valve; MVR = mitral valve replacement; PO = after operation; s = peak systole; SAM = systolic anterior motion of the anterior mitral leaflet; VS = ventricular septum; – = not applicable; other abbreviations as in Table 1.

Table 3. Hemodynamic and Angiographic Data Immediately Before and ≥6 Months After Valve Replacement in 11 Patients With Infective Endocarditis Complicating Hypertrophic Cardiomyopathy

Pt No.	Time of Cath (mo PO)	PA* (s/d)	RV* (s/d)	RA* (m)	Mean PAW*	LA* a	LA* v	LV* (s/d)	SA* (s/d)	LV-SA psg*	MR by LV Cine (0–4+)	AR by AA Cine (0–4+)	CAD by Cine	CI
1	Pre-VR	66/40	65/16	7	26	36	38	180/25	118/60	62	4+	—	—	3.8
	PO (6)	32/14	32/4	4	9	16	10	130/12	125/65	5	—	—	—	2.1
2	Pre-VR	80/40	80/18	18	45	AF	50	138/24	138/60	0	4+	1+	—	2.1
3	Pre-VR	88/40	88/14	11	32	32	44	140/30	114/65	26	4+	0	0	1.8
	PO (6)	44/20	44/6	4	14	16	12	150/14	158/88	0	0	0	—	3.3
4	Pre-VR	90/40	90/10	8	30	27	40	165/32	120/70	45	3+	—	0	2.0
5	Pre-VR†	50/25	50/10	5	15	—	—	245/40	160/90	85	3+	—	—	3.7
	PO (10)‡	—	120/30	19	35	23	55	130/24	130/65	0	2+	0	—	2.0
	PO (21)	60/25	60/9	11	24	—	32	—	—	—	—	—	—	2.5
6	Pre-VR	45/23	45/8	4	20	28	36	110/10	105/70	5	3+	—	—	2.5
	PO (6)	—	24/5	3	—	—	—	105/6	105/60	0	0	—	—	2.3
7	Pre-VR	50/25	50/5	6	31	AF	50	120/20	130/75	0	4+	—	§	1.5
8	Pre-VR	85/35	85/12	—	38	AF	55	120/14	120/60	0	4+	—	—	—
9	Pre-VR	50/25	50/15	6	27	40	45	164/34	86/40	78	1+	3+	0	—
	PO (12)	24/11	24/7	4	6	13	8	115/16	110/65	5	—	—	—	2.0
10	Pre-VR	60/30	65/15	9	20	10	22	200/28	130/68	70	1+	2+	0	3.1
	PO (8)	—	—	—	16	20	28	105/20	105/55	0	—	—	—	4.4
	PO (58)	30/12	30/5	6	12	—	—	—	120/70	—	—	—	—	—
11	Pre-VR	55/30	55/6	5	17	26	20	240/30	100/30	140	3+	3+	0	1.7
	PO (76)	75/35	75/16	15	31	28	44	150/24	145/85	5	3+	1+	0	2.1

*Pressures in mm Hg. †Cardiac catheterization (Cath) 36 months before valve replacement; ‡peribasilar bioprosthetic communication found by left ventricular cineangiography (Cine) and it was operatively closed after this cardiac catheterization procedure. §This patient was the only one with significant coronary narrowing and he had aortocoronary bypass grafting in addition to valve replacement (VR). a = a wave; AA = ascending aorta; AF = atrial fibrillation; AR = aortic regurgitation; CAD = coronary artery narrowing >50% in diameter of >1 major artery; CI = cardiac index in liters/min per m²; LA = left atrium; LV = left ventricle; MR = mitral regurgitation; PA = pulmonary artery; PAW = pulmonary artery wedge; PO = after operation (months); Pre = before; psg = peak systolic gradient; Pt = patient; RA = right atrium; RV = right ventricle; SA = systemic artery; s/d = peak systole/end-diastole; v = v wave.

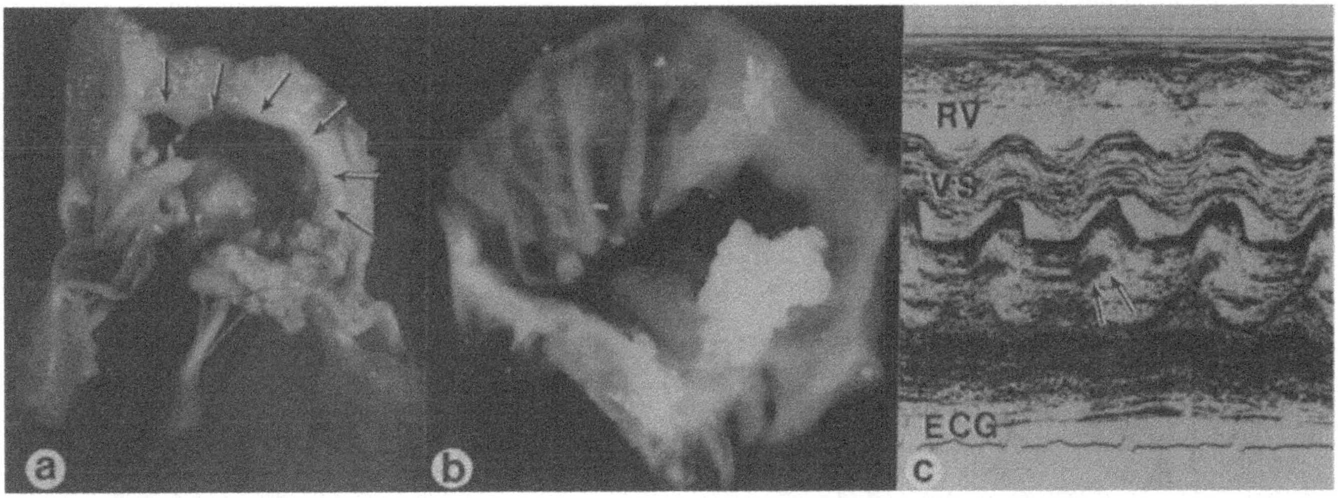

Figure 1 (above). Patient 1. Operatively excised mitral valve. **a,** Leaflets, chordae tendineae and attached papillary muscles showing loss of tissue in the posterior leaflet and absence of chordae tendineae (**arrows**). A large deposit of calcium is present and is better seen in **b,** a radiograph of the excised valve. **c,** M-mode echocardiogram taken shortly before mitral valve replacement, showing thickening and impaired mobility of the anterior mitral leaflet and fluttering (**arrows**) of the posterior leaflet. ECG = electrocardiogram; RV = right ventricular cavity; VS = ventricular septum.

Figure 2 (below). Patient 2. Operatively excised mitral valve (**a, b,** and **c**) and M-mode echocardiogram (**d**). **a,** Radiograph of the opened valve. The **arrows** point to a calcific deposit. **b** and **c,** Close-up views of the atrial aspect of a portion of both leaflets. The anterior leaflet contains two perforations (**solid arrows**) and the posterior leaflet one perforation (**dashed arrow**). **d,** Typical echocardiogram in hypertrophic cardiomyopathy with asymmetric thickening of the anterior ventricular septum (VS). The **arrows** point to dense echoes of the thickened anterior mitral leaflet, which contacts the ventricular septum in diastole. Mild mitral systolic anterior motion is present (*). PW = posterior wall; RV = right ventricular cavity.

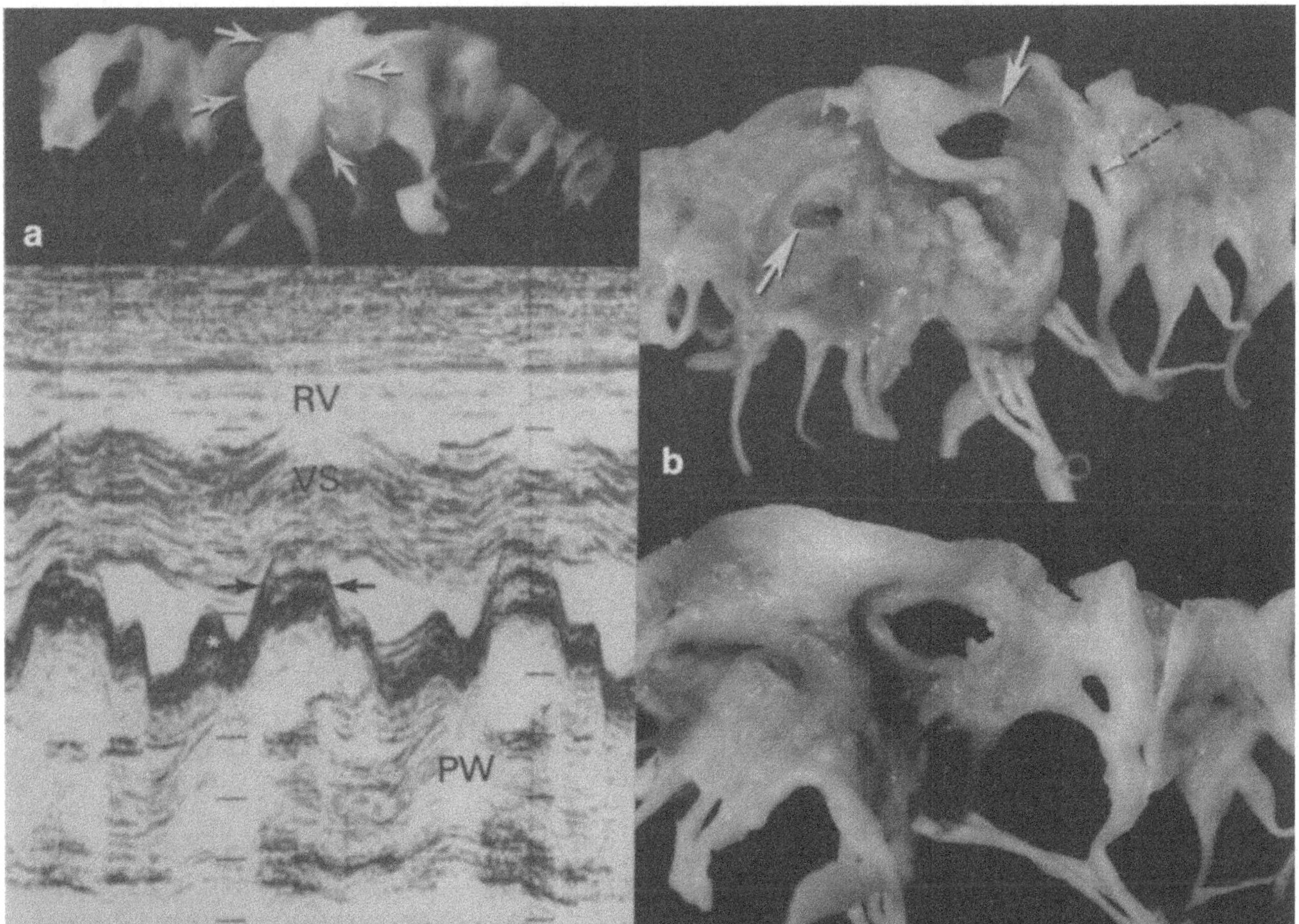

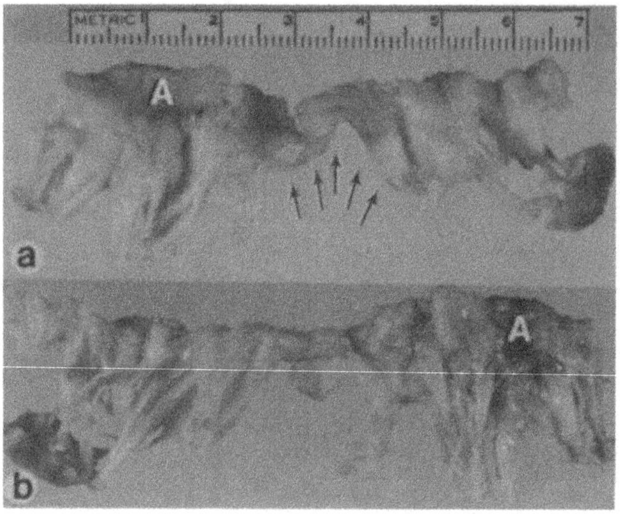

Figure 3. Patient 3. Opened mitral valve. **a,** Atrial surface. **b,** Ventricular surface. The **arrows** designate the area where chordae tendineae are missing (ruptured) and a site where a portion of the leaflet is absent (destroyed by the previous infection). A = anterior mitral leaflet.

ular cavity was of normal size on the echocardiogram immediately before valve replacement in nine of nine patients; left ventricular angiograms in the other two patients disclosed mild left ventricular cavity dilation in one of them. The degree of valvular regurgitation immediately before valve replacement in each of the 11 patients was severe: in the 7 patients with isolated mitral valve replacement, the degree of mitral regurgitation by left ventricular angiography was either 3+/4+ or 4+/4+; in the 3 patients with isolated aortic valve replacement, the degree of aortic regurgitation by aortic root angiography was 3+/4+ in 2 and 2+/4+ in 1; in the single patient with replacement of both left-sided cardiac valves, the degree of mitral regurgitation was 4+/4+ and aortic regurgitation, 1+/4+.

Effect of infective endocarditis on the left ventricular outflow pressure gradient. Active infective endocarditis involving the mitral valve was associated with a decrease in the peak systolic pressure gradient between the left ventricle and a systemic artery. In the three patients who had cardiac catheterization before and after active infective endocarditis, the peak systolic pressure gradient decreased from 90 to 62 mm Hg in Patient 1, from 100 to 5 mm Hg in Patient 4 and from 76 to 55 mm Hg in Patient 6.

Figure 4. Patient 5. Opened mitral valve from its atrial aspect, showing a large perforation (**arrow**) in the anterior leaflet (A) with adjacent focal calcific deposits. The perforation represents a site where vegetation had been present.

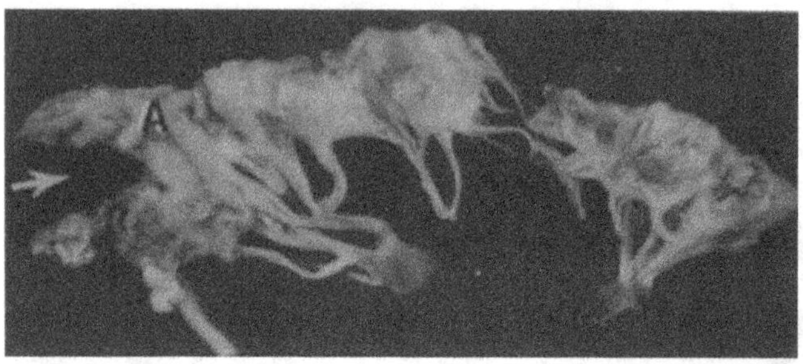

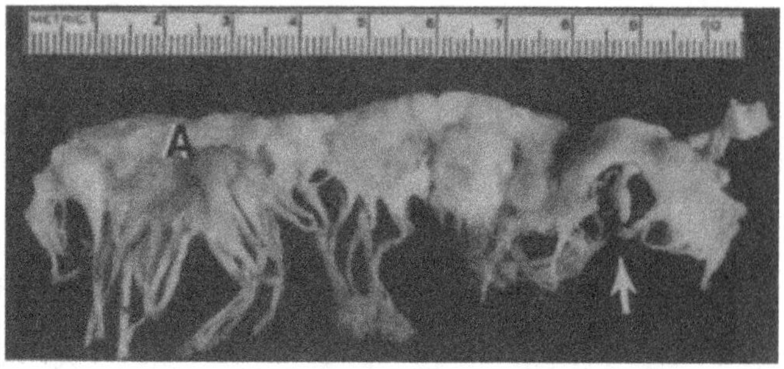

Figure 5. Patient 6. Opened mitral valve from its atrial aspect, showing a large indentation (**arrow**) in the posterior leaflet. Both anterior (A) and posterior leaflets are thickened by fibrous tissue. The indentation represents a site of previous vegetation.

Results of cardiac valve replacements. Valve replacement was successful in nine patients. The other two patients (Patients 7 and 11), each of whom died within 30 days of valve replacement, were the only patients who had had partial septectomy and septotomy before cardiac valve replacement. Of the nine hospital survivors after valve replacement (combined with partial septotomy and septectomy in four), eight were in functional class I or II and one was in class III when seen 6 to 21 months after valve replacement, whereas preoperatively three had been in functional class III and five in functional class IV. Cardiac catheterization was performed 6 to 21 months (mean 14) after valve replacement in seven of the nine long-term survivors (Table 3). In three of the seven patients, no left ventricular outflow tract obstruction was present preoperatively and the postoperative study disclosed no pressure gradient between the left ventricle and a systemic artery during peak systole. In the other four patients, the peak systolic pressure gradient before valve replacement (combined with partial septotomy and septectomy in three patients) decreased from an average of 74 mm Hg (range 62 to 85) preoperatively to ≤5 mm Hg postoperatively.

Discussion

Major findings of present study. Although 30 reports describing one or more patients (19 were single case studies) with hypertrophic cardiomyopathy and infective endocarditis have appeared (cases tabulated by Alessandri et al. [2]), the presence of infective endocarditis was confirmed anatomically (2–11) only in 15 of the reported 56 cases and in none was the type of valvular damage illustrated. The present study analyzed 11 patients from the same center with

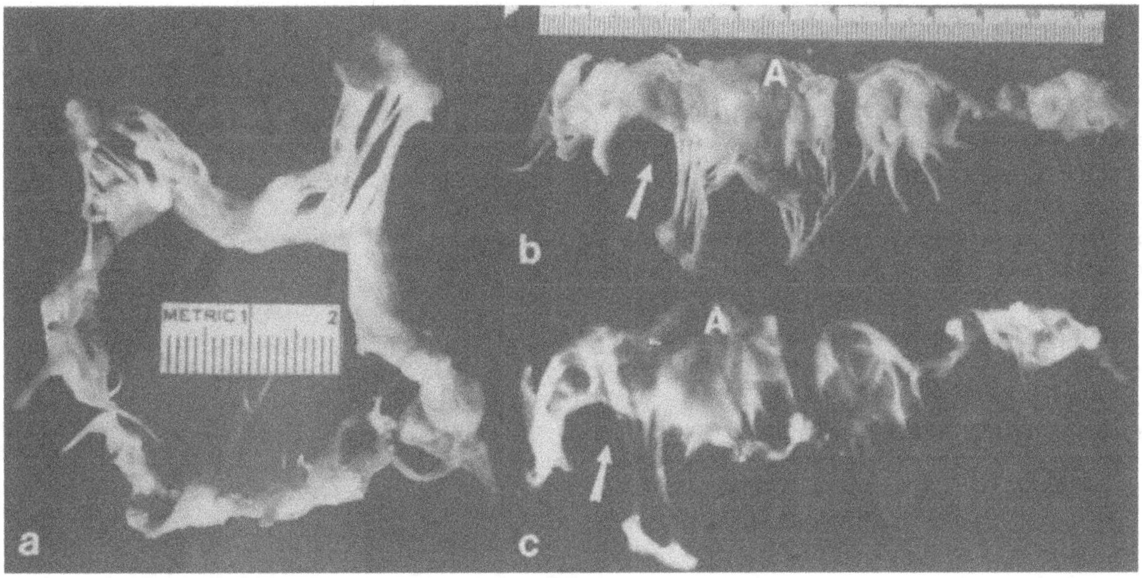

Figure 6. Patient 7. **a,** Unopened mitral valve. **b,** Opened mitral valve showing its atrial aspect. The **arrow** points to an indentation at the junction of the anterior (A) and posterior leaflets. Several chordae tendineae are missing (ruptured) at this site. **c,** Radiograph of the opened mitral valve. Several calcific deposits are present in the annular region of the posterior leaflet.

hypertrophic cardiomyopathy complicated by infective endocarditis necessitating replacement of one or more cardiac valves in each, and in each the operatively excised valve was studied. It is apparent that infective endocarditis should be recognized as a complication of hypertrophic cardiomyopathy and that the latter predisposes to infective endocarditis. The frequency with which the complication occurs is unclear. The present study suggests that among patients with hypertrophic cardiomyopathy with mitral or aortic valve regurgitation, or both, severe enough to warrant valve replacement, infective endocarditis often is responsible for the severe regurgitation. Of the 87 patients with hypertrophic cardiomyopathy who underwent valve replacement at our institution, 11 underwent this procedure because of damage by infective endocarditis. None of the other operatively excised valves had cusp perforations or tears or ruptured chordae tendineae and therefore it is unlikely that any of these other patients had had infective endocarditis at any time.

Location of the vegetations in infective endocarditis complicating hypertrophic cardiomyopathy. The most frequent site of vegetations in patients with hypertrophic cardiomyopathy is the mitral valve and specifically its anterior leaflet. It is this leaflet, of course, which tends to contact the mural endocardium of the ventricular septum during one or both phases of the cardiac cycle and it is likely that vegetations form at these contact sites. Of our 11 patients, 8 had vegetations that left telltale residua of infective endocarditis on the mitral valve (1 also had damage to the aortic valve, but the damage was not diagnostic of healed infective endocarditis [1]) and 3 had both clinical and anatomic evidence of damage to one or more aortic valve cusps by infective endocarditis. The vegetations on the anterior mitral leaflet appear to have been on their ventricular aspects, unlike those in most patients with active infective endocarditis involving the mitral valve. The mechanism of formation of aortic valve vegetations in patients with hypertrophic cardiomyopathy is unclear. In three of our four patients having aortic valve replacement, the left ventricular aortic

Figure 7. Patient 8. Three-cusped aortic valve with severe destruction of one of the three cusps by the infective process.

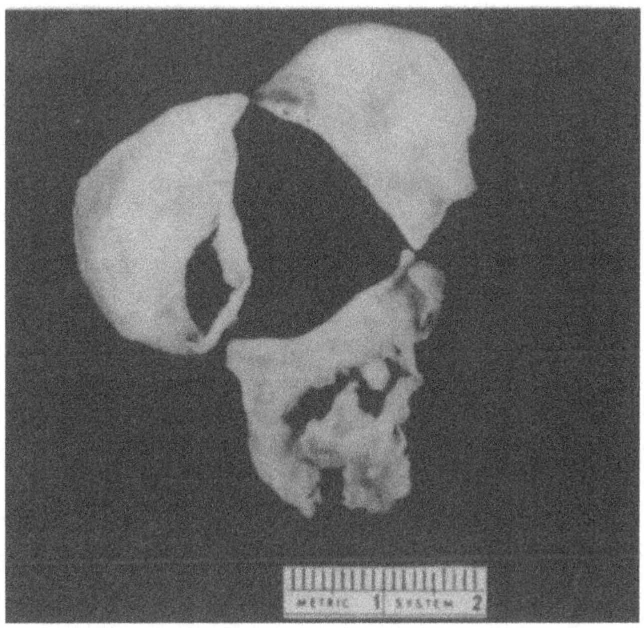

peak systolic pressure gradient was high (70, 78 and 140 mm Hg, respectively), whereas only one of the seven patients with isolated mitral valve replacement had a left ventricular outflow pressure gradient of this magnitude. The vegetations on the aortic valve appear to have been located on the ventricular aspects of these cusps, the usual location of vegetations on this valve.

Valvular regurgitation after infective endocarditis in hypertrophic cardiomyopathy. The present study shows that infective endocarditis complicating hypertrophic cardiomyopathy can result in serious consequences. In all 11 patients, the symptomatic status was unequivocally worsened by active infective endocarditis that healed. Additionally, the intensity of the precordial systolic murmur increased in the patients with infective endocarditis involving the mitral valve, and infective endocarditis involving the aortic valve caused the appearance of a murmur of aortic regurgitation, which was confirmed in each by angiography. The degree of valvular regurgitation was severe in all 11 patients; however, despite the severe degree of regurgitation, the left ventricular cavity immediately before valve replacement was not dilated in any patient on M-mode echocardiography and was only mildly dilated in one of two patients studied by angiography.

Benefit of valve replacement. Despite recognized potential complications of mitral valve replacement in patients with hypertrophic cardiomyopathy (12), the present study indicates that valve replacement for infective endocarditis complicating hypertrophic cardiomyopathy may result in a striking diminution or disappearance of previous symptoms of cardiac dysfunction.

References

1. Roberts WC, Buchbinder NA. Healed left-sided infective endocarditis: a clinicopathologic study of 59 patients. Am J Cardiol 1977;40:876–88.
2. Alessandri N, Pannarale G, del Monte F, Moretti F, Marino B, Reale A. Hypertrophic obstructive cardiomyopathy and infective endocarditis: a report of seven cases and a review of the literature. Eur Heart J 1990;11:1041–8.
3. Nagle JP. Idiopathic hypertrophic subaortic stenosis and bacterial endocarditis. JAMA 1967;200:643–5.
4. Vecht RJ, Oakley CM. Infective endocarditis in three patients with hypertrophic obstructive cardiomyopathy. Br Med J 1968;2:455–9.
5. Caramanian M, Joly F, Fouchard J, Guerinon J. Endocardite infectieuse sur stenose musculaire hypertrophique du ventricule gauche. Arch Mal Coeur 1971;64:1117–31.
6. Chretien EH, Limas C, Garagusi VF. Association of bacterial endocarditis in idiopathic hypertrophic subaortic stenosis. South Med J 1973;66:269–72.
7. Wang K, Gobel FL, Gleason DF. Bacterial endocarditis in idiopathic hypertrophic subaortic stenosis. Am Heart J 1975;89:359–65.
8. Heret JF, Jandin M, Rigaud M, et al. Endocardite a staphylocoque dore au cours d'une cardiomyopathic obstructive. Arch Mal Coeur 1977;70:1227–32.
9. Greenland P, Murphy GW. Acute valvular insufficiency complicating hypertrophic obstructive cardiomyopathy. Chest 1979;75:182–3.
10. LeJemtel TH, Factor SM, Koenigsberg M, O'Reilly M, Frater R, Sonnenblick EH. Mural vegetations at the site of endocardial trauma in infective endocarditis complicating idiopathic hypertrophic subaortic stenosis. Am J Cardiol 1979;44:569–74.
11. Pueyo JM, Shahin A, Benazet JM, Camaeno AM, San Miguel JG. Endocarditis infecciosa en estenosis subaortica hipertrofica idiopatica: a proposito de una observacion. Med Clin Barcelona 1981;76:129–31.
12. Roberts WC. Operative treatment of hypertrophic obstructive cardiomyopathy: the case against mitral valve replacement. Am J Cardiol 1973;32:377–81.

Reported Frequency of Coronary Arterial Narrowing by Angiogram in Patients with Valvular Aortic Stenosis

Gisela C. Mautner, MD, and William C. Roberts, MD

During the past 25 years most patients aged >40 years of age having aortic valve replacement have had coronary angiography preoperatively. At least 33 studies have reported the frequency of significant (>50% diameter reduction) coronary arterial narrowing in patients with valvular aortic stenosis, and most of these reported studies included only patients who had the stenotic valve replaced with a prosthesis or bioprosthesis[1-33] (Table I). Patients with mitral valve dysfunction usually were excluded. Analysis of the studies, which unfortunately also included a small percentage of patients <40 years of age, disclosed that 37% of the patients (1,302 of 3,509) had significant narrowing by angiogram of 1 or more major epicardial coronary arteries.

1. Linhart JW, de la Torre A, Ramsey HW, Wheat MW. The significance of coronary artery disease in aortic valve replacement. *J Thorac Cardiovasc Surg* 1968;55:811–819.
2. Harris CN, Kaplan MA, Parker DP, Dunne EF, Cowell HS, Ellestad MH. Aortic stenosis, angina, and coronary artery disease. Interrelations. *Br Heart J* 1975;37:656–661.

From the Pathology Branch, National Heart, Lung, and Blood Institute, National Institutes of Health, Bethesda, Maryland 20892. Manuscript received March 4, 1992, and accepted March 24.

3. Basta LL, Raines D, Najjar S, Kioschos JM. Clinical, haemodynamic, and coronary angiographic correlates of angina pectoris in patients with severe aortic valve disease. *Br Heart J* 1975;37:150–157.
4. Gross B, Mason DT, Amsterdam EA. Angina pectoris in aortic stenosis: clinical, hemodynamic and coronary angiographic correlates (abstr). *Circulation* 1975;51,52(suppl II):II-192.
5. Moraski RE, Russell RO, Mantle JA, Rackley CE. Aortic stenosis, angina pectoris, coronary artery disease. *Cathet Cardiovasc Diagn* 1976;2:157–164.
6. Mandal AB, Gray IR. Significance of angina pectoris in aortic valve stenosis. *Br Heart J* 1976;38:811–815.
7. Paquay PA, Anderson G, Diefenthal H, Nordstrom L, Richman HG, Gobel FL. Chest pain as a predictor of coronary artery disease in patients with obstructive aortic valve disease. *Am J Cardiol* 1976;38:863–869.
8. Hancock EW. Aortic stenosis, angina pectoris, and coronary artery disease. *Am Heart J* 1977;93:382–393.
9. Lacy J, Goodin R, McMartin D, Masden R, Flowers N. Coronary atherosclerosis in valvular heart disease. *Ann Thoracic Surg* 1977;23:429–435.
10. Graboys TB, Cohn PF. The prevalence of angina pectoris and abnormal coronary arteriograms in severe aortic valvular disease. *Am Heart J* 1977;93:683–686.
11. Swanton RH, Brooksby IAB, Jenkins BS, Coltart DJ, Webb-Peploe MM, Williams BT, Braimbridge MV. Determinants of angina in aortic stenosis and the importance of coronary arteriography. *Br Heart J* 1977;39:1347–1352.
12. Thompson RH, Ahmed MS, Mitchell AG, Towers MK, Yacoub MH. Angina, aortic stenosis and coronary heart disease. *Clin Cardiol* 1979;2:26–32.
13. Storstein O, Enge I. Angina pectoris in aortic valvular disease and its relation to coronary pathology. *Acta Med Scand* 1979;205:275–278.
14. Hakki AH, Kimbiris D, Iskandrian AS, Segal BL, Mintz GS, Bemis CE. Angina pectoris and coronary artery disease in patients with severe aortic valvular disease. *Am Heart J* 1980;100:441–449.
15. Bonow RO, Kent KM, Rosing DR, Lipson LC, Borer JS, McIntosh CL, Morrow AG, Epstein SE. Aortic valve replacement without myocardial revascu-

larization in patients with combined aortic valvular and coronary artery disease. *Circulation* 1981;63:243–251.

16. Bermudez GA, Abdelnur R, Midell A, DeMeester T. Coronary artery disease in aortic stenosis: importance of coronary arteriography and surgical implications. *Angiology* 1983;34:591–596.

17. Crochet D, Petitier H, de Laguerenne J, Wanlin P, Chiffoleau S, Grossète R, Godin JF. Adult aortic stenosis: value of catheterization for the study of associated lesions: a series of 137 cases. *Arch Mal Coeur* 1983;76:1057–1064.

18. Exadactylos N, Sugrue DD, Oakley CM. Prevalence of coronary artery disease in patients with isolated aortic valve stenosis. *Br Heart J* 1984;51:121–124.

19. Monsuez JJ, Drobinski G, Verdière C, Chollet D, Grosgogeat Y. Étude prospective de la fréquence de l' atteinte coronarienne en cas de rétrécissement aortique pur. *Ann Cardiol Angeiol (Paris)* 1985;34:65–69.

20. Abdulali SA, Baliga BG, Clayden AD, Smith DR. Coronary artery luminal diameter in aortic stenosis. *Am J Cardiol* 1985;55:450–453.

21. Green SJ, Pizzarello RA, Padmanabhan VT, Ong LY, Hall MH, Tortolani AJ. Relation of angina pectoris to coronary artery disease in aortic valve stenosis. *Am J Cardiol* 1985;55:1063–1065.

22. Turina J, Goebel N, Hess O, Krayenbühl HP. Indications for coronary arteriography in aortic valve disease. *Z Kardiol* 1986;75(suppl 2):68–72.

23. Sechtem U, Müller-Haake RC. Coronary artery disease in aortic stenosis. *Z Kardiol* 1986;75(suppl 2):86–89.

24. Lombard JT, Selzer A. Valvular aortic stenosis. A clinical and hemodynamic profile of patients. *Ann Intern Med* 1987;106:292–298.

25. Safford RE, Bove AA. Prediction of coronary artery disease by left ventricular regional wall motion abnormalities in patients with stenosis of the aortic valve. *Br Heart J* 1987;57:237–241.

26. Vandeplas A, Willems JL, Piessens J, de Geest H. Frequency of angina pectoris and coronary artery disease in severe isolated valvular aortic stenosis. *Am J Cardiol* 1988;62:117–120.

27. Bessone LN, Pupello DF, Hiro SP, Lopez-Cuenca E, Glatterer MS, Ebra G. Surgical management of aortic valve disease in the elderly: a longitudinal analysis. *Ann Thorac Surg* 1988;46:264–269.

28. Kishore AGR, Gupta SK, Reddy KN, Murthy JSN, Prasad SV, Abraham KA. Coronary artery disease in patients with isolated aortic valve stenosis. *Indian Heart J* 1988;40:481–484.

29. Chobadi R, Wurzel M, Teplitsky I, Menkes H, Tamari I. Coronary artery disease in patients 35 years of age or older with valvular aortic stenosis. *Am J Cardiol* 1989;64:811–812.

30. Vekshtein VI, Alexander RW, Yeung AC, Plappert T, St John Sutton MG, Ganz P, Selwyn AP, Bittl JA. Coronary atherosclerosis is associated with left ventricular dysfunction and dilatation in aortic stenosis. *Circulation* 1990;82: 2068–2074.

31. Lund O, Nielsen TT, Pilegaard HK, Magnussen K, Knudsen MA. The influence of coronary artery disease and bypass grafting on early and late survival after valve replacement for aortic stenosis. *J Thorac Cardiovasc Surg* 1990;100: 327–337.

32. Danielsen R, Nordrehaug JE, Vik-Mo H. Clinical and haemodynamic features in relation to severity of aortic stenosis in adults. *Eur Heart J* 1991; 12:791–795.

33. Mautner GC, Cannon RO III, Mautner SL, Hunsberger SA, Roberts WC. Clinical factors useful in predicting aortic valve structure in patients >40 years of age with isolated valvular aortic stenosis. Submitted to *Am J Cardiol* 1992; in press.

TABLE I Published Reports on the Frequency of Significant (≥ 50% diameter narrowing) Coronary Arterial Narrowing on Angiogram in Patients with Valvular Aortic Stenosis

First Author	Year of Publication	No. of Pts.	Age (years) Range (mean)	Men	Women	Mitral Valve Dysfunction	AVR	CA ↓ ≥ 50% in Diameter	CABG
1. Linhart	1968	52	19–68 (51)	41	11	0	33 (63%)	33/52 (63%)	—
2. Harris	1975	69	38–77 (58)	58	11	+	—	16*/69 (23%)	—
3. Basta	1975	68	34–77 (56)	50	18	—	68 (100%)	10/41 (24%)	—
4. Gross	1975	48	— (61)	—	—	—	—	16*/48 (33%)	—
5. Moraski	1976	88	31–81 (59)	67	21	—	81 (92%)	41/88 (47%)	19 (22%)
6. Mandal	1976	28	45–66 (58)	20	8	0	20 (71%)	14†/28 (50%)	8 (29%)
7. Paquay	1976	48	39–84 (60)	48	0	—	—	21*/48 (44%)	—
8. Hancock	1977	173	40–83 —	—	—	0	156 (90%)	97/173 (56%)	—
9. Lacy	1977	56	18–74 —	39	17	—	—	12/56 (21%)	—
10. Graboys	1977	19	47–76 (62)	12	7	0	19 (100%)	4*/19 (21%)	—
11. Swanton	1977	140	18–75 (60)	90	50	12	122 (87%)	32/140 (23%)	6 (4%)
12. Thompson	1979	139	30–79 —	—	—	—	127 (91%)	45‡/139 (32%)	36 (26%)
13. Storstein	1979	44	— —	—	—	—	—	13*/44 (30%)	—
14. Hakki	1980	39	43–79 (65)	26	13	0	—	18/39 (46%)	—
15. Bonow	1981	78	— (58)	—	—	0	78 (100%)	26/78 (33%)	0
16. Bermudez	1983	64	40–71 (55)	38	26	—	64 (100%)	32*/64 (50%)	—
17. Crochet	1983	137	— (63)	93	44	14	—	34/110 (31%)	—
18. Exadactylos	1984	88	38–77 (58)	64	24	0	88 (100%)	22/64 (34%)	—
19. Monsuez	1984	148	20–81 (62)	89	59	0	—	27/148 (18%)	—
20. Abdulali	1985	32	— (55)	26	6	—	—	11‡/32 (34%)	—
21. Green	1985	103	44–87 (66)	68	35	0	—	46‡/103 (45%)	—
22. Turina	1986	300	— (54)	—	—	—	300 (100%)	54/300 (18%)	—
23. Sechtem	1986	75	25–75 (59)	35	40	—	—	17/75 (23%)	12 (16%)
24. Lombard	1987	397	15–>80 (61)	276	121	0	—	135/234 (58%)	—
25. Safford	1987	83	33–85 (66)	65	18	—	—	55/83 (66%)	—
26. Vandeplas	1988	192	28–82 (59)	121	71	0	—	47/192 (24%)	—
27. Bessone	1988	219	70-88 (75)	132	87	+	219 (100%)	112‡/219 (51%)	107 (49%)
28. Kishore	1988	106	40–63 (48)	100	6	0	—	6/106 (6%)	—
29. Chobadi	1989	146	38–80 (63)	88	58	0	—	54/146 (37%)	—
30. Vekshtein	1990	78	— (74)	32	46	0	—	35/78 (45%)	—
31. Lund	1990	205	— —	—	—	—	205 (100%)	83/205 (40%)	55 (27%)
32. Danielsen	1991	100	41–79 (65)	64	36	3	—	54/100 (54%)	—
33. Mautner	1992	188	42–81 (61)	139	49	0	188 (100%)	80/188 (43%)	43 (23%)
Totals		3,750	15–88 (61)	1,881/ 2,763 (68%)	882/ 2,763 (32%)	29/ 2,500 (1%)	1,768/ 1,849 (96%)	1,302/ 3,509 (37%)	286/ 1,040 (28%)

*Coronary diameter narrowing > 75%.
†Coronary diameter narrowing > 60%.
‡Coronary diameter narrowing > 70%.
AVR = aortic valve replacement; CA ↓ = coronary artery narrowing; CABG = coronary artery bypass grafting.

Comparison of Active Infective Endocarditis Involving a Previously Stenotic Versus a Previously Nonstenotic Aortic Valve

William C. Roberts, MD, B. Olusola Oluwole, MB, BS, and Daniel J. Fernicola, MD

No previous studies, either clinical or morphologic, have compared findings in patients with active infective endocarditis (IE) involving a previously stenotic versus a previously nonstenotic aortic valve. Clinical and cardiac necropsy findings were analyzed in 96 patients with active IE involving the aortic valve. Of the 96 patients, 25 (26%) had active IE superimposed on a previously stenotic aortic valve and 71 (74%) on a previously nonstenotic aortic valve. The patients with stenotic aortic valves compared with those with nonstenotic aortic valves had significantly higher mean ages (61 vs 47 years), a higher percentage >60 years of age (52 vs 24%), a higher percentage of men (92 vs 73%), a higher frequency of an absent or unknown predisposing factor to infection (68 vs 38%), a lower frequency of a precordial murmur of aortic regurgitation (44 vs 79%), a lower percent with a long duration (>60 days) of signs and symptoms of active IE (4 vs 23%), a larger mean heart weight (594 vs 514 g), a higher percentage with aortic valve calcific deposits (100 vs 24%), and a higher frequency of associated ring abscess (84 vs 52%). Thus, active IE superimposed on a stenotic aortic valve differs in some features compared with active IE on a nonstenotic aortic valve. Because ring abscess is so common when active IE involves a stenotic aortic valve in adults, operative intervention at an early stage may be warranted.

(Am J Cardiol 1993;71:1082–1088)

From the Pathology Branch, National Heart, Lung, and Blood Institute, National Institutes of Health, Bethesda, Maryland. Manuscript received and accepted December 1, 1992 (see addendum).

Address for reprints: William C. Roberts, MD, Baylor Cardiovascular Institute, Baylor University Medical Center, 3500 Gaston Avenue, Dallas, Texas 75246.

Studies from this laboratory[1–31] and others indicate that the cardiac valve most likely to be involved by active infective endocarditis (IE) is the one which is anatomically abnormal but functionally normal. Next is the valve which is anatomically abnormal and which functions slightly abnormally. The usual functional disturbance in the latter situation is mild valvular regurgitation. IE superimposed on a severely regurgitant cardiac valve is extremely uncommon and indeed has not been encountered by us from a study of >200 cases of active IE involving 1 or more native cardiac valves at necropsy. Infective endocarditis involving a previously stenotic valve is relatively uncommon, and when it occurs the valve involved is most often the aortic one. The degree of valve stenosis may vary from mild to severe. When active IE involves a previously stenotic aortic valve the consequences may be quite different from that which occurs when active IE involves a previously nonstenotic valve, i.e., one that functioned normally or was only slightly regurgitant before the active IE appeared. To better understand these clinical and morphologic differences, we studied at necropsy 25 patients with active IE involving a previously stenotic aortic valve and compared the findings with those in 71 patients in whom active IE involved a previously nonstenotic aortic valve.

METHODS

Method of retrieving cases and exclusion criteria: Records of cases accessioned in the Pathology Branch, National Heart, Lung, and Blood Institute from 1954 until July 1, 1991, under the code "active infective endocarditis" were retrieved and examined. All cases had been classified originally by WCR. Cases in which the native aortic valve was not involved by active IE, i.e., no vegetations were present on the aortic valve, were excluded. The present study was limited to patients studied at necropsy in whom active IE involved the aortic valve. A total of 104 such cases were identified. To make comparisons among cases most meaningful, however, cases of active IE of the aortic valve in which other complicating conditions or circumstances were present were eliminated. Thus, the following cases were eliminated from further analysis: 2 patients with discrete subaortic stenosis, 1 patient with associated ventricular septal defect, 4 patients with associated mitral valve stenosis, and 1 patient who developed active IE shortly after "open" aortic valve commissurotomy. The remaining 96 patients with active IE were included in the present study. Although 21 (22%) of the 96 patients had aortic valve replacement during the period of active IE, all 96 patients had active IE of the native aortic valve.

TABLE I Clinical and Necropsy Observations in Active Infective Endocarditis Superimposed on Preexisting Aortic Valve Stenosis

Pt. No.	Age (year) & Sex	Diagnosis AS in Life	Diagnosis IE in Life	Infecting Organism	Murmur (intensity 1–6) AS	AR	Duration S & S of IE (days)	HB	PE	AVR	HW (g)	No. AV Cusps	AV Calcium (0–3+)	No. AV Cusps with V	V on MV	Ring Abscess	MAC (0–4+)	CA Embolus	AMI
1	21M	+ (CC)	+	*H. parainfluenzae*	+(−)	+(−)	21	+*	+(300 ml)	+	–	2	0	2	0	+	0	+	0
2	30M	+ (A)	+	*S. aureus*	+(4/6)	0	18	0	0	0	560	2	3+	2	0	+	0	0	0
3	45M	+ (E)	+	*α-Streptococcus*	0	0	12	0	+(150 ml)	0	920	2	2+	2	+	+	0	0	0
4	54M	+ (E)	+	*S. aureus*	+(2/6)	+(2/6)	35	0	0	0	480	2	2+	2	+	+	0	+	+
5	54M	+ (E)	+	*α-Streptococcus*	+(4/6)	+(3/6)	23	0	0	0	850	2	3+	2	+	+	0	0	0
6	55M	+ (A)	0	—	+(−)	0	2	0	—	0	600	2	2+	2	0	0	0	0	0
7	59M	+ (E)	+	—	+(−)	+(−)	—	0	—	+	315	2	2+	2	0	+	0	0	0
8	60M	+ (CC)	+	*Strept. pneumoniae*	+(−)	+(−)	7	+	—	0	540	2	3+	2	0	+	0	0	0
9	63M	+ (A)	+	*α-Streptococcus*	+(3/6)	+(2/6)	90	+	—	0	620	2	3+	2	0	+	0	0	0
10	71M	0	0	*S. epidermidis*	—	—	30	0	0	0	520	2	3+	2	0	+	0	+	+
11	31M	+ (A)	+	*H. parainfluenzae*	+(−)	+(−)	23	0	+(600 ml)	0	425	3	0	2	0	+	0	0	0
12	45F	+ (A)	+	—	+(−)	+(−)	—	–	0	0	490	3	2+	3	0	0	0	–	0
13	49M	+ (A)	+	*S. aureus*	+(4/6)	0	16	+*	0	0	580	3	2+	3	0	+	0	0	0
14	52M	+ (A)	+	*Gram -ve bacilli*	+(−)	+(−)	18	0	—	+	—	3	2+	—	0	+	0	0	0
15	53M	+ (E)	+	*Escherichia coli*	+(3/6)	0	42	0	+(1,000 ml)	0	—	3	3+	3	0	+	0	0	+
16	60M	+ (E)	+	*S. aureus*	+(3/6)	+(−)	60	+	—	0	580	3	2+	3	0	+	0	0	0
17	62M	+ (A)	+	*S. epidermidis*	+(−)	0	—	0	0	0	650	3	2+	3	+	0	2+	0	0
18	65M	+ (A)	+	*α-Streptococcus*	+(2/6)	0	28	0	+(100 ml)	0	610	3	3+	3	0	+	0	0	0
19	67M	+ (A)	+	*S. aureus*	+(2/6)	0	30	0	0	0	700	3	3+	2	0	0	0	+	+
20	70M	+ (A)	+	*β-Streptococcus*	+(3/6)	+(−)	42	0	—	0	560	3	3+	1	+	+	0	0	0
21	72M	0	+	*Strept. pneumoniae*	+(−)	0	7	—	—	0	700	3	3+	3	0	+	0	0	0
22	77F	+ (A)	+	*α-Streptococcus*	+(−)	0	14	0	—	0	450	3	3+	2	+	+	4+	0	0
23	77M	+ (A)	0	—	+(3/6)	0	—	0	—	0	590	3	3+	2	0	0	4+	0	0
24	83M	+ (A)	0	*Strept. pneumoniae*	+(−)	0	1	0	0	0	550	3	2+	3	0	+	2+	0	0
25	86M	+ (A)	0	—	+(−)	0	14	0	+(80 ml)	0	710	3	3+	1	0	+	0	0	0

*Second-degree heart block present.
A = auscultation; AMI = acute myocardial infarction; AR = aortic regurgitation; AS = aortic stenosis; AV = aortic valve; AVR = aortic replacement; CA = coronary artery; CC = cardiac catheterization; E = echocardiogram; HB = heart block; HW = heart weight; IE = infective endocarditis; MAC = mitral annular calcium; MV = mitral valve; PE = pericardial effusion; S and S = signs and symptoms; V = vegetation.

Sources of cases: The 96 patients included in this study had the autopsy performed at 23 different medical institutions: 12 institutions were local and 84 of the 96 cases came from them; the remaining 12 cases were submitted from 12 different nonlocal hospitals. Only 6 of the 96 cases had an autopsy performed at the Clinical Center of the National Institutes of Health. The hearts of all 96 patients were examined initially by WCR and classified by him. Photographs were prepared of the heart in 60 of the 96 cases and all were available for examination. Histologic sections of the heart including aortic valve were examined in 72 of the 96 patients; in the remaining 24 cases the reports of the necropsy findings were examined. The hearts in 32 of the 96 cases were reexamined for this study.

Division of cases: The 96 cases were divided into 2 groups based on whether or not there was evidence that the aortic valve was stenotic before the valve be-

TABLE II Comparison of Patients with Active Infective Endocarditis Involving Stenotic and Nonstenotic Aortic Valves

	Stenotic (n = 25)	Nonstenotic (n = 71)	p Value
1. Age (year): range (mean)	21–86 (61)	17–81 (47)	0.002
≤30	2 (8%)	12 (17%)	0.278
31–60	10 (44%)	42 (59%)	0.098
>60	13 (52%)	17 (24%)	0.009
2. Men: women	23 (92%): 2 (8%)	52 (73%): 19 (27%)	0.051
3. Diagnosis of AS in life	23 (92%)	—	—
4. Diagnosis of IE in life	20 (80%)	48 (68%)	0.241
5. Infecting organism			
Bacterium			
Staphylococcal	7 (28%)	20 (28%)	0.987
Streptococcal	9 (36%)	22 (31%)	0.645
Mixed	4 (16%)	10 (14%)	0.816
Fungus	0	2 (3%)	1.0
Unknown	5 (20%)	17 (24%)	0.687
6. Predisposing factor			
Alcoholism	5 (20%)	20 (28%)	0.424
Opiate addiction	0	11 (15%)	0.06
Dental procedure	2 (8%)	5 (7%)	0.874
Hemodialysis	1 (4%)	4 (6%)	0.752
Previous IE	0	4 (6%)	0.57
Unknown	17 (68%)	27 (38%)	0.010
7. Aortic regurgitation murmur	11 (44%)	56 (79%)	0.001
8. Duration of IE (days)			
≤60	20 (80%)	45 (63%)	0.126
>60	1 (4%)	16 (23%)	0.037
Uncertain	4 (16%)	10 (14%)	0.816
9. Complete heart block	3 (12%)	4 (6%)	0.292
10. Pericardial effusion (>50 ml)	6/15 (40%)	11/43 (26%)	0.446
11. Aortic valve replacement	3 (12%)	18 (26%)	0.165
12. Heart weight (g): range (mean)	315–920 (594)	240–980 (514)	0.013
Men (n = 62)	315–920 (604)	340–980 (549)	0.098
Women (n = 14)	490 and 500	240–570 (389)	—
13. Number of aortic valve cusps			
2	10 (40%)	21 (30%)	0.338
3	15 (60%)	47 (66%)	0.577
Uncertain	0	3 (4%)	0.533
14. Aortic valve calcium			
0–1+	2 (8%)	17 (24%)	0.0001
2+–3+	23 (92%)	0	0.0001
15. No. of cusps with vegetation			
Bicuspid aortic valves	10	21	—
1	0	4 (19%)	0.28
2	10 (100%)	15 (71%)	0.060
Uncertain	0	2 (10%)	0.548
Tricuspid aortic valve	15	47	—
1	2 (13%)	13 (28%)	0.471
2	4 (27%)	12 (26%)	0.930
3	8 (53%)	20 (42%)	0.465
Uncertain	1 (7%)	2 (4%)	—
16. Vegetation on mitral valve	6 (24%)	19 (22%)	0.787
17. Ring abscess	21 (84%)	37 (52%)	0.005
18. Mitral annular calcium	4 (16%)	6 (8%)	0.288
19. Coronary artery embolus	4 (16%)	5 (7%)	0.186
20. Acute myocardial infarct	4 (16%)	4 (6%)	0.107
21. Stroke	2 (8%)	5 (7%)	0.874

AS = aortic stenosis; IE = infective endocarditis.

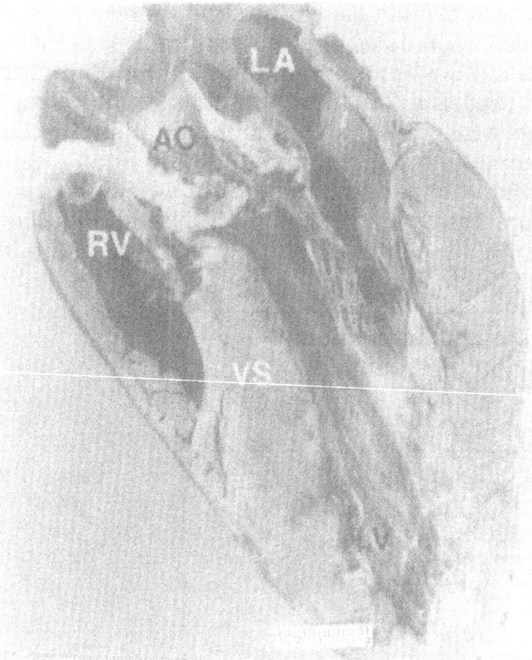

FIGURE 1. Case 1, Table I. Longitudinal view of heart (GT #76A-220) showing active infective endocarditis of a congenitally bicuspid and mildly stenotic aortic valve with extension of the infection into the right ventricular cavity via the ventricular septum (VS) and also with extension into the left atrial wall just cephalad to the anterior mitral leaflet. Left ventricular myocardium of the papillary muscle and of the subendocardial region is focally necrotic. Ao = aorta; LA = left atrium; LV = left ventricle; RV = right ventricle; VS = ventricular septum. (Reproduced with permission from Roberts WC, editor, Congenital Heart Disease in Adults, Philadelphia: FA Davis, 1979:422.)

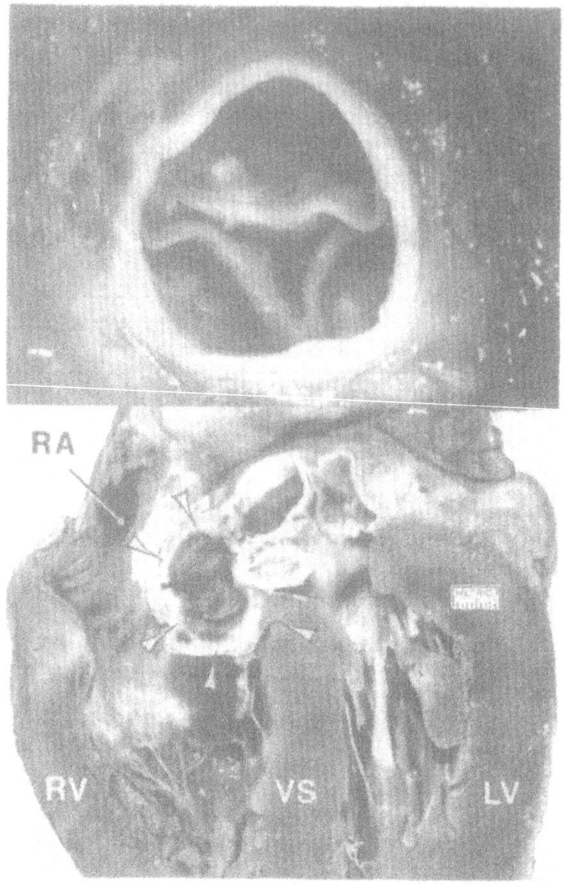

FIGURE 2. Case 6. *Top,* aortic valve seen from above (FSH# 4256). Each cusp is thickened and calcific deposits are present on their aortic surfaces. *Bottom:* longitudinal view of heart showing a large ring abscess *(arrows)* extending from the aortic valve toward the right atrial cavity. LV = left ventricular wall; RA = right atrial cavity; RV = right ventricular wall; VS = ventricular septum.

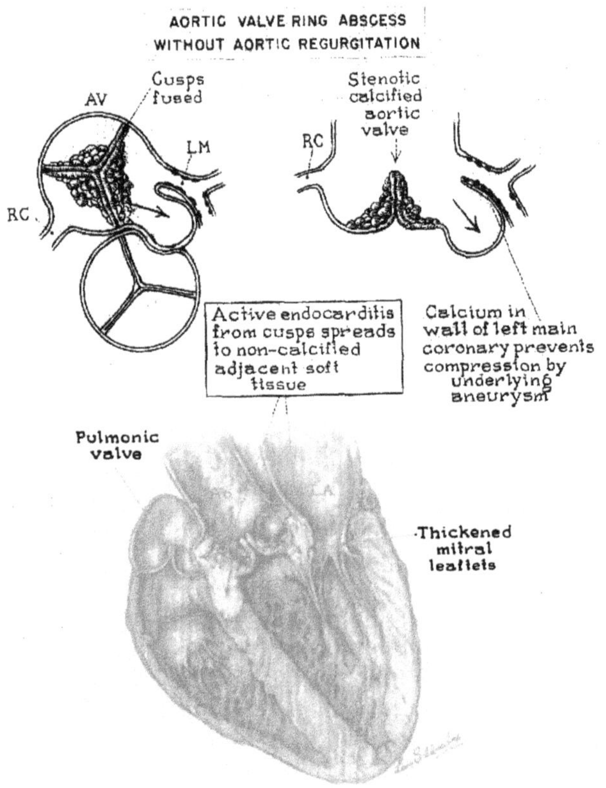

came the site of active IE. Of the 96 cases, 25 had preexisting aortic valve stenosis (Tables I and II) and 71 had nonstenotic aortic valves (Table II). The evidence of preexisting aortic stenosis was based on the finding at necropsy of heavy calcific deposits on the aortic aspects of the cusps resulting in loss of or severe reduction of mobility of the cusps leading to a clearly stenotic orifice. Twenty-three (92%) of the 25 patients had precordial ejection murmurs consistent with aortic valve stenosis, 6 had M-mode echocardiograms consistent with aortic valve stenosis, and 3 had cardiac catheterization with peak systolic pressure gradients recorded between the left ventricle and a systemic artery. Additionally, the presence of significant cardiomegaly without a history of systemic hypertension or the actual recording of an elevated systemic arterial diastolic blood pressure without

FIGURE 3. Case 8, Table I. Diagram of aortic valve (AV) (#33445) as seen from above *(upper left)* showing heavy calcific deposits and ring abscess *(arrow)* and longitudinal view of the valve *(upper right)* showing the ring abscess just beneath the left main (LM) coronary artery. *Lower,* longitudinal view showing large ring abscesses extending from the infection on the aortic valve. Ao = aorta; LA = left atrium; LV = left ventricle; RC = right coronary.

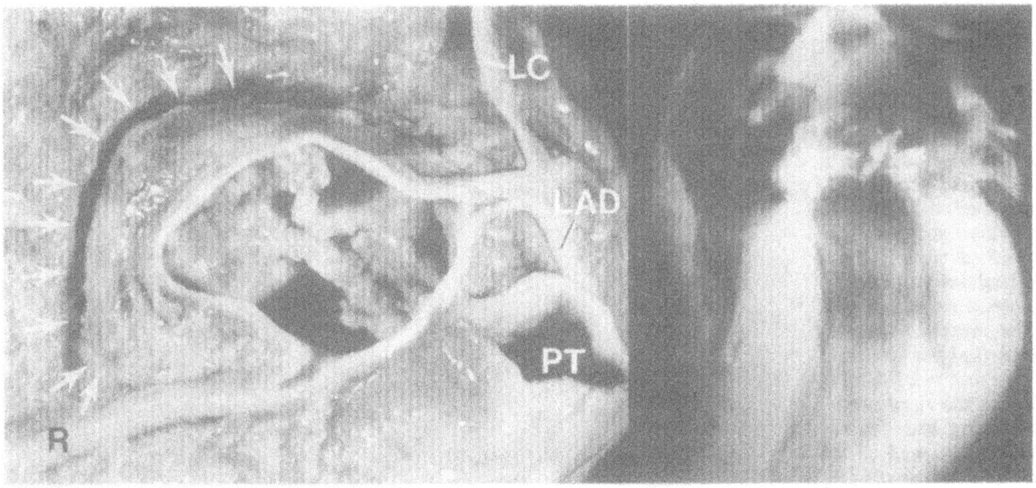

FIGURE 4. Case 9. ***Left,*** **Aortic valve (A75-55) seen from above showing a heavily calcified, severely stenotic valve with a large ring abscess *(arrows)* bulging toward the right atrium. LAD = left anterior descending; LC = left circumflex; PT = pulmonary trunk; R = right coronary arteries.** ***Right,*** **radiograph of the heart specimen showing heavy calcific deposits on the aortic valve.**

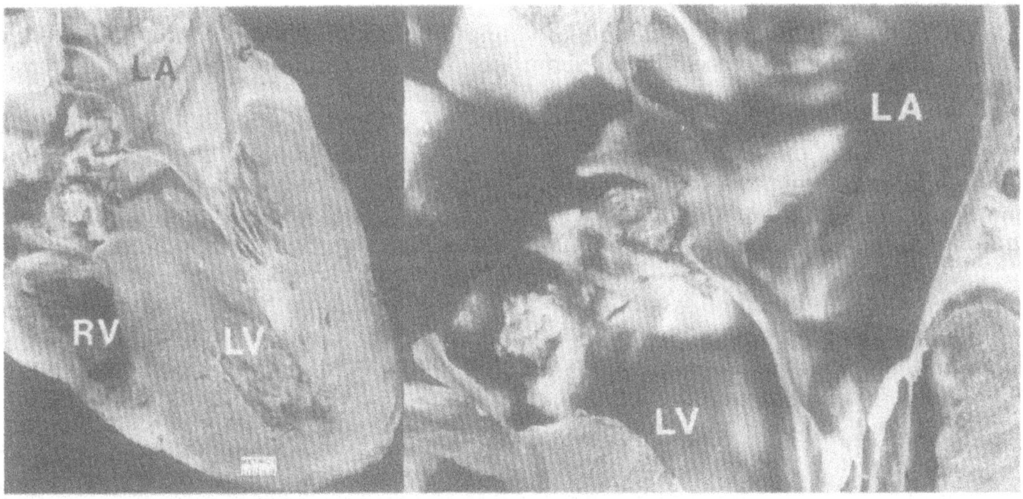

FIGURE 5. Case 15. ***Left,*** **longitudinal view of heart (FSH# A3965) showing active infective endocarditis of the aortic valve.** ***Right,*** **close-up view of the valve which is heavily calcified. Ring abscess is present in the area between aortic wall and wall of left atrium (LA). LV = left ventricle; RV = right ventricle.**

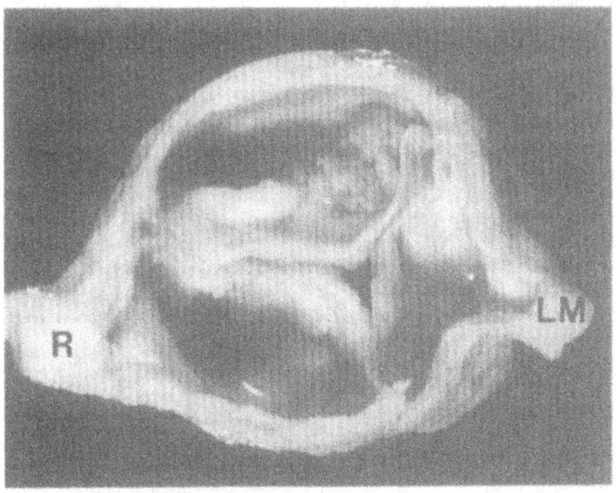

FIGURE 6. Case 20. Aortic valve (SH# A75-27) seen from above showing a small vegetation on the posterior cusp and calcific deposits in all 3 cusps. LM = left main; R = right coronary arteries.

significant aortic regurgitation supported the view of significant preexisting aortic valve stenosis.

Statistical analysis: Data were analyzed using SAS-PC, Stat View 512+, and MRTOD statistical software packages. Categorical comparisons were made with 2-tailed chi-squared analysis or with Fisher's exact test (where appropriate). Numerical comparisons were made using a 2-tailed paired *t* test. Frequency distributions were analyzed using the Stat View software package. Statistical significance was defined as $p < 0.05$.

RESULTS

Pertinent findings in each of the 25 patients with preexisting aortic valve stenosis are presented in Table I, and comparison of the findings in the 25 stenotic cases with those in the 71 nonstenotic cases are summarized in Table II. Some morphologic features of the active IE in the patients with preexisting aortic stenosis are illus-

FIGURE 7. Case 24. *Lower left,* diagram of the aortic and pulmonic valves seen from above *(left)* showing calcific deposits on the ventricular aspects of all 3 aortic valve cusps and the infection in the area between aortic and pulmonic valves causing compression of the wall of the pulmonic trunk. *Right,* longitudinal view (FSH# A4188) showing active infection of the aortic valve with extension of the infection into the most cephalad portion of the ventricular septum (VS) via a perforation of the right coronary cusp. The ring abscess extended also into the wall of the right atrium. LV = left ventricle; PT = pulmonary trunk; RV = right ventricle.

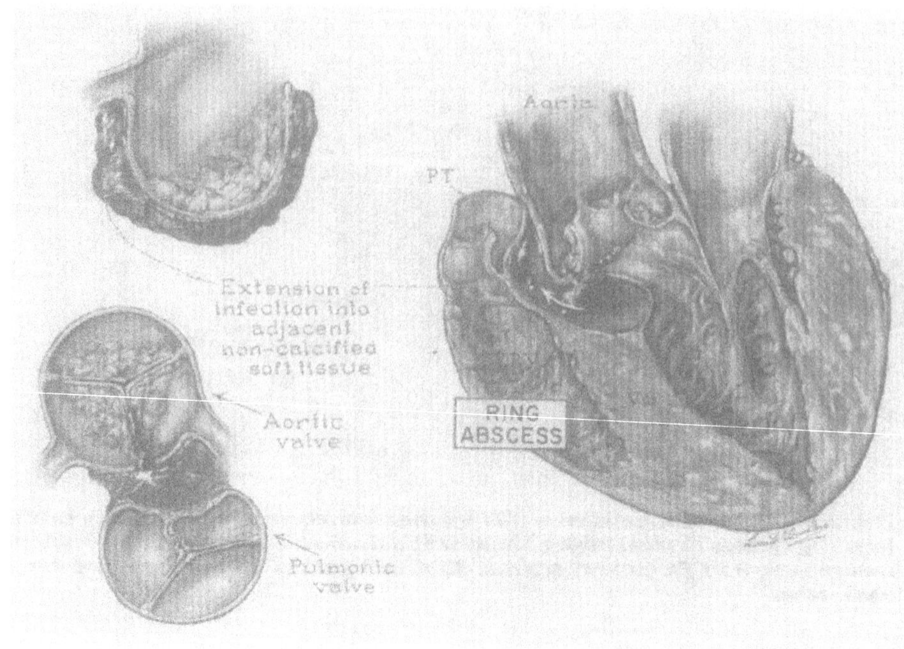

trated in Figures 1 to 7. The patients with stenotic aortic valves compared with those with nonstenotic aortic valves had significantly higher mean ages (61 vs 47 years), a higher percentage >60 years of age (52 vs 24%), a higher percentage of men (92 vs 73%), a higher frequency of an absent or unknown predisposing factor to infection (68 vs 38%), a lower frequency of a precordial murmur of aortic regurgitation (44 vs 79%), a lower percentage with a long duration (>60 days) of infection (4 vs 23%), a larger mean heart weight (594 vs 514 g), a higher percentage with aortic valve calcific deposits (100 vs 24%), and a higher frequency of associated ring abscess (84 vs 52%).

DISCUSSION

The present study indicates that active IE commonly affects previously stenotic aortic valves and that infection on previously stenotic aortic valves, in contrast to that involving previously nonstenotic ones, affects older patients (over 50% >60 years of age), mainly men (>90%), and that ring abscess is a frequent complication (>80%). Despite the presence of a ring abscess, associated aortic regurgitation occurred in less than half the patients with previously stenotic valves, whereas aortic regurgitation occurred in >80% of those with active IE involving a previously nonstenotic aortic valve.

Why is ring abscess significantly more common in patients with active IE superimposed on a previously stenotic valve than on a previously nonstenotic aortic valve? The answer probably is related to the presence of and amount of calcific deposits on the previously stenotic aortic valve. Microorganisms appear to grow poorly in calcific deposits ("rocks"), which were present in all patients with stenotic aortic valves and in <25%, and then of small size, of the patients with nonstenotic aortic valves. Because microorganisms appear to grow poorly in "rocks," the infective process spreads quickly to the adjacent noncalcific soft tissues and extension of the infection outside the aortic valve cusps results in ring abscess.

Because infection superimposed on a calcified aortic valve so often leads to the development of a ring abscess, which then makes valve replacement more difficult and decreases the frequency of a successful outcome, earlier operative intervention may be warranted in these patients compared with patients with active IE on previously nonstenotic aortic valves.

Although other publications have mentioned active IE complicating a previously stenotic aortic valve,[32–36] none have compared either clinical or necropsy findings in patients with previously stenotic to those with previously nonstenotic aortic valves. Indeed, review of 7 books on infective endocarditis disclosed no information on differences observed in patients with active IE superimposed on a previously stenotic valve compared with those on a previously nonstenotic aortic valve.[37–43]

1. Cooper T, Morrow AG, Roberts WC, Herman LG. Postoperative endocarditis due to Candida: clinical observations the experimental production of the lesion. *Surgery* 1961;50:341–346.
2. Andriole VT, Kravetz HM, Roberts WC, Utz JP. Candida endocarditis. Clinical and pathology studies. *Am J Med* 1962;32:251–285.
3. Roberts WC, Rabson AS. Focal glomerular lesions in fungal endocarditis. *Ann Intern Med* 1962;56:610–618.
4. Roberts WC, Braunwald E, Morrow AG. Acute severe mitral regurgitation secondary to ruptured chordae tendineae. Clinical, hemodynamic, and pathologic considerations. *Circulation* 1966;33:58–70.
5. Cohn LH, Roberts WC, Rockoff SD, Morrow AG. Bacterial endocarditis following aortic valve replacement. Clinical and pathologic correlations. *Circulation* 1966;33:209–217.
6. Archard HO, Roberts WC. Bacterial endocarditis after dental procedures in patients with aortic valve prostheses. *J Am Dent Assoc* 1966;72:648–652.
7. Roberts WC, Ewy GA, Glancy DL, Marcus FI. Valvular stenosis produced by active infective endocarditis. *Circulation* 1967;36:449–451.
8. Buchbinder NA, Roberts WC. Active infective endocarditis confined to mural endocardium. A study of six necropsy patients. *Arch Pathol* 1972;45:769–792.
9. Roberts WC, Buchbinder NA. Right-sided valvular infective endocarditis. A clinicopathologic study of twelve necropsy patients. *Am J Med* 1972;53:7–19.
10. Buchbinder NA, Roberts WC. Left-sided valvular active infective endocarditis. A study of forty-five necropsy patients. *Am J Med* 1972;53:20–35.

11. Buchbinder NA, Roberts WC. Alcoholism, an important but unemphasized factor predisposing to infective endocarditis. *Arch Intern Med* 1973;132:689–692.
12. Arnett EN, Roberts WC. Valve ring abscess in active infective endocarditis. Frequency, location, and clues to clinical diagnosis from the study of 95 necropsy patients. *Circulation* 1976;54:140–145.
13. Arnett EA, Roberts WC. Prosthetic valve endocarditis. Clinicopathologic analysis of 22 necropsy patients with comparison of observations in 74 necropsy patients with active infective endocarditis involving natural left-sided cardiac valves. *Am J Cardiol* 1976;38:281–292.
14. Arnett EN, Roberts WC. Active infective endocarditis: a clinicopathology analysis of 137 necropsy patients. *Curr Probl Cardiol* 1976;7:1–76.
15. Arnett EN, Roberts WC. Clinicopathology of prosthetic valve endocarditis. In: Duma RJ, ed. Infections of Prosthetic Heart Valves and Vascular Grafts. Prevention, Diagnosis, and Treatment. Baltimore: University Park Press, 1977:17–41.
16. Arnett EN, Kastl DG, Garvin AJ, Roberts WC. A conversation on prosthetic valve endocarditis. *Am Heart J* 1977;93:510–517.
17. Andy JJ, Shekh MU, Ali N, Barnes BO, Fox LM, Curry CL, Roberts WC. Echocardiographic observations in opiate addicts with active infective endocarditis. Frequency of involvement of the various valves and comparisons of echocardiographic features of right and left-sided cardiac valve endocarditis. *Am J Cardiol* 1977;40:17–23.
18. Roberts WC, Buchbinder NA. Healed left-sided infective endocarditis: a clinicopathologic study of 59 patients. *Am J Cardiol* 1977;40:876–888.
19. Roberts WC. Characteristics and consequences of infective endocarditis (active or healed or both) learned from morphologic studies. In: Rahimtoola SH, ed. Infective Endocarditis. New York: Grune & Stratton, 1978:55–123.
20. Breyer RH, Arnett EN, Spray TL, Roberts WC. Prosthetic valve endocarditis due to *Listeria monocytogenes*. *Am J Clin Pathol* 1978;69:186–187.
21. Ferrans VJ, Boyce SW, Billingham ME, Spray TL, Roberts WC. Infection of glutaraldehyde-preserved porcine valve heterografts. *Am J Cardiol* 1979;43:1123–1136.
22. Billingham ME, Ferrans VJ, Boyce SW, Spray TL, Roberts WC. Bacterial infection in implanted porcine valve heterografts: a histopathologic and ultrastructural study. In: Sebening F, Klovekorn WP, Meisner H, Struck E, eds. Proceedings of the Symposium on Bioprosthetic Cardiac Valves; Munich, April 5–7, 1979. Deutsches Herzzentrum Muncehn, Federal Republic of Germany, 1979:281–294.
23. Davis WA, Isner JM, Bracey AW, Roberts WC, Garagusi VF. Disseminated petriellidium boydiii and pacemaker endocarditis. *Am J Med* 1980;69:929–932.
24. Sheikh MU, Covarrubias EA, Ali N, Lee WR, Sheikh NM, Roberts WC. M-mode echocardiographic observations during and after healing of active bacterial endocarditis limited to the mitral valve. *Am Heart J* 1981;101:37–45.
25. Sheikh MU, Covarrubias EA, Ali N, Sheikh NM, Lee WR, Roberts WC. M-mode echocardiographic observations in active bacterial endocarditis limited to the aortic valve. *Am Heart J* 1981;102:66–75.
26. McManus BM, Katz NM, Blackbourne BD, Gottdiener JS, Wallace RB, Roberts WC. Acquired cor triatriatum (left ventricular false aneurysm): complication of active infective endocarditis of the aortic valve with ring abscess treated by valve replacement. *Am Heart J* 1982;104:312–314.
27. Arnett EN, Roberts WC. Pathology of active infective endocarditis: a necropsy analysis of 192 patients. *Thorac Cardiovasc Surg* 1982;30:327–335.
28. Silver MA, Roberts WC. Active infective endocarditis complicating idiopathic dilated cardiomyopathy. *Am J Cardiol* 1983;52:651–652.
29. Barbour DJ, Roberts WC. Valve excision only versus valve excision plus replacement for active infective endocarditis involving the tricuspid valve. *Am J Cardiol* 1986;57:475–478.
30. Dressler FA, Roberts WC. Infective endocarditis in opiate addicts: Analysis of 80 cases studied at necropsy. *Am J Cardiol* 1989;63:1240–1257.
31. Roberts WC, Kishel JC, McIntosh CL, Cannon RO III, Maron BJ. Severe mitral or aortic valve regurgitation, or both, requiring valve replacement for infective endocarditis complicating hypertrophic cardiomyopathy. *J Am Coll Cardiol* 1992;19:365–371.
32. Bayles TB, Lewis WH Jr. Subacute bacterial endocarditis in older people. *Ann Intern Med* 1940;13:2154–2163.
33. Gouley BA, Sickel E. Aortic regurgitation caused by dilatation of the aortic orifice and associated with a characteristic valvular lesion. *Am Heart J* 1943;26:24–38.
34. Seabury JH. Subacute bacterial endocarditis. Experiences during the past decade. *Arch Intern Med* 1947;79:1–21.
35. Lichtman P, Master AM. The incidence of valvular heart disease in people over fifty and penicillin prophylaxis of bacterial endocarditis. *NY State J Med* 1949;49:1693–1698.
36. Applefeld MM, Hornick RB. Infective endocarditis in patients over age 60. *Am Heart J* 1974;88:90–94.
37. Kerr A Jr. Subacute Bacterial Endocarditis. Springfield, IL: Charles C. Thomas, 1955:343.
38. Kay D, editor. Infective Endocarditis. Baltimore: University Park Press, 1976:272.
39. Kaplan EL, Taranta AV, editors. Infective Endocarditis. An American Heart Association Symposium. Dallas, Texas: The American Heart Association, Inc., 1977:95.
40. Rahimtoola SH, editor. Infective Endocarditis. New York: Grune & Stratton, 1978:386.
41. Freedman LR. Infective Endocarditis and Other Intravascular Infections. New York: Plenum Medical Book Co., 1982:243.
42. Sande MA, Kaye D, Root RK, editors. Endocarditis. New York: Churchill Livingstone, 1984:234.
43. Magilligan DJ Jr, Quinn EL. Endocarditis. Medical and Surgical Management. New York: Marcel Dekker, 1986:269.

ADDENDUM

The manuscript of this article had initially been sent to the *Journal of the American College of Cardiology* (JACC) (their #JAC921143) and it was declined by that journal because ". . . its priority is [was] too low to warrant publication in JACC."

The comments of the 2 JACC reviewers were as follows:

Reviewer #1

"A well conceived and presented paper giving new information regarding infective endocarditis. I have only two suggestions:

1. a reduction in the number of figures (2, 5, 6, 8 and 9) since I believe with the artistic drawings and the remaining specimens [present] the message you wish to transmit is accomplished;

2. with 52% of the non-stenotic valves having ring abscess, this group also warrants careful evaluation and believe paper would be strengthened by some comment about this. Dr. Roberts needs to decide if he is first or last author?"

Reviewer #2

"1. It should be made clear that since the information presented in this paper was derived from a study of necropsy cases, the data cannot necessarily be applied to the treatment of living patients. For example, the authors suggest that those patients with infectious endocarditis and aortic stenosis should be operated earlier because of the propensity of this group to develop ring abscesses. It may be correct, but, on the other hand, it may be that those patients with ring abscesses and aortic stenosis are those who came to autopsy. Unless one knew the denominator, i.e., the entire set of patients with aortic valve disease and infectious endocarditis, one could not justify this conclusion.

2. The observation that older men with large hearts are those with aortic stenosis is in keeping with the well know propensity for this group to have this pathology.

3. The explanation for the formation of ring abscesses in patients with aortic stenosis is extremely speculative and not substantiated by any fact. The suggestion that the micro-organisms do not grow well on 'rocks' and consequently spread out into the peri-aortic tissue is interesting but certainly not substantiated. One could easily speculate in the same way that the hemodynamics of aortic stenosis in some way influence the perivalvular tissue to make it less resistant to infection, but, again, this would be without evidence. The concept of bacteria seeking out a place to grow because one atmosphere is hostile is hard to substantiate.

4. The number of illustrations submitted is excessive. Many of them are redundant and could be eliminated."

Early descriptions of aortic valve stenosis

Steven N. Vaslef, MD, PhD,* and William C. Roberts, MD** *Bethesda, Md.*

Necropsy descriptions. Probably the earliest description of aortic stenosis (AS) was provided by the French physician, Lazare Rivière (1589-1655),[1] in 1663 (Fig. 1). He described a man whom he had seen in 1646 with cardiac palpitations and an irregular heart beat. Recognizing the symptoms of an "occluded artery," Rivière prescribed repeated bleedings and purgings. The patient's condition progressively worsened, breathing became difficult, the peripheral pulse disappeared, and the man died. At necropsy the left ventricle was enlarged, and round masses occluded the mouth of the aorta. Major[2] believed these "caruncle-like" masses described by Rivière to be vegetations of infective endocarditis on the aortic valve. Whatever the cause, the AS produced was possibly the first lesion of the aortic valve described at necropsy.

Theophile Bonet (1620-1689),[3] writing in his *Sepulchretum*, stated that Carolus Rayger (1641-1707) in 1672 had performed a necropsy on a middle-aged cobbler who had died suddenly and found hard, white ossific nodules on the three aortic valve cusps. Giovanni Maria Lancisi (1654-1720),[4] a papal physician noted for his work on aneurysms, wrote: "There are very many instances of the arteries and valves having become converted into a bony matter in those who have laboured under aneurysm of the heart." Giovanni Battista Morgagni (1682-1771)[5] (Fig. 2), who essentially established pathologic anatomy, described in *The Seats and Causes of Diseases* contracted and corregated semilunar valve cusps in a young man who had died suddenly.

Jean Nicolas Corvisart (1755-1821),[6] physician to Napoleon and author of one of the first treatises on cardiac disease, described AS and its consequences as follows: "When the indurated and ossified semi-lunar valves of the aorta stop a portion of this vessel, the obstacle which they form breaks the wave of blood propelled by the heart into the artery; strong and frequent palpitations supervene, because the heart is easily filled, but is difficulty emptied. . . ." In addition, Corvisart described an aortic valve "ossified and united so closely that the end of the little finger could scarcely be introduced. . . ." Joseph Hodgson (1788-1869)[7] reported in 1815: "Such depositions are indeed commonly called ossifications, although the

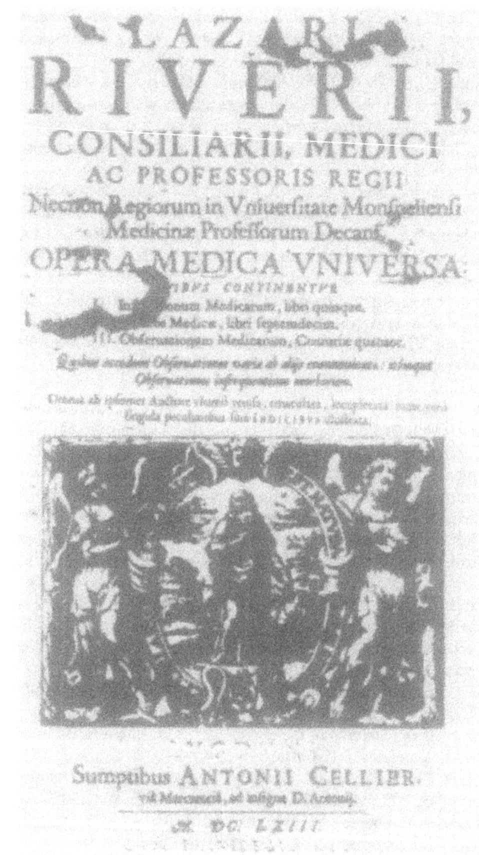

Fig. 1. Title page of Lazare Rivière's *Opera Medica Universa*, in which the first description of AS appeared. (From Rivière L. Opera Medica Universa. Lugduni: Sumptibus Antoni Cellier, 1663.)

From the Pathology Branch, National Heart, Lung, and Blood Institute, National Institutes of Health.

*Present address: Department of Surgery, Evanston Hospital.

**Present address: Baylor Cardiovascular Institute, Baylor University Medical Center.

Received for publication Oct. 12, 1992; accepted Nov. 4, 1992.

AM HEART J 1993;125:1465-1474.

4/1/44918

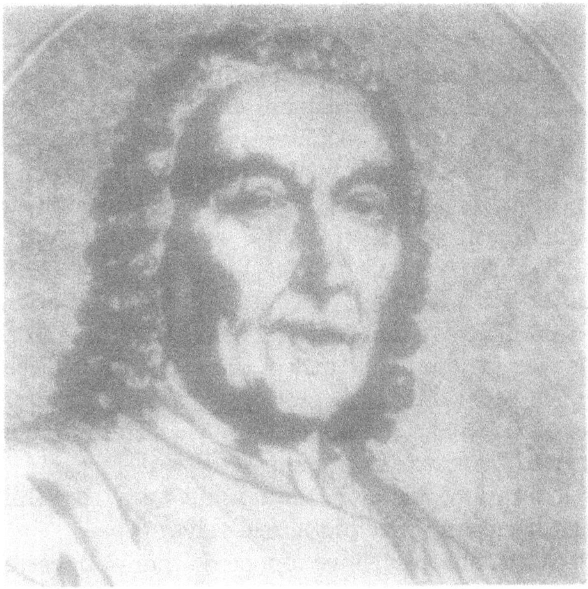

Fig. 2. Giovanni Battista Morgagni (1682-1771), a pathologist who described AS at necropsy. (From Major RH. Classic descriptions of disease. 3rd ed. Springfield, IL: Charles C Thomas, 1945. Reproduced with permission.)

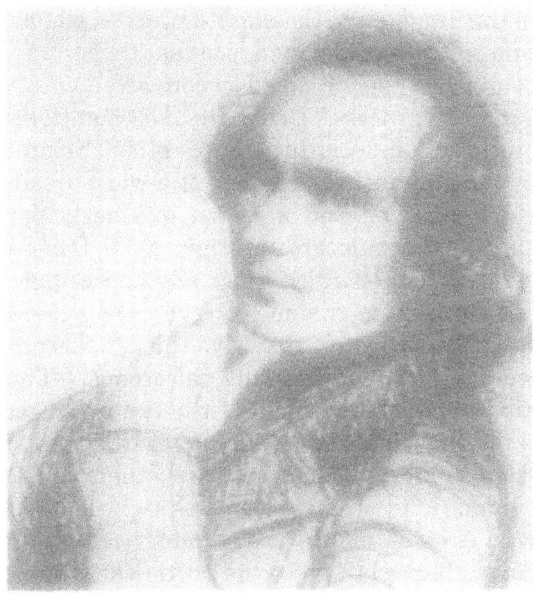

Fig. 4. William Stokes (1804-1878), who described certain diagnostic, prognostic, and etiologic aspects of AS. (From Major RH. Classic descriptions of disease. 3rd ed. Springfield, IL: Charles C Thomas, 1945. Reproduced with permission.)

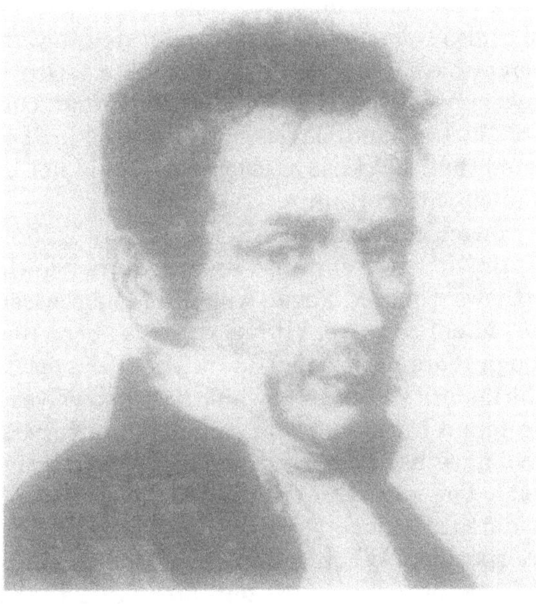

Fig. 3. Rene T. H. Laennec (1781-1826), inventor of the stethoscope. (From Major RH. Classic descriptions of disease. 3rd ed. Springfield, IL: Charles C Thomas, 1945. Reproduced with permission.)

phenomena of their formation bears no resemblance to that of bone." These depositions by chemical analysis consisted of 65% phosphate of lime and 35% "animal matter," mainly albumin.

Rene T. H. Laennec (1781-1826)[8] (Fig. 3), who invented the stethoscope, summed up in 1819 the postmortem manifestations of AS based on his observations and those of others: "The mitral and sigmoid valves of the aorta are subject to become the site of cartilaginous or bony productions, which increase their thickness, alter their shape, and obstruct, sometimes almost totally, the orifices in which they are placed. . . . These ossifications are never perfect bone; they are whiter and more opaque, more fragile, and evidently contain a greater proportion of phosphate of lime. . . ."

Etiology. One of the first persons to discuss the cause of AS was Jean Baptiste Bouillaud (1796-1881),[9] a clinical professor at the University of Paris, who described in 1835 a 37-year-old man who had fever, acute arthritis, endocarditis and died. At necropsy AS was found. Bouillaud believed AS to be caused by "endocarditis," which he defined merely as inflammation of the internal membrane of the heart and valves. Endocarditis coincident with acute articular rheumatism was considered the most important cause. Hasse[10] in 1846 challenged Bouillaud's theory by stating that, "ossification cannot invariably be ascribed to endocarditis." He described degenerative ossification.

In 1854 Stokes[11] (Fig. 4) observed: "We may divide cases of valvular disease into two classes, in one of which there is reason to believe that a carditis has been the first step in the morbid process, while in the second we are without evidence that the alteration of the valve has been in any way connected with an inflammatory process." Osler[12] in 1908 mentioned the sclerotic and endocarditic causes of AS. Sclerotic lesions, he maintained, are part of a widespread arterial degeneration and are seen in elderly persons. Regarding the endocarditic origin of AS, Osler wrote: "Following endocarditis from any cause, but more particularly from rheumatic fever, the vegetations organize, the edges of the valve thicken, become adherent, sclerotic, and finally calcareous." Thus investigators in the first half of the twentieth century debated the causes of AS. Some regarded AS as primarily degenerative in origin, and others considered it rheumatic in origin. Moenckeburg[13] claimed that calcific AS was due to the secondary deposition of calcium after sclerosis of the aortic valve cusps. He described two types of sclerosis, "ascending" and "descending": the former was characterized by changes that took place initially in the layers of the cusps facing the sinuses of Valsalva, and the degenerative process extended upward to the free margins of the cusps; the "descending" type was characterized by sclerotic changes that started in the aorta and descended to the valvular cusps and commissures. In contrast to Moenckeburg's views, the concept that calcific AS was associated primarily with a rheumatic cause was supported by many investigators, including Cabot,[14] Christian,[15] Dry and Willius,[16] and Karsner and Koletsky.[17]

A major study championing the rheumatic cause of AS was that by Karsner and Koletsky,[17] published in 1947. From a study of 200 necropsy patients, the investigators concluded, "... that calcific disease of the aortic valve is the result of previous inflammation, an inflammation of such character as to identify it as rheumatic." An analysis of their study today, however, led one of us (W. C. R.) to other conclusions. Compared with patients now considered to have rheumatic heart disease, the 200 patients studied by Karsner and Koletsky were generally older (mean age 61 years with 92% aged 40 years or more), mainly (72%) men with an infrequent (18%) history of acute rheumatic fever or chorea, a fairly frequent (32%) history of systemic hypertension (blood pressure > 160/95 mm Hg), and a fairly high (12%) occurrence of bicuspid aortic valves. Of the 200 patients, only 138 (69%) were considered by anatomic examination to have AS; three others had pure aortic regurgitation, and 59 patients (29%) had no anatomic evidence of either AS or aortic regurgitation. Of the 200 patients, 119 had anatomic disease limited to the aortic valve: three of them had a history of acute rheumatic fever, 16 had bicuspid aortic valves, and three had Aschoff nodules (criteria for diagnoses imprecise). The other 91 patients had gross anatomic disease of the mitral valve in addition to calcific deposits in the aortic valve cusps. Of the 91 patients with multivalve disease, 32 (35%) had a history of acute rheumatic fever or chorea, 48 (45%) had mitral stenosis (clearly a rheumatic lesion in > 99% of patients), and 17 (19%) had Aschoff bodies. Thus the cause of the valve disease in a high percentage of these 91 patients with multivalve involvement was rheumatic, but the case for a rheumatic cause of the aortic valve disease in the other 119 with grossly isolated aortic valve disease is weak. The majority in the latter group appear to belong to the "wear-and-tear" of aging (or degeneration) category and some to a congenital malformation (bicuspid aortic valve) type.

Others, however, have reported other or uncertain causes of AS. Sparks and Evans[18] indicated that in atherosclerosis the attached part of the valve was most likely to become calcified, whereas in rheumatic valvulitis the free edge was more likely to be site of calcific deposits. Sohval and Gross[19] provided histologic evidence of both degenerative and rheumatic causes. Clawson et al.,[20] Margolis et al.,[21] and Cohen et al.[22] also were among those who stated that the lesion may have a rheumatic basis in some patients and a degenerative basis in others. Berk and Dinnerstein[23] in 1938 and Davies and Steiner[24] in 1949 indicated that the cause of calcific AS could not be determined with certainty.

A congenital cause of AS was largely ignored by most previously mentioned investigators. Smith and Matthews[25] quoted Paget, who in 1844 discussed the bicuspid aortic valve: "It has never ... been noticed (though there need be no doubt about the fact) that in the majority of cases in which only two valves have been found in the aorta or pulmonary artery, these valves have been diseased and often extremely diseased." The nature of the disease, however, was not elucidated. Peacock (1886), who also was cited, was more specific: "When the whole of the segments are fused together or when two only are united, the valves not infrequently become the seat of chronic inflammation, by which they are rendered thick and unyielding and often become extremely ossified, thus inducing, first obstruction to the flow of blood from the ventricle into the aorta, and then incompetency."

Also in 1886 Osler[26] stated that the bicuspid condition may be the result of fetal endocarditis or a primary failure in development. He maintained that "the condition ... plays an important part in the history of aortic valve disease". Osler, however, did not mention the possibility that a congenitally bi-

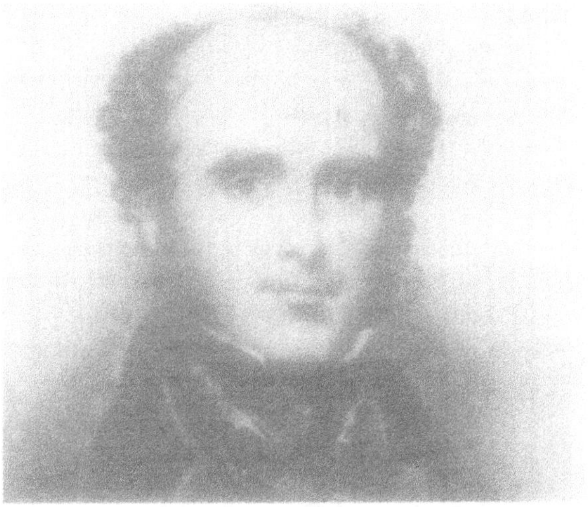

Fig. 5. James Hope (1801-1841), who provided detailed description of murmur produced by AS. (From Major RH. Classic descriptions of disease, 3rd ed. Springfield, IL: Charles C Thomas, 1945. Reproduced with permission.)

cuspid aortic valve could be the site of stenosis in addition to its being the site of infective endocarditis.

Abbott,[27] Koletsky,[28] Kiloh,[29] Campbell and Kauntze,[30] and Edwards[31] all recognized the tendency of the congenitally bicuspid aortic valve to become stenotic. Edwards proposed that the bicuspid valve was rarely stenotic at the time of birth but became stenotic as it became thickened by fibrous tissue and calcific deposits. A few years earlier[32] he had identified the congenitally unicommissural (one lateral attachment) aortic valve as a cause of AS and, in contrast to the bicuspid condition, he considered this type valve to be stenotic from the time of birth. Actually Chevers[33] in 1842 had described an aortic valve that appeared as a "mere funnel-shaped tube, with a slit at the apex through which the blood passes with difficulty." Perhaps this was an early description of a unicuspid aortic valve.

Although the debate on cause continued, it was generally agreed that calcific AS was more frequent in males than females. Cabot,[14] Christian,[15] Margolis et al.,[21] and McGinn and White[34] observed this trend, the latter investigators adding, however, that the incidence of noncalcareous AS was about equal in males and females.

Diagnosis. An early account of auscultation in a patient with AS was given in 1824 by René J. H. Bertin (1757-1828),[35] who perceived a murmur coincident with ventricular systole. James Hope (1801-1841)[36] (Fig. 5) provided a more detailed description in 1832: "One [murmur] is heard during the ventricular contraction (i.e., with the first sound) on the sternum, opposite to the lower margin of the third rib, and thence for about two inches or more upwards, along the course of the ascending aorta towards the right; and it is louder in these situations than below the level of the valves. Its pitch or key is usually that of a whispered r. . . ." Hope[36] went on to state the difficulty encountered in ascertaining whether or not the observed sounds were due to a diseased aorta, a diseased aortic valve, or a combination of the two. Moreover, discriminatory auscultation, Hope argued, could indicate the presence of aortic valve disease or mitral valve disease: "That a murmur is seated in the aorta or its valves, and not in the auricular valves, may be known by its sounding loud and near above the aortic valves, where an auricular murmur, if audible at all, sounds feeble, remote, and on low key like a whispered who."

William Stokes (1804-1878)[11] (Fig. 4), of Cheynes-Stokes respiration fame, in "two or three cases" observed: "Strong action of the left ventricle; extremely loud and musical murmur at the extent of the arterial tree. . . . The phenomena arise from extensive ossific disease of the aortic opening, which is rendered not only rigid, but singularly irregular, from the deposit of great quantities of earthy matter. . . . Under such circumstances we may safely make the diagnosis of extensive and irregular ossification of the aortic orifice, with contraction if the pulse be small and hard and without contraction if its ordinary volume be preserved." Stokes[11] described a man who dropped dead from extreme AS without showing any previous symptoms of heart disease. "It is generally believed that, organic disease being once established . . . is progressive . . . must end in death, either by rupture of the valves, organic disease of the remaining portion of the heart, or obstruction to the current of blood . . . but . . . this disorganizing process may be occasionally of singular slowness, so that the patient may live for many years in the enjoyment of good, or at least tolerable health, or that the diseased action is really arrested and the lesion becomes stationary." The prognosis then, according to Stokes, was variable and depended on (1) the severity of the obstruction, (2) the degree of cardiomegaly, (3) the regularity and intensity of the heartbeat, and (4) the duration of symptoms.

Others who discussed prognosis included Craigie,[37] who believed that AS constitutes "a reasonable proportion of the mortality of the adults of the human race," and Osler,[12] who believed the prognosis to be worse in younger persons because of associated complications of rheumatic fever rather than changes arising from sclerotic slow degeneration of the valvular cusps. Other investigators mentioned the occur-

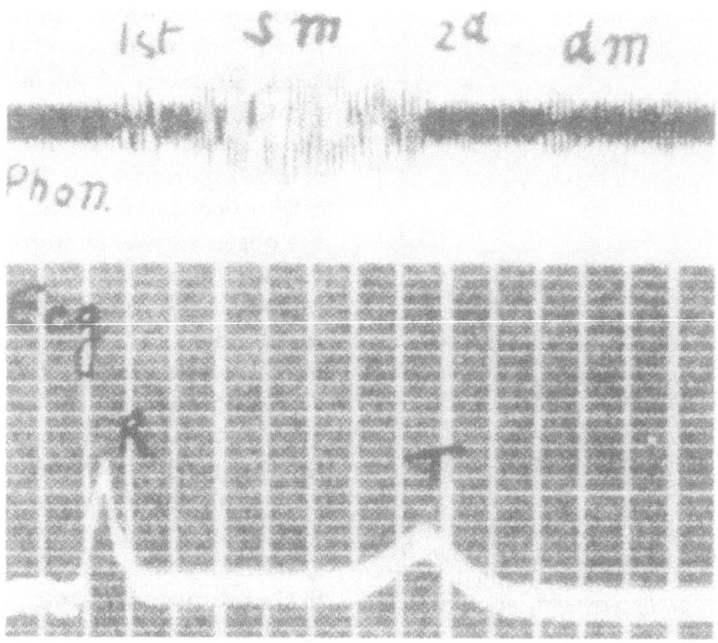

Fig. 6. Early phonocardiographic recording of diamond-shaped murmur of AS. (From Luisada AA. Clinical applications of phonocardiography. Arch Pediatr 1943;60:498-510. Reproduced with permission.)

rence of sudden death in association with the disease.[38-46]

Phonocardiography. Luisada[47] in 1943 stated that a typical phonocardiogram in AS demonstrated a maximum amplitude in midsystole and a progressively decreasing amplitude toward the end of systole (Fig. 6). Reinhold et al.[48] in 1955 described and recorded a loud early aortic systolic ejection sound at the apex in patients with congenital AS. Hancock,[49] in a 1966 study of 118 patients, reported that the ejection sound in AS was present uniformly in patients with noncalcific AS but in only about half of those with calcific AS and was uniformly absent in patients with subvalvular and supravalvular AS. McKusick[50] in 1958 observed the characteristic diamond-shaped contour of the oscillogram in AS at the cardiac base and often at the apex; he cautioned that the murmur of AS at the apex may be confused with that of mitral regurgitation.

Radiography. A new era in the diagnosis of AS was heralded by Roentgen's discovery of x-rays in 1895. Simmonds[51] in 1908 and Cutler and Sosman[52] in 1924 utilized x-rays to demonstrate valvular calcific deposits after death. Christian[53] in 1931 reported that the diagnosis of AS was made after Sosman first observed calcific deposits in the aortic valve in a living patient. In 1933 Sosman and Wosika[54] documented more cases of calcified aortic valves determined in vivo by x-rays.

Other investigators described cardiac dimensions in AS based on radiographic studies. Vaquez and Bordet[55] in 1913 observed that the left ventricular "hypertrophy" was greater in AS than in aortic regurgitation. Steel[56] in 1930 noted that in AS the radiographs demonstrated primarily left ventricular hypertrophy (change in shape), whereas in aortic regurgitation they demonstrated primarily left ventricular dilatation (change in size). Levene and Reid[57] in 1932 emphasized the utility of the x-ray in the differential diagnosis of heart disease.

Electrocardiography. ECG recordings were made in patients with AS as early as 1920 when Willius[58] observed negative T waves in leads I, II, or III in two patients. In 1927 he[59] reported atrial fibrillation, bundle branch block (both complete and incomplete), negative T waves, and conduction delays in patients with AS. Barnes and Whitten[60] at autopsy observed left ventricular hypertrophy and AS in a patient whose ECG showed negative T waves. Other investigators[21, 34] indicated the relatively uncommon occurrence of significant ECG abnormalities in AS. Boas[61] in 1935 observed left-axis deviation and transient bundle branch block in one patient and complete heart block with ventricular premature complexes in another patient with AS. Berk and Dinnerstein[23] demonstrated T wave negativity, left-axis deviation, left bundle branch block, and a prolonged QT interval in several patients with AS. In 1939 Dry and Willius[62] predicted and demonstrated that in left ventricular preponderance, as occurs in AS, the ECG will reflect left-axis deviation, and T wave negativity in lead I or in leads I and II. Other early studies of AS incorporating ECG findings include those by Schlomka and Dietz,[63] Friedberg and Sohval,[44] and Horan and Barnes.[45]

Catheterization and angiocardiography. Cardiac catheterization was first performed in 1929 by Forssmann,[64] who directed a catheter from an arm vein into the right side of the heart. Cournand and Ranges[65] in 1941 made pressure measurements in the right atrium after venous catheterization. Early accounts of left-sided cardiac catheterization[67, 68] were in patients with congenital abnormalities such as atrial septal defect or patent ductus arteriosus, which permitted passage of a catheter from the right to the left side of the heart or aorta. In 1953 Venner and Holling[68] measured left atrial and left ventricular pressures at operation by needle puncture. Gordon et al.[69] and Braunwald et al.[70] used this method to simultaneously measure left-sided cardiac pressures including the aortic pressure but not in patients with AS. Gorlin et al.[71] in 1955 estimated the aortic valve orifice area and the systolic pressure gradient across a stenotic valve based on postmortem perfusion studies. They also used venous catheterization to obtain hemodynamic data from patients with AS. They found "dynamically significant" AS when the orifice area was reduced to 0.5 cm^2 or less (normal = approximately 3 cm^2).

The procedure of Björk et al.[72] for measuring left atrial pressure by transthoracic left atrial needle puncture was expanded on[73] to include measurements of left ventricular and aortic pressures. This technique involved successively passing a catheter, introduced from the right paravertebral aspect area via a needle, from the left atrium to the left ventricle to the aorta. Fisher[74] in 1955 first used this method to measure a systolic gradient between the left ventricle and aorta. Schnabel et al.[75] also in 1955 simultaneously recorded pressures in both the left ventricle and aorta by means of different catheters to diagnose AS. One catheter was placed in the left ventricle after a transthoracic left atrial puncture, and a second catheter was introduced into the aorta via the femoral artery. Dexter et al.[76] correlated hemodynamic findings with the clinical manifestations of AS. Simultaneous pressure measurements were made in the left ventricle and brachial artery by means of a catheter and an indwelling needle, respectively. The catheter was inserted by the method of transthoracic left atrial puncture.

Arterial retrograde catheterization to determine left-sided cardiac pressures gained widespread use in the 1950s. Limón Lason et al.[77] reported in 1950 that they had measured left ventricular and aortic pressures in 17 patients by a catheter introduced via the radial artery. Salans et al.[78] measured aortic pressure in 1951 by a catheter inserted via the brachial artery. Porstmann et al.[79] guided a catheter into the left side of the heart from the common carotid artery and diagnosed AS. Hanson et al.[80] successfully performed retrograde catheterization via the radial artery to diagnose AS, whereas other retrograde attempts[81] failed to penetrate stenotic aortic valves. Lambert and Vlad[82] reported successful retrograde catheterization in 6 of 11 patients with AS. Honick et al.,[83] who developed an S-shaped catheter tip, were successful in 19 (79%) of 24 patients with AS.

Some investigators sought other ways to measure left-sided cardiac pressures. Morrow et al.[84] modified the transbronchial approach of Facquet et al.[85] and that of Allison and Linden[86, 87] to measure left ventricular pressures in patients including one with AS. Buchbinder and Katz[88] used an anterior thoracic approach to measure right and left ventricular pressures directly. Brock et al.[89] used this method to obtain left ventricular pressure to assess the severity of AS. Ross et al.[90, 91] devised a technique in which a transseptal left atrial puncture was performed. Radner[92, 93] used a suprasternal approach to reach the left atrium and aorta by needle puncture.

Although more useful in patients with AR, angiography was another method used to evaluate patients with AS. Grishman et al.[94] in 1947 used venous angiocardiography to see the dilated and/or hypertrophied left ventricle and thoracic aorta in patients with AS. Jönsson et al.[95] in 1949 injected contrast medium into the pulmonary artery by means of a catheter to observe the left atrium and left ventricle in AS. Kjellberg et al.[96] in 1955 observed during ventricular systole a dome-shaped stenotic aortic valve. Lehman et al.[97] injected contrast medium by transthoracic left ventricular needle puncture to view thickened aortic valve cusps. Ödman and Philipson[98] and Porstmann et al.[79] in 1958 used an arterial retrograde approach to inject contrast medium and visualize a stenotic aortic valve.

Echocardiography. Echocardiography has aided considerably in the diagnosis of many forms of cardiac disease. In 1970 Gramiak and Shah[99] observed that in calcific AS the cuspal echo intensity was greater than the wall intensity because of the presence of calcium. Yeh et al.[100] in 1973 used echocardiography to estimate aortic valve orifice dimensions in AS. Feizi et al.[101] in 1974 described impaired cuspal movement and dense echoes originating from calcific

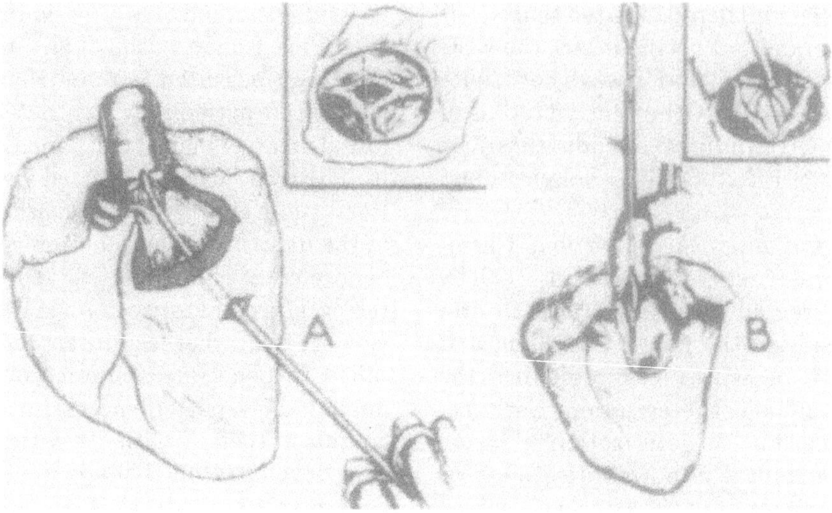

Fig. 7. Diagram showing left ventricular and aortic surgical approaches to AS. (From Glover RP, Bailey CP, O'Neill TTE. Surgery of stenotic valvular disease of the heart. JAMA 1950;144:1049. Reproduced with permission.)

deposits on the stenotic aortic valve. Bennett et al.[102] in 1975 estimated the systolic pressure gradient in AS by use of echocardiographic measurements. McDonald[103] in 1976 made echocardiographic measurements to study left ventricular size and contraction in AS and noted that increased wall thickness was related to the severity of the AS.

Surgical developments. The early part of the twentieth century witnessed initial attempts to surgically correct AS. In 1902 Brunton[104] proposed surgical intervention in patients with valvular stenosis. Seeing a man crippled by mitral stenosis he wrote: "It occurred to me that it was worth while for such a patient to run a risk, and even a very grave risk, in order to obtain such improvement or might enable him at least to stay at home." The idea was considered radical at the time, and 11 years passed before the first attempt to correct a stenotic valve was made by Doyen.[105]

In 1913 Tuffier[106] performed the first operation for AS. He intended to incise the stenosed valve but changed his mind and performed a digital dilation. The operation was a success and the patient, a young man, was reported to be doing well years later.

Surgical efforts in the 1920s to treat valvular stenosis were directed toward the mitral valve because of the common occurrence of mitral stenosis and because of the realatively easy accessibility of this valve. Cutler and Levine[107] and Cutler et al.[108, 109] were largely unsuccessful in treating mitral stenosis by valvulotomy or partial valvulectomy. Their work, however, prompted Powers[110] to suggest in 1932 that use of such procedures to treat mitral stenosis was dangerous because the regurgitation induced resulted in congestive heart failure and ultimately death. Only 2 of the 12 patients operated on from 1913 to 1928 to relieve valvular stenosis were alive in 1929. In 1948 Bailey[111] in Philadelphia, Harken et al.[112] in Boston, and Baker et al.[113] in London successfully performed commissurotomy for mitral stenosis.

Horace Smithy, a surgeon from Charleston, South Carolina, who himself had AS, began working in the late 1940s on a method of surgical repair. Smithy's death in 1948 encouraged Bailey to concentrate his efforts on devising an operation for AS. In 1950 an aortic valve commissurotomy was performed and described by Glover et al.[114] Their method differed from that of Tuffier[106] in that a dilating instrument not a finger was used, and the aortic valve was approached from the left ventricle in some patients, as well as from the aorta, as Tuffier had done 38 years earlier (Fig. 7).

The next important development in the surgical management of aortic valve disease was the successful implantation of a prosthesis by Hufnagel et al.[115, 116] in 1952. The operation, performed on a woman with aortic regurgitation, involved implanting a ball-type prosthesis into the descending thoracic aorta.

Swan and Kortz[117] in 1955 first performed a direct-vision operation on the aortic valve; an ice bath was used to induce hypothermia in a man whose stenotic aortic valve was widened by commissurotomy. Lewis et al.,[118] 1 month later, performed a similar direct-vision operation during hypothermia.

The development of the heart-lung machine[119-121] made it possible for Harken et al.[122] in 1960 to implant a prosthetic aortic valve in the anatomic position in a patient with aortic regurgitation. In 1961 Harken et al.[123] replaced a stenosed aortic valve with a caged-ball prosthesis, and since then more than 750,000 operations have been performed to replace defective cardiac valves.

REFERENCES

1. Rivière L. Opera Medica Universa. Observationum medicarum, centuria IV, observatio XXI, Cordis palpitatio pulsus inaequalitas. Lugduni: Sumptibus Antoni, Cellier, 1663:83.
2. Major RH. Notes on the history of endocarditis. Bull Hist Med 1945;17:351-9.
3. Bonet T. Sepulchretum; sive, anatomia practica, ex cadaveribos morbo denatis, proponens historias et observationes omnium humani corporis affectuum. Genevae: Sumptibus Leonardi Chouet, 1679:702.
4. Lancisi GM. De motu cordis et aneurysmatibus opus posthumun, in duas partes divisum. Romae: Apud Joannem Mariam Salvioni, 1728. In: Erichsen JE. Observations on aneurism. London: New Syndenham Society, 1844:63,65.
5. Morgagni JB. The seats and causes of diseases investigated by anatomy; in five books, containing a great variety of dissections, with remark. To which are added very accurate and copious indexes of the principal things and names therein contained. Translated from Latin by B. Alexander in 3 vols. "Facsimile of the London, 1769 edition." Vol. 1, Book II, Letter XXVII. New York: Hafner Publishing Co., 1960:840.
6. Corvisart JN. Essai sur les maladies et les lésions organiques du coeur. Paris, 1806. Translated by J. Gates, 1812. In: Willius FA, Keys TE. Cardiac classics. St. Louis: CV Mosby, 1941:285.
7. Hodgson J. A treatise on the diseases of arteries and views, containing the pathology and treatment of aneurisms and wounded arteries. London: J. Moyes, 1815:22.
8. Laennec RTH. A treatise on the disease of the chest. Paris, 1819. Translated by John Forbes, 1821. Published under auspices of the New York Academy of Medicine. New York: Hafner Publishing Co., 1962:236-8.
9. Bouillaud J. Traité clinique des maladies du coeur. vol. 2. Paris: Chez JB Baillière, 1835; 2nd ed., 1841:1,29-32.
10. Hasse CE. The diseases of the organs of circulation and respiration. London: C and J Adlard for the Syndenham Society, 1846:131.
11. Stokes W. The diseases of the heart and aorta. Extreme ossific disease of the aortic orifice. Dublin: Hodges and Smith, 1854:139-58.
12. Osler W. Modern medicine, its theory and practice. In 7 vols. vol. IV. Diseases of the Circulatory System—diseases of the blood—diseases of the spleen, thymus, and lymph glands. Philadelphia: Lea & Febiger, 1908:227-8.
13. Moenckeberg JG. Der normale histologische Bau und die Sklerose der Aortenklappen. Arch F Pathol Anat 1904;176:472-514.
14. Cabot RC: Facts on the heart. Philadelphia: WB Saunders. 1926:221.
15. Christian HA. Aortic stenosis with calcification of the cusps. JAMA 1931;97:158-61.
16. Dry TJ, Willius FA. Calcareous disease of the aortic valve. AM HEART J 1939;17:138-57.
17. Karsner HT, Koletsky S. Calcific disease of the aortic valve. Philadelphia: JB Lippincott: 1947.
18. Sparks JV, Evans C. Radiography of calcification in cardiac valves during life. Br J Radiol 1934;7:463-6.
19. Sohval AR, Gross L. Calcific sclerosis of the aortic valve (Mönckeberg type). Arch Pathol 1936;22:477-94.
20. Clawson BJ, Bell ET, Hartzell TB. Valvular diseases of the heart with special reference to the pathogenesis of old valvular defects. Am J Pathol 1926;2:193-234.
21. Margolis HM, Ziellessen FO, Barnes AR. Calcareous aortic valvular disease. AM HEART J 1931;6:349-74.
22. Cohen L, Gray I, Nash PI, Fink H. Calcareous aortic stenosis. Report of nine cases with autopsy findings. Ann Intern Med 1940;13:2091-2103.
23. Berk LH, Dinnerstein M. Calcific aortic stenosis. A clinical and electrocardiographic study. Arch Intern Med 1938; 61:781-97.
24. Davies CE, Steiner RE. Calcified aortic valve clinical and radiological features. Br Heart J 1949;11:126-39.
25. Smith DE, Matthews MB. Aortic valvular stenosis with coarctation of the aorta with special reference to the development of aortic stenosis upon congenital bicuspid valves. Br Heart J 1955;17:198-206.
26. Osler W. The bicuspid condition of the aortic valves. Trans Assoc Am Physicians 1886;1:185-92.
27. Abbott ME. On the relative incidence and clinical significance of a congenitally bicuspid aortic valve. Vol I. In: Libman Anniversary volumes, 3 vols. New York: The International Press, 1932:1-38.
28. Koletsky S. Congenital bicuspid aortic valves. Arch Intern Med 1941;67:129-76.
29. Kiloh GA. Pure aortic stenosis. Br Heart J 1950;12:33-44.
30. Campbell M, Kauntze R. Congenital aortic valvular stenosis. Br Heart J 1953;15:179-94.
31. Edwards JE. The congenital bicuspid aortic valve [editorial]. Circulation 1961;23:485-8.
32. Edwards JE. Pathologic aspects of cardiac valvular insufficiencies. Arch Surg 1958;77:634-49.
33. Chevers N. Observations on the diseases of the orifice and valves of the aorta. Guy's Hosp Rep 1842;7:387-452.
34. McGinn S, White PD. Clinical observations on aortic stenosis. Am J Med Sci 1934;188:1-15.
35. Bertin RJ. Treatise on the diseases of the heart and great vessels. Paris 1824. Translated by CW Chauncy. Philadelphia: Carey, Lea and Blanchard, 1833:224-5.
36. Hope J. A treatise on the diseases of the heart and great vessels, comprising a new view of the physiology of the heart's action. According to which the physical signs are explained. London: William Kidd, 1832:307-85.
37. Craigie D. Observations and cases illustrating the nature of false consecutive aneurysm of the heart. Edinburgh Med Surg J 1843;59:356-99.
38. Lloyd E. Aortic valvular disease. Trans Pathol Soc Lond 1846-8;1:67.
39. Wilks S, Moxon W. Lectures on pathological anatomy. 2nd ed. London: J & A Churchill, 1875:135.
40. Lutembacher R: La mort subite chez les cardiaques. Presse Méd 1921;29:203-4.
41. Marvin HM, Sullivan AG. Clinical observations upon syncope and sudden death in relation to aortic stenosis. AM HEART J 1935;10:705-35.
42. Contratto AW, Levine SA. Aortic stenosis with special reference to angina pectoris and syncope. Ann Intern Med 1937;10:1636-53.
43. DeVeer JA. Sudden death in aortic stenosis. Explanation on a mechanical basis. AM HEART J 1938;15:243-6.
44. Friedberg CK, Sohval AR. Nonrheumatic calcific aortic stenosis. AM HEART J 1939;17:452-69.
45. Horan MJ, Barnes AR. Calcareous aortic stenosis and coronary artery disease. Am J Med Sci 1948;215:451-5.
46. Bergeron J, Abelmann WH, Vazquez-Milan H, Ellis LB. Aortic stenosis—clinical manifestations and course of the disease. Arch Intern Med 1954;94:911-24.
47. Luisada AA. Clinical applications of phonocardiography. Arch Pediatr 1943;60:498-510.
48. Reinhold J, Rudhe U, Bonham-Carter RE. The heart sounds and the arterial pulse in congenital aortic stenosis. Br Heart J 1955;17:327-36.

49. Hancock EW. The ejection sound in aortic stenosis. Am J Med 1966;40:569-77.
50. McKusick VA. Cardiovascular sound in health and disease. Baltimore: Williams & Wilkins, 1958:261-9.
51. Simmonds M. Ueber den Nachweis von verkalkungen am Herzen durch das Roentgenverfahren. Fortsch Geb Roentgenstr 1908;12:371-3.
52. Cutler EC, Sosman MC. Calcification in the heart and pericardium. Am J Roentgenol Radium Ther 1924;12:312-20.
53. Christian HA. Aortic stenosis with calcification. Int Clin 1931;3:51-4.
54. Sosman MC, Wosika PH. Calcification in aortic and mitral valves with a report of twenty-three cases demonstrated in vivo by the roentgen ray. Am J Roentgenol Radium Ther 1933;30:328-48.
55. Vaquez H, Bordet E. Le coeur et l'aorte; etudes de radiologie clinique. Paris: JB Baillière, 1913:110-13.
56. Steel D. Roentgenological and pathological findings in some of the valvular lesions. Am J Roentgenol Radium Ther 1930;23:384-9.
57. Levene G, Reid WD. The differential diagnosis of organic heart disease by the roentgen ray. Am J Roentgenol Radium Ther 1932;28:466-80.
58. Willius FA. Observations on negativity of the final ventricular T wave of the electrocardiogram. Am J Med Sci 1920; 160:844-65.
59. Willius FA. A clinical study of aortic stenosis. Proc Staff Meet Mayo Clin 1927;2:123-4.
60. Barnes AR, Whitten MB. Study of T-wave negativity in predominant ventricular strain. AM HEART J 1929;5:14-67.
61. Boas EP. Angina pectoris and heart block, as symptoms of calcareous aortic stenosis. Am J Med Sci 1935;190:376-83.
62. Dry TJ, Willius FA. Interpretation of the electrocardiographic findings in calcareous stenosis of the aortic valve. Ann Intern Med 1939;13:143-50.
63. Schlomka G, Dietz EL. Beiträge zur klinischen Elektrokardiographie. III. Untersuchungen Über das Verhalten des Typs der Herzstromkurve bei Kranken mit Herzklappenfehlern. Z Klin Med 1936;129:572-84.
64. Forssmann W. Die Sondierung des rechten Herzens. Klin Wochenschr 1929;8:2085-7.
65. Cournand A, Ranges HA. Catheterization of the right auricle in man. Proc Soc Exp Biol Med 1941;46:462-6.
66. Cournand A, Motley HL, Himmelstein A, Dresdale D, Baldwin J. Recording of blood pressure from the left auricle and the pulmonary veins in human subjects with interauricular septal defect. Am J Physiol 1947;150:267-71.
67. Limón Lason R, Bouchard F, Rubio Alvarez V, Cahen P, Novelo S. El cateterismo intracardiaco. III. Persistencia del conducto arterioso con hallazgos clinicos atipicos. Presentacion de 8 casos, 5 de los cuales tenian cianosis. Pruebas de la existencia de "shunt" invertido y cruzado. Arch Inst Cardiol México 1950;20:147-81.
68. Venner A, Holling HE. Comparison of operation and clinical findings in mitral stenosis and incompetence. Br Heart J 1953;15:205-13.
69. Gordon AJ, Braunwald E, Ravitch MM. Simultaneous pressure pulses in the human left atrium, ventricle and aorta. Preliminary communication. Circ Res 1954;2:432-3.
70. Braunwald E, Moscovitz HL, Amram SS, Lasser RP, Sapin SO, Himmelstein A, Ravitch MM, Gordon AJ. The hemodynamics of the left side of the heart as studied by simultaneous left atrial, left ventricular, and aortic pressures; particular reference to mitral stenosis. Circulation 1955;12:69-81.
71. Gorlin R, McMillan IKR, Medd WE, Matthews MB, Daley R. Dynamics of the circulation in aortic valvular disease. Am J Med 1955;18:855-70.
72. Björk VO, Malmstrom G, Uggla LG. Left auricular pressure measurements in man. Ann Surg 1953;138:718-25.
73. Bjork VO. Direct pressure measurement in the left atrium and left ventricle and the aorta. Acta Chir Scand 1954;107:466-76.
74. Fisher DL. The use of pressure recordings obtained at transthoracic left heart catheterization in the diagnosis of valvular heart disease. J Thorac Surg 1955;30:379-96.
75. Schnabel TG Jr, Blakemore WS, Kuo PT, Langfield SB. Left heart catheterization in aortic and mitral disease. J Clin Invest 1955;34:915-23.
76. Dexter L, Harken DE, Cobb Jr LA, Novack P, Schlant RC, Phinney AO, Haynes FW. Aortic stenosis. Arch Intern Med 1958;101:254-66.
77. Limón Lason R, Rubio Alvarez V, Bouchard F. El cateterismo intracardiaco. V. Cateterización de las cavidades izquierdas en el hombre; registro simultaneo de presión y electrocardiograma intracavitarios. Arch Inst Cardiol Mex 1950;20:271-85.
78. Salans AH, Katz LN, Graham GR, Gordon A, Elisberg EI, Gerber A. A study of the central and peripheral arterial pressure pulse in man, correlation with simultaneously recorded electrokymograms. Circulation 1951;4:510-21.
79. Porstmann W, Geissler W, Wolf W. Die retrograde Lavokardiographie in Verbindung mit der intrakardialen Druckmessung. Fortschr Roentgenstr 1958;89:397-409.
80. Hanson HE, Jönsson G, Karnell J. Catheterization and selective roentgenographic demonstration of the left ventricle of the heart. Acta Radiol 1959;52:33-44.
81. Zimmerman HA, Scott RW, Becker NO. Catheterization of the left side of the heart in man. Circulation 1950;1:357-9.
82. Lambert EC, Vlad P. Retrograde arterial catheterization of the left heart: experience with 117 infants and children [Abstract]. Circulation 1959;20:724.
83. Honick GL, Cayler GG, Richardson WR, Taybi H. New type of catheter tip for retrograde catheterization of the left ventricle in congenital aortic stenosis. N Engl J Med 1962; 266:1101-3.
84. Morrow AG, Braunwald E, Haller JA, Sharp EH. Left heart catheterization by the transbronchial route: technic and applications in physiologic and diagnostic investigations. Circulation 1957;16:1033-9.
85. Facquet J, Lemoin JM, Alhomme P, Lefeboie J. La mesure de la pression auriculaire gauche par voie transbronchque. Arch Mal Coeur 1952;45:741-5.
86. Allison PR, Linden RJ. The bronchoscopic measurement of left auricular pressure. Circulation 1953;7:669-73.
87. Allison PR, Linden RJ. Bronchoscopic approach for measuring pressure in left auricle, pulmonary artery, and aorta. Lancet 1955;1:9-13.
88. Buchbinder WC, Katz LN. Intraventricular pressure curves of the human heart obtained by direct transthoracic puncture. Proc Soc Exp Biol Med 1949;71:673-5.
89. Brock R, Milstein BB, Ross DN. Percutaneous left ventricular puncture in the assessment of aortic stenosis. Thorax 1956;11:163-71.
90. Ross J, Braunwald E, Morrow AG. Transseptal left atrial puncture: new technique for the measurement of left atrial pressure in man. Am J Cardiol 1959;3:653-5.
91. Ross Jr J, Braunwald E, Morrow AG. Left heart catheterization by the transseptal route: a description of the technic and its applications. Circulation 1960;22:927-34.
92. Radner S. Method for recording aortic pressure pulses. Scand J Clin Lab Invest 1953;5:129-31.
93. Radner S. Suprasternal puncture of the left atrium for flow studies. Acta Med Scand 1954;148:57-60.
94. Grishman A, Steinberg MF, Sussman ML. Congenital aortic and subaortic stenosis with associated anomalies of the aorta. Med Clin North Am 1947;31:543-56.
95. Jönsson G, Brodén B, Karnell J. Selective angiocardiography. Acta Radiol 1949;32:486-97.
96. Kjellberg SR, Mannheimer E, Rudhe U, Jonsson B. Diagnosis of congenital heart disease. Chicago: Year Book Medical Publishers, Inc., 1955:496-515.
97. Lehman JS, Musser BG, Lykens HD. Cardiac ventriculography. Am J Roentgenol 1957;77:207-34.
98. Ödman P, Philipson J. Aortic valvular diseases studied by

percutaneous thoracic aortography. Acta Radiol 1958;suppl 172, 59 pp.

99. Gramiak R, Shah PM. Echocardiography of the normal and diseased aortic valve. Radiology 1970;96:1-8.

100. Yeh HC, Winsberg F, Mercer EM. Echocardiographic aortic valve orifice dimension: its use in evaluating aortic stenosis and cardiac output. J Clin Ultrasound 1973;1:182-9.

101. Feizi Ö, Symons C, Yacoub M. Echocardiography of the aortic valve. I. Studies of normal aortic valve, aortic stenosis, aortic regurgitation, and mixed aortic valve disease. Br Heart J 1974;36:341-51.

102. Bennett DH, Evans DW, Raj MVJ. Echocardiographic estimation of the systolic pressure gradient in aortic stenosis. Br Heart J 1975;37:557-63.

103. McDonald IG. Echocardiographic assessment of left ventricular function in aortic valve disease. Circulation 1976; 53:860-4.

104. Brunton L. Preliminary note on the possibility of treating mitral stenosis by surgical methods. Lancet 1902;1:352.

105. Doyen E. Chirurgie des malformations congénitales ou acquises du coeur. Presse Méd 1913;21:860-75.

106. Tuffier T. État actuel de la chirurgie intrathoracique. In: Transactions of the International Congress on Medicine 1913. London, 1914. Section 7, Surgery: 249; discussion: 326.

107. Cutler EC, Levine SA. Cardiotomy and valvulotomy for mitral stenosis. Boston: M and S J 1923;188:1023-7.

108. Cutler EC, Levine SA, Beck CS. The surgical treatment of mitral stenosis, experimental and clinical studies. Arch Surg 1924;9:689-821.

109. Cutler E, Beck CS. The present status of the surgical procedures in chronic valvular disease of the heart. Arch Surg 1929;18:403-16.

110. Powers JH. Surgical treatment of mitral stenosis. Arch Surg 1932;25:555-70.

111. Bailey CP. The surgical treatment of mitral stenosis (mitral commissurotomy). Dis Chest 1949;15:377-93.

112. Harken DE, Ellis LB, Ware PF, Norman LR. The surgical treatment of mitral stenosis. I. Valvuloplasty. N Engl J Med 1948;239:801-9.

113. Baker C, Brock RC, Campbell M. Valvulotomy for mitral stenosis; report of six successful cases. Br Med J 1950;1:1283-93.

114. Glover RP, Bailey CP, O'Neill TTE. Surgery of stenotic valvular disease of the heart. JAMA 1950;144:1049-57.

115. Hufnagel CA, Harvey WP. The surgical correction of aortic regurgitation: preliminary report. Bull Georgetown Univ Med Center 1953;6:60-1.

116. Hufnagel CA, Harvey WP, Rabil PJ, McDermott TF. Surgical correction of aortic insufficiency. Surgery 1954;35:673-83.

117. Swan H, Kortz AB. Direct vision transaortic approach to the aortic valve during hypothermia; experimental observations and report of successful clinical case. Ann Surg 1956;144:205-14.

118. Lewis FJ, Shumway NE, Niazi SA, Benjamin RB. Aortic valvulotomy under direct vision during hypothermia. J Thorac Surg 1956;32:481-92.

119. Gibbon JH. Artificial maintenance of circulation during experimental occlusion of pulmonary artery. Arch Surg 1937;34:1105-31.

120. Dennis C, Spreng DS, Nelson GE, Karlson KE, Nelson RM, Thomas JV, Eder WP, Varco RL. Development of a pump-oxygenator to replace the heart and lungs; an apparatus applicable to human patients, and application to one case. Ann Surg 1951;134:709-21.

121. Newman MH, Stuckey JH, Levowitz BS, Young LA, Dennis C, Fries C, Gorayeb EJ, Zuhdi M, Karlson KE, Adler S, Gliedman M. Complete and partial perfusion of animal and human subjects with the pump oxygenator; a study of factors yielding consistent survival; successful application to one case. Surgery 1955;38:30-7.

122. Harken DE, Soroff HS, Taylor WJ, Lefemine AA, Gupta SK, Lunzer S. Partial and complete prostheses in aortic insufficiency. J Thorac Cardiovasc Surg 1960;40:744-62.

123. Harken DE, Taylor WJ, Lefemine AA, Lunzer S, Low HBC, Cohen ML, Jacobey JA. Aortic valve replacement with a caged ball valve. Am J Cardiol 1962;9:292-9.

Clinical Factors Useful in Predicting Aortic Valve Structure in Patients >40 Years of Age with Isolated Valvular Aortic Stenosis

Gisela C. Mautner, MD, Susanne L. Mautner, MD, Richard O. Cannon III, MD, Sally A. Hunsberger, PhD, and William C. Roberts, MD

A number of reports have described the frequency of coronary arterial narrowing in patients with valvular aortic stenosis. No published reports have examined the structure of the stenotic aortic valve in adults and related the valve structure to variables, including coronary arterial narrowing, useful in predicting that structure. One hundred eighty-eight patients having aortic valve replacement for isolated valvular aortic stenosis were studied. All patients were >40 years of age at the time of aortic valve replacement, all had coronary angiograms preoperatively, and of 182 patients (97%) measurements of serum total cholesterol had been obtained and 184 (98%) had body mass index calculated. The structure of the operatively excised valve was classified as unicuspid or bicuspid (congenitally malformed), or tricuspid aortic valve. A logistic regression model was developed that found 4 factors (age, serum total cholesterol, angiographic coronary artery disease and body mass index) to be predictive of aortic valve structure: (1) Patients with at least 3 or all 4 factors high or present (i.e., age >65 years, serum total cholesterol >200 mg/dl, body mass index >29 kg/m² and coronary artery disease) had a low probability (10 to 29%) of having a congenitally malformed valve; (2) patients with at least 3 or all 4 factors low or absent (i.e., age ≤65 years, serum total cholesterol ≤200 mg/dl, body mass index ≤29 kg/m², and no coronary artery disease) had a high probability (72 to 90%) of having a congenitally malformed valve. Thus, the morphology of the operatively excised stenotic aortic valve can be predicted with knowledge of the age, serum total cholesterol, body mass index and coronary artery status of the patient.

(Am J Cardiol 1993;72:194–198)

From the Pathology, Cardiology, and Biostatistics Research Branches, National Heart, Lung, and Blood Institute, National Institutes of Health, Bethesda, Maryland. Manuscript received June 22, 1992; revised manuscript received and accepted February 8, 1993.

Address for reprints: Gisela C. Mautner, MD, Pathology Branch, National Heart, Lung, and Blood Institute, National Institutes of Health, Building 10, Room 2N258, Bethesda, Maryland 20892.

Aortic valve stenosis in adults is either congenital or acquired in origin. If congenital, the aortic valve is either unicuspid or bicuspid, and if acquired, it is tricuspid.[1–5] We asked if there were clinical factors that might help in predicting aortic valve structure, and, therefore, etiology in adults >40 years of age with aortic valve stenosis severe enough to warrant aortic valve replacement. The factors analyzed were age, gender, severity of the valve stenosis, serum total cholesterol, presence and extent of coronary arterial narrowing by angiogram, and presence of obesity. Such a study has not been performed previously.

METHODS

Sources of patients and inclusion criteria: A computer printout was obtained from the Cardiology Branch, National Heart, Lung, and Blood Institute, of 1,699 patients aged >40 years having cardiac valve replacement at the Clinical Center from 1960 to 1990. Of this number, 659 patients had isolated aortic valve replacement during this time period. Of the 659 patients, 299 were excluded from this study because the replacement was for pure aortic regurgitation, because there was associated mitral stenosis or moderate to severe mitral regurgitation, or because a previous aortic valve operation such as valvuloplasty had been performed. Of the remaining 360 patients with aortic stenosis, 172 were excluded because a left-sided cardiac catheterization or a coronary angiogram, or both, had not been performed. The remaining 188 patients who form the study group fulfilled the following criteria: (1) they had aortic stenosis (with or without associated aortic regurgitation) severe enough to warrant aortic valve replacement; (2) they were >40 years of age at the time of aortic valve replacement; (3) they had a normally functioning or only mildly regurgitant mitral valve; (4) preoperatively they had left-sided cardiac catheterization with measurement of both left ventricular and systemic arterial peak systolic pressures; and (5) preoperatively they had a coronary angiogram. The operatively excised aortic valve was examined by WCR and its structure was classified by him.

Variables analyzed: The medical records of the 188 patients were reviewed by GCM. The variables analyzed are listed in Table I. The coronary angiographic data were obtained from the coronary angiographic reports. The hemodynamic data in all patients were those obtained before aortic valve replacement, a mean of 34 days (range 0 to 385). The serum total cholesterol lev-

TABLE I Comparison of Clinical Features Among Men and Women with Congenitally Unicuspid or Bicuspid and Acquired Tricuspid Stenotic Aortic Valves

Variable	Men			Women			Totals
	Unicuspid	Bicuspid	Tricuspid	Unicuspid	Bicuspid	Tricuspid	
No. of patients	6	85	48	2	24	23	188
Age (years)	52 ± 7	59 ± 8	64 ± 9	42 ± 65	60 ± 8	67 ± 7	61 ± 9
Race							
White*	5	82 (96%)	45 (94%)	2	24 (100%)	23 (100%)	182 (97%)
Black*	1	3 (4%)	3 (6%)	0	0	0	6 (3%)
Systemic hypertension*	1	17 (22%)	12 (29%)	0	6 (29%)	6 (30%)	42 (22%)
Diabetes mellitus*	1	9 (11%)	7 (17%)	0	3 (14%)	7 (35%)	27 (14%)
LV-SA peak systolic gradient (mm Hg)	73 ± 39	71 ± 25	61 ± 25	86 & 70	86 ± 28	75 ± 30	71 ± 27
Aortic valve area (cm^2)/aortic valve index (cm^2/m^2 BSA)	0.7/0.4	0.6/0.3	0.6/0.3	0.4/0.3 0.9/0.5	0.5/0.3	0.6/0.3	0.6/0.3
Height (cm)/weight (kg)	171/71	172/75	171/78	160/61 175/65	157/64	160/71	168/74
Body mass index (kg/m^2)†	24	25	27	21 & 24	26	28	26
Body mass index (kg/m^2) > 29*	0	9 (11%)	11 (23%)	0	5 (21%)	9 (39%)	34 (18%)
Total cholesterol (mg/dl)‡	212 ± 23	210 ± 38	227 ± 37	228 & 250	223 ± 62	269 ± 67	224 ± 49
Total cholesterol > 200 (mg/dl)	3	47 (58%)	38 (79%)	2	14 (58%)	19 (86%)	123 (65%)
≥ 1 coronary artery narrowed > 50% in diameter angiographically*	2	33 (39%)	27 (56%)	0	7 (29%)	11 (48%)	80 (43%)
Patients having none or ≥ 1 coronary arteries narrowed 50% in diameter							
0	4	52 (61%)	21 (44%)	2	17 (71%)	12 (52%)	108 (57%)
1	1	18 (21%)	7 (15%)	0	4 (17%)	4 (17%)	34 (18%)
2	1	10 (12%)	11 (23%)	0	3 (13%)	4 (17%)	29 (15%)
3	0	5 (6%)	9 (19%)	0	0	2 (9%)	16 (9%)
4	0	0	0	0	0	1 (4%)	1 (1%)
Mean number of coronary arteries per patient narrowed > 50% in diameter	0.5	0.6	1.2	0	0.4	1.0	0.8
Mean number of coronary arteries narrowed > 50% in diameter in the patients with at least 1 artery so narrowed	1.5	1.6	2.0	0	1.4	2.0	1.8
Coronary bypass*	1	15 (18%)	14 (29%)	0	4 (17%)	9 (39%)	43 (23%)
Mean number of grafts in patients having coronary bypass	2	1.4	1.6	—	1.2	2	1.6

*Number of patients.
†Available in 184 of the 188 patients.
‡Available in 182 of the 188 patients.
BSA = body surface area; LV = left ventricular; SA = systemic artery.

els, available in 182 of the 188 patients, were obtained before aortic valve replacement from blood drawn usually at admission to the Clinical Center at the time of aortic valve replacement. Data to calculate the body mass index were obtained in 184 patients.

Statistics: A logistic regression model was used to model the probability of congenital valve disease given the predictor covariates. Initially, age, serum total cholesterol, body mass index, peak systolic pressure gradient across the stenotic aortic valve, sex and angiographic coronary artery narrowing were examined. The first 4 variables were examined to see if they should be included as continuous variables, but it was found that a binary relation existed between the variables and the probability of a congenitally malformed valve. The variables were modeled as follows: age ≤65 years or >65 years; serum total cholesterol ≤200 mg/dl or >200 mg/dl; body mass index ≤29 kg/m^2 or >29 kg/m^2; and peak systolic pressure gradient across the stenotic aortic valve ≤50 mm Hg or >50 mm Hg. Coronary artery narrowing was either present or absent.

The analysis was performed using PROC LOGISTIC in SAS V6. All first-order interactions were examined and none were found to be significant. The variables, sex and peak systolic pressure gradient, were found not to be significant and thus were not included in the model. The final model included age, serum total cholesterol, body mass index and coronary artery disease.

RESULTS

Characteristics of all patients studied: The major findings in the 188 patients are summarized in Table I and the types of stenotic aortic valves encountered are illustrated in Figure 1. Of the 188 patients, 109 (58%) had congenitally bicuspid aortic valves, 71 (38%) had tricuspid aortic valves, and 8 patients (4%) had unicuspid (also unicommissural) aortic valves. The average age of the 188 patients was 61 ± 9 years; 55 (38 men and 17 women) (29%) were >65 years of age and 133 (101 men and 32 women) (71%) were ≤65 years of age; 49 (26%) were women and 139 (74%) were men. Eighty patients (43%) by angiogram had narrowing of >50% in diameter of ≥1 major epicardial coronary arteries: 34 (18%) had only 1 artery so narrowed; 29 (15%), 2 arteries; and 16 (9%), 3 arteries so narrowed (mean 0.8 per patient). Of the 188 patients, 43 (23%) also had coronary artery bypass grafting at the time of aortic valve replacement. The average peak systolic pressure gradient

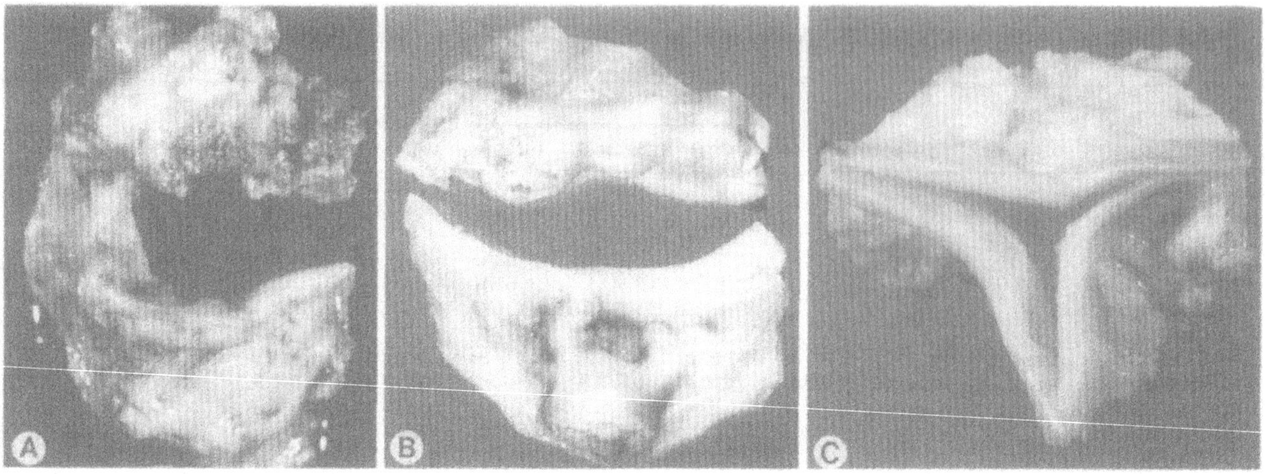

FIGURE 1. Operatively excised stenotic aortic valves from 3 different patients. *A*, congenitally unicuspid unicommissural valve from a 46-year-old man (NIH #S72-4126) with a peak systolic pressure gradient of 50 mm Hg across the aortic valve. *B*, congenitally bicuspid valve from a 71-year-old man (NIH #S89-46) with a peak systolic gradient of 60 mm Hg across the valve. *C*, tricuspid valve from a 68-year-old man (NIH #S83-82) with a peak systolic gradient of 50 mm Hg across the valve.

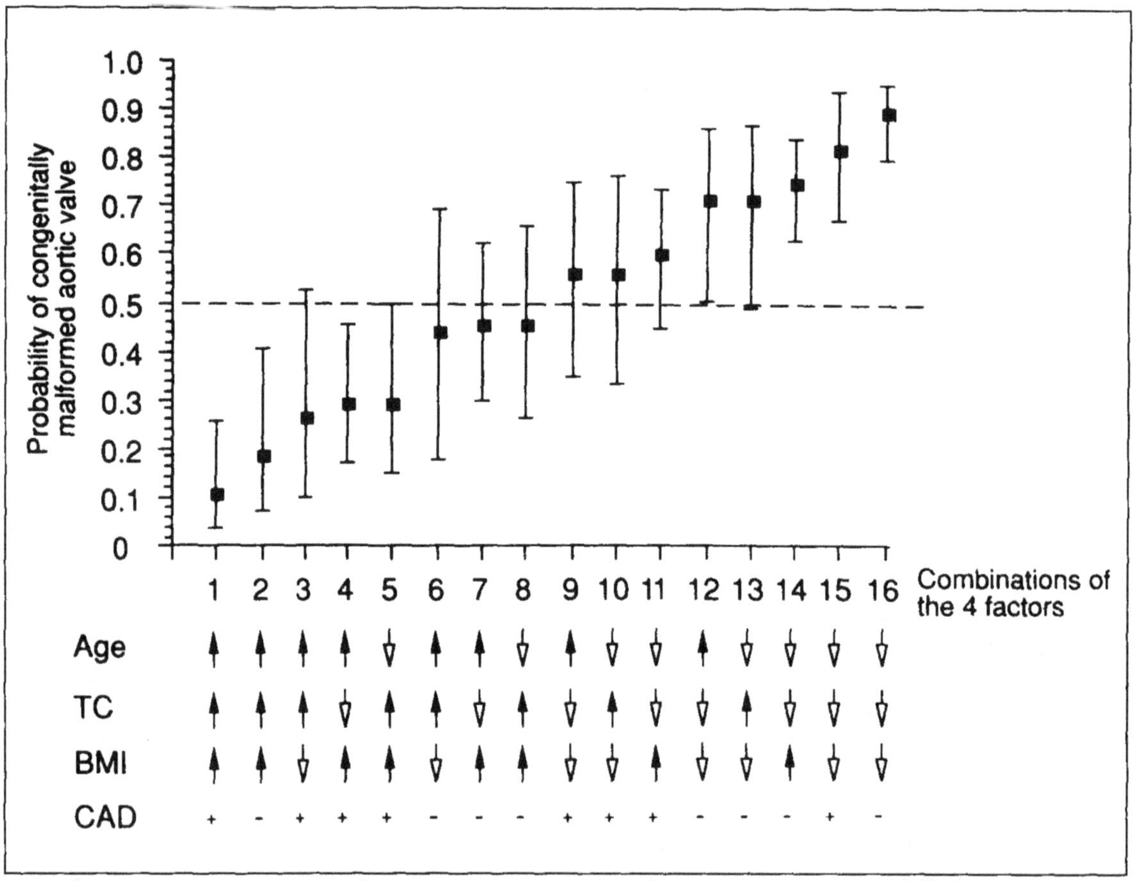

FIGURE 2. Illustration of the logistic regression model. The estimated probability *(black squares)* and 95% confidence intervals *(vertical lines)* for all combinations of predictor variables are provided. *Vertical lines* are the confidence intervals for each possible combination. If the *vertical lines* do not cross the *horizontal line* at 0.5, it is indicated that the combination of variables help predict the probability of the presence of a congenitally malformed valve better than could be done by guessing alone (i.e., the probability of 0.5 means a chance of 50% of having either a congenitally malformed valve or tricuspid valve). A probability close to 1 means a high chance of having a congenitally malformed valve, and, conversely, a probability closer to 0 means a low chance of having a congenitally malformed valve. Of the 16 possible combinations 10 were predictive: (1) patients with at least 3 or all 4 factors high *(solid arrow)* or present (+), i.e., age >65 years, total cholesterol (TC) >200 mg/dl, body mass index (BMI) >29 kg/m^2, and coronary artery disease (CAD) present, had a low probability (10 to 29%) of having a congenitally malformed valve; (2) patients with at least 3 or all 4 factors low *(open arrow)* or absent (−), i.e., age ≤65 years, total cholesterol ≤200 mg/dl, body mass index ≤29 kg/m^2, and coronary artery disease absent, had a high probability (72 to 90%) of having a congenitally malformed valve.

between left ventricle and a systemic artery was 71 ± 27 mm Hg (range 10 to 160 mm Hg). The mean serum total cholesterol was 224 ± 49 mg/dl and the value was >200 mg/dl in 123 patients (65%). Twenty-seven patients (14%) had a history of diabetes mellitus, and 42 patients (22%) had a history of systemic hypertension.

Comparison of findings in patients with the three types of aortic valve structure: The results of comparison of 18 variables among men and women with congenitally bicuspid or unicuspid and acquired tricuspid stenotic aortic valves are summarized in Table I. Compared to those with 3-cuspid valves in both men and women, the patients with congenitally malformed valves had younger mean ages (59 vs 64 years and 60 vs 67 years); higher average peak systolic pressure gradients across the stenotic valve (71 vs 61 mm Hg and 86 vs 75 mm Hg); lower mean serum total cholesterol levels (210 vs 227 mg/dl and 223 vs 269 mg/dl); a lower percentage of patients with serum total cholesterol levels >200 mg/dl (58 vs 79% and 58 vs 86%), and a lower mean number of coronary arteries narrowed >50% in diameter by angiogram (0.6 vs 1.2 and 0.4 vs 1.0). Body weight as measured by body mass index and percent with body mass index >29 kg/m^2 was lower in men with congenitally malformed valves than in those with 3-cuspid valves (25 vs 27 kg/m^2 and 11 vs 23%), and a similar trend was observed in women (26 vs 28 kg/m^2 and 21 vs 39%).

Usefulness of combination of factors for predicting whether the stenotic aortic valve is congenitally malformed, i.e., unicuspid or bicuspid, or whether it is tricuspid and therefore acquired in origin: In Figure 2, the estimated probability and 95% confidence intervals for all combinations of predictor variables are provided. The vertical lines are the confidence intervals for each possible combination. If the vertical lines do not cross the horizontal line at 0.5, it is indicated that the combination of variables help predict the probability of the presence of a congenitally malformed valve better than could be done by guessing alone, i.e., the probability of 0.5 means a chance of 50% of having either a congenitally malformed valve or tricuspid valve. A probability close to 1 means a very high chance of having a congenitally malformed valve, and, conversely, a probability closer to 0 means a very low chance of having a congenitally malformed valve. Of the 16 possible combinations, 10 proved to be predictive; when all 4 factors analyzed were at high levels or present (Figure 2, combination 1),

TABLE II Parameter Estimates, Standard Errors (SE) and p Values

Predictor	Estimate	SE	p Value
Age	−1.2943	0.3714	0.0005
Body mass index	−1.2888	0.4374	0.0032
Total cholesterol	−1.1170	0.3939	0.0046
Coronary artery disease	−0.6953	0.3411	0.0415

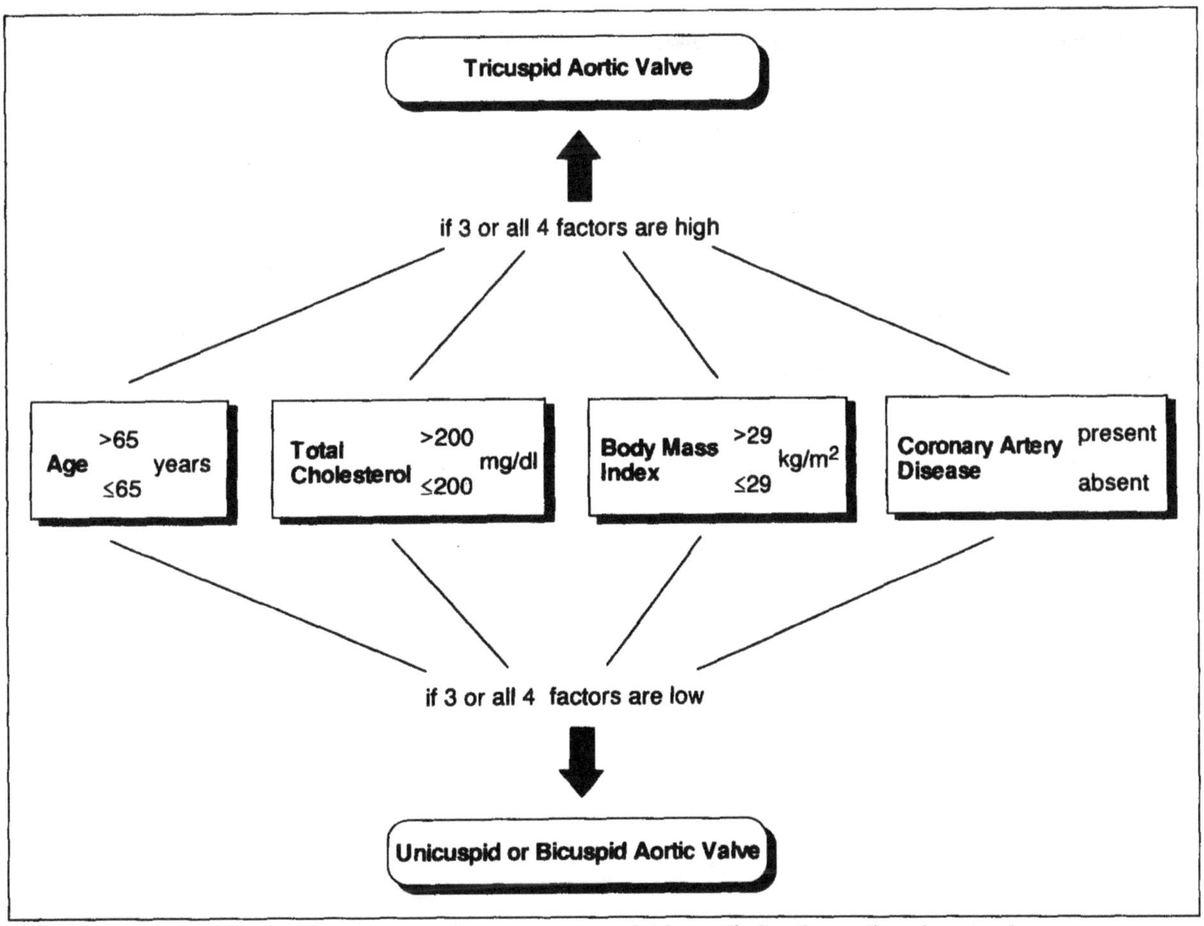

FIGURE 3. Illustration summarizing the 4 factors that proved useful in predicting the aortic valve structure.

i.e., old age (>65 years), elevated serum total cholesterol (>200 mg/dl), obesity (body mass index >29 kg/m^2), and significant angiographic coronary arterial narrowing (>50% reduction in diameter), the probability of a congenitally malformed aortic valve being present was low (10%). If 3 of the 4 variables were high or present but 1 variable was low or absent (Figure 2, combination 2–5), the probability of having a congenitally malformed aortic valve was 19 to 29%. If 2 of the 4 variables were low or absent (Figure 2, combination 6–11), it was not possible to predict the structure of the aortic valve. The likelihood of having a congenitally malformed aortic valve was between 72 and 82% when 3 variables were low or absent. For combination 16, in which all 4 factors were low or absent, i.e., age ≤65 years, serum total cholesterol ≤200 mg/dl, body mass index ≤29 kg/m^2, and no significant angiographic coronary arterial narrowing, the probability of having a congenitally malformed aortic valve was high (90%). Thus, the greater the number of examined factors that were low, the greater the probability that the patients had a congenitally malformed aortic valve and vice versa (Figure 3).

Table II gives the parameter estimates, standard errors of the estimates, and p value using a Wald test for testing the significance of each term. Age was the strongest predictor, total cholesterol and body mass index were about equally significant, and coronary artery disease was the least significant predictor.

DISCUSSION

Frequency of various valve structures and gender: All 188 patients included in this study had valvular aortic stenosis severe enough to warrant aortic valve replacement, all were >40 years of age at the time of aortic valve replacement, and none had associated mitral stenosis or significant mitral regurgitation. The 188 patients averaged 61 years of age, only 55 (29%) were >65 years of age, and 139 (74%) were men. A major finding was that a congenitally malformed valve, either unicuspid or bicuspid, was more common than a tricuspid aortic valve. Indeed, 117 of the 188 patients (62%) had a bicuspid or unicuspid valve and only 71 (38%) had a tricuspid valve. The reason that 1- and 2-cuspid valves were more frequent in the population studied may be: (1) because the population consisted of 3 times more men than women and 1- and 2-cuspid valves were present in 65% of the men and in only 53% of the women; and (2) because the percentage of the study patients >65 years of age was relatively small, and subjects who are older at the time of valve replacement usually have 3-cuspid aortic valves.

To predict the structure of the aortic valve in patients >40 years of age with severe aortic stenosis, a logistic regression model was developed and it proved useful. In the beginning, 6 factors were included, i.e., gender; age (>65 years or ≤65 years); serum total cholesterol level (>200 mg/dl or ≤200 mg/dl); coronary artery narrowing (>50% in diameter) by angiogram; peak systolic pressure gradient across the stenotic aortic valve (>50 mm Hg or ≤50 mm Hg), and body mass index (>29 kg/m^2 or ≤29 kg/m^2). As the peak systolic pressure gradient across the aortic valve and the gender were not useful they were excluded from the model. The other 4 variables were significant predictive factors (Figure 2). Of the 16 possible combinations 10 were predictive: (1) Patients who had 3 or all 4 factors high or present had a low probability of having a congenitally malformed valve (10 to 29%). (2) Conversely, patients who had 3 or all 4 factors low or absent had a high probability of having a congenitally malformed valve (72 to 90%).

Acknowledgment: We thank Vivian E. Norman and Michael W. Spencer for their secretarial and technical help.

1. Roberts WC. The structure of the aortic valve in clinically-isolated aortic stenosis. An autopsy study of 162 patients over 15 years of age. *Circulation* 1970;42:91–7.
2. Roberts WC. The congenitally bicuspid aortic valve. A study of 85 autopsy cases. *Am J Cardiol* 1970;26:72–83.
3. Roberts WC. Anatomically isolated aortic valvular disease. The case against its being of rheumatic origin. *Am J Med* 1970;49:151–9.
4. Roberts WC, Perloff JK, Constantino T. Severe valvular aortic stenosis in patients over 65 years of age. A clinicopathologic study. *Am J Cardiol* 1971;27:497–506.
5. Falcone MW, Roberts WC, Morrow AG, Perloff JK. Congenital aortic stenosis resulting from unicommissural valve. Clinical and anatomic features in twenty-one adult patients. *Circulation* 1971;44:272–80.

Congenitally Bicuspid Aortic Valve in Multiple Family Members

Brian N. Glick, MD,* and William C. Roberts, MD†

The congenitally bicuspid aortic valve has been the subject of numerous publications. Leonardo da Vinci in the 1400s drew the valve and provided some reasons why it might function abnormally.[1] In 1844, Paget[2] called attention to the peculiar liability of congenitally bicuspid aortic valves to disease, but their importance as something other than a pathologic curiosity was not appreciated. In 1858, Peacock[3] pointed out that bicuspid aortic valves tended to become "thick ... ossified ... inducing first obstruction ... and then incompetency." Osler[4] in 1886 first described the abnormal liability of the bicuspid aortic valve to develop infective endocarditis. It was not until the 1950s that the bicuspid condition was recognized to be a common underlying cause of aortic valve stenosis, and it was not until 1981 that it was recognized to be associated with pure aortic regurgitation unassociated with infective endocarditis.[5] The bicuspid aortic valve has been the subject, directly or indirectly, of ≥28 publications from this laboratory since 1962.[5,6–32]

Despite the frequency of the congenitally bicuspid aortic valve (possibly as high as 1% of the population), its occurrence in >1 family member is extremely uncommon. Only 4 reports have appeared describing 4 families (9 family members) with >1 member having a congenitally bicuspid aortic valve (Table I).[33–36] During the past 27 years, we have encountered 6 families (17 family members) in whom >1 member had aortic valve disease, with bicuspid valve confirmed at operation in 11. A description of certain findings in these 17 family members is the subject of this report.

The pedigree of the 6 families is shown in Figure 1. In 3 families (I, II and VI), a parent and ≥1 child were

From the Pathology Branch, National Heart, Lung, and Blood Institute, National Institutes of Health, Bethesda, Maryland 20892. Manuscript received April 16, 1993; revised manuscript received and accepted June 24, 1993.

*Cardiology Fellow, Georgetown University Medical Center, Washington, D.C.

†Current address: Baylor Cardiovascular Institute, Baylor University Medical Center, 3600 Gaston Avenue, Dallas, Texas 75246.

affected, and in 3 families (III, IV and V), ≥1 sibling only was affected. In 11 of 17 family members, the congenital bicuspid nature of the aortic valve was confirmed at the time of aortic valve replacement, and the operatively excised bicuspid aortic valves in 7 of these patients are shown in Figures 2 to 5. Another patient (number 10, family IV, Table II) also had aortic valve replacement, but the type of valve encountered was unknown to us. In the other 5 patients, the bicuspid nature of the aortic valve was demonstrated by echocardiogram in 2 (numbers 7 and 17; Table II) and strongly suggested by aortogram in 1 (number 2). The latter patient had significant aortic regurgitation by aortogram at age 10 years. Patients 11 and 12 were stated to have "aortic valve disease," but no other information regarding them was available to us. None of the 17 patients apparently had clinical evidence of mitral valve dysfunction.

Pertinent findings in each of the 17 patients are tabulated in Table II. Of the 17 patients, 10 had clinical evidence of aortic valve stenosis, with or without associated aortic regurgitation, including 6 in whom a

TABLE I Observations in Nine Previously Reported Patients (all men) with a Congenitally Biscuspid Aortic Valve in More Than One Family Member

Year of Publication	First Author	Case	Relation	Age (years) at Death	Age (years) at AVR	Year of AVR	AS	AR Murmur	Calcified AV (0–3)	LV-SA psg (mm Hg)	Type (size) of AV Prosthesis	BAV at AVR (+) or Necropsy (++)
1972	McKusick	1	Father*	—	44	—	−	+	2+	—	S-E	+
		2	Son*	19	—	—	−	+	—	—	—	++
1977	Gale	3	Brother†	—	38	1972	+	−	3+	—	§	+
		4	Brother†	—	44	1976	+	+	3+	40	B-S (23)	+
1987	Godden	5	Brother‡	—	57	1980	+	−	3+	60	C-E (27)	+
		6	Brother‡	61	57	1980	+	+	3+	65	B-S (23)	+
1989	McDonald	7	Brother	19	—	—	+	−	—	—	—	++
		8	Brother	—	23	—	+	−	—	80	SJM	+
		9	Brother	—	26	—	+	+	—	80	S-E	+

*Each had severe cystic medial necrosis of the ascending aorta. The father had dissection involving the entire aorta, which was not dilated; the son had a through-and-through fatal tear of a dilated ascending aorta with hemopericardium. Neither had skeletal features of the Marfan syndrome.
†Both have dilated ascending aortas. Case 4 had medial cystic necrosis confirmed by histologic study of portions of the excised ascending aorta. Neither patient had skeletal features of the Marfan syndrome.
‡Identical twins, probably monozygotic. Case 6 had infective endocarditis at 1 time.
§The type of substitute valve used is uncertain.
AR = aortic regurgitation; AS = aortic stenosis; AV = aortic valve; AVR = aortic valve replacement; BAV = biscuspid aortic valve; B-S = Bjork-Shirley; C-E = Carpentier-Edwards; LV = left ventricular; psg = peak systolic gradient; SA = systemic artery; s/d = peak systolic/end-diastolic; S-E = Starr-Edwards; SJM = St. Jude Medical; + = present or positive; 0 = absent or negative; — = information not available.

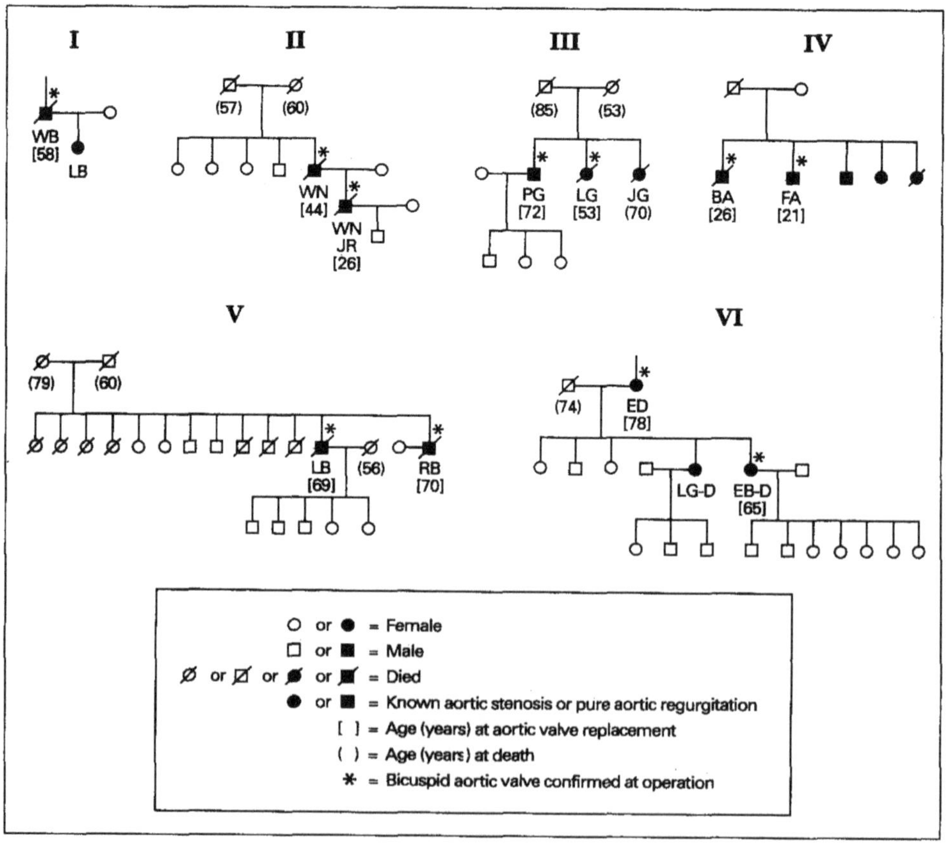

FIGURE 1. The pedigree of 6 families with >1 family member with a congenitally bicuspid aortic valve.

peak systolic pressure gradient ranging from 38 to 100 mm Hg was recorded at cardiac catheterization. Of the latter 6 patients, 5 had aortic valve replacement within 1 month of cardiac catheterization. The remaining patient (number 14, Table II) had a cardiac catheterization when she was aged 70 years, and now (April 1993), 9 months later, she has still not had aortic valve replacement, primarily because of noncardiac problems. Four of the 17 patients had pure aortic regurgitation, and 3 of them have had aortic valve replacement. In 3 patients (numbers 10, 11 and 12; Table II), the type of aortic valve dysfunction was unknown to us. Of the 6 families, all affected members in 3 families had aortic stenosis (with or without associated aortic regurgitation); in 2 families (numbers I and II, Table II), the father in each had aortic stenosis, and the child (1 daughter and 1 son) had pure aortic regurgitation, and in 1 family (number IV), it is likely but not proven that some family members had aortic stenosis and others pure aortic regurgitation.

In 2 families (numbers II and V, Table II), all affected members were men, in 1 family (number VI), all 3 affected members were women, and in 3 families (numbers I, III and IV; Table II), ≥1 affected member was male and ≥1 was female.

Infective endocarditis occurred in only 1 (number 8, Table II) of the 17 patients, and in this case, it caused severe aortic regurgitation and necessitated aortic valve replacement.

The hitherto described observations indicate that the bicuspid aortic valve may occur in >1 family member. Although approximately 75% of subjects with congenitally bicuspid aortic valves are male, female members of families are not immune to this congenital malformation. Of our 17 patients, only 9 (53%) were male; in 1 family (number VI), all 3 affected members were female. The type of valve dysfunction resulting from the bicuspid condition was variable. In some families, all affected members had aortic stenosis (with or without associated regurgitation), in some, all affected members

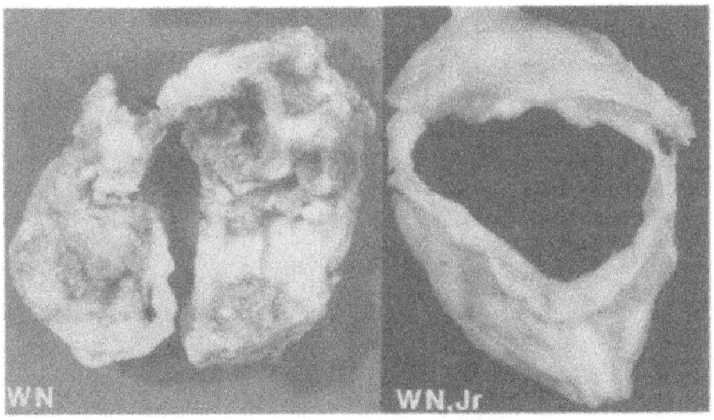

FIGURE 2. Patients 3 and 4 (Table II). Operatively excised aortic valves of patients WN (NIH# S67-3152) and WN Jr (NIH# S71-3019). The father, who was 44 years old at the time of aortic valve replacement, had aortic valve stenosis and a heavily calcified valve; the son, who was 26 years old at valve replacement, had pure aortic regurgitation and a noncalcified valve.

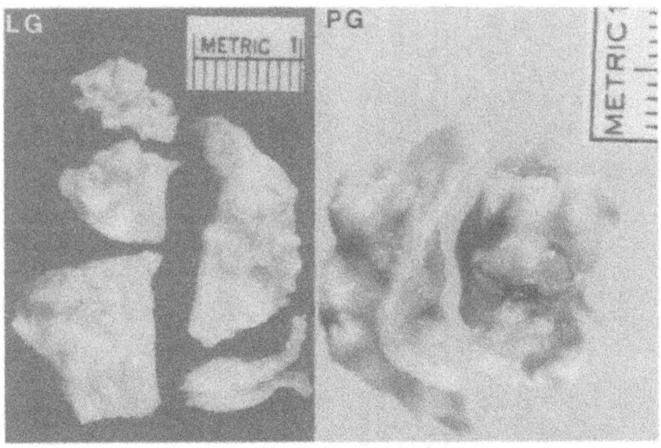

FIGURE 3. Patients 5 and 6 (Table II). Operatively excised aortic valves of patients LG (NIH# S78-43) and PG (NIH# S84-45). Patient LG was 53 years old, and PG was 72 at the time of valve replacement. Both patients had stenotic valves, but the older brother (PG) had considerably more calcific deposits in the valve than did the younger sister (LG).

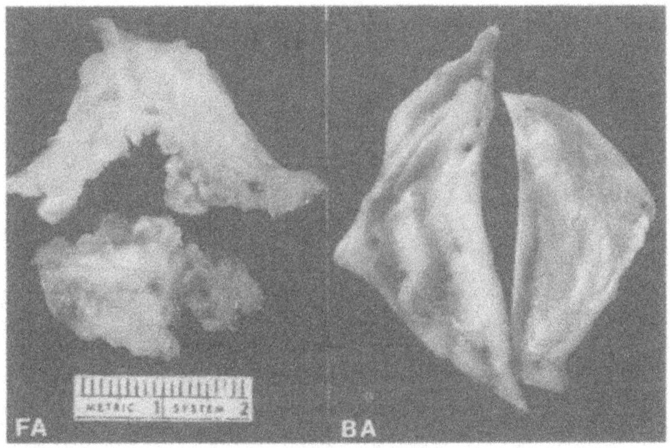

FIGURE 4. Patients 8 and 9 (Table II). Operatively excised aortic valves of patients FA (NIH# S79-30) and BA (NIH# 80-174). The valve of FA is focally calcified and was partially destroyed by active infective endocarditis approximately 1.5 years before valve replacement at age 21 years. The valve of patient BA is devoid of calcium, and it was purely regurgitant.

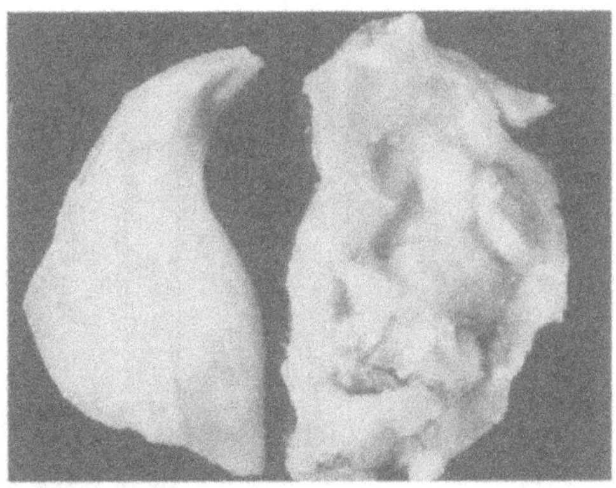

FIGURE 5. Patient 14 (Table II). Operatively excised aortic valve of patient LB (NIH# S89-50) who had valve replacement for aortic stenosis at age 69 years. One of the 2 cusps is heavily calcified, and the other one is devoid of calcium. The operatively excised valve weighed 4 g.

TABLE II Clinical Findings in the Six Families in Whom More Than One Member Had a Congenitally Bicuspid Aortic Valve

Family	Case	Patient's Initials	Relation	Age (years) at Death	Age (years) at AVR	Year of AVR	AS	AR Mumur	Calcified AV (0–3+)	LV (s/d) (mm Hg)	SA (s/d) (mm Hg)	LV-SA psg (mm Hg)	AR by AA Angiogram (0–4+)	CI	AVA (cm^2)	Type (size) of AV Prosthesis	CAD by Angiogram	BAV Confirmed at AVR	Serum TC (mg/dl)
I	1	WB	Father	58	58	1966	+	0	3+	205/8	120/55	85	0	2.6	0.6	S-E (8A)	–	+	—
	2	LB	Daughter	—	—	—	0	+	—	135/5§	135/55§	0§	3+§	4.9§	—	—	–	0	—
II	3	WN	Father	58	44	1967	+	+	3+	180/20	130/52	50	3+	3.3	—	S-E (12A)	–	+	181
	4	WN Jr	Son	26	26	1971	0	+	0	145/26	145/65	0	3+	4.0	—	S-E (11A)	–	+	189
III	5	LG	Sister	60	53	1978	+	0	3+	135/30	80/55	55	—	2.7	0.5	B-S (19)	+¶	+	253
	6	PG	Brother	—	72	1984	+	+	3+	240/37	180/70	60	2+	2.2	—	B-S (19)	+	+	236
	7	JG	Sister	70	—	—	+	–	3+	—	—	—	—	—	—	—	–	0	—
IV	8	FA	Brother	—	21	1979	0	+	1+	—	120/40	—	4+	2.4	—	Hancock (23)	–	+	122
	9	BA	Brother	26	26	1980	0	+	0	140/13	140/60	0	4+	3.4	—	S-E (9A)	–	+	201
	10	—	Sister*	—	—	—	–	–	—	—	—	—	—	—	—	+*	–	–	—
	11	—	Sister†	—	—	—	–	–	—	—	—	—	—	—	—	—	–	–	—
	12	—	Brother†	—	—	—	–	–	—	—	—	—	—	—	—	—	–	–	—
V	13	RB	Brother	80	70	1981	+	–	—	—	—	—	—	—	—	+‖	–	+	—
	14	LB	Brother	73	69	1989	+	–	3+	180/18	142/80	38	—	2.3	0.6	SJM (25)	0	+	262
VI	15	ED	Mother	—	78	1982	+	–	—	—	—	—	—	—	—	+‖	–	+	—
	16	EBD	Daughter	—	65	1989	+	0	3+	—	180/90	100	—	—	—	C-E (21)	+	+	232
	17	LGD	Daughter	—	—‡	—	+	0	3+	190/16	140/70	50	—	—	—	—	0	0	207

*This patient died at the time of aortic valve replacement. The type of valve dysfunction, and the number of aortic valve cusps are unknown to us.
†The only information available in these 2 subjects is that each was described in the medical records of FA and BA as having "aortic valve disease."
‡This woman was aged 70 years at cardiac catheterization, and by publication, she will be 71.
§These data were collected when the patient was 10 years old (1966).
‖Aortic valve replacement was performed. The type of substitute valve used is unknown.
¶Coronary artery bypass surgery.
AA = ascending aorta; AVA = aortic valve area; CAD = coronary artery disease; CI = cardiac index (L/min/m^2); TC = total cholesterol; other abbreviations as n Table I.

had pure aortic regurgitation (no element of stenosis), and in others, ≥1 family member had aortic stenosis and ≥1 had pure aortic regurgitation.

The frequency in which a congenitally bicuspid aortic valve occurs in >1 family member is unclear. Although our study includes a relatively large number of families in which >1 family member had a bicuspid aortic valve found at the time of aortic valve replacement, we do not know how many other operatively excised congenitally bicuspid aortic valves we have seen in which only 1 family member had a congenitally bicuspid aortic valve. Some information regarding this frequency question, however, has been provided by Emanuel and associates.[37] These authors examined 188 living, first-degree relatives of 41 patients (41 different families) who had malfunctioning congenitally bicuspid aortic valves excised at operation. By precordial examination, chest radiograph and electrocardiogram in all 188 relatives, and by M-mode echocardiogram in 52 (28%), 8 of the 188 relatives (4%) from 7 of the 41 families (17%) had evidence of "aortic valve disease." Thus, of 229 family members examined in 41 families, 49 (21%) had clinical or operative evidence of aortic valve disease (the bicuspid condition probably in all of them). Of the 71 family members in our 6 families, 17 (24%) had evidence of aortic valve disease (most likely a bicuspid aortic valve in all of them). This high percentage is not surprising, because each of the 6 families that provided the 71 family members had ≥2 members with aortic valve disease. Of the 71 family members in our 6 families, aortic valve disease was present in 8 of 46 living members (17%) and in 9 of 25 dead members (36%). In the study by Emanuel and colleagues,[37] only 2 of 229 patients were stated to be dead (assuming that each of the 41 patients having aortic valve replacement are alive), and both of them had aortic valve disease; of the 227 presumably living patients, 47 (21%) had evidence of aortic valve disease.

In conclusion, the bicuspid aortic valve is clearly more common in first-degree relatives of subjects with a bicuspid aortic valve than in those of subjects with a tricuspid aortic valve. It appears reasonable to recommend a good precordial examination and possibly an echocardiogram in first-degree relatives of subjects clearly identified as having a congenitally bicuspid aortic valve.

1. O'Malley CD, Saunders CM. Leonardo da Vinci on the Human Body. New York: H. Wolff Company, 1952:506.
2. Paget J. On obstruction of the branches of the pulmonary artery. *Med-Chir Trans* 1884;27:162–188.
3. Peacock TB. On Malformations of the Human Heart. 2nd ed. London: Churchill, 1858:204.
4. Osler W. The bicuspid condition of the aortic valves. *Trans Assoc Am Physicians* 1886;2:185–192.
5. Roberts WC, Morrow AG, McIntosh CL, Jones M, Epstein SE. Congenitally bicuspid aortic valve causing severe, pure aortic regurgitation without superimposed infective endocarditis. Analysis of 13 patients requiring aortic valve replacement. *Am J Cardiol* 1981;47:206–209.
6. Roberts WC, Morrow AG, Braunwald E. Complete interruption of the aortic arch. *Circulation* 1962;26:39–59.
7. Roberts WC, Morrow AG. Cardiac valves and the surgical pathologist. *Arch Pathol* 1966;82:309–313.
8. Roberts WC, Elliott L. Lesions complicating the congenitally bicuspid aortic valve. Anatomic and radiographic features. *Radiol Clin North Am* 1968;6:408–421.
9. Roberts WC. The structure of the aortic valve in clinically-isolated aortic stenosis. An autopsy study of 162 patients over 15 years of age. *Circulation* 1970;42:91–97.
10. Roberts WC. The congenitally bicuspid aortic valve. A study of 85 cases. *Am J Cardiol* 1970;26:72–83.
11. Roberts WC. Anatomically isolated aortic valvular disease. The case against its being of rheumatic etiology. *Am J Med* 1970;49:151–159.
12. Roberts WC, Perloff JK, Costantino T. Severe valvular aortic stenosis in patients over 65 years of age. A clinicopathologic study. *Am J Cardiol* 1971;27:497–506.
13. Buchbinder NA, Roberts WC. Left-sided valvular active infective endocarditis. A study of forty-five necropsy patients. *Am J Med* 1972;53:20–35.
14. Roberts WC. Valvular, subvalvular, and supravalvular aortic stenosis: morphologic features. *Cardiol Clin* 1973;5:97–126.
15. Roberts WC, Dangel JC, Bulkley BH. Non-rheumatic valvular cardiac disease: a clinicopathologic survey of 27 different conditions causing valvular dysfunction. *Cardiol Clin* 1973;5:333–446.
16. Arnett EN, Roberts WC. Valve ring abscess in active infective endocarditis. Frequency, location, and clues to clinical diagnosis from the study of 95 necropsy patients. *Circulation* 1976;54:140–145.
17. McReynolds RA, Ali NO, Cuadra M, Roberts WC. Combined acute rheumatic fever and congenitally bicuspid aortic valve. A hitherto unconfirmed combination. *Chest* 1976;70:98–100.
18. Arnett EN, Roberts WC. Active infective endocarditis: a clinicopathology analysis of 137 necropsy patients. *Curr Probl Cardiol* 1976;1:1–76.
19. Roberts WC, Buchbinder NA. Healed left-sided infective endocarditis: a clinicopathologic study of 59 patients. *Am J Cardiol* 1977;40:876–888.
20. Shemin RJ, Kent KM, Roberts WC. Syndrome of valvular pulmonary stenosis and valvular aortic stenosis with atrial septal defect. *Br Heart J* 1979;42:442–446.
21. Roberts WC. Aortic dissection: anatomy, consequences, and causes. *Am Heart J* 1981;101:195–214.
22. Roberts WC, Arnett EA, Cabin HS, McIntosh CL, Aisner SC. Documented development of severe stenoses of previous confirmed normally functioning aortic valves. *Am Heart J* 1982;104:306–308.
23. Arnett EA, Roberts WC. Pathology of active infective endocarditis: a necropsy analysis of 192 patients. *Thorac Cardiovasc Surg* 1982;30:327–335.
24. Glancy DL, Morrow AG, Simon AL, Roberts WC. Juxtaductal aortic coarctation. Analysis of 84 patients studied hemodynamically, angiographically and morphologically after age 1 year. *Am J Cardiol* 1983;51:537–551.
25. Roberts WC. Congenital cardiovascular abnormalities usually silent until adulthood. In: Roberts WC, ed. Adult Congenital Heart Diseases. Philadelphia: FA Davis, 1987:631–691.
26. Roberts WC, McIntosh CL, Wallace RB. Aortic valve perforation with calcific aortic valve stenosis and without infective endocarditis or significant aortic regurgitation. *Am J Cardiol* 1987;59:476–478.
27. Roberts WC. Examining operative excised cardiac valves. *Am J Cardiol* 1987; 59:1434–1436.
28. Mann JM, McIntosh CL, Katz NM, Roberts WC. Cardiac valve replacement for stenotic bicuspid aortic valve in husband and for purely regurgitant prolapsed mitral valve in wife. *Am J Cardiol* 1987;60:401–402.
29. Kalan JM, McIntosh CL, Bonow RO, Roberts WC. Development of severe stenosis in a previously purely regurgitant, congenitally bicuspid aortic valve. *Am J Cardiol* 1988;62:988–989.
30. Dressler FA, Roberts WC. Infective endocarditis in opiate addicts: analysis of 80 cases studied at necropsy. *Am J Cardiol* 1989;63:1240–1257.
31. Roberts WC. Living with a congenitally bicuspid aortic valve. *Am J Cardiol* 1989;64:1408–1409.
32. Brown PS Jr, Roberts CS, McIntosh CL, Roberts WC, Clark RE. Combined obstructive hypertrophic cardiomyopathy and stenotic congenitally bicuspid aortic valve. *Am J Cardiol* 1990;66:1368–1372.
33. McKusick V. Association of congenital bicuspid aortic valve and Erdheim's cystic medial necrosis. *Lancet* 1972;1:1026–1027.
34. Gale AN, McKusick VA, Hutchins GH, Gott VL. Familial congenital bicuspid aortic valve. *Chest* 1977;72:5:668–670.
35. Godden DJ, Sandhu PS, Kerr F. Stenosed bicuspid aortic valves in twins. *Eur Heart J* 1987;8:316–318.
36. McDonald K, Maurer BJ. Familial aortic valve disease: evidence for a genetic influence? *Eur Heart J* 1989;10:676–677.
37. Emanuel R, Withers R, O'Brien K, Ross P, Feizi O. Congenitally bicuspid aortic valve. Clinicogenetic study of 41 families. *Br Heart J* 1978;40:1402–1407.

Pure Mitral Regurgitation Associated with a Malfunctioning Congenitally Bicuspid Aortic Valve Necessitating Combined Mitral and Aortic Valve Replacement

Daniel J. Fernicola, MD,* and William C. Roberts, MD†

Some patients with clinically significant aortic valve dysfunction have associated pure mitral regurgitation (no element of mitral stenosis), but usually the mitral regurgitation is of minimal or mild degree. On occasion, however, the degree of pure mitral regurgitation associated with clinically significant aortic valve dysfunction is considerable (i.e., severe enough to result in associated mitral valve repair or replacement at the time of aortic valve replacement). In the present study, we sought to determine the etiology of pure mitral regurgitation in a group of patients who had aortic valve replacement because of a dysfunctioning congenitally bicuspid aortic valve and simultaneous mitral valve replacement because of associated mitral regurgitation.

From the Pathology Branch, National Heart, Lung, and Blood Institute, National Institutes of Health, Bethesda, Maryland. Manuscript received January 4, 1994; revised manuscript received and accepted March 21, 1994.

*Division of Cardiology, Department of Medicine, Georgetown University, Washington, D.C. 20058.
†Baylor Cardiovascular Institute, Baylor University Medical Center, 3500 Gaston Avenue, Dallas, Texas 75246.

The surgical files of the Pathology Branch, National Heart, Lung, and Blood Institute, were reviewed to identify patients who had simultaneous replacement of both native mitral and aortic valves. A total of 115 cases were identified. Of them, 103 patients (90%) had 3-cuspid aortic valves, and 12 (10%) had congenitally bicuspid aortic valves. Of the latter 12 patients, 1 had associated congenital mitral stenosis and was therefore excluded from this study.[1] The other 11 patients with congenitally bicuspid aortic valves had associated pure mitral regurgitation. The 11 operatively excised congenitally bicuspid aortic valves and the simultaneously excised mitral valves were retrieved and reexamined. Certain clinical and cardiac morphologic features in each of the 11 patients are tabulated in Table I and illustrated in Figures 1 to 8.

All 11 patients were men, aged 25 to 77 years (mean 56). Four (cases 1 to 4, Table I) had pure aortic regurgitation and their mean age was younger than that of the 7 patients (cases 5 to 11, Table I) with some degree of aortic valve stenosis (with or without associated aortic regurgitation) (45 vs 63 years). Of the 7 patients with aortic stenosis, 6 had cardiac catheterization, and their

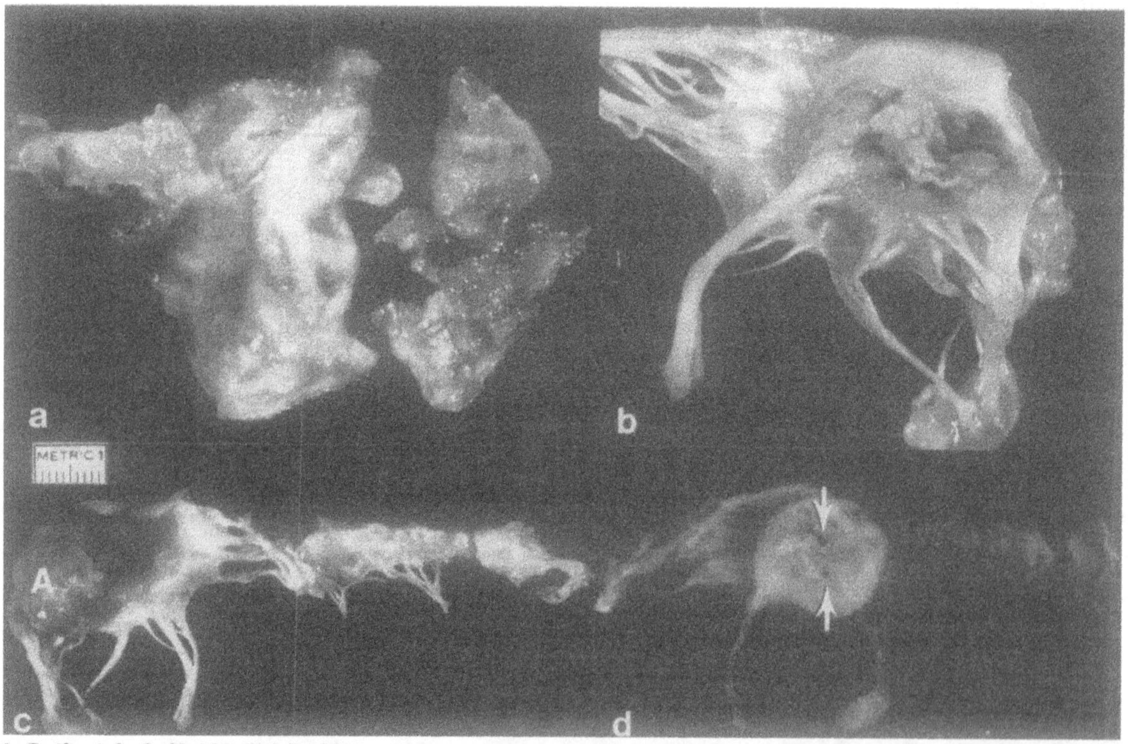

FIGURE 1. Patient 1. G. H. (GT #83-S-1910), a 25-year-old man, developed signs and symptoms of *Streptococcus bovis* endocarditis 4 months before valve replacement. Later he developed acute pulmonary edema due to severe aortic and mitral regurgitation. Both native left-sided cardiac valves were replaced with Carpentier-Edwards bioprostheses. *a*, excised aortic valve. Infective material is located on both cusps. *b*, ventricular aspect of anterior mitral leaflet. Infective material fills an aneurysm of the leaflet. *c*, opened mitral valve showing both leaflets. The large aneurysm (A) bulges toward the left atrium. *d*, radiograph of the mitral valve showing 2 perforations *(arrows)* in the aneurysm.

peak systolic pressure gradient ranged from 10 to 130 mm Hg (average 60). All 11 patients had pulmonary hypertension, with peak systolic pressures ranging from 37 to 90 mm Hg (average 64). Ten of the 11 patients had elevated mean pulmonary artery wedge pressures ranging from 24 to 35 mm Hg (average 29). The pulmonary artery V wave was >35 mm Hg in 7 of the 8 patients in whom this datum was available. The left ventricular angiogram in 8 patients indicated that the mitral regurgitation was 4+/4+ in 3, 3+/4+ in 3, and 2+/4+ in 2. In 4 patients with pure aortic regurgitation, aortic root angiogram indicated the regurgitation to be either 3+/4+ or 4+/4+. The left ventricular cavity was dilated, either by echocardiogram or left ventriculogram, in 9 of the 10 patients in whom either of these procedures

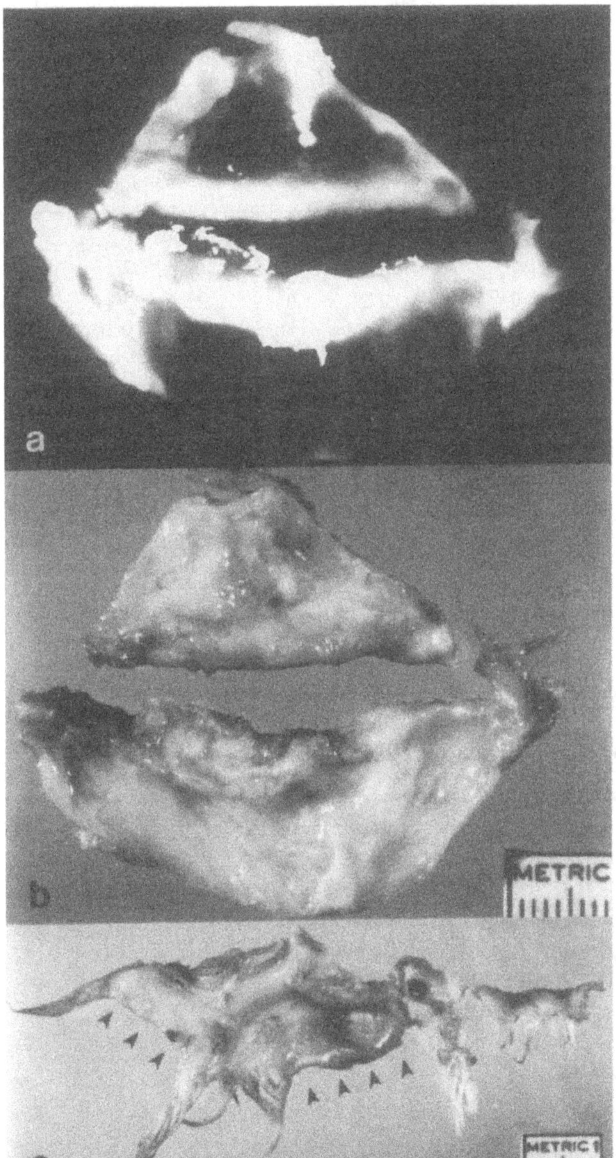

FIGURE 2. Patient 2. A. L. (NIH #S84-105), a 48-year-old man, had aortic regurgitation noted at age 38 years. He developed active infective endocarditis at age 44. A second episode of active infective endocarditis occurred 4 months before valve replacement. Within 3 months, the patient went from New York Heart Association functional class II to functional class IV. *a,* radiograph of the excised aortic valve showing small calcific deposits. *b,* excised aortic valve. The 2 cusps are of unequal size. *c,* excised mitral valve. Most chordae tendineae to the anterior mitral leaflet are ruptured (missing) *(arrowheads).*

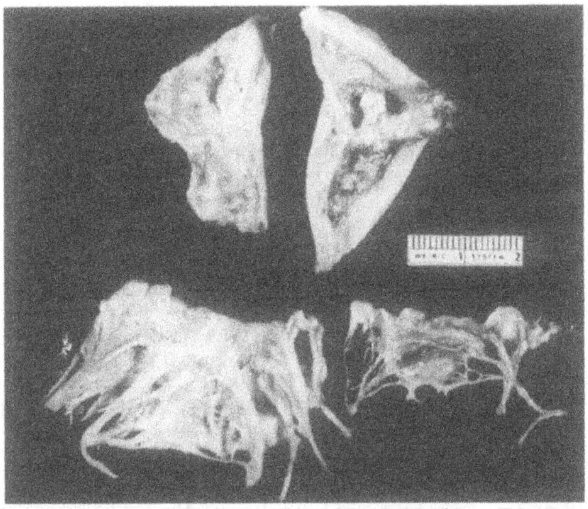

FIGURE 3. Patient 3. D. U. (NIH #S72-4111), a 51-year-old man, was first noted to have a precordial murmur at age 23 years. Symptoms began at age 50 years, approximately 1 year before valve replacement. The excised aortic valve *(top)* is diffusely thickened with a focal calcific deposit limited to the raphe. The excised mitral valve leaflets *(bottom)* are essentially normal.

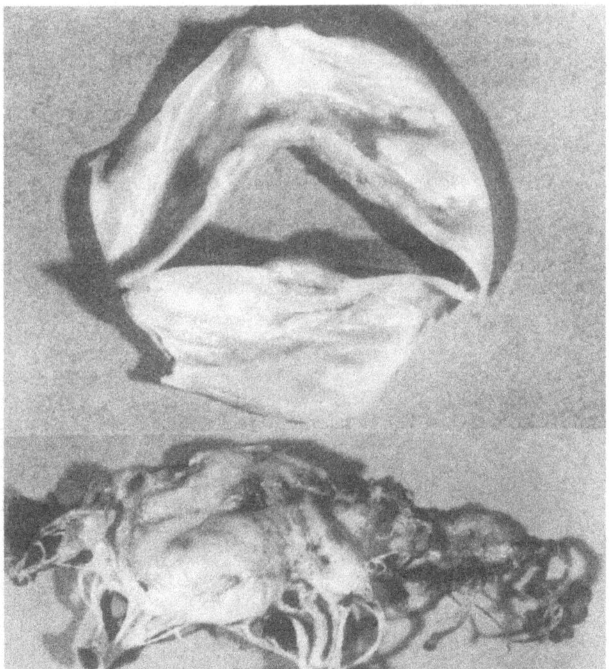

FIGURE 4. Patient 4. M. W. (NIH #S70-3100), a 55-year-old man, was noted to have a murmur of aortic regurgitation at the age of 47. The patient remained asymptomatic until 6 weeks before surgery when he developed acute pulmonary edema. The excised aortic valve *(top)* is mildly and diffusely fibrotic and purely regurgitant. The anterior leaflet of the mitral valve *(bottom)* is greatly thickened by fibrous tissue. The chordae tendineae to the anterior mitral leaflet are thickened by fibrous tissue and are very short. The commissure between the anterior and posterior leaflets is abnormal but not fused.

TABLE I Clinical and Morphologic Features of 11 Men with a Malfunctioning Bicuspid Aortic Valve and Associated Pure Mitral Regurgitation and Operative Excision of Both Valves

Case No.	Age at operation (years)	Interval (days) CC to VR	Pressures (mm Hg) RV (s/d)	PA (s/d)	PAW Mean	PAW V Wave	LV (s/d)	SA (s/d)	LV-SA psg	Angiogram MR (1+−4+)	Angiogram AR (1+−4+)	No. CA >50%
1	25	1	—	50/20	25	—	120/30	120/60	0	2+	4+	—
2	48	30	50/12	45/24	29	41	100/35	110/45	0	3+	4+	0
3	51	4	80/10	80/35	30	65	125/22	125/55	0	3+	3+	—
4	55	21	65/10	65/25	25	65	120/24	120/55	0	4+	4+	—
5	52	30	56/10	55/30	30	36	120/25	110/65	10	2+**	2+	0
6	54	5	70/11	70/30	30	—	220/30	110/60	100	—	—	—
7	56	—	38/11	37/15	24	—	145/10	95/65	50	4+	0	0
8	58	4	—	70/25	35	45	—	118/50	—	—	—	1
9	71	14	90/4	90/40	35	38	210/20	90/60	130	—	—	0
10	71	—	80/15	80/25	10	16	140/16	100/70	40	4+	0	0
11	77	18	44/12	44/19	25	41	126/12	99/57	27	3+	—	3§§

Case No.	Cavity Size (mm) by Echocardiogram LV_s	LV_d	LA	Year of VR	Prosthesis in AV Position Type	Size	Prosthesis in MV Position Type	Size	Calcium (0−4+) AV	MV	BA-DM Length (cm) AML	PML	Etiology of MR IE	MVP	Ruptured MV CT
1	—		—	1983	CE	25	CE	29	0	0	1.4	0.7	+ (A)	0	0
2	51	75	45	1984	SE	24A*	SE	30M†	1+	0	2	—	+ (H)	0	+
3	—‡		—	1972	SE	27A§	SE	32M‖	1+	0	2	1.5	0	0	0
4	—‡		—	1970	SE	26A¶	SE	30M†	0	1+	2.5	1.0	+ (H)	0	0
5	60	65	53	1986	SE	24A*	SE	30M†	3+	1+	1.4	—	0††	0††	0††
6	—		33	1979	Ha	21	Ha	31	4+	0	2.2	1.7	0	0	0††
7	42	61	63	1989	SJM	21	SJM	29	2+	1+	1.8	—	+ (H)††	0††	0
8	62	69	56	1980	SE	24A*	SE	32M‖	3+	0	2.0	1.0	0	0	0
9	60	70	56	1983	Ha	21	Ha	29	4+	0	2.2	1.0	+ (H)	0	+
10	34	52	58	1991	MH	25	MH	31	3+	1+	2	2	0	+	+
11	—	58	40	1992	CE	23	CE	31	2+	1+	2	—	0	0	0

*Old terminology is 10A.
†Old terminology is 3M.
‡Left ventricle very large by left ventricular angiogram.
§Old terminology is 12A.
‖Old terminology is 4M.
¶Old terminology is 11A.
**No mitral regurgitation, however, by Doppler echocardiogram.
††Only the anterior mitral leaflet excised at operation.
§§Coronary artery bypass surgery performed at time of valve replacement.
A = active; AML = anterior mitral leaflet; AR = aortic regurgitation (by aortic root cineangiogram); AV = aortic valve; BA = basal attachment; CA = coronary artery; CC = cardiac catheterization; CE = Carpentier-Edwards bioprosthesis; CT = chordae tendineae; DM = distal margin; H = healed; Ha = Hancock bioprosthesis; IE = infective endocarditis; LA = left atrium; LV = left ventricle; LV_s = left ventricular (cavity size in systole); LV_d = left ventricular (cavity size in diastole); MH = Medtronic-Hall mechanical prosthesis; MR = mitral regurgitation (by left ventriculogram); MV = mitral valve; MVP = mitral valve prolapse; PA = pulmonary artery; PAW = pulmonary artery wedge; PML = posterior mitral leaflet; psg = peak systolic gradient; RV = right ventricle; SA = systemic artery; SE = Starr-Edwards mechanical prosthesis; s/d = peak systole/end-diastole; SJM = Saint Jude mechanical prosthesis; VR = valve replacement.

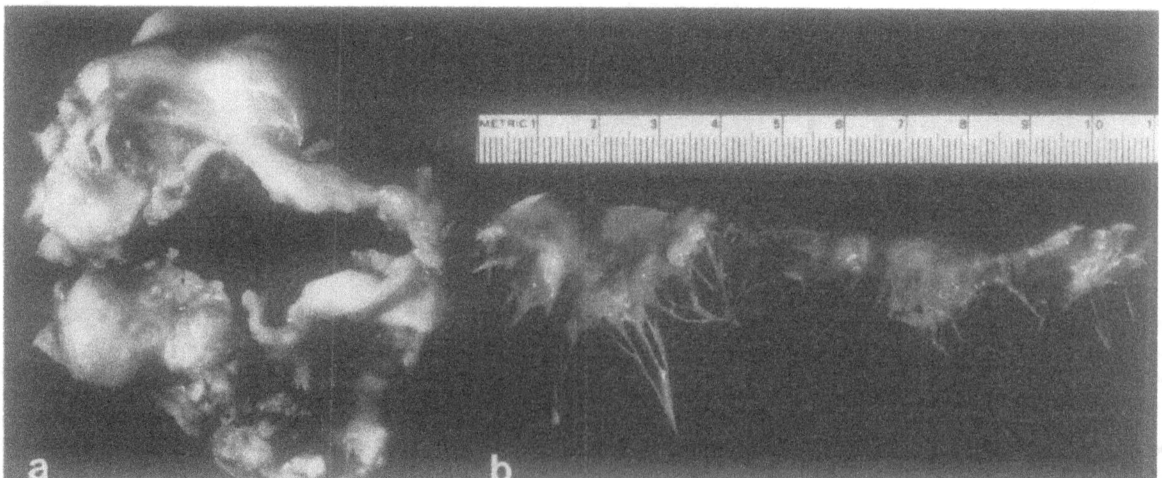

FIGURE 5. Patient 6. B. O. (NIH #S79-142) was a 54-year-old man in whom a precordial murmur was noted at age 43 years. At age 51, the peak systolic pressure gradient between left ventricle and aorta was 65 mm Hg. Over the next 2 years, congestive heart failure progressed. At the time of valve replacement, the peak systolic gradient across the aortic valve was 100 mm Hg. The patient died 12 days after operation from sepsis. *a*, excised heavily calcified aortic valve. *b*, opened mitral valve. Some segments of the posterior mitral leaflet are elongated.

was performed; the 1 patient (case 1, Table I) without cavity dilation had aortic regurgitation secondary to active infective endocarditis of short duration. The 1 patient who did not have either an echocardiogram or a left ventriculogram had an ejection fraction of 20%, and chest radiogram showed a large cardiac silhouette.

Infective endocarditis, either active (case 1) or healed (cases 2, 4, 7, and 9), was the etiology of the mitral regurgitation in 5 patients (45%). In 2 of the 4 patients with healed infective endocarditis, several chordae tendineae in each had ruptured (Figures 2 and 7). In the other 2 patients the diagnosis of infective endocarditis was made by a history of positive blood cultures. In 1 patient (case 4) the excised anterior mitral leaflet was diffusely thickened by fibrous tissue without calcific deposits, the attached chordae tendineae were thickened and short, and the posterior mitral leaflet was smaller than expected. The etiology of this distorted anatomy is uncertain, but infective endocarditis that healed and was not diagnosed clinically may have caused the local fibrous thickening. In 1 patient mitral valve prolapse was present and some chordae tendineae from the posterior mitral leaflet had ruptured. In 4 patients the excised mitral leaflets and chordae tendineae were anatomically normal, but the left ventricular cavities were very dilated.

In the 4 patients with purely regurgitant aortic valves, calcific deposits, determined by x-ray of the excised valves, were either absent or minute. In each of the 7 stenotic aortic valves, large calcific deposits were present. Of the 11 excised mitral valves, 5 had minute calcific deposits, confined to the annular region in 4.

Although most persons with a congenitally bicuspid aortic valve have a normally functioning mitral valve, the present study indicates that associated mitral regurgitation not only may occur, but also may be severe enough to warrant mitral valve replacement at the time of aortic valve replacement. It is well appreciated that the congenitally bicuspid aortic valve has a high propensity to be the site of infective endocarditis.[1–12] Furthermore, when active endocarditis of the aortic valve leads to aortic regurgitation, vegetations on the aortic valve may be dislodged retrogradely by the regurgitant jet and the vegetations may adhere to mitral chordae tendineae causing their rupture, or to the anterior mitral leaflet causing it to perforate or to become aneurysmal. The latter scenario appears to have been responsible for the mitral regurgitation in 5, and possibly 6, of the 11 patients in the present study.

Mitral valve prolapse without superimposed infective endocarditis was responsible for the mitral regurgitation

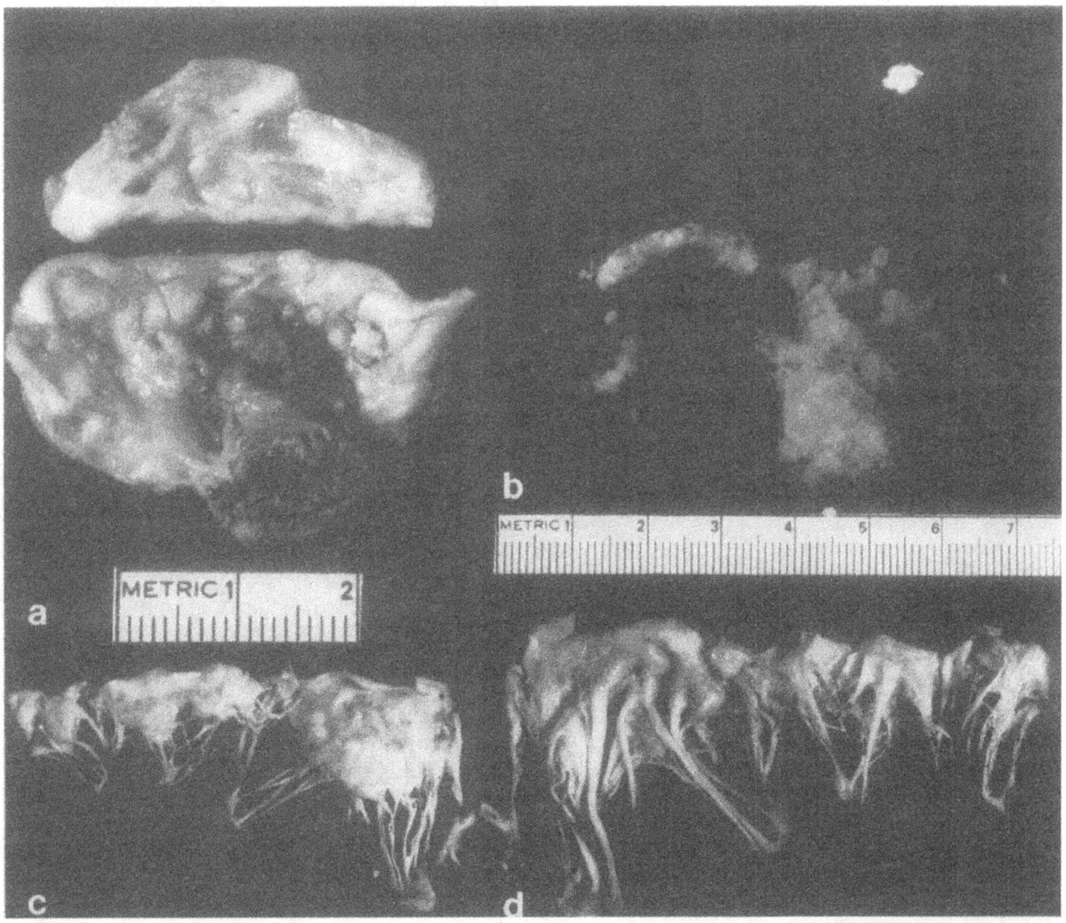

FIGURE 6. Patient 8. J. M. (NIH #S80-75), a 58-year-old man, had a precordial murmur since at least age 19 years. He remained asymptomatic until age 51 when he had an acute myocardial infarction. He developed acute pulmonary edema 2 weeks before valve replacement. *a*, excised aortic valve. *b*, radiograph of the aortic valve. The cusps are of different sizes and calcium is virtually limited to the largest cusp. *c and d*, excised mitral valve. Atrial *(c)* and ventricular *(d)* views of the excised mitral leaflets. Both leaflets are moderately thickened. Portions of the posterior leaflet are elongated.

in only 1 patient.[13–16] It is surprising that mitral valve prolapse (unassociated with infective endocarditis) is not seen more often in patients with congenitally bicuspid aortic valves, because mitral valve prolapse may occur in as many as 5% of the adult population, and the bicuspid aortic valve in as many as 1% of the population.[17] In 4 patients, the mitral leaflets and chordae tendineae were normal but the mitral annulae were quite dilated. Today, these latter 4 patients would probably have had mitral annuloplasty rather than replacement.

Although all 11 patients had pure mitral regurgitation, the type of aortic valve dysfunction was variable. Four patients had pure aortic regurgitation, in 3 due to superimposed infective endocarditis or at least worsened by the endocarditis, and in 1 patient due entirely to the bicuspid condition of the valve. Seven patients had stenotic aortic valves. Of the 4 purely regurgitant aortic valves, 3 had superimposed infective endocarditis; of the 7 stenotic aortic valves, 2 had superimposed infective endocarditis.

In summary, some patients with severely dysfunctioning congenitally bicuspid aortic valves develop pure mitral regurgitation severe enough to warrant mitral valve replacement or repair. The most common cause of the associated mitral regurgitation is leaflet and chordal damage from infective endocarditis.

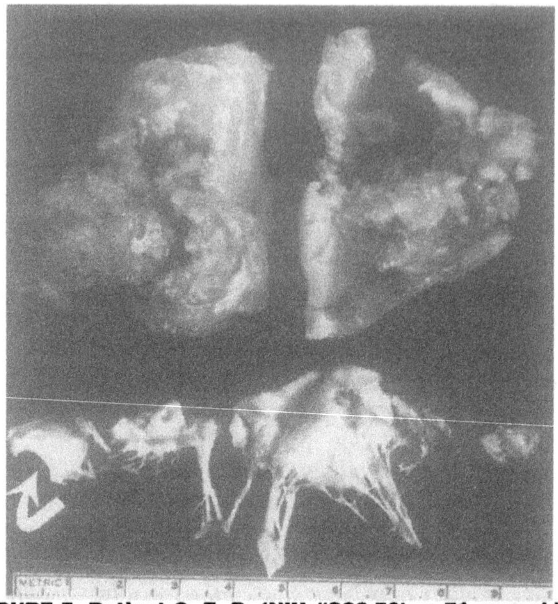

FIGURE 7. Patient 9. E. P. (NIH #S83-56), a 71-year-old man who developed congestive heart failure 9 months before valve replacement. Four months before valve replacement, he was treated with ampicillin for bronchitis. *Top*, excised aortic valve showing heavy calcific deposits. *Bottom*, excised mitral valve. A portion of posterior leaflet is indented *(arrow)* with missing chordae tendineae at this site. These latter findings are consistent with healed infective endocarditis.

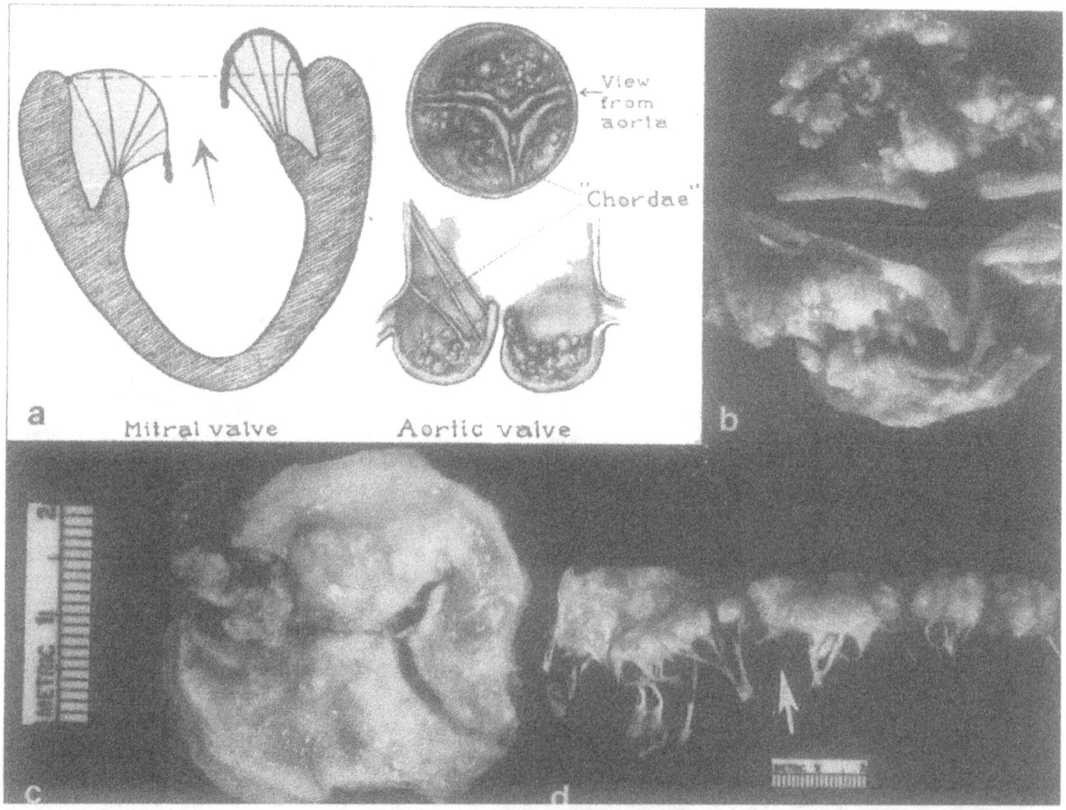

FIGURE 8. Patient 10. A. S. (GT #91S-6903), a 71-year-old man, developed acute pulmonary edema and severe mitral regurgitation 2 weeks before valve replacement. The patient had been in New York Heart Association functional class II before the development of severe mitral regurgitation. *a*, illustration of the mitral and aortic valves as they probably appeared in life. "Chordae" were present from the raphe of the aortic valve cusps to the wall of the aorta. *b*, excised aortic valve from the aortic aspect. *c*, aortic valve from the ventricular side. *d*, excised mitral valve showing "missing" chordae tendineae *(arrows)*. An adjacent portion of posterior leaflet is hooded.

1. Roberts WC. The congenitally bicuspid aortic valve. A study of 85 autopsy cases. *Am J Cardiol* 1970;26:72–83.

2. Arnett EN, Roberts WC. Valve ring abscess in active infective endocarditis. Frequency, location, and clues to clinical diagnosis from the study of 95 necropsy patients. *Circulation* 1976;54:140–145.

3. Arnett EN, Roberts WC. Prosthetic valve endocarditis. Clinicopathologic analysis of 22 necropsy patients with comparison of observations in 74 necropsy patients with active infective endocarditis involving natural left-sided cardiac valves. *Am J Cardiol* 1976;38:281–292.

4. Arnett EN, Roberts WC. Active infective endocarditis: a clinicopathology analysis of 137 necropsy patients. *Curr Probl Cardiol* 1976;1:1–76.

5. Roberts WC, Buchbinger NA. Healed left-sided infective endocarditis: a clinicopathologic study of 59 patients. *Am J Cardiol* 1977:72:757–761.

6. Roberts WC, Morrow AG, McIntosh CL, Jones M, Epstein SE. Congenitally bicuspid aortic valve causing severe, pure aortic regurgitation without superimposed infective endocarditis. Analysis of 13 patients requiring aortic valve replacement. *Am J Cardiol* 1981;47:206–209.

7. Roberts WC, McIntosh CL, Wallace RB. Aortic valve perforation with calcific aortic valve stenosis and without infective endocarditis or significant aortic regurgitation. *Am J Cardiol* 1987;59:476–478.

8. Dressler FA, Roberts WC. Infective endocarditis in opiate addicts: analysis of 80 cases studied at necropsy. *Am J Cardiol* 1989;63:1240–1257.

9. Roberts WC. Living with a congenitally bicuspid aortic valve. *Am J Cardiol* 1989;64:1408–1409.

10. Brown PS Jr, Roberts CS, McIntosh CL, Roberts WC, Clark RE. Combined obstructive hypertrophic cardiomyopathy and stenotic congenitally bicuspid aortic valve. *Am J Cardiol* 1990;66:1273–1275.

11. Roberts WC. Morphologic aspects of cardiac valve dysfunction. *Am Heart J* 1992:123:1610–1632.

12. Roberts WC, Oluwole BO, Fernicola DJ. Comparison of active infective endocarditis involving a previously stenotic versus a previously nonstenotic aortic valve. *Am J Cardiol* 1993;71:1082–1088.

13. Rippe JM, Slors LJ, Angoff G, Alpert JS. Mitral valve prolapse in adults with congenital heart disease. *Am Heart J* 1979;97:561–573.

14. Chisholm JC. Mitral valve prolapse syndrome associated with congenital bicuspid aortic valve. *JAMA* 1981;73:921–923.

15. Roberts WC, McIntosh CL, Wallace RB. Mechanisms of severe mitral regurgitation in mitral valve prolapse determined from analysis of operatively excised valves. *Am Heart J* 1987;113:1316–1323.

16. Dollar AL, Roberts WC. Morphologic comparison of patients with mitral valve prolapse who died suddenly with patients who died from severe valvular dysfunction or other conditions. *J Am Coll Cardiol* 1991;17:921–931.

17. Roberts WC. The 2 most common congenital heart diseases. *Am J Cardiol* 1984;53:1198.

Comparison of Age, Gender, Number of Aortic Valve Cusps, Concomitant Coronary Artery Bypass Grafting, and Magnitude of Left Ventricular–Systemic Arterial Peak Systolic Gradient in Adults Having Aortic Valve Replacement for Isolated Aortic Valve Stenosis

Phillip J. Stephan, BS, A. Carl Henry III, MD, Robert F. Hebeler, Jr., MD, Lonnie Whiddon, MD, and William C. Roberts, MD

Correlation of the structure of the operatively excised aortic valve with various clinical variables has received relatively little attention. This report describes certain observations in 115 patients aged >30 years (mean age 70) who had aortic valve replacement for aortic valve stenosis unassociated with mitral valve dysfunction. The operatively excised aortic valve was congenitally unicuspid in 3 patients (3%), congenitally bicuspid in 54 patients (47%), tricuspid in 57 patients (50%), and of uncertain structure in 1. Of the 87 patients (76%) aged ≥65 years (Medicare population), 36 (41%) had congenitally malformed valves (bicuspid in each), and of the 28 patients (24%) aged <65 years, 21 (75%) had congenitally malformed valves. A higher percentage of patients with congenitally malformed valves had peak systolic pressure gradients across the valve >50 mm Hg than did patients with tricuspid valves (57% vs 43%). Concomitant coronary artery bypass grafting (CABG) was performed in 52 patients (45%) (34 men and 18 women), and they had average peak systolic pressure gradients across the valve significantly lower than patients without coronary bypass (46 vs 64 mm Hg): 39% of the 57 patients with congenitally malformed valves and 53% of the 57 patients with tricuspid valves had concomitant coronary bypass (insignificant difference). Thus, in a relatively older population of 115 patients having aortic valve replacement for isolated aortic valve stenosis, with or without associated aortic regurgitation, one half had congenitally malformed valves (either unicuspid or bicuspid valves) and one half had tricuspid valves. Patients having concomitant CABG had significantly smaller gradients across the stenotic valves than those who had no CABG.

(Am J Cardiol 1997;79:166–172)

Of the life-threatening cardiovascular conditions in the Western world, systemic hypertension and atherosclerosis are the most common and aortic valve stenosis is the third most common. The first 2 receive far more attention in medical publications — and rightfully so — than does the third. Among cardiac operations, aortic valve replacement is second only to coronary artery bypass grafting (CABG). Morphologic features of aortic valve stenosis have been a focus of interest at necropsy for about 60 years.[1–17] Opportunity to study the aortic valve after operative excision has been available for 36 years, but only in recent years have features of the operatively excised aortic valve received much attention.[18–26] The present study again examines aortic valve structure in operatively excised aortic valves in isolated aortic valve stenosis (with or without associated aortic regurgitation), but in contrast to previous studies[18–26] this article also correlates the valvular structure to 5 clinical variables (those mentioned in the title).

From the Baylor Cardiovascular Institute, Baylor University Medical Center, Dallas, Texas. Dr. Stephan is a Sophomore Medical Student, University of Texas Southwestern Medical School, Dallas, Texas. Dr. Stephan was supported by the Chilton Foundation. Manuscript received June 5, 1996; revised manuscript received and accepted October 10, 1996.

Address reprint requests to: William C. Roberts, MD, Baylor Cardiovascular Institute, Baylor University Medical Center, 3500 Gaston Avenue, Dallas, Texas 75246.

METHODS

Patients: A list was obtained from the Baylor University Medical Center patient database of patients having aortic valve replacement from January 1993 through July 1995. During this period, 169 patients underwent replacement of a malfunctioning *native* aortic valve, and 12 underwent replacement of a malfunctioning *prosthetic* or *bioprosthetic* valve in the aortic valve position. The latter 12 patients were eliminated from further study. Of the other 169 patients, 19 were eliminated from further analysis because both mitral and aortic valves were replaced in each of them. Of the remaining 150 patients, 32 had aortic valve replacement because of pure aortic regurgitation (no element of aortic valve stenosis) and they too were eliminated from further analysis. Of the remaining 118 patients, 3 were eliminated from

TABLE I Isolated Aortic Valve Stenosis: Comparison of Five Variables in Patients <65 Years Versus ≥65 Years of Age

Variable	Totals (n = 115)	Age <65 Years (n = 28)	Age ≥65 Years (n = 87)	p Value
1. Men/women	65/50	18/10	47/40	0.39
2. Number of aortic valve cusps				
1	3 } (50%)	3 } (75%)	0 } (41%)	
2	54 }	18 }	36 }	0.002
3	57 (50%)	6 (21%)	51 (59%)	0.002
Uncertain	1 (<1%)	1 (4%)	0	
3. Coronary artery bypass grafting	52 (45%)	10 (19%)	42 (81%)	0.28
4. LV-SA psg (mm Hg) Range (average)	18–133 (56)	18–107 (58)	18–133 (55)	0.70
5. Aortic valve area (cm^2) Range (mean)	0.2–1.8 (.67)	0.4–1.2 (.76)	0.2–1.8 (0.65)	0.07

LV = left ventricular; psg = peak systolic gradient; SA = systemic artery.

TABLE II Isolated Aortic Valve Stenosis: Comparison of Five Variables in Men Versus Women

Variable	Totals (n = 115)	Men (n = 65) (57%)	Women (n = 50) (43%)	p Value
1. Ages range (mean) (yr)	33–89 (70)	36–86 (68)	33–89 (71)	
≥65 years	87 (76%)	47 (72%)	40 (80%)	0.12
<65 years	28 (24%)	18 (28%)	10 (20%)	0.34
2. Number of aortic valve cusps				
1	3 (3%)	2 } (51%)	1 } (48%)	
2	54 (47%)	31 }	23 }	0.86
3	57 (49%)	31 (48%)	26 (52%)	0.65
Uncertain	1 (1%)	1 (1%)	0	
3. Coronary artery bypass	52 (45%)	34 (52%)	18 (36%)	0.08
4. LV-SA psg (mm Hg) Range (average)	18–133 (56)	21–120 (54)	18–133 (59)	0.39
5. Aortic valve area (cm^2) Range (mean)	0.2–1.8 (0.67)	0.2–1.8 (0.72)	0.3–1.2 (0.62)	<0.05

Abbreviations as in Table I.

TABLE III Isolated Aortic Valve Stenosis: Comparison of Five Variables in Patients Having Versus Patients Not Having Simultaneous Coronary Artery Bypass Grafting

		Coronary Artery Bypass Grafting		
Variable	Total (n = 115)	+ (n = 52) (45%)	0 (n = 63) (55%)	p Value
1. Age range (mean) (yr)	33–89 (70)	51–89 (72)	33–86 (68)	
≥65 years	87 (76%)	42 (81%)	45 (71%)	0.08
<65 years	28 (24%)	10 (19%)	18 (29%)	0.25
2. Men/women	65 (57%)/49 (43%)	34 (65%)/18 (35%)	31 (49%)/32 (51%)	0.08
3. Number of aortic valve cusps				
1	3 (3%)	1 } (42%)	2 } (55%)	
2	54 (47%)	21 }	33 }	0.20
3	57 (49%)	30 (58%)	27 (43%)	0.11
Uncertain	1 (1%)	0	1 (2%)	
4. LV-SA psg (mm Hg) Range (mean)	18–133 (56)	18–108 (46)	18–133 (64)	0.001
5. Aortic valve area (cm^2) Range (mean)	0.2–1.8 (0.67)	0.3–1.4 (0.70)	0.2–1.8 (0.65)	0.38

Abbreviations as in Tables I.

further analysis because 2 of them had aortic valvulotomy during childhood and 1 was eliminated because of associated mitral stenosis (a mitral commissurotomy had been performed at the time of aortic valve replacement). The remaining 115 patients are the subjects of the present analysis. In summary, each of these 115 study patients had (1) aortic valve stenosis (with left ventricular–aortic peak systolic pressure gradients ranging from 18 to 133 mm Hg); (2) none had associated mitral stenosis; (3) none had a concomitant or previous mitral valve operation; (4) none had a previous aortic valve opera-

TABLE IV Isolated Aortic Valve Stenosis: Comparison of Five Variables in Patients With Left Ventricular to Systemic Artery Peak Systolic Pressure Gradients ≤50 mm Hg Versus >50 mm Hg

Variable	Totals (n = 97)	LV–SA Peak Systolic Gradient (mm Hg) ≤50 (n = 48)	>50 (n = 49)	p Value
1. Age range (mean) (yr)	3–89 (69)	33–86 (69)	36–89 (70)	
≥65 years	74 (76%)	38 (79%)	36 (73%)	0.83
<65 years	23 (24%)	10 (21%)	13 (27%)	0.51
2. Men/women	52 (54%)–45 (46%)	29 (60%)/19 (40%)	23 (47%)/26 (53%)	0.18
3. Number aortic valve cusps				
1	3 (3%)	2} (37%)	1} (57%)	
2	43 (44%)	16}	27}	0.031
3	51 (53%)	30 (63%)	21 (43%)	0.053
4. Coronary artery bypass	44 (45%)	30 (63%)	14 (29%)	0.0008
5. Aortic valve area (cm^2) Range (mean)	0.30–1.40 (0.67)	0.3–1.4 (0.76)	0.2–1.8 (0.57)	0.0001

Abbreviations as in Table I.

TABLE V Isolated Aortic Valve Stenosis: Comparison of Five Variables in Patients with Unicuspid and Bicuspid Versus Tricuspid Aortic Valves

Variable	Totals (n = 114)	Unicuspid (3) and Bicuspid Valves (54) (n = 57)	Tricuspid Valve (n = 57)	p Value
1. Age range (mean) (yr)	33–89 (71)	33–89 (67)	58–86 (73)	
≥65 years	87 (76%)	36 (63%)	51 (89%)	0.001
<65 years	27 (23%)	21 (37%)	6 (11%)	0.0009
2. Men/women	62 (56%)/50 (44%)	33 (58%)/24 (42%)	31 (54%)/26 (46%)	0.71
3. Coronary artery bypass	52 (46%)	22 (39%)	30 (53%)	0.13
4. LV–SA psg (mm Hg) Range (average)	18–133 (56)	20–133 (59)	18–125 (53)	0.22
5. Aortic valve area (cm^2) Range (mean)	0.2–1.8 (.67)	0.3–1.2 (0.64)	0.2–1.8 (0.70)	0.27

Abbreviations as in Table I.

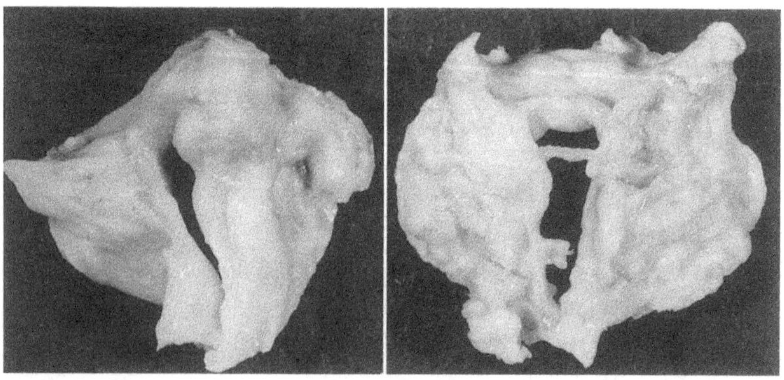

FIGURE 1. Operatively excised congenitally unicuspid aortic valves from 2 patients. *Left,* a 63-year-old man whose peak systolic gradient across the valve was 44 mm Hg. The coronary arteries were angiographically normal. *Right,* a 51-year-old man with a pressure gradient across the valve of 107 mm Hg. He had concomitant coronary artery bypass grafting.

tion; (5) all were aged >30 years at the time of aortic valve replacement; and (6) none had a purely regurgitant aortic valve.

Hemodynamic and angiographic data were sought from the Baylor Heart's Computer Center in each of the 115 study patients with aortic stenosis and in each of the 32 patients with pure aortic regurgitation (all 32 were subsequently eliminated from this analysis). Of the 115 study patients with aortic stenosis, left-sided cardiac catheterization data were available in 108; the medical records were reviewed in the other 7 patients to see if cardiac catheterization had been performed before the patient came to Baylor University Medical Center. Some left-sided hemodynamic data were available in 111 patients (97%); in 1 of the 4 patients without available left-sided cardiac catheterization data, Doppler echocardiogram disclosed the left ventricular–aortic peak systolic pressure gradient to be 120 mm Hg and the aortic valve area to be 0.5 cm^2. Each of the 3 patients without available hemodynamic data had had cardiac catheterization elsewhere and were referred to Baylor University Medical Center because of documented aortic stenosis.

Coronary angiography was performed in 112 (97%) of the 115 patients, and the presence of narrowing of >50% in diameter was recorded in each of the 3 major coronary systems (right, left anterior descending, and left circumflex). Additionally, 75 patients (65%) had left ventricular angiograms and 53 patients (46%), aortic "root" angiograms.

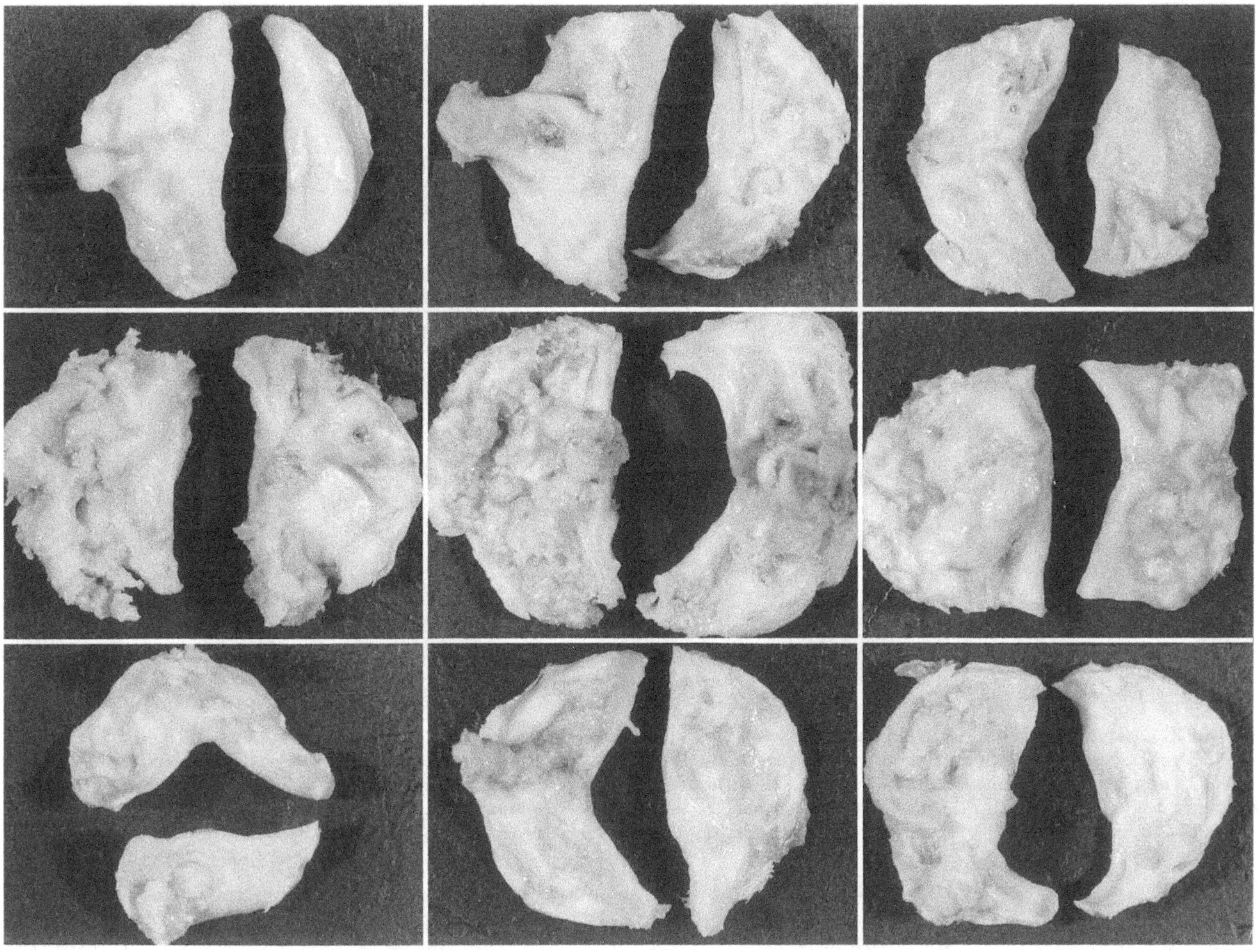

FIGURE 2. Operatively excised congenitally bicuspid aortic valves from 6 patients. The *top 2 rows* illustrate valves from patients who did not have concomitant coronary bypass grafting. Their ages *(left to right)* at the time of valve replacement were 33, 66, 69, 51, 74, and 74, respectively, and the peak systolic pressure gradients across the valves were 24, 38, 41, 57, 120, and 133 mm Hg, respectively. Each of the 3 patients whose valves are shown in the *bottom row* had concomitant coronary bypass grafting. Their ages *(left to right)* were 78, 65, and 72 years, respectively, and the peak pressure gradients were 23, 51, and 53 mm Hg, respectively.

The patients' age and gender at the time of aortic valve replacement was obtained from Baylor's central computer database, and the name of the operating surgeon from the cardiovascular surgery database. Although 14 surgeons performed aortic valve replacements in the 115 patients, 39 (34%) were performed by A.C.H. III, 22 (19%) by R.F.H., Jr., 12 (10%) by L.W., and the remaining 11 surgeons performed 1 to 8 valve replacements (mean 4) during the 31 months of this study.

The structure of the operatively excised aortic valve was determined from its examination by one of us (W.C.R.) in 98 (85%) of the 115 patients. In the other 17 patients the structure was determined from examination of the operative report and also the Pathology Department's surgical report. Fortunately, nearly all of the valves had been excised intact or nearly so, so the judgment as to the number of cusps present usually was not difficult.

Statistics: For each continuous variable and median and mean ± SD, and for each noncontinuous variable, frequency and percentage were reported. Student's *t* test was used to calculate the significance of the difference between variables. Differences were considered significant at $p < 0.05$.

RESULTS

Results of analysis of 5 variables are summarized in Tables I to V. One significant difference was noted when comparing the 28 patients aged <65 years with the 87 patients aged ≥65 years (Table I): the younger group had a larger percentage of congenitally malformed valves (75% vs 41%) and a smaller percentage of 3-cuspid aortic valves (21% vs 59%). The only significant difference among the 5 variables in the 65 men (57%) and in the 50 women (43%) was a larger aortic valve area in men than women (0.72 cm^2 vs 0.62 cm^2) (Table II). When we compared the 52 patients (45%) having CABG with the 63 patients (55%) not having CABG, the latter group had smaller average left ventricular to systemic arterial peak systolic pressure gradients (46 vs 64 mm Hg, respectively) (Table III). The 48 patients (49%) with left ventricular–systemic arterial pressure gradients ≤50 mm Hg compared with the 49 patients (51%) with gradients >50 mm Hg were more likely to have

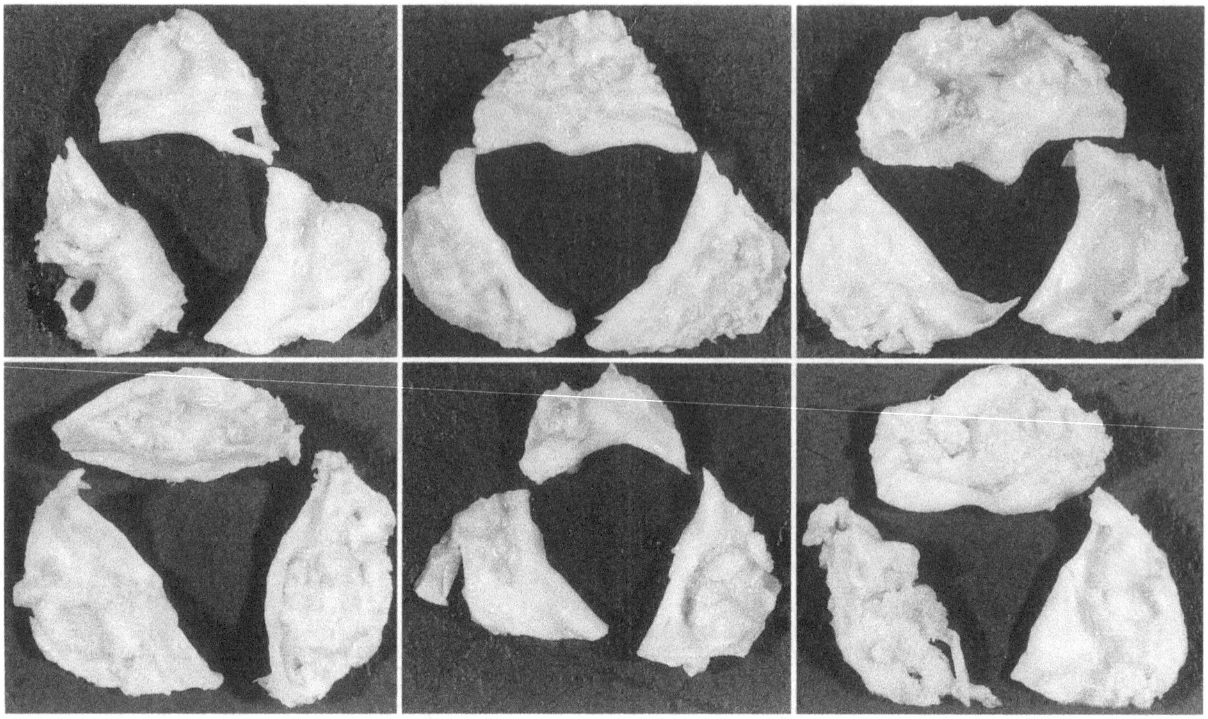

FIGURE 3. Operatively excised 3-cuspid aortic valves in 6 patients. The 3 on the *top row (left to right)* were from women aged 64, 79, and 73 years, respectively, at the time of valve replacement, and the peak systolic pressure gradients across the valve were 96, 120, and 125 mm Hg, respectively. None had concomitant coronary artery bypass grafting. The 3 valves in the *bottom row* were from 2 men and 1 woman aged 70, 71, and 79 years, respectively, and the peak systolic pressure gradients across the valves *(left to right)* were 28, 40, and 69 mm Hg, respectively. Each of these 3 patients had concomitant coronary artery bypass grafting.

tricuspid aortic valves (63% vs 43%) and less likely to have unicuspid or bicuspid valves (37% vs 57%), and were more likely to have concomitant CABG (63% vs 29%) and higher aortic valve areas (0.76 cm^2 vs 0.58 cm^2) (Table IV). The 57 patients (50%) with congenitally unicuspid (3 patients) or bicuspid (54 patients) aortic valves compared with the 57 patients (50%) with tricuspid aortic valves were significantly younger (mean age 68 vs 73 years, respectively), fewer were aged ≥65 years (63% vs 89%) and more were aged <65 years (37% vs 11%).

DISCUSSION

The major findings in this study could be the following: aortic valve stenosis when unassociated with mitral stenosis or significant mitral regurgitation is primarily a condition affecting older persons: (76% of the 115 patients were aged ≥65 years [the Medicare population]); 50% had congenitally malformed valves, including 36 (41%) of the 87 patients aged ≥65 years and 21 (75%) of the 28 patients aged <65 years; stenotic 3-cuspid aortic valves were observed primarily in patients aged ≥65 years (51 [89%] of 57 patients). Nearly half (45%) of the 115 patients had CABG at the time of aortic valve replacement. Of the latter 52 patients, 41 (81%) were aged ≥65 years, including 34 (65%) men and 18 (35%) women. In contrast, of the 63 patients not having concomitant CABG, 50% were men and 50% were women. The magnitude of the aortic stenosis was significantly less in the 52 patients having CABG than in the 63 patients not having concomitant CABG (average peak systolic gradient 46 vs 64 mm Hg). Of the 44 patients having CABG and pressure gradients available, 30 (63%) were ≤50 mm Hg (range 18 to 49) and 14 (29%) were >50 mm Hg (range 51 to 108); only 2 patients (14%) had gradients >100 mm Hg and only 4 (29%), >75 mm Hg. In contrast, of the 53 patients not having CABG but available pressure tracings, 18 (34%) had gradients ≤50 mm Hg, and 35 (66%) had gradients >50 mm Hg; 6 (17%) were >100 mm Hg and 16 (46%) were >75 mm Hg. Thus, of the 97 patients with left ventricular outflow pressure gradients available, only 4 (9%) of the 44 having CABG had gradients >50 mm Hg, whereas 35 (66%) of the 53 patients not having CABG had gradients >50 mm Hg.

One might question the indication for aortic valve replacement in the 18 patients with peak systolic pressure gradients ≤50 mm Hg and insignificant coronary arterial narrowing by angiogram. Although the peak systolic pressure gradients in these 18 patients ranged from 18 to 50 mm Hg (average 36), the aortic valve areas ranged from 0.4 to 1.2 cm^2 (mean 0.75) and the aortic valve area indexes from 0.22 to 0.74 cm^2/m^2 (mean 0.40). The estimated degree of stenosis in the operatively excised aortic valve and at necropsy appears to correlate better with the peak systolic pressure gradient across the valve than with the calculated aortic valve area. Only 3 of these 18 patients had associated significant aortic regurgitation.

It is reasonable to believe that aortic stenosis in patients aged ≥65 years and a tricuspid aortic valve is the result of atherosclerosis. The basis for this belief

TABLE VI Previously Reported Studies of Operatively Excised Stenotic Aortic Valves for Comparison With the Present Study

First Author	Year of Publication	Number of Patients	Ages (yr) Range (mean)	Number of Aortic Valve Cusps				Associated Mitral Valve Disease	Years of Valve Replacement	Authors Combined Cases of AS With Those of Pure AR	Authors Combined Cases of "Pure AS" With Those of AS Plus AR	CABG
				1	2	3	Uncertain					
1. Subramanian[19]	1984	374	21–91 (60)	21 (6%)	171 (46%)	168 (45%)	14 (3%)	42 (11%)*	1965, 1970, 1975, 1980	0	0†	—
2. Subramanian[20]	1985	213	18–85 (55)	14 (7%)	43 (20%)	152 (71%)	4 (2%)‡	98 (46%)§	1965, 1970, 1975, 1980	0	0	—
3. Peterson[21]	1985	109	"adults"	1 (1%)	53 (49%)	55 (50%)	0	—‖	1979–1983	0	+	—
4. Roberts[22]	1987	393	17–74 (–)	28 (7%)	203 (52%)	101 (26%)	61 (15%)	0	1962–1982	0	+	—
5. Passik[23]	1987	646	9–91 (67)	10 (2%)	248 (38%)	377 (58%)	11 (2%)	+¶	1081–1985	0	0†	—
6. Turri[24]	1990	348	3–86 (50)#	0	65 (19%)	283 (81%)	—	—**	1981–1987	+	+	—
7. Dare[25]	1993	178	20–92 (70)	0	59 (33%)	119 (67%)	—	—**	1990 only	+	+	—
8. Davies[26]	1996	465	31–95 (68)	7 (2%)	308 (66%)	150 (32%)	—	0	1986–1995	0	+	122 (28%)
9. Present study	1996	115	33–89 (70)	3 (3%)	54 (47%)	57 (49%)	1 (1%)	0	1993–1995	0	+	52 (45%)

* The mitral valve was stenotic (with or without associated regurgitation) in 25 and purely regurgitant in 17. In 31 of the 42 patients mitral valve replacement was performed.

† Although the authors characterized all of their 374 and 646 cases as "pure aortic stenosis" it is clear from examination of some of their photographs of excised aortic valves that the valve orifices were fixed in an open position and therefore some degree of aortic regurgitation had to be present. Furthermore, the authors stated that some patients had "mildly regurgitant valves."

‡ One patient had a quadricuspid aortic valve.

§ The mitral valve was stenotic in 72 (73%) of the 98 patients, purely regurgitant in 14 (14%), and functionally abnormal in the other 12, but the type of dysfunction was not stated. Of the 98 patients, 76, and maybe 81, had mitral valve replacement.

‖ Although the authors made no comments in their article about the mitral valve, the article's "tone" suggests that none or few of the patients had associated mitral valve disease.

¶ Number not stated. The authors included in their study "all patients" who had had aortic valve replacement at their institution in a 5-year period, so it is certain that some of their patients had associated mitral valve disease and mitral valve replacement as well.

\# Also includes ages of 254 patients with pure aortic regurgitation.

** Although the authors did not mention associated mitral valve disease, it is likely that many patients did indeed have associated mitral disease because the authors included "all" aortic valves excised during the period of the study.

AR = aortic regurgitation; AS = aortic stenosis; CABG = coronary artery bypass grafting; I = indeterminate; O = other.

resides in the observation that most of these patients have associated coronary arterial atherosclerosis and often also calcific deposits in the mitral annular region; persons with homozygous familial hypercholesterolemia with serum total cholesterol levels >800 mg/dl develop aortic stenosis usually by the time of puberty and their aortic valves are tricuspid, and persons residing in areas of the world where serum total cholesterol levels are <150 mg/dl rarely have calcific deposits in their valves and, therefore, infrequently develop aortic valve stenosis (unless there is associated rheumatic mitral disease). Of the 57 patients in the present study with 3-cuspid aortic valves, 51 (89%) patients were aged ≥65 years and 30 (53%) had concomitant CABG. How then does one explain the presence of aortic stenosis in the 6 patients with 3-cuspid aortic valves and ages <65 years? Three of the 6 patients (aged 58 to 64 years [mean 61]) also had concomitant CABG and thus associated severe coronary narrowing; their peak systolic pressure gradients across the aortic valve were 18, 41, and 42 mm Hg, respectively. The remaining 3 patients had insignificant coronary narrowing by angiogram and large peak systolic pressure gradients of 67, 84, and 96 mm Hg, respectively. The etiology of the aortic stenosis in these 3 patients is unclear.

Patients with congenitally bicuspid aortic valves, of course, were not immune to atherosclerosis, but they clearly had less severe coronary artery disease than did patients with tricuspid aortic valves. Of the 57 patients with congenitally unicuspid or bicuspid aortic valves, 22 (39%) had concomitant CABG: 7 (33%) of 21 patients aged <65 years and 15 (42%) of 36 patients aged ≥65 years. Of the 57 patients with tricuspid aortic valves, 30 (53%) had concomitant CABG: 3 of 6 patients aged <65 years, and 27 (53%) of 51 patients aged ≥65 years.

Other previously published studies examining operatively excised stenotic aortic valves are summarized in Table VI. None of the 8 previously reported studies provided hemodynamic data and only 1[26] discussed associated CABG procedures. Two studies[24,25] also included cases of pure aortic regurgitation with their cases of aortic stenosis. Also, in contrast to the present study, 2 of the previously reported studies[19,20] definitely included cases with associated mitral valve disease with or without mitral valve replacement, and 3 other studies[23–25] almost certainly also included patients with associated mitral valve disease. If the mitral cases are included with the aortic valve cases, the frequency of 3-cuspid aortic valves is higher and the frequency of congenitally bicuspid valves is lower than in studies limited to aortic valve stenosis with or without associated aortic regurgitation. The previously published studies that most closely correspond to the present one was by Peterson and associates[21] and by Davies and associates.[26] The findings in the study of Peterson et al were identical to those of the present study, i.e., 50% of the patients had congenitally malformed valves (unicuspid in 1% and bicuspid in 49%), and 50% of the patients had tricuspid valves. The present study, however, appears to be the first to correlate hemodynamic findings with valve structure. The study of Davies et al is the first to correlate the presence or absence of concomitant CABG with the structure of the operatively excised stenotic aortic valve. Of their 465 patients, 122 (26%) had concomitant CABG: 66 (21%) of 308 patients with bicuspid valves and 56 (37%) of 150 patients with tricuspid valves.

Acknowledgment: We are indebted to J. Carolyn Banks, PhD, for providing statistical support, Edward L. Bond, PhD, for providing numerous individual patient data printouts, and John F. Dixon, MSN, RN, for creating a patient database program for analyzing data.

1. Dry TJ, Willius FA. Calcareous disease of the aortic valve. A study of two hundred twenty-eight cases. *Am Heart J* 1939;17:138–157.
2. Karsner HT, Koletsky S. Calcific Disease of the Aortic Valve. Philadelphia: J.B. Lippincott, 1947:111.
3. Kumpe CW, Bean WB. Aortic stenosis: a study of the clinical and pathologic aspects of 107 proved cases. *Medicine* 1948;27:139–185.
4. Anderson MW, Kelsey JR Jr, Edwards JE. Clinical and pathological considerations in cases of calcific aortic stenosis. *JAMA* 1952;149:9–15.
5. Smith DE, Matthews MB. Aortic valvular stenosis with coarctation of the aorta. With special reference to the development of aortic stenosis upon congenital bicuspid valves. *Br Heart J* 1955;17:198–206.
6. Bacon APC, Matthews MB. Congenital bicuspid aortic valves and the aetiology of isolated aortic valvular stenosis. *Quart J Med* 1959;28:545–560.
7. Braunwald E, Roberts WC, Goldblatt A, Aygen MM, Rockoff SD, Gilbert JW. Aortic stenosis: physiological, pathological, and clinical concepts. Combined clinical staff conference at the National Institutes of Health. *Ann Intern Med* 1963;58:494–522.
8. Roberts WC, Morrow AG. Congenital aortic stenosis produced by an unicommissural valve. *Br Heart J* 1965;27:505–510.
9. Morrow AG, Roberts WC, Ross J Jr, Fisher RD, Behrendt DM, Mason DT, Braunwald E. Obstruction to left ventricular outflow. Current concepts of management and operative treatment. *Ann Intern Med* 1968;69:1255–1286.
10. Storstein O. Etiology of aortic valvular disease. *Acta Med Scand* 1969;185:17–2
11. Roberts WC. The structure of the aortic valve in clinically-isolated aortic stenosis. An autopsy study of 162 patients over 15 years of age. *Circulation* 1970;42:91–97.
12. Roberts WC. The congenitally bicuspid aortic valve. A study of 85 autopsy cases. *Am J Cardiol* 1970;26:72–83.
13. Roberts WC. Anatomically isolated aortic valvular disease. The case against its being of rheumatic etiology. *Am J Med* 1970;49:151–159.
14. Roberts WC, Perloff JK, Costantino T. Severe valvular aortic stenosis in patients over 65 years of age. A clinicopathologic study. *Am J Cardiol* 1971;27:497–506.
15. Falcone MW, Roberts WC, Morrow AG, Perloff JK. Congenital aortic stenosis resulting from unicommissural valve. Clinical and anatomic features in twenty-one adult patients. *Circulation* 1971;44:272–280.
16. Roberts WC, Dangel JC, Bulkley BH. Non-rheumatic valvular cardiac disease: a clinicopathologic survey of 27 different conditions causing valvular dysfunction. *Cardiovasc Clin* 1973;5:333–446.
17. Roberts WC, McIntosh CL, Wallace RB. Aortic valve perforation with calcific aortic valve stenosis and without infective endocarditis or significant aortic regurgitation. *Am J Cardiol* 1987;59:476–478.
18. Mautner GC, Mautner SL, Cannon RO III, Hunsberger SA, Roberts WC. Clinical factors useful in predicting aortic valve structure in patients >40 years of age with isolated valvular aortic stenosis. *Am J Cardiol* 1993;72:194–198.
19. Subramanian R, Olson LJ, Edwards WD. Surgical pathology of pure aortic stenosis: a study of 374 cases. *Mayo Clin Proc* 1984;59:683–690.
20. Subramanian R, Olson LJ, Edwards WD. Surgical pathology of combined aortic stenosis and insufficiency: a study of 213 cases. *Mayo Clin Proc* 1985;60:247–254.
21. Peterson MD, Roach RM, Edwards JE. Types of aortic stenosis in surgically removed valves. *Arch Pathol Lab Med* 1985;109:829–832.
22. Roberts WC. Congenital cardiovascular abnormalities usually silent until adulthood. In: Roberts WC, ed. Adult Congenital Heart Disease. Philadelphia: FA Davis, 1987:631–691.
23. Passik CS, Ackermann DM, Pluth JR, Edwards WD. Temporal changes in the causes of aortic stenosis: a surgical pathological study of 646 cases. *Mayo Clin Proc* 1987;62:119–123.
24. Turri M, Thiene G, Bortolotti U, Milano A, Mazzucco A, Gallucci V. Surgical pathology of aortic valve disease. A study based on 602 specimens. *Eur J Cardiothoracic Surg* 1990;4:556–560.
25. Dare AJ, Veinot JP, Edwards WD, Tazelaar HD, Schaff HV. New observations on the etiology of aortic valve disease: a surgical pathologic study of 236 cases from 1990. *Human Pathol* 1993;24:1330–1338.
26. Davies MJ, Treasure T, Parker DJ. Demographic characteristics of patients undergoing aortic valve replacement for stenosis: relation to valve morphology. *Heart* 1996;75:174–178.

Observations on the Heart

William C. Roberts, MD, Section Editor, Baylor Cardiovascular Institute, Baylor University Medical Center, Dallas, TX

Congenitally Bicuspid Stenotic Aortic Valves in Octogenarians

Stuart R. Lander, MD; Jeff E. Taylor, MD; William C. Roberts, MD
From the Baylor Cardiovascular Institute, Baylor University Medical Center, Dallas, TX

An 84-year-old white woman was apparently asymptomatic until about 2 months before aortic valve replacement when she went to her physician because of developing exertional dyspnea and chest tightness. A transthoracic echocardiogram showed a normally contracting left ventricle, a normal sized left ventricular cavity, and an estimated aortic valve area of 0.6 cm^2. The possibility of aortic valve replacement was discussed with the patient but she declined operative intervention.

She was then in her usual state until nearly 2 months later when the dyspnea and chest tightness worsened and she came to the hospital's emergency room. Precordial examination disclosed a grade 3/6 systolic ejection type murmur heard best along the left sternal border with radiation into the neck. No diastolic murmur was heard. Electrocardiogram disclosed sinus rhythm, nonspecific ST, T wave changes, and total 12 lead QRS voltage of 184 mm (10 mm=1 mV) (normal ≤ 175 mm).[1] Chest radiograph disclosed bilateral pleural effusions and mild cardiomegaly; no calcium was seen in either the mitral valve region or in the aortic valve cusps. Cardiac catheterization disclosed the following pressures: left ventricle 173/19 mm Hg; aorta 122/54 mm Hg, yielding a peak systolic pressure gradient of 51; pulmonary artery, 33/14 mm Hg (mean 20), and pulmonary artery wedge mean 12. The aortic valve area was calculated to be 0.51 cm^2 and the valve area index, 0.3 cm^2/body surface area. The patient weighed 145 lbs (68 kg) and was 63 inches tall (160 cm). Coronary angiogram disclosed a dominant right coronary system. The distal left anterior descending coronary artery was narrowed up to 70% in diameter, the left circumflex up to 30%, and the right coronary artery <20%. The left main was normal.

On January 12, 1999, the aortic valve was excised and replaced with a Baxter parietal pericardial 21 mm bioprosthesis. Coronary bypass also was performed. The operatively excised valve was congenitally bicuspid (Figure). Early postoperatively the patient was transiently confused, developed atrial fibrillation, and had mild elevation in blood urea nitrogen. She went home the eleventh postoperative day. By that time she was again in sinus rhythm, mentally alert, and had normal renal function. Eight months after operation she was asymptomatic, and cared for herself living alone.

The above case indicates that a congenitally bicuspid aortic valve can be seen in octogenarians and that a stenotic one can be successfully replaced. The oldest reported patient having aortic valve replacement for congenitally stenotic aortic valve was a 92-year-old man.[2] The present patient was

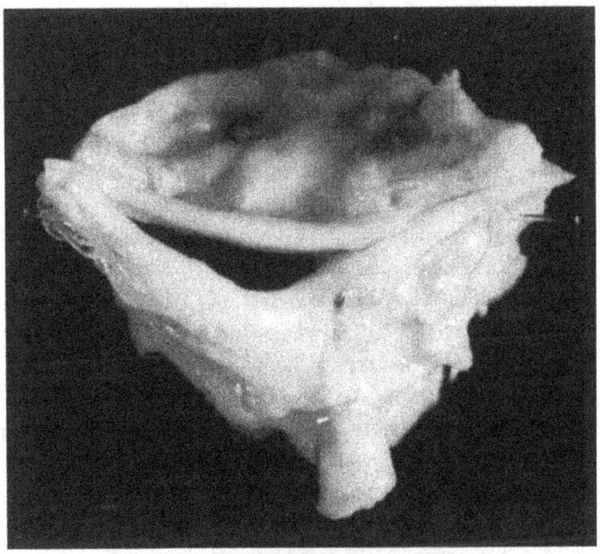

Figure. Operatively excised congenitally bicuspid stenotic aortic valve in the 84-year-old patient described herein.

Table. Published Reports of Aortic Valve Replacement With and Without Coronary Artery Bypass in Octogenarians

First Author (Year)	Number of Patients	Age (Mean)	Procedure (Number of Patients)	Operative Mortality	30 Day Mortality (%)	Actuarial Survival (Years) 1	3	5
Aranki (1983)	188	80–95 (-)	AVR (83)	4%	—	—	—	—
			AVR + CABG (105)	9%	—	—	—	—
Elayda (1983)	152	80–91 (93)	AVR (77)	5%				
			AVR + CABG (75)	24%	18%	84%	79%	57%
Deiwick (1997)	37	80–92 (81)	AVR (23)	—				
			AVR & CABG (14)	—	8%	88%	79%*	73%
Schmitz (1998)	52	>80 (-)	AVR (33)	3%	—	—	—	87%
			AVR + CABG (19)	22%	—	—	—	59%

*2 year postoperative follow up; AVR=aortic valve replacement; CABG=coronary bypass grafting.

asymptomatic until just a few weeks before aortic valve replacement. A recent study from the Mayo Clinic[3] described 527 patients >20 years of age with operative excision of congenitally bicuspid aortic valves including stenotic ones (444 patients), purely regurgitant ones without infection (67 patients), and infected ones (16 patients). Of the 527 patients >20 years of age, 28 (5.3%) were octogenarians. At Baylor University Medical Center since January 1993, 397 patients >20 years of age have undergone isolated aortic valve replacement (no replacement of the mitral valve) (115 were described elsewhere[4]): the aortic valve in 169 (43%) was congenitally bicuspid; in 13 (3%) it was unicuspid; in 211 (53%) it was tricuspid; and in 4 (1%) the valve structure was unclear. Of the 169 patients with a congenitally bicuspid aortic valve, 60 (36%) were <65 years of age and 109 (64%) were aged 65 or over including 19 (11%) who were octogenarians.

Only one major coronary artery in the above described patient was narrowed >50% in diameter. As a rule, the cleaner the coronary arteries in older individuals the greater the chance that a stenotic aortic valve will be congenitally bicuspid.[5]

Recent reports of octogenarians undergoing isolated aortic valve replacement with or without coronary artery bypass are reviewed in the Table.[6–9] Operative mortality of combined valve replacement and coronary bypass was relatively high. Of the 52 patients reported by Schmidtz et al,[9] 81% of the early survivors stated that their functional status had improved and 97% stated that the operation was worthwhile.

Finally, as the population continues to age the frequency of aortic valve stenosis will almost certainly increase. Congenital heart disease is not limited to the younger population but indeed may occur in the elderly.

References

1 Odom H II, Davis JL, Dinh H, Baker BJ, Roberts WC, Murphy ML. QRS voltage measurements in autopsied men free of cardiopulmonary disease: A basis for evaluating total QRS voltage as an index of left ventricular hypertrophy. *Am J Cardiol.* 1986;58:801–804.

2 Karalis DG, Wahl JM, Mintz GS, Chandrasekaran K. Severe stenosis involving a congenitally bicuspid aortic valve in the tenth decade of life. *Am J Cardiol.* 1990;65:264–265.

3 Sabet HY, Edwards WD, Tazelaar HD, Daly RC. Congenitally bicuspid aortic valves: A surgical pathology study of 542 cases (1991 through 1996) and a literature review of 2,715 additional cases. *Mayo Clin Proc.* 1999;74:14–26.

4 Stephan PJ, Henry III AC, Hebeler Jr RF, Whiddon L, Roberts WC. Comparison of age, gender, number of aortic valve cusps, concomitant coronary artery bypass grafting, and magnitude of left ventricular-systemic arterial peak systolic gradient in adults having aortic valve replacement for isolated aortic valve stenosis. *Am J Cardiol.* 1997;79:166–172.

5 Mautner GC, Mautner SL, Cannon RO III, Hunsberger SA, Roberts WC. Clinical factors useful in predicting aortic valve structure in patients >40 years of age with isolated valvular aortic stenosis. *Am J Cardiol.* 1993;72:194–198.

6 Aranki SF, Rizzo RJ, Couper GS, Adams DH, Collins Jr JJ, Gildea JS, Kinchla NM, Cohn LH.

Aortic valve replacement in the elderly. Effect of gender and coronary artery disease on operative mortality. *Circulation.* 1993;88:17–23.

7 Elayda MAA, Hall RJ, Reul RM, Alonzo DM, Gillette N, Reul Jr, GJ, Cooley DA. Aortic valve replacement in patients 80 years and older. Operative risks and long-term results. *Circulation.* 1993;88:11–16.

8 Deiwick M, Tandler R, Mollhoff T, Kerber S, Rotker J, Roeder N, Scheld HH. Heart surgery in patients aged eighty years and above: Determinants of morbidity and mortality. *Thorac Cardiovasc Surg.* 1997;45:119–126.

9 Schmitz C, Welz A, Reichart B. Is cardiac surgery justified in patients in the ninth decade of life? *J Card Surg.* 1998;13:113–119.

Weights of Operatively-Excised Stenotic Unicuspid, Bicuspid, and Tricuspid Aortic Valves and Their Relation to Age, Sex, Body Mass Index, and Presence or Absence of Concomitant Coronary Artery Bypass Grafting

William Clifford Roberts, MD, and Jong Mi Ko, BA

This study was designed to evaluate weights of operatively-excised stenotic aortic valves and to compare them with age, sex, body mass index, and presence or absence of concomitant coronary artery bypass grafting. Weights of operatively-excised stenotic aortic valves have not been previously reported. We weighed operatively-excised stenotic valves in 499 patients (aged 19 to 91 years, mean 70), none of whom had mitral valve replacement. The 499 aortic valves ranged in weight from 0.45 to 11.30 g (mean 2.67). The mean weights of the unicuspid and bicuspid valves were heavier than those of the tricuspid valves (4.36 vs 3.34 vs 2.04 g, $p < 0.05$). Mean valve weights were greater in the 304 men than in the 195 women (3.19 vs 1.87 g, $p < 0.001$), in the younger patients than in the older patients (3.13 g in patients ≤40 years old vs 2.89 g in patients 41 to 70 years old and 2.47 g in patients 71 to 91 years old, $p < 0.05$), and in the 230 patients who did not undergo simultaneous coronary artery bypass grafting compared with the 269 patients who had this additional procedure (2.94 vs 2.45 g, $p < 0.001$). The mean weights of the valves were similar in patients whose body mass index was <25, 25 to 30, and >30 kg/m^2 (2.62 vs 2.76 vs 2.57 g). Weights of operatively-excised stenotic aortic valves provide objective evidence of valvular stenosis.

(Am J Cardiol 2003;92:1057–1065)

No reports have appeared describing weights of operatively-excised stenotic aortic valves or their relation to age, sex, body mass index, or to the presence or absence of concomitant coronary artery bypass grafting. Such is the purpose of this study.

METHODS

From January 28, 1998, to December 31, 2002 (59 months), cardiac valve tissue from 1,131 patients who underwent cardiac valve replacement or repair was submitted to the Pathology Department of Baylor University Medical Center (Figure 1). Of these 1,131 cases, 714 patients underwent aortic valve replacement. Of these, 504 had isolated aortic valve replacement for aortic stenosis (with or without associated aortic regurgitation), 135 patients had aortic valve replacement for pure aortic regurgitation (no element of stenosis), and 60 patients had double valve replacements (59 patients had aortic and mitral valves replaced and 1 patient had mitral and tricuspid valves replaced). The present study is limited to the patients who had replacement of the aortic valve for aortic stenosis (with or without associated aortic regurgitation) but without associated mitral valve replacement. Of these 504 patients with isolated aortic valve stenosis, 499 had the valve weighed by 1 of us (WCR), and this study is limited to these 499 patients. Five other specimens were excluded from the study because 1 of the cusps or the whole specimen was missing.

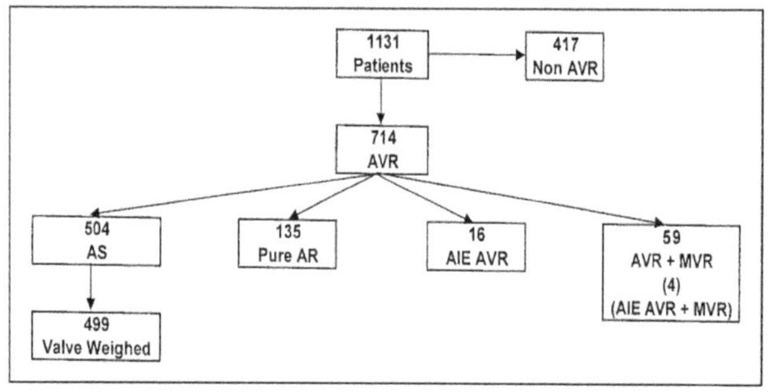

FIGURE 1. Algorithm showing breakdown of the 1,132 patients who underwent valve replacement or repair at Baylor University Medical Center in a 59-month period and the origin of the 499 cases included in the present study. AIE = active infective endocarditis; AR = aortic regurgitation; AS = aortic stenosis; AVR = aortic valve replacement; MVR = mitral valve replacement.

Each operatively-excised cardiac valve arrived in the surgical pathology unit in a container filled with formaldehyde. The valve was removed from the container, placed on absorbing paper to absorb excess formaldehyde, and then weighed on a Ohaus scale

From the Baylor Heart & Vascular Institute and the Departments of Pathology and Medicine, Baylor University Medical Center, Dallas, Texas. Manuscript received June 23, 2003; revised manuscript received and accepted July 29, 2003.

Address for reprints: William C. Roberts, MD, Baylor Heart & Vascular Institute, Baylor University Medical Center, 3500 Gaston Avenue, Dallas, Texas 75246. E-mail: wc.roberts@baylorhealth.edu.

TABLE 1 Gender, Ages, Body Mass Index, Concomitant Coronary Bypass, and Aortic Valve Weights According to Type of Valve Structure

Valve Structure	No. of Patients	Men : Women	Ages (Years)	Body Mass Index (kg/m^2)	Coronary Bypass	Aortic Valve Weights (g)
Unicuspid	14 (2%)	12 : 2 (86% : 14%)	29–65 (45)	21–46 (29)	1 (7%)	1.35–8.00 (4.36)
Bicuspid	218 (44%)	155 : 63 (71% : 29%)	19–91 (66)	17–58 (28)	107 (49%)	0.79–11.30 (3.34)
Tricuspid	267 (54%)	137 : 130 (51% : 49%)	28–90 (74)	17–51 (28)	161 (60%)	0.45–6.60 (2.04)
Totals	499 (100%)	304 : 195 (61% : 39%)	19–91 (70)	17–58 (28)	269 (54%)	0.45–11.30 (2.67)

TABLE 2 Ages, Body Mass Index, Concomitant Coronary Bypass, and Aortic Valve Weights in Men Versus Women According to Aortic Valve Structure

Gender	Valve Structure	No. of Patients	Ages (Years)	Body Mass Index (kg/m^2)	Coronary Bypass	Aortic Valve Weights (g)
Men	Unicuspid	12 (4%)	29–57 (45)	21–46 (30)	1 (8%)	2.12–8.00 (4.60)
	Bicuspid	155 (51%)	32–91 (66)	17–51 (28)	82 (53%)	1.03–11.30 (3.71)
	Tricuspid	137 (45%)	47–90 (74)	18–49 (27)	83 (61%)	1.10–6.60 (2.47)
	Subtotals	304 (61%)	29–91 (69)	17–51 (28)	166 (55%)	1.03–11.30 (3.19)
Women	Unicuspid	2 (1%)	33 & 65 (49)	26 & 26 (26)	0	1.35 & 4.50 (2.93)
	Bicuspid	63 (32%)	19–85 (66)	18–58 (28)	25 (40%)	0.79–4.97 (2.42)
	Tricuspid	130 (67%)	28–90 (74)	17–51 (29)	78 (60%)	0.45–4.81 (1.59)
	Subtotals	195 (39%)	19–90 (71)	17–58 (29)	103 (53%)	0.45–4.97 (1.87)

(Ohaus Corporation, Florham Park, New Jersey), which has an accuracy to 0.01 g. Ages and sex of the patients were obtained from the patient demographics displayed on the submitting surgical slip and confirmed from the patient identification label pasted on the container submitted from the operating room. Whether the patient had aortic stenosis was first determined by the surgical slip and examination by WCR. It was then confirmed again from the hemodynamic data from the catheterization report or the echocardiogram data, or both.

The body mass index (kilograms per square meter) immediately before aortic valve replacement in each patient was calculated from the body weight and height obtained from the cardiac catheterization report or from the medical record. Whether or not the patient had concomitant coronary artery bypass grafting was obtained from the patient's medical record.

Statistical analysis was performed using SigmaStat, Version 2.0 (SPSS Inc., Chicago, Illinois). Parametric tests were used for analysis of the data that passed the assumption tests of normality and equal variance. For continuous variables, the unpaired *t* test was performed for 2 variable comparisons and 1-way analysis of variance was used for >2 variable comparisons. When the data did not pass the assumption tests, nonparametric tests (i.e., Mann-Whitney rank-sum test and Kruskal-Wallis 1-way analysis of variance on the rank test) were performed to find the significant differences in 2 and >2 continuous variable comparisons, respectively. For categorical variables, the chi-square test or Fisher's exact test was used as appropriate for analysis of the proportions of the observations found in different categories. To find the correlation coefficient (r), Pearson's product moment test or the Spearman's rank order test was used, as appropriate. A p value <0.05 was considered statistically significant.

In all 499 patients the number of aortic valve cusps was determined by 1 of us (WCR).

The Baylor University Medical Center committee on human research approved the protocol for this study.

RESULTS

The stenotic aortic valves ranged in weight from 0.45 to 11.30 g (mean 2.67), a 25-fold difference between the smallest and the largest (Table 1). In general, the fewer the number of aortic valve cusps, the heavier the valves. The mean weights of the 14 unicuspid valves were 4.36 g, the 218 bicuspid valves, 3.34 g, and the 267 tricuspid valves, 2.04 g (unicuspid vs tricuspid and bicuspid vs tricuspid, p <0.05).

The mean weights of the stenotic aortic valves were larger in the men than in the women (Table 2). The valves in the 304 men ranged from 1.03 to 11.30 g (mean 3.19), an 11-fold difference, and the valves in the 195 women ranged from 0.45 to 4.97 g (mean 1.87), also an 11-fold difference (p <0.001). Additionally, the mean weights of each of the 3 valve structures were greater in the men than in the women: (1) unicuspid, 4.60 (12 men) versus 2.93 g (2 women) (p = 0.302); (2) bicuspid, 3.71 versus 2.42 g (p <0.001), and (3) tricuspid, 2.47 versus 1.59 g (p <0.001). The valve weights in each of the 304 men and of the 195 women are displayed in Figure 2. The

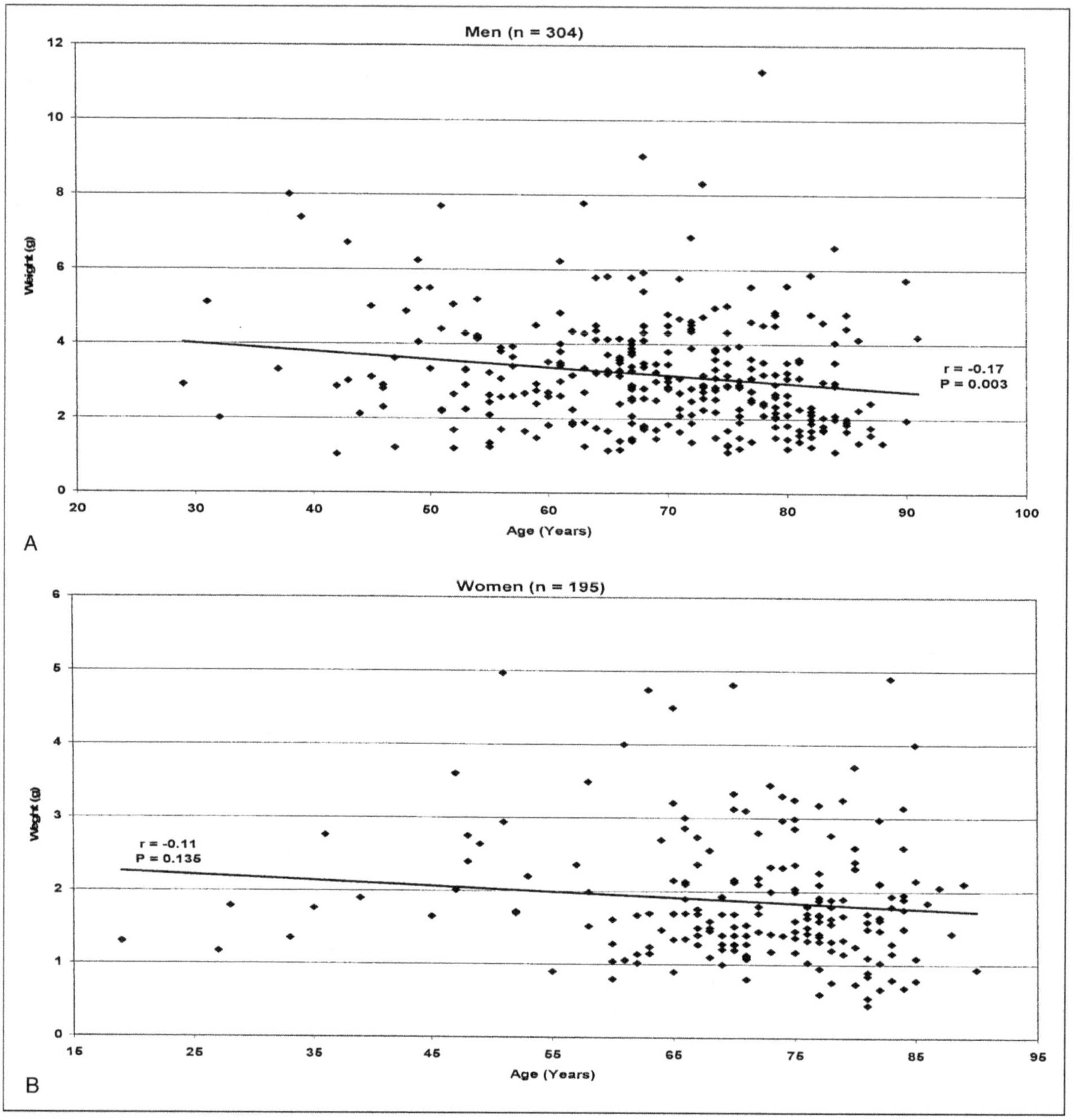

FIGURE 2. Relation of aortic valve weights (in grams) to ages (in years) at the time of aortic valve replacement *(A)* in the 304 men and *(B)* in the 195 women. Valve weight did not correlate with ages in these adults.

mean valve weights in men and women in each of 7 decades are displayed in Figure 3.

The younger patients tended to have heavier aortic valves than the older patients (Table 3). The aortic valves in the 13 patients ≤40 years of age ranged from 1.17 to 8.00 g (mean 3.13), a 7-fold difference; those in the 224 patients aged 41 to 70 years ranged from 0.80 to 9.04 g (mean 2.89), an 11-fold difference; and the valves in the 262 patients aged 71 to 91 years weighed from 0.45 to 11.30 g (mean 2.47), a 25-fold difference. The difference in mean weights in the patients ≤40 years of age compared with those aged 41 to 70 years was not significant, but the differences in valve weights between the intermediate (aged 41 to 70 years) and oldest groups (aged 71 to 91 years) were significant ($p < 0.05$). Of the 267 three-cuspid aortic valves, no association between patient age and the valve weight was found (Figure 4).

The mean weights of the stenotic aortic valves were not significantly different among patients divided into 3 groups by body mass index (Table 4). The aortic valves in the 139 patients with body mass indexes <25 kg/m^2 ranged from 0.55 to 9.04 g (mean 2.62), a 16-fold difference; those in the 233 patients with body mass indexes from 25 to 30 kg/m^2 ranged from 0.45 to 11.30 g (mean 2.76), a 25-fold differ-

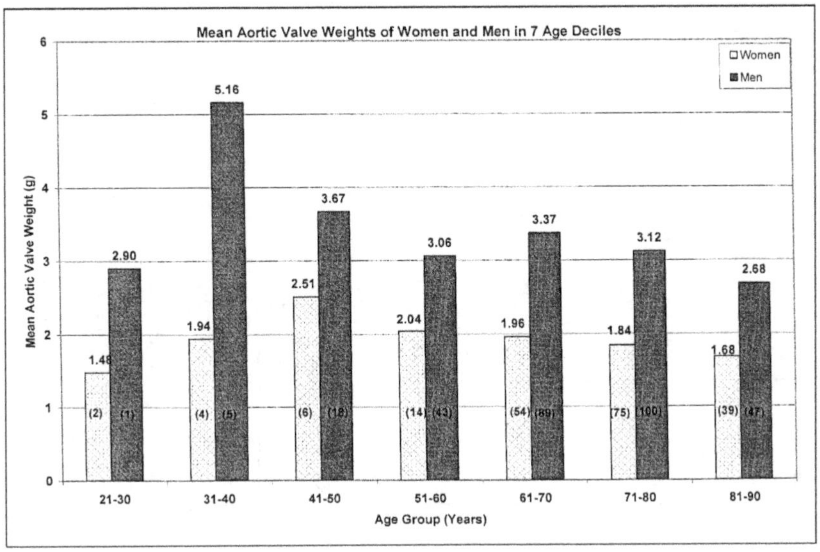

FIGURE 3. Bar graph showing mean aortic valve weights in women and men in each of 7 decades. The 1 patient who was <20 years old and the 1 patient who was >90 years of age are not included in this graph.

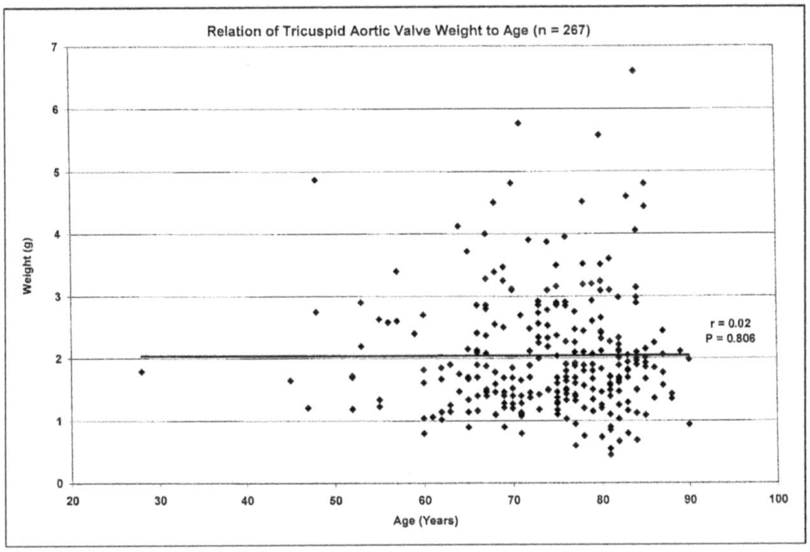

FIGURE 4. Relation of aortic valve weight to age in the 267 patients with stenotic 3-cuspid aortic valves.

ence; and the 127 patients with body mass indexes >30 kg/m^2 had aortic valves that ranged in weight from 0.69 to 7.70 g (mean 2.57), an 11-fold difference.

The stenotic aortic valves in the 230 patients who did not undergo simultaneous coronary artery bypass grafting were significantly ($p < 0.001$) heavier than in the 269 patients who underwent coronary bypass during the operation in which the stenotic aortic valve was operatively excised (Table 5). The weights of the 230 aortic valves in the patients who did not undergo bypass ranged from 0.67 to 11.30 g (mean 2.94), a 17-fold difference, and the 269 valves in the patients who underwent simultaneous coronary bypass ranged from 0.45 to 8.30 g (mean 2.45), an 18-fold difference (mean 2.94 vs 2.45, $p < 0.001$).

Table 6 shows the numbers of patients, sex, ages, body mass indexes, and whether coronary bypass was performed according to 6 aortic valve weight categories. Table 7 compares the 18 patients with valves weighing ≤1 g with the 12 patients who had valves weighing >6 g; it discloses the following: mean age 77 vs 60 years ($p = 0.004$); women (18 of 18) versus men (12 of 12) ($p < 0.001$); mean body mass index 28 vs 27 kg/m^2 ($p = 0.983$); and concomitant coronary artery bypass grafting (12 of 18 patients [67%] vs 4 of 12 [25%]) ($p = 0.156$).

Photographs of operatively-excised unicuspid, bicuspid, and tricuspid valves in 34 of the 499 patients are illustrated in Figures 5 to 7, respectively, and the pertinent data for each of the 34 patients whose valves are illustrated are listed in Table 8.

DISCUSSION

This study of 499 adults who underwent aortic valve replacement because of aortic valve stenosis with or without associated aortic regurgitation and without mitral valve replacement showed a huge range of aortic valve weights, from 0.45 to 11.30 g, a 25-fold difference between the smallest and the largest. The mean weights of the congenitally malformed valves (either unicuspid or bicuspid) were heavier than those of the 3-cuspid aortic valves. Men had heavier valves than the women. Younger adults had heavier valves than older adults, a consequence of a higher frequency of congenitally malformed valves in the younger group. Body mass index had insignificant effect on valve weight. The patients who underwent concomitant coronary artery bypass grafting had smaller valve weights than the patients who did not have this additional procedure (2.45 vs 2.94 g, $p < 0.001$).

Some data are available on the weights of normal aortic valves in adults studied at necropsy. Silver and Roberts[1] excised 100 normal aortic valves (each 3-cuspid) at necropsy in patients aged 18 to 100 years, and all but 1 weighed ≤1 g. The valve weights increased with age ($p < 0.001$), with heart weight ($p < 0.001$), with the sum of the area of the 3 cusps ($p < 0.001$), with the volume of the 3 sinuses of Valsalva

TABLE 3 Gender, Body Mass Index, Concomitant Coronary Bypass, and Aortic Valve Weights in Three Age Groups According to Aortic Valve Structure

Ages (Years)	Valve Structure	No. of Patients	Men : Women	Body Mass Index (kg/m²)	Coronary Bypass	Aortic Valve Weights (g)
≤40	Unicuspid	5 (38%)	4 : 1 (80% : 20%)	23–42 (28)	0	1.35–8.00 (4.95)
	Bicuspid	7 (54%)	2 : 5 (29% : 71%)	22–52 (33)	0	1.17–3.30 (2.03)
	Tricuspid	1 (8%)	0 : 1 (0% : 100%)	19	0	1.79
	Subtotals	13 (2%)	6 : 7 (46% : 54%)	19–52 (30)	0	1.17–8.00 (3.13)
41–70	Unicuspid	9 (4%)	8 : 1 (89% : 11%)	21–46 (30)	1 (11%)	2.12–7.70 (4.03)
	Bicuspid	131 (58%)	96 : 35 (73% : 27%)	17–58 (29)	54 (41%)	0.90–9.04 (3.36)
	Tricuspid	84 (38%)	42 : 42 (50% : 50%)	19–51 (30)	41 (49%)	0.80–4.87 (2.04)
	Subtotals	224 (45%)	146 : 78 (65% : 35%)	17–58 (29)	96 (43%)	0.80–9.04 (2.89)
71–91	Unicuspid	0 (0%)	0	—	0	—
	Bicuspid	80 (31%)	53 : 27 (66% : 34%)	19–40 (26)	53 (66%)	0.79–11.30 (3.42)
	Tricuspid	182 (69%)	95 : 87 (52% : 48%)	17–47 (27)	120 (66%)	0.45–6.60 (2.05)
	Subtotals	262 (53%)	148 : 114 (56% : 44%)	17–47 (27)	173 (66%)	0.45–11.30 (2.47)

TABLE 4 Gender, Ages, Body Mass Index (BMI), Concomitant Coronary Bypass, and Aortic Valve Weights in Three Body Mass Index Groups According to Aortic Valve Structure

BMI (kg/m²)	Valve Structure	No. of Patients	Men : Women	Ages (Years)	Coronary Bypass	Aortic Valve Weights (g)
<25	Unicuspid	3 (2%)	3 : 0 (100% : 0%)	31–49 (42)	0	2.89–5.10 (4.01)
	Bicuspid	56 (40%)	35 : 21 (63% : 37%)	27–91 (69)	30 (54%)	0.79–9.04 (3.38)
	Tricuspid	80 (58%)	42 : 38 (53% : 47%)	28–90 (74)	49 (61%)	0.55–6.60 (2.04)
	Subtotals	139 (28%)	80 : 59 (58% : 42%)	27–91 (72)	79 (57%)	0.55–9.04 (2.62)
25–30	Unicuspid	6 (3%)	4 : 2 (67% : 33%)	33–65 (46)	1 (17%)	1.35–8.00 (4.95)
	Bicuspid	106 (45%)	81 : 25 (76% : 24%)	36–86 (66)	54 (51%)	1.20–11.30 (3.41)
	Tricuspid	121 (52%)	70 : 51 (58% : 42%)	47–89 (75)	73 (60%)	0.45–5.77 (2.10)
	Subtotals	233 (47%)	155 : 78 (67% : 33%)	33–89 (70)	128 (55%)	0.45–11.30 (2.76)
>30	Unicuspid	5 (4%)	5 : 0 (100% : 0%)	29–57 (47)	0	2.90–7.70 (4.29)
	Bicuspid	56 (44%)	39 : 17 (70% : 30%)	19–77 (61)	23 (41%)	0.90–6.72 (3.14)
	Tricuspid	66 (52%)	25 : 41 (38% : 62%)	52–86 (71)	39 (59%)	0.69–4.81 (1.95)
	Subtotals	127 (25%)	69 : 58 (54% : 46%)	19–86 (66)	62 (49%)	0.69–7.70 (2.57)

TABLE 5 Ages, Body Mass Index, and Aortic Valve Weights in Patients Without Versus Patients With Concomitant Coronary Bypass Grafting (CABG) According to Aortic Valve Structure

CABG	Valve Structure	No. of Patients	Men : Women	Ages (Years)	Body Mass Index (kg/m²)	Aortic Valve Weights (g)
0	Unicuspid	13 (6%)	11 : 2 (85% : 15%)	29–65 (45)	21–46 (30)	1.35–8.00 (4.53)
	Bicuspid	111 (48%)	73 : 38 (66% : 34%)	19–90 (62)	18–58 (28)	0.90–11.30 (3.46)
	Tricuspid	106 (46%)	54 : 52 (51% : 49%)	28–89 (72)	19–51 (28)	0.67–5.77 (2.19)
	Subtotals	230 (46%)	138 : 92 (60% : 40%)	19–90 (65)	18–58 (28)	0.67–11.30 (2.94)
+	Unicuspid	1 (<1%)	1 : 0 (100% : 0%)	44	26	2.12
	Bicuspid	107 (40%)	82 : 25 (77% : 23%)	49–91 (70)	17–51 (27)	0.79–8.30 (3.21)
	Tricuspid	161 (60%)	83 : 78 (52% : 48%)	52–90 (75)	17–51 (28)	0.45–6.60 (1.95)
	Subtotals	269 (54%)	166 : 103 (62% : 38%)	44–91 (73)	17–51 (27)	0.45–8.30 (2.45)

($p < 0.001$), and with the aortic area at the sinotubular junction ($p < 0.001$). In the present study, 18 valves weighed ≤1 g and none of them had significant associated aortic regurgitation. All 18 patients were women (mean age 77 years); 16 (89%) had 3-cuspid aortic valves and 12 (67%) had concomitant coronary artery bypass grafting. The reasons for aortic valve replacement in the 6 patients who did not have concomitant coronary artery bypass grafting and valves weighing ≤1 g are unclear.

In most centers in the United States, operatively-excised aortic valves are examined in surgical pathol-

TABLE 6 Gender, Ages, Body Mass Index, and Concomitant Coronary Bypass in Seven Aortic Valve Weight Groups

Aortic Valve Weight (g)	Valve Structure	No. of Patients	Aortic Valve Weight (g) Range (mean)	Men : Women	Ages (Years)	Body Mass Index (kg/m²)	Coronary Bypass
≤1	Unicuspid	0	—	—	—	—	—
	Bicuspid	2 (11%)	0.79–0.90 (0.85)	0 : 2	55–85 (70)	24–42 (33)	1 (50%)
	Tricuspid	16 (89%)	0.45–0.95 (0.77)	0 : 16	60–90 (78)	21–47 (27)	11 (69%)
>1–2	Unicuspid	1 (<1%)	1.35	0 : 1	33	26	0
	Bicuspid	38 (21%)	1.03–2.00 (1.60)	13 : 25	19–84 (63)	19–58 (29)	19 (50%)
	Tricuspid	143 (79%)	1.02–2.00 (1.52)	54 : 89	28–90 (73)	17–51 (28)	90 (63%)
>2–3	Unicuspid	3 (2%)	2.12–2.90 (2.64)	3 : 0	29–46 (40)	21–42 (30)	1 (33%)
	Bicuspid	59 (44%)	2.01–3.00 (2.57)	39 : 20	36–84 (65)	18–51 (28)	31 (53%)
	Tricuspid	72 (54%)	2.01–2.98 (2.45)	50 : 22	48–89 (74)	18–51 (28)	42 (58%)
>3–4	Unicuspid	3 (3%)	3.33–3.93 (3.62)	3 : 0	47–57 (51)	32–46 (37)	0
	Bicuspid	59 (69%)	3.01–4.00 (3.44)	46 : 13	37–85 (67)	17–40 (28)	29 (49%)
	Tricuspid	24 (28%)	3.09–4.00 (3.41)	22 : 2	57–84 (74)	17–40 (27)	13 (54%)
>4–5	Unicuspid	3 (6%)	4.05–4.50 (4.24)	2 : 1	49–65 (56)	24–26 (25)	0
	Bicuspid	39 (76%)	4.01–5.00 (4.48)	36 : 3	45–91 (68)	19–42 (27)	20 (51%)
	Tricuspid	9 (18%)	4.05–4.87 (4.52)	8 : 1	48–85 (74)	19–39 (26)	4 (44%)
>5–6	Unicuspid	1 (6%)	5.10	1 : 0	31	23	0
	Bicuspid	13 (81%)	5.03–5.93 (5.56)	13 : 0	49–90 (66)	24–36 (28)	4 (31%)
	Tricuspid	2 (13%)	5.58–5.77 (5.68)	2 : 0	71–80 (76)	26–27 (27)	0
>6	Unicuspid	3 (25%)	7.39–8.00 (7.70)	3 : 0	38–51 (43)	25–37 (29)	0
	Bicuspid	8 (67%)	6.23–11.30 (7.81)	8 : 0	43–78 (63)	21–32 (27)	3 (38%)
	Tricuspid	1 (8%)	6.60	1 : 0	84	24	1 (100%)
Totals		499	0.45–11.30 (2.67)	304 : 195	19–91 (70)	17–58 (28)	269

TABLE 7 Comparison of 18 Operatively-Excised Stenotic Aortic Valves Weighing ≤1 g to 12 Aortic Valves Weighing >6 g

Cases	Aortic Valve Weight (g) Range (mean)	Age (Years) Range (mean)	Female	Male	Body Mass Index (kg/m²) Range (mean)	Coronary Bypass	Tricuspid Aortic Valve
18	0.45–0.95 (0.78)	55–90 (77)	18	0	21–47 (28)	12 (67%)	16 (89%)
12	6.23–11.3 (7.68)	38–84 (60)	0	12	21–37 (27)	4 (33%)	1 (8%)
p Value	<0.001	0.004	<0.001		0.983	0.156	<0.001

ogy departments in a manner similar to that used for examination of other types of tissues. Portions of ≥1 cusps are submitted for histologic study, a procedure that destroys much of the valvular tissue, and useful information is rarely provided from examination of the histologic sections. We submit that weighing and photographing the valves provide more meaningful information, the type that can be correlated with the various clinical findings.[2]

Most of the weight in stenotic aortic valves is the result of that contributed by calcific deposits. Thus, the heavier valves in the present study were heavier than the lighter ones because of the larger quantity of calcium deposited on and in them. Glancy and colleagues[3] determined the amount of calcium as seen on lateral chest radiograph in dysfunctional aortic valves. Those with no calcium either had pure aortic regurgitation or an average transvalvular peak systolic pressure gradient of 10 mm Hg. The average peak systolic transvalvular gradient in those with 1+ calcium by radiograph was 45 mm Hg; those with 2+ calcium, 58 mm Hg, and those with 3+ calcium, 84 mm Hg. Thus, the larger the calcific deposits, the higher the transvalvular pressure gradient.

Acknowledgment: The 499 patients who had aortic valve replacement and were included in this study were operated on by 12 surgeons. The numbers of cases done by each surgeon were: Gregory J. Matter = 159 (32%); Baron L. Hamman = 88 (18%); A. Carl Henry III = 85 (17%); Robert F. Hebeler = 71 (14%); Richard E. Wood = 36 (7%); Edson H. Cheung = 15 (3%); Thomas P. Meyers = 15 (3%); Thomas Hoang = 14 (3%); Lonnie L. Whiddon = 7 (1%); Derrick D. McElroy = 5 (1%); W. Steves Ring = 3 (<1%); and Harry Kourlis = 1 (<1%).

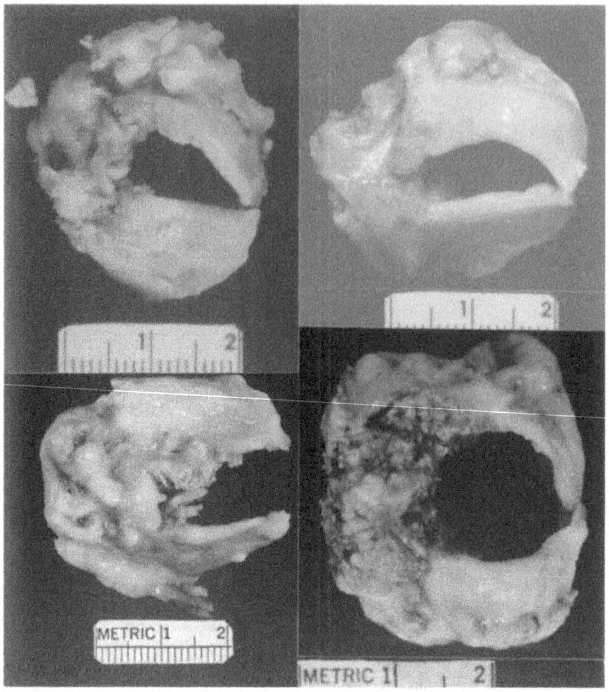

FIGURE 5. Photographs of operatively-excised congenitally unicuspid unicommissural aortic valves in 4 patients (see Table 8 for pertinent details in each patient). The valve weights progressively increase from top left across to bottom right across. (Photographs by Bonnie Martinez.)

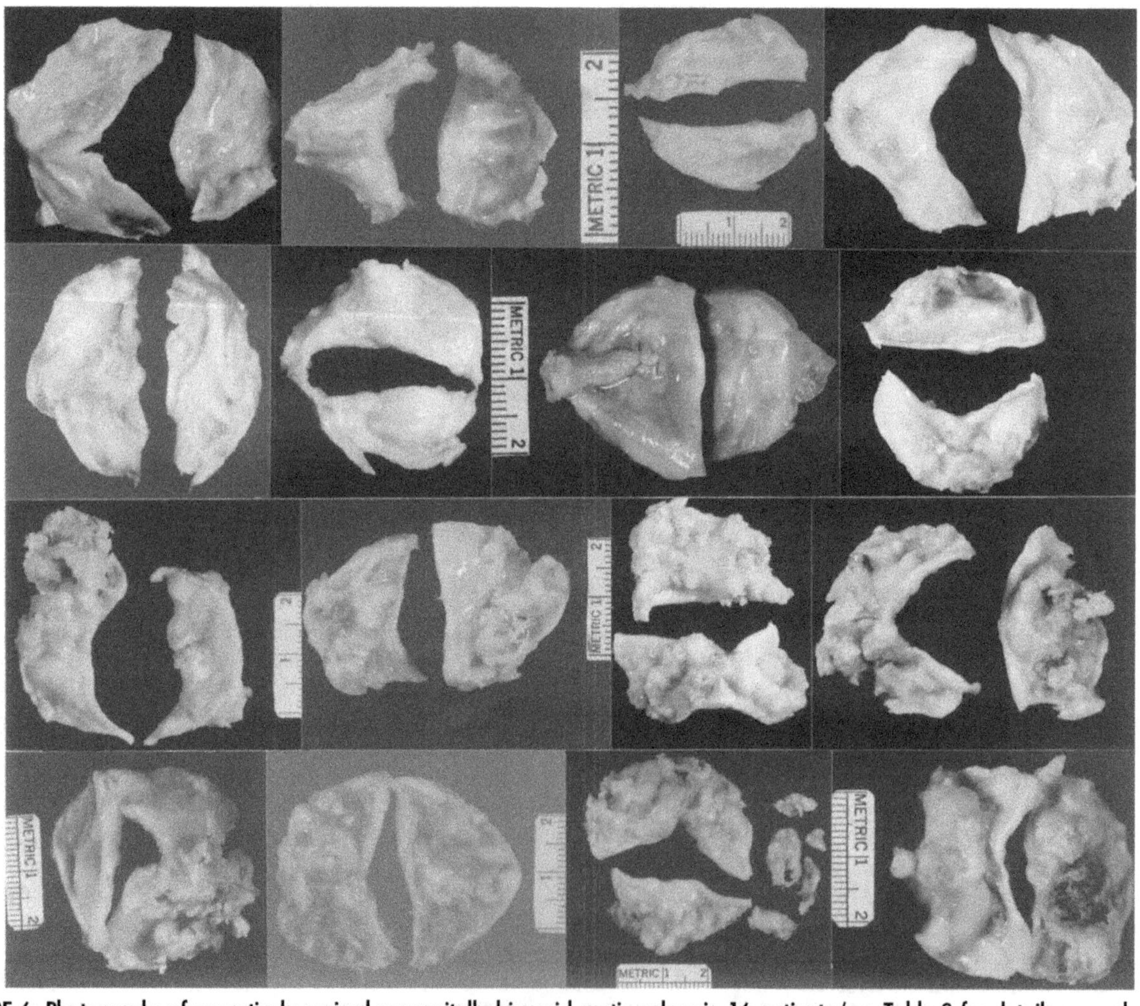

FIGURE 6. Photographs of operatively-excised congenitally bicuspid aortic valves in 16 patients (see Table 8 for details on each patient). The valve weights progressively increase from top left across to bottom right across. (Photographs by Bonnie Martinez.)

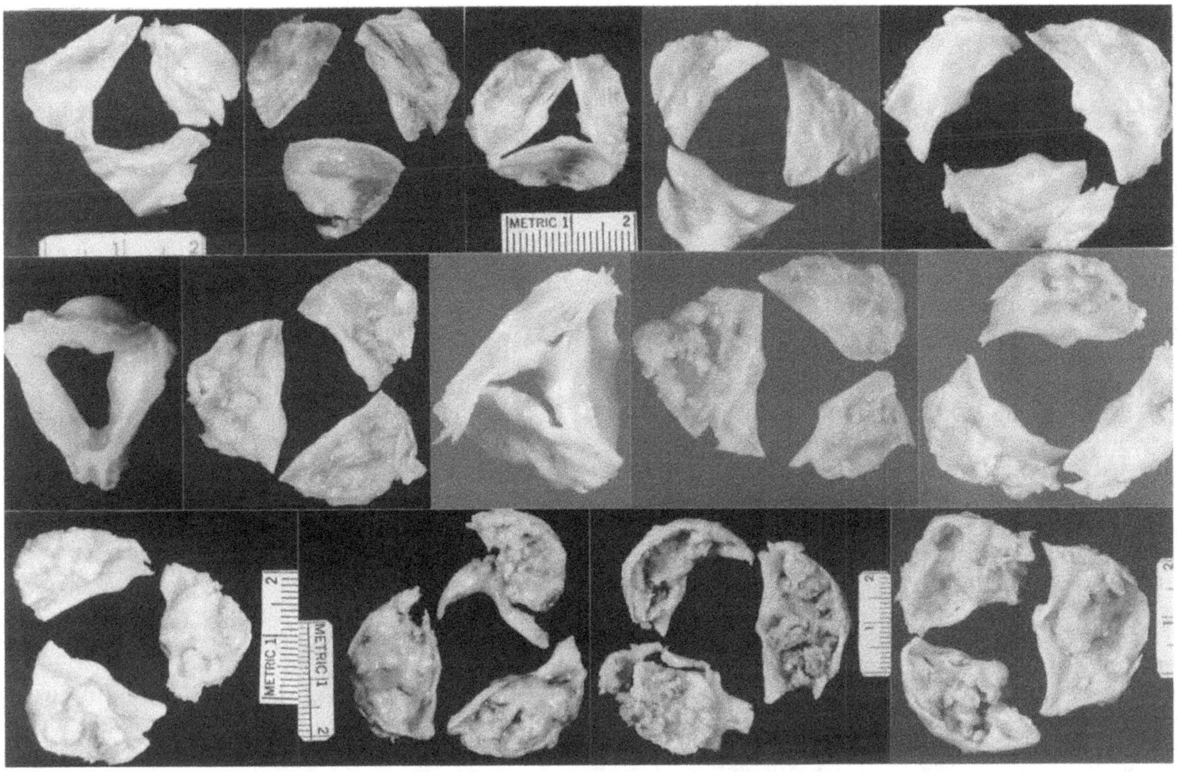

FIGURE 7. Photographs of operatively-excised tricuspid aortic valves in 14 patients (see Table 8 for details on each case). The valve weights progressively increase from top left across to bottom right across. (Photographs by Bonnie Martinez.)

TABLE 8 Aortic Valve Weights, Ages, Sex, and Presence or Absence of Simultaneous Coronary Artery Bypass Grafting in the Patients Whose Aortic Valves Are Illustrated in Figures 5 to 7

Figure Number	Patient	No. of Aortic Valve Cusps	Weight (g) of Excised Aortic Valve	Age/(Years) Sex	Concomitant Coronary Bypass
5	1	Unicuspid	3.61	47 M	0
	2	Unicuspid	3.93	57 M	0
	3	Unicuspid	5.10	31 M	0
	4	Unicuspid	7.39	39 M	0
6	5	Bicuspid	1.27	70 F	+
	6	Bicuspid	1.28	70 F	+
	7	Bicuspid	1.66	58 M	0
	8	Bicuspid	1.93	69 F	+
	9	Bicuspid	2.00	73 F	0
	10	Bicuspid	2.00	32 M	0
	11	Bicuspid	2.01	47 F	0
	12	Bicuspid	3.00	70 M	+
	13	Bicuspid	4.74	63 F	0
	14	Bicuspid	4.97	51 F	+
	15	Bicuspid	5.03	75 M	+
	16	Bicuspid	5.93	68 M	0
	17	Bicuspid	6.72	43 M	0
	18	Bicuspid	6.87	72 M	+
	19	Bicuspid	7.78	63 M	0
	20	Bicuspid	9.04	68 M	0
7	21	Tricuspid	0.45	81 F	+
	22	Tricuspid	0.69	84 F	+
	23	Tricuspid	0.74	80 F	0
	24	Tricuspid	0.80	83 F	+
	25	Tricuspid	0.85	81 F	0
	26	Tricuspid	1.02	62 F	0
	27	Tricuspid	1.14	65 M	+
	28	Tricuspid	1.21	47 M	0
	29	Tricuspid	1.85	86 F	+
	30	Tricuspid	2.00	73 F	0
	31	Tricuspid	3.14	84 F	+
	32	Tricuspid	4.81	70 F	0
	33	Tricuspid	5.77	71 M	0
	34	Tricuspid	6.87	72 M	+

1. Silver MA, Roberts WC. Detailed anatomy of the normally functioning aortic valve in hearts of normal and increased weight. *Am J Cardiol* 1985;55:454–461.
2. Roberts WC, Morrow AG. Cardiac valves and the surgical pathologist. *Arch Pathol* 1966;82:309–313.
3. Glancy DL, Freed TA, O'Brien KP, Epstein SE. Calcium in the aortic valve. Roentgenologic and hemodynamic correlations in 148 patients. *Ann Intern Med* 1969;71:245–250.

ADDENDUM

The manuscript of the enclosed article initially was sent to another medical journal and declined. The comments of the 2 reviewers and our responses to them follow.

Reviewer #1

(1) "Correlation with historical or catheterization data. The valve weights alone may not appear to justify valve replacement; however, when combined with additional clinical information the appropriateness of valve surgery may be more apparent. It seems inappropriate to indicate that valve surgery should not be done below a given valve weight without these considerations."

The manuscript initially stated "that valve replacement may not have been indicated when the aortic valve weights were <1 gram in the absence of significant aortic regurgitation." This statement was deleted from the revised manuscript.

(2) "Aortic regurgitation. As the authors concentrated on aortic stenosis and valve weight, how do the authors adjust for patients with mixed valve disease where aortic regurgitation may have required surgical intervention before the stenosis was 'mature'?"

No patient included in this study had moderately severe or severe associated aortic regurgitation.

(3) "Coronary artery disease. Is it possible that the surgeries at low valve weights were necessitated by severe CAD requiring bypass surgery before the aortic stenosis was severe?"

In 1 table we indicated that the valves were smaller in general in the patients who had concomitant coronary artery bypass grafting, and indeed, the operation in many of those cases was done primarily for coronary disease and not for aortic stenosis. We believe that the reviewer overlooked this observation in our manuscript.

(4) "Histopathology. Is there a difference in the histopathology of tricuspid versus unicuspid or bicuspid valves? In view of the increased calcium content of the congenital valves, and the younger age of unicuspid and bicuspid surgical patients, does aortic sclerosis differ from calcific aortic stenosis? Would there be a correlation of valve weight with age if only tricuspid valves were considered?"

Our article is not one on the histology of aortic valves. Yes, aortic sclerosis does differ from calcific aortic stenosis. That differentiation is easy to determine by gross inspection. We added Table 5 to show that there was no correlation between aortic valve weight and age among the 267 patients with aortic valve replacement and 3 cuspid aortic valves.

(5) "How would the findings of this study alter current medical practice?"

They would not. If that were a requirement, many medical manuscripts would not be accepted.

Reviewer #2

(1) "There is no clear hypothesis."

A hypothesis is an explanation that accounts for a set of facts that can be tested by further investigation. We think our manuscript fulfills this definition.

(2) "The clinical implications of the study are not clear."

That is debatable. Excision of aortic valves that weigh <1 gram in the absence of significant aortic regurgitation might bother some physicians. The reviewer, however, is correct.

(3) "The conclusion that valve surgery is not warranted for valves weighing <1 gram is not warranted as very little clinical data and no outcome data is provided."

The sentence referencing this point was deleted from the revised manuscript.

(4) "The authors mention that hemodynamic data was available (cath or echo). Is there any correlation between hemodynamic severity and valve weight?"

Yes, but that is not the topic of this manuscript.

(5) "The authors imply that heavier valves had more calcification but no data on valve composition is provided. How was fibrosis distinguished from calcification?"

Calcification is a process that cannot be seen. Calcific deposits are readily distinguished by gross inspection from fibrotic valves. The reasons some valves were heavier than others was because there were more calcific deposits in them.

(6) "Is it possible that the trileaflet valves were not excised as completely as the unicuspid and bicuspid valves, leading to the impression that valve weights differ?"

Highly unlikely.

(7) "Were any of the valves removed for mild-moderate aortic stenosis at the time of bypass grafting?"

Yes.

(8) "There is an excessive number of tables with redundant data."

Table 7 is redundant, but the contrast between the lightest and heaviest valves might be overlooked otherwise.

Before it was initially submitted to the other journal, our manuscript was sent to Dr. D. Luke Glancy for his comments. Dr. Glancy found an incorrect number in Figure 3, which was corrected.

Weights of Individual Cusps in Operatively-Excised Congenitally Bicuspid Stenotic Aortic Valves

William C. Roberts, MD, and Jong Mi Ko, BA

We weighed each cusp separately in 200 operatively excised stenotic congenitally bicuspid aortic valves. It was found in 152 patients (76%) that the cusps differed (by >0.2 g) in weight and in 48 patients (24%) that the cusps were of similar (a ≤0.2 g difference) weights. In 161 of the 200 patients (80%), raphes were present in 1 cusp; the raphe and nonraphe cusps differed in weight in 120 patients (74%), with the raphe cusps being larger in 89 patients (74%), and were of similar weights in 41 patients (26%). Of the 39 patients with raphes in neither cusp, 32 cusps (82%) differed in weight and 7 (18%) were of similar weights. The weight of each cusp differed more as the total valve weights increased. ©2004 by Excerpta Medica, Inc.

(Am J Cardiol 2004;94:678–681)

Recently, we reported the total weights of operatively excised stenotic unicuspid, bicuspid, and tricuspid aortic valves.[1] In this report, we describe, for the first time, the weights of each cusp in 200 patients who had their congenitally bicuspid stenotic aortic valves excised at the time of aortic valve replacement.

• • •

From January 1, 1998, to December 31, 2003 (6 years), at Baylor University Medical Center, 1,405 patients had replacement or repair of ≥1 cardiac valves (Figure 1). Of the 1,366 without active infective endocarditis, 64 had replacement of aortic and mitral valves, and 807 had replacement of only the aortic valve, without the replacement of another cardiac valve. Of the latter 807 patients, 650 had aortic stenosis with or without associated aortic regurgitation, and 157 had pure aortic regurgitation (no element of stenosis). Of the 650 with aortic stenosis, 281 had congenitally bicuspid stenotic aortic valves, 52 of which had the fusion of 1 or both true commissures, so that neither cusp could be weighed separately. Of the 229 without the fusion of either true commissure, 29 valves were excluded from this study because the valves had been excised in several pieces (21 patients), because a previous aortic valvulotomy had been done (1 patient), or because each cusp had not been weighed separately (7 patients). Thus, 200 patients remained, and they form the basis of this study. None of them had the fusion of either true commissure, and each cusp was weighed separately. Because the mean weights of operatively excised stenotic aortic valves in adults differ significantly in men and women,[1] the weights of each cusp were analyzed separately in men and women.

Of the 200 patients with congenitally bicuspid stenotic aortic valves without the fusion of 1 or both true commissures, 52 (26%) were women and 148 (74%) were men. The women ranged in age from 47 to 86 years (mean 68) and the men, from 32 to 91 years (mean 67).

Each operatively excised aortic valve arrived in the surgical pathology unit in a container filled with formaldehyde. The valve was removed from the container, placed on absorbing paper to absorb excess formaldehyde, and then weighed by 1 of us (WCR) on an

From the Baylor Heart & Vascular Institute and the Departments of Pathology and Medicine, Baylor University Medical Center, Dallas, Texas. Dr. Roberts' address is: Baylor Heart & Vascular Institute, Baylor University Medical Center, 3500 Gaston Avenue, Dallas, Texas 75246. E-mail: wc.roberts@baylorhealth.edu. Manuscript received April 14, 2004; revised manuscript received and accepted May 20, 2004.

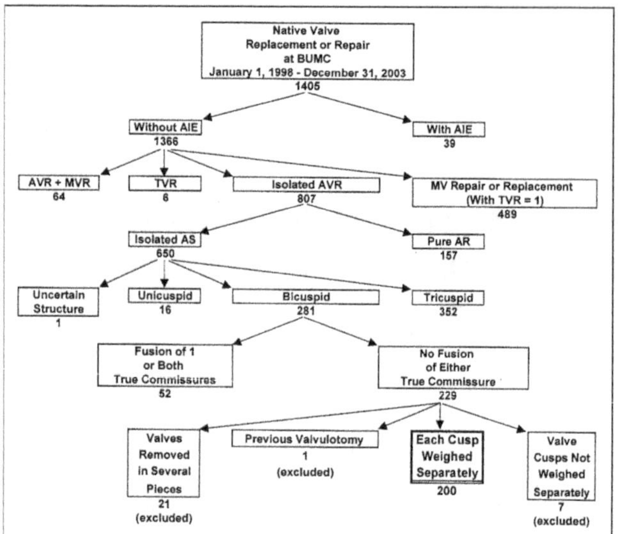

FIGURE 1. Algorithm showing the breakdown of 1,405 patients having valve replacement or repair at Baylor University Medical Center (BUMC) in a 6-year period and the origin of the 200 patients included in the present study. AIE = active infective endocarditis; AR = aortic regurgitation; AS = aortic stenosis; AVR = aortic valve replacement; MVR = mitral valve replacement; TVR = tricuspid valve replacement.

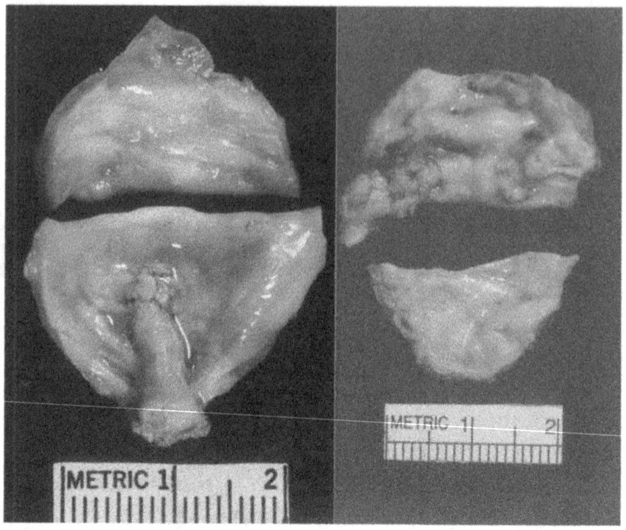

FIGURE 2. Photographs of 2 operatively excised congenitally bicuspid stenotic aortic valves. *Left,* valve weighing 1.92 g in a 47-year-old woman. A raphe, which is calcified, is present in 1 cusp. The raphe cusp weighed 1.27 g and the nonraphe cusp 0.65 g. *Right,* valve weighing 2.37 g in an 86-year-old woman. Neither cusp contains a raphe. One cusp weighed 1.76 g and the other 0.61 g. (Photographs were taken by Bonnie Martinez.)

TABLE 1 Total Valve Weights in Patients With Stenotic Congenitally Bicuspid Aortic Valves, Subdivided by Those With Fusion of 1 or Both True Commissures Verses Those Without Fusion of Either True Commissure and Also Subdivided by Gender

		Fusion of 1 or Both True Commissures		
	Number	0	+	p Value
Total	252	200 (79%)	52 (21%)	<0.001
		0.79–11.30 (3.24)	1.14–8.26 (3.33)	0.576
Men	176	148 (84%)	28 (16%)	<0.001
		0.89–11.30 (3.59)*	1.90–8.26 (3.90)*	0.269
Women	76	52 (68%)	24 (32%)	0.007
		0.79–4.97 (2.22)*	1.14–4.94 (2.66)*	0.069

*Range (mean), grams.

Ohaus scale (Ohaus Corporation, Florham Park, New Jersey), which has an accuracy to 0.01 g.

The z test was used to compare the percentages in 2 different groups (Tables 1 to 4). The parametric unpaired *t* test was used for comparison of the total valve weights in the 52 women without fusion of 1 or both true commissures with those in the 24 women with fusion of ≥1 true commissure (Table 1). The nonparametric Mann-Whitney rank sum test was used for comparison of the total valve weights in the 200 patients without fusion of 1 or both true commissures with those in the 52 patients with fusion of ≥1 true commissure (Table 1), for comparison of the total valve weights in men without fusion of 1 or both true commissures with those in men with fusion of ≥1 true commissure (Table 1), and for comparison of the weights of the raphe and nonraphe cusps (Table 5). A p value <0.05 was considered statistically significant. Statistical analysis was performed using SigmaStat version 2.0 (SPSS, Inc., Chicago, Illinois).

The mean weights of the excised valves were similar (a ≤0.2 g difference) in the 200 patients without fusion of either true commissure and in the 52 patients with fusion of 1 or both true commissures (3.24 vs 3.33 g, p = 0.576; Table 1). The remainder of this study focuses exclusively on the 200 patients in whom each cusp of the congenitally bicuspid stenotic aortic valve was weighed separately.

Of the 200 patients, the 2 cusps differed (by >0.2 g) in weight in 152 (76%) and were similar in weight in 48 (24%) (a ≤0.2 g difference; Table 2 and Figure 2). This difference was similar in the 148 men and the 52 women and whether or not a raphe was present in 1 of the 2 cusps (Table 2).

The raphe cusps overall were heavier than the nonraphe cusps (Table 3). Of the 161 patients with raphes in 1 of the 2 cusps, 120 had differences in cuspal weights: in 89 of them (74%), the raphe cusps were heavier than the nonraphe cusps, and in 31 (26%), the raphe cusps were lighter than the nonraphe cusps (Table 3).

The weights of each cusp in the entire group and in men and women are listed in Table 4 and 5. As expected, the mean weights of the entire cusps were heavier in the men than the women (3.59 vs 2.22 g, p <0.001), and the mean weights of the raphe cusps in the entire

TABLE 2 Cases of Operatively Excised Congenitally Bicuspid Aortic Valve Displaying Whether Each of the 2 Cusps Was of Similar or Dissimilar Weight and Subdivided by the Presence or Absence of a Raphe in 1 Cusp and by Gender

		Cuspal Weight		Raphe in 1 of 2 Cusps		No Raphe in Either Cusp	
	Cases	Each Different	Each Similar	Weights* Different	Weights Similar	Weights Different	Weights Similar
Total	200 (100%)	152 (76%)†	48 (24%)†	120 (74%)‡	41 (26%)†	32 (82%)‡	7 (18%)‡
Men	148 (74%)	117 (79%)†	31 (21%)†	91 (77%)†	27 (23%)†	26 (87%)§	4 (13%)§
Women	52 (26%)	35 (67%)‖	17 (33%)‖	29 (68%)¶	14 (32%)¶	6 (67%)#	3 (33%)#

*See Table 3; †Across $p < 0.001$; ‡$p = 0.004$; §$p = 0.008$; ‖$p = 0.04$; ¶$p = 0.08$; #$p = 0.80$.

TABLE 3 Operatively Excised Congenitally Bicuspid Stenotic Aortic Valves Displaying Relative Weights of Raphe and Nonraphe Cusps and Subdivided by Gender

	Total Cases	Raphe in 1 Cusp	Raphe Cusp Heavier Than Nonraphe Cusp	Raphe Cusp Lighter Than Nonraphe Cusp	Raphe and Nonraphe Cusps of Similar Weights
Total	200	161	89 (55%)*	31 (19%)*	41 (26%)
Men	148	118	71 (60%)*	20 (17%)*	27 (23%)
Women	52	43	18 (42%)†	11 (26%)†	14 (32%)

*Across $p < 0.001$; †$p = 0.38$.

TABLE 4 Relation of Whether the Individual Cusps Were of Different (>0.2 g) or Similar (a ≤0.2 g Difference) Weights, Subdivided Into 4 Groups According to the Total Weight of the Congenitally Bicuspid Stenotic Aortic Valves

Total Valve Weights (g)	Number	Cuspal Weights: Each Different	Cuspal Weights: Each Similar	p Value
≤2.0	18 Men	11 (61%)	7 (39%)	0.669
	24 Women	12 (50%)	12 (50%)	0.683
>2.0–4.0	82 Men	65 (79%)	17 (21%)	<0.001
	25 Women	21 (84%)	4 (16%)	0.028
>4.0–6.0	40 Men	33 (83%)	7 (17%)	0.002
	3 Women	2	1	—
>6.0	8 Men	8* (100%)	0	—
	— Women	—	—	—

*See Table 6 for data on each of these 8 cases.

group and in the men were heavier than the mean weights of the nonraphe cusps (1.73 vs 1.38 g and 1.95 vs 1.50 g, $p < 0.001$).

The relation of the patient cuspal weights—whether different or similar—to the total valve weights subdivided into 4 weight groups is listed in Table 4. The greater the total cuspal weights, the greater the chance that the 2 cusps differed in weight. Of the 8 valves, for example, weighing >6.0 g, the cusps differed in weight in all 8 (100%). In contrast, of the 42 valves weighing ≤2.0 g, only 23 (55%) had cusps that differed in weight.

The differences in cuspal weights in each of the 8 men with stenotic valves weighing >6 g are listed in Table 6. The 2 cusps differed in weight in these 8 patients from 0.24 to 5.05 g (mean 2.56, median 2.96). In 5 of these 8 patients, 1 cusp weighed ≥70% of the total weight of the valve, and in the other 3 patients, neither cusp weighed >55% of the valve's total weight. In all 8 patients, the difference in weight between the 2 cusps was always >0.2 g.

• • •

Whether or not 2 cusps differ in weight is dependent, of course, on the definition of "difference." In this study, we defined "difference" as >0.2 g in weight between the 2 cusps. In the 200 patients with congenitally bicuspid stenotic aortic valves, 152 (76%) had cusps that differed in weight by >0.2 g. If we had defined "difference" as >0.1 g between the cusps, then 167 of the 200 valves (83%) would have had cusps that differed in weight. To picture what these numbers represent, 2 drops from a plastic transfer Pipette (manufactured by Allegiance Healthcare Corporation, Cypress, California) roughly equal 0.1 g, and 4 drops roughly equal 0.2 g.

Why do the 2 cusps of a congenitally bicuspid stenotic aortic valve usually differ in weight irrespective of whether or not a raphe is present? The most likely explanation would appear to be that the cusps differ in size, that is, in surface area, from the time of birth. The cusp with the largest surface area has, of course, the larger area on which calcium can be deposited, and the weight of a cusp is determined primarily by the amount of calcium deposited on its aortic surface.

TABLE 5 Weights of Operatively Excised Congenitally Bicuspid Aortic Valves and of Each Cusp, Subdivided by the Presence or Absence of a Raphe in 1 Cusp and by Gender

	Number	Total Valve Weights (g), Range (mean)	Weight (g)* of Each Cusp, Range (mean)		Weight (g)† of Each Cusp When Neither Contained a Raphe, Range (mean)
			Raphe Cusp	Nonraphe Cusp	
Total	200 (100%)	0.79–11.30 (3.24)	0.40–7.08 (1.73)‡	0.25–4.81 (1.38)‡	0.31–8.10 (1.58)
Men	148 (74%)	0.89–11.30 (3.59)	0.42–7.08 (1.95)‡	0.25–4.81 (1.50)‡	0.31–8.10 (1.69)
Women	52 (26%)	0.79–4.97 (2.22)	0.40–2.83 (1.11)§	0.32–2.33 (1.05)§	0.38–1.99 (1.20)

*161 cases, 322 cusps; †39 cases, 78 cusps; ‡across $p < 0.001$; §$p = 0.46$.

TABLE 6 Weights of Each Cusp in the 8 Patients in Whom Total Valve Weight Was >6 g

No.	Age (yrs)	Total Valve Weight (g)	Weight (g) of Each Cusp	Cuspal Weight Difference (g)
1	49	6.09	4.47 (73%):1.62 (27%)	2.85
2	63	6.45	4.87 (76%) (R):1.58 (24%)	3.29
3	54	6.64	3.20 (48%) (R):3.44 (52%)	0.24
4	72	6.85	3.63 (53%) (R):3.22 (47%)	0.41
6	40	7.19	5.13 (71%) (R):2.06 (29%)	3.07
5	68	8.76	3.95 (45%) (R):4.81 (55%)	0.86
7	90	9.11	7.08 (78%) (R):2.03 (22%)	5.05
8	78	11.50	8.10 (70%):3.40 (30%)	4.70

R = raphe.

Acknowledgment: The 200 patients having aortic valve replacement and included in this study were operated on by 11 surgeons. The numbers of cases done by each surgeon were as follows: Gregory J. Matter, 52 cases (26%); A. Carl Henry III, 44 cases (22%); Baron L. Hamman, 34 cases (17%); Robert F. Hebeler, 30 cases (15%); Richard E. Wood, 12 cases (6%); Thomas Hoang, 10 cases (5%); Lonnie L. Whiddon, 7 cases (4%); Edson H. Cheung, 4 cases (2%); Thomas P. Meyers, 4 cases (2%); Derrick D. McElroy, 2 cases (1%); and Harry Kourlis, Jr., 1 case (<1%).

1. Roberts WC, Ko JM. Weights of operatively-excised stenotic unicuspid, bicuspid, and tricuspid aortic valves and their relation to age, sex, body mass index, and presence or absence of concomitant coronary artery bypass grafting. *Am J Cardiol* 2003:92:1057–1065.

Weights of Individual Cusps in Operatively-Excised Stenotic Three-Cuspid Aortic Valves

William C. Roberts, MD, and Jong Mi Ko, BA

We weighed each cusp separately in 260 operatively excised stenotic 3-cuspid aortic valves. All 3 cusps differed (by >0.1 g) in weight in 69 patients (26%); all 3 cusps were similar (a ≤0.1 g difference) in weight in 33 patients (13%); and 1 cusp differed from either of the other 2 cusps, which were similar in weight, in 158 patients (61%). The weight differences appeared to be caused by differing quantities of calcium on the aortic surfaces of the cusps. ©2004 by Excerpta Medica, Inc.

(Am J Cardiol 2004;94:681–684)

From the Baylor Heart & Vascular Institute and the Departments of Pathology and Medicine, Baylor University Medical Center, Dallas, Texas. Dr. Roberts's address is: Baylor Heart & Vascular Institute, Baylor University Medical Center, 3500 Gaston Avenue, Dallas, Texas 75246. E-mail: wc.roberts@baylorhealth.edu. Manuscript received April 14, 2004; revised manuscript received and accepted May 20, 2004.

In another study in this issue,[1] we reported the weights of each cusp of congenitally bicuspid stenotic aortic valves. In this report, we describe for the first time the weights of each cusp in 260 patients who had their stenotic 3-cuspid aortic valves excised at the time of aortic valve replacement.

• • •

From January 1, 1998, to December 31, 2003 (6 years), at Baylor University Medical Center, 1,405 patients had replacement or repair of ≥1 cardiac valves (Figure 1). Of the 1,366 without active infective endocarditis, 64 had replacement of aortic and mitral valves and 807 had replacement of only the aortic valve, without replacement of another cardiac valve. Of the latter 807 patients, 650 had aortic stenosis, with or without associated aortic regurgitation, and 157 had pure aortic regurgitation. Of the 650 with aortic stenosis, 352 had stenotic tricuspid aortic valves. Of them, 64 had fusion of ≥1 commissures, so that the cusps could not be weighed individually. The remaining 288 patients had no fusion at any of the 3

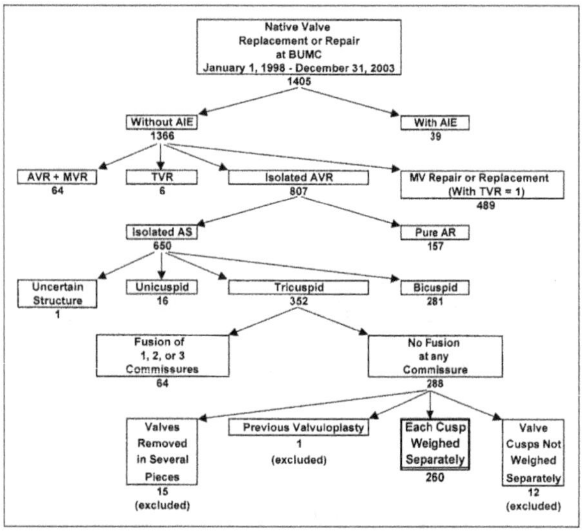

FIGURE 1. Algorithm showing the breakdown of the 1,405 patients having valve replacement or repair at Baylor University Medical Center (BUMC) in a 6-year period and the origin of the 260 patients included in the present study. AIE = active infective endocarditis; AR = aortic regurgitation; AS = aortic stenosis; AVR = aortic valve replacement; MVR = mitral valve replacement; TVR = tricuspid valve replacement.

TABLE 1 Total Valve Weights in Patients With Stenotic Tricuspid Aortic Valves, Subdivided by Those With Fusion of 1, 2, or 3 Commissures Versus Those Without Fusion at Any Commissure and Also Subdivided by Gender

		Fusion of 1, 2, or 3 Commissures		
	Number	0	+	p Value
Total	324	260 (80%) 0.45–6.60 (2.02)*	64 (20%) 0.55–4.87 (2.16)*	<0.001 0.227
Men	175	143 (82%) 1.12–6.60 (2.41)*	32 (18%) 1.20–4.87 (2.63)*	<0.001 0.174
Women	149	117 (79%) 0.45–4.81 (1.58)*	32 (21%) 0.55–3.12 (1.70)*	<0.001 0.238

*Range (mean), grams.

commissures, but of them, 28 were excluded for varying reasons (see Figure 1). The remaining 260 patients are the subjects of this report. None of these 260 patients had fusion of any commissure, and each cusp was weighed separately. Because the mean weights of operatively excised stenotic aortic valves in adults differ significantly in men and women,[2] the weight of each cusp was analyzed separately in men and women. The women ranged in age from 28 to 90 years (mean 74) and the men from 52 to 90 years (mean 75).

Each operatively excised aortic valve arrived in the surgical pathology unit in a container filled with formaldehyde. The valve was removed from the container, placed on absorbing paper to absorb excess formaldehyde, and then weighed by 1 of us (WCR) on an Ohaus scale (Ohaus Corporation, Florham Park, New Jersey), which has an accuracy to 0.01 g.

The z test was used to compare the percentages in 2 different groups (Table 1). The nonparametric Mann-Whitney rank sum test was used to compare the total valve weights in the 260 patients without cuspal fusion at any of the 3 commissures with those of the 64 patients with fusion of ≥1 commissure (Table 1). The nonparametric Kruskal-Wallis 1-way analysis of variance on ranks was used to compare total weights in the 260 patients without cuspal fusion at any of the 3 commissures, in the 64 patients with cuspal fusion at ≥1 commissure, and in the 15 patients in whom the valves were excised in several pieces. A p value <0.05 was considered statistically significant. Statistical analysis was performed using SigmaStat version 2.0 (SPSS, Inc., Chicago, Illinois).

We compared the total weights of the operatively excised stenotic valves in the 260 patients without cuspal fusion at any of the 3 commissures, in the 64 patients with cuspal fusion at ≥1 commissure, and in the 15 patients in whom the valves were excised in several pieces (Figure 1 and Table 1). The mean total valve weights were insignificantly different among the 3 groups (2.02 vs 2.16 vs 2.26 g, p = 0.20).

We defined cuspal weight difference as >0.1 g. As listed in Table 2, in the 260 patients, all 3 cusps differed (by >0.1 g) in weight in 71 patients (27%), all 3 cusps were similar (a ≤0.1 g difference) in weight in 33 patients (13%), and 1 cusp differed in weight from each of the other 2 similarly sized cusps in 156 patients (60%). Similar breakdowns were observed in men and women (Table 2). When the total aortic valve weights were divided into 4 groups (≤1, >1 to 2, >2 to 3, and >3 g), differences in cuspal weights were more evident in the heavier valves compared with the lighter valves.

The weights of each aortic valve cusp in each of the 33 patients in whom the total valve weights were >3 g are listed in Table 3. Differences and similarities in patient cuspal weights are listed.

• • •

This study shows in adults with operatively excised stenotic 3-cuspid aortic valves without cuspal fusion at any of the 3 commissures that cuspal differences in weight were common: the most common scenario was valves in which 2 cusps were similar in weight and 1 cusp differed in weight from either or both of them (156 patients [60%]); the least common scenario was valves in which all 3 cusps were similar in weight (33 patients [13%]), and the intermediate group included those patients in whom all 3 cusps differed in weight (71 patients [27%]).

In contrast to the study of congenitally bicuspid aortic valves, in the present study, we used a weight of 0.1 g to indicate a difference between cuspal weights.[1] We used this smaller weight difference because the total weights of the operatively excised 3-cuspid valves were considerably and significantly smaller

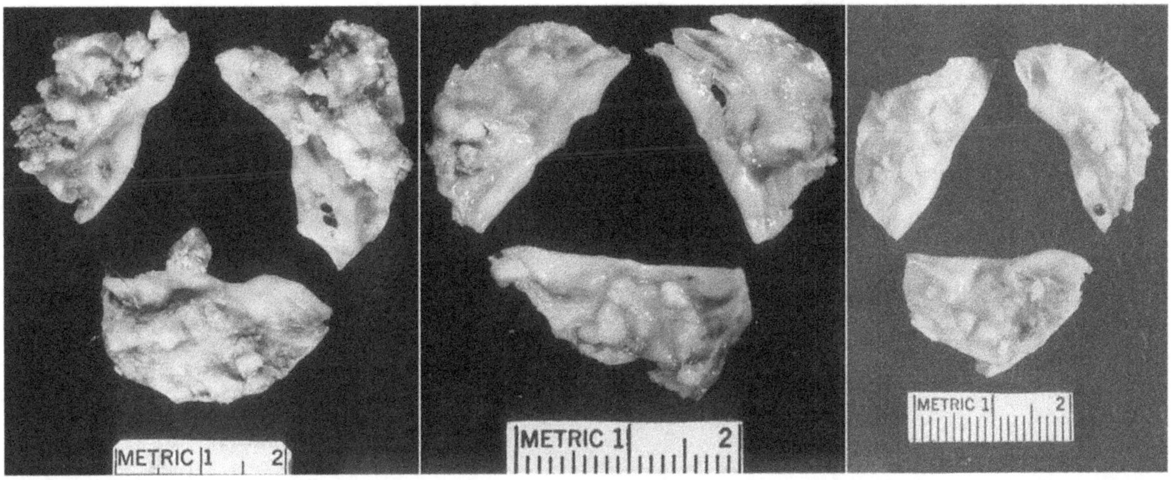

FIGURE 2. Photographs of 3 operatively excised stenotic 3-cuspid aortic valves. *Left,* valve weighing 3.08 g in a 77-year-old man. All 3 cusps differed in weight (1.16 vs 1.04 vs 0.87 g). *Middle,* valve weighing 1.22 g in an 81-year-old woman. All 3 cusps were similar in weight (0.41 vs 0.42 vs 0.32 g). *Right,* valve weighing 1.57 g in a 58-year-old man. One cusp was different in weight from 1 of the other 2 similar cusps (0.43 vs 0.45 vs 0.68 g). (Photographs by Bonnie Martinez.)

TABLE 2 Relation of Whether the Individual Cusps Were of Different (>0.1 g) or Similar (a ≤ 0.1-g difference) Weights, Subdivided Into 4 Groups According to the Total Weight of the Stenotic 3-Cuspid Aortic Valves

			Cuspal Weight		
Total Valve Weights (g)	Gender	Number	All 3 Different	All 3 Similar	1 Different from Either of the Other 2 Similar Cusps
≤1	Men	—	—	—	—
	Women	16	1 (6%)	5 (31%)	10 (63%)
>1–2	Men	61	14 (23%)	8 (13%)	39 (64%)
	Women	79	16 (20%)	13 (16%)	50 (64%)
>2–3	Men	52	13 (25%)	4 (8%)	35 (67%)
	Women	19	8 (42%)	1 (5%)	10 (53%)
>3	Men	30*	16 (53%)	2 (7%)	12 (40%)
	Women	3*	3	—	—
Total		260 (100%)	71 (27%)	33 (13%)	156 (60%)
Men		143 (55%)	43 (30%)	14 (10%)	86 (60%)
Women		117 (45%)	28 (24%)	19 (16%)	70 (60%)

*See Table 3 for data on each of these 30 men and 3 women.

than those in the congenitally bicuspid aortic valves.[2] Had we used >0.2 g as the indicator of a difference between cuspal weights, only 20 of the 260 patients (8%) would have had differences among all 3 cusps; 94 patients (36%) would have had similar weights of all 3 cusps, and 146 patients (56%) would have had 1 cusp different from either or both of the 2 similarly weighed cusps (see Table 2 for comparisons when using a 0.1-g difference).

Why might cusps differ in weight in patients with operatively excised stenotic 3-cuspid aortic valves unassociated with mitral valve disease requiring mitral valve replacement? Although most patients included in this study had the stenotic aortic valve excised intact, some had small calcific deposits excised separately, and it was not possible to determine from which cusp the small calcific fragment had been excised. That scenario, however, is unlikely to explain the weight differences between cusps in most patients. It has been demonstrated previously that the posterior (noncoronary) aortic valve cusp normally has a larger surface area than the left or right aortic valve cusp.[3] The larger the cuspal surface area, the greater the area for calcific deposits, and it is the latter that is the major determinant of cuspal weight. None of the 3 separately excised aortic valve cusps in the present study, however, had the particular cusp identified by the surgeon, so we had no way of knowing which cusp had been located in which aortic sinus of Valsalva (Figure 2).

Acknowledgment: The 260 patients having aortic valve replacement and included in this study were operated on by 12 surgeons. The numbers of cases done by each surgeon were as follows: Gregory J. Matter, 78 cases (30%); Baron L. Hamman, 51 cases (20%); A. Carl Henry III, 44 (17%); Robert F. He-

TABLE 3 Weights of Individual Cusps in the 30 Men and 3 Women in Whom Total Valve Weights Were >3 g								
		Total Valve	Weights (g) of Individual Cusps*			Differences in Cuspal Weights (g)		
Case	Age (yrs)	Weight (g)*	1	2	3	1 vs 2	1 vs 3	2 vs 3
				Men				
1	80	3.09	0.95	0.89	1.21	0.06	0.26	0.32
2	70	3.10	1.19	1.05	0.86	0.14	0.33	0.19
3	68	3.13	1.13	1.03	0.96	0.10	0.17	0.07
4	75	3.16	1.12	1.06	1.02	0.06	0.10	0.04
5	78	3.19	1.21	1.00	0.92	0.21	0.29	0.08
6	79	3.20	1.27	0.95	0.48	0.32	0.79	0.47
7	69	3.25	1.15	0.95	0.83	0.20	0.32	0.12
8	67	3.28	1.36	0.96	0.81	0.40	0.55	0.15
9	84	3.31	1.22	0.98	0.90	0.24	0.32	0.08
10	68	3.39	1.28	1.16	1.00	0.12	0.28	0.16
11	80	3.42	1.63	1.09	0.70	0.54	0.93	0.39
12	75	3.50	1.26	1.20	0.86	0.06	0.40	0.34
13	80	3.51	1.09	0.99	0.44	0.10	0.65	0.55
14	78	3.53	1.20	1.17	1.17	0.03	0.03	0.00
15	81	3.60	1.76	1.24	0.53	0.52	1.23	0.71
16	80	3.61	1.80	0.95	0.84	0.85	0.96	0.11
17	78	3.85	1.73	1.20	0.90	0.53	0.83	0.30
18	74	3.87	1.30	1.51	1.07	0.21	0.23	0.44
19	72	3.90	1.21	0.93	0.77	0.28	0.44	0.16
20	76	3.95	1.86	1.09	1.03	0.77	0.83	0.06
21	67	4.00	1.56	1.47	0.88	0.09	0.68	0.59
22	84	4.05	1.84	1.21	1.00	0.63	0.84	0.21
23	85	4.43	1.73	1.69	0.99	0.04	0.74	0.70
24	68	4.50	2.44	1.09	1.06	1.35	1.38	0.03
25	78	4.51	1.60	1.50	1.30	0.10	0.30	0.20
26	67	4.58	1.93	1.43	1.20	0.50	0.73	0.23
27	83	4.59	1.74	1.47	1.35	0.27	0.39	0.12
28	80	5.58	2.21	2.11	1.07	0.10	1.14	1.04
29	71	5.77	2.69	1.68	1.39	1.01	1.30	0.29
30	84	6.60	3.02	1.96	1.63	1.06	1.39	0.33
				Women				
1	84	3.07	1.46	0.96	0.62	0.50	0.84	0.34
2	73	3.14	1.20	1.02	0.84	0.18	0.36	0.18
3	70	4.81	2.03	1.48	1.37	0.55	0.66	0.11

*The differences in the total valve weights and the sum of the weights of each of the 3 cusps represent the weights of small calcific fragments excised separately.

beler, 41 cases (16%); Richard E. Wood, 16 cases (6%); Thomas Hoang, 10 cases (4%); Edson H. Cheung, 8 cases (3%); Thomas P. Meyers, 6 cases (2%); Lonnie L. Whiddon, 1 case (<1%); Derrick D. McElroy, 2 cases (<1%); W. Steves Ring, 2 cases (<1%); and Harry Kourlis, Jr., 1 case (<1%).

1. Roberts WC, Ko JM. Weights of individual cusps in operatively-excised congenitally bicuspid stenotic aortic valves. *Am J Cardiol* 2004;94:678–681.

2. Roberts WC, Ko JM. Weights of operatively-excised stenotic unicuspid, bicuspid, and tricuspid aortic valves and their relation to age, sex, body mass index, and presence or absence of concomitant coronary artery bypass grafting. *Am J Cardiol* 2003;92:1057–1065.

3. Silver MA, Roberts WC. Detailed anatomy of the normally functioning aortic valve in hearts of normal and increased weight. *Am J Cardiol* 1985;55:454–461.

ROBERT OGDEN BONOW, MD: a conversation with the editor on valvular heart disease and indications for operative intervention

Bob Bonow (*Figure*) was born in Camden, New Jersey, on March 11, 1947, and grew up in the suburbs of New York City. He graduated magna cum laude from Lehigh University in chemical engineering in 1969 and from the University of Pennsylvania School of Medicine in 1973. His medical internship and residency were at the Hospital of the University of Pennsylvania. From 1976 until 1992, Dr. Bonow was in the Cardiology Branch of the National Heart, Lung, and Blood Institute in Bethesda, Maryland. In 1992 he moved to Chicago to be the Goldberg Distinguished Professor of Cardiology and chief of the Division of Cardiology in the Department of Medicine of the Northwestern University Feinberg School of Medicine. He recently was president of the American Heart Association.

Dr. Bonow is one of the world's outstanding cardiologists. He is a superb clinician, a splendid clinical investigator, and a marvelous teacher. He is the author of numerous articles in peer-reviewed publications and recently became one of the 4 editors of Braunwald's *Heart Disease* textbook. He was the chair of the first and second American College of Cardiology (ACC)/American Heart Association (AHA) committees for writing guidelines for management of patients with valvular heart disease. Dr. Bonow gave medical ground rounds at Baylor University Medical Center (BUMC) on September 14, 2004, and discussed indications for operative therapy in patients with aortic stenosis, aortic regurgitation, and mitral regurgitation. Thereafter, Bob and I had a discussion on valvular heart disease.

William Clifford Roberts, MD (hereafter, WCR): *Bob, I appreciate your willingness to talk to me and therefore to the readers of* BUMC Proceedings. *To start, could you discuss valvular heart disease in general, the magnitude of the problem, and your general guidelines for recommending a cardiac valve operation?*

Robert Ogden Bonow, MD (hereafter, ROB): Bill, first it's an honor for me to visit BUMC, to give grand rounds, and to spend time with you. We are seeing more and more patients with valvular heart disease because of our aging population. General internists and even cardiovascular specialists are a bit uncertain about the most appropriate evaluation and treatment for patients with valvular heart disease. Unlike coronary heart disease and heart failure, where results of many trials allow specific guidelines for management, there are no prospective randomized trials with definitive results for patients with valvular heart disease, and therefore the guidelines are based only upon consensus of experts. As cardiovascular specialists we expect evidence to guide our decisions, but the evidence in patients with valvular heart disease is primarily retrospective from individual medical centers and based on relatively small numbers of patients. Unfortunately, there are wide differences in opinion among experts in management of these patients. As a consequence, the threshold for proceeding with a valve operation may vary tremendously from place to place depending upon the expected results of the surgeons as well as the skill of the referring cardiologists.

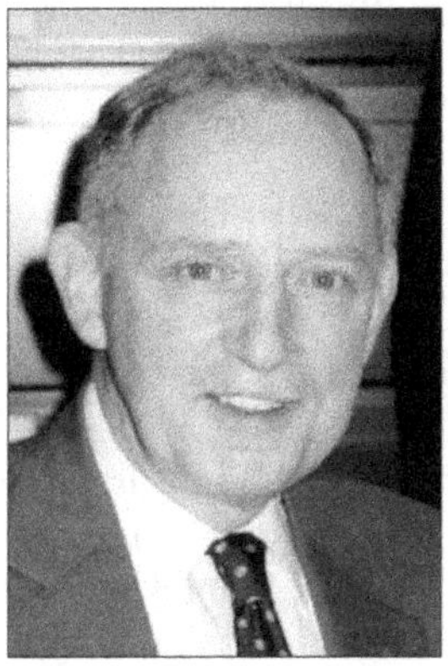

Figure. Dr. Robert Bonow during the interview.

WCR: *You were the chair for development of the latest ACC/AHA guidelines for operative intervention in valvular heart disease. How did that endeavor come about, how was the committee formed, and who made up that committee?*

ROB: It came about in the mid 1990s when the ACC/AHA guidelines task force began moving from procedure-driven guidelines to disease-based guidelines. In the future we'll be seeing fewer procedure-related guidelines and more patient management guidelines. We realized from the beginning that formulating guidelines for valvular heart disease would be a challenge because of the lack of data from randomized clinical trials. The committee was composed initially of 10 to 12 physicians appointed by the chair of the guidelines task force, which also appointed the chair of the writing group. The committee consisted of very knowledgeable and influential physicians who had written extensively on valvular heart disease. The committee included one pediatric cardiologist (Michael Freed), one family practitioner (Brad Fedderly), and one cardiac surgeon (Hank Edmonds); the remainder of the members were adult cardiologists, including both echocardiographers and interventionalists. The committee consisted of a good balance of physicians.

WCR: *How many meetings did you have?*

ROB: Initially, the plan was for the committee to meet a few times and complete the written document in 18 months. We realized early on, however, that that timetable was unrealistic.

From Division of Cardiology, Department of Medicine, Northwestern University Medical School, Chicago, Illinois (Bonow) and Baylor Heart and Vascular Institute, Baylor University Medical Center, Dallas, Texas (Roberts).

Corresponding author: Robert O. Bonow, MD, Division of Cardiology, Northwestern University Medical School, 201 East Huron Street, Galter 10-240, Chicago, Illinois 60611 (e-mail: r-bonow@northwestern.edu).

We found ourselves arguing, for example, for 3 hours on the definition of *severe* aortic valve stenosis. Should the definition be based on valve area, the transvalvular gradient, or the echo Doppler velocity across the valve? That definition was important because several committee members believed that valve replacement should not be recommended unless the degree of stenosis was severe. Was severe aortic stenosis a valve area of 1.0 or 0.8 cm^2? Ultimately, we decided it didn't matter too much because the real indication for operation for aortic stenosis was not how tight the valve was but what effect the obstruction had on the left ventricle and on the patient. An asymptomatic patient with normal left ventricular function was not a candidate for aortic valve replacement irrespective of the severity of the obstruction. Once the symptom status of the patient and the presence or absence of normal left ventricular function were settled, we returned to the question of the severity of the obstruction.

The committee members could discuss a single item for hours. The discussions took several meetings, usually in Chicago (a central location), and they generally lasted 1½ days. We then assigned a specific topic to each committee member. As the manuscripts were submitted, they were circulated to other committee members for comments. Thus, thereafter we had drafts to discuss at the meetings. Not everybody got their drafts in on the specified date, but that individual lateness proved helpful because it allowed focus on the individual components rather than on the whole document. The process took about 2½ years to complete. We're now revising the guidelines, which were formulated in 1998. The revision has been in progress for about 1½ years, and we're hoping to complete this revision in the fall of 2004 and have it published in the spring of 2005.

WCR: *In the 1998 guidelines, which section of the initial draft did you prepare?*

ROB: The one on aortic regurgitation. The committee actually voted on who wrote which portion initially. Every section, however, had input from all committee members. Every line, every nuance, was carefully reviewed. The 1998 guidelines were the lengthiest ones in any area up to that time. The document consisted of 102 pages in the *Journal of the American College of Cardiology*, including over 730 references! I'm not suggesting that length represents excellence. Guidelines ideally contain concise bullet points such that physicians can put them in their pocket or Palm Pilot and memorize them for patient management. Our guidelines in 1998 were based on consensus, not on large-scale clinical trials, and, therefore, we believed it important to discuss, sometimes at length, why a certain recommendation was being made. We included lots of information about natural history, pathophysiology, and whatever clinical evidence was available. Although we created a very lengthy document, we also had an executive summary that distilled the huge amount of information into a pocket guide. In essence, we wrote a textbook on valvular heart disease.

WCR: *As chair of the committee, you went over every word multiple times?*

ROB: Yes, I did. Since each section was prepared by a different committee member, the document had many different styles. I tried to make it more cohesive, and that took much editing and rewriting. That created lots of e-mails and conference calls. Each committee member had a chance to go over every word. I read it several times.

WCR: *Who paid the expenses of the committee: flights, hotels, secretarial assistance, etc.?*

ROB: The expenses were covered by a budget created jointly by the AHA and ACC. Both organizations had decided in the 1980s to focus on quality—not only for their members but also for the American public, for managed care, and for everyone involved in the medical enterprise. Both organizations have invested substantially in a very rigorous guidelines process. In fact, the process itself was well articulated in a 2-part review article in *Circulation* in 2003 by Ray Gibbons, the outgoing chair; Elliott Antman, the current chair; and Sid Smith, the incoming chair of the ACC/AHA task force.

WCR: *When you went to the National Heart, Lung, and Blood Institute in 1976, cardiac valve replacement was the number one operation being done there. The studies you did on aortic regurgitation there were the first attempt to put science into the process of managing patients with valvular heart disease.*

ROB: I think that's a fair assessment, Bill. I arrived at the National Institutes of Health (NIH) when the foundations for this effort were already in place. Your laboratory was studying valve diseases extensively and had written lots on the topic. Stephen Epstein, Walt Henry, and Jeff Borer had created some prospective protocols to enlist patients with aortic valve disease and mitral valve disease. I cannot take credit for devising these protocols. Although some protocols were already in place, others were not. Two major groups of patients were studied. One group consisted of patients who had already had valve replacement, and we examined preoperative characteristics that would predict outcome. To define the natural history, the second group consisted of patients who had not had valve operations. At that time, echocardiography was brand new. This new technique could not only evaluate the valve but could also determine left ventricular dimensions and function.

At that time, little was known about predicting outcomes in patients with valve disease. In the 1970s, we waited for patients to have symptoms before recommending valve operations because the results of valve replacement were not as fully developed as they are currently. Outcome after valve replacement depended on the type of substitute valve inserted, on the operative skill and technique of the surgeon, and on the functional status of the patient preoperatively. We learned that if we always waited for symptoms to develop, the outcome was not ideal. Indeed, some patients were not improved by technically "successful" valve replacement. It became apparent that waiting for symptoms as the only indication for surgery, at least in some patients, was waiting too long. Echocardiography not only allowed preoperative evaluation but also served as an excellent tool to follow patients postoperatively.

The first study that Walt Henry and I did (Walt was the first author of the first couple of papers) demonstrated that echocardiography in both aortic stenosis and aortic regurgitation could identify a group of symptomatic patients undergoing surgery in whom the postoperative outcome was poor. The patients with increased mortality after valve replacement were those who preoperatively had left ventricular systolic dysfunction (that is, impaired pump function), such as a low ejection fraction, and increased end-systolic and end-diastolic left ventricular dimensions. Although the findings were true of both aortic stenosis and aortic regurgitation, they were more predictive in the latter group than in the former group. We found a very high risk subset in the aortic regurgitation group. We were the first to publish the predictive value of either ejection fraction or fractional shortening, which we measured by the echocardiogram.

Others confirmed our findings. Not all other investigators confirmed the same threshold values that we found or the particular numbers that we found predictive for ejection fraction or end-systolic left ventricular dimension, but those 2 parameters have stood the test of time. One reason others found different thresholds was that they studied less sick patients. Cardiologists now tend to refer patients earlier for valve replacement or repair. Presently, we recommend valve operation when the ejection fraction begins to fall or the left ventricular end-systolic dimension begins to increase. As a consequence, the results of the valvular operations now are better than in earlier years.

WCR: *You're talking about pure aortic regurgitation?*

ROB: Right. That was an important series of studies. The other series of studies also was quite important. That involved an examination of the natural history of the disease and the predictors of symptoms. These turned out to be the same variables, namely left ventricular systolic dysfunction as determined by left ventricular ejection fraction and left ventricular end-systolic dimensions. The patients with the larger left ventricles and the lower ejection fractions were the ones who developed symptoms, particularly when those 2 factors worsened over time. When we started operating sooner in patients with aortic regurgitation because of evidence of left ventricular systolic dysfunction by echocardiogram, the patients had better outcomes postoperatively. The duration of the left ventricular systolic dysfunction also was an important predictor of outcome after valve replacement.

WCR: *Your patients were asymptomatic when you initially studied them?*

ROB: That's right. Some developed symptoms with time and then they were included in the surgical group.

WCR: *The ejection fractions in those early studies were determined by echocardiogram?*

ROB: They were determined initially by left ventricular angiography and then, as echocardiography became available, by this latter method. The protocols that we developed were really pristine. (One reason the intramural programs at NIH need to be preserved is because the protocols created there can be very tight and rigorous.) For example, all of our preoperative patients had an echocardiogram, an electrocardiogram, and a cardiac catheterization with angiography. Six months after valve replacement, the patients returned, and all of those studies were repeated. Then, after that, they would have an echocardiogram every year. When other techniques came along in the later 1970s, such as radionuclide angiography, then every patient had that study as well. Initially the ejection fractions in the preoperative patients were predominantly determined by echocardiogram because this was the method by which patients were followed postoperatively. By the 1980s, however, radionuclide angiograms became the gold standard for ejection fraction.

WCR: *The cut-offs for normal vs abnormal left ventricular ejection fraction by either echocardiogram or angiogram seem to vary considerably. I have observed that one reader would estimate the ejection fraction to be 65%, another 50%, and another 40%. If you use 60% as the cut-off for proceeding to valve operation, these interpretations must be accurate. The variation in estimating ejection fraction worries me a good bit.*

ROB: It worries me too. We all see patients who have a 55% ejection fraction but may have had this level of left ventricular function for the last 10 years. In patients like that, I would not recommend valve surgery, but I would recommend valve operation if the ejection fraction had been 75% earlier. I agree that many times the ejection fraction is under- or overestimated. I saw a patient recently with aortic regurgitation who had good left ventricular systolic function by serial echocardiograms over the last 6 years, and the end-diastolic dimension measured by different people ranged from 58 to 68 mm with no particular trend and considerable scatter within this range. I explained to the patient that the left ventricle is shaped like a strawberry and that the measurements obtained depend upon whether the measurement was along a true short axis or not. These measurements do vary depending on location of the measurement, not to mention the physiologic variations in ventricular size depending upon blood pressure, amount of regurgitation, and heart rate. There's much variability in the measurement and also in the physiology.

The message here is that an important decision, like whether to perform a valve operation, should not be based upon a single measurement. There's always time to repeat the measurement or obtain the ejection fraction by a different technique such as radionuclide angiography, which can be quite precise. Magnetic resonance imaging (MRI) will probably be used more in the future because it can determine chamber volumes, ejection fractions, and dimensions very accurately. I've been recommending more studies of MRI to all physicians involved in imaging research in valve disease. When the left ventricle enlarges, it doesn't always do so in the same way. In some patients it elongates; in others it becomes more spherical. MRI can do a much better job of sizing up ventricular volume and function than either 2-dimensional echocardiography or angiography. Three-dimensional echocardiography also will provide more precise measurements than either 2-dimensional echocardiography or angiography.

We have a series of protocols now in our lab using both 3-dimensional echocardiography and MRI in patients with valve disease, trying to replicate what we did in the 1970s. Such protocols are much more difficult to perform now. In the 1970s, we simply followed patients until symptoms occurred. It was a straightforward decision-making process. Now in a large, complex medical center with >50 cardiologists managing their patients, each one has a different threshold for proceeding. We can't control when and how each cardiologist sends his or her valve patient to operation. We can look at patients who are going to surgery, evaluate their left ventricular function, and examine the result of the operative procedure, but it is more difficult now to have a homogenous group of patients or to define natural history.

WCR: *Your discussion here of aortic regurgitation concerns only patients with chronic and not acute aortic regurgitation?*

ROB: Correct. Our guidelines, however, also consider acute aortic regurgitation, and the criteria for valve replacement in that circumstance are different.

WCR: *You mentioned in your presentation earlier today that aortic regurgitation, in contrast to aortic stenosis, has a number of different etiologies. Sometimes it's due to an abnormality of the valve, sometimes to an abnormality entirely of the ascending aorta, and, on occasion, to both. Are your criteria for operation the same regardless of etiology?*

ROB: That's a very important point because today we see more and more patients whose aortic regurgitation is due entirely to disease of the aorta. For example, high blood pressure can lead to aortic regurgitation. Patients with congenitally bicuspid aortic valves also often have dilated ascending aortas due to medial deficiencies. In many patients, the valve condition alone causes regurgitation, but associated aortic root enlargement makes the valve malfunction more severe. Whether the aortic regurgitation is due to valve disease or to disease of the aorta or to both does not change the effect of aortic regurgitation on the left ventricle and therefore the need or the lack thereof for valve replacement.

In some cases, though, the principal concern is the disease of the aorta, and the ascending aorta needs to be replaced or repaired because it is enlarging too much even though the degree of aortic regurgitation is relatively mild. The criteria for operative intervention on the aorta is a dimension of 50 to 55 mm in diameter measured just above the sinotubular junction. There are other issues in these patients. Should they exercise? Should they be on beta-blockers? We have no information. Proper recommendations regarding pregnancy, which may further enlarge the aortic root, are also difficult to formulate because of lack of a strong evidence base.

WCR: *Replacing a portion of ascending aorta makes for a much more complex operation than replacing only the aortic valve. The frequency of replacing both has clearly increased in recent years both in patients with pure aortic regurgitation and in patients with aortic valve stenosis. Whether 50 or 55 mm is the proper criterion for aortic replacement in these patients is unclear to me. To use these same numbers for a 100-pound woman and a 220-pound man seems inappropriate. I think the move to excise and replace a portion of ascending aorta has gone too far in recent years. What is your view?*

ROB: I agree that we don't really know what the right threshold is, and body size or body mass index has not been evaluated thoroughly in this area. I think either subconsciously or by correction of these measurements to body surface area, we make these assessments when we're managing individual patients. Certainly, a small woman normally has different ventricular and aortic sizes than a huge man.

WCR: *Do you think that body surface area ought to be replaced by body mass index?*

ROB: I don't know, but probably. Body surface area has never for me been a very good correction factor. I haven't used it. Body mass index may be better, but we don't have data yet on it.

WCR: *Could you summarize then the indications for aortic valve operation with or without simultaneous replacement of the ascending aorta in patients with pure aortic regurgitation?*

ROB: The guidelines provide a very complex table of class I, IIA, and IIB indications. There are 4 or 5 bullet-point take-home messages. Symptoms are the most important indication for valve surgery. One of the most important tests we do is to take a careful history. It's complex because many patients with aortic regurgitation have mild symptoms that do not warrant surgery. It's rare to find a patient with significant aortic regurgitation who is unequivocally asymptomatic, as many note fatigue or mild dyspnea. Sometimes an exercise stress test is helpful in eliciting unrecognized symptoms in a sedentary individual. Without symptoms I would recommend surgery if the ejection fraction is <50%, if the left ventricular end-systolic dimension is >55 mm, or if the end-diastolic dimension is >75 mm. Body size must be kept in mind for all of these dimensions. The 75-mm diastolic dimension was based upon data in which 80 mm preoperatively led to poor results. But in the current era, we rarely see dimensions close to those figures as we tend to operate before the left ventricle dilates to this degree.

When using these numbers, we run the risk of waiting too long in patients, even though I'm concerned that we may be operating too early in others. In patients who are being followed carefully with good measurements—and those numbers progressively increase or the ejection fraction progressively decreases, or both—these fixed numbers do not have to be reached if the patient is getting close to these thresholds and the surgical expertise in that hospital setting is superb. Guidelines are created as helpful recommendations to improve quality. Every physician, however, has to make decisions that are sometimes quite difficult. Do guidelines set the highest bar or the lowest bar or in between? Are we trying to set the standard which we know everybody can achieve and therefore everybody would accept? Or, are we trying to set the goal at a higher level of quality? Wouldn't it be good if we could all achieve that higher level? But, then you're running the risk that not every center can achieve these results.

Getting back to aortic regurgitation, the final bullet point is related to the aortic root. Is the aortic root enlarged or enlarging? The current recommendation is a threshold of a 50-mm diameter, realizing that it's a consensus. There are few good data. Some physicians would use a higher or lower threshold. The whole issue of body size must be considered.

WCR: *Let's discuss aortic stenosis. It obviously is more common than pure aortic regurgitation. At the NIH, patients with valve disease were divided into 2 categories: those with "predominant regurgitation" and those with "predominant stenosis." I've never liked that arbitrary classification because "predominant regurgitation" means that there is some stenosis and thus the valve cusps are unequivocally structurally abnormal, whereas in pure regurgitation the valve structure may be entirely normal. If a patient has wide-open aortic regurgitation but a peak systolic transvalvular gradient of 20 mm Hg, how do you classify that patient?*

ROB: That sounds like pure aortic regurgitation because if the regurgitation is severe you might anticipate some degree of outflow pressure gradient because of the enormous forward stroke volume against what may be a structurally normal valve. Then again, a small transvalvular gradient may reflect some stenosis although the lesion appears to be mostly aortic regurgitation.

WCR: *I have never seen a structurally normal valve in a patient whose transvalvular peak systolic pressure gradient is >10 mm Hg.*

ROB: During exercise, huge stroke volumes may cross the aortic valves, and a 10- to 20-mm Hg transvalvular gradient may be the consequence. Usually these large volumes in themselves do not produce a precordial systolic murmur. Patients with pure aortic regurgitation, however, always have a systolic murmur, presumably because of the huge stroke volume going across the valve during ventricular systole. In fact, the systolic murmur is often easier to hear than the diastolic murmur.

WCR: *You include patients in your studies with "pure aortic regurgitation" if the peak transvalvular systolic gradient is ≤30 mm Hg?*

ROB: Yes, it was ≤30 mm Hg. Thus, we did include patients who had mild aortic stenosis. Many patients, of course, have both aortic regurgitation and stenosis. The guidelines we just discussed for patients with aortic regurgitation do not necessarily apply to patients with both regurgitation and stenosis. Guidelines for patients with both mitral and aortic valve disease are even more difficult to develop, although we attempted to do so.

WCR: *What are your criteria for operation in adults with aortic stenosis?*

ROB: The guidelines also have a section for adolescents. We did not deal with a preadolescent pediatric population.

WCR: *Essentially, your guidelines concern patients >10 years of age?*

ROB: Yes. The very young are quite different, and they tend to be seen by a different group of physicians. The best methods to assess the severity of aortic stenosis have varied. In those ≤10 years of age, the peak transvalvular pressure gradient is the most commonly used measurement, whereas in adults it is the mean transvalvular gradient or the valve area. The pediatric cardiologists have defined the natural history of aortic stenosis using the peak-to-peak gradient, but that measurement is not really physiologic since those peaks occur at separate times during ejection.

What gradient to use in evaluating the severity of aortic stenosis in adolescent patients with congenital aortic stenosis created much discussion in the guidelines committee. We distributed our recommendation widely through the American pediatric cardiologic community. Although only one pediatric cardiologist was on the committee, we had a lot of input. In addition to weighing the pieces of evidence and going over them word for word, the committee sent the guidelines to a number of outside consultants. Unlike an original manuscript submitted for publication, in which you get 2 or 3 reviews that authors respond to, it's not uncommon in guidelines development to have 50 or 60 reviewers with extensive comments. Sometimes the reviewers were chosen because they were experts in a specific area. Although they might have been asked to read the entire document, we really wanted their comments only on a specific area. Although we had only 1 surgeon on the committee, we had input from a number of well-known cardiac surgeons, and they often disagreed with our recommendations and even with each other, and we had to address those differences. Then we revised the guidelines appropriately.

WCR: *To develop the first guidelines, you and your colleagues spent 2½ years, with numerous e-mails, a lot of your secretarial time to type what you had dictated or written, and huge amounts of editing time. You were responsible for the whole thing and you made it read like it came from a single author. Were you paid anything for your efforts?*

ROB: No, I wasn't paid. All committee members were volunteers. Furthermore, the president of the American Heart Association and its other officers were not paid.

WCR: *I think it's important for lawyers and others who use these guidelines to know that they were prepared free of charge by physicians using their professional time, their family time, their university time, or whatever to do them.*

ROB: That's true.

WCR: *Now back to aortic stenosis. The aortic valves are like fingerprints. No two are alike. Let me return to the problem of the best way to determine the severity of the stenosis. You mentioned the peak-to-peak transvalvular gradient, the mean gradient, and the valve area. You also mentioned in your presentation that patients with so-called "low cardiac output—low gradients" nevertheless can have severe aortic stenosis. With peak transvalvular gradient, you've got a single measurement, whereas with valve area there are several variables including heart rate, ejection fraction, a constant, etc. Dallas is a valve-area town. I've seen operatively excised aortic valves in patients not having simultaneous coronary bypass with small valve areas (<0.8 cm²) but peak gradients of <20 mm Hg. It appears that the valve area may be less accurate when the peak gradient is small. I'm referring to patients with normal cardiac outputs and ejection fractions. Your comments?*

ROB: Those are excellent points. The complexity of evaluating individual patients makes writing guidelines difficult. All these factors need to be considered. If we accept the view that the valve area is really what is going on physiologically—assuming it is measured accurately—then recommendations can start there. That makes a lot of sense. But, how you get there is something else. If things do not fit together properly for an individual patient, I would try to look at the big picture as best I could. If the valve area was 0.9 cm², the cardiac output was normal, and the peak gradient was only 16 mm Hg, then these variables do not fit together very well. I either need more information or I'm going to ignore one of those variables. If the patient is asymptomatic with normal left ventricular function, that patient doesn't need surgery regardless of the valve area. If the patient has symptoms, then it's something else because then you want to know whether the symptoms are caused by the aortic stenosis or whether valve replacement would not only improve the symptoms but also prolong life. Then, I think you do need more information to get a feeling for how tight that valve really is.

WCR: *With aortic stenosis, if the patient is asymptomatic you don't operate except under very unusual circumstances. What about the 50-year-old man who runs 15 to 20 miles a week (he has a loud ejection murmur typical of aortic stenosis), and by echocardiogram, lo and behold, the calculated peak transvalvular gradient is >110 mm Hg. Is anybody really asymptomatic with that degree of obstruction?*

ROB: Well, these are also good points. You and I just made the statement that you wouldn't operate upon asymptomatic individuals except in very unusual circumstances. Sometimes unusual circumstances are kind of usual. The natural history studies often do not include patients with peak transvalvular gradients >100 mm Hg. In the Mayo Clinic series, for example, nobody with aortic stenosis died without first developing symptoms. They excluded a number of patients, however, who went directly to surgery. The patients who went directly to surgery were those patients with very high transvalvular gradients. This raises the possibility that the outcomes were good in that asymptomatic group because the clinicians had made the correct decision to operate on the ones with the most severe stenosis. The overall mortality of asymptomatic patients with aortic stenosis (defined as a valve area <1.0 cm²) is <1% per year! This has to be balanced against the operative mortality rate of >1% for aortic valve replacement in this country.

However, I too am concerned about an individual patient who has very severe stenosis. Perhaps exercise tests in the young or middle-aged athletic man might be useful. Some patients who claim to be asymptomatic will for the first time develop symptoms during exercise stress testing. That was shown by Dawson and coworkers. Twenty-five percent of their patients developed symptoms "for the first time" on a treadmill. They were either denying symptoms or just weren't pushing themselves during normal activities. You can also observe the blood pressure response to exercise treadmill testing, and other variables can be assessed during echocardiographic stress testing. We do recommend that valve replacement is reasonable if the blood pressure fails to increase or actually decreases with exercise. I'll admit that I've got some patients with a valve so tight that I'm very nervous. If the person is very vigorous and athletic I might recommend valve replacement earlier.

We actually do make recommendations in the guidelines, totally based on consensus, as to what degree of aortic stenosis by itself would be enough to recommend aortic valve replacement. We couldn't decide on anything higher than a valve area of 0.6 cm^2, which is a very stenotic valve. We also considered other measurements of stenotic severity, such as the peak aortic valve gradient, the mean gradient, or the peak left ventricular systolic pressure. There was enough consensus that severe aortic stenosis in and of itself would be an indication for valve replacement, but we did not come up with rigid guidelines that everyone would agree upon other than a valve area of ≤0.6 cm^2. Other than that, it's a decision we have to make in individual patients. We did agree that if the degree of obstruction is severe enough to cause left ventricular systolic dysfunction (an ejection fraction <50%), surgery should be performed.

WCR: *In your presentation, you mentioned the article by Ross and Braunwald in 1968 on the natural history of aortic stenosis. That article of course has been hugely quoted. As I recall, the number of patients in their study was only 15 or 16, a very small number, but each of them had had cardiac catheterization, so they knew the severity of the stenosis. That was the unique feature. But surely you wouldn't base the natural history of many diseases on only 15 patients!*

ROB: Yes, we all have had that figure implanted in our mind, and most of us have a slide from their article. Other studies, however, have confirmed their findings. Kelly and coworkers at the University of Virginia reported another natural history study that demonstrated that in asymptomatic patients with aortic stenosis the outcome is good, in that patients don't die before they develop symptoms. They had 2 deaths among their patients, and both patients developed symptoms first. (There are a few patients who fell through the cracks who retrospectively did develop symptoms before they died, but they died before surgery could be performed. That's why patients with aortic stenosis must be followed very carefully when they have severe aortic stenosis.) But to address your point, Kelly et al also reported a second group of symptomatic patients with severe aortic stenosis who did not undergo surgery (for whatever reason). The mortality rate in them over the course of 2 to 3 years was 50%! They replicated the Ross and Braunwald diagram 20 years later.

WCR: *You mentioned that once a person with aortic stenosis develops symptoms it is time to operate. Is the prognosis similar or different with the 3 symptoms—dyspnea, chest pain, and syncope?*

ROB: It's difficult to know for certain. The Ross and Braunwald schematic has different slopes for each of the 3 different symptoms: heart failure has a deeper slope than angina pectoris, which has a deeper slope than presyncope. I tend to treat them as equal culprits. With any symptom I recommend surgery. Now having said that, what do you do with a patient who's only mildly dyspneic? It's much trickier because it's not overt heart failure, which was what Ross and Braunwald were talking about: 50% mortality in 2 years if you had severe heart failure. The patients of Ross and Braunwald had severe heart failure. Is the mild dyspnea the result of aortic stenosis or the consequence of growing older and becoming more out of shape? The mild dyspnea might not even be recognized by the patient; the patient may attribute it to being out of shape and may not report it to the physician. We all have patients like that. It's a clinical judgment of how much dyspnea is enough to convince you that it's coming from the heart and therefore is significant enough to warrant valve replacement. A stress test in this circumstance might be helpful, although everybody gets dyspneic on a treadmill sooner or later.

WCR: *You tell a patient with aortic stenosis that his or her aortic valve has some degree of obstruction, and, although there are no symptoms now, once symptoms develop, aortic valve replacement will be recommended. After hearing that message, that individual is going to attribute any symptoms that he or she develops in the next 2 years to the valve stenosis irrespective of the degree of the transvalvular gradient.*

ROB: That's a real issue in practice, but it works the opposite way too. If the patient does not want surgery, he or she may not inform the physician when symptoms develop. This is where everything else has to come into play too. Mild symptoms are more eminent when they develop in a patient with a valve area of 0.7 cm^2 compared with one with an area of 1.2 cm^2. First and foremost, we need time to talk to patients. Unfortunately, in the current era we are spread thin and often are not able to spend much time talking with our patients. A good physician with sufficient time can often talk through these things and figure out what's going on.

WCR: *At the NIH, Dr. Eugene Braunwald advised his colleagues in the cardiac catheterization laboratory to try for up to 45 minutes to get the catheter across a stenotic aortic valve. When the echocardiogram came along, many quit trying to get the catheter across the stenotic valve and settled for coronary angiography alone. How many patients with aortic stenosis do you actually send to cardiac catheterization now to determine the severity of the obstruction as well as the status of the coronary arteries?*

ROB: In the current era, echo Doppler is what we use. A hemodynamic study is not needed to characterize the valve in most patients. Cardiac catheterization is useful when the echocardiographic data are discrepant or imprecise in some way. The problem with the catheterization data is that the valve area calculations are critically dependent on the flow measurements. I'm not sure we always get accurate cardiac output measurements. In a busy cath lab, no one spends 45 minutes anymore trying to cross a stenotic valve. The main reason to perform cardiac catheterization in a patient with aortic stenosis is to determine the status of the coronary arteries.

WCR: *If your patient has good left ventricular function, you will try to get across the aortic valve at the time of cardiac catheterization?*

ROB: Certainly.

WCR: *Could you summarize your indications for doing aortic valve replacement in patients with aortic stenosis (unassociated with mitral valve disease)?*

ROB: Symptoms are the most important determinant. Second, in an asymptomatic person or a minimally symptomatic person, valve replacement is recommended if there is evidence of a declining ejection fraction.

WCR: *If you do 2 studies to get the left ventricular ejection fraction what is the usual difference between them?*

ROB: It depends on the technique. With echocardiography, you get about 8% variability. Thus, 50% and 58% are essentially the same. With radionuclide angiography, the variability is about 5%. Thus, 50% and 55% are the same. With contrast left ventriculography, the variability is greater.

WCR: *Eight percent could make a huge difference in your decision making.*

ROB: Absolutely. If a person really has no symptoms and the decision for or against operation is based on the ejection fraction measurement, you want to be sure that it really is low. If there is any question, you can repeat it or verify it by a different technique. That's why I say "below normal." If it goes from 55% to 50%, that could be physiologic variation only. It's also rare for a patient with aortic stenosis to have true left ventricular systolic dysfunction and be asymptomatic. If that circumstance occurs, I would worry about associated coronary heart disease for its cause.

That brings up a third indication for surgery for aortic stenosis: the patient with severe stenosis who is undergoing coronary bypass surgery. What severity of aortic stenosis warrants aortic valve replacement in the patient whose symptoms appear to be the consequence of coronary artery disease and who is to have coronary bypass surgery? The decision is easy if the aortic stenosis is severe: the valve should be replaced. If, however, the stenosis is only mild, the decision regarding valve replacement is much more difficult. Predicting when the aortic stenosis will progress rather rapidly is imprecise. We tend to make the decision on the basis of the peak transvalvular gradient. If it is >30 mm Hg, then the valve is replaced at the time of the coronary bypass. It is unclear what to recommend in patients with milder degrees of stenosis. The stenosis in patients with heavily calcified aortic valves tends to progress more rapidly than in those with only mildly calcified valves. Thus, assessing the quantity of calcific deposits on the valve in a patient with a low gradient may be helpful.

Beyond these 3 criteria for surgery (symptoms, left ventricular dysfunction, and patients undergoing coronary bypass surgery), the other criteria for aortic valve replacement are a little bit looser: IIA and IIB indications. I'm not sure how many of these we are going to keep in the next revision of the guidelines because it's not clear how helpful they are. One is the blood pressure response to exercise. Another factor is the degree of left ventricular hypertrophy. Runs of ventricular tachycardia by Holter monitoring may also tilt the decision toward valve replacement.

WCR: *When we were both at NIH, peak systolic gradients >80 mm Hg in patients with aortic stenosis were common. Today, I rarely see an operatively excised stenotic aortic valve with a peak gradient >80 mm Hg. The severity of the stenosis now is certainly less than it was in the 1960s and 1970s.*

Let's move to mitral regurgitation. The indications for mitral valve operation in patients with mitral regurgitation secondary to left ventricular ischemia or infarction must be considerably different from those resulting from nonischemic mitral regurgitation. Your comments?

ROB: It's an easier discussion and more difficult in the same breath because the physiology differs so much depending on etiology. Is the mitral regurgitation secondary to cardiomyopathy? Is it secondary to myocardial ischemia, in which case left ventricular dysfunction is always present? Patients with left ventricular dysfunction do poorly no matter what you do. The operative approach is also unclear in those patients. They represent a high-risk group with bad outcomes because outcome is influenced primarily by the left ventricular dysfunction whether or not the mitral valve is replaced or repaired.

Let us focus on the conditions in which the valve itself causes the mitral regurgitation. Mitral valve prolapse is the major cause in this country of mitral regurgitation secondary to valve disease, and the mitral valve can often be repaired rather than replaced in this circumstance. The reason I said the decision is both easy and difficult is that it's been suggested that since the valve can usually be repaired, the threshold for operation should be lowered. Thus, the argument is that operation might be indicated for severe mitral regurgitation alone in the absence of symptoms. The analogy that is often made is atrial septal defect, which can be repaired successfully with low risk. We prevent the complications of atrial septal defect in later life by closing the defect in all patients in early life. The problem here is that in this country most patients with mitral regurgitation secondary to mitral valve prolapse end up having mitral valve replacement rather than repair!

The outcome of mitral valve repair is not reported in every center. The reports we see are from those centers that get great results—mainly the large centers with large volumes of patients. Establishing guidelines when results of surgery vary so much from one center to the next can be a problem. Do we set the lowest or highest common denominator? Should every patient with severe mitral regurgitation be referred for operation if repair can be performed? Or, do we not operate unless there are symptoms or evidence of declining left ventricular function or pulmonary hypertension or some other objective parameter? If we do that, then we tie the hands of those centers that are leading the field and perhaps showing what we could and should achieve. We don't want the guidelines to imply that these centers are doing things they shouldn't be doing because actually they may be setting new standards for the rest of us. We're going to try to make that point in the revision. If your center can achieve excellent results in individual patients based upon your own track record, and you know you can achieve a satisfactory repair with a very high likelihood, then maybe it's okay to recommend an early repair in a patient with severe mitral regurgitation. But, that action is appropriate only if you can achieve those superb results.

WCR: *One of my children is a cardiovascular surgeon, and he tells me that the average cardiovascular surgeon in the USA does about 10 valve replacements or repairs a year. Doing only 10 valve operations a year, the surgeon could not be comfortable doing either procedure, much less repair. You're talking about centers where the* *average surgeons do 100 valve operations a year and therefore become good at the repair procedure.*

ROB: That's absolutely right. It's a difficult issue, but I think each physician has an absolute obligation to do what's best for each patient independent of the physician's referral pattern and location. In our program in Chicago, we have had a couple of different surgical teams since I've been there. We had a great surgeon who did terrific valve repairs but he left for personal reasons. We were left for a while without a surgeon who could repair valves, and consequently I referred some patients to other institutions. Then, we recruited successfully and now we perform superb valve repairs again at the medical center in which I work. Those out-referring decisions are difficult because we all want to be loyal to the team we work with day in and day out. But, we must do what is best for every patient.

We have difficulty writing guidelines for cardiologists as well as cardiac surgeons who see relatively few patients with valve conditions. Surgeons need sufficient volume to be proficient at both valve replacement and repair, but more so with the latter than the former. We have not achieved uniform standards nationwide on the surgical side on this point, nor do we have uniform standards regarding when to recommend valve repair. I've followed patients for over a decade now who have got enough mitral regurgitation that some centers undoubtedly would have operated on them 10 years ago, and they're still doing fine.

WCR: *Braunwald used to say that if you're going to have one valve lesion then mitral regurgitation is the best one to have because it is more compatible with long-term survival than the other left-sided valve lesions. What do you know about the edge-to-edge operation for mitral regurgitation?*

ROB: That's another Pandora's box. That's the procedure in which the posterior and anterior leaflets are brought together in the central portion of the mitral orifice, and it results in a double-orifice mitral valve. A mitral anular ring is also usually inserted at the same time. That procedure is not the one of choice because it usually results in some residual mitral regurgitation. It is not good to leave any mitral regurgitation behind, as a number of surgical series indicate that any degree of residual mitral regurgitation after repair puts a patient at higher risk of needing a second operation over the next 5 to 10 years.

WCR: *Are any good follow-up studies available on that procedure postoperatively?*

ROB: No. There are no reproducible results on that procedure as there are with other types of mitral repair. This procedure is now being done via the percutaneous route using an investigational device at a few centers. The percutaneous procedure worries me because once it gets in the community it's going to be even more difficult to put a break on the excitement about this new opportunity for intervening in patients, some of whom may not need intervention at all. Another worry is that if the edge-to-edge procedure is ineffective, it may prevent a more definitive repair procedure from being done later. Before these new devices get approved, careful scrutiny is needed as well as long-term clinical trials to be sure they are effective. The edge-to-edge procedure may be helpful in a patient who's very sick and potentially could not tolerate a long operation.

WCR: *It's my understanding that most people with mitral valve prolapse, at least in the USA, are women. Of those persons with mitral valve prolapse who die suddenly, most are women. The ones who develop enough mitral regurgitation to warrant mitral valve repair or replacement, however, are mostly men. Why is that?*

ROB: That's my impression too. I agree with you. The people who get into trouble and develop endocarditis, ruptured chordae, or mitral regurgitation are mainly men >45 years of age. Men in that age group tend to have more severe myxomatous changes. I don't know why that is. There may be a genetic polymorphism that is more common in men, or maybe other factors influence the phenotypic expression of mitral valve prolapse in men and not in women.

WCR: *Let's say your daughter had mitral valve prolapse at age 20. What would be your recommendations to her in an attempt to prevent any mitral operation years later? What can be done to slow its progression?*

ROB: I'm not aware of anything to slow its progression.

WCR: *You would certainly want to make sure her blood pressure stays down.*

ROB: Oh, yes. Blood pressure is important. We certainly want to control hypertension if present.

WCR: *In a nutshell, when would you recommend operative intervention in patients with mitral stenosis unassociated with aortic valve disease?*

ROB: When patients have symptoms or develop pulmonary hypertension. Balloon valvulotomy is a good procedure for patients with no or minimal calcific deposits in the valve and no or only mild mitral regurgitation.

WCR: *Why do you think atrial fibrillation occurs more frequently in patients with mitral stenosis than in patients with mitral regurgitation secondary to mitral valve prolapse?*

ROB: That's a good question because the atria tend to be quite big with both. I don't know the answer. Atrial fibrillation clearly is a devastating component of mitral stenosis. I guess I would put that into my equation also, getting back to my indications for balloon valvulotomy. If the patient is a candidate for a balloon valvulotomy and the patient is having atrial fibrillation, I might move earlier. As mitral stenosis is almost always the result of rheumatic heart disease, it may be that inflammation or scarring of the atrial wall increases susceptibility to atrial fibrillation. What do you think?

WCR: *I think rheumatic heart disease involves the atrial wall. Inflammation may be present during acute rheumatic fever, but later the amount of fibrous tissue, mainly occurring between myofibers, in patients with chronic mitral stenosis is considerable. Patients with mitral valve prolapse have essentially normal atrial walls.*

I certainly agree that the expertise among both cardiologists and cardiac surgeons regarding cardiac valve disease is less now than in the past. Surgeons now are doing fewer valve operations during their training, and, therefore, they are not good valve surgeons upon completion of their training.

ROB: Yes, it's a real problem.

WCR: *With so many cardiologists, the expertise is being diffused.*

ROB: Yes, I agree. This is an area that requires more attention in our educational and training programs.

WCR: *Bob, thank you so much. I really appreciate your coming to BUMC. You did a fantastic job.*

ROB: Thank you, Bill.

Bonow RO, Carabello B, de Leon AC, Edmunds LH Jr, Fedderly BJ, Freed MD, Gaasch WH, McKay CR, Nishimura RA, O'Gara PT, O'Rourke RA, Rahimtoola SH. ACC/AHA guidelines for the management of patients with valvular heart disease. A report of the American College of Cardiology/American Heart Association Task Force on Practice Guidelines (Committee on Management of Patients with Valvular Heart Disease). *J Am Coll Cardiol* 1998;32:1486–1588.

Gibbons RJ, Smith S, Antman E; American College of Cardiology; American Heart Association. American College of Cardiology/American Heart Association clinical practice guidelines: Part I: where do they come from? *Circulation* 2003;107:2979–2986.

Pellikka PA, Nishimura RA, Bailey KR, Tajik AJ. The natural history of adults with asymptomatic, hemodynamically significant aortic stenosis. *J Am Coll Cardiol* 1990;15:1012–1017.

Kelly TA, Rothbart RM, Cooper CM, Kaiser DL, Smucker ML, Gibson RS. Comparison of outcome of asymptomatic to symptomatic patients older than 20 years of age with valvular aortic stenosis. *Am J Cardiol* 1988;61:123–130.

Ross J Jr, Braunwald E. Aortic stenosis. *Circulation* 1968;38(1 suppl):61–67.

Frequency by Decades of Unicuspid, Bicuspid, and Tricuspid Aortic Valves in Adults Having Isolated Aortic Valve Replacement for Aortic Stenosis, With or Without Associated Aortic Regurgitation

William C. Roberts, MD; Jong M. Ko, BA

Background—Aortic valve stenosis (with or without aortic regurgitation and without associated mitral stenosis) in adults in the Western world has been considered in recent years to most commonly be the result of degenerative or atherosclerotic disease.

Methods and Results—We examined operatively excised, stenotic aortic valves from 932 patients aged 26 to 91 years (mean±SD, 70±12), and none had associated mitral valve replacement or evidence of mitral stenosis: A total of 504 (54%) had congenitally malformed valves (unicuspid in 46 [unicommissural in 42; acommissural in 4] and bicuspid in 458); 417 (45%) had tricuspid valves (either absent or minimal commissural fusion); and 11 (1%) had valves of undetermined type. It is likely that the latter 11 valves also had been congenitally malformed. Of the 584 men, 343 (59%) had either a unicuspid or a bicuspid valve; of the 348 women, 161 (46%) had either a unicuspid or a bicuspid aortic valve.

Conclusions—The data from this large study of adults having isolated aortic valve replacement for aortic stenosis (with or without associated aortic regurgitation) and without associated mitral stenosis or mitral valve replacement strongly suggest that an underlying congenitally malformed valve, at least in men, is more common than a tricuspid aortic valve.
(*Circulation*. 2005;111:920-925.)

Key Words: aorta ■ heart defects, congenital ■ valves ■ regurgitation

The most common cardiac operation today, of course, is coronary artery bypass grafting. The second most common is aortic valve replacement for aortic valve stenosis. During the past 11 years, we have examined 932 operatively excised, stenotic aortic valves from adults. This study describes the frequency of the various aortic valve structures (unicuspid, bicuspid, and tricuspid) in each of 8 decades of life in a group of patients who had isolated aortic valve replacement. This study differs from previously reported similar analyses in that children and patients with concomitant mitral valve replacement or associated mitral stenosis were excluded. The hypothesis was that if cases of rheumatic heart disease could be excluded, then the frequency of an underlying congenital heart disease of those undergoing aortic valve replacement would be higher than previously realized.

See p 832

Methods

From January 1993 through June 2004, every cardiac valve operatively excised at Baylor University Medical Center and submitted to the surgical pathology department of the same medical center has been examined by one of us (W.C.R.). Among the valves examined during this >11-year period were 932 aortic valves that had some degree of stenosis (a peak left ventricular to aortic systolic pressure gradient ≥10 mm Hg or clear anatomic evidence of aortic valve stenosis) with or without some degree of aortic regurgitation. Excluded from this study were patients having combined aortic and mitral valve replacement, patients with mitral stenosis whether or not the mitral valve was excised or the patient had a mitral valvuloplasty, patients ≤20 years of age at the time of aortic valve replacement, patients who had had a previous aortic valvulotomy, and patients who also had hypertrophic cardiomyopathy. Thus, patients included herein were those in whom only the aortic valve was excised and the aortic valve had some degree of stenosis.

Each stenotic aortic valve was received in the surgical pathology department in a container of formaldehyde. The valve structure in all cases was determined by one of us (W.C.R.). In recent years, the operatively excised stenotic valve was weighed. The age and sex of each patient was recorded from the surgical slip accompanying the operatively excised aortic valve. The preoperative cardiac catheterization and echocardiographic reports were obtained from either the respective laboratory or the patient's medical chart or, in more recent years, from the Apollo cardiovascular database of Baylor University Medical Center.

Hemodynamic data from cardiac catheterization was available for 689 (74%) patients, 43 of whom had transvalvular peak pressure

TABLE 1. Aortic Valve Structure in 584 Men and 348 Women Aged 26 to 91 Years With Operatively Excised Stenotic Aortic Valves Unassociated With Mitral Valve Disease and Excised From 1993 to 2004

Aortic Valve Structure	Cases, n (%)	Ages (y) of Patients by Decades at Time of Aortic Valve Replacement							
		21–30	31–40	41–50	51–60	61–70	71–80	81–90	91–100
Men									
Unicuspid	34 (6)	3	4	11	8	4	4	0	0
Bicuspid	309 (53)	1	4	20	54	111	94	24	1
Tricuspid	234 (40)	0	0	0	14	50	119	51	0
Uncertain	7 (1)	0	0	0	0	3	2	2	0
Subtotals, n (%)	584 (100)	4 (<1)	8 (1)	31 (5)	76 (13)	168 (29)	219 (38)	77 (13)	1 (<1)
Women									
Unicuspid	12 (3)	1	2	3	1	4	1	0	0
Bicuspid	149 (43)	1	5	10	20	44	55	14	0
Tricuspid	183 (53)	0	0	2	11	43	79	47	1
Uncertain	4 (1)	0	0	1	0	0	3	0	0
Subtotals, n (%)	348 (100)	2 (<1)	7 (2)	16 (5)	32 (9)	91 (26)	138 (46)	61 (18)	1 (<1)

Values in parentheses are percentages.

gradients between 10 and 20 mm Hg. Nearly all of the remaining 243 patients also had undergone cardiac catheterization, but those studies were performed before the patient was referred to Baylor University Medical Center, and the data were not available to us. Another 111 patients had echocardiographic data available but no cardiac catheterization data available. Thus, for 800 (86%) of the 932 patients, either cardiac catheterization data or echocardiographic data before aortic valve replacement were available. The transvalvular peak systolic pressure gradients ranged from 10 to 141 mm Hg (mean±SD, 53±25); in the patients not having simultaneous coronary bypass surgery, the peak gradients ranged from 10 to 141 mm Hg (mean±SD, 57±26), and in those patients having coronary bypass surgery at the time of aortic valve replacement, from 10 to 133 mm Hg (mean±SD, 49±24; $P<0.001$). Aortic valve areas (637 patients) ranged from 0.18 to 1.90 cm^2 (mean±SD, 0.74±0.25) and were significantly different in those having versus those not having simultaneous coronary bypass surgery (mean±SD, 0.72±0.25 versus 0.76±0.25; $P=0.037$). All 932 patients had structurally abnormal aortic valves including calcific deposits, including those patients with peak transvalvular pressure gradients as low as 10 mm Hg.

Statistical analysis was performed with SigmaStat version 2.0 software (SPSS Inc). To compare the percentages in 2 different groups, the z test was used. To compare the mean transvalvular peak systolic pressure gradients and the mean aortic valve areas in patients with and without simultaneous coronary bypass surgery, the nonparametric Mann-Whitney rank-sum test was used instead of a parametric test because the data to be analyzed did not pass the normality and equal-variance assumption tests. To compare the mean ages among patient groups with unicuspid, bicuspid, and tricuspid valves, the nonparametric Kruskal-Wallis 1-way ANOVA on ranks test was used. A probability value <0.05 was considered statistically significant. The institutional review board of Baylor University Medical Center approved the study protocol.

Results

The numbers and percentages of patients in each of the 8 decades subdivided by aortic valve structure and sex are shown in Table 1. Among the 932 patients, 46 (5%) had unicuspid unicommissural valves, 458 (49%) had bicuspid valves, 417 (45%) had 3-cuspid aortic valves, and 11 (1%) had valves excised in several pieces, such that the underlying valve structure was not clearly discernible. (We believe that these 11 valves with uncertain structure were also congenitally malformed because they all contained a very large amount of calcific deposits.) More men than women had congenitally malformed valves (59% versus 46%, $P=0.008$; Table 1), and fewer men than women had tricuspid aortic valves (40% versus 53%, $P=0.011$; Table 1).

The unicuspid aortic valves were all heavily calcified, and their cusps were rigid. Of these 46 valves, 42 had a single, unfused commissure, and the valve orifice was linear (similar to an exclamation point), eccentrically triangular, or oval (Figure 1); the other 4 had triangular, more central orifices, and 3 "undeveloped commissures" (Figure 2).

The bicuspid aortic valves were of 2 types (Figure 3). All had been excised in 2 pieces. In 432, the free margins of both cusps were relatively linear in appearance, or the margins of one of the 2 cusps had a V-shaped configuration, with the apex of the V pointing toward a raphe (false commissure). In

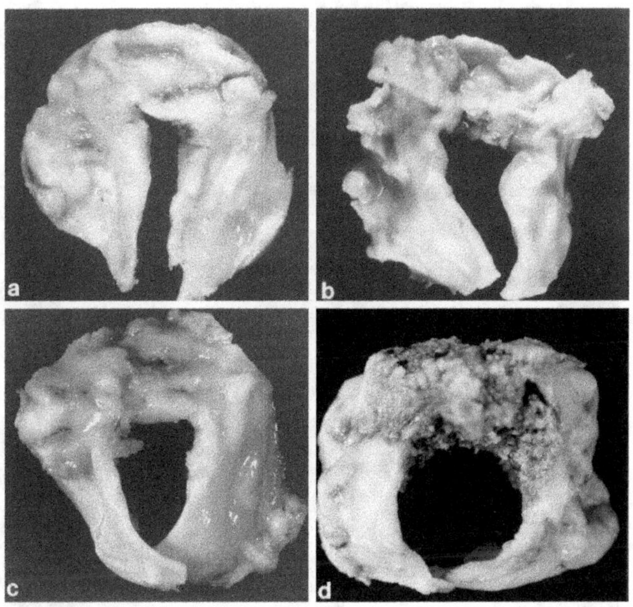

Figure 1. Unicuspid unicommissural aortic valves. See Table 3.

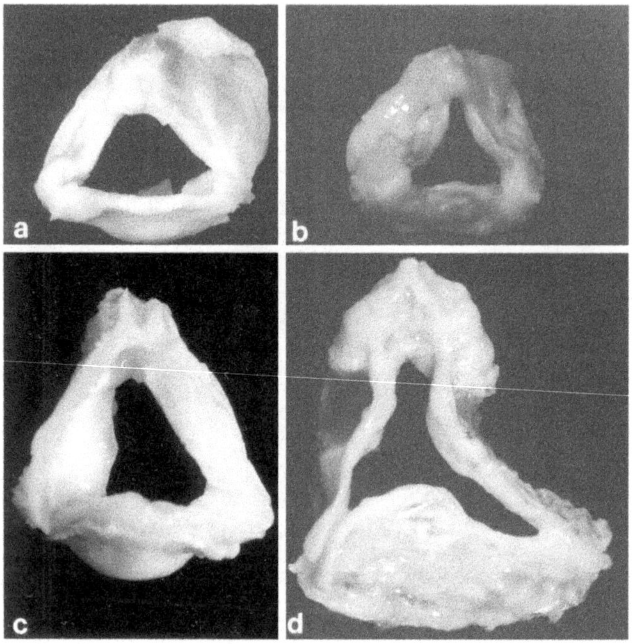

Figure 2. Unicuspid acommissural aortic valves. See Table 3.

the latter situation, the free margins of the raphe cusp were concave, and the free margins of the nonraphe cusp were convex, such that the valvular orifices were nevertheless usually competent. The ventricular aspect of the valve beneath the raphe in all instances was flat or nearly so. Furthermore, on the aortic aspect at the site of the raphe, the V-shaped cuspal margins were not visible in the raphe. The cephalad extension of the raphe was always less than that of

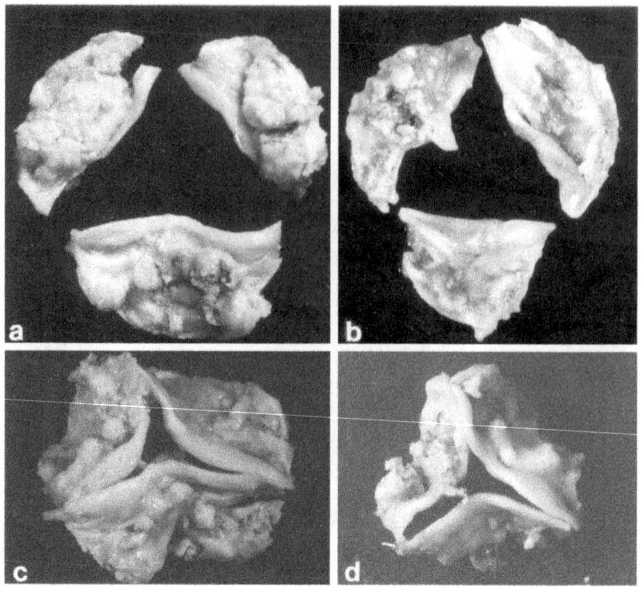

Figure 4. Three-cuspid aortic valves. See Table 3.

the 2 true commissures. In the remaining 26 valves classified as bicuspid, the cusps were fused at one commissure, and the length of the fusion was $\geq$4 mm and usually $\approx$10 mm. In these circumstances, the free margins were visible cephalad to the cuspal fusion, which was located caudal to the margins. The fused cusps beneath the visible free margins (which extended to the aortic wall) were either flat or not. Additionally, the cephalad extension of the fused commissure appeared to be on the same horizontal plane as the other 2 commissures.

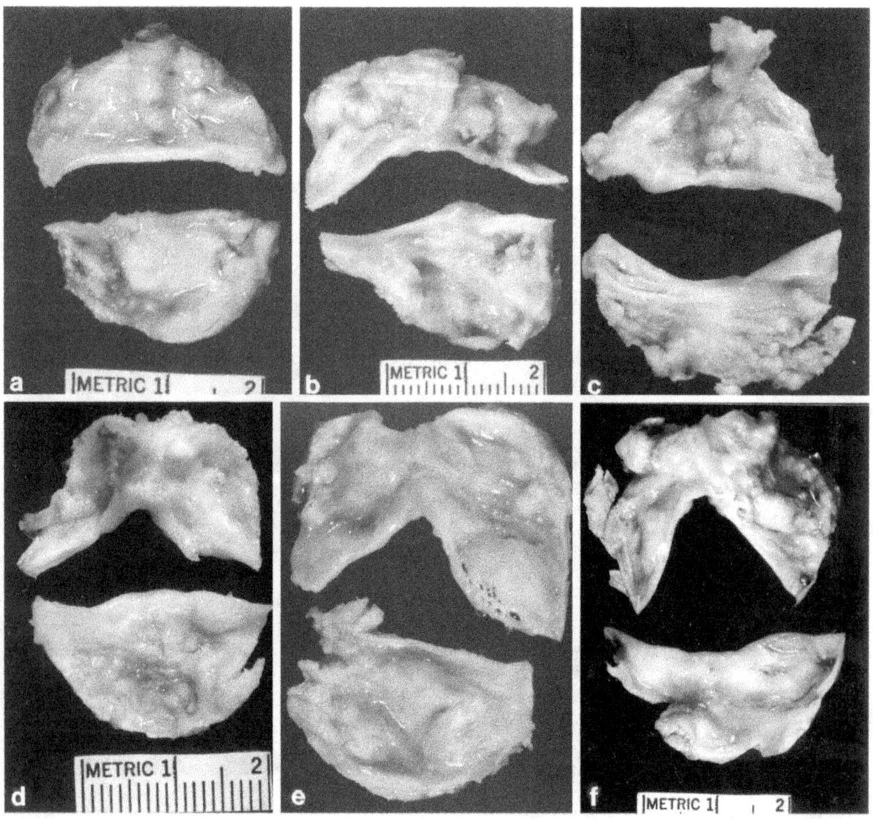

Figure 3. Congenitally bicuspid aortic valve. See Table 3.

TABLE 2. Aortic Valve Structure in Patients With Isolated Aortic Stenosis Subdivided Into Those With and Without Concomitant Coronary Artery Bypass Grafting

		Ages (y) of Patients by Decades at Time of Aortic Valve Replacement							
Aortic Valve Structure	Cases	21–30	31–40	41–50	51–60	61–70	71–80	81–90	91–100
Without coronary artery bypass grafting									
Men									
Unicuspid	28	3	4	10	6	3	2	0	0
Bicuspid	151	1	4	15	31	50	41	8	1
Tricuspid	76	0	0	0	3	19	37	17	0
Uncertain	4	0	0	0	0	2	1	1	0
Women									
Unicuspid	11	1	1	3	1	4	1	0	0
Bicuspid	96	1	5	6	13	30	33	8	0
Tricuspid	73	0	0	2	6	16	30	19	0
Uncertain	3	0	0	1	0	0	2	0	0
Totals, n (%)	442 (100)	6 (1)	14 (3)	37 (8)	60 (14)	124 (28)	147 (33)	53 (12)	1 (<1)
With coronary artery bypass grafting									
Men									
Unicuspid	6	0	0	1	2	1	2	0	0
Bicuspid	158	0	0	5	23	61	53	16	0
Tricuspid	158	0	0	0	11	31	82	34	0
Uncertain	3	0	0	0	0	1	1	1	0
Women									
Unicuspid	1	0	1	0	0	0	0	0	0
Bicuspid	53	0	0	4	7	14	22	6	0
Tricuspid	110	0	0	0	5	27	49	28	1
Uncertain	1	0	0	0	0	0	1	0	0
Totals, n (%)	490 (100)	0 (0)	1 (<1)	10 (2)	48 (10)	135 (28)	210 (43)	85 (17)	1 (<1)

Values in parentheses are percentages.

The tricuspid aortic valves were of 2 types (Figure 4). None of the 3 commissures were fused, such that each cusp was excised separately (340 cases), or there was slight (≤3 mm) fusion of one or more commissures (77 cases); in nearly all cases, the fusion extended for only 1 or 2 mm.

The fewer the number of aortic valve cusps, the younger was the patient. Patients with 3-cuspid aortic valves had higher mean ages than did patients with fewer cusps. The ages of the 46 patients with unicuspid valves ranged from 26 to 75 years (mean±SD, 51±14); that of the 458 patients with bicuspid valves, from 27 to 91 years (mean±SD, 67±11); and that of the 417 patients with 3-cuspid valves, from 45 to 91 years (mean±SD, 74±8; $P<0.001$). Of the 932 patients, 176 (19%) were in the 4 younger decades (21 to 60 years), and 756 (81%) were in the 4 older decades (61 to 100 years). Nearly two thirds (66%) of the 932 patients were aged 61 to 80 years at the time of aortic valve replacement. Of the 46 patients with unicuspid valves, 33 (72%) were in the 4 younger decades, and the other 13 were in the next 2 older decades (61 to 80 years). Of the 458 patients with bicuspid valves, 115 (25%) were in the 4 younger decades (21 to 60 years), and 343 (75%) were in the 4 older decades (61 to 100 years). Of the 417 patients with tricuspid aortic valves, 27 (6%) were in the 4 younger decades (21 to 60 years; 25 of the 27 in the sixth decade); the other 390 (94%) were in the 4 older decades (61 to 100 years). Of the 176 patients in the 4 younger decades, the aortic valves in 33 (19%) were unicuspid; in 115 (65%), bicuspid; and in 27 (15%), tricuspid. In contrast, of the 756 patients in the 4 older decades (61 to 100 years), the aortic valves were unicuspid in 13 (2%); bicuspid in 343 (45%); and tricuspid in 390 (52%).

The age range of the 932 patients was 26 to 91 years (mean±SD, 70±12). The 584 men ranged in age from 26 to 91 years (mean±SD, 69±11), and the 348 women, from 27 to 91 years (mean±SD, 71±11). Of the 584 men, 119 (20%) were in the 4 younger decades (21 to 60 years), and 465 (80%) were in the 4 older decades (61 to 100 years); of the 348 women, 57 (16%) were in the 4 younger decades, and 291 (84%) were in the 4 older decades.

Of the 932 patients, 490 (53%) also had coronary artery bypass grafting at the time of aortic valve replacement (Table 2). Coronary artery bypass grafting was performed in 7 (15%) of the 46 patients with unicuspid valves, in 211 (46%) of the 458 patients with bicuspid valves, in 268 (64%) of the 417 patients with tricuspid aortic valves, and in 4 (36%) of the 11 with undetermined valve structure. Of the 176 patients in the 4 younger decades (21 to 60 years), 59 (34%) had concomitant coronary bypass surgery; of the 756 patients in the 4

TABLE 3. Data in Patients Whose Stenotic Aortic Valves Are Shown in Figures 1–4

Aortic Valve Structure	Age, y	Sex	LV-Aorta PSG (S/D), mm Hg	LV-Aorta Mean Gradient (S/D), mm Hg	Aortic Valve Area, cm^2	Aortic Valve Weight, g
Unicuspid (unicommissural)						
Figure 1a	41	F	...	...	1.10	2.50
Figure 1b	48	M	23	23	1.40	5.84
Figure 1c	43	M	...	28	...	...
Figure 1d	39	M	41	...	1.00	7.39
Unicuspid (acommissural)						
Figure 2a	30	F	42	35	0.84	2.07
Figure 2b	75	F	53	54	0.57	1.67
Figure 2c	62	F	22	19	0.62	1.02
Figure 2d	73	M	25	32	1.12	2.73
Bicuspid						
Figure 3a	60	F	80	64	0.66	2.09
Figure 3b	72	M	46	46	0.88	3.46
Figure 3c	80	M	37	31	0.58	3.72
Figure 3d	63	M	71	...	0.70	1.61
Figure 3e	68	M	...	...	...	2.55
Figure 3f	69	M	...	25	...	2.97
Tricuspid						
Figure 4a	78	M	77	57	0.41	3.93
Figure 4b	53	M	...	...	...	2.90
Figure 4c	68	M	97	42	0.80	2.62
Figure 4d	85	F	82	...	0.50	1.69

LV indicates left ventricular; PSG, peak systolic gradient; and S/D, peak systole/end diastole.

older decades, 431 (57%) had concomitant coronary bypass surgery.

Discussion

The present study of 932 stenotic aortic valves operatively excised from 1993 to 2004 in patients >20 years of age has demonstrated that slightly more patients had congenitally malformed aortic valves (either unicuspid or bicuspid) than tricuspid aortic valves (54% versus 45%; indeterminate structure=1%). Among the 46 patients with unicuspid aortic valves, 42 (91%) had valves with 2 rudimentary commissures and 1 true commissure (Figure 1): Four had valves with 3 rudimentary commissures and no true commissures (Figure 2). We classify these latter 4 cases as unicuspid acommissural aortic valves. These 4 cases in the past would have been classified by most investigators, we suspect, as rheumatic in origin. We, however, searched the medical records thoroughly for evidence of mitral valve disease in these 4 cases and found none. It is possible, of course, in rheumatic heart disease for aortic valve disease to be clinically apparent before the appearance of clinical evidence of mitral disease, and that could be the situation in these 4 cases. It is also possible that the cuspal fusion at each of the 3 rudimentary commissures was present at the time of birth, and therefore, this multifusion represents congenital heart disease. Lack of separation of each of 3 cusps before birth appears to us a more reasonable explanation of the valve disease in these 4 cases than rheumatic heart disease manifesting itself clinically as isolated aortic valve disease.

Although the patients with unicuspid or bicuspid aortic valves clearly had congenital heart disease underlying their aortic stenosis, the cause of the aortic stenosis in the patients with 3-cuspid aortic valves is almost certainly acquired in origin. Although stenosis involving a 3-cuspid aortic valve unassociated with mitral valve disease has in the past most commonly been called "degenerative" in origin—a consequence of aging—we prefer to call these stenotic, 3-cuspid aortic valves (unassociated with mitral disease) "atherosclerotic" in origin. The evidence for attributing the calcific and other deposits on the aortic aspects of the 3 cusps in these patients to atherosclerosis is the following: (1) Patients with homozygous familial hypercholesterolemia (individuals with serum total cholesterol levels >800 mg/dL from the time of birth) develop aortic stenosis by the teenage years (without lipid-lowering therapy)[1]; (2) patients >65 years of age with aortic stenosis involving a 3-cuspid aortic valve (unassociated with mitral valve disease) usually have extensive atherosclerosis involving the major epicardial coronary arteries and usually other arterial systems[2,3]; (3) serum total cholesterol levels tend to be higher in patients with aortic stenosis involving a 3-cuspid aortic valve than in patients of similar age and sex without aortic stenosis[4]; (4) the use of lipid-lowering therapy (statins) has been demonstrated to slow the progression of aortic valve stenosis[5]; and (5) histological study of 3-cuspid, stenotic aortic valves has demonstrated that these valves have features similar to those in arterial atherosclerotic plaques. It has been demonstrated that the cusps of congenitally bicuspid, stenotic valves are usually of unequal size; ie, that they differ in weight.[6] Likewise, the cusps of 3-cuspid, stenotic aortic valves also often differ in weight. Roberts and Ko[7] weighed 260 operatively excised, stenotic 3-cuspid aortic valves from patients having no evidence of mitral valve disease and found that all 3 cusps differed (by >0.1 g) in weight in 69 patients (26%), that one cusp differed in weight from the other 2 in 158 patients (61%), and that in only 33 patients (13%) were all 3 cusps of similar weight.

The first institution where a large number of operatively excised stenotic aortic valves were examined was the Mayo Clinic. Subramanian and colleagues[8] in 1984 described 374 valves with "pure aortic stenosis" (no associated aortic regurgitation or only mild regurgitation); Passik and colleagues[9] in 1987 examined another 646 operatively excised valves with "pure aortic stenosis"; and Subramanian et al[10] in 1985 examined another group of operatively excised valves with "combined aortic stenosis and insufficiency." The difficulty in comparing their findings with those in the present study is that the former also included patients with coexistent mitral disease and children. Combining the findings of the 3 studies from the Mayo Clinic together indicated that 44 (4%) of their 1219 patients with operatively excised, stenotic aortic valves had unicuspid valves, 459 (38%) had bicuspid valves, 431 (35%) had "postinflammatory" valves, 257 (21%) had "degenerative" valves, and 28 (2%) had valves of indeterminate structure. Their inclusion of children appeared to increase the likelihood of congenitally malformed valves. These authors also intermixed etiology with structure, a process that prevented us from being entirely clear about valve structure in their cases. Their patients as a group were younger than those included in the present study because the earlier studies included both children and patients with unambiguous rheumatic heart disease. The present study, in contrast, made every reasonable attempt to exclude patients whose valve disease was of rheumatic etiology.

Turri and colleagues[11] in 1990 described operatively excised aortic valves from 602 patients having valve replacement, but these authors combined data from patients with pure regurgitation and those with some degree of aortic stenosis. That study also included patients who had concomitant mitral valve disease, and indeed, the most common cause of aortic stenosis (≈348 patients) in their patients was rheumatic heart disease (undefined; in 172 [49%]). Only 17 (5%) of their patients had congenitally bicuspid aortic valves, and only 44 (13%) had the "senile" type of stenotic valve, presumably 3-cuspid ones. Although it was not possible to separate the ages of their patients with stenotic valves from those with purely regurgitant valves, the mean ages of their stenotic cases were clearly much younger than patients included in the present study (mean age, ≈50 versus 70 years).

Agozzino and associates[12] in 1992 described operatively excised aortic valves from 912 patients having valve replacement in the 1980s: A total of 787 valves had some degree of stenosis, but there was no attempt to describe valve structure. These authors also included patients with associated mitral valve disease, and indeed, rheumatic heart disease was the most common etiology of the aortic valve stenosis (573 of 787 [73%]). "Degenerative calcification" was the explanation for the stenosis in the other 214 patients (27%). These authors also included children in their study. The mean ages of their patients with aortic stenosis was 47 years.

Several features of the present study make it different from previous studies on operatively excised, stenotic aortic valves. First, the study was limited to adults >20 years of age and excluded those patients who had had a previous aortic valvulotomy. Second, it excluded patients with associated mitral stenosis, which in adults is virtually always of rheumatic origin, and it also excluded patients having mitral valve replacement for any reason. Third, it included only patients whose stenotic aortic valve was excised in the last decade of the 20th century or the first decade of the 21st century. Fourth, the structure of the operatively excised stenotic aortic valve was determined by a single physician (W.C.R.), who has studied the aortic valve for >40 years. Fifth, it made no attempt to separate stenotic valves into those that were purely stenotic versus those that were both stenotic and regurgitant, a division that is fraught with error unless an aortogram or echocardiogram has been used for this determination.

References

1. Sprecher DL, Schaefer EJ, Kent KM, Gregg RE, Zech LA, Hoeg JM, McManus B, Roberts WC, Brewer HB Jr. Cardiovascular features of homozygous familial hypercholesterolemia: analysis of 16 patients. *Am J Cardiol.* 1984;54:20–30.
2. Roberts WC. The senile cardiac calcification syndrome. *Am J Cardiol.* 1986;58:572–574.
3. Mautner GC, Roberts WC. Reported frequency of coronary arterial narrowing by angiogram in patients with valvular aortic stenosis. *Am J Cardiol.* 1992;70:539–540.
4. Chui MC, Newby DE, Panarelli M, Bloomfield P, Boon NA. Association between calcific aortic stenosis and hypercholesterolemia: is there a need for a randomized controlled trial of cholesterol-lowering therapy?. *Clin Cardiol.* 2001;24:52–55.
5. Bellamy MF, Pellikka PA, Klarich KW, Tajik AJ, Enriquez-Sarano M. Association of cholesterol levels, hydroxymethylglutaryl coenzyme-A reductase inhibitor treatment, and progression of aortic stenosis in the community. *J Am Coll Cardiol.* 2002;40:1723–1730.
6. Roberts WC, Ko JM. Weights of individual cusps in operatively-excised congenitally bicuspid stenotic aortic valves. *Am J Cardiol.* 2004;94:678–681.
7. Roberts WC, Ko JM. Weights of individual cusps in operatively-excised stenotic three-cuspid aortic valves. *Am J Cardiol.* 2004;94:681–684.
8. Subramanian R, Olson LJ, Edwards WD. Surgical pathology of pure aortic stenosis: a study of 374 cases. *Mayo Clin Proc.* 1984;59:683–690.
9. Passik CS, Ackermann DM, Pluth JR, Edwards WD. Temporal changes in the causes of aortic stenosis: a surgical pathologic study of 646 cases. *Mayo Clin Proc.* 1987;62:119–123.
10. Subramanian R, Olson LJ, Edwards WD. Surgical pathology of combined aortic stenosis and insufficiency: a study of 213 cases. *Mayo Clin Proc.* 1985;60:247–254.
11. Turri M, Thiene G, Bortolotti U, Milano A, Mazzucco A, Gallucci V. Surgical pathology of aortic valve disease: a study based on 602 specimens. *Eur J Cardiothorac Surg.* 1990;4:556–560.
12. Agozzino L, Falco A, De Luca Tupputi Schinosa L, De Vivo F, Esposito S, Cotrufo M. Aortic valve pathology: a study on 912 surgically excised aortic valves. *G Ital Cardiol.* 1992;22:1169–1177.

Comparison of Valve Structure, Valve Weight, and Severity of the Valve Obstruction in 1849 Patients Having Isolated Aortic Valve Replacement for Aortic Valve Stenosis (With or Without Associated Aortic Regurgitation) Studied at 3 Different Medical Centers in 2 Different Time Periods

William Clifford Roberts, MD; Jong Mi Ko, BA; Cody Hamilton, PhD

Background—Aortic valve replacement (AVR) for patients with aortic stenosis (AS) has now been available for 45 years. During this period, indications for the procedure have changed.

Methods and Results—Operatively excised stenotic aortic valves (with or without associated aortic regurgitation and without associated mitral valve disease) from 3 different medical centers (National Institutes of Health, Georgetown University Medical Center, and Baylor University Medical Center) were examined during 2 different time periods by the same physician to compare aortic valve structure, valve weight, age at operation, preoperative transvalvular peak pressure gradient, calculated aortic valve area, and whether simultaneous coronary artery bypass grafting (CABG) was performed. Compared with the first 3 decades (1961–1990) of AVR, patients having this operation during the fourth and fifth decades (1991–2004) had a lower frequency of congenitally malformed aortic valves, a higher frequency of tricuspid aortic valves, an older age, valves of lighter weight and lower transvalvular peak pressure gradients, and more often simultaneous CABG.

Conclusions—Although patients having isolated AVR for AS in the present and last decade were older than in the first 3 decades of valve replacement surgery, congenitally malformed aortic valves continue to be more common than tricuspid aortic valves, but the degree of AS and therefore, valve weight was significantly lower than in the earlier decades. **(*Circulation*. 2005;112:3919-3929.)**

Key Words: aortic valve stenosis ■ bypass ■ coronary disease ■ surgery ■ valvuloplasty

In the early years of cardiac valve replacement, this operation was usually restricted to patients with severe forms of valve disease. In recent times, less sick and even asymptomatic patients have undergone cardiac valve replacement or repair. During the past 40+ years, one of us (W.C.R.) has examined operatively excised cardiac valves at 3 different medical centers during at least 2 different time periods in patients who had isolated aortic valve replacement (AVR) for aortic stenosis (AS) with or without associated aortic regurgitation. Comparison of the aortic valve structure, valve weight, and severity of the valve obstruction at these 3 institutions is the purpose of this report. The hypothesis is that aortic valves excised in the earlier periods would have higher transvalvular peak pressure gradients across them, more calcific deposits, and therefore, larger weights and more often were congenitally malformed structures than those excised and replaced in more recent times, the implication being that the indications for AVR earlier may have been too restrictive and now are too lenient.

Clinical Perspective p 3929

Methods

One of us (W.C.R.) was at the National Institutes of Health (NIH) in Bethesda, Md, from July 1959 until March 1993. From July 1963 onward, all tissues excised by cardiac surgeons at the NIH were examined by W.C.R. From 1969 through 1992, nearly all cardiac valves excised at the time of valve replacement at Georgetown University Medical Center (GUMC) also were submitted to the Pathology Branch, National Heart, Lung, and Blood Institute (NHLBI), and examined by W.C.R. When W.C.R. moved to Baylor University Medical Center (BUMC) in March 1993, the gross photographs of the NHLBI and GUMC operatively excised valves were transported to BUMC in Dallas, Tex. Since March 1993 until

TABLE 1. Comparison of Valve Structure, Valve Weights, and Transvalvular Peak Systolic Pressure Gradients (PSPGs) and Demographies in Patients Having Isolated AVR for AS at 3 Different Medical Centers (1963–2004)

Aortic Valve Structure	Cases, n (%)	Age, y	Aortic Valve Weight, g	LV-Aorta PSPG, mm Hg	Aortic Valve Area, cm^2	Cardiac Index, $L \cdot min^{-1} \cdot m^{-2}$	Simultaneous CABG, n (%)
NIH (1963–1989; n=489)							
Men							
Unicuspid	84 (25)	21–78 (47)	1.53–10.2 (4.27)	10–135 (68)	0.30–0.93 (0.61)	1.80–4.50 (2.78)	2
Bicuspid	158 (46)	24–76 (56)	1.00–9.90 (4.14)	10–130 (66)	0.30–1.90 (0.70)	1.10–5.00 (2.61)	12
Tricuspid	47 (14)	28–82 (62)	0.70–6.50 (2.75)	30–136 (63)	0.35–1.30 (0.65)	1.30–3.65 (2.40)	7
Indeterminate	53 (15)	31–80 (54)	2.50–10.0 (5.17)	20–145 (90)	0.20–1.52 (0.66)	1.70–3.40 (2.53)	0
Subtotal	342 (100)	21–82 (54)	0.70–10.2 (4.05)	10–145 (69)	0.20–1.90 (0.66)	1.10–5.00 (2.58)	21 (9)
		333*	182*	139*	71*	113*	238*
Women							
Unicuspid	14 (13)	33–66 (53)	1.49–3.45 (2.92)	30–86 (63)	0.44, 0.70 (0.57)	2.10–4.20 (2.84)	0
Bicuspid	53 (48)	35–86 (55)	1.00–5.50 (3.12)	10–165 (86)	0.30–1.10 (0.54)	2.00–4.50 (2.76)	1
Tricuspid	28 (25)	35–78 (64)	0.55–5.50 (2.27)	20–125 (71)	0.30–1.10 (0.56)	1.80–4.20 (2.59)	3
Indeterminate	15 (14)	45–79 (57)	1.33–5.00 (3.09)	20–130 (67)	0.23–0.70 (0.43)	1.60–3.60 (2.46)	2
Subtotal	110 (100)	33–86 (57)	0.55–5.50 (2.80)	10–165 (76)	0.23–1.10 (0.53)	1.60–4.50 (2.68)	6 (8)
		104*	61*	56*	33*	39*	74*
GUMC (1969–1992; n=403)							
Men							
Unicuspid	56 (22)	33–73 (56)	1.60–9.50 (4.91)	10–160 (74)	0.40–1.23 (0.71)	2.06–4.30 (3.01)	10
Bicuspid	129 (50)	24–84 (63)	1.60–11.00 (4.46)	10–140 (69)	0.27–1.97 (0.76)	1.00–7.30 (2.95)	35
Tricuspid	63 (25)	40–88 (71)	1.20–6.00 (3.55)	17–120 (64)	0.30–1.20 (0.69)	1.50–3.30 (2.50)	30
Indeterminate	7 (3)	48–73 (60)	1.50–5.00 (3.50)	50–100 (68)	0.60, 1.90 (1.25)	2.15–2.80 (2.52)	2
Subtotal	255 (100)	24–88 (64)	1.20–11.0 (4.36)	10–160 (69)	0.27–1.97 (0.75)	1.00–7.30 (2.87)	77 (39)
		251*	161*	181*	113*	84*	198*
Women							
Unicuspid	24 (17)	34–81 (58)	1.46–6.70 (3.81)	34–135 (88)	0.30–0.65 (0.48)	1.60–3.00 (2.22)	3
Bicuspid	68 (47)	22–84 (66)	1.40–5.45 (3.22)	30–170 (86)	0.20–1.30 (0.58)	2.00–6.20 (2.92)	7
Tricuspid	48 (33)	46–89 (73)	0.40–5.30 (2.16)	35–120 (69)	0.21–1.09 (0.58)	1.67–3.90 (2.67)	17
Indeterminate	5 (3)	63–78 (69)	5.80	50–170 (113)	0.34, 0.60 (0.47)	4.30	2
Subtotal	145 (100)	22–89 (67)	0.40–6.70 (3.02)	30–170 (81)	0.20–1.30 (0.57)	1.60–6.20 (2.79)	29 (25)
		142*	87*	104*	70*	43*	118*
BUMC (1993–2004; n=957)						Ejection Fraction, %	
Men							
Unicuspid	36 (6)	25–75 (50)	1.82–8.00 (4.19)	21–141 (61)	0.40–1.82 (0.84)	20–75 (54)	6
Bicuspid	316 (53)	27–91 (67)	0.89–11.30 (3.57)	13–121 (55)	0.30–1.66 (0.76)	10–75 (48)	160
Tricuspid	242 (40)	51–90 (75)	1.03–6.60 (2.40)	10–100 (48)	0.20–1.90 (0.81)	10–85 (49)	163
Indeterminate	7 (1)	63–87 (74)	1.77, 2.89 (2.33)	18–99 (46)	0.39–1.11 (0.81)	47–69 (58)	3
Subtotal	601 (100)	25–91 (69)	0.89–11.30 (3.11)	10–141 (52)	0.20–1.90 (0.78)	10–85 (49)	332 (55)
		601*	441*	384*	402*	267*	601*
Women							
Unicuspid	12 (4)	30–75 (52)	1.02–4.50 (2.44)	22–72 (47)	0.30–0.88 (0.64)	33–80 (58)	1
Bicuspid	153 (43)	27–89 (67)	0.73–4.97 (2.30)	13–133 (61)	0.23–1.20 (0.62)	10–70 (54)	54
Tricuspid	186 (52)	45–91 (74)	0.45–4.81 (1.56)	10–125 (49)	0.18–1.49 (0.71)	15–85 (54)	111
Indeterminate	5 (1)	49–77 (70)	0.95–3.04 (2.03)	26–89 (58)	0.27–0.79 (0.49)	45	1
Subtotal	356 (100)	27–91 (70)	0.45–4.97 (1.89)	10–133 (54)	0.18–1.49 (0.67)	10–85 (54)	167 (47)
		356*	269*	247*	249*	173*	356*

LV indicates left ventricle. Values are range (mean) unless otherwise specified.
*No. of cases with data.

the present, W.C.R. has examined and dictated reports on all valves and other cardiovascular tissues excised at the time of cardiovascular operations at BUMC. Furthermore, all operatively excised valves examined by W.C.R. at NHLBI, GUMC, and BUMC were photographed, and hemodynamic and demographic data were made available to W.C.R. for most patients.

Each valve operatively excised at each of the 3 institutions was received in a container of formaldehyde. The valve structure was described, and usually the valve was weighed after blotting off excess formaldehyde with dry paper towels.[1] Hemodynamic data at NIH were obtained from the cardiac catheterization records. Hemodynamic data from GUMC were usually provided by a cardiology fellow who was responsible for presenting the case at the cardiac pathology conference that was conducted at GUMC by W.C.R. The preoperative cardiac catheterization and echocardiographic reports in the BUMC cases were obtained either from the patient's medical chart or, in more recent years, from the Apollo cardiovascular database of BUMC.

The 1849 patients included in this study represent 94% of the cases having isolated AVR for AS (with or without aortic regurgitation) at the NHLBI from 1963 to 1989, 97% of the cases having AVR at GUMC from 1969 through 1992, and 100% of the cases having AVR for AS (with or without aortic regurgitation) at BUMC from March 1993 through September 30, 2004. The few cases not included at NHLBI or GUMC did not have their operatively excised aortic valve examined by W.C.R.

This study was limited to patients >20 years of age having replacement only of the aortic valve, which was judged to be stenotic on the basis the cusps' having been made rigid or relatively rigid by calcific deposits (mainly on their aortic aspects) and/or by a measured transvalvular peak systolic pressure gradient ≥10 mm Hg. Patients ≤20 years of age, those with associated mitral stenosis, those having replacement of either the tricuspid and/or mitral valve, and those having a previous aortic valvulotomy or discrete subaortic stenosis or hypertrophic cardiomyopathy were excluded.

All continuous measures (age, valve weight, transvalvular peak gradient, valve area, and cardiac index) were analyzed as a function of time by a linear model. For each of these dependent measures, a test for time trend was performed after adjusting for differences across facilities (NIH, GUMC, and BUMC). When necessary (based on a likelihood-ratio test), an interaction term was added to the model to allow the trend over time to vary by facility. Similarly, an interaction term between time and sex was added when the trend varied significantly between men and women. The residual error was estimated separately for each facility to allow the residual variability to vary by facility. The tests for trends in aortic valve area, valve weight, and cardiac index were adjusted for age, sex, and number of cusps (unicuspid, bicuspid, tricuspid, indeterminate). The trend per year (including a 95% confidence interval [CI]) for each measure was estimated on the basis of the corresponding model. When the trend varied by facility, trends were reported on a by-facility basis.

Binary measures were modeled by logistic regression. These measures included sex, coronary artery bypass grafting (CABG; yes/no), and congenital malformation of the aortic valve (yes/no). A facility term was included in the model to account for facility-to-facility differences, and an interaction term was added when necessary to allow the trend to vary by facility. For the analyses of CABG and congenital malformation of the aortic valve, an interaction term was included to account for varying trends by sex when appropriate. The test for trend in CABG was adjusted for sex, number of cusps, and age. The analysis for the congenital malformations of the aortic valve was adjusted for age and sex. The yearly increase/decrease in each measure and the corresponding 95% CI were estimated on the basis of the appropriate model. As stated earlier, this increase/decrease was reported on a by-facility basis when a difference in trend across facilities was detected.

Because CABG was not performed during the entire length of time included in this study, the analysis for trend in the frequency of CABG was restricted to NIH data from 1974 onward and to GUMC data from 1978 onward. These are the years in which the first valve

TABLE 2. Cases From 3 Different Medical Centers Subdivided by Ages During Which AVR Took Place*

		Age (y) in Decade of AVR							
Valve Structure	No. of Cases	21–30	31–40	41–50	51–60	61–70	71–80	81–90	91–100
NIH (1963–1989)									
Unicuspid	94 (22)	7 (58)	18 (46)	29 (34)	24 (15)	15 (14)	1 (3)	0 (0)	0 (0)
Bicuspid	204 (47)	4 (33)	12 (31)	39 (46)	82 (52)	54 (51)	12 (35)	1 (33)	0 (0)
Tricuspid	71 (16)	1 (9)	3 (8)	3 (4)	19 (12)	27 (25)	16 (47)	2 (67)	0 (0)
Indeterminate	68 (15)	0 (0)	6 (15)	14 (16)	32 (21)	11 (10)	5 (15)	0 (0)	0 (0)
Subtotal	437 (100)	12 (3)	39 (9)	85 (19)	157 (36)	107 (24)	34 (8)	3 (<1)	0 (0)
GUMC (1969–1992)									
Unicuspid	78 (20)	0 (0)	8 (61)	15 (47)	22 (27)	25 (20)	7 (6)	1 (4)	0 (0)
Bicuspid	193 (49)	2 (100)	4 (31)	12 (38)	47 (58)	74 (58)	48 (42)	6 (25)	0 (0)
Tricuspid	111 (28)	0 (0)	1 (8)	4 (12)	10 (12)	23 (18)	56 (50)	17 (71)	0 (0)
Indeterminate	11 (3)	0 (0)	0 (0)	1 (3)	2 (3)	6 (4)	2 (2)	0 (0)	0 (0)
Subtotal	393 (100)	2 (<1)	13 (3)	32 (8)	81 (21)	128 (33)	113 (29)	24 (6)	0 (0)
BUMC (1993–2004)									
Unicuspid	48 (5)	5 (71)	6 (38)	14 (30)	9 (8)	9 (3)	5 (1)	0 (0)	0 (0)
Bicuspid	469 (49)	2 (29)	10 (62)	30 (64)	77 (68)	158 (60)	152 (41)	39 (28)	1 (50)
Tricuspid	428 (45)	0 (0)	0 (0)	2 (4)	27 (24)	93 (36)	205 (56)	101 (71)	1 (50)
Indeterminate	12 (1)	0 (0)	0 (0)	1 (2)	0 (0)	3 (1)	6 (2)	2 (1)	0 (0)
Subtotal	957 (100)	7 (<1)	16 (2)	47 (5)	113 (12)	263 (27)	368 (38)	141 (15)	2 (<1)

Values are n (%)

*Of the total 1849 patients, the ages were uncertain, other than knowing that they were adults, in 22 (1%), indicating that the ages at operation were available in 1827.

TABLE 3. Differences in the 8 Variables Analyzed for the 3 Institutions*

Variables	NIH	GUMC	BUMC	P† Men	P† Women
Valve structure, n/N (%)				<0.0001	<0.0001
Unicuspid					
Men	84/342 (25)	56/255 (22)	36/601 (6)		
Women	14/110 (13)	24/145 (17)	12/356 (4)		
Bicuspid					
Men	158/342 (46)	129/255 (50)	316/601 (53)		
Women	53/110 (48)	68/145 (47)	153/356 (43)		
Tricuspid					
Men	47/342 (14)	63/255 (25)	242/601 (40)		
Women	28/110 (25)	48/145 (33)	186/356 (52)		
Indeterminate					
Men	53/342 (15)	7/255 (3)	7/601 (1)		
Women	15/110 (14)	5/145 (3)	5/356 (1)		
Age, y				<0.0001	<0.0001
Men, range (mean±SD)	21–82 (54±12)	24–88 (64±11)	25–91 (69±12)		
Men ≥65, n/N (%)	62/331 (19)	124/251 (49)	424/601 (71)		
Women, range (mean±SD)	33–86 (57±11)	22–89 (67±12)	27–91 (70±11)		
Women ≥65, n/N (%)	27/104 (26)	94/142 (66)	273/356 (77)		
Sex, n/N (%)				<0.0001‡	
Men	342/452 (76)	255/400 (64)	601/957 (63)		
Women	110/452 (24)	145/400 (36)	356/957 (37)		
Aortic valve weight, g; range (mean±SD)				<0.0001	<0.0001
Men	0.70–10.2 (4.05±1.91)	1.20–11.0 (4.36±1.83)	0.89–11.30 (3.11±1.51)		
Women	0.55–5.50 (2.80±1.26)	0.40–6.70 (3.02±1.26)	0.45–4.97 (1.89±0.87)		
Left ventricular to aortic peak systolic gradient, mm Hg; range (mean±SD)				<0.0001	<0.0001
Men	10–145 (69±30)	10–160 (69±25)	10–141 (52±23)		
Women	10–165 (76±34)	30–170 (81±32)	10–133 (54±28)		
Aortic valve area, cm^2; range (mean±SD)				0.0023	<0.0001
Men	0.20–1.90 (0.66±0.32)	0.27–1.97 (0.75±0.31)	0.20–1.90 (0.78±0.26)		
Women	0.23–1.10 (0.53±0.21)	0.20–1.30 (0.57±0.21)	0.18–1.49 (0.67±0.22)		
Cardiac index, L · min^{-1} · m^{-2}; range (mean±SD)				0.0167	0.2115
Men	1.10–5.00 (2.58±0.72)	1.00–7.30 (2.87±0.93)	...		
Women	1.60–4.50 (2.68±0.69)	1.60–6.20 (2.79±0.81)	...		
Simultaneous CABG, n/N (%)				<0.0001	<0.0001
Men	21/238 (9)	77/198 (39)	332/601 (55)		
Women	6/74 (8)	29/118 (25)	167/356 (47)		

*See Table 1 for the numbers of patients in each category for whom data were available.

†*P* value based on a test for differences in the outcome measure across facilities by sex. The χ^2 test was used for categorical outcomes, and the ANOVA *F* test was used for continuous outcomes.

‡*P* value based on chi-square test for differences in sex across facilities.

replacement with concurrent CABG were recorded at each facility. Because CABG was common practice by 1993, no date restrictions were placed on the BUMC data. All statistical analyses were performed with SAS version 9.1. The study protocol was approved by the institutional review board of BUMC.

Results

The aortic valve structure, patient age at operation, aortic valve weight, preoperative transvalvular (left ventricular to aortic) peak pressure gradient, calculated aortic valve area, cardiac index, and whether simultaneous CABG was performed in men compared with women at each of the 3 medical centers are presented in Table 1. The aortic valve structures in each of 8 age decades during which the stenotic aortic valve was replaced are displayed in Table 2. The peak decade for AVR at NIH was 51 to 60 years (36% of cases); at GUMC, 61 to 70 years (33% of cases); and at BUMC, 71 to 80 years (38% of cases). The percentage of cases having AVR in the sixth decade was 36% at NIH, 21% at GUMC, and 12% at BUMC; the percentage of cases having AVR in the eighth decade was 8% at NIH, 29% at GUMC, and 38% at BUMC. The frequency of congenitally malformed aortic valves (either unicuspid or bicuspid) in the first 4 decades (21

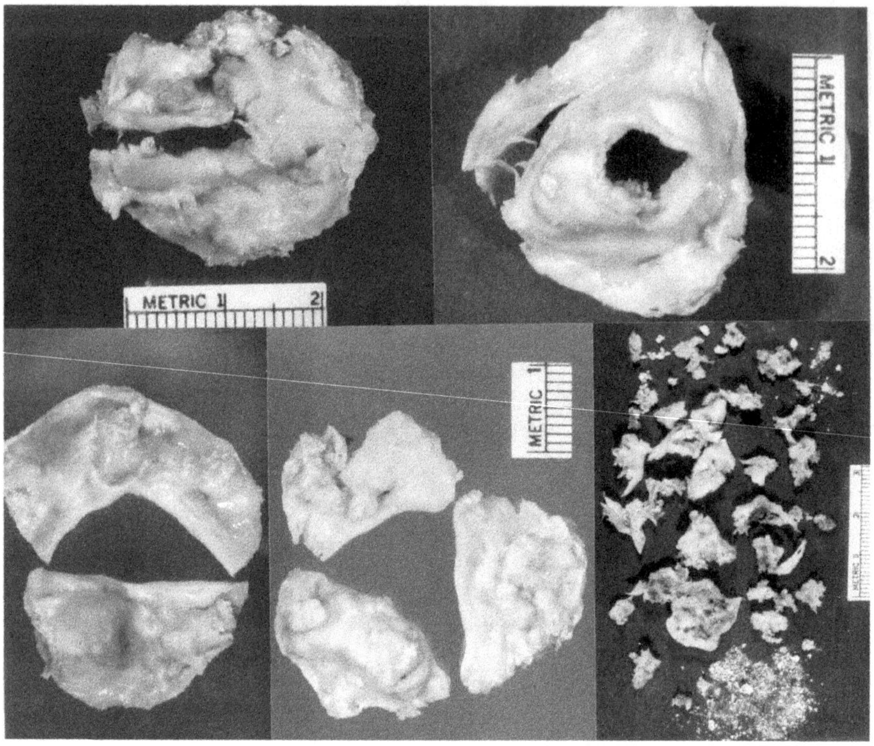

Figure 1. Photographs of operatively excised stenotic aortic valves. Upper left, Unicuspid, unicommissural valve from a 53-year-old man. Upper right, Unicuspid, acommissural valve from a 51-year-old woman. Lower left, Congenitally bicuspid valve from a 58-year-old man. Lower center, Tricuspid valve from an 86-year-old woman. Lower right, Valve of indeterminate structure (excised in multiple pieces) from a 31-year-old man.

to 60 years) compared with the latter 4 decades (61 to 100 years) at NIH was 73% (215/293) versus 58% (83/144); at GUMC, 86% (110/128) versus 61% (161/265); and at BUMC, 84% (153/183) versus 47% (364/774).

The similarities and differences in the 8 variables analyzed for the 3 medical centers are summarized in Table 3. The data on aortic valve structure were available for all 1849 patients. The data for men and women are presented separately in each of the 3 medical center groups so that men in 1 medical center could be compared with men in the other 2 centers and the same for women. The various valve structures are illustrated in Figure 1. Plots of each outcome over time by facility are presented in Figures 2 through 9. Results from the statistical models are contained in Table 4.

The frequency of tricuspid valves increased in both sexes from NIH to GUMC to BUMC: in men, from 14% to 25% to 40%, and in women, from 25% to 33% to 52%, respectively (see Table 3 for significance). After adjusting for sex, the estimated average patient age increased significantly by 0.478 years per year at NIH (95% CI, 0.339, 0.617) and by 0.628 years per year at GUMC (95% CI, 0.359, 0.897). Estimated patient age did not increase significantly at BUMC. This is not surprising, given the older mean patient age at BUMC (>69 years), introducing greater likelihood of a "ceiling" effect that would limit a further increase. The estimated percentage of female patients did not increase significantly over time. Based on the regression model, estimated average aortic valve weight decreased by 0.058 g per year (95% CI, −0.084, −0.032) over the time period analyzed. This trend did not vary by facility. No statistically significant trend in transvalvular peak systolic pressure gradient was detected at NIH or at GUMC (see Table 4). There was, however, a

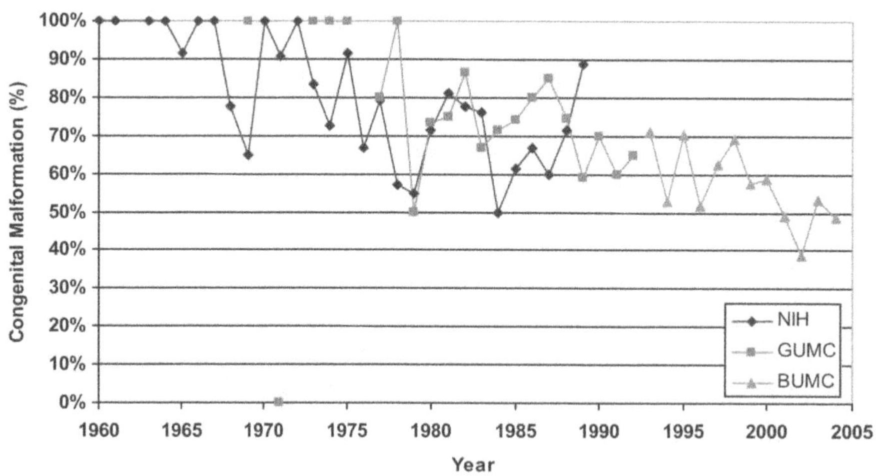

Figure 2. Change in frequency of congenitally malformed aortic valves excised over time by facility.

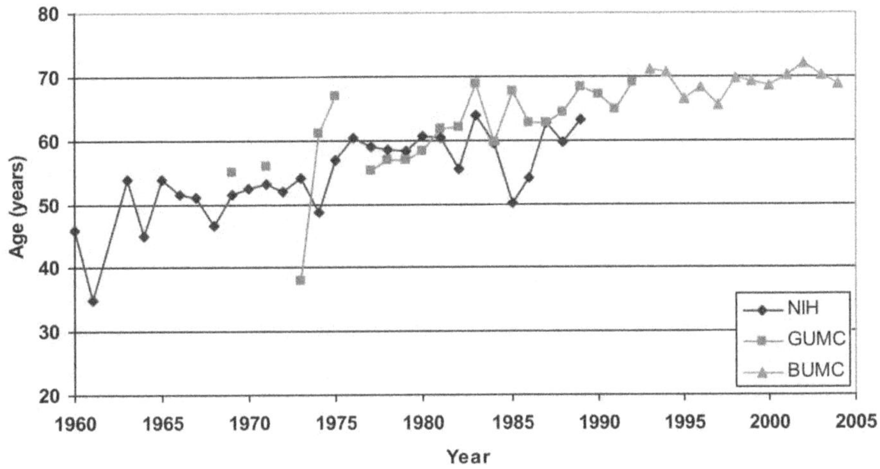

Figure 3. Change in age of the patients at the time of AVR over time by facility.

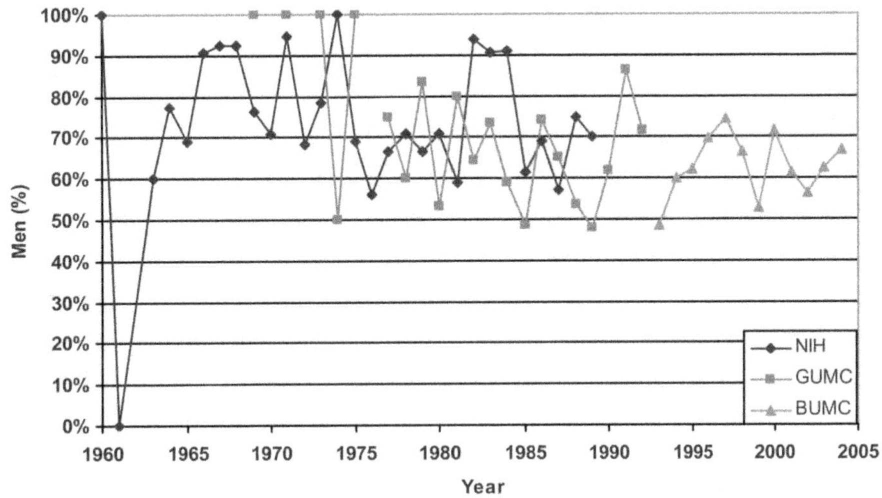

Figure 4. Change in the percentage in men undergoing AVR over time by facility.

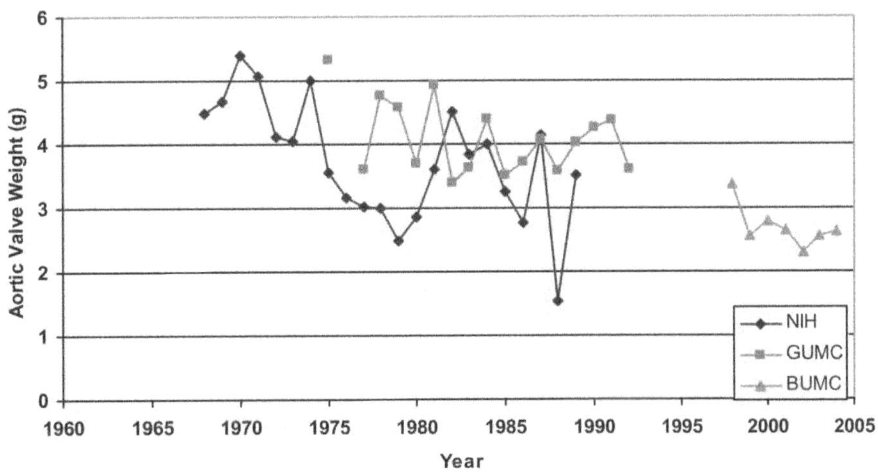

Figure 5. Change in operatively excised aortic valve weight over time by facility.

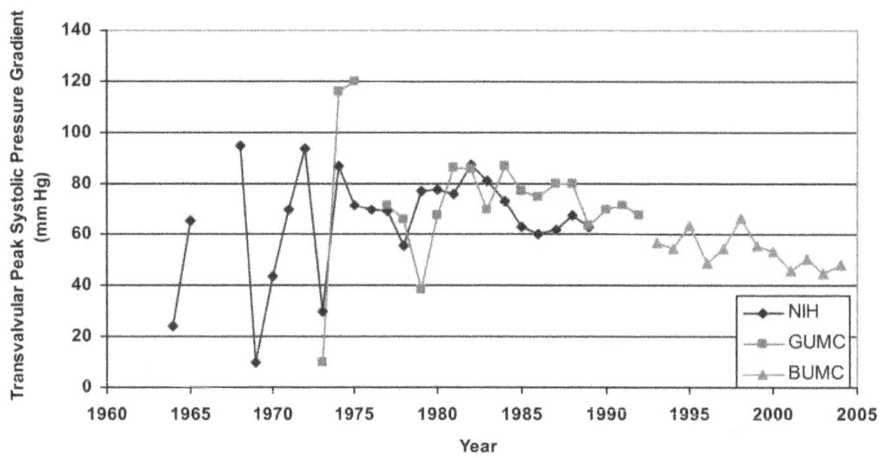

Figure 6. Change in transvalvular peak systolic pressure gradient over time by facility.

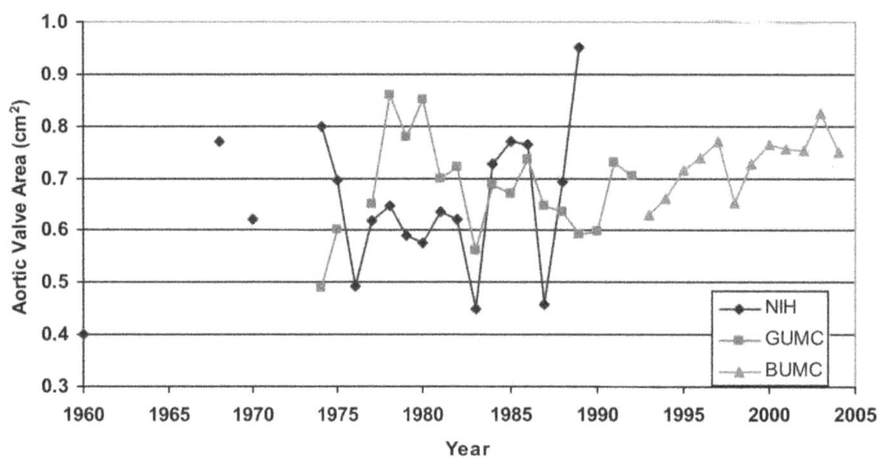

Figure 7. Change in aortic valve area over time by facility.

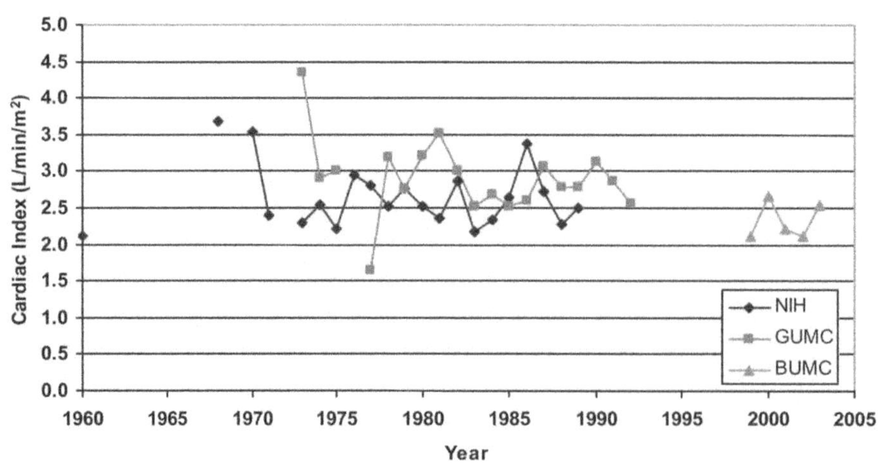

Figure 8. Change in cardiac index over time by facility.

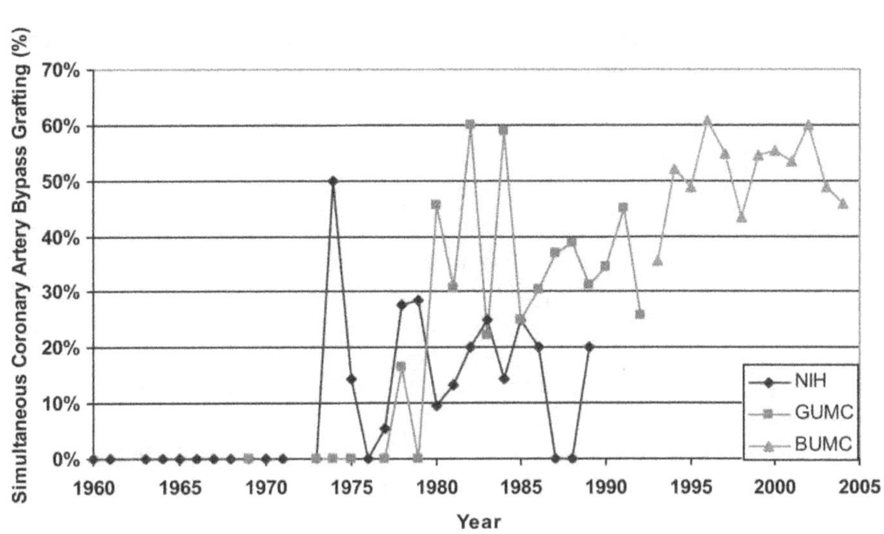

Figure 9. Change in frequency of simultaneous CABG over time by facility.

significant decrease in the transvalvular pressure gradient for both men and women at BUMC between 1993 and 2004. The estimated change in peak systolic gradient for men at BUMC was −0.801 mm Hg per year (95% CI, −1.420, −0.182). A change of −1.217 mm Hg per year (95% CI, −1.864, −0.571) was estimated for women. There was a significant increase of 0.011 cm^2 per year (95% CI, 0.006, 0.017) in aortic valve area at BUMC, whereas the trends in valve area over time were not significant at the other 2 facilities (see Table 4). The valve areas were calculated from hemodynamic data garnered during cardiac catheterization. Ejection fractions, more available in the BUMC cases than were cardiac index values, were ≥40% in 82% (360/440): in men, 79% (210/267) and in women, 87% (150/173). The ejection frac-

TABLE 4. Trends in Characteristics of Patients Undergoing AVR for AS Between 1963 and 2004

Variables	Cases*	Sex†	Facility†	Change per Year (95% CI)‡
Aortic valve structure, % tricuspid	1696	Combined	Combined	0.946 (0.920, 0.972)§
Age, y	1787	Combined	NIH	0.478 (0.339, 0.617)§
			GUMC	0.628 (0.359, 0.897)§
			BUMC	0.161 (−0.075, 0.396)
Sex, % female	1809	Combined	Combined	1.012 (0.991, 1.034)
Aortic valve weight, g	1187	Combined	Combined	−0.058 (−0.084, −0.032)§
Peak systolic pressure gradient, mm Hg	1110	Men	NIH	0.576 (−0.370, 1.522)
			GUMC	−0.371 (−1.141, 0.399)
			BUMC	−0.801 (−1.420, −0.182)§
		Women	NIH	0.160 (−0.838, 1.158)
			GUMC	−0.787 (−1.603, 0.028)
			BUMC	−1.217 (−1.864, −0.571)§
Aortic valve area, cm^2	936	Combined	NIH	0.007 (−0.005, 0.020)
			GUMC	−0.002 (−0.011, 0.007)
			BUMC	0.011 (0.006, 0.017)§
Cardiac index, $L \cdot min^{-1} \cdot m^{-2}$	296	Combined	NIH	−0.015 (−0.039, 0.008)
			GUMC	−0.015 (−0.050, 0.019)
			BUMC	−0.076 (−0.311, 0.159)
Simultaneous CABG, %	1435	Combined	Combined	0.989 (0.955, 1.023)

*No. of patients included in the analysis for the given measure. Some patients were excluded because of missing covariates in the regression model.

†Trends are reported at the sex or facility level only for those variables for which trends varied significantly by sex or facility.

‡Based on time parameters from the appropriate regression model. For dichotomous outcomes, odds ratios are reported.

§$P<0.01$.

TABLE 5. Numbers of Patients Having Transvalvular Peak Systolic Pressure Gradients (PSPGs) From 10 to 25 mm Hg and Frequency of Associated Severe Aortic Regurgitation (AR), Simultaneous CABG, Valve Type, and Valve Weight

Medical Center	Total Cases	Cases Having PSPG Measured	Cases Having PSPG 10–25 mm Hg	AR (3–4+)	CABG	Ages, y; Range (Mean)	No. of Men	Aortic Valve Structure U	B	T	I	Valve Weight, g; Range (Median)
NIH	489	195	15 (8)	5/15*	3 (20)	44–80 (60)	12 (80)	2	10	1	2	0.64–4.40 (2.80)
GUMC	403	285	8 (3)	2/4*	4 (50)	38–72 (61)	8 (100)	3	2	3	0	2.00–5.20 (3.20)
BUMC	957	631	85 (13)	8/21*	55 (65)	33–89 (70)	45 (53)	5	28	51	1	0.74–5.84 (1.53)

B indicates bicuspid; I, indeterminate; T, tricuspid; and U, unicuspid.

*Denominator is the number of patients with transvalvular PSPGs of 10 to 25 mm Hg and for whom aortic root angiography was performed.

tions at BUMC averaged 49±16% in men and 54±14% in women. There was no significant change over time in cardiac index within the 3 facilities (see Table 4). Although the rate of concomitant CABG varied by facility, there was no significant trend in this rate within each facility (see Table 4). Concomitant CABG at NIH, GUMC, and BUMC in men was 9%, 39%, and 55%, respectively, and in women, 8%, 25%, and 47%, respectively.

Aortic valve stenosis was defined herein as a peak transvalvular gradient of ≥10 mm Hg. This number was chosen from earlier experiences indicating that a gradient of this degree was indicative of a structural abnormality of the aortic valve. Of course, some patients with low transvalvular gradients also had significant aortic regurgitation, and others underwent the operation primarily for the purpose of CABG and the aortic valve was replaced at the same time, presumably to prevent further progression of the AS and the need for a later AVR in the setting of a previous CABG, a circumstance that increases operative mortality.

Table 5 summarizes the 108 patients at the 3 institutions with transvalvular peak systolic gradients of 10 to 25 mm Hg, a frequency of 10% among the 1111 patients having this gradient measured at cardiac catheterization. Of the 40 patients with aortograms and transvalvular peak gradients from 10 to 25 mm Hg, 15 (38%) had 3+ to 4+/4+ aortic regurgitation. Additionally, 62 (57%) of the 108 patients had simultaneous CABG at the time of AVR.

Discussion

The present study presents demographic and hemodynamic data in the first 3 decades (1960s, 1970s, and 1980s) of valve replacement for AS (with or without associated aortic regurgitation and without associated mitral stenosis or other valve replacement) at 2 medical centers (NIH [1963–1989] and GUMC [1969–1992]) and data from 1 medical center (BUMC [1993–2004]) collected in the fourth (1990s) and fifth (2000s) decades of valve replacement. The unique feature of this study is that all operatively excised stenotic valves at the 3 medical centers were examined and classified by the same physician, namely, W.C.R. The analyses demonstrated a significant decrease in the frequency of congenitally malformed aortic valves, an increase of tricuspid aortic valves, and a decrease in aortic valve weight. The age of patients increased significantly during the first 3 decades of AVR. Additionally, a significant decrease in peak systolic gradient and an increase in aortic valve area were apparent at BUMC. Data for many of the BUMC cases have been published previously.[2]

The proportion of congenitally malformed valves (unicuspid or bicuspid) at the 3 medical centers changed during the 5 decades. At NIH, GUMC, and BUMC, the proportion in men was 71%, 72%, and 59%, respectively, and in women, 61%, 64%, and 47%, respectively. If the valves with indeterminate structure are included among the congenitally malformed ones (almost surely the situation), the proportion of definitely congenitally malformed valves at NIH, GUMC, and BUMC in men would be 86%, 75%, and 60%, respectively, and in women, 75%, 67%, and 48%, respectively.

Although the data in the present study have been separated according to the 3 institutions from which they originated, there was some overlap of time periods among the 3 institutions. Table 6 shows the results of sorting the data by the decade during which AVR was performed, irrespective of institution. Longitudinal trends in the data over time and by facility can be viewed in Figures 2 through 9.

Although it started in the late 1950s, cardiac valve replacement became predictably successful in the early 1960s with the introduction of the caged-ball prosthesis. Collection of data in the present study began in 1963 and continued through 2004. In the early years of valve replacement, the procedure was reserved primarily for very symptomatic patients and those with considerable degrees of valvular stenosis and/or severe degrees of valvular regurgitation. In contrast to patients with mitral stenosis, virtually always in adults the consequence of rheumatic heart disease, which had been successfully treated by commissurotomy since 1948, aortic valve commissurotomy, begun in the late 1950s, proved predictably unsuccessful in adults with calcific AS. As a consequence, when AVR became predictably successful in the early 1960s, a large number of adults with AS suddenly were available for operation. Criteria for AVR in the early 1960s were quite stringent and rightly so, because the procedure was new and operative and postoperative procedures were evolving. Additionally, CABG was not initiated until 1967, and indeed, coronary angiography was infrequently performed until the late 1960s. Even after CABG became available, some centers limited its performance in patients with combined AS and coronary artery disease because of fear that the CABG procedure would prolong cardiopulmonary bypass time and aortic cross-clamp time significantly and, as a consequence, reduce the chance of successful AVR. Technical developments (myocardial pres-

TABLE 6. **Trends and Changes in 5 Decades of AVR After Combining Data From the 3 Institutions***

Variables	Decades, y 1961–1970 (n=169)	1971–1980 (n=241)	1981–1990 (n=425)	1991–2000 (n=580)	2001–2004 (n=433)
Valve structure, n/N (%)					
Unicuspid					
Men	40/130 (31)	35/152 (23)	55/271 (20)	35/378 (9)	11/267 (4)
Women	6/34 (17)	7/62 (11)	24/146 (16)	6/203 (3)	7/166 (4)
Bicuspid					
Men	60/130 (46)	71/152 (47)	137/271 (51)	208/378 (55)	127/267 (48)
Women	18/34 (53)	30/62 (48)	69/146 (47)	97/203 (48)	60/166 (36)
Tricuspid					
Men	5/130 (4)	26/152 (17)	67/271 (25)	126/378 (33)	128/267 (48)
Women	5/34 (15)	17/62 (28)	46/146 (32)	97/203 (48)	97/166 (59)
Indeterminate					
Men	25/130 (19)	20/152 (13)	12/271 (4)	9/378 (2)	1/267 (<1)
Women	5/34 (15)	8/62 (13)	7/146 (5)	3/203 (1)	2/166 (1)
Ages, y; mean±SD					
Men	50±10	56±10	62±12	67±12	71±11
Men ≥65, n/N (%)	8/130 (6)	30/142 (21)	127/269 (47)	249/377 (66)	198/267 (74)
Women	53±7	59±11	66±13	71±11	70±12
Women ≥65, n/N (%)	2/34 (6)	19/59 (32)	88/140 (63)	165/203 (81)	119/166 (72)
Sex, n/N (%)					
Men	130/164 (79)	152/214 (71)	271/417 (65)	378/581 (65)	267/433 (62)
Women	34/164 (21)	62/214 (29)	146/417 (35)	203/581 (35)	166/433 (38)
Aortic valve weight, g; mean±SD					
Men	5.34±2.11	3.86±1.60	4.21±1.94	3.48±1.64	2.99±1.48
Women	4.09±1.45	2.72±1.20	3.00±1.24	2.09±0.92	1.78±0.83
Left ventricular to aortic peak systolic gradient, mm Hg; mean±SD					
Men	59±41	66±29	71±26	56±24	47±22
Women	...	75±33	82±32	60±30	48±25
Aortic valve area, cm^2; mean±SD					
Men	0.60±0.19	0.72±0.36	0.71±0.31	0.76±0.26	0.82±0.26
Women	...	0.53±0.20	0.55±0.20	0.64±0.21	0.71±0.24
Simultaneous CABG, n/N (%)					
Men	0/130 (0)	11/80 (14)	71/200 (36)	197/376 (52)	151/267 (57)
Women	0/34 (0)	7/36 (19)	26/115 (23)	94/203 (46)	75/166 (45)

*See Table 1 for the numbers of patients in each category for whom data were available.

ervation, etc) and greater experience have obviated this approach in the current era.

One explanation for the lower transvalvular gradients, lower valve weights, and older ages in the patients having AVR for AS in the more recent decades compared with the earlier ones is the much higher frequency of having CABG at the time of valve replacement in more recent decades compared with the earlier ones. Symptomatic patients with combined AS and coronary artery disease are more likely to have AVR for relatively small degrees of stenosis because of fear that the valve stenosis will progress.[3] The risk of AVR some time after isolated CABG is much higher than the chance of complications, including death, after the first operation.

Were some of the differences in patient demographics and hemodynamics at the 3 institutions the result of referral biases? Certainly, the referral patterns were a bit different. All patients with AS presenting at NIH were referred directly to the Cardiology Branch, and nearly all patients referred had cardiac catheterization performed at that branch, whether or not it had been performed earlier at a different hospital. Older patients often were not accepted at NIH, and unless significant aortic regurgitation was present, the peak transvalvular gradient across the aortic valve usually had to be >50 mm Hg for the patient to be considered for AVR. Furthermore, CABG, which was performed for the first time elsewhere in 1967, was not done in the patients having AVR at NIH until the 1970s. The criteria for isolated AVR at GUMC appear to have been similar to those at NIH, despite the fact that many GUMC referring physicians were in private practice. Patients referred to GUMC were not limited by age, as was frequently the cases at NIH, and CABG was far more frequently performed at GUMC than at NIH. The pool of physicians referring patients to BUMC was much larger than at GUMC, and not infrequently, patients were referred by non-BUMC physicians directly to cardiovascular surgeons at BUMC, a referral method never done at NIH and probably infrequently done at GUMC. Additionally, the pool of private cardiologists at BUMC was and is large, and the number of patients with AS seen by any one cardiologist is therefore not particularly large. As a consequence, expertise in valvular heart disease among cardiologists may be diminishing. Also, the hemodynamic and angiographic data collected by BUMC cardiologists were less standardized than those collected by NIH cardiologists and probably also by GUMC cardiologists. Moreover, in the 1980s, echocardiography became more widespread and, at least in younger patients, often substituted for hemodynamic data collected at cardiac catheterization. In patients >40 years of age who had echocardiograms, cardiac catheterization often was used only for coronary angiography without measuring left ventricular outflow pressure gradients and/or valve areas. Lastly, there has been a push in recent years to perform AVR in patients who are less symptomatic or even asymptomatic than in the earlier decades.

There are limitations to the present study. The main one was that individual patient data were missing for some patients, including sex (2%; 39/1849); exact ages (3%; 61/1849); aortic valve weights (35%; 647/1849); transvalvular peak systolic pressure gradients (40%; 736/1849); and aortic valve areas (49%; 911/1849). Nevertheless, the numbers are large enough that the missing data almost certainly had little effect on the totals or the conclusions of this study.

Disclosures

None.

References

1. Roberts WC, Ko JM. Weights of operatively excised stenotic unicuspid, bicuspid, and tricuspid aortic valves and their relation to age, sex, body mass index, and presence or absence of concomitant coronary artery bypass grafting. *Am J Cardiol*. 2003;92:1057–1065.
2. Roberts WC, Ko JM. Frequency by decades of unicuspid, bicuspid, and tricuspid aortic valves in adults having isolated aortic valve replacement for aortic stenosis, with or without associated aortic regurgitation. *Circulation*. 2005;111:920–925.
3. Stephan PJ, Henry AC III, Hebeler RF Jr, Whiddon L, Roberts WC. Comparison of age, gender, number of aortic valve cusps, concomitant coronary artery bypass grafting, and magnitude of left ventricular-systemic arterial peak systolic gradient in adults having aortic valve replacement for isolated aortic valve stenosis. *Am J Cardiol*. 1997;79:166–172.

CLINICAL PERSPECTIVE

How can the information provided in this report be useful clinically? First, it shows that isolated AS (unassociated with mitral valve disease) more often involves a congenitally malformed valve than a tricuspid one, and therefore, it is unlikely that AS will become less frequent in the Western world as has rheumatic heart disease. Second, this report shows that the degree of AS in patients having isolated AVR in the last decade or so is, as a rule, considerably less than in earlier decades. Some of the less stringent criteria for AVR in recent times have been necessitated by the need for CABG more than for the need for AVR. Even without simultaneous CABG, the degree of AS today in patients having AVR is considerably less than in previous decades. Probably the criteria for AVR in patients with AS today are more lenient than they ought to be.

Sudden Onset of "Cardiac" Symptoms, (?) Mild or Severe Aortic Valve Stenosis Involving a Congenitally Bicuspid Aortic Valve, and Nearly Normal Coronary Arteries in an Octogenarian

William C. Roberts, MD;[1,2,3] Paul A. Grayburn, MD[1,3]
From the Departments of Internal Medicine, Division of Cardiology;[1] and Pathology;[2] and the Baylor Heart and Vascular Institute,[3] Baylor University Medical Center, Dallas, TX
Address for correspondence: William C. Roberts, MD, Baylor Heart and Vascular Institute, Baylor University Medical Center, 621 North Hall Street, Suite H-030, Dallas, TX 75226
E-mail: wc.roberts@baylorhealth.edu

An 86-year-old woman who lived alone was in good health until one evening, just after cleaning the kitchen, she suddenly noted palpitations, dizziness, weakness, and cool clammy skin while sitting. She called an ambulance service and was brought to a hospital. The symptoms resolved spontaneously after a few minutes. She was 61 inches tall and weighed 158 lb (body mass index, 29.8 kg/m^2). A grade 2–3/6 systolic ejection murmur was heard over the precordium and best at the cardiac base and into both carotid arteries. An ECG showed sinus rhythm, atrial premature complexes, and no ST-segment or T-wave abnormalities. An echocardiogram (Figure 1) disclosed the following dimensions in centimeters: left ventricle end diastole was 4.3 and peak systole was 3.7, left ventricular and ventricular septal walls were each 1.3, and the left atrial cavity was 3.1. The calculated peak transvalvular aortic gradient was 47 mm Hg; blood hematocrit was 33% and hemoglobin was 10.9 g/dL. Serum total cholesterol was 260 mm Hg, low-density lipoprotein cholesterol 177 mm Hg, high-density lipoprotein cholesterol 88 mm Hg, and triglycerides 62 mg/dL. Troponins and creatine kinase levels were normal.

Cardiac catheterization disclosed the following pressures: pulmonary artery wedge A wave 29, V wave 36, mean 25; pulmonary artery, 54/26; right ventricle, 62/23; left ventricle, 206/33; and ascending aorta, 183/80 mm Hg. The peak transaortic valve gradient was 23 and the mean gradient was 29 mm Hg, the calculated aortic valve area was 0.61 cm^2 (index, 0.36 cm^2/m^2), and the left ventricular ejection fraction was 60%. The cardiac index was 2.2 L/min/m^2. Coronary angiogram disclosed no significant narrowings.

The aortic valve at operation was found to be congenitally bicuspid (Figure 2). It was excised virtually intact. It weighed 2.51 g: the raphe cusp weighed 1.74 g and the nonraphe cusp, 0.69 g.[1,2] Her postoperative course was uneventful.

COMMENTS

The above-described elderly woman who was known to have a precordial murmur for many years was asymptomatic until a single near-syncopal episode prompted hospitalization and cardiac evaluation. The transvalvular peak systolic pressure gradient across her aortic valve was only 23 mm Hg (mean gradient, 29 mm Hg) in the absence of associated aortic regurgitation and in the presence of a normal ejection fraction (60%), but the calculated aortic valve area was 0.61 cm^2. The valve area would, of course, indicate severe aortic valve stenosis, but the peak transvalvular gradient would indicate only mild aortic stenosis. Which is correct? Could the measured transvalvular gradient be incorrect or the calculated aortic

www.lejacq.com ID: 5267

Table. Echocardiographic and Catheterization Data		
VARIABLE	ECHOCARDIOGRAPHY	CATHETERIZATION
Peak aortic velocity (m/sec)	3.8	—
Peak transvalvular gradient (mm Hg)*	58	23
Mean transvalvular gradient (mm Hg)	36	29
Aortic valve area (cm²)	0.6	0.6
Aortic regurgitation	Mild	—

*Peak gradient by Doppler represents the greatest difference in pressure between the left ventricle and aorta at any point in time. Peak gradient by catheterization represents the difference between the peak left ventricular pressure and the peak aortic pressure, which do not occur simultaneously due to a temporal delay in the peak aortic pressure (tardus). This explains why the peak gradient is less than the mean gradient at catheterization in this case.

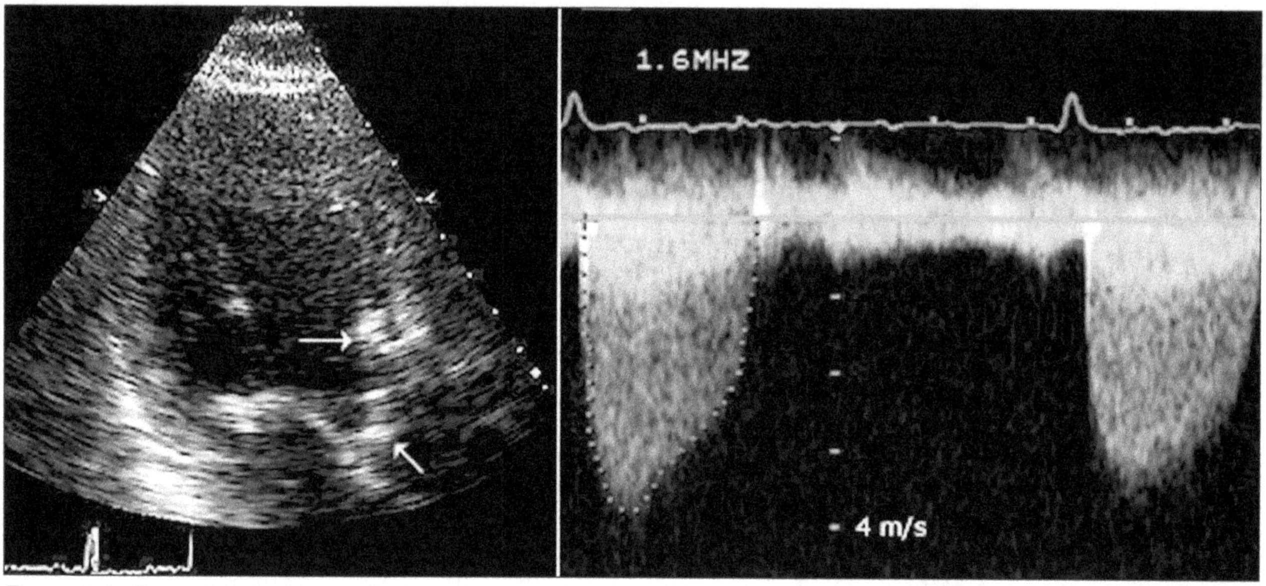

Figure 1. Left panel: Apical long-axis view showing extensive calcium along the ventricular septum (horizontal arrow) and the aortic valve leaflets (diagonal arrow). Right panel: Continuous wave Doppler spectral velocity signal across the aortic valve. The peak velocity was 3.8 m/sec and the mean transvalvular gradient was calculated as 36 mm Hg.

valve area be incorrectly calculated? Although the patient's peak systolic left ventricular and aortic peak systolic pressures were high (206 and 183 mm Hg, respectively, indicating isolated systolic hypertension), her A peak-to-peak pressure gradient was only 23 mm Hg.[3]

There is some evidence that the calculated aortic valve area is not as accurate in patients with low transvalvular aortic pressure gradients as it is in patients with high transvalvular pressure gradients. Roberts and Ko[4] found that the peak transaortic pressure gradient correlated much better with the weight of the operatively excised stenotic aortic valve than did the calculated aortic valve area. Among women in whom the operatively excised stenotic aortic valve weighed ≤1 g, the peak transvalvular aortic pressure gradient averaged 28 mm Hg and the aortic valve area 0.83 cm²; of valves weighing >2–3 g (as in the present patient), the peak gradient averaged 63 mm Hg and the area, 0.58 cm²; of valves weighing >3–4 g, the peak gradient averaged 85 mm Hg and the valve area 0.51 cm². Thus, caution is needed in relying on the calculated aortic valve area in patients with small peak systolic pressure gradients.

In this patient, both echocardiography and catheterization yielded similar mean gradients and identical aortic valve areas in the setting of a low cardiac index (Table). This suggests that the low calculated valve area was an artifact of a low flow state rather than a technical error. Importantly, aortic valve area is notoriously misleading in the setting of a low transvalvular gradient.[5] Dobutamine challenge is recommended to recalculate both the mean gradient and aortic valve area at a higher level of flow (the numerator in both the Gorlin and continuity equations).[6] Given that the valve was only moderately abnormal by pathologic examination, it is likely that dobutamine would have resulted in a higher aortic valve area without an increased gradient, and surgery might have been avoided. The single episode of syncope, which prompted surgery, was probably not caused by aortic stenosis in this case. It must be remembered that syncope has many other causes, including vagal episodes, conduction system disease, and noncardiac etiologies. The echocardiogram showed large calcific deposits of the ventricular septum, which could indicate conduction system disease.

The above-described patient also raises the issue of the frequency of bicuspid aortic valves in octogenarians with aortic valve stenosis unassociated with significant mitral valve disease. Of 190 patients aged 80–89 years who had isolated aortic valve replacement for aortic valve stenosis in the past 12 years (1993–2005) at Baylor University Medical Center (Dallas, TX), 54 (28%) had congenitally bicuspid aortic valves.[7] Of them, 20 (37%) were women (such as the present patient) and 34 (63%) were men.

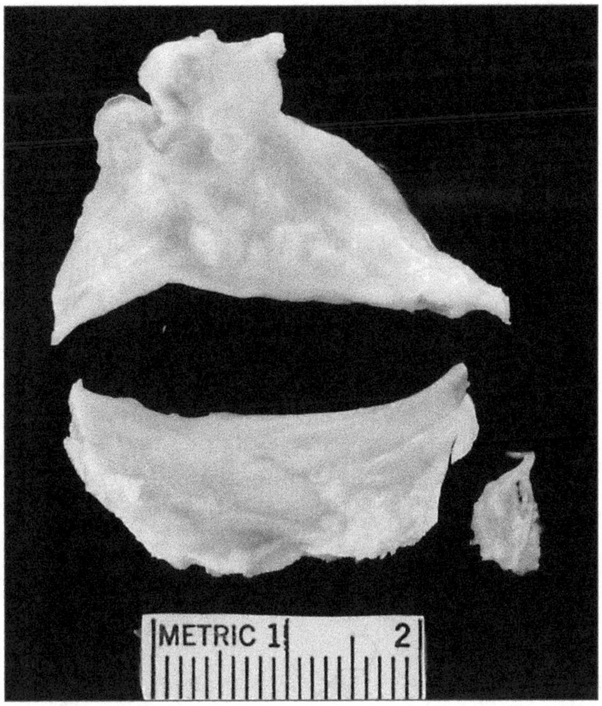

Figure 2. Photograph of the congenitally bicuspid aortic valve. Focal calcific deposits are present in each cusp.

References

1 Roberts WC, Ko JM. Weights of operatively-excised stenotic unicuspid, bicuspid, and tricuspid aortic valves and their relation to age, sex, body mass index, and presence or absence of concomitant coronary artery bypass grafting. *Am J Cardiol.* 2003;92:1057–1065.

2 Roberts WC, Ko JM. Weights of individual cusps in operatively-excised stenotic congenitally bicuspid aortic valves. *Am J Cardiol.* 2004;94:678–681.

3 Roberts WC, Perloff JK, Costantino T. Severe valvular aortic stenosis in patients over 65 years of age. A clinicopathologic study. *Am J Cardiol.* 1971;27:497–506.

4 Roberts WC, Ko JM. Relation of weights of operatively excised stenotic aortic valves to preoperative transvalvular peak systolic pressure gradients and to calculated aortic valve areas. *J Am Coll Cardiol.* 2004;44:1847–1855.

5 Carabello BA. Evaluation and management of patients with aortic stenosis. *Circulation.* 2002;105:1746–1750.

6 Grayburn PA, Eichhorn EJ. Dobutamine challenge for low gradient aortic stenosis. *Circulation.* 2002;106:763–765.

7 Roberts WC, Ko JM. Frequency by decade of unicuspid, bicuspid, and tricuspid aortic valves in adults having isolated aortic valve replacement for aortic stenosis, with or without associated aortic regurgitation. *Circulation.* 2005;111:920–925.

Aortic Valve Replacement for Aortic Stenosis in Nonagenarians

William Clifford Roberts, MD[a,b,d,*], Jong Mi Ko, BA[d], and Gregory John Matter, MD[c,d]

We reviewed certain clinical and morphologic findings in 9 patients who had aortic valve replacement (AVR) for aortic stenosis (AS) when ≥90 years of age. All had AVR from February 2000 to April 2006. The aortic valve areas ranged from 0.41 to 1.00 cm^2, and the transvalvular peak systolic gradients ranged from 20 to 110 mm Hg. The left ventricular ejection fractions were ≥50% in 6 of the 9 patients. The aortic valve was congenitally bicuspid in 3 patients, and the operatively excised valves in them weighed 4.20, 5.73, and 9.75 g, respectively (mean 6.56). The other 6 patients had 3-cuspid valves without commissural fusion, and the operatively excised valves in them weighed 0.43, 0.94, 1.08, 1.51, 1.98, and 4.43 g, respectively (median 1.30, mean 1.73). Coronary artery bypass grafting (CABG) was performed at the time of AVR in 8 of the patients. One patient died a day postoperatively and 2 others died 874 and 1,011 days, respectively, after operation. Two were in skilled nursing units postoperatively for several weeks. In conclusion, AS can be severe in nonagenarians and may be superimposed on a congenitally bicuspid aortic valve. **(Am J Cardiol 2006;98:1251–1253)**

Numerous reports have appeared describing clinical and operative results of aortic valve replacement (AVR) for aortic stenosis (AS) in octogenarians.[1–9] In contrast, few reports are available describing clinical or other features of nonagenarians having AVR for AS. Such is the purpose of this report.

Methods and Results

Cases having isolated AVR for AS from March 1993 to April 2006 at Baylor University Medical Center (BUMC) were reviewed. A total of 1,157 patients had isolated AVR for AS during this 13-year period and 9 (0.8%) of them were ≥90 years of age at the time of AVR. All 9 had AVR from 2000 to 2006 and none had AVR in the 1990s. This study focuses exclusively on observations in these 9 patients. Certain clinical and morphologic aortic valve findings in them are summarized in Table 1, and the operatively excised aortic valves are illustrated in Figures 1 and 2. Of the 6 men, 3 had congenitally bicuspid aortic valves that weighed 4.20, 5.73, and 9.75 g, respectively (mean 6.56). Each of the 3 women and the 3 other men had 3-cuspid aortic valves ranging in weight from 0.43 to 4.43 g (median 1.30, mean 1.73).

The calculated aortic valve areas ranged preoperatively from 0.41 to 1.00 cm^2 (mean 0.68). The transvalvular peak systolic gradients (6 patients) ranged from 20 to 110 mm Hg (average 58, median 60) and the transvalvular mean gradients (8 patients) ranged from 15 to 75 mm Hg (average 44). The left ventricular ejection fractions were ≥ 50% in 6 of the 9 patients.

[a]Departments of Internal Medicine (Division of Cardiology), [b]Pathology, and [c]Cardiothoracic Surgery, and [d]Baylor Heart and Vascular Institute, Baylor University Medical Center, Dallas, Texas 75246.

*Corresponding author: Tel: 214-820-7911; fax: 214-820-7533.

E-mail address: wc.roberts@baylorhealth.edu (W.C. Roberts).

Table 1
Data in eight nonagenarians having aortic valve replacement for aortic valve stenosis

Case No.	Age at AVR Years/ Sex	LV (s/d) (mm Hg)	Aorta (s/d) (mm Hg)	LV-Aortic PSG (mm Hg)	LV-Aortic MSG (mm Hg)	Aortic Valve Area (cm^2)	EF (%)	No. of Aortic Valve Cusps	Valve Weight (g)	CABG	Date of AVR	Days in Hospital After AVR	Status 3/27/2006 (days after AVR)
1	91M	—	—	—	40	0.60	75*	2	4.20	+	11/5/2001	9	Died (1,011)
2	90M	207/15	157/60	50	57	0.64	50	2	5.73	0	5/14/2002	8	Alive (1,413)
3	90M	—	146/58	110*	75*	0.55*	65	2	9.75	+	10/10/2003	10	Alive (899)
4	90F	156/19	136/55	20	30	0.82	70	3	0.43	+	2/8/2005	1	Died (1)
5	90F	—	133/76	—	—	0.50*	25*	3	0.94	+	11/12/2002	9	Alive (1,231)
6	91M	—	—	—	15	1.00	50	3	1.08	+	4/3/2006	25	Alive (27 as of 4/30/06)
7	91F	237/32	168/61	69	54	0.66	74*	3	1.51	+	3/19/2004	6	Alive (738)
8	90M	95/14	64/30	31	25	0.91	30	3	1.98	+	2/17/2000	7	Alive (2230)
9	91M	187/28	118/62	69	52	0.41	15	3	4.43	+	7/6/2000	14	Died (874)

* From echocardiogram.

Ao = aorta; AR = aortic regurgitation; AVR = aortic valve replacement; EF = ejection fraction; LV = left ventricular; MSG = mean systolic gradient; PO = postoperation; PSG = peak systolic gradient; s/d = peak systole/end diastole.

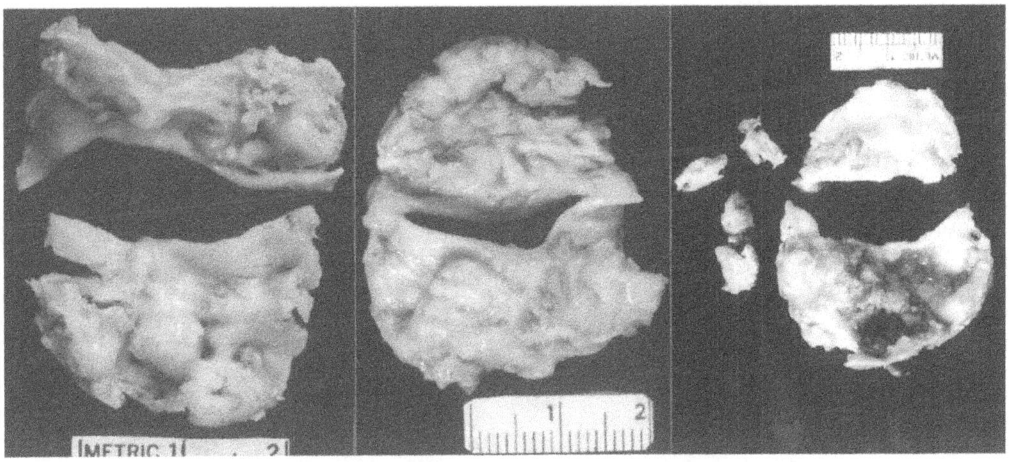

Figure 1. Congenitally bicuspid aortic valves (see Table 1). *Left*, case 1; *middle*, case 2; and *right*, case 3.

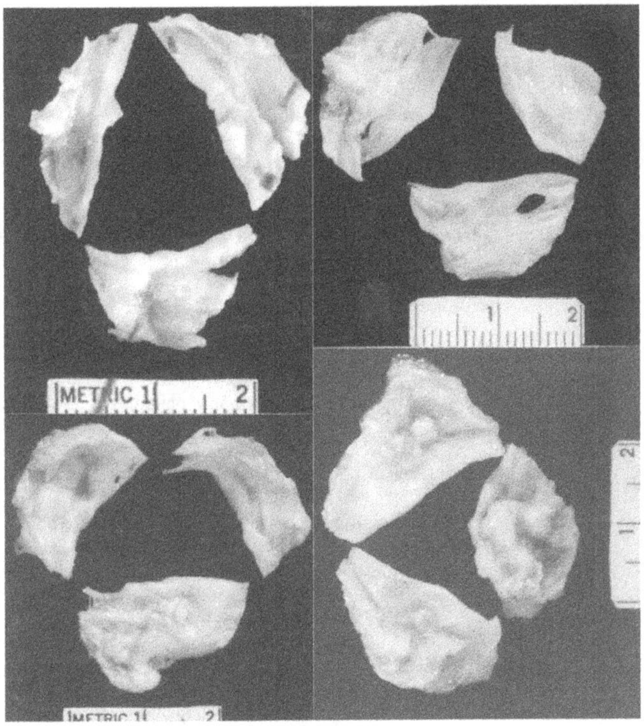

Figure 2. Tricuspid aortic valves (see Table 1). *Upper left*, case 4; *upper right*, case 5; *lower left*, case 6; and *lower right*, case 7.

One patient died 1 day postoperatively and 2 others died 874 and 1,011 days, respectively, after operation. Of the 6 living patients, 5 remain alive from 738 to 2,230 days postoperatively as of March 27, 2006, and the remaining 1 patient is alive 27 days postoperatively as of April 30, 2006. Two patients were in the rehabilitation hospital for several weeks postoperatively.

Eight of the 9 patients had coronary artery bypass grafting (CABG) at the time of AVR.

Discussion

Of the 9 nonagenarians included in this study, all but 1 survived the operative period, another died 874 days postoperatively, and another 1,011 days postoperatively. The exact cause of death in these patients is unclear and a necropsy was not performed in any of them. The other 6 patients are alive 27, 738, 899, 1,231, 1,413, and 2,230 days, respectively, postoperatively.

A surprise finding in the 9 patients was the presence of a congenitally bicuspid aortic valve in 3 of them. As described previously, the operatively excised stenotic congenitally bicuspid aortic valves are, as a rule, much heavier than are the operatively excised stenotic 3-cuspid aortic valves. All 3 patients with congenitally bicuspid aortic valves were men and 3 of the 6 patients with operatively excised stenotic 3-cuspid aortic valves were men. Men, irrespective of valve structure, tend to have heavier valves than do women of similar age.[10] The valve weight in the stenotic valves is determined primarily by the quantity of calcium on the aortic aspects of the cusps, and men tend to have larger deposits of calcium on their stenotic valves than women. The quantity of calcium in stenotic congenitally bicuspid aortic valves tends to be much larger than in patients with stenotic 3-cuspid aortic valves (when comparing adults of similar age) and that fact accounts for the heavier weights in the patients with bicuspid valves.

Few reports have described patients ≥90 years of age having AVR with or without simultaneous CABG. Samuel and colleagues,[11] in 1996, described 6 nonagenarians (4 women, 2 men). All survived the perioperative period: 1 died 4 months, another 31 months, and another 73 months postoperatively: the remaining 3 patients were alive 24, 44, and 62 months, respectively, postoperatively. The structure of the operatively excised stenotic aortic valves in these 6 patients was not described.

Blanche and associates,[12] in 1997, briefly described 17 nonagenarians who had AVR, 10 with and 7 without simultaneous CABG. Because these 17 patients were included among 13 others who had CABG without AVR, details of outcomes and other findings in the group having AVR could not be determined. The structure of the operatively excised stenotic aortic valves was not described. The authors noted that the average hospital cost of isolated AVR in their nonagenarians was \$60,000, whereas those having combined AVR and CABG was \$51,000, figures considerably higher than in their younger patients having these proce-

Table 2
Frequency of unicuspid, bicuspid, and tricuspid valves operatively excised at the Baylor University Medical Center (Dallas) from 1993 to 2006 in septuagenarians, octogenarians, and nonagenarians

Age Group (Years)	Mean Age (Years)	Number of Patients	Aortic Valve Structure				Aortic Valve Weight (g)			
			Unicuspid	Bicuspid	Tricuspid	Indeterminate	Unicuspid	Bicuspid	Tricuspid	Indeterminate
70–79										
Men	74.6	259	6 (2%)	113 (44%)	138 (53%)	2 (1%)	2.71–3.40 (2.95)	1.20–11.3 (3.42)	0.76–5.77 (2.40)	—
Women	74.9	182	1 (1%)	71 (39%)	106 (58%)	4 (2%)	1.67	0.98–3.97 (2.27)	0.60–4.81 (1.54)	0.95–2.10 (2.03)
80–89										
Men	82.7	121	0	37 (31%)	82 (68%)	2 (1%)	—	0.81–7.84 (3.69)	1.03–6.60 (2.32)	1.77, 2.89 (2.33)
Women	83.1	87	0	23 (26%)	64 (73%)	0	—	0.79–4.90 (2.58)	0.45–3.14 (1.55)	—
90–99										
Men	90.5	6	0	3 (50%)	3 (50%)	0	—	4.20–9.75 (6.56)	1.08–4.43 (2.50)	—
Women	90.3	3	0	0	3 (100%)	0	—	—	0.43–1.51 (0.96)	—

dures. Bacchetta and colleagues,[13] in 2003, described findings in 18 nonagenarians who underwent AVR: 5 had isolated AVR, 10 had AVR and CABG, and 3 had AVR, mitral valve replacement, and CABG. All 18 appeared to have survived 30 days postoperatively, but their courses thereafter are unclear. The structure of the operatively excised aortic valves in these 18 patients was not described.

Comparison of the frequency of the congenitally bicuspid aortic valve among septuagenarians, octogenarians, and nonagenarians who had isolated AVR for AS (with or without associated aortic valve regurgitation) at BUMC from 1993 through 2006 are shown in Table 2. The frequency of the congenitally bicuspid aortic valve among patients with isolated AVR for AS was 42% (184 of 441) in the septuagenarians, 29% (60 of 208) in the octogenarians, and 33% (3 of 9) in the nonagenarians.

1. Deleuze P, Loisance DY, Besnainou F, Hillion ML, Aubry P, Bloch G, Cachera JP. Severe aortic stenosis in octogenarians: is operation an acceptable alternative? *Ann Thorac Surg* 1990;50:226–229.
2. Culliford AT, Galloway AC, Colvin SB, Grossi EA, Baumann FG, Esposito R, Ribakove GH, Spencer FC. Aortic valve replacement for aortic stenosis in persons aged 80 years and over. *Am J Cardiol* 1991;67:1256–1260.
3. Kleikamp G, Minami K, Breymann T, Samar U, Luth JU, Reichelt W, Gleichmann U, Korfer R. Aortic valve replacement in octogenarians. *J Heart Valve Dis* 1992;1:196–200.
4. Elayda MA, Hall RJ, Reul RM, Alonzo DM, Gillette N, Reul GJ Jr, Cooley DA. Aortic valve replacement in patients 80 years and older. Operative risks and long-term results. *Circulation* 1993;88:II11–II16.
5. Aranki SF, Rizzo RJ, Couper GS, Adams DH, Collins JJ Jr, Gildea JS, Kinchla NM, Cohn LH. Aortic valve replacement in the elderly. Effect of gender and coronary artery disease on operative mortality. *Circulation* 1993;88:II17–23.
6. Straumann E, Kiowski W, Langer I, Gradel E, Stulz P, Burckhardt D, Pfisterer M, Burkart F. Aortic valve replacement in elderly patients with aortic stenosis. *Br Heart J* 1994;71:449–453.
7. Logeais Y, Roussin R, Langanay T, Sevray B, Chaperon J, Leguerrier A, Rioux C, Corbineau H, Lelong B, Valla J. Aortic valve replacement for aortic stenosis in 200 consecutive octogenarians. *J Heart Valve Dis* 1995;4(suppl 1):S64–S71.
8. Rossi MS. The octogenarian cardiac surgery patient. *J Cardiovasc Nurs* 1995;9:75–95.
9. Levin IL, Olivecrona GK, Thulin LI, Olsson SB. Aortic valve replacement in patients older than 85 years: outcomes and the effect on their quality of life. *Coron Artery Dis* 1998;9:373–380.
10. Roberts WC, Ko JM. Weights of operatively-excised stenotic unicuspid, bicuspid, and tricuspid aortic valves and their relation to age, sex, body mass index, and presence or absence of concomitant coronary artery bypass grafting. *Am J Cardiol* 2003:92:1057–1065.
11. Samuels LE, Sharma S, Morris RJ, Kuretu MLR, Grunewald KE, Strong MD III, Brockman SK. Cardiac surgery in nonagenarians. *J Card Surg* 1996;11:121–127.
12. Blanche C, Matloff JM, Denton TA, Khan SS, DeRobertis MA, Nessim S, Chaux A. Cardiac operations in patients 90 years of age and older. *Ann Thorac Surg* 1997;63:1685–1690.
13. Bacchetta MD, Ko W, Girardi LN, Mack CA, Krieger KH, Isom OW, Lee LY. Outcomes of cardiac surgery in nonagenarians: a 10-year experience. *Ann Thorac Surg* 2003;75:1215–1220.

Isolated Aortic Valve Replacement Without Coronary Bypass for Aortic Valve Stenosis Involving a Congenitally Bicuspid Aortic Valve in a Nonagenarian

William C. Roberts, MD;[1,2,4] Jong Mi Ko, BA;[4] Gregory John Matter, MD[3]
From the Departments of Internal Medicine, Division of Cardiology,[1] Pathology,[2] and Cardiothoracic Surgery,[3] and the Baylor Heart and Vascular Institute,[4] Baylor University Medical Center, Dallas, TX
Address for correspondence: William C. Roberts, MD, Baylor Heart and Vascular Institute, Baylor University Medical Center, 621 North Hall Street, Suite H-030, Dallas, TX 75226
E-mail: wc.roberts@baylorhealth.edu

A 90-year-old man sought care because of rapidly progressing dyspnea and an episode of near syncope. Examination found him to be 71 inches tall and to weigh 180 lb (body mass index, 25 kg/m^2). A grade 5/6 harsh systolic ejection precordial murmur was present, loudest over the right second intercostal space. A murmur of aortic regurgitation was not described. The blood hematocrit was 39%. Cardiac catheterization disclosed the following pressures (mm Hg): left ventricle, 207/15; aorta, 157/60; and peak transvalvular systolic pressure gradient, 50. The left ventricular ejection fraction was 50%, and the calculated aortic valve area was 0.64 cm^2. Angiogram disclosed wide open coronary arteries. The aortic valve was replaced with a 25-mm pericardial bioprosthesis (Baxter, Deerfield, IL). His postoperative course was uncomplicated. The operatively excised aortic valve was congenitally bicuspid, heavily calcified, and rigid, and it weighed 5.73 g. The patient was known to be alive 1507 days after valve replacement.

COMMENTS

The hitherto described patient had congenital heart disease, specifically a bicuspid aortic valve. Symptoms of aortic valve stenosis, namely those of heart failure and near syncope, did not develop until 90 years after birth. By this time, the bicuspid aortic valve was heavily calcified, quite stenotic, and replaced. The operatively excised valve was very heavy (5.73 g [normal, 0.5 g])[1] and immobile[2] (Figure).

Aortic stenosis, of course, is fairly common in older individuals, but it usually manifests itself symptomatically long before the age of 90, particularly when the stenosis involves a congenitally malformed valve. From 1993 to 2006, we studied operatively excised stenotic aortic valves in 9 nonagenarians: 3 had congenitally bicuspid aortic valves, including the present patient, and 6 had 3-cuspid aortic valves.[3] All but 1 patient survived the operative period; 1 died 874 days and 1 died 1011 days after valve replacement; 6 others have survived from 787 to 2324 days postoperatively as of June 29, 2006. The hitherto described patient is doing well 1507 days after valve replacement.

Why some patients with a congenitally bicuspid stenotic valve do not become symptomatic until their 90s and why others become symptomatic in early life is unclear. The stenosis is primarily the result of calcific deposits on the aortic aspects of the cusps. Those with higher serum cholesterol levels may develop calcific deposits on the valve cusps at an earlier age than the patients with lower serum cholesterol numbers. Unfortunately, we were unable to obtain the cholesterol values in the above-described patient. The fact that his coronary arteries were virtually free of plaque as determined by angiography suggests that his serum cholesterol levels were relatively low.

www.lejacq.com ID: 5268

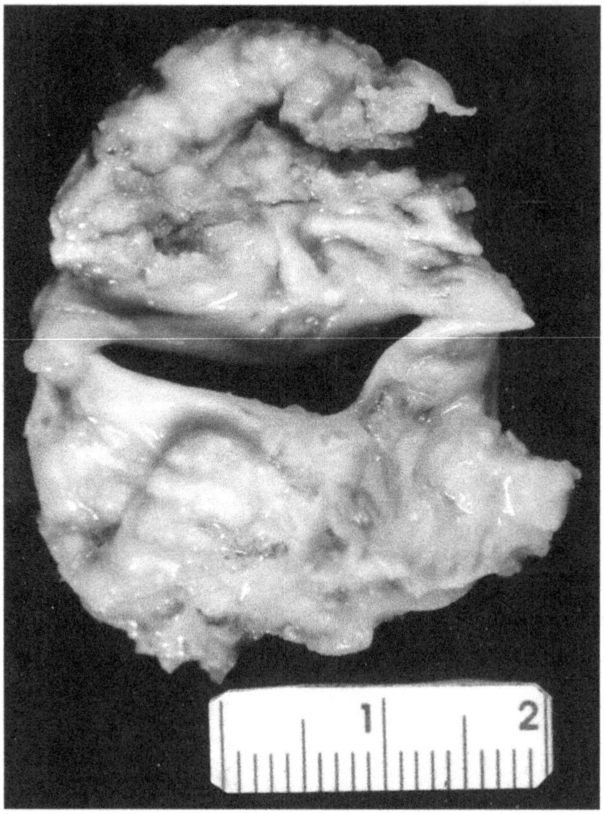

Figure. Congenitally bicuspid aortic valve in the 90-year-old patient described.

In patients with isolated aortic valve stenosis unassociated with mitral valve dysfunction, the absence of coronary narrowing by angiogram suggests that the underlying structure of the aortic valve is bicuspid rather than tricuspid, at least in patients aged 40–70 years.[4] Among 3 patients aged 90–91 years with isolated aortic stenosis and bicuspid aortic valves, 2 by angiogram had 1 or more epicardial coronary arteries narrowed >50% in diameter. In contrast, of 6 patients aged 90–91 years with isolated aortic valve stenosis superimposed on a 3-cuspid aortic valve, all had severe narrowing of 1 or more major epicardial coronary arteries by angiogram. Mautner and colleagues[4] examined the structure of stenotic aortic valves in adults and related the valve structure to several variables, including coronary arterial narrowing, useful in predicting that structure. One hundred eighty-eight patients having aortic valve replacement for isolated valvular aortic stenosis were studied. All patients were older than 40 years at the time of aortic valve replacement; all had coronary angiograms preoperatively; 182 (97%) had measurements of serum total cholesterol; and 184 (98%) had body mass index calculated. The structure of the operatively excised valve was classified as unicuspid or bicuspid (congenitally malformed) or as a tricuspid aortic valve. A logistic regression model was developed that found 4 factors (age, serum total cholesterol, angiographic coronary artery disease, and body mass index) to be predictive of aortic valve structure.[1] Patients with at least 3 or all 4 factors high or present (ie, age older than 65 years, serum total cholesterol >200 mg/dL, body mass index >29 kg/m^2, and coronary artery disease) had a low probability (10%–29%) of having a congenitally malformed valve[2] and patients with at least 3 or all 4 factors low or absent (ie, age 65 years or younger, serum total cholesterol ≤200 mg/dL, body mass index ≤29 kg/m^2, and no coronary artery disease) had a high probability (72%–90%) of having a congenitally malformed valve. Thus, the morphology of the operatively excised stenotic aortic valve can be predicted with knowledge of the age, serum total cholesterol, body mass index, and coronary artery status of the patient.

The presence of an elevated systolic systemic arterial pressure in an older person should not be interpreted to mean absent or only minimal or mild aortic valve stenosis. The peak systemic systolic pressure in the present patient at cardiac catheterization was 157 mm Hg and yet the peak left ventricular pressure was 207 mm Hg. We have observed the peak systemic systolic pressure to be as high as 200 mm Hg and yet the degree of aortic stenosis was severe, with a peak left ventricular systolic pressure of 300 mm Hg and a peak transvalvular gradient of 100 mm Hg.[5]

Aortic valve replacement even in nonagenarians is the procedure of choice for severe aortic stenosis. Bacchetta and associates[6] reported 18 patients aged 90 years or older who had aortic valve replacement for aortic stenosis, 13 of whom also had simultaneous coronary bypass grafting. All patients survived the 30-day operative period and, although the data are scant, at least up to 2.5 years postoperatively. Among 9 nonagenarians having aortic valve replacement for aortic stenosis at Baylor University Medical Center (Dallas, TX), all but 1 survived the 30-day postoperative period, 2 died nearly 2+ years later, and the others are alive up to 6+ years postoperatively.

References

1 Silver MA, Roberts WC. Detailed anatomy of the normally functioning aortic valve in hearts of normal and increased weight. *Am J Cardiol.* 1985;55:454–461.

2 Roberts WC, Ko JM, Hamilton C. Comparison of valve structure, valve weight, and severity of the valve obstruction in 1849 patients having isolated aortic valve

replacement for aortic valve stenosis (with or without associated aortic regurgitation) studied at 3 different medical centers in 2 different time periods. *Circulation.* 2005;112:3919–3929.

3 Roberts WC, Ko JM, Matter GJ. Aortic valve replacement for aortic stenosis in nonagenarians. *Am J Cardiol.* In press.

4 Mautner GC, Mautner SL, Cannon RO III, et al. Clinical factors useful in predicting aortic valve structure in patients > 40 years of age with isolated valvular aortic stenosis. *Am J Cardiol.* 1993;72:194–198.

5 Roberts WC, Perloff JK, Costantino T. Severe valvular aortic stenosis in patients over 65 years of age. A clinicopathologic study. *Am J Cardiol.* 1971;27:497–506.

6 Bacchetta MD, Ko W, Girardi LN, et al. Outcomes of cardiac surgery in nonagenarians: a 10-year experience. *Ann Thorac Surg.* 2003;75:1215–1220.

Valve Structure and Survival in *Octogenarians* Having Aortic Valve Replacement for Aortic Stenosis (± Aortic Regurgitation) With Versus Without Coronary Artery Bypass Grafting at a Single US Medical Center (1993 to 2005)

William Clifford Roberts, MD[a,b,d,*], Jong Mi Ko, BA[d], William Lance Garner, MD[a], Giovanni Filardo, PhD, MPH[e,f], Albert Carl Henry, MD[c], Robert Frederick Hebeler, Jr., MD[c], Gregory John Matter, MD[c], and Baron Lloyd Hamman, MD[c]

The purpose of this study was to determine the effect of simultaneous coronary artery bypass grafting (CABG) and valve structure on both early and late survival in octogenarians having aortic valve replacement (AVR) for aortic stenosis (AS) (with or without aortic regurgitation). Although a number of reports are available in octogenarians having AVR for AS, none have described aortic valve structure. Most have limited numbers of patients and few have described late results. We analyzed survival and valve structure in 196 octogenarians having AVR for AS from 1993 to 2005 at Baylor University Medical Center, including 118 (60%) with and 78 (40%) without simultaneous CABG. Sixty-day mortality, which was identical to 30-day mortality, was similar (10% and 11%) in the groups with and without simultaneous CABG. Unadjusted analysis of late survival (up to 13 year follow-up) was not affected by gender (male vs female), aortic valve structure (bicuspid vs tricuspid) or preoperative severity of the AS (transvalvular peak pressure gradient > 50 vs ≤50 mm Hg), or by performance of CABG. Of the 196 patients, 54 (28%) had a congenitally bicuspid aortic valve, and 142 (72%) had a tricuspid aortic valve. In conclusion, gender, valve structure, preoperative severity of the AS, or performance of simultaneous CABG did not effect survival in octogenarians having AVR for AS. **(Am J Cardiol 2007;100:489–495)**

A number of articles have appeared in recent years describing survival in octogenarians having various cardiac operations.[1–21] Some reports have focused exclusively on results of isolated coronary artery bypass grafting (CABG), others on results of aortic valve replacement (AVR) or mitral valve replacement with or without simultaneous CABG. None have described the structure of the operatively excised aortic valve, and relatively few have long-term follow-up. In this report, we compare survival and valve structure in octogenarians having AVR for aortic stenosis (AS) with versus without simultaneous CABG at Baylor University Medical Center in a recent 13-year period.

Methods

From January 1993 to December 2005, a total of 1,112 patients had AVR with or without simultaneous CABG and without mitral valve replacement at Baylor University Medical Center (BUMC). Of the 1,112 patients, 196 (18%) were aged 80 to 89 years, and they are the subject of this report. The operatively excised aortic valve in each patient was submitted to the surgical pathology section, and all 196 valves were examined and described by 1 of us (WCR). In 2, the valves had been excised in multiple fragments and the structure could not be determined by WCR. The structure in these 2 cases was that provided by the operating cardiac surgeon. The valves were photographed by JMK. Additionally, since 1998, all operatively excised valves have been weighed by 1 of us (WCR).

The echocardiographic and hemodynamic data in the 196 octogenarians was collected by JMK and WLG from the cardiovascular computer database (Apollo Advance C/S, version 4.2.13, Lumdx Corp., Oakland, California) and from the medical records. Whether simultaneous CABG was performed at the time of AVR was also obtained from either the computer database or from the medical records. Information regarding death of any patient was obtained from 2 sources: (1) early death information was obtained from the medical record, and (2) post-hospital death information was obtained from the Social Security Death Index. The hospital death information also was reconfirmed from the Social Security Death Index.

Echocardiographic data were preoperatively available to us in 69 patients (35%). Cardiac catheterization data were available to us in most patients: peak transvalvular pressure gradient in 119 patients (61%); mean transvalvular pressure

Departments of [a]Internal Medicine (Division of Cardiology), [b]Pathology, and [c]Cardiothoracic Surgery and the [d]Baylor Heart & Vascular Institute, Baylor University Medical Center; [e]Institute for Health Care Research and Improvement, Baylor Health Care System, and the [f]Department of Statistical Science, Southern Methodist University, Dallas, Texas. Manuscript received January 26,; revised manuscript received and accepted March 6, 2007.

*Corresponding author: Tel: 214-820-7911; fax: 214-820-7533.

E-mail address: wc.roberts@baylorhealth.edu (W.C. Roberts).

Table 1

Clinical and valve structure information in the 196 octogenarians having aortic valve replacement for isolated aortic stenosis with or without simultaneous coronary artery bypass grafting

Year	Number of AVRs for AS at BUMC	Number of Octogenarians	Age (year) Range (mean)	Men	Women	Coronary Artery Bypass Grafting	Hospital Stay (days)* AVR→DC Range (mean ± SD)	Died ≤60 days†	Died >60 days
1993	31	7	80–85 (82)	1	6	3	8–17 (11.5 ± 3.9)	1	6
1994	50	7	80–89 (84)	3	4	4	5–18 (9 ± 5.2)	2	5
1995	44	3	80–81 (80)	3	0	3	5	2	0
1996	56	5	80–85 (82)	5	0	4	5–8 (6.6 ± 1.1)	0	3
1997	51	7	80–88 (82)	6	1	5	6–35 (13 ± 11.8)	2	4
1998	68	15	80–86 (83)	6	9	7	4–24 (9 ± 5.5)	1	7
1999	110	15	80–87 (82)	6	9	8	4–23 (10.8 ± 6.0)	0	8
2000	112	20	80–88 (83)	15	5	14	5–19 (8.7 ± 3.7)	2	10
2001	98	23	80–87 (83)	14	9	17	5–25 (11.1 ± 5.4)	3	6
2002	110	29	80–89 (83)	15	14	22	5–23 (11.4 ± 4.4)	2	5
2003	136	29	80–89 (83)	18	11	13	3–28 (10.4 ± 6.1)	1	1
2004	120	15	80–88 (82)	11	4	6	6–29 (12.3 ± 7.4)	0	3
2005	126	21	80–89 (84)	10	11	12	6–15 (9.8 ± 3.4)	5	0
	1112	196 (18%)	80–89 (83)	113 (58%)	83 (42%)	118 (60%)	3–35 (10.4 ± 5.5)	21 (11%)	58 (30%)

* Includes only patients surviving >60 days after valve replacement.

† Thirty- and 60-day mortality were the same.

‡ Number of patients in whom the valve was weighted.

AS = aortic stenosis; AVR = aortic valve replacement; BUMC = Baylor University Medical Center; DC = discharge; M = man; W = woman; —, not information or not applicable.

gradient in 113 (58%); aortic valve area in 125 patients (64%); and left ventricular ejection fraction in 93 patients (47%). Most patients in whom cardiac catheterization data were not available to WCR and JMK were referred directly to a cardiovascular surgeon. These patients had coronary angiographic studies before being referred to BUMC, but the data were not available to us.

Means, standard deviations (SDs), and percentages were calculated to describe the study cohort (n = 196). Unadjusted relative risks (RR) and 95% confidence intervals (95% CIs) were estimated to describe short-term mortality. To investigate late survival, we excluded patients who died within 60 days from AVR (n = 21) and subjects with missing survival time (n = 1). This left 174 patients for the late survival analysis. Log-rank test statistics were computed to compare unadjusted survival curves for the variables of interest. Lastly, the actuarial survival of the isolated AVR and AVR with simultaneous CABG groups, unadjusted for other factors, was described by a Kaplan-Meier plot.

Statistical analysis was performed using SigmaStat Version 2.0 (SPSS Inc., Chicago, Illinois) and SAS version 9.1 (SAS Institute, Cary, North Carolina).

This study was approved by Institutional Review Board at BUMC.

Results

Pertinent data in the 196 octogenarians are summarized in Tables 1 and 2. The native stenotic aortic valve in 188 (96%) patients was replaced with a bioprosthesis and in the remaining 8 (4%) patients, with a mechanical prosthesis. Of the 196 patients, 113 (58%) were men and 83 (42%) were women. Simultaneous CABG was performed in 118 (60%) patients (Figure 1). Of the 196 patients having AVR from January 1993 to December 2005, as of December 2006, 117 (60%) have survived from 1.04 to 11.03 years (mean 4.58 ± 2.26, median 4.19) (Figure 2). As of December 2006, of the 17 patients having AVR in 1993 to 1995, 1 (6%) is alive; of the 62 patients having AVR from 1996 to 2000, 25 (40%) are alive; of the 117 patients having AVR from 2001 to 2005, 91 (78%) are alive. Of the 196 patients, 131 (67%) have been followed for ≥3 years (including those patients having AVR from 1993 to 2002), and 62 (47%) of them were alive as of December 2006. Overall, 117 (60%) of the 196 patients were alive as of December 2006. Thirty- and 60-day mortality were identical; 21 (11%) deaths occurred within 30 days of AVR and none from 31 to 60 days after AVR.

The median survival time for those patients included in the *late survival analysis* (n=174) was 6.6 years (95% CI 6 to 9.9): median survival time for men was 6.6 years (95% CI 6.1 to 13.3), and women, 7.8 years (95% CI 5.4 to 8.9); patients with bicuspid valves, 6.5 years (95% CI 4.8, NA), and with 3-cuspid valves, 6.6 years (95% CI 6 to 13.3); patients with peak transvalvular gradients ≤50 mm Hg, 7.8 years, (95% CI 5.8 to 13.3) and patients with higher gradients, 6 years (95% CI 5.4 to 8); patients having simultaneous CABG, 7.4 years (95% CI 6.4 to 13.3); and for patients not having CABG, 6 years (95% CI 5.4 to 8.9). Log-rank test results indicated that *late survival* curves were statistically equivalent for men and women (p = 0.45, n = 174), for patients with a bicuspid and tricuspid valve structure (p = 0.42, n = 174), for patients with low peak transvalvular gradient (≤50 mm Hg) and high peak trans-

Table 1
(continued)

Interval (years) AVR→Death* Range (mean ± SD)	Aortic Valve Structure		Aortic Valve Weight (g) Range (Mean)			
	Bicuspid (M:W)	Tricuspid (M:W)	Bicuspid		Tricuspid	
			Men	Women	Men	Women
0.21–13.36 (4.33 ± 4.85)	5 (0:5)	2 (1:1)	—	—	—	—
3.88–8.92 (6.28 ± 2.17)	4 (3:1)	3 (0:3)	—	—	—	—
—	1 (1:0)	2 (2:0)	—	—	—	—
6.00–7.47 (6.61 ± 0.77)	2 (2:0)	3 (3:0)	—	—	—	—
6.55–7.82 (7.10 ± 0.62)	2 (2:0)	5 (4:1)	—	—	—	—
2.93–6.18 (4.43 ± 1.28)	4 (1:3)	11 (5:6)	—	1.50–4.00 (3.07)	1.69–5.58 (2.70)	1.50–2.32 (1.84)
1.69–5.57 (4.23 ± 1.23)	7 (4:3)	8 (2:6)	1.20–4.80 (3.45)	1.76–4.90 (3.09)	3.24	0.85–2.41 (1.55)
2.39–6.43 (4.39 ± 1.37)	4 (3:1)	16 (12:4)	1.72–5.87 (3.71)	2.60	1.35–4.43 (2.38)	0.80–2.12 (1.40)
2.22–5.56 (4.04 ± 1.35)	3 (3:0)	20 (11:9)	2.65–3.52 (3.23)	—	1.36–6.60 (2.60)	0.45–2.98 (1.56)
1.00–4.03 (3.04 ± 1.21)	3 (2:1)	26 (13:13)	1.52, 4.13 (2.83)	0.79	1.12–4.59 (2.15)	0.55–3.14 (1.48)
1.75	9 (5:4)	20 (13:7)	3.03–5.24 (4.58)	1.64–4.27 (2.64)	1.21–3.61 (2.36)	1.03–2.85 (1.80)
1.31–2.30 (1.69 ± 0.53)	3 (3:0)	12 (8:4)	3.72–7.84 (5.48)	—	1.03–4.53 (1.91)	1.22–2.63 (1.70)
—	7 (4:3)	14 (6:8)	0.81–3.65 (2.34)	0.81–2.51 (1.84)	2.12–3.29 (2.65)	0.57–1.86 (1.31)
0.21–13.36 (4.10 ± 2.36)	54 (33:21) (28%)	142 (80:62) (72%)	0.81–7.84 (3.71) 24‡	0.79–4.90 (2.53) 15‡	1.03–6.60 (2.37) 69‡	0.45–3.14 (1.56) 57‡

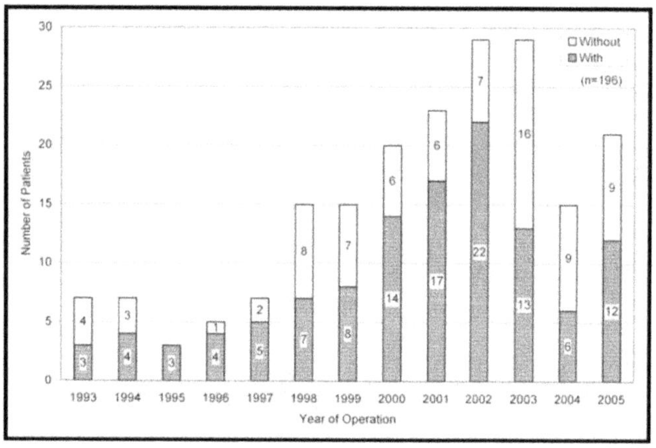

Figure 1. Number of octogenarians having aortic valve replacement for aortic valve stenosis at BUMC 1993 to 2005 with versus without simultaneous coronary bypass grafting.

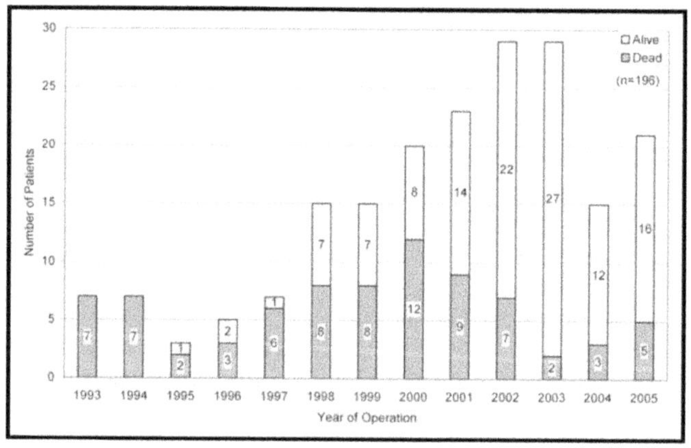

Figure 2. Number of octogenarians surviving and not surviving aortic valve replacement for aortic stenosis (with or without simultaneous coronary artery bypass grafting) at BUMC 1993 to 2005 (follow-up to December 30, 2006). Most of the deaths occurred ≥1 years after the year of operation.

valvular gradient (>50 mm Hg) (p = 0.35, n = 106), and for patients receiving simultaneous CABG and not having CABG (p = 0.06, n = 174; see Figure 3).

Likewise, the unadjusted analysis of short-term mortality indicated that *simultaneous CABG* was not associated with decreased 60-day mortality (RR 0.96, 95% CI 0.54 to 1.70). In total, 21 (11%) patients died ≤60 days of AVR and another 58 patients (30%) at later periods. Of the 21 patients who died within 60 days after AVR with (13 patients) or without (8 patients) simultaneous CABG, only 1 died in the operating room; the other 20 died from 1 to 24 days (mean 11; median 12.5).

Length of stay in the hospital in the 175 patients who survived the operative period ranged from 3 to 35 days (mean 10.4), and in the 21 who died early from 0 to 24 days (mean 9.52) (p = NS). Simultaneous CABG had no effect on length of hospital stay. Length of stay in the 105 of 118 patients with CABG who survived the operative period ranged from 3 to 35 days (mean 10.6±5.6), and in the 70 of 78 patients without CABG, the length of hospitalization ranged from 3 to 29 days (mean 10.2 ± 5.5). Of the 13 patients with CABG who died early, the length of hospitalization before death ranged from 1 to 22 days (mean 11 ± 7); of the 8 patients without CABG who died early, the length of hospitalization ranged from 0 to13 days (mean 7 ± 4).

The *severity of the AS* was similar in the patients with and without simultaneous CABG. The transvalvular *peak* systolic pressure gradients in the patients with versus without CABG ranged from 14 to 105 mm Hg (average 49) and 11 to 103 mm Hg (average 49), respectively; the mean

Table 2
Comparison of the 196 octogenarians having aortic valve replacement for aortic stenosis without versus with simultaneous coronary artery bypass grafting

Year	Without Coronary Artery Bypass Grafting						
	Number Having AVR (M:W)	Length of Stay* (days) Range (Mean ± SD)	Died			BAV (M:W)	TAV (M:W)
			Total (M:W)	≤60 days[†] (M:W)	>60 days (M:W)		
1993	4 (0:4)	8, 10 (9 ± 1.4)	4 (0:4)	0	4 (0:4)	3 (0:3)	1 (0:1)
1994	3 (1:2)	5, 6, 9 (6.7 ± 2.1)	3 (1:2)	0	3 (1:2)	1 (1:0)	2 (0:2)
1995	—	—	—	—	—	—	—
1996	1 (1:0)	8	1 (1:0)	0	1 (1:0)	1 (1:0)	—
1997	2 (2:0)	6, 8 (7 ± 1.4)	1 (1:0)	0	1 (1:0)	—	2 (2:0)
1998	8 (3:5)	4–24 (10.5 ± 6.8)	6 (3:3)	1 (0:1)	5 (3:2)	3 (0:3)	5 (3:2)
1999	7 (4:3)	5–20 (8.8 ± 6.3)	4 (2:2)	0	4 (2:2)	3 (2:1)	4 (2:2)
2000	6 (5:1)	5, 8, 19 (10.7 ± 7.4)	4 (3:1)	2 (2:0)	2 (1:1)	1 (1:0)	5 (4:1)
2001	6 (3:3)	5–12 (8 ± 3.2)	3 (2:1)	1 (1:0)	2 (1:1)	1 (1:0)	5 (2:3)
2002	7 (2:5)	9–23 (14.3 ± 4.4)	3 (2:1)	1 (1:0)	2 (1:1)	0	7 (2:5)
2003	16 (9:7)	3–24 (9.4 ± 5.4)	0	0	0	6 (3:3)	10 (6:4)
2004	9 (7:2)	7–29 (11.7 ± 7.6)	2 (1:1)	0	2 (1:1)	2 (2:0)	7 (5:2)
2005	9 (2:7)	7–15 (11.2 ± 3.2)	3 (0:3)	3 (0:3)	0	4 (1:3)	5 (1:4)
	78 (39:39) (40%)	3–29 (10.2 ± 5.5)	34 (16:18) (44%)	8 (4:4) (10%)	26 (12:14) (33%)	25 (12:13) (32%)	53 (27:26) (68%)

* This data only include early survivors.
[†] Thirty- and 60-day mortality were the same.
— = no information available or not applicable; AVR = aortic valve replacement; BAV = bicuspid aortic valve; M = man; TAV = tricuspid aortic valve; W = woman.

systolic pressure gradients, from 11 to 88 (average 40) and 5 to 84 (average 39), respectively; the calculated aortic valve area, from 0.18 to 1.43 cm^2 (mean 0.72) and 0.23 to 1.82 cm^2 (mean 0.68), respectively, and the left ventricular ejection fractions from 10 to 85% (mean 50%) and 25 to 80% (mean 55%), respectively.

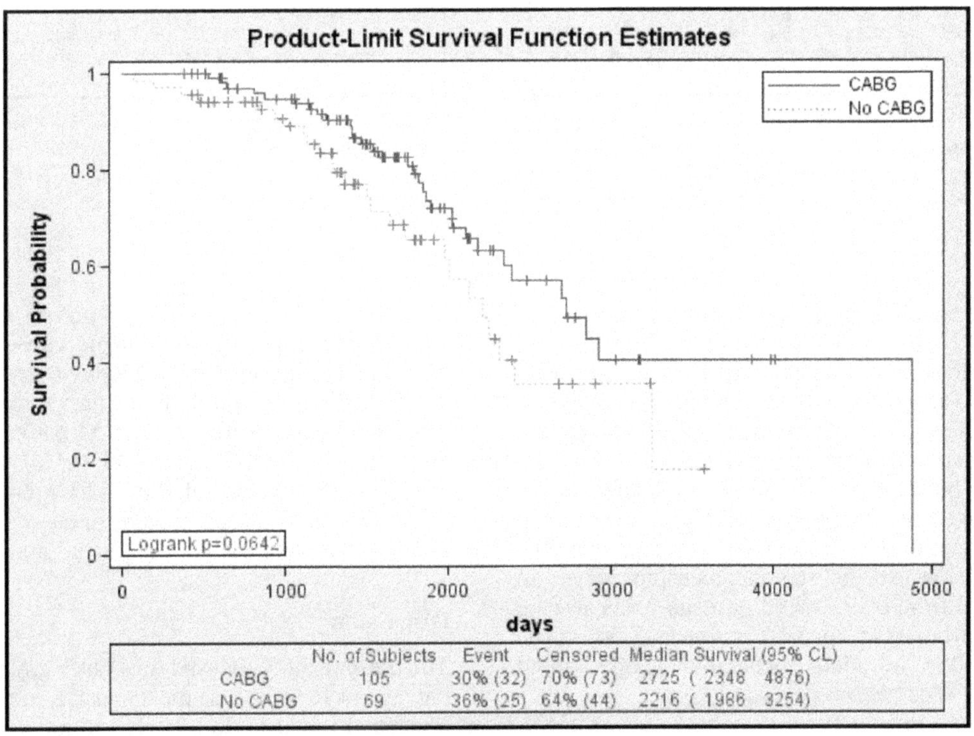

Figure 3. Kaplan-Meier survival curves comparing patients not having simultaneous coronary bypass to the patients having simultaneous coronary bypass.

Table 2
(*continued*)

With Coronary Artery Bypass Grafting						
Number Having AVR (M:W)	Length of Stay* (days) Range (Mean ± SD)	Died			BAV (M:W)	TAV (M:W)
		Total (M:W)	≤60 days† (M:W)	>60 days (M:W)		
3 (1:2)	11, 17 (14 ± 4.2)	3 (1:2)	1 (0:1)	2 (1:1)	2 (0:2)	1 (1:0)
4 (2:2)	7, 18 (12.5 ± 7.8)	4 (2:2)	2 (2:0)	2 (0:2)	3 (2:1)	1 (0:1)
3 (3:0)	5	2 (2:0)	2 (2:0)	0	1 (1:0)	2 (2:0)
4 (4:0)	5–7 (6.3 ± 1.0)	2 (2:0)	0	2 (2:0)	1 (1:0)	3 (3:0)
5 (4:1)	6–35 (16.5 ± 13.8)	5 (4:1)	2 (2:0)	3 (2:1)	2 (2:0)	3 (2:1)
7 (3:4)	4–13 (7.3 ± 2.9)	2 (1:1)	0	2 (1:1)	1 (1:0)	6 (2:4)
8 (2:6)	4–23 (12 ± 5.9)	4 (1:3)	0	4 (1:3)	4 (2:2)	4 (0:4)
14 (10:4)	5–14 (8.3 ± 2.7)	8 (6:2)	0	8 (6:2)	3 (2:1)	11 (8:3)
17 (11:6)	5–25 (12.1 ± 5.7)	6 (5:1)	2 (2:0)	4 (3:1)	2 (2:0)	15 (9:6)
22 (13:9)	5–20 (10.4 ± 4.1)	4 (2:2)	1 (0:1)	3 (2:1)	3 (2:1)	19 (11:8)
13 (9:4)	3–28 (11.6 ± 6.9)	2 (1:1)	1 (1:0)	1 (0:1)	3 (2:1)	10 (7:3)
6 (4:2)	6–27 (13.2 ± 7.8)	1 (0:1)	0	1 (0:1)	1 (1:0)	5 (3:2)
12 (8:4)	6–15 (9 ± 3.3)	2 (2:0)	2 (2:0)	0	3 (3:0)	9 (5:4)
118 (74:44) (60%)	3–35 (10.6 ± 5.6)	45 (29:16) (38%)	13 (11:2) (11%)	32 (18:14) (27%)	29 (21:8) (25%)	89 (53:36) (75%)

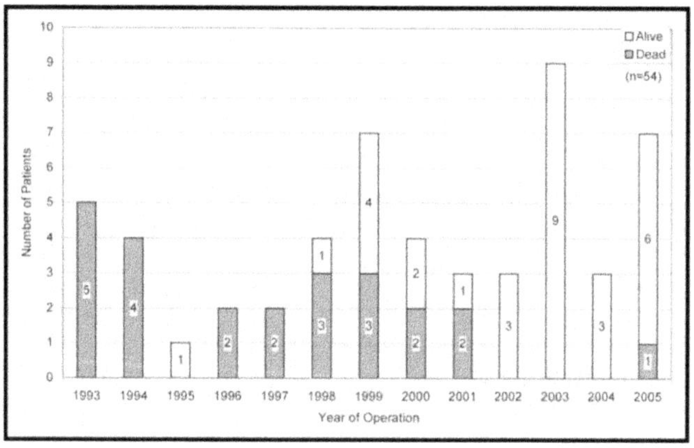

Figure 4. Number of octogenarians surviving and not surviving aortic valve replacement for aortic stenosis involving a bicuspid aortic valve (± simultaneous coronary artery bypass grafting) at BUMC 1993 to 2005 (follow-up to December 30, 2006). Most of the deaths occurred ≥1 years after the year of operation.

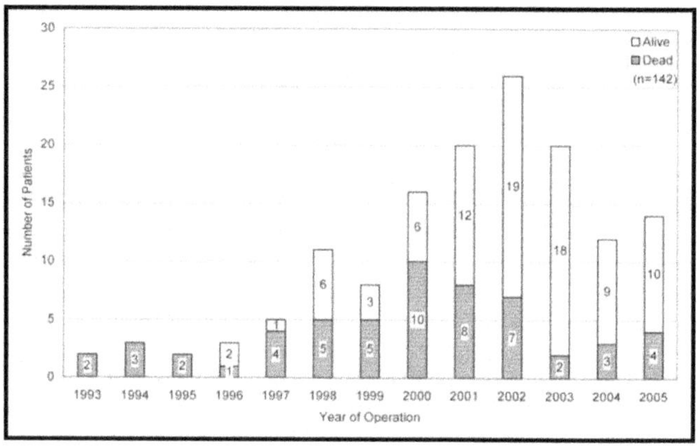

Figure 5. Number of octogenarians surviving and not surviving aortic valve replacement for aortic stenosis involving a tricuspid aortic valve (± simultaneous coronary artery bypass grafting) at BUMC 1993 to 2005 (follow-up to December 30, 2006). Most of the deaths occurred ≥1 years after the year of operation.

Another tool providing some evidence of the severity of the AS is gained by the *weight of the operatively excised valves.*[22–25] (Previous studies have indicated that men with AS have heavier valves than do women and that congenitally unicuspid and bicuspid stenotic aortic valves are heavier than 3-cuspid stenotic aortic valves.[22–25]) The operatively excised bicuspid aortic valves in the men in the present study ranged in weight from 0.81 to 7.84 g (mean 3.71) and the 3-cuspid valves in the men from 1.03 to 6.60 g (mean 2.36). In contrast, the stenotic bicuspid valves in the women ranged from 0.79 to 4.90 g (mean 2.65) and the 3-cuspid valves from 0.45 to 3.14 g (mean 1.56). (The normal aortic valve in adults generally weighs about 0.50 g.[26])

Aortic valve structure in the 196 patients was the following: bicuspid in 54 (28%) patients and tricuspid in the remaining 142 (72%) (Figures 4 and 5). Of the 113 men, 33 (29%) had a congenitally bicuspid valve (Figure 6), and 80 (71%) had a tricuspid valve (Figure 6); of the 83 women, 21 (25%) had a congenitally bicuspid valve, and 62 (75%) had a 3-cuspid aortic valve. Of the 54 patients with a congenitally bicuspid aortic valve, 33 (61%) were men and 21 (39%) were women. Of the 142 patients with a tricuspid aortic valve, 80 (56%) were men and 62 (44%) were women. No patient had a unicuspid aortic valve.

Discussion

The present study focused on a large group of octogenarians having AVR for AS at the same US medical center during a recent 13-year period. Early mortality was 10% and similar in the patients with and without simultaneous CABG.

Table 3
Previously reported studies of octogenarians having aortic valve replacement for aortic stenosis with or without simultaneous coronary artery bypass grafting

First Author	Reference Number	Year of Publication	Total	AVR Without CABG	AVR With CABG	Early Deaths	Follow-up (months) Range (mean)
Edmunds	1	1988	50	33	17	14	12–142 (41 ± 28)
Levinson	2	1989	60	31	29	6	1–157 (28 ± 5)
Kleikamp	3	1992	48	25	23	2	12–48 (22)
Olsson	4	1992	44	22	22	2	6–96 (median 6)
Logeais	5	1995	199	187	12	23	1–132 (36 ± 24)
Gehlot	6	1996	298	162	136	14	—–180 (46)
Olsson	7	1996	32	20	12	3	—–— (—)
Akins	8	1997	216	105	111	15	—–— (38)
Kirsch	9	1998	136	110	26	31	0–73 (22 ± 21)
Medalion	10	1998	248	99	149	22	—–— (48)
Khan	11	1998	49	30*	19*	7	6–95 (median 30)
Kolh	12	1999	83	62	21	11	—–— (27)
Craver	13	1999	144	71	73	11	—–— (36 ± 24)
Kolh	14	2001	100	70	30	14	—–— (_)
Caus	15	2002	101	80	21	7	—–— (36)
Brunvand	16	2002	94	42	52	8	0–84 (—)
Mistiaen	17	2004	60	18*	42*	6	—–— (_)
Chiappini	18	2004	115	71	44	10	3–132 (37 ± 32)
Collart	19	2005	159	116	43	14	—–— (_)
Collart	20	2005	154	115	39	12*	—–— (_)
Chukwuemeka	21	2006	95	48	47	4	—–— (61 ± 37)
			2485	1517 (61%)	968 (39%)	236 (9.5%)	

* Educated guess.
— = no information available.

Gender (male vs female), severity of the AS (peak transvalvular gradient ≤50 vs >50 mm Hg), and structure of the aortic valve (bicuspid or tricuspid), or receiving simultaneous CABG (yes vs no) had insignificant effect on survival.

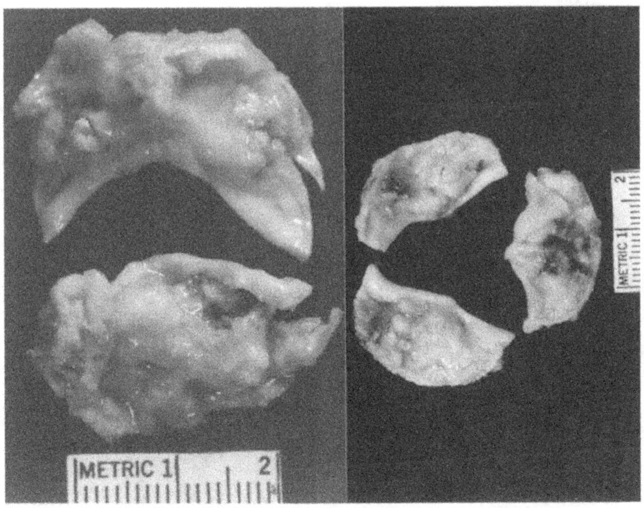

Figure 6. Photographs of 2 operatively excised stenotic aortic valve: congenitally bicuspid (*left*) and tricuspid (*right*). The bicuspid valve was excised from an 87-year-old man in whom the peak transvalvular peak systolic gradient was 81 mm Hg, the calculated aortic valve area 0.42 cm^2, and the valve weight, 4.24 g. The tricuspid aortic valve was excised from an 83-year-old man whose peak transvalvular gradient was 52 mm Hg, aortic valve area 0.88 cm^2, and valve weight 4.59 g.

Previously reported early results in cases of AVR for AS in octogenarians are summarized in Table 3 (includes only studies involving >30 patients).[1–21] In contrast to the present study where 60% of our octogenarians had simultaneous CABG, of the 2,485 previously reported octogenarians having AVR for AS and summarized in Table 3, 968 (39%) had simultaneous CABG. The early (usually 30 day) mortality was 9.5% (236 of 2,485), virtually identical to that in the present study.

None of the previously reported studies (Table 3) on AVR for AS in octogenarians described the aortic valve structure encountered at operation or in a surgical pathology unit. Among our 196 patients, 54 (28%) had a congenitally bicuspid aortic valve, and 142 (72%), a tricuspid aortic valve. Because mitral valve function in our patients was either normal or only mildly abnormal (mild regurgitation), the AS involving the tricuspid aortic valves can reasonably be attributed to an atherosclerotic process, something that potentially could lessen as serum cholesterol levels continue to fall. The bicuspid condition, in contrast, is, of course, a congenital malformation that reasonably will persist at a similar rate for decades to come.

Although hemodynamic data were available in most of our octogenarians, most (165 of 196 [84%]) also had the operatively excised valve weighed on extremely accurate scales. Previously reported studies have demonstrated that stenotic aortic valves in adults are up to 30 times the normal aortic valve weight, and if stenotic valves are separated by gender, that the valve weight correlates well with the peak transvalvular gradient.[22–25] Unicuspid and bicuspid stenotic valves also, as a rule, are much heavier than stenotic tricuspid aortic valves.[22–25] In our patients, in women, the bicuspid valve weight averaged 2.53 g and in men, 3.71 g; in women, the tricuspid valves averaged 1.56 g and in men, 2.37 g.

The positive features of the present study include a large number of octogenarians, relatively long post-AVR follow-up, preoperative hemodynamic data in most patients, and full knowledge of aortic valve structure and weight. The negative features of the present study include lack of information on preoperative and postoperative symptoms and functional class, on early postoperative complications, comorbidities, late quality of life, numbers of epicardial coronary arteries narrowed > 50% in diameter, and causes of death late postoperatively.

1. Edmunds LH Jr, Stephenson LW, Edie RN, Ratcliffe MB. Open-heart surgery in octogenarians. *N Engl J Med* 1988;131–136.
2. Levinson JR, Akins CW, Buckley MJ, Newell JB, Palacios IF, Block PC, Fifer MA. Octogenarians with aortic stenosis. Outcome after aortic valve replacement. *Circulation* 1989;80:I-49–I-56.
3. Kleikamp G, Minami K, Breymann T, Samar U, Luth J-U, Reichelt W, Gleichmann U, Korfer R. Aortic valve replacement in octogenarians. *J Heart Valve Dis* 1992;1:196–200.
4. Olsson M, Granstrom L, Lindblom D, Rosenqvist M, Ryden L. Aortic valve replacement in octogenarians with aortic stenosis: a case-control study. *J Am Coll Cardiol* 1992;20:1512–1516.
5. Logeais Y, Roussin R, Langanay T, Sevray B, Chaperon J, Leguerrier A, Rioux C, Corbineau H, Lelong B, Valla J. Aortic valve replacement for aortic stenosis in 200 consecutive octogenarians. *J Heart Valve Dis* 1995;4:S64–S71.
6. Gehlot A, Mullany CJ, Ilstrup D, Schaff HV, Orszulak TA, Morris JJ, Daly RC. Aortic valve replacement in patients aged eighty years and older: early and long-term results. *J Thorac Cardiovasc Surg* 1996; 111:1026–1036.
7. Olsson M, Janfjall H, Orth-Gomer K, Unden A, Rosenqvist M. Quality of life in octogenarians after valve replacement due to aortic stenosis. *Eur Heart J* 1996;17:583–589.
8. Akins CW, Daggett WM, Vlahakes GJ, Hilgenbert AD, Torchiana DF, Madsen JC, Buckley MJ. Cardiac operations in patients 80 years old and older. *Ann Thorac Surg* 1997;64:606–615.
9. Kirsch M, Guesnier L, LeBesnerais P, Hillion M-L, Debauchez M, Seguin J, Loisance DY. Cardiac operations in octogenarians: perioperative risk factors for death and impaired autonomy. *Ann Thorac Surg* 1998;66:60–67.
10. Medalion B, Lytle BW, McCarthy PM, Stewart RW, Arheart KL, Arnold JH, Loop FD, Cosgrove DM III. Aortic valve replacement for octogenarians: are small valves bad? *Ann Thorac Surg* 1998;66:699–706.
11. Khan JH, McElhinney DB, Hall TS, Merrick SH. Cardiac valve surgery in octogenarians. Improving quality of life and functional status. *Arch Surg* 1998;133:887–893.
12. Kolh P, Lahaye L, Gerard P, Limet R. Aortic valve replacement in the octogenarians: perioperative outcome and clinical follow-up. *Eur J Cardiothorac Surg* 1999;16:68–73.
13. Craver JM, Puskas JD, Weintraub WW, Shen Y, Guyton RA, Gott JP, Jones EL. 601 octogenarians undergoing cardiac surgery: outcome and comparison with younger age groups. *Ann Thorac Surg* 1999;67: 1104–1110.
14. Kolh P, Kerzmann A, Lahaye L, Gerard P, Limet R. Cardiac surgery in octogenarians. Peri-operative outcome and long-term results. *Eur Heart J* 2001;22:1235–1243.
15. Caus T, Calon D, Collart F, Marin P, Seree Y, Mesana T. Parsonnet's risk score predicts late survival but not late functional results after aortic valve replacement in octogenarians. *J Heart Valve Dis* 2002; 11:498–503.
16. Brunvand H, Offstad J, Nitter-Hauge S, Svennevig JL. Coronary artery bypass grafting combined with aortic valve replacement in healthy octogenarians does not increase postoperative risk. *Scand Cardiovasc J* 2002;36:297–301.
17. Mistiaen W, Cauwelaert PV, Muylaert P, Wuyts F, Harrisson F, Bortier H. Risk factors and survival after aortic valve replacement in octogenarians. *J Heart Valve Dis* 2004;13:538–544.
18. Chiappini B, Camurri N, Loforte A, Marco LD, Bartolomeo RD, Marinelli G. Outcome after aortic valve replacement in octogenarians. *Ann Thorac Surg* 2004;78:85–89.
19. Collart F, Feier H, Kerbaul F, Mouly-Bandini A, Riberi A, Mesana TG, Metras D. Valvular surgery in octogenarians: operative risks factors, evaluation of Euroscore and long term results. *Eur J Cardiothorac Surg* 2005;27:276–280.
20. Collart F, Feier H, Kerbaul F, Mouly-Bandini A, Riberi A, Stephano ED, Seree Y, Mesana TG, Metras D. Primary valvular surgery in octogenarians: perioperative outcome. *J Heart Valve Dis* 2005;14: 238–242.
21. Chukwuemeka A, Borger MA, Ivanov J, Armstrong S, Feindel CM, David TE. Valve surgery in octogenarians: a safe option with good medium-term results. *J Heart Valve Dis* 2006;15:191–196.
22. Roberts WC, Ko JM. Weights of operatively excised stenotic unicuspid, bicuspid, and tricuspid aortic valves and their relation to age, sex, body mass index, and presence or absence of concomitant coronary artery bypass grafting. *Am J Cardiol* 2003;92:1057–1065.
23. Roberts WC, Ko JM. Relation of weights of operatively excised stenotic aortic valves to preoperative transvalvular peak systolic pressure gradients and to calculated aortic valve areas. *J Am Coll Cardiol* 2004;44:1847–1855.
24. Roberts WC, Ko JM. Frequency by decades of unicuspid, bicuspid, and tricuspid aortic valves in adults having isolated aortic valve replacement for aortic stenosis, with or without associated aortic regurgitation. *Circulation* 2005;111:920–925.
25. Roberts WC, Ko JM, Hamilton C. Comparison of valve structure, valve weight, and severity of the valve obstruction in 1849 patients having isolated aortic valve replacement for aortic valve stenosis (with or without associated aortic regurgitation) studied at 3 different medical centers in 2 different time periods. *Circulation* 2006;114:422–429.
26. Silver MA, Roberts WC. Detailed anatomy of the normally functioning aortic valve in hearts of normal and increased weight. *Am J Cardiol* 1985;55:454–461.

Clinical and Morphologic Features of the Congenitally Unicuspid Acommissural Stenotic and Regurgitant Aortic Valve

William Clifford Roberts[a–c] Jong Mi Ko[c]

[a]Department of Internal Medicine, Division of Cardiology, [b]Department of Pathology, and [c]Baylor Heart & Vascular Institute, Baylor University Medical Center, Dallas, Tex., USA

Key Words
Aortic stenosis · Aortic valve replacement · Congenitally unicuspid acommissural valve

Abstract
Five adults, aged 30–75 years, are described with stenotic and regurgitant unicuspid acommissural aortic valves. Because none of these patients had clinical, echocardiographic or hemodynamic evidence of mitral valve disease, a case is made that these valves were congenitally malformed and not the result of an acquired condition.

Introduction

In 1958, Edwards [1] described a stenotic aortic valve which had a single valve commissure and an orifice shaped like an exclamation point. He designated the valve as unicuspid unicommissural and observed that it was the most common type of aortic valve structure in infants and young children with congenital aortic stenosis. Subsequently, a number of adults with aortic valve stenosis were observed to have a unicuspid unicommissural valve [2–8]. Edwards [1] also pointed out that most patients with pulmonic valve stenosis unassociated with a ventricular septal defect had a dome-shaped pulmonic valve with a central orifice with or without rudimentary commissures. We have encountered several patients with stenotic aortic valves with more or less triangular-shaped central orifices and 3 commissures which were fused over a relatively long distance (>5 mm). In the past, these valves almost certainly would have been called rheumatic. We present 5 such cases and try to make a case that these valves actually are congenitally malformed valves from birth rather than valves where commissural fusion was acquired later in life.

Methods and Results

From January 1993 to March 2006, W.C.R. examined all cardiovascular tissues submitted to the surgical pathology section of Baylor University Medical Center. During these 13 years, we examined 1,144 stenotic aortic valves from patients in whom no procedure was performed on the mitral valve and where there was no clinical, echocardiographic or hemodynamic evidence of mitral stenosis. Among these 1,144 patients having aortic valve replacement for aortic valve stenosis with or without aortic regurgitation, 64 patients had unicuspid, 551 patients bicuspid and 514 patients tricuspid valves; 1 patient had a quadricuspid valve, and 14 patients had valves of uncertain structure. Among the 64 patients with unicuspid aortic valves, the valve was unicommissural in 59

Table 1. Data in 5 patients with unicuspid acommissural stenotic and regurgitant aortic valves and normally functioning mitral valves

Patient	Age (years)	Gender	Pressure, mm Hg				Valve area (cm^2)	AR (0–4+)	EF (%)	MS/MR	Number of coronary arteries narrowed >50% in diameter by angiogram	Valve weight (g)
			LV (s/d)	aorta (s/d)	LV-aorta PSG	LV-aorta mean gradient						
1	30	F	187/37	145/79	42	35	0.84	4	60	0/0	0	2.07
2	62	F	144/15	122/48	22	19	0.62	–	40	0/0	0	1.02
3	75	F	242/29	169/46	73	65	0.33	–	55	0/0	0	1.19
4	75	F	199/27	146/53	53	54	0.57	2	80	0/0	0	1.67
5	73	M	203/34	178/58	25	32	1.12	4	50	0/0	0	2.73

LV = Left ventricular; s/d = peak systolic/end diastolic; PSG = peak systolic gradient; AR = aortic regurgitation; EF = ejection fraction; F = female; M = male; MR = mitral regurgitation; MS = mitral stenosis.

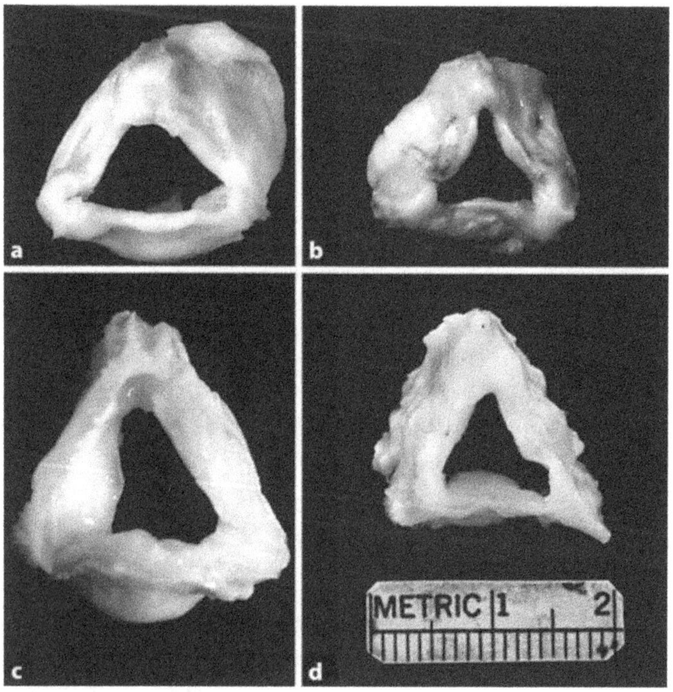

Fig. 1. Acommissural unicuspid aortic valves of case 1 (**a**), case 4 (**b**), case 2 (**c**) and case 3 (**d**). Reproduced with permission from Roberts and Ko [7].

patients and acommissural in 5 patients. This report focuses on the 5 patients in whom the aortic valve was unicuspid and acommissural. Certain demographic, hemodynamic, angiographic and morphologic features are summarized in table 1, and photographs of the operatively excised aortic valves in 4 of the 5 patients are shown in figure 1.

Discussion

Although aortic valve disease is more common in men than in women (about 8:1 with pure aortic regurgitation, 3:1 with aortic stenosis involving a congenitally bicuspid aortic valve, and about 6:4 with aortic stenosis involving a 3-cuspid aortic valve), 4 of our 5 cases with acommissural unicuspid aortic valves were women [8]. The degree of aortic valve stenosis was quite variable (peak transvalvular gradients ranging from 22 to 73 mm Hg, average 43). The operatively excised valve in each of the 5 patients not only showed the valve orifice to be stenotic, but the triangular-shaped orifice remained open in ventricular diastole, and therefore, each had some degree of aortic regurgitation. Injection of contrast material into the ascending aorta in 3 of the 5 patients disclosed severe (4+/4+) aortic regurgitation in 2 and moderate (2+/4+) regurgitation in 1 patient.

Although generally unicuspid unicommissural stenotic aortic valves are the heaviest of all stenotic aortic valves (due to the presence of the most calcific deposits and the fact that most patients are males, and men have heavier valves than women) [6], the weights of the operatively excised unicuspid acommissural aortic valves were relatively small, ranging from 1.02 to 2.73 g (mean 1.73) (fig. 1), a finding in part due to the fact that 4 of the 5 patients were women.

The medical records, echocardiographic and hemodynamic reports were searched thoroughly for evidence of mitral valve disease; none had any evidence of mitral stenosis, and mitral regurgitation, if present, was no more than minimal. Additionally, coronary angiography showed normal or virtually normal coronary arteries, a finding further suggesting the congenital nature of the aortic valve disease in each of the 5 patients [9].

Acquired causes of the aortic valve disease in each of our 5 patients certainly deserve consideration. Of course, some patients with rheumatic heart disease have aortic valve disease, either stenosis or pure regurgitation or both, without clinical evidence of mitral valve disease [4, 10]. W.C.R. has defined rheumatic heart disease as a disease of the mitral valve; other valves may be involved, but at least anatomically, the mitral valve is always involved. The mitral disease consists of either diffuse (100%) thickening of the leaflets, with or without chordal thickening (a circumstance always present in mitral stenosis), or thickening by fibrous tissue of the entire free margins of each of the 2 cusps [11]. The latter circumstance may be associated with some degree of pure mitral regurgitation or it may simply be an anatomic change without functional consequence. (One may have a large scar on the forearm without a dysfunction of the arm.) In the present 5 patients, the latter circumstance, i.e. margin leaflet scarring, could have been present, but we are unable to disprove this thesis because we do not have the mitral valves to examine anatomically. However, by echocardiogram, the mitral leaflets were normal. Rheumatic heart disease is certainly uncommon in patients >70 years of age, and 3 of our 5 patients were in their eighth decade of life. Although rheumatic mitral disease is more common in women than in men, combined rheumatic disease of both the mitral and aortic valves is more common in men, whereas 4 of our 5 patients were women. Although a history of acute rheumatic fever is not essential for a diagnosis of rheumatic heart disease, none of our 5 patients had a history compatible with acute rheumatic fever.

Healed infective endocarditis might be considered. By history, none of our 5 patients had had an episode compatible with active infective endocarditis. To our knowledge, this condition does not result in near symmetrical fusion of each of the 3 aortic valve commissures, a circumstance which would have to exist if infective endocarditis were the culprit [12]. Thus, this possibility appears highly unlikely.

Systemic lupus erythematosus can result in aortic valve stenosis, but when lupus erythematosus is the cause of aortic valve stenosis, other signs of this systemic disease are also present [13], and none of our 5 patients had an illness compatible with lupus erythematosus.

Thus, it is most reasonable to conclude that the aortic valves in the 5 patients described were malformed from birth rather than due to a condition acquired after birth. The presence of a precordial murmur early in life would support the congenital etiology, but unfortunately, we have no reliable information in any of the 5 patients on this point. Incidentally, we have seen numerous clearly congenitally bicuspid aortic valves in patients in their 80s and even their 90s [8, 14]; therefore, the older ages in 4 of our 5 patients are not against our thesis of a congenital origin of their aortic valve disease.

References

1 Edwards JE: Pathologic aspects of cardiac valvular insufficiencies. AMA Arch Surg 1958;77:634–649.
2 Roberts WC, Morrow AG: Congenital aortic stenosis produced by a unicommissural valve. Br Heart J 1965;27:505–510.
3 Roberts WC: The structure of the aortic valve in clinically isolated aortic stenosis. An autopsy study of 162 patients over 15 years of age. Circulation 1970;42:91–97.
4 Roberts WC: Anatomically isolated aortic valvular disease. The case against its being of rheumatic etiology. Am J Med 1970;49:151–159.
5 Falcone MW, Roberts WC, Morrow AG, Perloff JK: Congenital aortic stenosis resulting from unicommissural valve. Clinical and anatomic features in twenty-one adult patients. Circulation 1971;44:272–280.
6 Roberts WC, Ko JM: Weights of operatively-excised stenotic unicuspid, bicuspid, and tricuspid aortic valves and their relation to age, sex, body mass index, and presence or absence of concomitant coronary artery bypass grafting. Am J Cardiol 2003;92:1057–1065.
7 Roberts WC, Ko JM: Frequency by decades of unicuspid, bicuspid, and tricuspid aortic valves in adults having isolated aortic valve replacement for aortic stenosis, with or without associated aortic regurgitation. Circulation 2005;111:920–925.
8 Roberts WC, Ko JM, Hamilton C: Comparison of valve structure, valve weight, and severity of the valve obstruction in 1,849 patients having isolated aortic valve replacement for aortic valve stenosis (with or without associated aortic regurgitation) studied at 3 different medical centers in 2 different time periods. Circulation 2005;112:3919–3929.
9 Mautner GC, Mautner SL, Cannon RO 3rd, Hunsberger SA, Roberts WC: Clinical factors useful in predicting aortic valve structure in patients >40 years of age with isolated valvular aortic stenosis. Am J Cardiol 1993; 72:194–198.
10 Roberts WC, Perloff JK: Mitral valvular disease. A clinicopathologic survey of the conditions causing the mitral valve to function abnormally. Ann Intern Med 1972;77:939–975.
11 Roberts WC: Morphologic features of the normal and abnormal mitral valve. Am J Cardiol 1983;51:1005–1028.
12 Roberts WC, Buchbinger NA: Healed left-sided infective endocarditis: a clinicopathologic study of 59 patients. Am J Cardiol 1977; 40:876–888.
13 Roberts WC, High ST: The heart in systemic lupus erythematosus. Curr Probl Cardiol 1999;24:1–56.
14 Roberts WC, Ko JM, Matter GJ: Aortic valve replacement for aortic stenosis in nonagenarians. Am J Cardiol, in press.

Sudden Collapse in Aortic Stenosis

William Clifford Roberts, MD;[1,2,3] Jong Mi Ko, BA;[3] Jeffrey M. Schussler, MD[1]
From the Department of Internal Medicine, the Division of Cardiology,[1] and the Department of Pathology,[2] and the Baylor Heart and Vascular Institute,[3] Baylor University Medical Center, Dallas, TX
Address for correspondence: William Clifford Roberts, MD, Baylor Heart and Vascular Institute, Baylor University Medical Center, 621 North Hall Street, Suite H-030, Dallas, TX 75226
E-mail: wc.roberts@baylorhealth.edu

A 78-year-old woman, who was born on May 3, 1928, and died on November 22, 2006, had been in her usual state of health until November 6, 2002, when, at age 74 years, she noted sudden left-sided weakness and was hospitalized. On examination, a right-gaze preference and left facial droop were noted as well as systemic hypertension (blood pressure 160/75 mm Hg), atrial fibrillation, and a grade 3/6 ejection-type murmur over the base of the precordium. A computed tomographic scan showed hyperdensity of the right middle cerebral artery. A thrombolytic agent was administered intra-arterially and the previously occluded artery opened to normal caliber. Echocardiography at the time disclosed a mass (thrombus) in the left atrial appendage, normal left ventricular function, and aortic valve stenosis (AS), with an estimated peak transvalvular gradient of 65 mm Hg and an aortic valve orifice area estimated at $\leq$0.4 cm^2 (Figure 1). At the time there were no symptoms of heart failure, syncope, or chest pain. She was started on warfarin sodium and lisinopril.

Thereafter, she was lost to follow-up until November 22, 2006 (age 78), when she was found on the floor of her home by her husband and was taken to the emergency room. On arrival, she was responsive but had left-sided weakness and slurred speech. Chest radiograph was consistent with heart failure. An electrocardiogram showed ventricular premature complexes. An echocardiogram showed severe AS and a low (20%) ejection fraction. None of the aortic valve cusps moved in either phase of the cardiac cycle. During the recording of the echocardiogram she became pulseless and resuscitative efforts were unsuccessful. The interval from the time she was found on the floor to the fatal cardiac arrest was 2.6 hours.

www.lejacq.com ID: 6223

At necropsy, the heart weighed 440 g. The ventricular septum and left ventricular free wall were thickened (each 2.2 cm) but free of foci of fibrosis and necrosis. The 3 aortic valve cusps were severely thickened by both fibrous tissue and heavy calcific deposits and each was immobile; the posterior and left cusps were fused over a distance of 1.2 cm (Figure 2). All major epicardial coronary arteries were focally calcified, and the lumens of the right, left anterior descending, and left circumflex each were narrowed from 51% to 75% in cross-sectional area by plaque. Small calcific deposits were also present in the mitral annulus. The mitral leaflets and chordae were normal except for aging changes. The brain was grossly normal.

COMMENTS

The patient described had severe AS. Her first symptom of the valvular problem appears to have been her last symptom, namely cardiac arrest. There had never been previous syncope, or chest pain, or dyspnea. Because the major epicardial coronary arteries were not severely narrowed, it is reasonable to attribute the sudden collapse to the AS.

In patients with severe AS, sudden death is a well-recognized consequence. Most patients with AS who die suddenly have had symptoms that could logically be attributed to the AS. Indeed, Braunwald[1] has emphasized "...that operative treatment is the most common cause of sudden death in asymptomatic patients with aortic stenosis.... Such patients should, in general, not be referred for surgical therapy but should be followed-up frequently and carefully. On the other hand, there has never been much argument that surgical treatment should be carried out

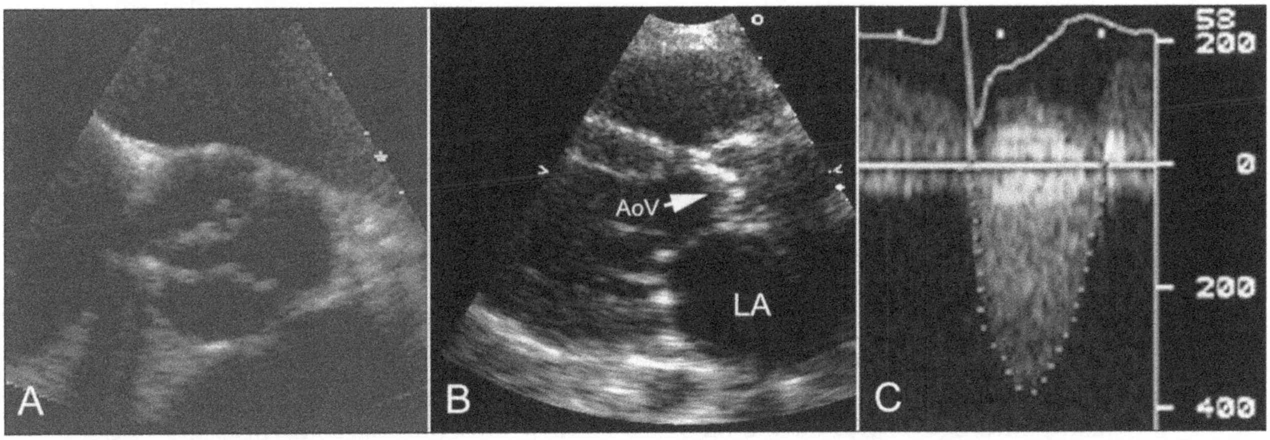

Figure 1. A, Transesophageal echocardiogram demonstrating thickened aortic valve leaflets and reduced aortic valve (AoV) orifice. B, During systole, the AoV leaflets have a significantly reduced opening. C, High velocity of the blood flowing through the AoV during systole is measured by Doppler interrogation during echocardiography. LA indicates left atrium.

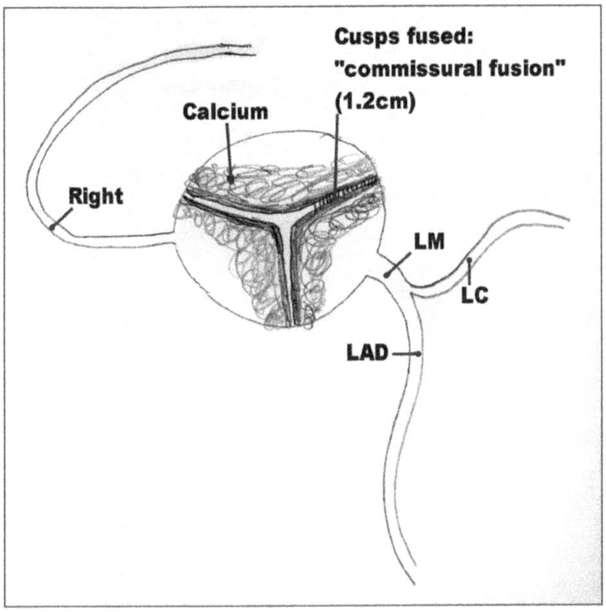

Figure 2. Tricuspid aortic valve, severely thickened by both fibrous tissue and heavy calcific deposits. Each cusp was immobile, and 2 cusps were fused at 1 commissural fusion (1.2 cm). LM indicates left main artery; LC, left circumflex artery; and LAD, left anterior descending artery.

promptly, as soon as the patient develops symptoms secondary to aortic stenosis."

Current guidelines for the management of patients with severe AS recommend valve replacement for patients who exhibit symptoms that can be related to the AS (chest pain, dyspnea, or syncope). In patients who have equivocal symptoms, stress testing can be performed to quantify their exercise response. Abnormal response to exercise in an otherwise asymptomatic individual with severe AS is an indication for valve replacement. In the truly asymptomatic individual, close clinical follow-up and at least a yearly echocardiogram is the current recommendation.[2]

One of us (WCR) has had an opportunity to study at necropsy 192 patients older than 15 years of age with AS unassociated with morphologic disease of the mitral valve (other than aging changes ± mitral annular calcium) and not treated operatively. Of the 192 patients, 47 (24%) died suddenly and unexpectedly. Of the 42 patients (of the 47) in whom good information was available on symptoms, 10 (24%) were considered asymptomatic before the sudden cardiac arrest. Of the 47 patients, the AS was considered to be severe in 36 (77%) and moderate (4 patients) or mild (7 patients) in the others. Of these 47 patients, 28 (60%) had a congenitally bicuspid aortic valve; 2 (4%) had a unicuspid acommissural valve, and 17 (36%) had a tricuspid valve. The patient described herein had a functionally bicuspid aortic valve because 2 of the 3 cusps were fused together at one commissure over a distance of 1.2 cm.

In summary, a patient with severe AS unassociated with significant mitral valve disease or severe coronary artery disease is presented whose symptom of AS was sudden death. Such cases are very uncommon.

References

1 Braunwald E. On the natural history of severe aortic stenosis. *J Am Coll Cardiol.* 1990;15:1018–1020.

2 Bonow RO, Carabello BA, Chatterjee K, et al. ACC/AHA 2006 guidelines for the management of patients with valvular heart disease: a report of the American College of Cardiology/American Heart Association Task Force on Practice Guidelines (writing Committee to Revise the 1998 guidelines for the management of patients with valvular heart disease) developed in collaboration with the Society of Cardiovascular Anesthesiologists endorsed by the Society for Cardiovascular Angiography and Interventions and the Society of Thoracic Surgeons. *J Am Coll Cardiol.* 2006;48:e1–e148.

Valve Structure and Survival in *Septuagenarians* Having Aortic Valve Replacement for Aortic Stenosis (±Aortic Regurgitation) With Versus Without Coronary Artery Bypass Grafting at a Single US Medical Center (1993 to 2005)

William Clifford Roberts, MD[a,b,d,*], Jong Mi Ko, BA[d], Giovanni Filardo, PhD, MPH[e,f], Albert Carl Henry, MD[c], Robert Frederick Hebeler, Jr., MD[c], Edson Hoi-Kam Cheung, MD[c], Gregory John Matter, MD[c], and Baron Lloyd Hamman, MD[c]

The purpose of this study was to determine the effect of simultaneous coronary artery bypass grafting (CABG) and the influence of valve structure on both early and late survival in septuagenarians having aortic valve replacement (AVR) for aortic stenosis (AS) (with or without aortic regurgitation). We analyzed valve structure in 424 septuagenarians having AVR for AS from 1993 through 2005 at Baylor University Medical Center, including 254 (60%) with and 170 (40%) without simultaneous CABG. Of the 424 patients, 8 (2%) had a congenitally unicuspid aortic valve, 179 (42%), a congenitally bicuspid aortic valve, 235 (55%), a 3-cuspid valve, and in 2 patients (1%) the valve structure was indeterminate. Survival data were available in 418 of the 424 patients: 23 (5.5%) died within 30 days of AVR and 9 other patients from 31 to 60 days after AVR (7.7% 60-day mortality). Sixty-day mortality was not affected by congenital valve abnormality (unicuspid/bicuspid 8.5% vs tricuspid 7.0%). In contrast, late survival (up to 13-year follow-up) was affected by valve structure: it was longer in the unicuspid/bicuspid valve structure group than in the tricuspid valve structure (hazard ratio 0.54, 95% confidence intervals 0.36 to 0.81). The hazard ratio was estimated after adjusting for concomitant CABG. In conclusion, aortic valve structure affected late, but not early survival in septuagenarians undergoing AVR for AS. **(Am J Cardiol 2007;100:1157–1165)**

Although a number of articles have appeared describing results of various cardiac operations in octogenarians,[1] only 7 published reports have appeared describing results of aortic valve replacement (AVR) for aortic stenosis (AS) in septuagenarians.[2–8] The numbers of patients included in these 7 reports was ≤25 in 5, 101 patients in 1, and 208 patients in another. None of the 7 reports described aortic valve structure. This report describes the structure of operatively excised aortic valves in 424 patients and compares survival and valve structure in septuagenarians having AVR for AS with versus without simultaneous coronary artery bypass grafting (CABG) at 1 institute in a recent 13-year period.

[a]Departments of Internal Medicine (Division of Cardiology), [b]Pathology and [c]Cardiothoracic Surgery, and the [d]Baylor Heart and Vascular Institute, Baylor University Medical Center; the [e]Institute for Health Care Research and Improvement, Baylor Health Care System; and the [f]Department of Statistical Science, Southern Methodist University, Dallas, Texas. Manuscript received June 1, 2007; revised manuscript received and accepted June 20, 2007.

*Corresponding author: Telephone: 214-820-7911; fax: 214-820-7533.

E-mail address: wc.roberts@baylorhealth.edu (W.C. Roberts).

Methods

From January 1993 through December 2005, a total of 1,112 patients underwent AVR for AS (with or without aortic regurgitation) with or without simultaneous CABG and without mitral valve replacement at Baylor University Medical Center. Of the 1,112 patients, 424 (38%) were aged 70 to 79, and they are the subject of this report. The operatively excised aortic valve in each patient was submitted to the surgical pathology section, and all 424 valves were examined and described by 1 author (WCR). In 6, the valves had been excised in multiple fragments and the structure could not be determined. The structure in 4 of the 6 cases was that provided by the operating cardiac surgeon. The valves were photographed by JMK. Since 1998, all operatively excised valves have been weighed by 1 of us (WCR).

The echocardiographic and hemodynamic data in the 424 septuagenarians was collected by JMK from the cardiovascular computer database (Apollo Advance C/S, version 4.2.13, LUMEDX Corp., Oakland, California) and from the medical records. Information regarding death of any patient was obtained from 2 sources: (1) early death information was obtained from the medical record, and (2) post-hospital death information was obtained and confirmed from the Social Security Death Index.

Table 1
Clinical and valve structure information in the 424 septuagenarians having aortic valve replacement for isolated aortic stenosis with or without coronary artery bypass grafting

Year	Number of AVRs for AS at BUMC	Number of Septuagenarians	Age (years) Range (Mean)	Men	Women	Coronary Artery Bypass Grafting	Hospital Stay (days)* AVR→DC Range (mean±SD)	Died		Interval (years) AVR→Death* Range (mean±SD)	Aortic Valve Structure				Aortic Valve Weight (g) Range (Mean)			
															Bicuspid		Tricuspid	
								≤60 days	>60 days		Unicuspid (M:W)	Bicuspid (M:W)	Tricuspid (M:W)	Indeterminate (M:W)	Men	Women	Men	Women
1993	31	14	70–79 (75)	5	9	4	6–27 (10.7±6.5)	1	6	2.83–12.95 (8.48±3.26)	0	9 (3:6)	5 (2:3)	0	—	—	—	—
1994	50	22	70–79 (76)	15	7	13	5–60 (12.0±11.9)	0	15	0.30–9.40 (4.14±3.19)	0	6 (4:2)	15 (10:5)	1 (1:0)	—	—	—	—
1995	44	15	70–79 (75)	8	7	8	5–70 (13.6±16.6)	0	9	0.35–11.45 (5.71±3.48)	2 (2:0)	8 (2:6)	5 (4:1)	0	—	—	—	—
1996	56	27	70–79 (75)	19	8	14	4–21 (7.4±3.5)	0	16	0.92–10.55 (6.59±3.00)	0	9 (7:2)	18 (12:6)	0	—	—	—	—
1997	51	18	70–77 (74)	12	6	15	5–56 (13.1±12.6)	1	4	3.33–9.35 (5.43±2.83)	1 (1:0)	7 (5:2)	10 (6:4)	0	—	—	—	—
1998	68	25	70–79 (74)	16	9	12	4–37 (8.5±6.9)	1	10	2.40–8.01 (5.04±2.49)	0	16 (11:5)	8 (4:4)	1 (1:0)	2.85–11.3 (4.47)	2.00–3.30 (2.49)	2.07–3.90 (3.02)	1.34–1.80 (1.59)
1999	110	44	70–79 (75)	20	24	31	3–44 (10.6±8.5)	3	15	0.18–6.87 (2.80±2.20)	0	19 (10:9)	25 (10:15)	0	2.09–5.55 (3.73)	1.40–3.25 (2.31)	1.10–3.20 (2.15)	1.03–2.86 (1.66)
2000	112	36	70–79 (74)	21	15	25	3–22 (9.5±4.6)	1	5	0.38–5.63 (2.31±2.09)	1 (1:0)	20 (14:6)	15 (6:9)	0	1.37–8.30 (3.88)	1.28–3.45 (2.79)	1.27–2.91 (2.36)	0.60–1.88 (1.38)
2001	98	34	70–79 (75)	19	15	18	4–26 (9±4.5)	6	4	2.83–5.25 (3.96±1.16)	0	17 (10:7)	17 (9:8)	0	2.04–4.79 (3.49)	1.27–3.12 (2.01)	1.39–3.95 (2.57)	1.17–2.37 (1.45)
2002	110	41	70–79 (74)	25	16	30	4–32 (9.6±6.3)	3	7	0.35–3.34 (1.85±1.21)	0	13 (9:4)	28 (16:12)	0	1.20–4.86 (2.90)	1.32–2.77 (1.94)	1.49–5.77 (2.85)	0.80–4.81 (1.74)
2003	136	53	70–79 (74)	31	22	30	4–35 (10.4±7.8)	5	6	0.19–2.76 (1.71±0.99)	1 (0:1)	26 (18:8)	26 (13:13)	0	1.24–5.01 (2.91)	1.10–3.18 (2.08)	1.50–3.85 (2.40)	0.74–3.07 (1.66)
2004	120	50	70–79 (75)	35	15	29	5–45 (11.4±9.4)	6	8	0.25–2.37 (0.92±0.73)	1 (1:0)	18 (9:9)	31 (25:6)	0	1.82–4.66 (2.98)	1.00–3.86 (2.63)	1.26–3.68 (2.32)	0.88–1.97 (1.40)
2005	126	45	70–79 (75)	26	19	25	4–51 (10.1±9.4)	5	3	0.18–1.85 (0.93±0.78)	2 (1:1)	11 (7:4)	32 (18:14)	0	1.48–4.17 (2.76)	0.98–1.57 (1.24)	0.76–3.68 (2.17)	0.77–2.20 (1.48)
	1,112	424	70–79 (75)	252	172	254	3–70 (10.2±8.4)	32/418	108/418	0.18–12.95 (4.09±3.19)	8 (6:2)	179 (109:70)	235 (135:100)	(2:0)	1.20–11.3 (3.41)	0.98–3.86 (2.25)	0.76–5.77 (2.42)	0.60–4.81 (1.57)
		(38%)		(59%)	(41%)	(60%)		(8%)	(26%)		(2%)	(42%)	(55%)	(<1%)	89†	52†	100†	81†

* Includes only patients surviving >60 days after valve replacement.
† Number of patients in whom the valve was weighed.
AS = aortic stenosis; AVR = aortic valve replacement; BUMC = Baylor University Medical Center; DC = discharge; M = man; W = woman. — = no information available or not applicable.

Echocardiographic data preoperatively was available to us in 100 patients (24%). Cardiac catheterization data were available to us in most patients: peak transvalvular pressure gradients in 286 patients (67%); mean transvalvular pressure gradients in 255 (60%); aortic valve areas in 284 patients (67%), and left ventricular ejection fractions in 182 patients (43%). Most patients in whom cardiac catheterization data were not available to WCR and JMK were referred directly to a cardiovascular surgeon. These patients had coronary angiographic studies before being referred to BUMC, but the data were not available to us.

Means, SDs, and percentages were calculated to describe the study cohort (n = 424). Due to the low unicuspid (n = 8) counts, patients with unicuspid and bicuspid valve structure were grouped together in the analysis investigating short- and long-term mortality. Unadjusted relative risk (RR) and 95% confidence intervals (95% CI) were estimated to describe the relation between valve structure and short-term mortality. To investigate late survival, we excluded patients who died within 60 days from AVR (n = 32) and subjects with missing survival time (n = 8). This left 384 patients for the late survival analysis. Log-rank test statistics were computed to compare unadjusted survival curves for the variables of interest. Moreover, a Cox proportional hazards model was fitted to estimate the adjusted relation of aortic valve structure with mortality. All those risk factors shown to be confounders of the association between aortic valve structure and mortality were included in the final adjusted model. Assumptions for the final model were assessed, and the model was tested for the need of any pairwise interaction with aortic valve structure using a likelihood ratio test. Finally, the adjusted hazard ratio (HR) and 95% CI describing the association between aortic valve structure and risk of death at up to 13 years from the date of operation (based on the Cox models) was estimated and unadjusted (Kaplan-Meier) and adjusted survival curves were generated. Statistical analysis was performed using SigmaStat Version 2.0 (SPSS Inc., Chicago, Illinois) and SAS version 9.1 (SAS Institute, Cary, North Carolina).

This study was approved by Institutional Review Board at Baylor University Medical Center.

Results

Pertinent data in the 424 septuagenarians are summarized in Tables 1 and 2. The native stenotic aortic valve was replaced with a bioprosthesis in 361 (86%) patients and with a mechanical prosthesis in the remaining 57 (14%) patients. Of the 424 patients, 252 (59%) were men and 172 (41%) were women. Simultaneous CABG was performed in 254 (60%) patients (Figure 1). Of the 32 patients dying within 60 days of AVR, 23 (5.5%) died within 30 days and 9 patients from 31 to 60 days (7.7% 60-day mortality). The unadjusted analysis of 60-day mortality indicated that it was not affected by valve structure (RR 0.81, 95% CI 0.41 to 1.58). Likewise, having concomitant CABG did not affect crude mortality (RR 0.77, 95% CI 0.38 to 1.56). In total, 32 (7.7%)

Table 2
Comparison of the 424 septuagenarians having aortic valve replacement for aortic stenosis without versus with simultaneous coronary artery bypass grafting

Year	Without Coronary Artery Bypass Grafting									With Coronary Artery Bypass Grafting								
	Number Having AVR (M:W)	Length of Stay* (days) Range (mean±SD)	Died			UAV (M:W)	BAV (M:W)	TAV (M:W)	I (M:W)	Number Having AVR (M:W)	Length of Stay* (days) Range (Mean±SD)	Died			UAV (M:W)	BAV (M:W)	TAV (M:W)	I (M:W)
			Total (M:W)	≤60 days (M:W)	>60 days (M:W)							Total (M:W)	≤60 days (M:W)	>60 days (M:W)				
1993	10 (3:7)	6–19 (8.7±4.0)	5 (2:3)	0	5 (2:3)	0	7 (2:5)	3 (1:2)	0	4 (2:2)	10, 27 (18.5±12)	2 (0:2)	1 (0:1)	1 (0:1)	0	2 (1:1)	2 (1:1)	0
1994	9 (6:3)	5–60 (15.6±17.5)	6 (6:0)	0	6 (6:0)	0	4 (2:2)	5 (4:1)	0	13 (9:4)	5–19 (9.3±4.2)	9 (6:3)	0	9 (6:3)	0	2 (2:0)	10 (6:4)	1 (1:0)
1995	7 (2:5)	6–70 (17.4±23.4)	4 (1:3)	0	4 (1:3)	1 (1:0)	4 (0:4)	2 (1:1)	0	8 (6:2)	5–15 (9.7±3.9)	5 (5:0)	0	5 (5:0)	1 (1:0)	4 (2:2)	3 (3:0)	0
1996	13 (8:5)	4–14 (7.5±2.9)	7 (3:4)	0	7 (3:4)	0	7 (5:2)	6 (3:3)	0	14 (11:3)	5–21 (7.4±4.1)	9 (7:2)	0	9 (7:2)	0	2 (2:0)	12 (9:3)	0
1997	3 (2:1)	6–11 (8.5±3.5)	2 (1:1)	1 (0:1)	1 (1:0)	0	1 (1:0)	2 (1:1)	0	15 (10:5)	5–56 (13.7±13.3)	3 (2:1)	0	3 (2:1)	1 (1:0)	6 (4:2)	8 (5:3)	0
1998	13 (7:6)	4–37 (8.9±8.6)	6 (3:3)	0	6 (3:3)	0	8 (4:4)	4 (2:2)	1 (1:0)	12 (9:3)	4–18 (7.9±4.1)	5 (4:1)	1 (1:0)	4 (3:1)	0	8 (7:1)	4 (2:2)	0
1999	13 (5:8)	3–14 (7.8±3.1)	5 (2:3)	0	5 (2:3)	0	6 (2:4)	7 (3:4)	0	31 (15:16)	5–44 (11.9±9.9)	13 (4:9)	3 (0:3)	10 (4:6)	0	13 (8:5)	18 (7:11)	0
2000	11 (7:4)	3–22 (8.8±5.5)	3 (1:2)	1 (0:1)	2 (1:1)	1 (1:0)	5 (4:1)	5 (2:3)	0	25 (14:11)	4–22 (9.8±4.2)	3 (1:2)	0	3 (1:2)	0	15 (10:5)	10 (4:6)	0
2001	16 (10:6)	4–15 (7.6±3.3)	4 (2:2)	2 (0:2)	2 (2:0)	0	6 (4:2)	10 (6:4)	0	18 (9:9)	5–26 (10.4±5.2)	6 (2:4)	4 (2:2)	2 (0:2)	0	11 (6:5)	7 (3:4)	0
2002	11 (8:3)	4–16 (8.1±3.6)	3 (2:1)	1 (0:1)	2 (2:0)	0	3 (3:0)	8 (5:3)	0	30 (17:13)	4–32 (10.1±7.0)	7 (4:3)	2 (1:1)	5 (3:2)	0	10 (6:4)	20 (11:9)	0
2003	23 (10:13)	4–30 (9.6±7.3)	3 (1:2)	1 (0:1)	2 (1:1)	1 (0:1)	13 (6:7)	9 (4:5)	0	30 (2:9)	5–35 (11.1±8.2)	8 (4:4)	4 (2:2)	4 (2:2)	0	13 (12:1)	17 (9:8)	0
2004	21 (11:10)	5–26 (8.6±4.6)	3 (2:1)	2 (1:1)	1 (1:0)	1 (1:0)	12 (5:7)	8 (5:3)	0	29 (24:5)	5–45 (13.5±11.5)	11 (10:1)	4 (3:1)	7 (7:0)	0	6 (4:2)	23 (20:3)	0
2005	20 (9:11)	4–45 (9.5±9.7)	4 (1:3)	3 (1:2)	1 (0:1)	1 (0:1)	5 (2:3)	14 (7:7)	0	25 (17:8)	4–51 (10.5±9.4)	4 (3:1)	2 (1:1)	2 (2:0)	1 (1:0)	6 (5:1)	18 (11:7)	0
	170 (88:82)	3–70 (9.4±8.6)	55/168	11/168	44/168	5 (3:2)	81 (40:41)	83 (44:39)	1 (1:0)	254 (164:90)	4–56 (10.8±8.3)	85/250	21/250	64/250	3 (3:0)	98 (69:29)	152 (91:61)	1 (1:0)
			(27:28)	(2:9)	(25:19)							(10:11)	(10:11)	(42:22)				
	(40%)		(33%)	(7%)	(26%)	(3%)	(48%)	(49%)	(<1%)	(60%)		(34%)	(8%)	(26%)	(1%)	(39%)	(60%)	(<1%)

* This data only include early survivors.

AVR = aortic valve replacement; BAV = bicuspid aortic valve; I = indeterminate; M = man; W = woman; TAV = tricuspid aortic valve; UAV = unicuspid aortic valve.

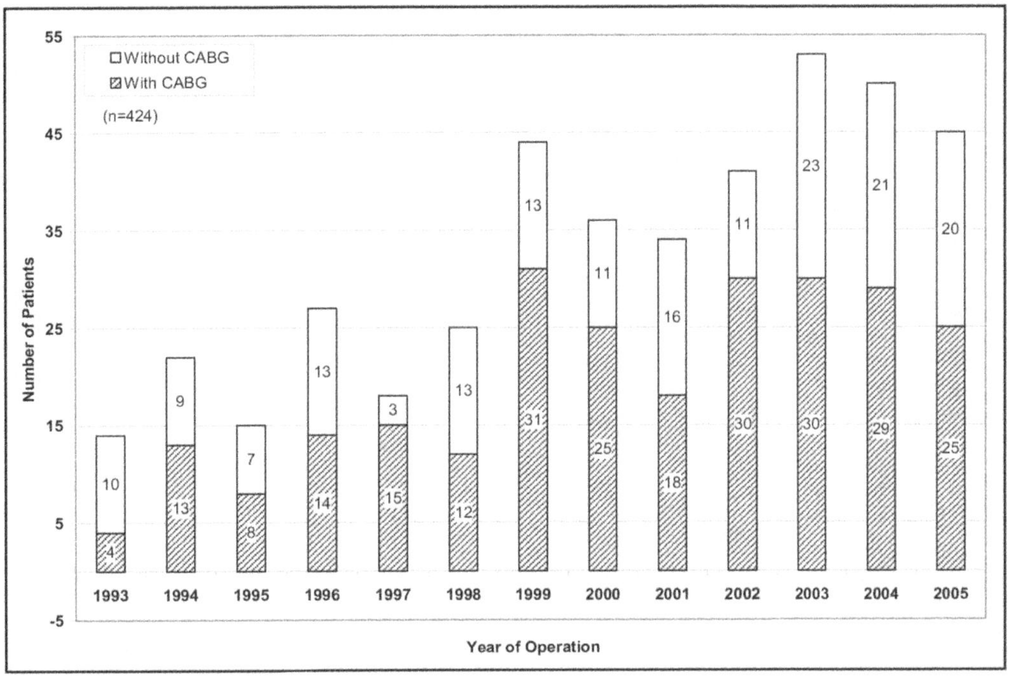

Figure 1. Number of septuagenarians having aortic valve replacement for aortic valve stenosis at BUMC from 1993 to 2005 with versus without simultaneous coronary bypass grafting (CABG).

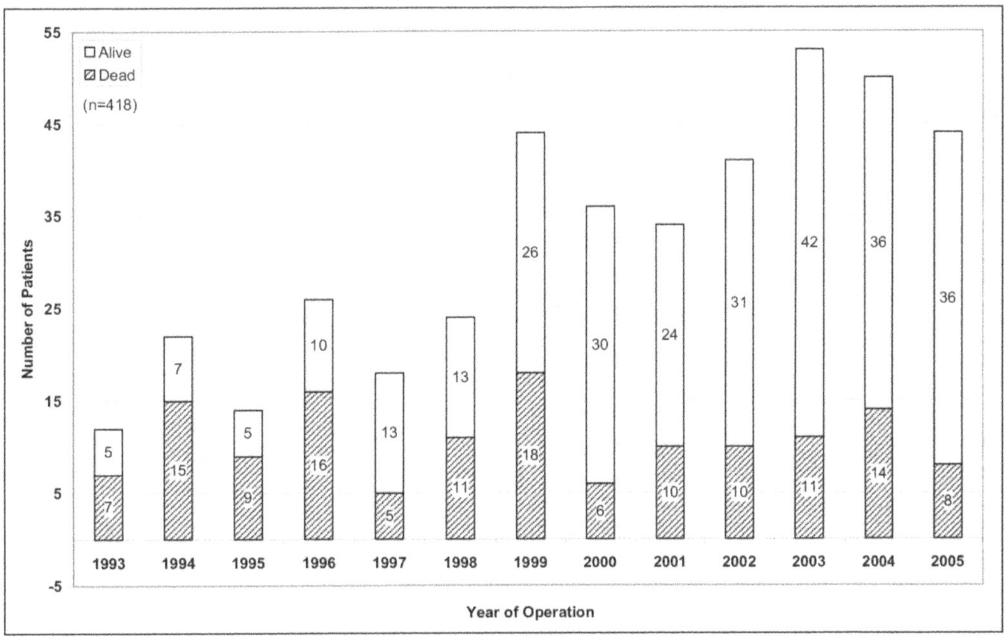

Figure 2. Number of septuagenarians surviving and not surviving aortic valve replacement for aortic stenosis (with or without simultaneous coronary artery bypass grafting) at BUMC from 1993 to 2005 (follow-up to 30 December 2006). The deaths include both early and late mortality. Most of the deaths occurred 1 or more years after the year of operation. Note trend of better AVR ± CABG survival over the 13-year period.

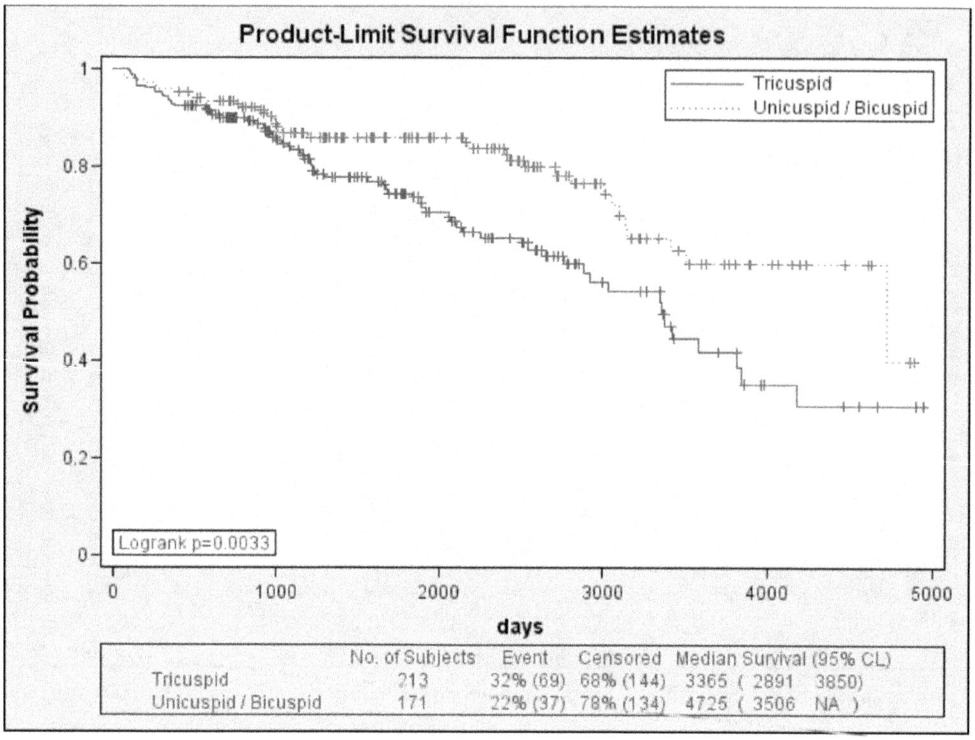

Figure 3. Kaplan-Meier survival curves comparing patients with unicuspid/bicuspid valve structure to the patients having tricuspid structure.

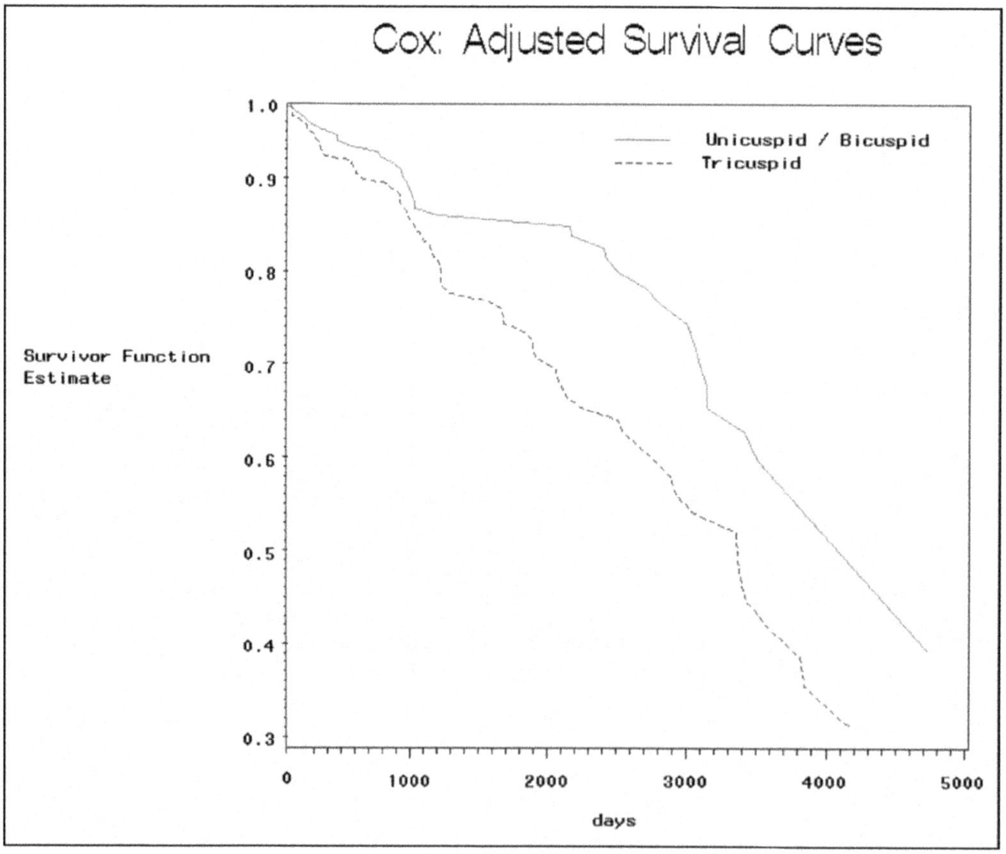

Figure 4. Adjusted survival curves based on the Cox model developed to describe the association between valve structure and mortality during the 13-year follow-up. Model covariates included gender, and simultaneous execution of CABG (Yes, No) during operation.

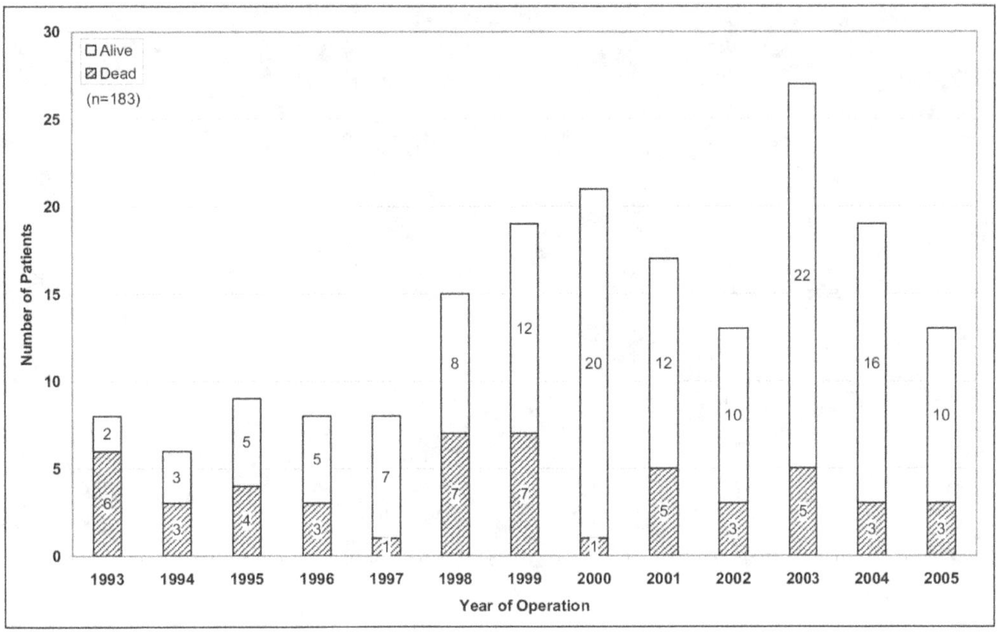

Figure 5. Number of septuagenarians surviving and not surviving aortic valve replacement for aortic stenosis involving a unicuspid and bicuspid aortic valve (± simultaneous coronary artery bypass grafting) at BUMC from 1993 to 2005 (follow-up to 30 December 2006). The deaths include both early and late mortality. Most of the deaths occurred 1 or more years after the year of operation.

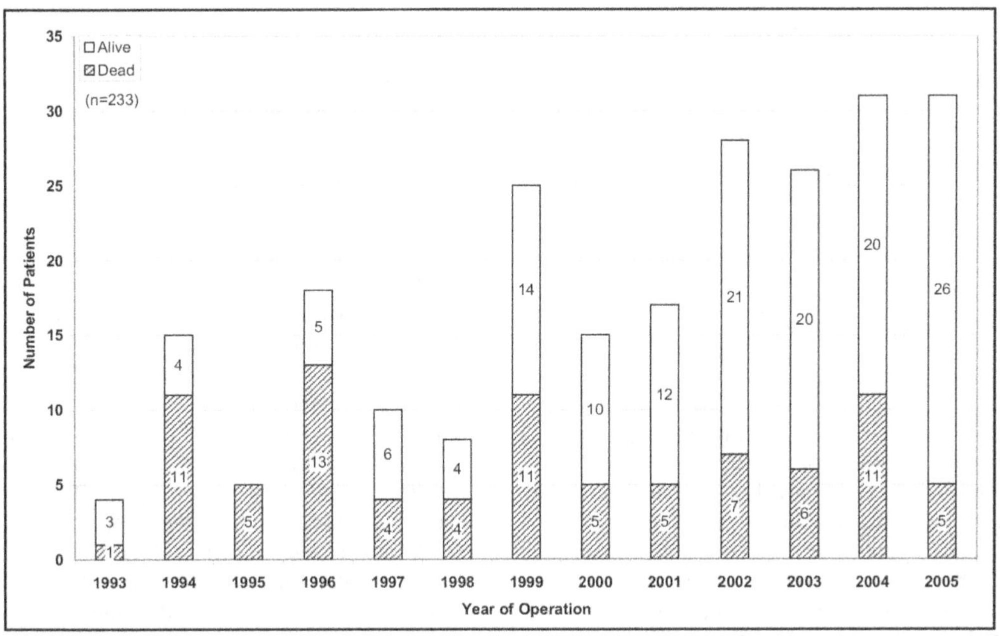

Figure 6. Number of septuagenarians surviving and not surviving aortic valve replacement for aortic stenosis involving a tricuspid aortic valve (± simultaneous coronary artery bypass grafting) at BUMC from 1993 to 2005 (follow-up to 30 December 2006). The deaths include both early and late mortality. Most of the deaths occurred 1 or more years after the year of operation.

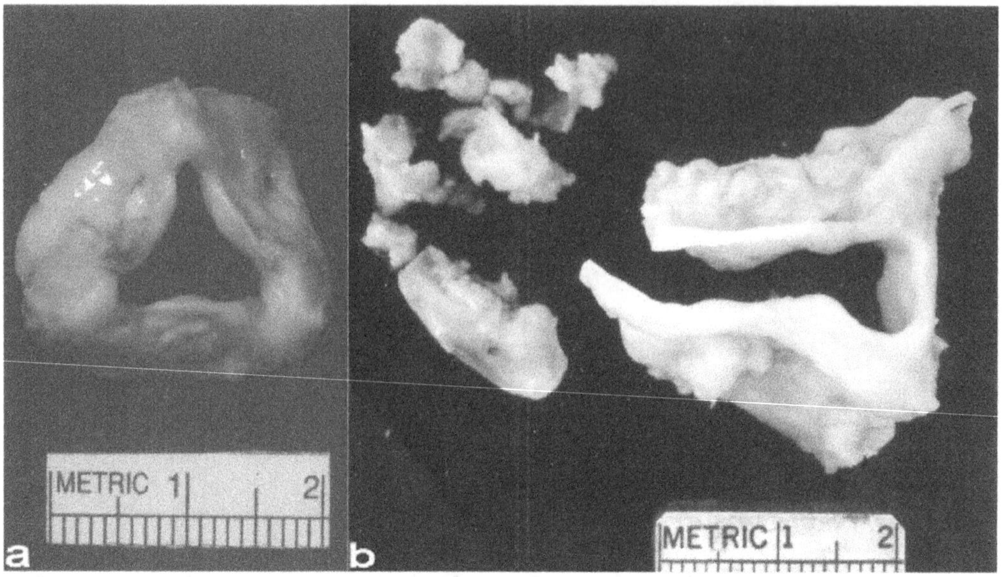

Figure 7. Photographs of 2 operatively excised stenotic congenitally *unicuspid* aortic valves: *(A)* The acommissural unicuspid valve was excised from a 75-year-old woman in whom the peak transvalvular systolic gradient was 53 mm Hg, the calculated aortic valve area 0.57 cm^2, and the valve weight, 1.67 g. (Reprinted with permission from Roberts and Ko,[11] with permission.) (The following reference describes the acommissural unicuspid aortic valve. *Cardiology* 2007;108:79–81) *(B)* The unicommissural unicuspid valve was excised from a 75-year-old man in whom the valve weight was 2.71 g.

patients died ≤60 days after AVR and another 108 patients (26%) at later periods. Of the 392 patients surviving >60 days, follow-up information was available in 384 patients. As of December 2006, 278 (71%) survived from 1.10 to 13.54 years (mean 5.42 ± 3.08, median 4.89) (Figure 2). The median survival time for those patients included in the late survival analysis (n = 384) was 10.45 years: median survival time for men was 9.82 years, and women, 12.97 years; patients with bicuspid valves, 12.94 years, and with 3-cuspid valves, 9.21 years; patients with peak transvalvular gradients ≤50 mm Hg, 10.45 years, and patients with higher gradients, 9.60; patients having simultaneous CABG, 10.54 years, and for patients not having CABG, 9.26 years. Log-rank test results indicated that *late survival* curves were statistically equivalent for men and women (p = 0.63, n = 384), for patients with low peak transvalvular gradient (≤50 mm Hg) and high peak transvalvular gradient (>50 mm Hg) (p = 0.58, n = 260), and for patients receiving simultaneous CABG and not having CABG (p = 0.97, n = 384). In contrast, the unadjusted analysis suggested that late survival curves were statistically different for patients with an unicuspid/bicuspid and tricuspid valve structure (p = 0.003, n = 384). The Kaplan-Meier plot (see Figure 3) indicated that patients with unicuspid/bicuspid valve structure had better survival. The adjusted Cox model confirmed the results obtained through the unadjusted analysis. Late survival was significantly better in the unicuspid/bicuspid valve structure group than in the tricuspid valve group (HR 0.54, 95% CI 0.36 to 0.81; see Figure 4).

Length of stay in the hospital in the 384 patients who survived the operative period ranged from 3 to 70 days (mean 10.3) and in the 32 who died early from 0 to 53 days (mean 10.6). Simultaneous CABG increased length to 1.7 days on average (*crude* p = 0.046). Length of stay in the 227 patients with CABG who survived the operative period ranged from 4 to 56 days (mean 10.9 ± 8.3), and in the 157 patients without CABG, from 3 to 70 days (mean 9.2 ± 8.6). Of the 21 patients with CABG who died early (≤60 days), the length of hospitalization before death ranged from 0 to 53 days (mean 9.8 ± 13.2); of the 11 patients without CABG who died early, the length of hospitalization ranged from 2 to 29 days (mean 12.1 ± 7.6).

The transvalvular *peak* systolic pressure gradient on average was higher in patients without simultaneous CABG (range 10 to 133 mm Hg, mean 57 ± 27) than in patients receiving concomitant CABG (range 10 to 133 mm Hg, mean 42 ± 23) (*crude* p = 0.003); the mean systolic pressure gradients, ranged from 1 to 103 (average 46) and 8 to 100 (average 39) (*crude* p = 0.001), respectively; the calculated aortic valve area, from 0.20 to 2.51 cm^2 (mean 0.71) and from 0.27 to 1.44 cm^2 (mean 0.76) (*crude* p = 0.11), respectively; and the left ventricular ejection fractions from 15% to 80% (mean 54%) and from 15% to 85% (mean 50%) (*crude* p = 0.09), respectively.

Another tool providing some evidence of the severity of the AS is gained by the *weight of the operatively excised valves.*[9–12] (Previous studies have shown that men with AS have heavier valves than women and that congenitally unicuspid and bicuspid stenotic aortic valves are heavier than 3-cuspid stenotic aortic valves.[9–12]) The operatively excised unicuspid aortic valves in the 3 men in the present study weighed 2.71, 2.73, and 3.40 g (mean 2.95); the bicuspid valves in the 89 men, from 1.20 to 11.3 g (mean 3.41), and the tricuspid aortic valves in the 100 men, from 0.76 to 5.77 g (mean 2.42). In contrast, the 2 unicuspid valves in women weighed 1.19 and 1.67 g, respectively; the bicuspid valves in the 52 women, from 0.98 to 3.86 g (mean 2.25),

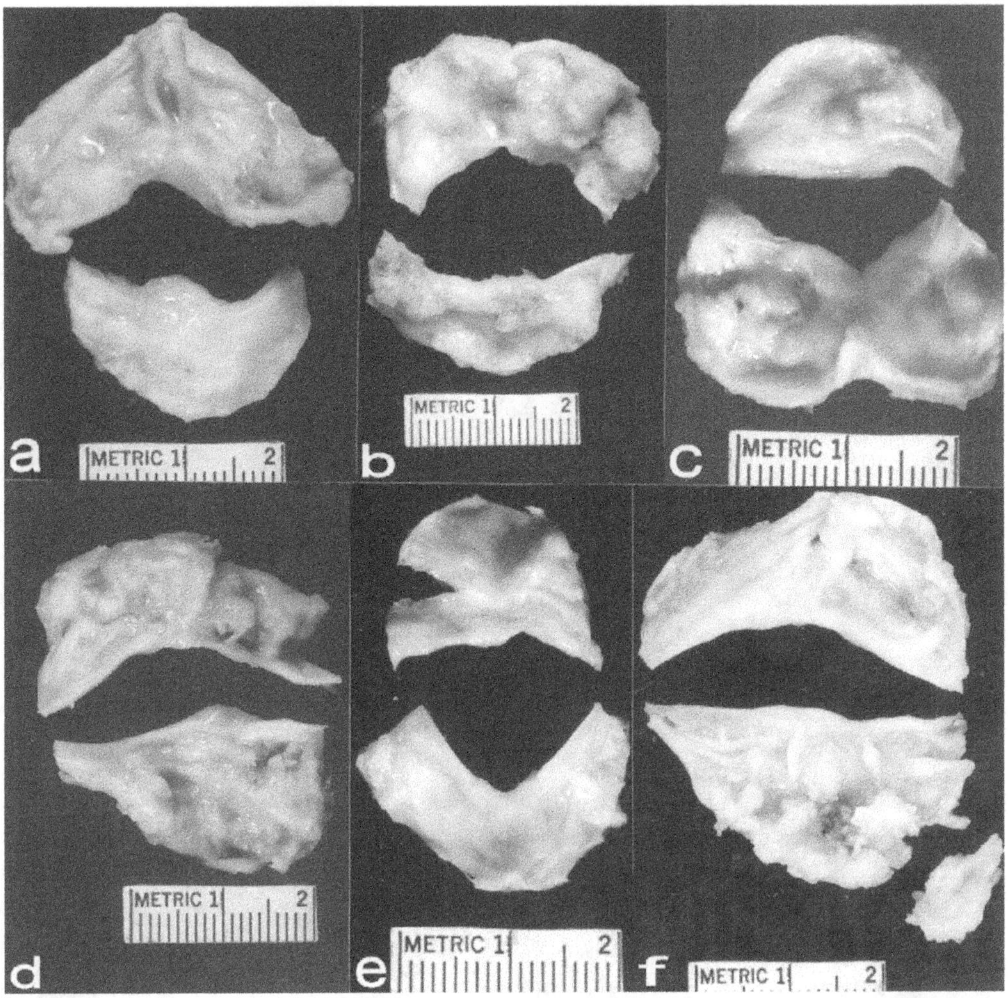

Figure 8. Photographs of 6 operatively excised stenotic congenitally *bicuspid* aortic valves: *(A)* The valve was excised from a 71-year-old woman in whom the peak transvalvular systolic gradient was 38 mm Hg and the valve weight, 3.51 g. *(B)* The valve was excised from a 71-year-old man in whom the peak transvalvular systolic gradient was 105 mm Hg, the calculated aortic valve area 0.42 cm^2, and the valve weight, 4.66 g. *(C)* The valve was excised from a 74-year-old woman in whom the peak transvalvular systolic gradient was 60 mm Hg, the calculated aortic valve area 0.70 cm^2, and the valve weight, 2.58 g. *(D)* The valve was excised from a 72-year-old man in whom the peak transvalvular systolic gradient was 46, the calculated aortic valve area 0.88 cm^2, and the valve weight, 3.46 g. *(E)* The valve was excised from a 76-year-old woman in whom the valve weight was 1.0 g. *(F)* The valve was excised from a 79-year-old woman in whom the peak transvalvular systolic gradient was 31 mm Hg, the calculated aortic valve area 0.67 cm^2, and the valve weight, 3.41 g.

and the tricuspid aortic valves in the 81 women, from 0.60 to 4.81 g (mean 1.57). *Aortic valve structure* in the 424 patients was the following: unicuspid in 8 (2%); bicuspid in 179 (42%); 3-cuspid in 235 (55%), and indeterminate in 2 (<1%) (Figures 5 to 9).

Discussion

The present study focused on a large group of septuagenarians having AVR for AS at the same US medical center during a recent 13-year period. Early mortality (≤60 days) was 7.5% and similar in the patients with unicuspid/bicuspid and tricuspid valves. Late mortality was significantly less in the patients having unicuspid/bicuspid valves than in patients with tricuspid aortic valves.

The positive features of the present study include a large number of septuagenarians, relatively long post-AVR follow-up, preoperative hemodynamic data in most patients, and knowledge of aortic valve structure and weight. That all valves were examined by the same individual (WCR) produced uniformity not available if valve structure was that recorded in the operative note by a number of different cardiac surgeons, each of whom might have different views of what constituted a congenitally malformed or a 3-cuspid aortic valve with fusion of ≥1 aortic valve commissures. (WCR has been a student of aortic valve structure for >40 years.) The negative features of the present study include lack of information on preoperative and postoperative symptoms and functional class, on early postoperative complications, comorbidities, late quality of life, numbers of epicardial coronary arteries narrowed >50% in diameter, and causes of death late postoperatively.

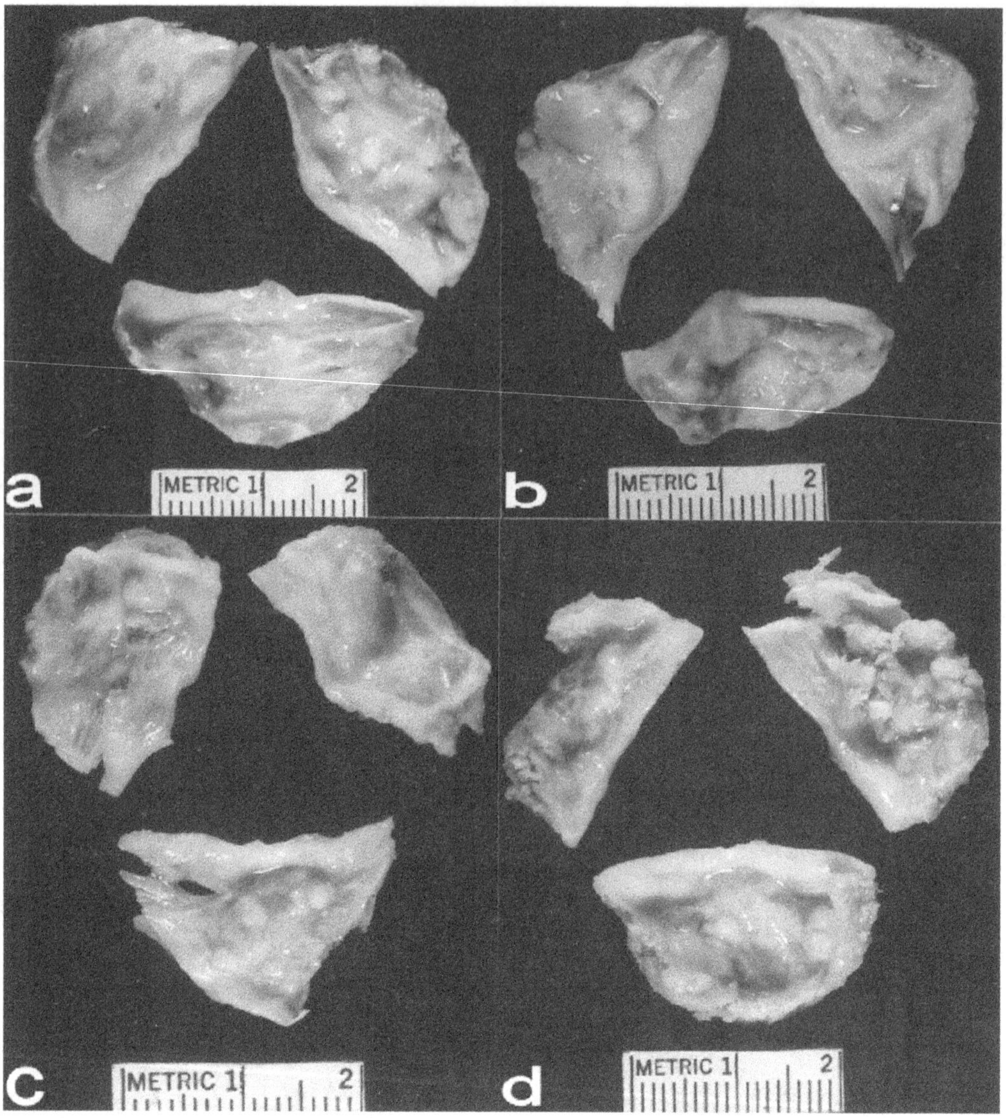

Figure 9. Photographs of 4 operatively excised stenotic *tricuspid* aortic valves: *(A)* The valve was excised from a 75-year-old man in whom the valve weight was 2.26 g. *(B)* The valve was excised from a 77-year-old man in whom the peak transvalvular systolic gradient was 35 mm Hg, the calculated aortic valve area 0.90 cm^2, and the valve weight, 2.44 g. *(C)* The valve was excised from a 78-year-old man in whom the peak transvalvular systolic gradient was 21 mm Hg, the calculated aortic valve area 0.91 cm^2, and the valve weight, 1.85 g. *(D)* The valve was excised from a 79-year-old man in whom the peak transvalvular systolic gradient was 44 mm Hg, the calculated aortic valve area 0.94 cm, and the valve weight, 3.14 g.

1. Roberts WC, Ko JM, Garner WL, Filardo G, Henry AC, Hebeler RF JR, Matter GJ, Hamman BL. Valve structure and survival in octogenarians having aortic valve replacement for aortic stenosis (± aortic regurgitation) with vs without coronary artery bypass grafting at a single US medical center (1993 to 2005). *Am J Cardiol* 2007 (in press).
2. Wisoff BG, Hartstein ML, Aintalian A. Hamby RI. Results of open heart surgery in the septuagenarian. *J Gerontol* 1976;31:275–277.
3. Hines GL, Boal BH, Reed GE. Safety of aortic valve replacement in septuagenarians. *N Y State J Med* 1977;77:1285–1288.
4. Tsai TP, Matloff JM, Chaux A, Kass RM, Lee ME, Czer LSC, DeRobertis MA, Gray RJ. Combined valve and coronary artery bypass procedures in septuagenarians and octogenarians: results in 120 patients. *Ann Thorac Surg* 1986;42:681–684.
5. Grondin CM, Thornton JC, Engle JC, Schreiber H, Cross FS. Cardiac surgery in septuagenarians: is there a difference in mortality and morbidity? *J Thorac Cardiovasc Surg* 1989;98:908–914.
6. Lindblom D, Lindblom U, Ivert T. Heart valve replacement in septuagenarians. *Scand J Thor Cardiovasc Surg* 1989;23:29–32.
7. Lund O, Nielsen TT, Magnussen K, Pilegaard HK, Knudsen MA. Valve replacement for calcified aortic stenosis in septuagenarians infers normal life-length. *Scand J Thor Cardiovasc Surg* 1991;25:37–44.
8. Kawachi Y, Arinaga K, Nakashima A, Toshima Y, Kawano H, Kosuga T. Aortic valve replacement in patients age 70 years and older: early and late results. *Artif Organs* 2002;26:706–710.
9. Roberts WC, Ko JM. Weights of operatively excised stenotic unicuspid, bicuspid, and tricuspid aortic valves and their relation to age, sex, body mass index, and presence or absence of concomitant coronary artery bypass grafting. *Am J Cardiol* 2003:92:1057–1065.
10. Roberts WC, Ko JM. Relation of weights of operatively excised stenotic aortic valves to preoperative transvalvular peak systolic pressure gradients and to calculated aortic valve areas. *J Am Coll Cardiol* 2004;44:1847–1855.
11. Roberts WC, Ko JM. Frequency by decades of unicuspid, bicuspid, and tricuspid aortic valves in adults having isolated aortic valve replacement for aortic stenosis, with or without associated aortic regurgitation. *Circulation* 2005;111:920–925.
12. Roberts WC, Ko JM, Hamilton C. Comparison of valve structure, valve weight, and severity of the valve obstruction in 1849 patients having isolated aortic valve replacement for aortic valve stenosis (with or without associated aortic regurgitation) studied at 3 different medical centers in 2 different time periods. *Circulation* 2006;114:422–429.

Valve Structure and Survival in *Sexagenarians* Having Aortic Valve Replacement for Aortic Stenosis (±Aortic Regurgitation) With Versus Without Coronary Artery Bypass Grafting at a Single US Medical Center (1993 to 2005)

William Clifford Roberts, MD[a,b,d,*], Jong Mi Ko, BA[d], Giovanni Filardo, PhD, MPH[e,f], Albert Carl Henry, MD[c], Robert Frederick Hebeler, Jr., MD[c], Edson Hoi-Kam Cheung, MD[c], Gregory John Matter, MD[c], and Baron Lloyd Hamman, MD[c]

The purpose of this study was to determine the effect of simultaneous coronary artery bypass grafting (CABG) and the influence of valve structure on both early and late survival in sexagenarians having aortic valve replacement (AVR) for aortic stenosis (AS) (with or without aortic regurgitation). We analyzed survival and valve structure in 289 sexagenarians having AVR for AS from 1993 through 2005 at Baylor University Medical Center, including 147 (51%) with and 142 (49%) without simultaneous CABG. Of the 282 patients with information available, 13 (4.6%) died within 30 days of operation and 1 additional patient, from 31 to 60 days after operation (5.0% 60-day mortality). Sixty-day mortality was similar (6% and 4%) in the groups with and without simultaneous CABG. A total of 66 patients (23%) died from >60 days up to 13 years postoperatively. The unadjusted survival analysis showed that late survival was not affected by gender (male versus female), aortic valve structure (unicuspid, bicuspid, and quadricuspid versus tricuspid) or preoperative severity of the AS (transvalvular peak pressure gradient >50 mm Hg versus ≤50 mm Hg), or by performance of CABG. The aortic valve was congenitally unicuspid in 10 patients (3%), congenitally bicuspid in 170 (59%), 3-cuspid in 107 (37%), congenitally quadricuspid in 1 patient, and the valve structure was indeterminate in 1 patient. In conclusion, gender, valve structure, preoperative severity of the AS, or performance of simultaneous CABG did not effect unadjusted survival in sexagenarians undergoing AVR for AS. **(Am J Cardiol 2007;100:1286–1292)**

We recently described aortic valve structure and early and late survival in 196 *octogenarians* and in 424 *septuagenarians* having aortic valve replacement (AVR) for aortic stenosis (AS) at Baylor University Medical Center from 1993 to 2005.[1,2] The present report focuses on aortic valve structure and survival in 289 *sexagenarians* having AVR for AS at the same medical center in the same time frame.

Methods

From January 1993 through December 2005, a total of 1,112 patients underwent AVR for AS (with or without aortic regurgitation) with or without simultaneous CABG and without mitral valve replacement at Baylor University Medical Center. Of the 1,112 patients, 289 (26%) were aged 60 to 69 years, and they are the subject of this report. The operatively excised aortic valve in each patient was submitted to the surgical pathology section and all 289 valves were examined and described by 1 author (WCR). In 5, the valves had been excised in multiple fragments and the structure could not be determined. The structure in 4 of the 5 cases was that provided by the operating cardiac surgeon. The valves were photographed by JMK. Since 1998, all operatively excised valves have been weighed by 1 of us (WCR).

The echocardiographic and hemodynamic data in the 289 sexagenarians were collected by JMK from the cardiovascular computer database (Apollo Advance C/S, version 4.2.13, LUMEDX Corp., Oakland, California) and from the medical records. Information regarding death of any patient was obtained from 2 sources: (1) early death information was obtained from the medical record, and (2) post-hospital death information was obtained and confirmed from the Social Security Death Index.

Echocardiographic data preoperatively was available to us in 94 patients (33%). Cardiac catheterization data were available to us in most patients: peak transvalvular pressure gradients in 188 patients (65%); mean transvalvular pressure gradients in 179 (62%); aortic valve area in 191 patients (66%), and left ventricular ejection fraction in 133 patients (46%). Most patients in whom cardiac catheterization data were not available to WCR and JMK were referred directly to a cardiovascular surgeon. These patients had

Departments of [a]Internal Medicine (Division of Cardiology), [b]Pathology, and [c]Cardiothoracic Surgery and the [d]Baylor Heart and Vascular Institute, Baylor University Medical Center; the [e]Institute for Health Care Research and Improvement, Baylor Health Care System; and the [f]Department of Statistical Science, Southern Methodist University, Dallas Texas. Manuscript received June 1, 2007; revised manuscript received and accepted June 29, 2007.

*Corresponding author: Telepone: 214-820-7911; fax: 214-820-7533.
E-mail address: wc.roberts@baylorhealth.edu.

Table 1
Clinical and valve structure information in the 289 sexagenarians having aortic valve replacement for isolated aortic stenosis with or without simultaneous coronary artery bypass grafting

Year	Number of AVRs for AS at BUMC	Number of Sexagenarians	Age (years) Range (Mean)	Men	Women	Coronary Artery Bypass Grafting	Died		Interval (years) AVR→Death* Range (mean±SD)	Aortic Valve Structure†			Aortic Valve Weight (g) Range (Mean)			
													Bicuspid		Tricuspid	
							≤60 days	>60 days		UAV (M:W)	BAV (M:W)	TAV (M:W)	Men	Women	Men	Women
1993	31	6	60–69 (65)	5	1	5	0	1	7.17	0	4 (4:0)	2 (1:1)	—	—	—	—
1994	50	18	60–69 (65)	11	7	9	0	7	1.03–11.23 (7.31±3.36)	1 (1:0)	12 (9:3)	5 (1:4)	—	—	—	—
1995	44	16	60–69 (65)	10	6	7	0	6	1.65–11.21 (5.21±3.17)	0	12 (8:4)	3 (1:2)	—	—	—	—
1996	56	13	60–68 (64)	8	5	8	0	6	0.31–10.38 (4.16±3.88)	1 (1:0)	6 (3:3)	6 (4:2)	—	—	—	—
1997	51	13	60–69 (66)	11	2	6	1	2	5.92–6.14 (6.03±0.16)	1 (1:0)	8 (7:1)	4 (3:1)	—	—	—	—
1998	68	19	61–69 (66)	15	4	7	2	8	1.39–6.01 (3.76±1.61)	2 (1:1)	15 (12:3)	2 (2:0)	1.72–5.83 (4.12)	1.70–4.00 (2.90)	2.50, 4.00 (3.25)	—
1999	110	34	61–69 (66)	18	16	16	3	11	0.71–7.35 (3.78±2.35)	2 (0:2)	17 (12:5)	15 (6:9)	1.90–4.29 (3.43)	1.50–3.20 (2.33)	1.40–4.50 (2.17)	0.90–2.10 (1.44)
2000	112	32	60–69 (66)	24	8	19	0	9	0.21–6.89 (2.79±2.42)	0	21 (17:4)	11 (7:4)	1.78–4.84 (3.26)	1.35–4.74 (2.69)	1.16–3.72 (2.10)	1.15–2.86 (1.93)
2001	98	25	60–69 (65)	17	8	15	1	4	1.40–4.02 (2.72±1.28)	0	12 (11:1)	13 (6:7)	1.70–9.04 (4.37)	1.69	1.14–2.80 (1.76)	0.93–2.13 (1.46)
2002	110	23	60–69 (64)	12	11	7	2	4	1.57–3.89 (2.95±1.08)	0	13 (8:5)	10 (4:6)	2.56–5.93 (3.53)	1.24–1.76 (1.45)	2.41–3.39 (2.98)	0.85–1.69 (1.32)
2003	136	32	61–69 (65)	24	8	22	1	6	0.37–3.07 (1.80±1.14)	0	19 (13:6)	13 (11:2)	1.49–8.26 (3.12)	1.28–2.38 (1.84)	1.33–4.58 (2.47)	0.87, 1.07 (0.97)
2004	120	27	60–69 (65)	16	11	13	3	1	0.52	1 (1:0)	14 (10:4)	12 (5:7)	2.00–14.30 (4.70)	1.36–3.16 (2.07)	1.99–5.04 (2.79)	0.87–2.81 (1.66)
2005	126	31	60–69 (65)	20	11	13	1	1	0.39	2 (0:2)	17 (12:5)	11 (8:3)	1.49–6.16 (3.22)	0.82–2.79 (1.70)	1.47–3.41 (2.12)	0.74–2.42 (1.43)
	1,112	289 (26%)	60–69 (65)	191 (66%)	98 (34%)	147 (51%)	14‡/282 (5%)	66/282 (23%)	0.21–11.23 (3.91±2.80)	10 (5:5) (3%)	170 (126:44) (59%)	107 (59:48) (37%)	1.49–14.30 (3.67) 94§	0.82–4.74 (2.06) 33§	1.14–5.04 (2.35) 48§	0.74–2.86 (1.49) 38§

* Includes only patients surviving >60 days after valve replacement.
† One valve was quadricuspid and the structure in 1 other valve was indeterminate.
‡ Thirteen of the patients died ≤30 days after operation and the other patient, 35 days postoperatively.
§ Number of patients in whom the valve was weighted.
AS = aortic stenosis; AVR = aortic valve replacement; BAV = bicuspid; BUMC = Baylor University Medical Center; DC = discharge; I = Indeterminate; M = man; TAV = tricuspid; UAV = unicuspid; W = woman; — = no information available or not applicable.

hemodynamic and coronary angiographic studies before being referred to BUMC, but the data were not available to us.

Means, SDs, and percentages were calculated to describe the study cohort (n = 289). Due to the low unicuspid (n = 10) and quadricuspid (n = 1) counts, patients with unicuspid, bicuspid, and quadricuspid valve structure were grouped together in the analysis investigating short- and long-term mortality. Unadjusted relative risk (RR) and 95% confidence intervals (95% CI) were estimated to describe the relation between short-term mortality and performance of simultaneous CABG and number of aortic valve cusps. To investigate *late survival,* we excluded patients who died within 60 days of AVR (n = 14) and subjects with missing survival time (n = 9). This left 266 patients for the late survival analysis. Log-rank test statistics were computed to compare unadjusted survival curves for the variables of interest. Unadjusted plot (Kaplan-Meier) was also generated. Statistical analysis was performed using SigmaStat® Version 2.0 (SPSS Inc., Chicago, Illinois) and SAS version 9.1 (SAS Institute, Cary, North Carolina).

This study was approved by Institutional Review Board at Baylor University Medical Center.

Results

Pertinent data in the 289 sexagenarians are summarized in Tables 1 and 2. The native stenotic aortic valve was replaced with a bioprosthesis in 154 of 281 (55%) patients and with a mechanical prosthesis in the remaining 127 of 281 (45%) patients. Of the 289 patients, 191 (66%) were men and 98 (34%) were women. Simultaneous CABG was performed in 147 (51%) patients (Figure 1). Of the 14 patients dying within 60 days of AVR, 13 died within 30 days and 1 patient from 31 to 60 days. The unadjusted analysis of 60-day mortality indicated that it was not affected by valve structure (tricuspid vs uni-bi-quadricuspid RR 0.95, 95% CI 0.30 to 2.90). Likewise, having concomitant CABG did not affect crude mortality (RR 1.31, 95% CI 0.44 to 3.88). In total, 14 (5%) patients died ≤60 days of AVR and another 66 patients (23%) at later periods. Of the patients surviving >60 days, follow-up information was available in 266 patients. As of December 2006, 200 (75%) have survived from 1.04 to 13.58 years (mean 5.66 ± 3.24) (Figure 2). Log-rank test results indicated that *late survival* curves were statistically equivalent for men and women (p = 0.68, n = 266), for patients with low peak transvalvular gradient (≤50 mm Hg) and high peak transvalvular gradient (>50 mm Hg) (p = 0.62, n = 174), for patients receiving simultaneous CABG and patients not receiving CABG (p = 0.11, n = 266), and for patients with an unicuspid/bicuspid/quadricuspid and tricuspid valve structure (p = 0.92, n = 265). Figures 3 and 4 show the unadjusted survival Kaplan-Meier plots comparing patients receiving simultaneous CABG to patients not receiving it and comparing patients across valve structures.

Length of stay in the hospital in the 266 patients who survived the operative period ranged from 3 to 75 days (mean 8.75) and in the 14 who died early (from 0 to 30 days, mean 7.86). Simultaneous CABG increased length of 3 days on average (*crude* p = 0.08). Length of stay in the 134 patients with CABG who survived the operative period

Table 2

Comparison of the 289 sexagenarians having aortic valve replacement for aortic stenosis without versus with simultaneous coronary artery bypass grafting

Year	Without Coronary Artery Bypass Grafting							
	Number Having AVR (M:W)	Length of Stay* (days) Range (Mean±SD)	Died			UAV (M:W)	BAV (M:W)	TAV (M:W)
			Total (M:W)	≤60 days (M:W)	>60 days (M:W)			
1993	1 (1:0)	—	0	—	—	0	0	1 (1:0)
1994	9 (4:5)	6–10 (7.75±1.75)	3 (3:0)	0	3 (3:0)	1 (1:0)	5 (3:2)	3 (0:3)
1995	9 (6:3)	3–9 (5.33±1.87)	3 (3:0)	0	3 (3:0)	0	9 (6:3)	0
1996	5 (4:1)	4–27 (9.40±9.86)	2 (2:0)	0	2 (2:0)	0	3 (2:1)	2 (2:0)
1997	7 (5:2)	4–18 (7.67±5.20)	2 (1:1)	1 (0:1)	1 (1:0)	1 (1:0)	5 (4:1)	1 (0:1)
1998	12 (8:4)	4–14 (8.90±3.14)	7 (4:3)	2 (1:1)	5 (3:2)	2 (1:1)	8 (5:3)	2 (2:0)
1999	18 (7:11)	4–36 (10.71±8.44)	5 (1:4)	1 (0:1)	4 (1:3)	2 (0:2)	10 (5:5)	6 (2:4)
2000	13 (10:3)	3–9 (6.15±1.82)	3 (3:0)	0	3 (3:0)	0	10 (8:2)	3 (2:1)
2001	10 (6:4)	3–16 (7.33±4.03)	2 (2:0)	0	2 (2:0)	0	5 (4:1)	5 (2:3)
2002	16 (8:8)	3–11 (6.33±2.47)	3 (0:3)	1 (0:1)	2 (0:2)	0	11 (7:4)	5 (1:4)
2003	10 (6:4)	3–14 (6.80±3.08)	2 (2:0)	0	2 (2:0)	0	8 (4:4)	2 (2:0)
2004	14 (8:6)	4–15 (7.92±4.03)	1 (0:1)	1 (0:1)	0	0	9 (6:3)	5 (2:3)
2005	18 (9:9)	5–43 (9.94±8.70)	0	—	—	2 (0:2)	10 (5:5)	6 (4:2)
	142 (82:60)	3–43 (8.01±5.51)	33/139 (21:12)	6/139 (1:5)	27/139 (20:7)	8 (3:5)	93 (59:34)	41 (20:21)
	(49%)		(24%)	(4%)	(19%)	(6%)	(65%)	(29%)

Year	With Coronary Artery Bypass Grafting							
	Number Having AVR (M:W)	Length of Stay* (days) Range (Mean±SD)	Died			UAV (M:W)	BAV (M:W)	TAV (M:W)
			Total (M:W)	≤60 days (M:W)	>60 days (M:W)			
1993	5 (4:1)	7–16 (12.0±4.24)	1 (1:0)	0	1 (1:0)	0	4 (4:0)	1 (0:1)
1994	9 (7:2)	7–24 (13.67±7.74)	4 (2:2)	0	4 (2:2)	0	7 (6:1)	2 (1:1)
1995	7 (4:3)	6–8 (6.83±0.75)	3 (2:1)	0	3 (2:1)	0	3 (2:1)	3 (1:2)
1996	8 (4:4)	4–22 (9.50±5.86)	4 (2:2)	0	4 (2:2)	1 (1:0)	3 (1:2)	4 (2:2)
1997	6 (6:0)	5–11 (6.83±2.14)	1 (1:0)	0	1 (1:0)	0	3 (3:0)	3 (3:0)
1998	7 (7:0)	4–13 (7.57±3.31)	3 (3:0)	0	3 (3:0)	0	7 (7:0)	0
1999	16 (11:5)	3–26 (8.57±5.42)	9 (4:5)	2 (0:2)	7 (4:3)	0	7 (7:0)	9 (4:5)
2000	19 (14:5)	5–75 (12.74±15.61)	6 (5:1)	0	6 (5:1)	0	11 (9:2)	8 (5:3)
2001	15 (11:4)	5–38 (10.07±8.59)	3 (2:1)	1 (0:1)	2 (2:0)	0	7 (7:0)	8 (4:4)
2002	7 (4:3)	4–10 (7.33±2.34)	3 (1:2)	1 (0:1)	2 (1:1)	0	2 (1:1)	5 (3:2)
2003	22 (18:4)	4–27 (9.67±5.94)	5 (3:2)	1 (1:0)	4 (2:2)	0	11 (9:2)	11 (9:2)
2004	13 (8:5)	3–11 (7.36±2.54)	3 (2:1)	2 (1:1)	1 (1:0)	1 (1:0)	5 (4:1)	7 (3:4)
2005	13 (11:2)	4–19 (8.25±4.16)	2 (1:1)	1 (0:1)	1 (1:0)	0	7 (7:0)	5 (4:1)
	147 (109:38)	3–75 (9.49±7.73)	47/143 (29:18)	8/143 (2:6)	39/143 (27:12)	2 (2:0)	77 (67:10)	66 (39:27)
	(51%)		(33%)	(6%)	(27%)	(1%)	(52%)	(46%)

* This data only include early survivors.

AVR = aortic valve replacement; BAV = bicuspid aortic valve; M = man; UAV = unicuspid aortic valve; W = woman; TAV = tricuspid aortic valve; — = no information available or not applicable.

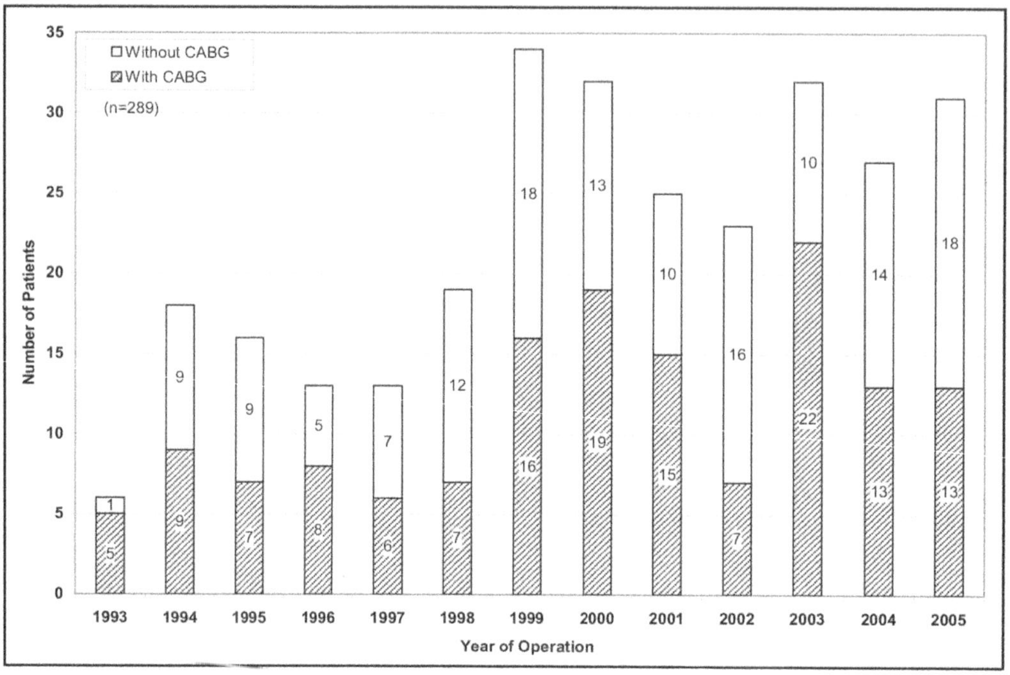

Figure 1. Number of sexagenarians having aortic valve replacement for aortic valve stenosis at Baylor University Medical Center 1993 to 2005 with versus without simultaneous coronary bypass grafting.

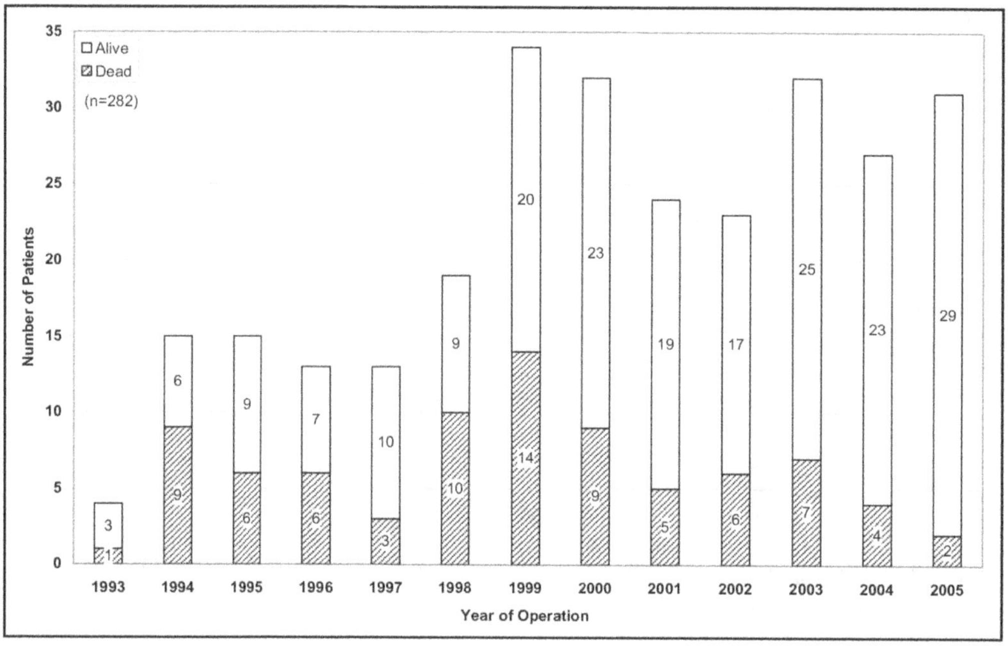

Figure 2. Number of sexagenarians surviving and not surviving aortic valve replacement for aortic stenosis (with or without simultaneous coronary artery bypass grafting) at Baylor University Medical Center 1993 to 2005 (follow-up to 30 December 2006). The deaths include both early and late mortality. Most of the deaths occurred 1 or more years after the year of operation. Note trend of better aortic valve replacement ± coronary artery bypass grafting survival over the 13-year period.

ranged from 3 to 75 days (mean 9.5 ± 7.7), and in the 133 patients without CABG, from 3 to 43 days (mean 8.0 ± 5.5). Of the 8 patients with CABG who died early (≤60 days), the length of hospitalization before death ranged from 0 to 30 days (mean 10.6 ± 10.0); of the 6 patients without CABG who died early, the length of hospitalization ranged from 0 to 8 days (mean 4.2 ± 3.3).

The transvalvular *peak* systolic pressure gradient on average was higher in patients without simultaneous CABG (range 14 to 131 mm Hg, mean 57 ± 24) than in patients receiving concomitant CABG (range 10 to 113 mm Hg, mean 50 ± 24) (*crude* p = 0.03); the mean systolic pressure gradients, ranged from 11 to 128 mm Hg (average 47) and 10 to 90 (average 40) (*crude* p = 0.02), respectively; the calculated aortic valve area, from 0.28 to 1.28 cm^2 (mean 0.72) and from 0.30 to 1.90 cm^2 (mean 0.80) (*crude* p =

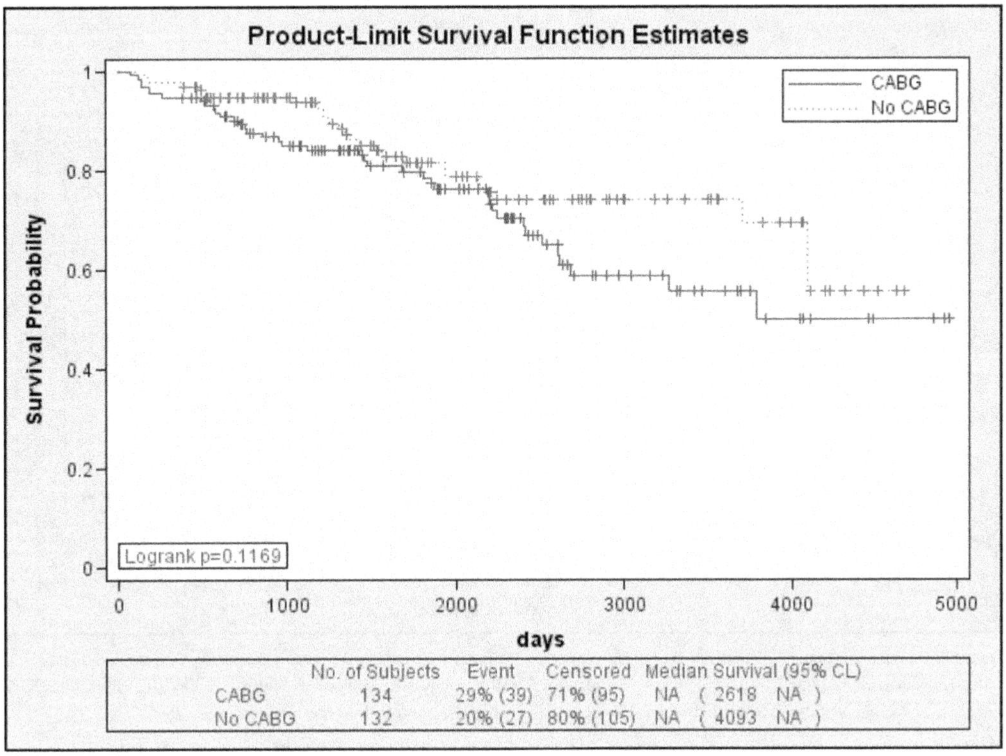

Figure 3. Kaplan-Meier survival curves comparing patients receiving simultaneous coronary artery bypass grafting to patients not receiving it.

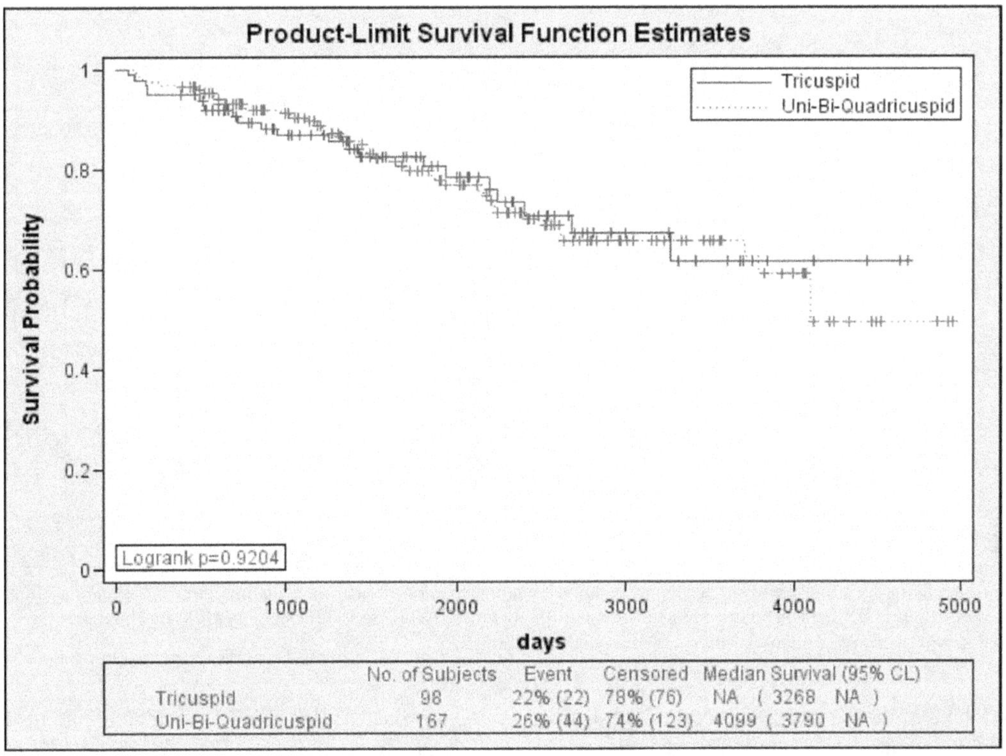

Figure 4. Kaplan-Meier survival curves comparing patients with uni-bi-quadricuspid and patients with tricuspid valve structures.

0.03), respectively; and the left ventricular ejection fraction from 15% to 75% (mean 53%) and from 10% to 80% (mean 47%) (*crude* p = 0.04), respectively.

Another tool providing some evidence of the severity of the AS is gained by the *weight of the operatively excised valves.*[3–6] (Previous studies have shown that men with AS have heavier valves than women and that congenitally unicuspid and bicuspid stenotic aortic valves are heavier than 3-cuspid stenotic aortic valves.[3–6]) The operatively excised unicuspid aortic valves in the 2 men in the present study

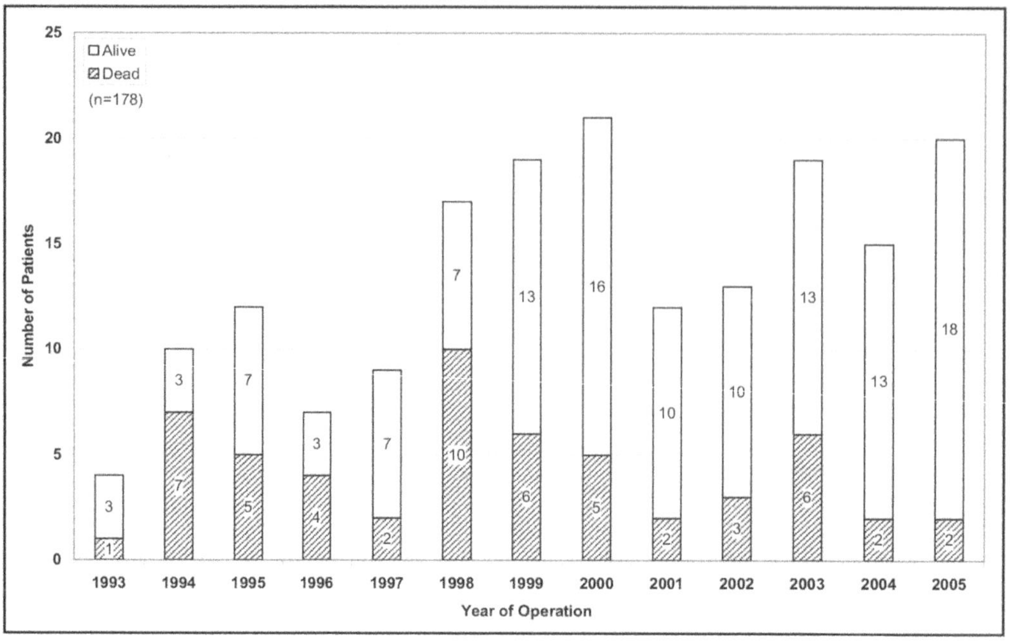

Figure 5. Number of sexagenarians surviving and not surviving aortic valve replacement for aortic stenosis involving a *unicuspid, bicuspid, and quadricuspid* aortic valve (± simultaneous coronary artery bypass grafting) at Baylor University Medical Center 1993 to 2005 (follow-up to 30 December 2006). The deaths include both early and late mortality. Most of the deaths occurred 1 or more years after the year of operation.

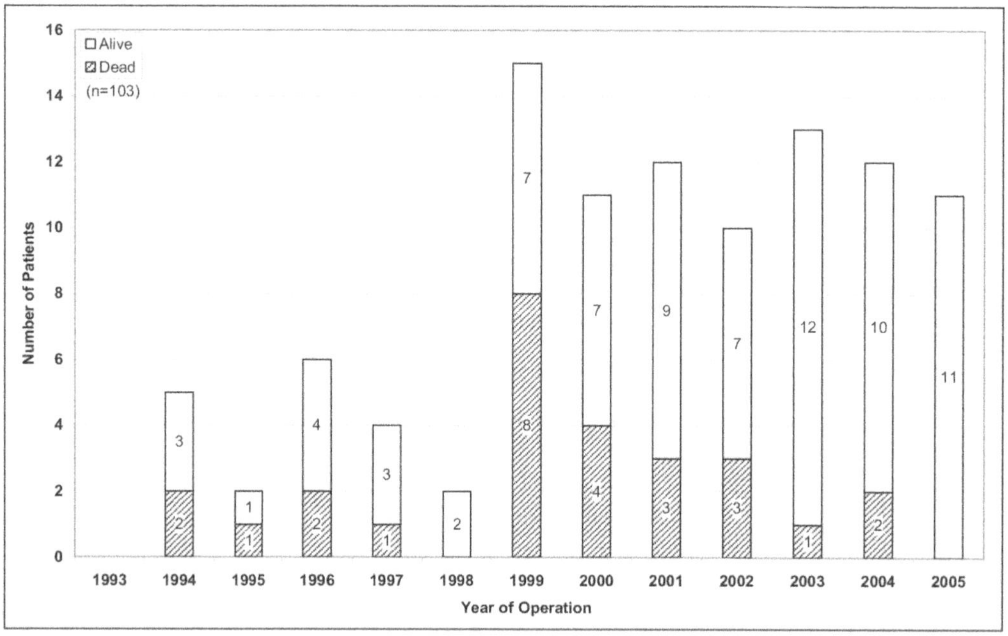

Figure 6. Number of sexagenarians surviving and not surviving aortic valve replacement for aortic stenosis involving a *tricuspid* aortic valve (± simultaneous coronary artery bypass grafting) at Baylor University Medical Center 1993 to 2005 (follow-up to 30 December 2006). The deaths include both early and late mortality. Most of the deaths occurred 1 or more years after the year of operation.

weighed 2.27 and 4.12 g; the bicuspid valves in the 94 men, from 1.49 to 14.3 g (mean 3.67), and the tricuspid aortic valves in the 48 men, from 1.14 to 5.04 g (mean 2.35). In contrast, the 5 unicuspid valves in women weighed from 1.02 to 4.50 g (mean 2.44); the bicuspid valves in the 33 women, from 0.82 to 4.74 g (mean 2.06), and the tricuspid aortic valves in the 38 women, from 0.74 to 2.86 g (mean 1.49). *Aortic valve structure* in the 289 patients was the following: unicuspid in 10 (3%); bicuspid in 170 (59%); 3-cuspid in 107 (37%), quadricuspid in 1 (<1%), and indeterminate in 1 (<1%) (Figures 5 and 6).

Discussion

The present study focused on a large group of sexagenarians having AVR for AS at the same US medical center during a recent 13-year period. Early mortality (≤60 days) was 5% and similar in the patients with unicuspid/bicuspid and tricuspid valves. Likewise, the unadjusted analysis of *late survival* indicated that gender, valve structure, preoperative severity of the AS, or performance of simultaneous CABG did not effect *late survival* in sexagenarians undergoing AVR for AS.

The positive features of the present study include a large number of sexagenarians, relatively long post-AVR follow-up, preoperative hemodynamic data in most patients, and knowledge of aortic valve structure and weight. That all valves were examined by the same individual (WCR) produced uniformity not available if valve structure was that recorded in the operative note by a number of different cardiac surgeons, each of whom might have different views of what constituted a congenitally malformed or a 3-cuspid aortic valve with fusion of ≥1 aortic valve commissures. (WCR has been a student of aortic valve structure for >40 years.) The negative features of the present study include lack of information on preoperative and postoperative symptoms and functional class, on early postoperative complications, co-morbidities, late quality of life, numbers of epicardial coronary arteries narrowed >50% in diameter, and causes of death late postoperatively.

1. Roberts WC, Ko JM, Garner WL, Filardo G, Henry AC, Hebeler RF JR, Matter GJ, Hamman BL. Valve structure and survival in octogenarians having aortic valve replacement for aortic stenosis (±aortic regurgitation) with versus without coronary artery bypass grafting at a single US medical center (1993 to 2005). *Am J Cardiol* 2007 (in press).
2. Roberts WC, Ko JM, Filardo G, Henry AC, Hebeler RF JR, Cheung EH, Matter GJ, Hamman BL. Valve structure and survival in septuagenarians having aortic valve replacement for aortic stenosis (±aortic regurgitation) with versus without coronary artery bypass grafting at a single US medical center (1993 to 2005). *Am J Cardiol* 2007 (in press).
3. Roberts WC, Ko JM. Weights of operatively excised stenotic unicuspid, bicuspid, and tricuspid aortic valves and their relation to age, sex, body mass index, and presence or absence of concomitant coronary artery bypass grafting. *Am J Cardiol* 2003:92:1057–1065.
4. Roberts WC, Ko JM. Relation of weights of operatively excised stenotic aortic valves to preoperative transvalvular peak systolic pressure gradients and to calculated aortic valve areas. *J Am Coll Cardiol* 2004;44: 1847–1855.
5. Roberts WC, Ko JM. Frequency by decades of unicuspid, bicuspid, and tricuspid aortic valves in adults having isolated aortic valve replacement for aortic stenosis, with or without associated aortic regurgitation. *Circulation* 2005;111:920–925.
6. Roberts WC, Ko JM, Hamilton C. Comparison of valve structure, valve weight, and severity of the valve obstruction in 1849 patients having isolated aortic valve replacement for aortic valve stenosis (with or without associated aortic regurgitation) studied at 3 different medical centers in 2 different time periods. *Circulation* 2006;114:422–429.

Valve Structure and Survival in *Quinquagenarians* Having Aortic Valve Replacement for Aortic Stenosis (±Aortic Regurgitation) With Versus Without Coronary Artery Bypass Grafting at a Single US Medical Center (1993 to 2005)

William Clifford Roberts, MD[a,b,d,*], Jong Mi Ko, BA[d], Giovanni Filardo, PhD, MPH[e,f], Albert Carl Henry, MD[c], Robert Frederick Hebeler, Jr, MD[c], Edson Hoi-Kam Cheung, MD[c], Gregory John Matter, MD[c], and Baron Lloyd Hamman, MD[c]

The purpose of this study was to determine the effect of simultaneous coronary artery bypass grafting (CABG) and the influence of valve structure on both early and late survival in quinquagenarians having aortic valve replacement (AVR) for aortic stenosis (AS) (with or without aortic regurgitation). We analyzed survival and valve structure in 120 quinquagenarians having AVR for AS from 1993 through 2005 at Baylor University Medical Center, including 44 (37%) with and 76 (63%) without simultaneous CABG. Of the 120 patients, 2 (2%) died within 30 days of operation and none from 31 to 60 days postoperatively. Fifteen other patients (13%) died from >60 days to up to 13 years postoperatively. The unadjusted survival analysis showed that late survival was significantly better in the unicuspid/bicuspid valve structure group than in the tricuspid valve structure group (log-rank test p = 0.001), but that it was not affected by gender (male vs female), preoperative severity of the AS (transvalvular peak pressure gradient >50 vs ≤50 mm Hg), or by performance of CABG. The aortic valve was congenitally unicuspid in 18 patients (15%), congenitally bicuspid in 84 (70%), and 3-cuspid in 18 (15%). In conclusion, aortic valve structure affected the unadjusted late survival in quinquagenarians undergoing AVR for AS, but concomitant CABG, gender, and transvalvular peak systolic gradient had no effect. **(Am J Cardiol 2007;100:1584–1591)**

We recently described aortic valve structure and early and late survival in 9 *nonagenarians*, in 196 *octogenarians*, in 424 *septuagenarians*, and in 289 *sexagenarians* having aortic valve replacement (AVR) for aortic stenosis (AS) at Baylor University Medical Center from 1993 to 2005.[1–4] The present report focuses on aortic valve structure and survival in 120 *quinquagenarians* having AVR for AS at the same medical center in the same time frame.

Methods

From January 1993 through December 2005, a total of 1,112 patients underwent AVR for AS (with or without aortic regurgitation) with or without simultaneous CABG and without mitral valve replacement at Baylor University Medical Center. Of the 1,112 patients, 120 (11%) were aged 50 to 59, and they are the subject of this report. The operatively excised aortic valve in each patient was submitted to the surgical pathology section and all 120 valves were examined and described by 1 of us (WCR). The valves were photographed by JMK. Since 1998, all operatively excised valves have been weighed by 1 of us (WCR).

The echocardiographic and hemodynamic data in the 120 quinquagenarians were collected by JMK from the cardiovascular computer database (Apollo Advance C/S, version 4.2.13, LUMEDX Corp., Oakland, California) and from the medical records. Information regarding death of any patient was obtained from 2 sources: (1) early death information was obtained from the medical record, and (2) post-hospital death information was obtained and confirmed from the Social Security Death Index.

Echocardiographic data preoperatively were available to us in 50 patients (42%). Cardiac catheterization data were available to us in most patients: peak transvalvular pressure gradients in 74 patients (62%), mean transvalvular pressure gradients in 70 (58%), aortic valve area in 76 patients (63%), and left ventricular ejection fraction in 56 patients (47%). Most patients in whom cardiac catheterization data were not available to WCR and JMK were referred directly to a cardiovascular surgeon. These patients had hemodynamic and coronary angiographic studies before being referred to Baylor University Medical Center, but the data are not available to us.

Means, standard deviations (SD), and percentages were calculated to describe the study cohort (n = 120). Due to the low number of deaths (n = 2), short-term mortality analysis was not conducted. To investigate *late survival*, we excluded patients who died within 60 days of AVR (n = 2). This left 118 patients for analysis of late survival. Patients with unicuspid and bicuspid valve structure were grouped together in the analysis of long-term mortality. Log-rank test statistics were computed to compare unadjusted sur-

[a]Departments of Internal Medicine (Division of Cardiology), [b]Pathology, and [c]Cardiothoracic Surgery, and the [d]Baylor Heart and Vascular Institute, Baylor University Medical Center, Dallas, Texas 75246; and the [e]Institute for Health Care Research and Improvement, Baylor Health Care System and the [f]Department of Statistical Science, Southern Methodist University, Dallas, Texas. Manuscript received July 27, 2007; revised manuscript received and accepted August 6, 2007.

*Corresponding author: Tel: 214-820-7911, Fax: 214-820-7533.

E-mail: wc.roberts@baylorhealth.edu (W.C. Roberts).

Table 1
Clinical and valve structure information in the 120 quinquagenarians having aortic valve replacement for isolated aortic stenosis with or without simultaneous coronary artery bypass grafting

Year	Number of AVRs for AS at BUMC	Number of Quinguagenarians	Age (year) Range (mean)	Men	Women	Coronary Artery Bypass Grafting	Died		Interval (years) AVR-Death* Range (mean ± SD)
							≤60 days	>60 days	
1993	31	2	52, 53 (53)	2	0	0	0	0	—
1994	50	1	51	1	0	0	0	0	—
1995	44	6	51–59 (56)	6	0	5	0	2	9.19, 11.53 (10.36 ± 1.65)
1996	56	8	51–59 (56)	4	4	4	0	1	3.83
1997	51	8	50–58 (54)	5	3	3	1	2	6.95, 9.60 (8.28 ± 1.87)
1998	68	6	51–59 (55)	5	1	3	1	0	—
1999	110	11	50–57 (54)	9	2	2	0	2	6.59, 7.02 (6.81 ± 0.30)
2000	112	14	51–59 (55)	11	3	8	0	4	2.79–5.79 (4.63 ± 1.42)
2001	98	8	51–59 (54)	6	2	4	0	2	0.18, 0.31 (0.25 ± 0.09)
2002	110	9	52–58 (55)	7	2	2	0	0	—
2003	136	15	50–59 (55)	7	8	4	0	1	0.36
2004	120	17	50–59 (55)	9	8	5	0	0	—
2005	126	15	50–59 (55)	12	3	4	0	1	0.21
	1,112	120 (11%)	50–59 (55)	84 (70%)	36 (30%)	44 (37%)	2† (2%)	15 (13%)	0.18–11.53 (4.95)

*Includes only patients surviving >60 days after valve replacement.
†Two patients died 11 and 12 days after operation.
‡Number of patients in whom the valve was weighed.
AS = aortic stenosis; AVR = aortic valve replacement; BAV = bicuspid; BUMC = Baylor University Medical Center; DC = discharge; I = indeterminate; M = man; TAV = tricuspid; UAV = unicuspid; W = woman.

Table 2
Comparison of the 120 quinquagenarians having aortic valve replacement for aortic stenosis without-vs-with simultaneous coronary artery bypass grafting

Year	Without Coronary Artery Bypass Grafting							
	Number Having AVR (M:W)	Length of Stay* (days) Range (mean ± SD)	Died			UAV (M:W)	BAV (M:W)	TAV (M:W)
			Total (M:W)	≤60 days (M:W)	>60 days (M:W)			
1993	2 (2:0)	7, 8 (7.50 ± 0.71)	0	—	—	0	2 (2:0)	0
1994	1 (1:0)	6	0	—	—	0	1 (1:0)	0
1995	1 (1:0)	7	0	—	—	0	1 (1:0)	0
1996	4 (3:1)	5–14 (7.50 ± 4.36)	1 (1:0)	0	1 (1:0)	1 (1:0)	3 (2:1)	0
1997	5 (3:2)	5–31 (12.50 ± 12.48)	3 (2:1)	1 (1:0)	2 (1:1)	3 (2:1)	1 (0:1)	1 (1:0)
1998	3 (3:0)	4–5 (4.33 ± 0.58)	0	—	—	1 (1:0)	2 (2:0)	0
1999	9 (7:2)	3–7 (5.22 ± 1.30)	2 (2:0)	0	2 (2:0)	1 (1:0)	8 (6:2)	0
2000	6 (4:2)	3–14 (7.67 ± 4.08)	1 (0:1)	0	1 (0:1)	0	4 (3:1)	2 (1:1)
2001	4 (4:0)	4–5 (4.50 ± 0.58)	0	—	—	2 (2:0)	2 (2:0)	0
2002	7 (5:2)	4–13 (7.43 ± 3.10)	0	—	—	0	7 (5:2)	0
2003	11 (5:6)	4–11 (6.82 ± 2.56)	0	—	—	1 (1:0)	7 (2:5)	3 (2:1)
2004	12 (6:6)	4–11 (5.58 ± 2.11)	0	—	—	3 (1:2)	9 (5:4)	0
2005	11 (9:2)	3–8 (5.00 ± 1.55)	0	—	—	2 (2:0)	9 (7:2)	0
	76 (53:23) (63%)	3–31 (6.41 ± 3.80)	7 (5:2) (9%)	1 (1:0) (1%)	6 (4:2) (8%)	14 (11:3) (18%)	56 (38:18) (74%)	6 (4:2) (8%)

*These data only include early survivors.
— = no information available or not applicable; AVR = aortic valve replacement; M = man; W = woman.

vival curves for the variables of interest. Unadjusted (Kaplan-Meier) plots were also generated. Statistical analysis was performed using SigmaStat Version 2.0 (SPSS Inc., Chicago, Illinois) and SAS version 9.1 (SAS Institute, Cary, North Carolina).

This study was approved by Institutional Review Board at Baylor University Medical Center.

Results

Data in the 120 quinquagenarians are summarized in Tables 1 and 2. The native stenotic aortic valve was replaced with a bioprosthesis in 30 (25%) patients and with a mechanical prosthesis in the remaining 90 (75%) patients. Of the 120 patients, 84 (70%) were men and 36 (30%) were women.

Table 1
(continued)

Aortic Value Structure			Aortic Value Weight (g) Range (mean)					
UAV (M:W)	BAV (M:W)	TAV (M:W)	Unicuspid		Bicuspid		Tricuspid	
			Men	Women	Men	Women	Men	Women
0	2 (2:0)	0	—	—	—	—	—	—
0	1 (1:0)	0	—	—	—	—	—	—
2 (2:0)	1 (1:0)	3 (3:0)	—	—	—	—	—	—
1 (1:0)	7 (3:4)	0	—	—	—	—	—	—
3 (2:1)	4 (2:2)	1 (1:0)	—	—	—	—	—	—
1 (1:0)	4 (4:0)	1 (0:1)	7.70	—	2.44–4.50 (3.18)	—	—	1.70
1 (1:0)	10 (8:2)	0	3.33	—	2.10–5.50 (3.54)	0.90, 2.36 (1.63)	—	—
0	10 (8:2)	4 (3:1)	—	—	1.34–4.40 (2.62)	2.94, 3.49 (3.22)	1.23–2.63 (1.81)	1.72
2 (2:0)	4 (3:1)	2 (1:1)	3.93, 4.17 (4.05)	—	2.65–4.14 (3.24)	4.97	1.19	2.20
0	9 (7:2)	0	—	—	1.69–5.06 (3.48)	1.52, 1.99 (1.76)	—	—
1 (1:0)	9 (3:6)	5 (3:2)	4.07	—	0.89–2.20 (1.61)	1.12–4.94 (2.38)	1.71–1.77 (1.75)	1.74, 1.80 (1.77)
4 (1:3)	11 (6:5)	2 (2:0)	5.03	2.22–4.30 (3.18)	1.85–4.25 (3.58)	0.73–2.99 (1.86)	1.48, 1.57 (1.53)	—
3 (3:0)	12 (9:3)	0	1.72–5.44 (3.58)	—	0.90–6.44 (3.15)	1.53–2.04 (1.74)	—	—
18 (14:4) (15%)	84 (57:27) (70%)	18 (13:5) (15%)	1.72–7.70 (4.33) 9‡	2.22–4.30 (3.18) 3‡	0.89–6.44 (3.14) 47‡	0.73–4.97 (2.23) 21‡	1.19–2.63 (1.66) 9‡	1.70–2.20 (1.83) 5‡

Table 2
(continued)

With Coronary Artery Bypass Grafting							
Number Having AVR (M:W)	Length of Stay* (days) Range (mean ± SD)	Died			UAV (M:W)	BAV (M:W)	TAV (M:W)
		Total (M:W)	≤60 days (M:W)	>60 days (M:W)			
0	—	—	—	—	—	—	—
0	—	—	—	—	—	—	—
5 (5:0)	4–7 (5.80 ± 1.30)	2 (2:0)	0	2 (2:0)	2 (2:0)	0	3 (3:0)
4 (1:3)	5–11 (6.75 ± 2.87)	0	—	—	0	4 (1:3)	0
3 (2:1)	4–6 (5.00 ± 1.00)	0	—	—	0	3 (2:1)	0
3 (2:1)	4–7 (5.50 ± 2.12)	1 (1:0)	1 (1:0)	0	0	2 (2:0)	1 (0:1)
2 (2:0)	5, 12 (8.50 ± 4.95)	0	—	—	0	2 (2:0)	0
8 (7:1)	5–21 (9.63 ± 6.63)	3 (3:0)	0	3 (3:0)	0	6 (5:1)	2 (2:0)
4 (2:2)	9–61 (27.75 ± 24.38)	2 (1:1)	0	2 (1:1)	0	2 (1:1)	2 (1:1)
2 (2:0)	6, 13 (9.50 ± 4.95)	0	—	—	0	2 (2:0)	0
4 (2:2)	4–8 (6.00 ± 1.83)	1 (0:1)	0	1 (0:1)	0	2 (1:1)	2 (1:1)
5 (3:2)	6–19 (10.40 ± 5.03)	0	—	—	1 (0:1)	2 (1:1)	2 (2:0)
4 (3:1)	7–12 (9.00 ± 2.16)	1 (0:1)	0	1 (0:1)	1 (1:0)	3 (2:1)	0
44 (31:13) (37%)	4–61 (9.72 ± 9.61)	10 (7:3) (23%)	1 (1:0) (2%)	9 (6:3) (20%)	4 (3:1) (9%)	28 (19:9) (64%)	12 (9:3) (27%)

Simultaneous CABG was performed in 44 (37%) patients (Figure 1). Of the 2 patients dying within 60 days of AVR, 1 died 11 days and the other patient 12 days after the operation. In total, 2 (2%) patients died ≤60 days of AVR and an additional 15 patients (13%) at later periods. Of the patients surviving >60 days, follow-up information was available in all 118 patients. As of December 2006, 103 (86%) have survived from 1.05 to 13.52 years (mean 5.53 ± 3.33) (Figure 2). Log-rank test results indicated that *late survival* curves were statistically equivalent for men and women ($p = 0.43$, $n = 118$), for patients with low peak transvalvular gradient (≤50 mm Hg) and high peak transvalvular gradients (>50 mm Hg) ($p = 0.08$, $n = 73$), and for patients having simultaneous CABG and patients not

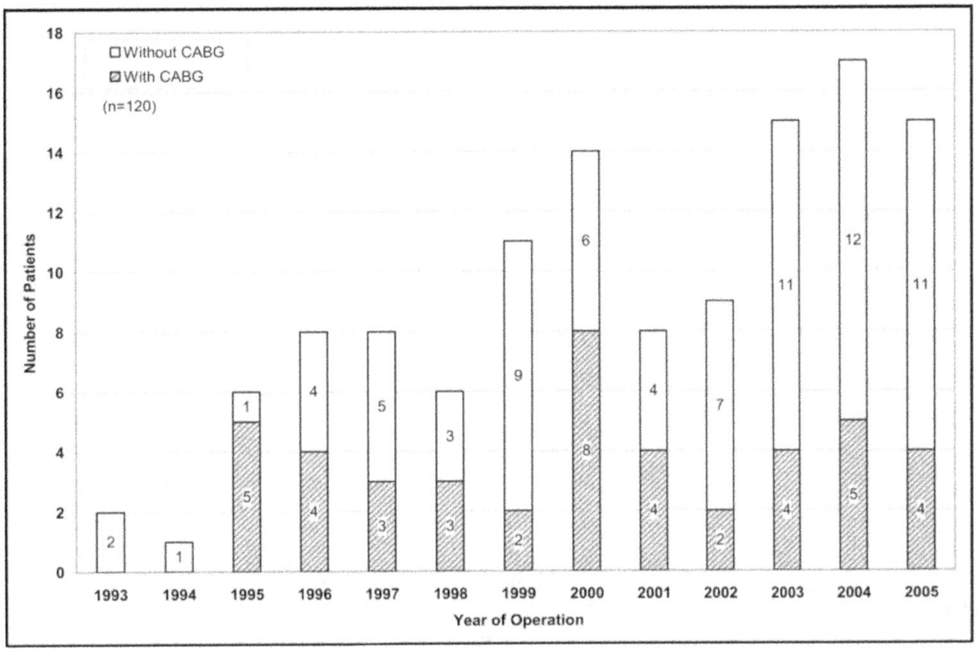

Figure 1. Number of quinquagenarians having aortic valve replacement for aortic valve stenosis at Baylor University Medical Center 1993 to 2005 with versus without simultaneous coronary bypass grafting.

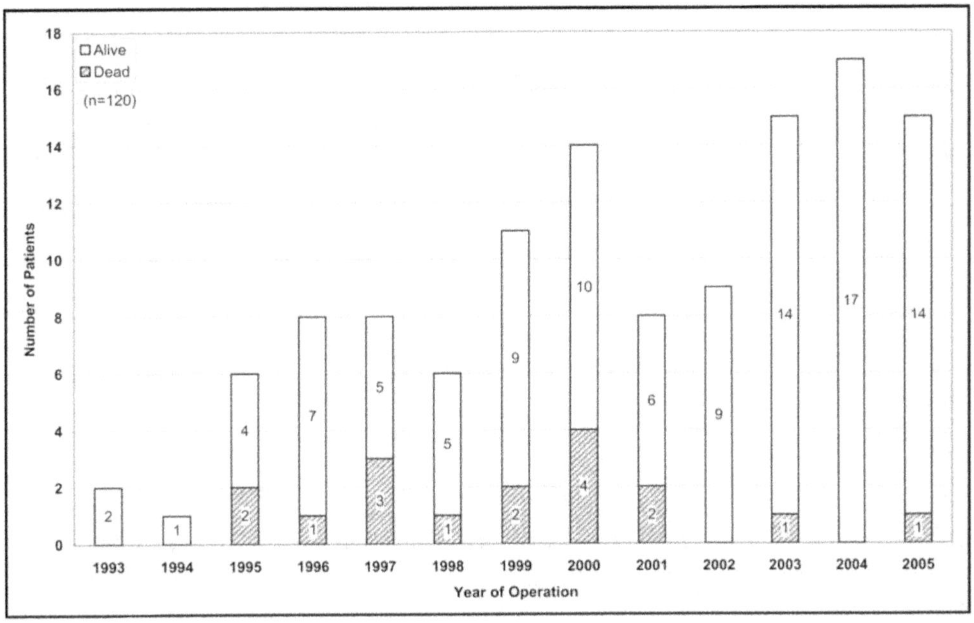

Figure 2. Number of quinquagenarians surviving and not surviving aortic valve replacement for aortic stenosis (with or without simultaneous coronary artery bypass grafting) at Baylor University Medical Center 1993 to 2005 (follow-up to 30 December 2006). Most of the deaths occurred 1 or more years after the year of operation.

having CABG ($p = 0.35$, $n = 118$). The unadjusted analysis indicated that late survival curves were statistically different for patients with a unicuspid/bicuspid and tricuspid valve structure ($p = 0.001$, $n = 118$). Figures 3 and 4 show the unadjusted survival Kaplan-Meier plots comparing patients with versus without simultaneous CABG and those with unicuspid/bicuspid versus 3-cuspid aortic valves.

Length of stay in the hospital in the 118 patients who survived the operative period ranged from 3 to 61 days (mean 7.62) and in the 2 who died early, 11 and 12 days, respectively. Hospital stay in 43 having simultaneous CABG averaged 3 days longer than in the 75 not having CABG (4 to 61 days [mean 9.72 ± 9.61] vs 3 to 31 days [mean 6.41 ± 3.80], respectively, *crude* $p = 0.001$).

The transvalvular *peak* systolic pressure gradient in the patients without simultaneous CABG averaged 62 ± 27 mm Hg and in patients having concomitant CABG, 50 ± 24 mm Hg, (*crude* $p = 0.45$); the mean systolic pressure gradients ranged from 13 to 91 mm Hg (average 50) and 10 to 77 mm Hg (average 40) (*crude* $p = 0.52$), respectively; the calcu-

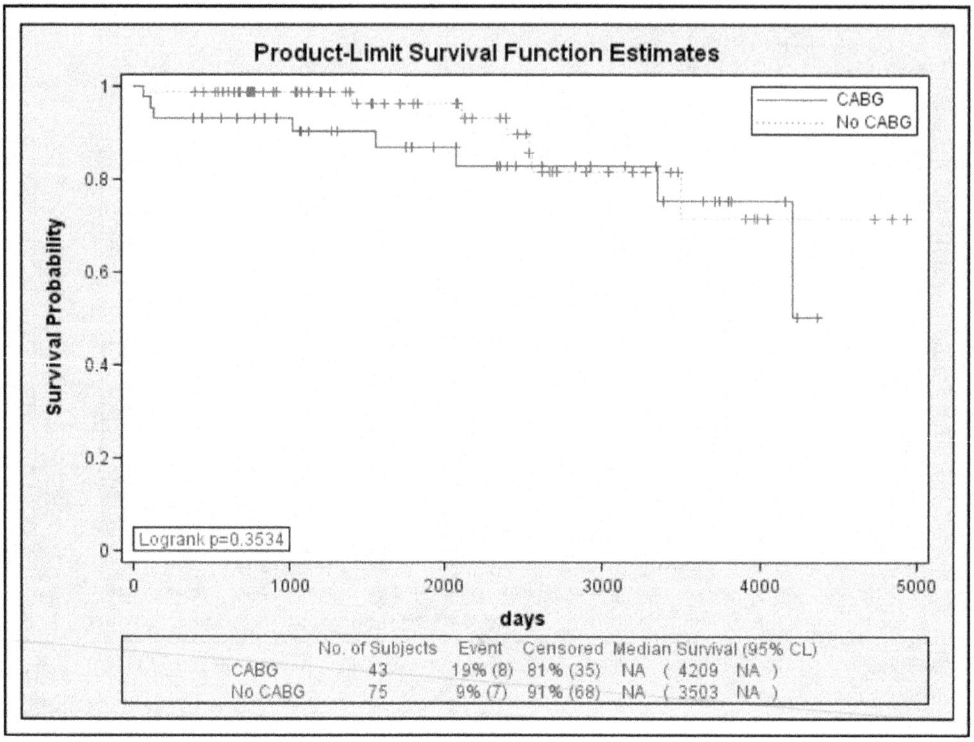

Figure 3. Kaplan-Meier survival curves comparing patients receiving simultaneous coronary artery bypass grafting with patients not receiving it.

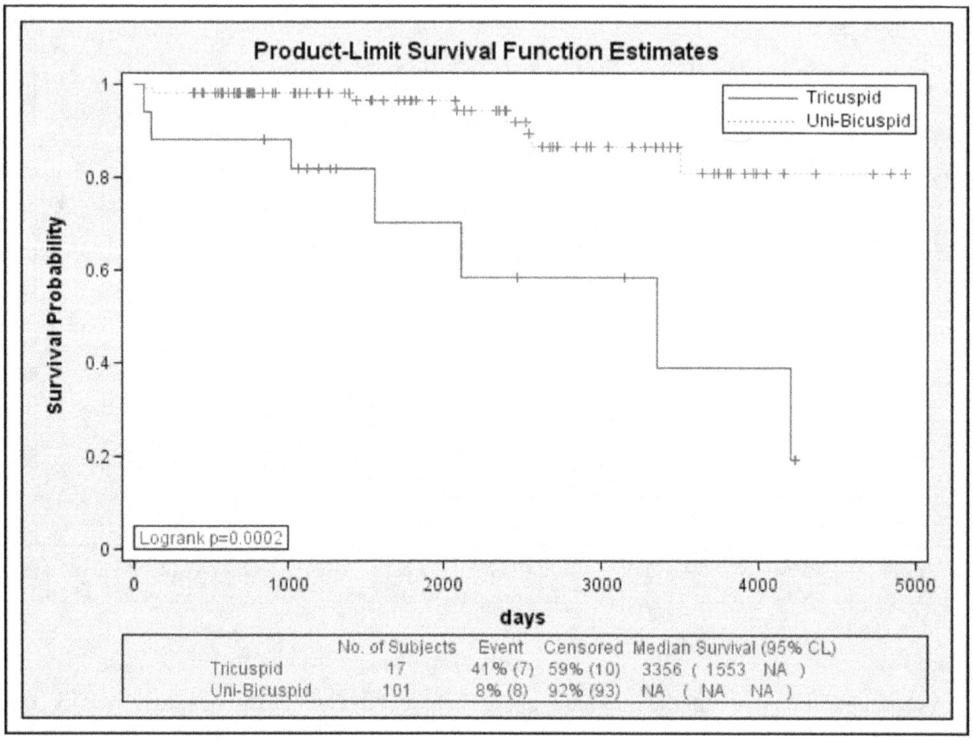

Figure 4. Kaplan-Meier survival curves comparing patients with uni/bicuspid and patients with tricuspid valve structures.

lated aortic valve area, from 0.40 to 1.66 cm^2 (mean 0.75) and from 0.40 to 1.24 cm^2 (mean 0.79) (*crude* p = 0.04), respectively; and the left ventricular ejection fraction from 10% to 75% (mean 53) and from 15% to 68% (mean 49) (*crude* p = 0.34), respectively.

Another tool providing some evidence of the severity of the AS is gained by the *weight of the operatively excised valves*.[5–8] (Previous studies have shown that men with AS have heavier valves than women and that congenitally unicuspid and bicuspid stenotic aortic valves are heavier than 3-cuspid stenotic aortic valves.[5–8]) The operatively excised unicuspid aortic valves in the 9 men in the present study

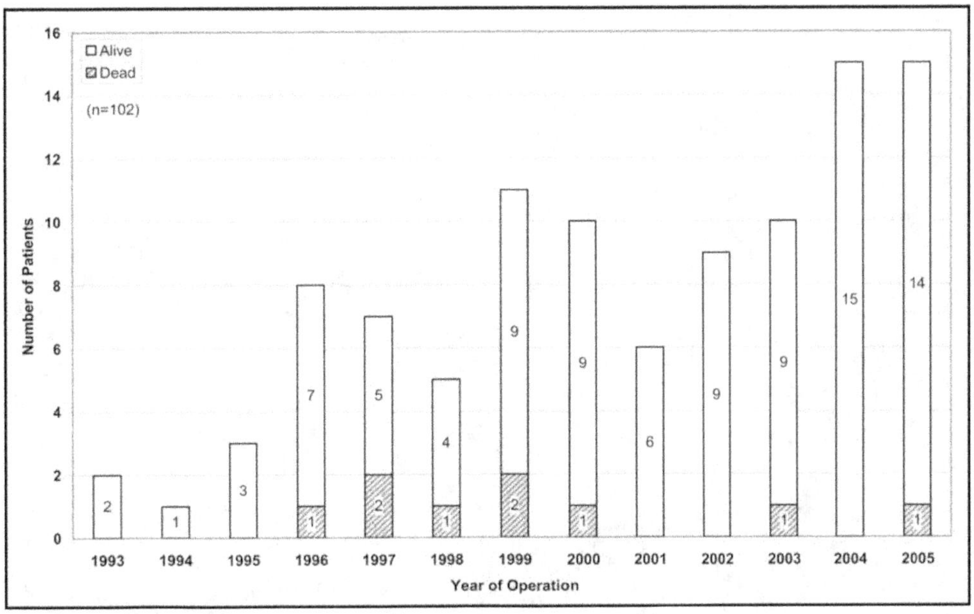

Figure 5. Number of quinquagenarians surviving and not surviving aortic valve replacement for aortic stenosis involving a *unicuspid and bicuspid* aortic valve (± simultaneous coronary artery bypass grafting) at Baylor University Medical Center 1993 to 2005 (follow-up to 30 December 2006). Most of the deaths occurred 1 or more years after the year of operation.

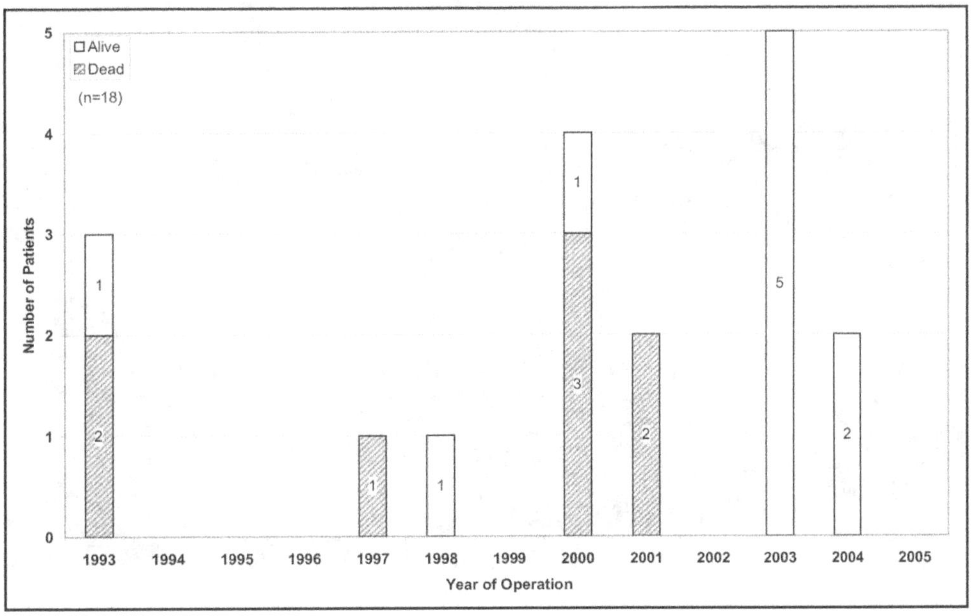

Figure 6. Number of quinquagenarians surviving and not surviving aortic valve replacement for aortic stenosis involving a *tricuspid* aortic valve (± simultaneous coronary artery bypass grafting) at Baylor University Medical Center 1993 to 2005 (follow-up to 30 December 2006). Most of the deaths occurred 1 or more years after the year of operation.

ranged from 1.72 to 7.70 g (mean 4.33); the bicuspid valves in the 47 men, from 0.89 to 6.44 g (mean 3.14), and the tricuspid aortic valves in the 9 men, from 1.19 to 2.63 g (mean 1.66). In contrast, the 3 unicuspid valves in women weighed 2.22, 3.03, and 4.30 g (mean 3.18); the bicuspid valves in the 21 women, from 0.73 to 4.97 g (mean 2.23), and the tricuspid aortic valves in the 5 women, from 1.70 to 2.20 g (mean 1.83). Of the 120 patients, 18 (15%) had congenitally unicuspid aortic valves, 84 (70%) congenitally bicuspid, and 18 (15%), 3-cuspid valves (Figures 5 to 7).

Discussion

The present study focused on a large group of *quinquagenarians* having AVR for AS at the same US medical center during a recent 13-year period. Early mortality analysis (≤60 days) was not possible because only 2 of the 120 patients died early. Unadjusted analysis indicated that gender, preoperative severity of the AS, or performance of simultaneous CABG had no effect on *late survival*. Late survival, however, was significantly better in patients with

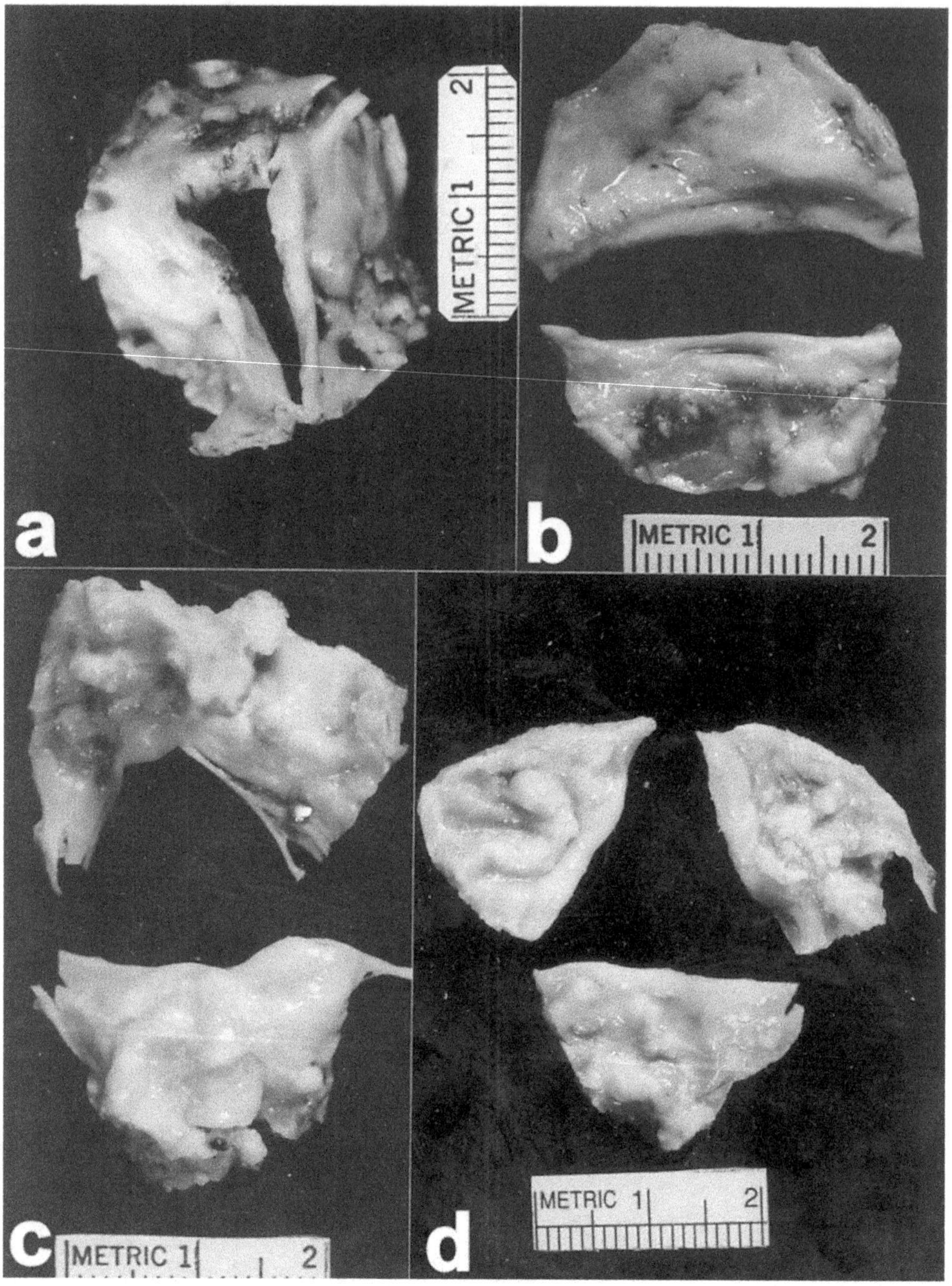

Figure 7. Photographs of 4 operatively excised stenotic aortic valves: *(A)* Congenitally unicuspid valve from a 50-year-old man in whom the mean systolic gradient was 60 mm Hg, the calculated aortic valve area, 0.90 cm^2, and the valve weight, 4.07 g. *(B)* Congenitally bicuspid valve from a 50-year-old man in whom the valve weighed 1.75 g. *(C)* Congenitally bicuspid valve from 59-year-old man in whom the peak systolic gradient was 18 mm Hg, the calculated aortic valve area, 0.74 cm^2, and the valve weight, 2.20 g. *(D)* Tricuspid valve from a 59-year-old man in whom the peak systolic gradient was 38 mm Hg, the calculated aortic valve area, 0.89 cm^2, and the valve weight, 1.76 g.

unicuspid/bicuspid valves than in patients with tricuspid aortic valves.

The positive features of the present study include a relatively large number of quinquagenarians, relatively long post-AVR follow-up, preoperative hemodynamic data in most patients, and knowledge of aortic valve structure and weight. That all valves were examined by the same individual (WCR) produced uniformity not available if valve structure was that recorded in the operative note by a number of different cardiac surgeons, each of whom might have different views of what constituted a congenitally malformed or a 3-cuspid aortic valve with fusion of 1 or more aortic valve commissures. (WCR has been a student of aortic valve structure for >40 years.) The negative features of the present study include lack of information on preoperative and postoperative symptoms and functional class, on early postoperative complications, co-morbidities, late quality of life, numbers of epicardial coronary arteries narrowed >50% in diameter, and causes of late death postoperatively.

1. Roberts WC. Ko JM. Matter GJ. Aortic valve replacement for aortic stenosis in nonagenarians. *Am J Cardiol* 2006;98:1251–1253.
2. Roberts WC, Ko JM, Garner WL, Filardo G, Henry AC, Hebeler RF Jr, Matter GJ, Hamman BL. Valve structure and survival in octogenarians having aortic valve replacement for aortic stenosis (±aortic regurgitation) with versus without coronary artery bypass grafting at a single US medical center (1993 to 2005). *Am J Cardiol* 2007;100:489–495.
3. Roberts WC, Ko JM, Filardo G, Henry AC, Hebeler RF JR, Cheung EH, Matter GJ, Hamman BL. Valve structure and survival in septuagenarians having aortic valve replacement for aortic stenosis (±aortic regurgitation) with versus without coronary artery bypass grafting at a single US medical center (1993 to 2005). *Am J Cardiol* 2007:100:1157–1165.
4. Roberts WC, Ko JM, Filardo G, Henry AC, Hebeler RF JR, Cheung EH, Matter GJ, Hamman BL. Valve structure and survival in sexagenarians having aortic valve replacement for aortic stenosis (±aortic regurgitation) with versus without coronary artery bypass grafting at a single US medical center (1993 to 2005). *Am J Cardiol* 2007;100:1286–1292.
5. Roberts WC, Ko JM. Weights of operatively excised stenotic unicuspid, bicuspid, and tricuspid aortic valves and their relation to age, sex, body mass index, and presence or absence of concomitant coronary artery bypass grafting. *Am J Cardiol* 2003;92:1057–1065.
6. Roberts WC, Ko JM. Relation of weights of operatively excised stenotic aortic valves to preoperative transvalvular peak systolic pressure gradients and to calculated aortic valve areas. *J Am Coll Cardiol* 2004;44: 1847–1855.
7. Roberts WC, Ko JM. Frequency by decades of unicuspid, bicuspid, and tricuspid aortic valves in adults having isolated aortic valve replacement for aortic stenosis, with or without associated aortic regurgitation. *Circulation* 2005;111:920–925.
8. Roberts WC, Ko JM, Hamilton C. Comparison of valve structure, valve weight, and severity of the valve obstruction in 1849 patients having isolated aortic valve replacement for aortic valve stenosis (with or without associated aortic regurgitation) studied at 3 different medical centers in 2 different time periods. *Circulation* 2006;114:422–429.

Valve Structure and Survival in *Quadragenarians* Having Aortic Valve Replacement for Aortic Stenosis (±Aortic Regurgitation) With Versus Without Coronary Artery Bypass Grafting at a Single US Medical Center (1993 to 2005)

William Clifford Roberts, MD[a,b,d,*], Jong Mi Ko, BA[d], Giovanni Filardo, PhD, MPH[e,f], Benjamin L. Kitchens[g], Albert Carl Henry, MD[c], Robert Frederick Hebeler, Jr., MD[c], Edson Hoi-Kam Cheung, MD[c], Gregory John Matter, MD[c], and Baron Lloyd Hamman, MD[c]

The purpose of this study was to determine the effect of simultaneous coronary artery bypass grafting (CABG) and the influence of valve structure on both early and late survival in quadragenarians having aortic valve replacement (AVR) for aortic stenosis (AS) (with or without aortic regurgitation). We analyzed survival and valve structure in 48 adults (12 women), aged 40 to 49 years, having AVR for AS from 1993 through 2005 at Baylor University Medical Center, including 7 (15%) with and 41 (85%) without simultaneous CABG. Of the 48 quadragenarians, none died within 60 days of operation. Assessment of the relation between long-term survival and gender, aortic valve structure, preoperative severity of the AS, and concomitant CABG was not possible due to the low mortality. Four patients (9%) died >60 days after AVR: at 1.8, 6.3, 7.1, and 9.9 years, respectively. The aortic valve was congenitally unicuspid in 15 patients (31%), congenitally bicuspid in 32 (67%), and 3-cuspid in 1 (2%). In conclusion, of the 48 quadragenarians having AVR for AS, 47 (98%) had a congenitally malformed aortic valve, 60-day mortality was zero, and late mortality was low (8%). **(Am J Cardiol 2007; 100:1683–1690)**

We recently described aortic valve structure and early and late survival in 9 *nonagenarians*, in 196 *octogenarians*, in 424 *septuagenarians*, in 289 *sexagenarians*, and in 120 *quinquagenarians* having aortic valve replacement (AVR) for aortic stenosis (AS) at Baylor University Medical Center (BUMC) from 1993 to 2005.[1–5] The present report focuses on aortic valve structure and survival in 48 *quadragenarians* having AVR for AS at the same medical center in the same time frame.

Methods

From January 1993 through December 2005, a total of 1,112 patients underwent AVR for AS (with or without aortic regurgitation) with or without simultaneous coronary artery bypass grafting (CABG) and without mitral valve replacement at BUMC. Of the 1,112 patients, 48 (4%) were aged 40 to 49 years, and they are the subject of this report.

The operatively excised aortic valve in each patient was submitted to the surgical pathology section, and all 48 valves were examined and described by 1 author (WCR). The valves were photographed by JMK. Since 1998, all operatively excised valves have been weighed by 1 of us (WCR). Six of the 48 patients also had partial resection of the ascending aorta.

The echocardiographic and hemodynamic data in the 48 quadragenarians were collected by BLK from the cardiovascular computer database (Apollo Advance C/S, version 4.2.13, LUMEDX Corp., Oakland, California) and from the medical records. Information regarding death of any patient was obtained from 2 sources: (1) early death information was obtained from the medical record, and (2) post-hospital death information was obtained and confirmed from the Social Security Death Index.

Echocardiographic data preoperatively were available to us in 21 patients (44%). Cardiac catheterization data were available to us in most patients: peak transvalvular pressure gradients in 28 patients (58%), mean transvalvular pressure gradients in 26 (54%), aortic valve area in 33 patients (69%), and left ventricular ejection fraction in 25 patients (52%). Most patients in whom cardiac catheterization data were not available to WCR and BLK were referred directly to a cardiovascular surgeon. These patients had hemodynamic and coronary angiographic studies before being referred to BUMC, but the data are not available to us.

[a]Departments of Internal Medicine (Division of Cardiology), [b]Pathology, and [c]Cardiothoracic Surgery, and the [d]Baylor Heart and Vascular Institute, Baylor University Medical Center, Dallas, Texas 75246; the [e]Institute for Health Care Research and Improvement, Baylor Health Care System, and the [f]Department of Statistical Science, Southern Methodist University, Dallas, Texas; and [g]New York University, New York, New York.

*Corresponding author: Tel: 214-820-7911; Fax: 214-820-7533.

E-mail address: wc.roberts@baylorhealth.edu (W.C. Roberts).

Table 1
Clinical and valve structure information in the 48 quadragenarians having aortic valve replacement for isolated aortic stenosis with or without simultaneous coronary artery bypass grafting

Year	Number of AVRs for AS at BUMC	Number of Quadra-genarians	Age (year) Range (mean)	Men	Women	Coronary Artery Bypass Grafting	Died		Interval (years) AVR to Death* Range (mean ± SD)	Aortic Valve Structure			Aortic Valve Weight (g) Range (Mean)				
													Unicuspid		Bicuspid		Tricuspid
							≤60 Days	>60 Days		UAV (M:W)	BAV (M:W)	TAV (M:W)	Men	Women	Men	Women	Women
1993	31	1	49	1	0	0	0	0	—	0	1(1:0)	0	—	—	—	—	—
1994	50	1	45	0	1	0	0	1	9.94	0	1(0:1)	0	—	—	—	—	—
1995	44	3	41–44 (43)	1	2	1	0	1	7.07	0	3(1:2)	0	—	—	—	—	—
1996	56	2	43,47 (45)	2	0	0	0	0	—	1(1:0)	1(1:0)	0	—	—	—	—	—
1997	51	2	40,41 (41)	2	0	0	0	0	—	1(1:0)	1(1:0)	0	—	—	—	—	—
1998	68	0	—	—	—	—	—	—	—	0	0	0	—	—	—	—	—
1999	110	4	43–46 (45)	4	0	0	0	1	6.31	0	4(4:0)	0	—	—	2.3–5.00 (3.28)	—	—
2000	112	8	42–49 (46)	7	1	0	0	0	—	3(3:0)	5(4:1)	0	1.82–4.05 (3.16)	—	2.86–6.72 (4.55)	3.60	—
2001	98	5	47–49 (48)	2	3	1	0	0	—	0	5(2:3)	0	—	—	4.87,6.24 (5.56)	2.01–2.64 (2.35)	—
2002	110	2	44,45 (45)	1	1	1	0	0	—	0	1(1:0)	1(0:1)	—	—	2.12	—	1.65
2003	136	5	40–49 (44)	4	1	2	0	1	1.79	1(1:0)	4(4:0)	0	—	—	1.16–9.68 (4.20)	—	—
2004	120	7	40–48 (45)	5	2	1	0	0	—	4(3:1)	3(2:1)	0	2.36–5.84 (3.57)	2.50	1.47, 2.20 (1.84)	2.50	—
2005	126	8	41–47 (45)	7	1	1	0	0	—	5(4:1)	3(3:0)	0	1.97–4.44 (3.38)	3.41	2.12–5.04 (3.17)	—	—
	1,112	48	40–49 (45)	36	12	7	0/47	4/47	1.79–9.94 (6.28 ± 3.38)	15(12:3)	32(25:7)	1(0:1)	1.82–5.84 (3.06)	2.50, 3.41 (2.96)	1.16–9.68 (3.90)	2.01–3.60 (2.63)	1.65
		(4%)		(75%)	(25%)	(15%)	(0%)	(9%)		(31%)	(67%)	(2%)	10[†]	2[†]	20[†]	5[†]	1[†]

* Includes only patients surviving >60 days after valve replacement.
[†] Number of patients in whom the valve was weighted.
— = no information available or not applicable; AS = aortic stenosis; AVR = aortic valve replacement; BAV = bicuspid aortic valve; BUMC = Baylor University Medical Center; M = man; TAV = tricuspid aortic valve; UAV = unicuspid aortic valve; W = woman.

Table 2

Comparison of the 48 quadragenarians having aortic valve replacement for aortic stenosis without versus with simultaneous coronary artery bypass grafting

Year	Without Coronary Artery Bypass Grafting									With Coronary Artery Bypass Grafting								
	Number Having AVR (M:W)	Length of Stay* (days) Range (mean±SD)	Died			UAV (M:W)	BAV (M:W)	TAV (M:W)	Number Having AVR (M:W)	Length of Stay* (days) Range (mean±SD)	Died			UAV (M:W)	BAV (M:W)	TAV (M:W)
			Total (M:W)	≤60 days (M:W)	>60 days (M:W)						Total (M:W)	≤60 days (M:W)	>60 days (M:W)			
1993	1(1:0)	6	0	0	0	0	1(1:0)	0	0(0:0)	—	—	—	—	—	—	—
1994	1(0:1)	12	1(0:1)	0	1(0:1)	0	1(0:1)	0	0(0:0)	—	—	—	—	—	—	—
1995	2(1:1)	6	1(1:0)	0	1(0:1)	0	2(1:1)	0	1(0:1)	6	0	0	0	0	1(0:1)	0
1996	2(2:0)	8	0	0	0	1(1:0)	1(1:0)	0	0(0:0)	—	—	—	—	—	—	—
1997	2(2:0)	4,5 (4.5±0.71)	0	0	0	1(1:0)	1(1:0)	0	0(0:0)	—	—	—	—	—	—	—
1999	4(4:0)	4–5 (4.25±0.50)	1(1:0)	0	1(1:0)	0	4(4:0)	0	0(0:0)	—	—	—	—	—	—	—
2000	8(7:1)	3–11 (6.63±2.89)	0	0	0	3(3:0)	5(4:1)	0	0(0:0)	—	—	—	—	—	—	—
2001	4(2:2)	4–7 (5.25±1.26)	0	0	0	0	4(2:2)	0	1(0:1)	8	0	0	0	0	1(0:1)	0
2002	1(0:1)	4	0	0	0	0	0	1(0:1)	1(1:0)	7	0	0	0	0	1(1:0)	0
2003	3(2:1)	5–12 (7.33±4.04)	0	0	0	1(0:1)	2(2:0)	0	2(2:0)	5	1(1:0)	0	1(1:0)	0	2(2:0)	0
2004	6(4:2)	5–11 (7.00±2.76)	0	0	0	4(3:1)	2(1:1)	0	1(1:0)	5	0	0	0	0	1(1:0)	0
2005	7(6:1)	3–7 (4.71±1.25)	0	0	0	4(3:1)	2(1:1)	0	1(1:0)	4	0	0	0	0(1:0)	0	0
	41(31:10) (85%)	3–12 (5.98±2.44)	3/40 (8%)	0/40 (0%)	3/40 (8%)	14(11:3) (34%)	26(20:6) (63%)	1(0:1) (2%)	7(5:2) (15%)	4–8 (5.83±1.38)	1/7 (14%)	0/7 (0%)	1/7 (14%)	1(1:0) (14%)	6(4:2) (86%)	0 (0%)

* This data only include early survivors.

— = no information available or not applicable; AVR = aortic valve replacement; BAV = bicuspid aortic valve; M = man; TAV = tricuspid aortic valve; UAV = unicuspid aortic valve; W = woman.

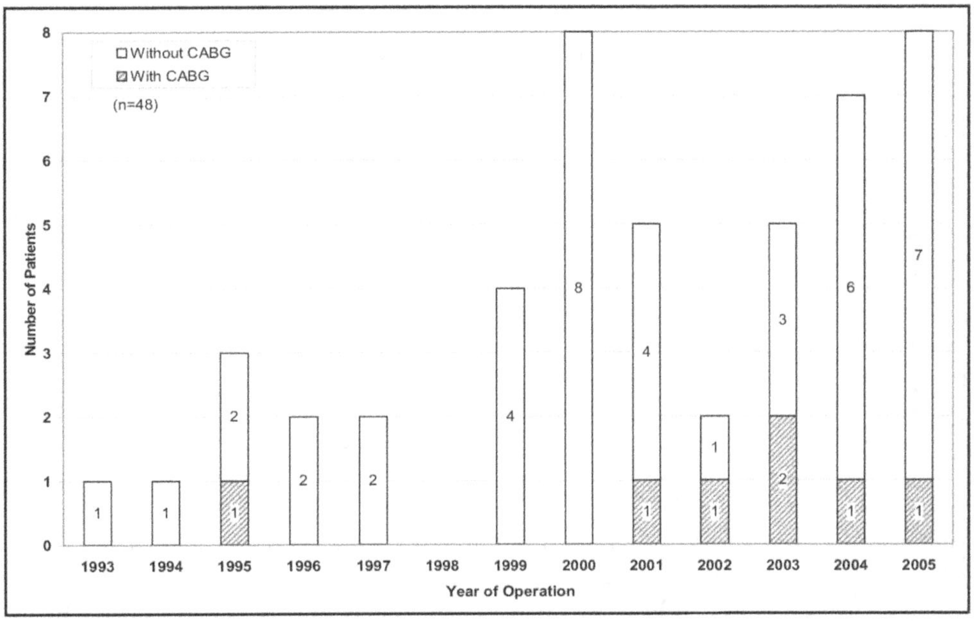

Figure 1. Number of quadragenarians having aortic valve replacement for aortic valve stenosis at Baylor University Medical Center 1993 to 2005 with versus without simultaneous coronary bypass grafting.

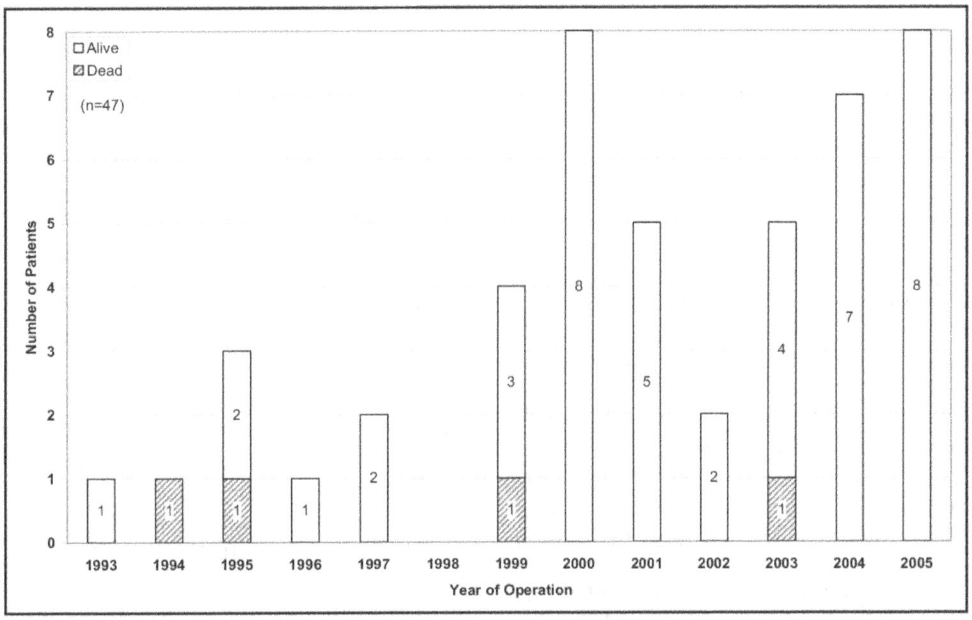

Figure 2. Number of quadragenarians surviving and not surviving aortic valve replacement for aortic stenosis (with or without simultaneous coronary artery bypass grafting) at Baylor University Medical Center 1993 to 2005 (follow-up to December 30, 2006). All deaths occurred ≥1 year after the year of operation. Note trend of better aortic valve replacement with or without coronary artery bypass grafting survival over the 13-year period.

Due to the low number of deaths (n = 4), short- and long-term mortality analyses were not conducted. Means, standard deviations (SDs), and percentages were calculated to describe the study cohort (n = 48), and a Kaplan-Meier plot was generated to describe late survival in this cohort of quadragenarians having AVR for AS (with or without aortic regurgitation). SigmaStat Version 2.0 (SPSS Inc., Chicago, Illinois) and SAS version 9.1 (SAS Institute, Cary, North Carolina) were used to perform the descriptive analysis. This study was approved by Institutional Review Board at BUMC.

Results

Pertinent data in the 48 quadragenarians are summarized in Tables 1 and 2. The native stenotic aortic valve was replaced with a bioprosthesis in 9 (19%) patients, with a

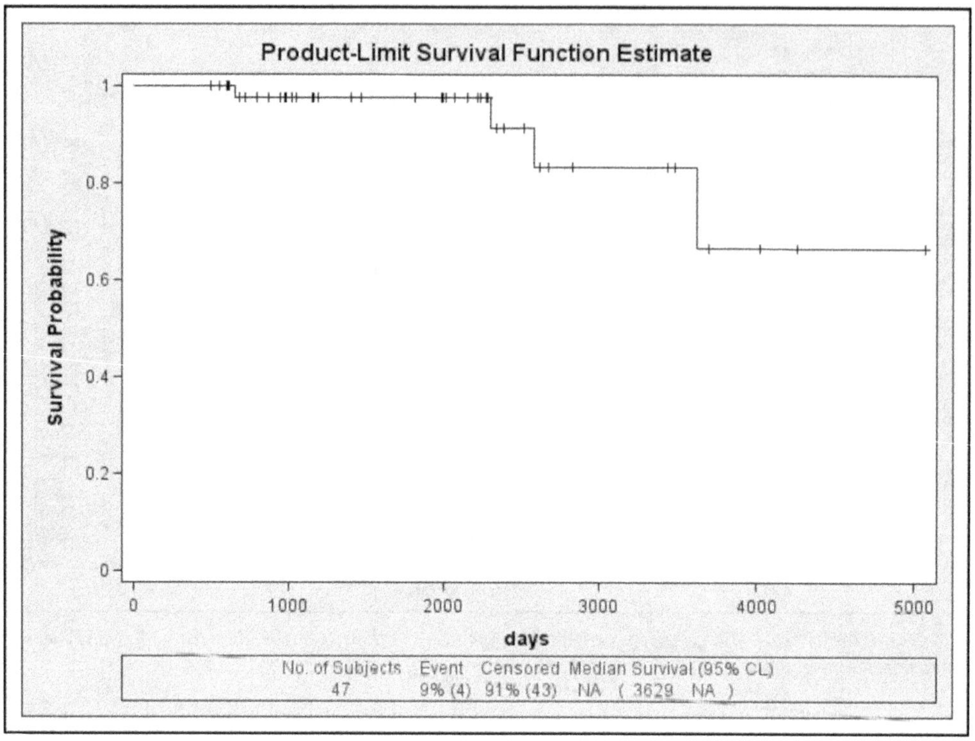

Figure 3. Kaplan-Meier survival curves describing survival in 47 quadragenarians having AVR for AS (with or without aortic regurgitation).

mechanical prosthesis in 35 (74%) patients, and a Ross procedure was done in 3 patients. Of the 48 patients, 36 (75%) were men and 12 (25%) were women. Simultaneous CABG was performed in 7 (15%) patients (Figure 1). There were no deaths in the first 60 days postoperatively. Four patients (9%) died >60 days of AVR: at 1.8, 6.3, 7.1, and 9.9 years, respectively (Figure 2). Of the 48 patients surviving > 60 days, as of December 2006, 43 (90%) were alive and have survived from 1.35 to 13.90 years (mean 5.14 ± 3.10) (Figure 3). One patient was lost to follow up.

Length of stay in the hospital in the 48 patients, all of whom survived the operative period, ranged from 3 to 12 days (mean 5.94 ± 2.31). Length of stay in the 7 patients with CABG ranged from 4 to 8 days (mean 5.71 ± 1.38), and in the 41 patients without CABG, from 3 to 12 days (mean 5.98 ± 2.44).

The transvalvular *peak* systolic pressure gradient in the patients without simultaneous CABG ranged from 15 to 119 mm Hg (mean 58 ± 32) and in patients receiving concomitant CABG, from 27 to 107 mm Hg (mean 55 ± 45); the *mean* systolic pressure gradients ranged from 14 to 85 mm Hg (average 47 ± 21) and 19 to 77 mm Hg (average 42 ±31), respectively; the calculated aortic valve area, from 0.46 to 1.82 cm^2 (mean 0.91 ± 0.33) and from 0.50 to 1.64 cm^2 (mean 0.90 ± 0.43), respectively.

Another tool providing some evidence of the severity of the AS is gained by the *weight of the operatively excised valves*.[6–9] (Previous studies have shown that men with AS have heavier valves than women, and that congenitally unicuspid and bicuspid stenotic aortic valves are heavier than 3-cuspid stenotic aortic valves.[6–9]) The operatively excised unicuspid aortic valves in the 11 men in the present study weighed from 1.82 to 5.84 g (mean 3.06), and the bicuspid valves in the 20 men, from 1.16 to 9.68 g (mean 3.90). In contrast, the 2 unicuspid valves in women weighed 2.50 and 3.41 g (mean 2.96); the bicuspid valves in the 5 women, from 2.01 to 3.60 g (mean 2.63), and the tricuspid aortic valve in the 1 woman, 1.65 g. *Aortic valve structure* in the 48 patients was the following: unicuspid in 15 (31%), bicuspid in 32 (67%), and 3-cuspid in 1 (2%) (Figures 4 to 7).

Of the 6 patients who also had simultaneous excision of the ascending aorta, histologic examination disclosed that the configuration and number of elastic fibers in the media in 5 were normal and in 1 the number of fibers was mildly decreased (cystic medial necrosis grade 1/4). By echocardiography preoperatively, the largest diameter of ascending aorta ranged from 3.4 to 6.0 cm (mean 5.0). The operatively excised aortas ranged in weight from 6.3 to 27.2 g (mean 15.1). In these 6 patients, the aortic valve was unicuspid in 4 and bicuspid in 2. Five were men and 1, a woman.

Discussion

The present study focused on a group of quadragenarians having AVR for AS at the same US medical center during a recent 13-year period. None died early (≤60 days), and 4 died late. The relatively low number of deaths did not allow for assessment of the relation between *late survival* and gender, valve structure, preoperative severity of the AS, or performance of simultaneous CABG. The low frequency of associated significant coronary artery disease in most (85%)

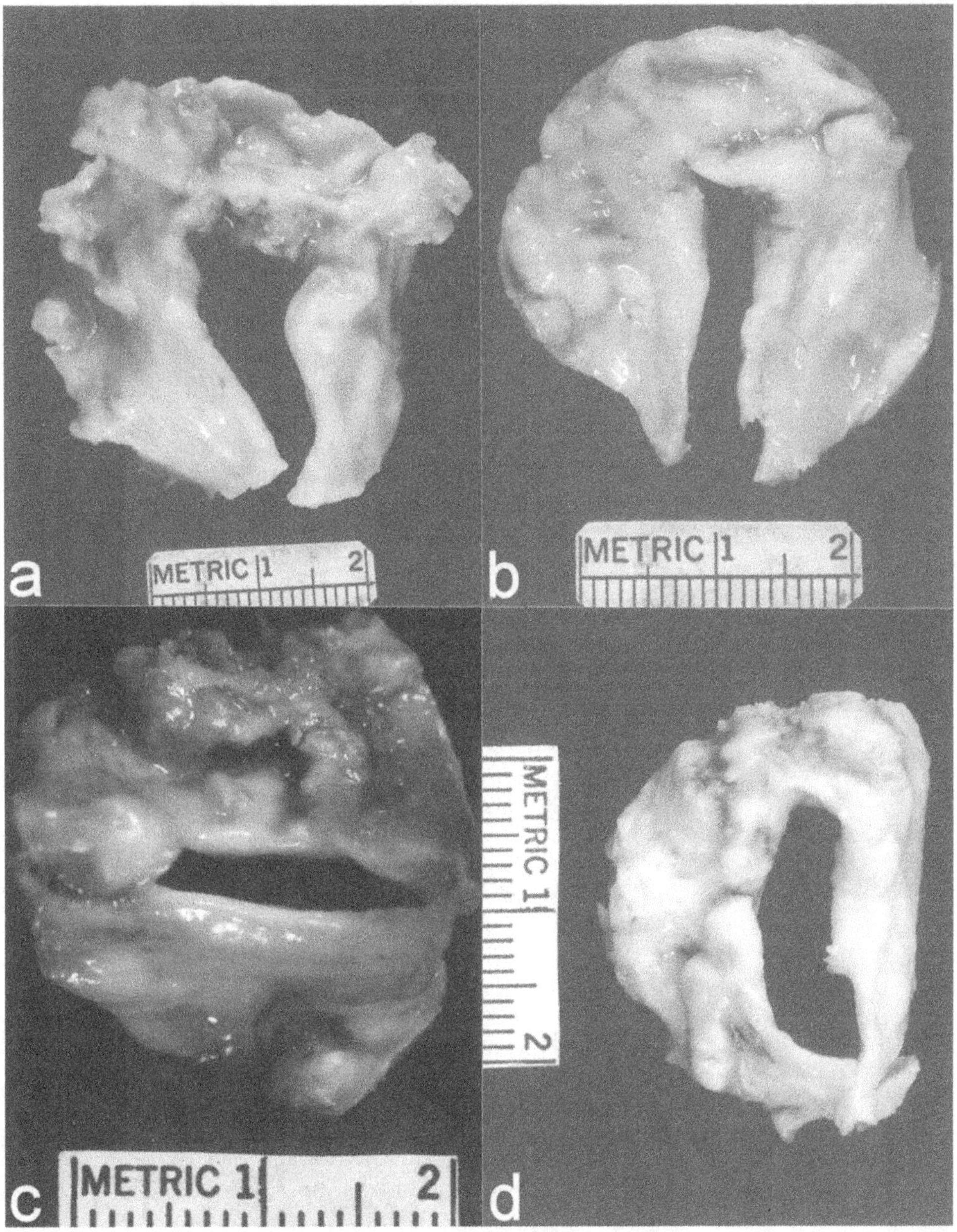

Figure 4. Photographs of 4 operatively excised stenotic congenitally *unicuspid* aortic valves: *(A)* valve from a 48-year-old man in whom the peak transvalvular systolic gradient was 23 mm Hg, the calculated aortic valve area 1.4 cm^2, and the valve weight, 5.84 g. *(B)* Valve from a 41-year-old woman in whom the calculated aortic valve area was 1.1 cm^2 and the valve weight, 2.5 g. *(C)* Valve from a 48-year-old woman in whom the peak transvalvular systolic gradient was 68 mm Hg, the calculated aortic valve area 0.46 cm^2, and the valve weight, 2.4 g. *(D)* Valve from a 44-year-old man in whom the calculated aortic valve area was 0.8 cm^2 and the valve weight, 2.12 g.

of the quadragenarians may explain at least in part the excellent survival rates in these patients.

The positive features of the present study include a relatively long post-AVR follow-up, preoperative hemodynamic data in most patients, and knowledge of aortic valve structure and weight. That all valves were examined by the same individual (WCR) produces uniformity not available if valve structure was that recorded in the operative note by a number of different cardiac surgeons, each of whom might have different views of what constituted a congenitally malformed or a 3-cuspid aortic valve with fusion of ≥ 1 aortic valve commissures. The negative features of the present study include lack of information on preoperative and postoperative symptoms and functional class, on early postoperative complications, co-morbidities, late quality of life, numbers of epicardial coronary arteries narrowed $>50\%$ in diameter, and causes of death late postoperatively.

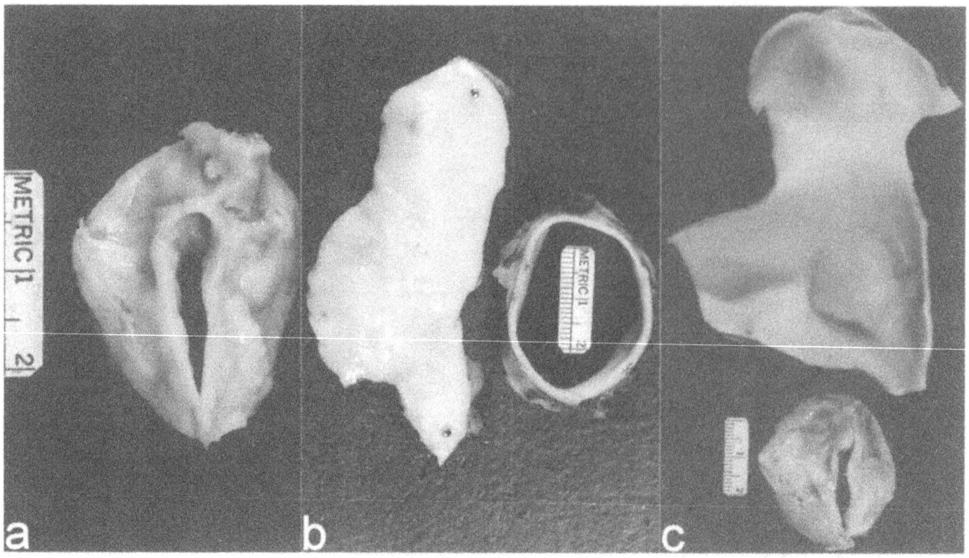

Figure 5. Photographs of 2 operatively excised stenotic congenitally *unicuspid* aortic valves and their concomitantly resected aortas: *(A)* valve from a 47-year-old man in whom the peak transvalvular systolic gradient was 21 mm Hg, the calculated aortic valve area 0.8 cm^2, and the valve weight, 2.36 g. The simultaneously removed *(B)* aorta weighed 12.51 g and the aortic diameter measured up to 5.5 cm. *(C)* The valve and ascending aorta from a 46 year old man in whom the peak transvalvular gradient was 26 mm Hg, the calculated aortic valve area 1.82, and the valve weight, 1.82 g.

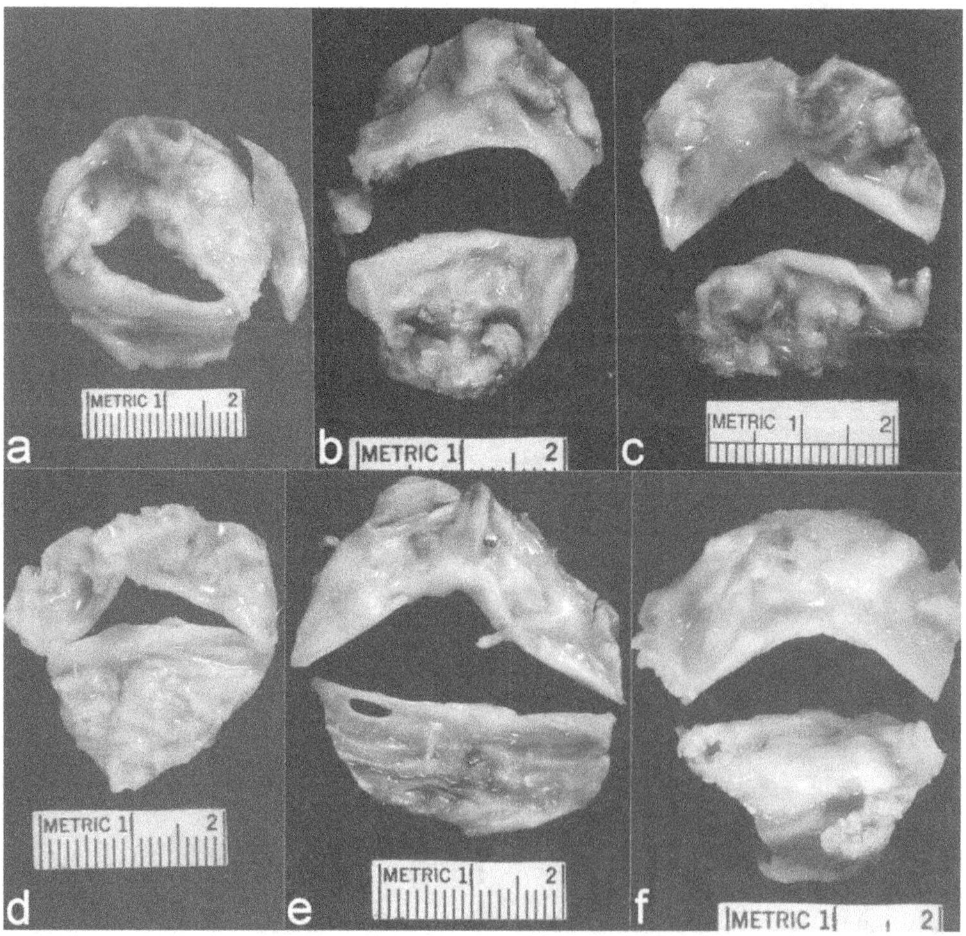

Figure 6. Photographs of 6 operatively excised congenitally *bicuspid* aortic valves: *(A)* valve from a 43-year-old man in whom the peak transvalvular gradient was 31 mm Hg, the calculated aortic valve area 1.05 cm^2, and the valve weight, 2.51 g. *(B)* The valve was excised from a 46-year-old woman in whom the valve weight was 2.50 g. *(C)* Valve from a 49-year-old man in whom the calculated aortic valve area was 0.7 cm^2 and the valve weight, 3.45 g. *(D)* Valve from a 48-year-old man in whom the peak transvalvular systolic gradient was 31 mm Hg, the calculated aortic valve area 0.87 cm^2, and the valve weight, 1.47 g. *(E)* Valve from a 44-year-old man in whom the valve weight was 1.16 g. *(F)* Valve from a 49-year-old woman in whom valve weight was 2.64 g.

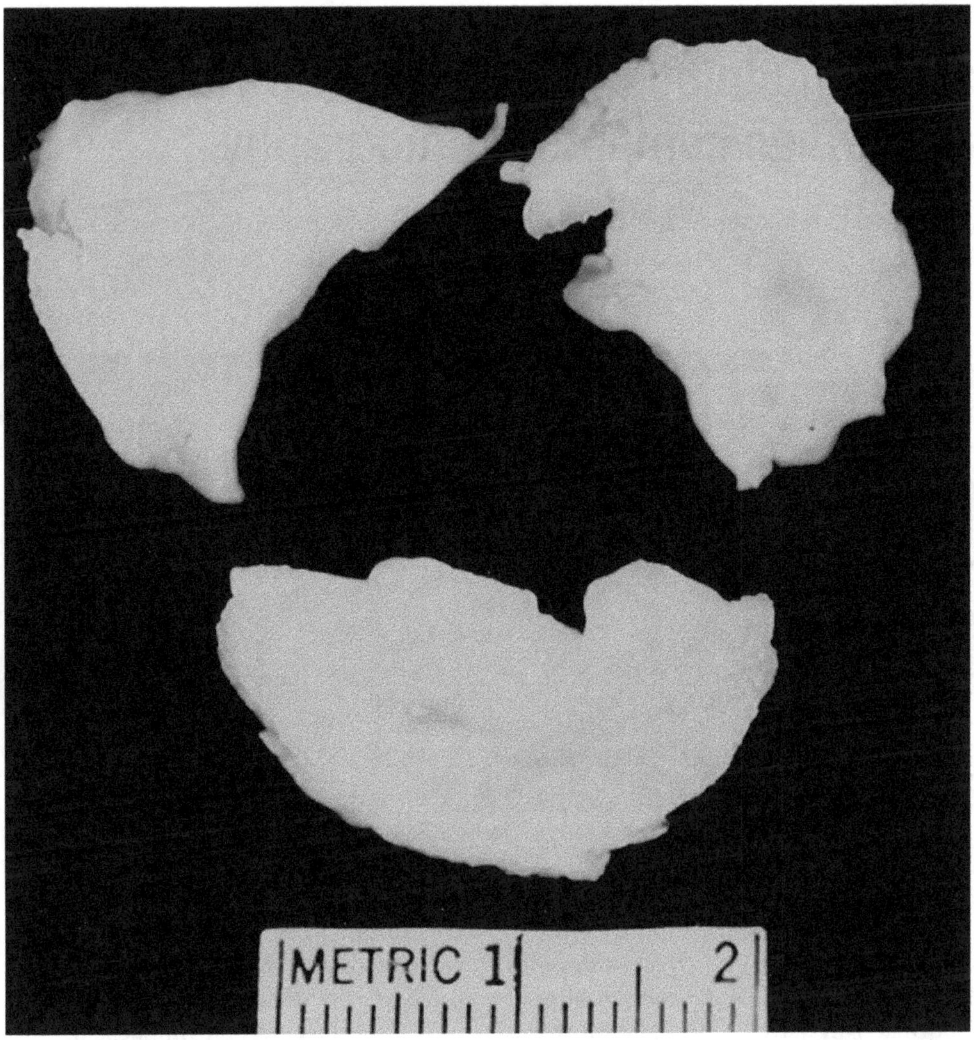

Figure 7. Photograph of the only operatively excised *tricuspid* aortic valve in the study. The valve was from a 45-year-old woman, and the valve weighed 1.65 g. Mitral valve function was entirely normal, and by echocardiogram the mitral leaflets were not thickened. The cause of the diffuse cuspal thickening in the present patient was not established.

1. Roberts WC, Ko JM, Matter GJ. Aortic valve replacement for aortic stenosis in nonagenarians. *Am J Cardiol* 2006;98:1251–1253.
2. Roberts WC, Ko JM, Garner WL, Filardo G, Henry AC, Hebeler RF JR, Matter GJ, Hamman BL. Valve structure and survival in octogenarians having aortic valve replacement for aortic stenosis (±aortic regurgitation) with versus without coronary artery bypass grafting at a single US medical center (1993 to 2005). *Am J Cardiol* 2007;100:489–495.
3. Roberts WC, Ko JM, Filardo G, Henry AC, Hebeler RF JR, Cheung EH, Matter GJ, Hamman BL. Valve structure and survival in septuagenarians having aortic valve replacement for aortic stenosis (±aortic regurgitation) with versus without coronary artery bypass grafting at a single US medical center (1993 to 2005). *Am J Cardiol* 2007;100:1157–1165.
4. Roberts WC, Ko JM, Filardo G, Henry AC, Hebeler RF JR, Cheung EH, Matter GJ, Hamman BL. Valve structure and survival in sexagenarians having aortic valve replacement for aortic stenosis (±aortic regurgitation) with versus without coronary artery bypass grafting at a single US medical center (1993 to 2005). *Am J Cardiol* 2007;100:1286–1292.
5. Roberts WC, Ko JM, Filardo G, Henry AC, Hebeler RF Jr, Cheung EH, Matter GJ, Hamman BL. Valve structure and survival in quinquagenarians having aortic valve replacement for aortic stenosis (±aortic regurgitation) with versus without coronary artery bypass grafting at a single US medical center (1993 to 2005). *Am J Cardiol* 2007;100:1584–1591.
6. Roberts WC, Ko JM. Weights of operatively excised stenotic unicuspid, bicuspid, and tricuspid aortic valves and their relation to age, sex, body mass index, and presence or absence of concomitant coronary artery bypass grafting. *Am J Cardiol* 2003:92:1057–1065.
7. Roberts WC, Ko JM. Relation of weights of operatively excised stenotic aortic valves to preoperative transvalvular peak systolic pressure gradients and to calculated aortic valve areas. *J Am Coll Cardiol* 2004;44:1847–1855.
8. Roberts WC, Ko JM. Frequency by decades of unicuspid, bicuspid, and tricuspid aortic valves in adults having isolated aortic valve replacement for aortic stenosis, with or without associated aortic regurgitation. *Circulation* 2005;111:920–925.
9. Roberts WC, Ko JM, Hamilton C. Comparison of valve structure, valve weight, and severity of the valve obstruction in 1849 patients having isolated aortic valve replacement for aortic valve stenosis (with or without associated aortic regurgitation) studied at 3 different medical centers in 2 different time periods. *Circulation* 2006;114:422–429.

Diagnosis of congenital unicuspid aortic valve by 64-slice cardiac computed tomography

Wende N. Gibbs, MD, Baron L. Hamman, MD, William C. Roberts, MD, and Jeffrey M. Schussler, MD

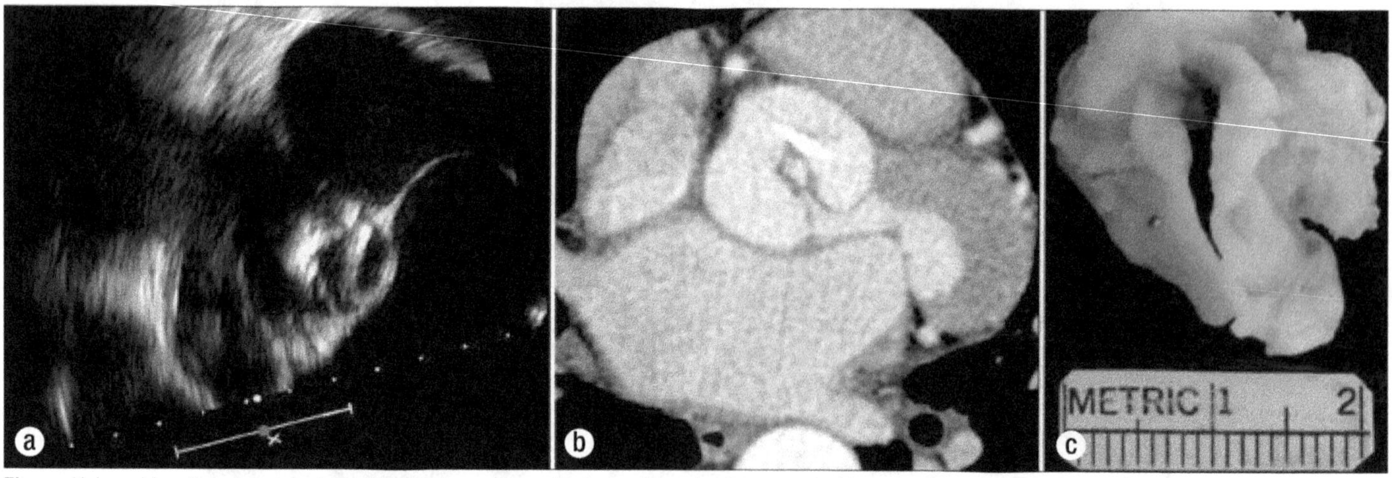

Figure. Unicuspid aortic valve evaluated with **(a)** transesophageal echocardiography, **(b)** computed tomography, and **(c)** gross pathology.

A 28-year-old man presented to our hospital with 3 days of intermittent, escalating dyspnea and chest tightness. He reported that he often experienced dyspnea when smoking, chewing tobacco, or exerting himself beyond the level of normal daily activity. His discomfort was partially relieved by his albuterol inhaler, which he used ≥10 times per day. As a child, he was told that he had a precordial murmur, but he had not sought medical attention. Five years prior to this evaluation, he was having similar symptoms and was treated with antibiotics. He was told at that time that he had mild asthma.

On examination, the patient was mildly dyspneic, with a harsh systolic murmur at the right upper sternal border. Transthoracic echocardiogram revealed left ventricular thickening with normal systolic and diastolic function and a left ventricular ejection fraction of 65%. A peak gradient of >4 meters per second was noted, with a calculated aortic valve area of <0.9 cm^2. The morphology of the valve was not clearly seen, but a unicuspid valve was suspected.

Transesophageal echocardiogram demonstrated a heavily calcified unicuspid aortic valve with reduced cuspid excursion and moderate to severe aortic regurgitation *(Figure 1a)*. Preoperative 64-slice computed tomographic coronary angiography (Lightspeed VCT, GE Healthcare) confirmed the valve morphology and demonstrated no significant coronary narrowing *(Figure 1b)*.

At operation, the valve was found to be unicuspid with one true unfused commissure. The free edge traversed the cusps without contact with the aortic wall *(Figure 1c)*. The patient received a St. Jude medical mechanical prosthesis, and his postoperative course was uncomplicated.

The estimated incidence of unicuspid aortic valve is 0.02% (1–3). During development, the aortic valve is formed from three tubercles, which each develop a cusp and sinus of Valsalva. Fusion of the cusps results in a unicuspid valve. Unicommissural unicuspid valves, as in our case, have one lateral attachment and an eccentric orifice. Acommissural unicuspid valves have no lateral attachment to the aorta.

1. Novaro GM, Mishra M, Griffin BP. Incidence and echocardiographic features of congenital unicuspid aortic valve in an adult population. *J Heart Valve Dis* 2003;12(6):674–678.
2. Roberts WC, Ko JM. Frequency by decades of unicuspid, bicuspid, and tricuspid aortic valves in adults having isolated aortic valve replacement for aortic stenosis, with or without associated aortic regurgitation. *Circulation* 2005;111(7):920–925.
3. Roberts WC, Ko JM. Clinical and morphologic features of the congenitally unicuspid acommissural stenotic and regurgitant aortic valve. *Cardiology* 2007;108(2):79–81

From the Department of Internal Medicine (Gibbs), Department of Thoracic Surgery (Hamman), Department of Pathology (Roberts), and Division of Cardiology (Schussler), Baylor University Medical Center, Dallas, Texas.

Corresponding author: Jeffrey M. Schussler, MD, 621 North Hall Street, Suite 500, Dallas, TX 75226 (e-mail: Jeffrey.Schussler@heartplace.com).

Some observations on mitral and aortic valve disease

William Clifford Roberts, MD, and Jong Mi Ko, BA

SOURCES FOR MORPHOLOGIC STUDIES

Before 1960, the only source for studying the heart was the autopsy. The early years of cardiac valve replacement provided a rich source of necropsy "material" until valve techniques and artificial heart valves became more refined. In the 1950s and 1960s, most physicians attributed valvular heart disease in adults to rheumatic heart disease. During the 1960s and 1970s, many thousands of patients with rheumatic heart disease underwent replacement of one or more cardiac valves. By the 1980s, most of this rheumatic heart disease pool of patients had undergone operation; in addition, the frequency of rheumatic fever and subsequently rheumatic heart disease had dropped dramatically. By the 1970s, the congenitally malformed aortic valve was found to be frequent in adults with aortic stenosis (AS), and mitral valve prolapse (MVP) was being recognized as a common cause of pure (no associated stenosis) mitral regurgitation (MR). By the 1990s, the frequency of autopsies in US hospitals had dropped enormously compared with the 1950s, and operatively excised cardiac valves were becoming the major source of anatomic study. Although established by the 1980s, cardiac transplantation was rarely performed in patients with valvular heart disease.

Table 1. Functional and anatomic classification of valvular heart disease in 1010 necropsy patients aged ≥15 years*

		Anatomic class				
Functional class	**Patients (%)**	**AV**	**MV**	**MV-AV**	**TV-MV**	**TV-MV-AV**
1. Aortic stenosis (AS)	292 (29%)	256 (88%)	0	35 (12%)	0	1 (0.3%)
2. Mitral stenosis (MS)	189 (19%)	0	117 (62%)	40 (21%)	13 (7%)	19 (10%)
3. MS + AS	152 (15%)	0	0	120 (79%)	0	32 (21%)
4. Aortic regurgitation (AR)†	119 (12%)	107 (90%)	0	10 (8%)	0	2 (2%)
5. Mitral regurgitation (MR)	97 (10%)	0	85 (88%)	8 (8%)	1 (1%)	3 (3%)
6. MS + AR	65 (6%)	0	52 (80%)	0	0	13 (20%)
7. MR + AR	45 (4%)	0	0	39 (87%)	0	6 (13%)
8. AS + MR	23 (2%)	0	0	21 (91%)	0	2 (9%)
9. Tricuspid stenosis + MS ± AS	28 (3%)	0	0	0	4 (14%)	24 (86%)
Totals	1010 (100%)‡	363 (36%)	254 (25%)	273 (27%)	18 (2%)	102 (10%)

* Excludes patients with mitral regurgitation secondary to coronary heart disease (papillary muscle dysfunction), carcinoid heart disease, hypertrophic cardiomyopathy, and those with infective endocarditis limited to one or both right-sided cardiac valves. Tricuspid valve regurgitation was present in many patients in most of the nine functional groups. All patients were in functional class III or IV (New York Heart Association), and more than half had one or more cardiac operations.

† In many patients, the aortic valve cusps were normal or nearly normal and the regurgitation was the result of disease of the aorta (the Marfan and Marfan-like syndrome, syphilis, systemic hypertension, healed aortic dissection).

‡ The hearts in all 1010 patients were examined and classified by WCR.

From Roberts WC, 1987 (1); reproduced with permission from Roberts WC, 1983 (39).

AV indicates aortic valve; MV, mitral valve; TV, tricuspid valve.

FREQUENCY OF VARIOUS VALVULAR DISORDERS IN NECROPSY STUDIES

Roberts (1) personally studied 1010 hearts at necropsy in patients with fatal valvular heart disease *(Table 1)*. All had died between 1955 and 1980 and the specimens were retrieved from a number of different hospitals, most of which were located in the Washington, DC, area. As shown in Table 1, these cases were given both a *functional* (valve stenosis ± regurgitation or pure regurgitation [no element of stenosis]) and an *anatomic* classification. A number of these patients had only one dysfunctional valve but in addition had one or more anatomically abnormal valves (normal function). (A valve may be anatomically abnormal yet function normally.) AS was the most common functional

From the Baylor Heart and Vascular Institute and the Departments of Pathology and Medicine (Cardiology), Baylor University Medical Center, Dallas, Texas.

Corresponding author: William C. Roberts, MD, Baylor Heart and Vascular Institute, Baylor University Medical Center, 621 North Hall Street, Dallas, Texas 75226 (e-mail: wc.roberts@BaylorHealth.edu).

Table 2. Type of valvular dysfunction in patients* having aortic valve replacement and/or mitral valve replacement or repair at Baylor University Medical Center at Dallas (1993–2006)

Valve dysfunction	Patients (%)
1. Aortic stenosis (AS)	985 (53%)
2. Mitral stenosis (MS)	129 (7%)
3. MS + AS	54 (3%)
4. Aortic regurgitation (AR)†	326 (17%)
5. Mitral regurgitation (MR)*	313 (17%)
6. MS + AR	10 (<1%)
7. MR + AR	28 (1%)
8. AS + MR	27 (1%)
9. Tricuspid stenosis + MS + AS	0
Totals	1872 (100%)‡

*Excludes patients with mitral regurgitation secondary to coronary heart disease (papillary muscle dysfunction), carcinoid heart disease, hypertrophic cardiomyopathy, and those with infective endocarditis limited to one or both right-sided cardiac valves. Tricuspid valve regurgitation was present in many patients in most of the nine functional groups.

† In many patients, the aortic valve cusps were normal or nearly normal and the regurgitation was the result of disease of the aorta (the Marfan and Marfan-like syndrome, syphilis, systemic hypertension, healed aortic dissection).

‡The operatively excised valves in the 1872 patients were examined and classified by WCR.

disorder (29%); in 35 (12%) of these 292 patients, the mitral leaflets were diffusely thickened (rheumatic heart disease) but there was no clinical evidence of mitral dysfunction. Most of the 256 patients with AS and anatomically normal mitral valves had congenitally unicuspid or bicuspid aortic valves.

Mitral stenosis (MS) was the next most common functional valve disease, but 72 (38%) of these 189 patients also had anatomic involvement of one or more other cardiac valves. All patients with MS, whether isolated or associated with a functional disorder of another cardiac valve, had the valvular disease attributed to rheumatic heart disease.

Combined MS and AS was the third most common functional valvular disease (15%), and 32 (21%) of these 152 cases also had anatomic disease of the tricuspid valve leaflets. The purely regurgitant lesions (aortic regurgitation [AR], MR, or both) were less common. Tricuspid stenosis of rheumatic etiology occurred in only 3% of the 1010 cases, and all had associated MS with or without associated AS. No other large series of patients with valvular heart disease studied at necropsy has been reported in the last 25 years, and it is unlikely that such a large series, all studied by a single physician, will be accumulated in the future because of the low autopsy rates in most hospitals today and because few specimens are retained indefinitely after autopsy.

CHANGING FREQUENCY OF VARIOUS VALVULAR DISORDERS IN RECENT DECADES IN THE WESTERN WORLD

Today the most frequently studied operatively excised valve is the stenotic aortic valve, followed by a portion of posterior mitral leaflet in patients with MR excised secondary to MVP *(Table 2)*. Operatively excised purely regurgitant aortic valves with or without excision of portions of ascending aorta are also common. Purely regurgitant mitral valves that are replaced usually yield only anterior mitral leaflets as specimens; the posterior leaflet is usually not excised. Tricuspid valves are rarely excised today.

The remainder of this article discusses specific mitral and aortic valvular disorders.

AORTIC STENOSIS (± REGURGITATION)

Frequency and causes

If systemic hypertension is not considered, AS is the second most common potentially fatal or fatal heart disease after coronary heart disease. There are three major causes of AS: *atherosclerosis* (formerly called degenerative), *congenitally malformed valves*, and *rheumatic heart disease.*

That atherosclerosis is a cause of AS is derived primarily from five pieces of evidence:

1. Patients with familial homozygous hyperlipidemia (serum total cholesterol levels >800 mg/dL from birth) usually develop calcific deposits on the aortic aspects of their aortic valve cusps early in life, usually by the teenage years (2).
2. Progression of AS can be slowed by lowering total and low-density lipoprotein cholesterol levels by statins (3).
3. Patients >65 years of age with AS involving a three-cuspid aortic valve (unassociated with mitral valve disease) usually have extensive atherosclerosis involving the major epicardial coronary arteries and usually other systemic arterial systems (4).
4. Serum total cholesterol levels and concomitant coronary bypass grafting tend to be higher in patients with AS involving three-cuspid aortic valves than in patients of similar age and sex without AS or with congenitally bicuspid aortic valves (5).
5. Histologic study of three-cuspid stenotic aortic valves demonstrates features similar to those in atherosclerotic plaques (2).

The unicuspid aortic valve appears to be stenotic from birth (6, 7). The congenitally bicuspid valve, however, is infrequently stenotic at birth but becomes stenotic as calcific deposits form on the aortic aspects of the cusps (8). Rheumatic heart disease never involves the aortic valve anatomically without also involving the mitral valve (9). Although the mitral valve may be diffusely abnormal anatomically, its function can be normal. Consequently, a patient with rheumatic heart disease can present initially with only aortic valve dysfunction, and therefore rheumatic heart disease has to be considered a cause of functionally isolated AS (± AR) or pure AR (9).

Valve structure

In patients with isolated AS (± AR) (only cardiac valve anatomically abnormal) the aortic valve may be unicuspid, bicuspid, tricuspid, or quadricuspid. The congenitally *unicuspid valve* is of two types: acommissural and unicommissural (7, 10). The acommissural valve, which represents <10% of the unicuspid valves, has a central orifice and no distinct commissures. The

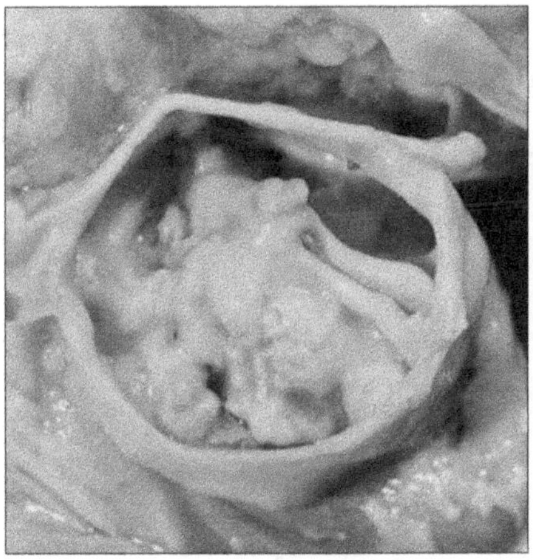

Figure 1. Aortic stenosis. *Congenitally unicuspid unicommissural aortic valve* in a 48-year-old man. The heart weighed 750 g. Reproduced with permission from Falcone MW et al, 1971 (7).

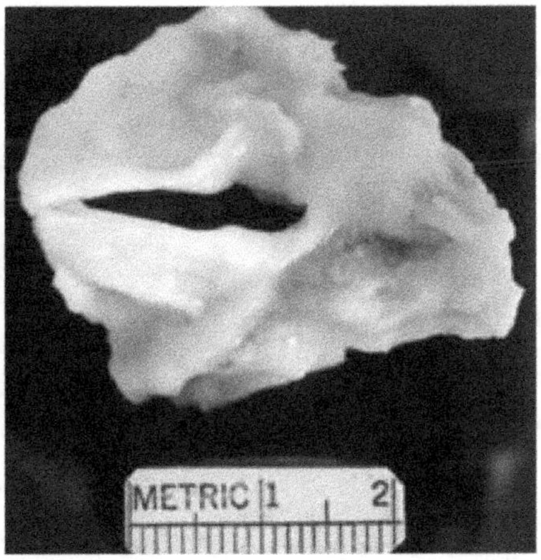

Figure 2. Aortic stenosis. Operatively excised *unicuspid unicommissural aortic valve* in a 41-year-old man. The valve weighed 5.42 g. The mean transvalvular pressure gradient was 51 mm Hg.

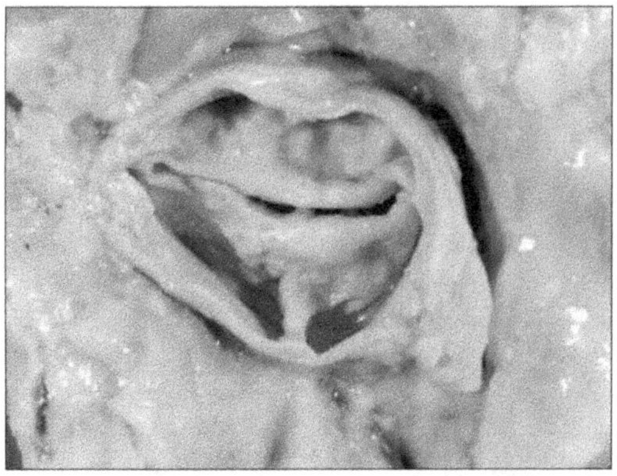

Figure 3. Aortic stenosis. *Congenitally bicuspid aortic valve* in a 61-year-old man. At catheterization 2 years before his death, the peak systolic transvalvular pressure gradient was 45 mm Hg when the cardiac index was 2.6 L/min/m². He had complete heart block secondary to destruction of the atrioventricular bundle by calcium. The heart weighed 700 g.

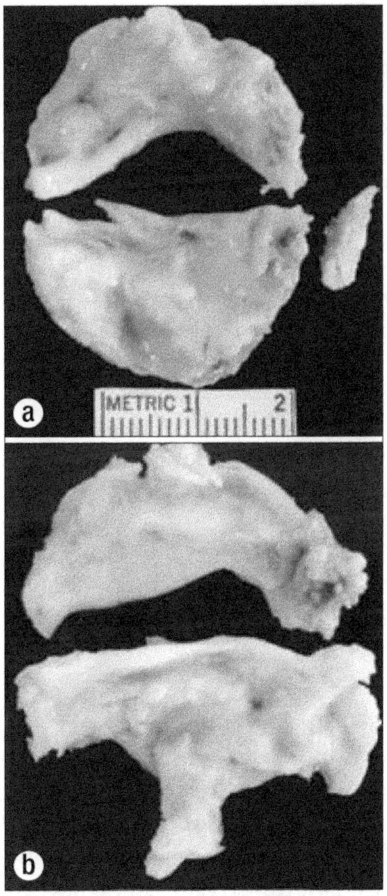

Figure 4. Aortic stenosis. Two operatively excised *congenitally bicuspid aortic valves.* **(a)** Valve in a 60-year-old man with severe heart failure. The valve weighed 4.65 g. **(b)** Valve in a 66-year-old man. The valve weighed 4.79 g and the peak systolic transvalvular gradient was 84 mm Hg.

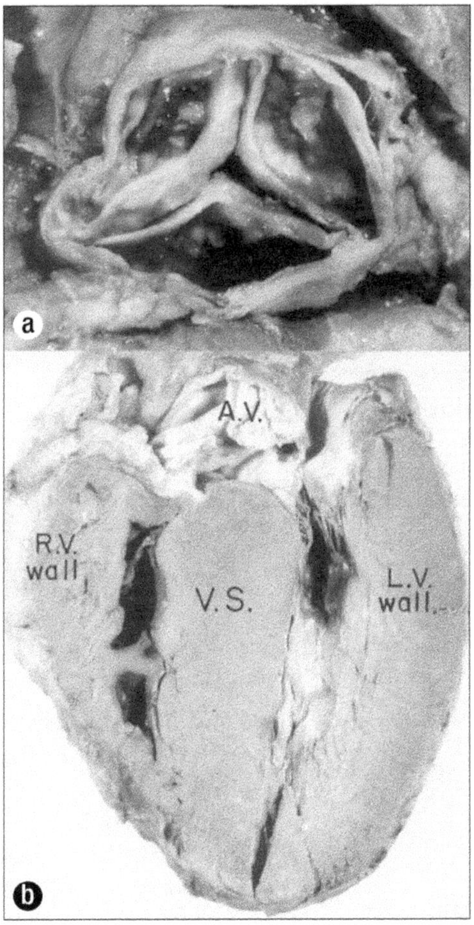

Figure 5. Aortic stenosis. **(a)** Three-cuspid aortic valve and **(b)** longitudinal section of the heart in an 89-year-old man whose heart weighed 440 g. None of the three aortic valve commissures are fused. The mitral annulus contains calcific deposits. Reproduced with permission from Roberts WC et al, 1971 (4).

unicommissural valve, which constitutes most of the unicuspid valves, has one commissure and usually two other rudimentary commissures (raphae) and a vertical orifice extending from the only true commissure *(Figures 1 and 2)* (9).

The *congenitally bicuspid valve (Figures 3 and 4)* of course has two cusps, and they are usually of slightly unequal size in both cuspal surface area and weight. Usually one of the two cusps contains a raphe in its central portion. Often the raphe cusp has free margins that are V-shaped with the apex of the V pointing to the raphe, producing a concave configuration. The nonraphe cusp in this circumstance commonly has a convex configuration that fits nicely into the concave shape of the raphe cusp such that associated regurgitation is absent or minimal. These bicuspid valves with a concave configuration of the raphe cusp and a convex appearance of free margin of the nonraphe cusp are often confused with tricuspid valves with fusion of one of three commissures. In other bicuspid valves the free margins of both cusps are relatively straight.

The *tricuspid aortic valve* is common in older patients with AS (atherosclerotic origin) and in patients in whom the AS is of rheumatic etiology. (These latter patients always have mitral leaflets that are diffusely fibrotic [with or without focal calcific deposits], or at least the margins of both leaflets are everywhere thickened by fibrous tissue.) In patients with AS of rheumatic etiology, one or more of the three commissures are often fused and the cusps may be either diffusely or focally fibrotic with or without commissural fusion or calcific deposits. The stenotic tricuspid aortic valve in older persons contains calcific deposits on the aortic surfaces, usually involving the sites of cuspal attachments, and the commissures characteristically are not fused *(Figure 5)*. Thus, operative excision produces three cusps, none of which is attached to another *(Figure 6)*. Older patients with AS often

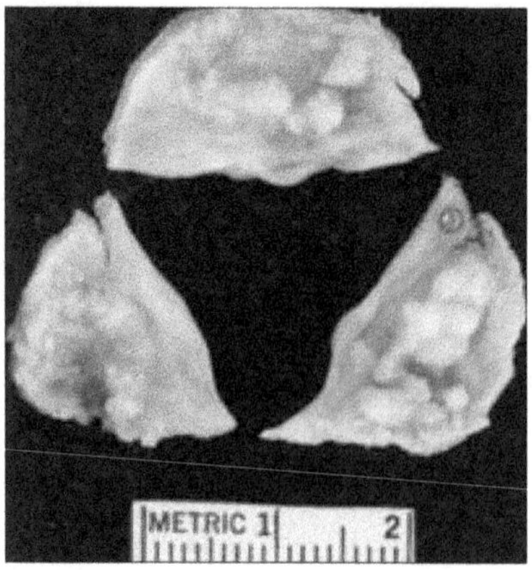

Figure 6. Aortic stenosis. Operatively excised aortic valve in a 70-year-old man. The valve weighed 1.69 g, the peak systolic transvalvular gradient was 55 mm Hg, and left ventricular function was normal (ejection fraction = 60%).

also have calcified mitral anomaly. *Figure 7* shows how calcium might develop in both the aortic valve and the mitral annulus.

The *quadricuspid aortic valve* is rare (12). When present and if dysfunctional, the dysfunction is usually pure AR. AS with a quadricuspid valve is exceedingly rare, seen by Roberts (13) in 1 of 1118 operatively excised stenotic aortic valves.

Necropsy studies of patients with isolated aortic stenosis (± AR) and never a cardiac operation—natural history

During a 32-year period at the National Institutes of Health (NIH), Roberts collected (mainly from hospitals in the Washington, DC, area) the hearts of 192 adults (aged 16–99 years) with isolated AS; none of them had ever had a cardiac operation (unpublished data). Of the 192 patients, 139 (72%) were men and 53 (28%) were women *(Table 3)*. The average age of the men was 61 years, and that of the women, 71 years, the same average ages of death as in coronary heart disease. The weight of the hearts was 610 ± 135 g (normal, <400 g) in the men and 486 ± 111 g (normal, <350 g) in the women. The aortic valve was congenitally unicuspid in 17 patients (9%), congenitally bicuspid in 89 patients (46%), and tricuspid in 86 (45%) *(Table 4)*. Other observations in these 192 patients are shown in Tables 3 and 4.

Table 3. Findings at necropsy in unoperated isolated aortic valve stenosis in men vs women (n = 192)

Variable	Men (n = 139)		Women (n = 53)	
Age (years): range (mean)	16–99 (61)		32–90 (71)	
Symptomatic	103/129 (80%)		41/49 (84%)	
Total cholesterol (mg/dL)	206 ± 63		161± 26	
Severity of stenosis				
1+	24 (17%)		7 (13%)	
2+	22 (16%)		9 (17%)	
3+	93 (67%)		37 (70%)	
Coronary narrowing				
0	73 (53%)		20 (38%)	
≥1	66 (47%)		33 (62%)	
Mitral annular calcium				
0	101 (73%)		23 (43%)	
1+–3+	38 (27%)		30 (57%)	
Heart weight (g)	610 ± 135		486 ± 111	
Aortic valve				
Unicuspid	16 (12%)	59%	1 (2%)	45%
Bicuspid	66 (47%)		23 (43%)	
Tricuspid	57 (41%)		29 (55%)	
Left ventricular				
Fibrosis	57 (41%)		13 (25%)	
Necrosis	13 (9%)		5 (9%)	

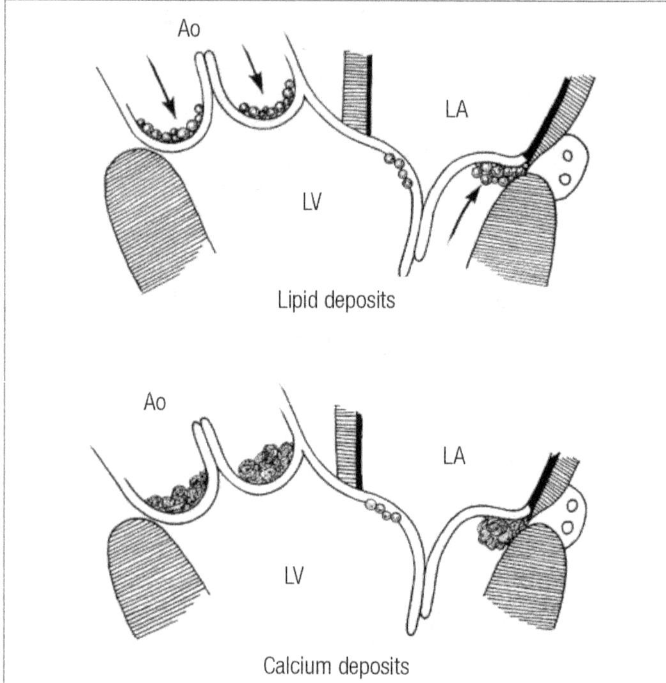

Figure 7. Aortic valve and mitral annular calcium. Commonly calcific deposits are present in the aortic valve cusps, mitral annulus, and epicardial coronary arteries. Roberts has referred to this condition as "the senile cardiac calcification syndrome" (11). The cause of the deposits is speculative, but atherosclerosis seems to be the most reasonable. In younger individuals lipid deposits are usually present on the aortic aspects of the aortic valve cusps and on the ventricular aspects of the posterior mitral leaflet and, to a much lesser extent, on the ventricular aspect of the anterior mitral leaflet. The lipid in these locations is usually both intracellular and extracellular. Degeneration of the lipid probably leads to the calcific deposits in these locations.

Weights of operatively excised stenotic aortic valves

The weight of operatively excised stenotic aortic valves is useful in quantitating the severity of the stenosis because the weight is determined primarily by the quantity of calcific deposits and the larger the calcific deposits, the greater the transvalvular pressure gradient (13–24). Roberts and colleagues (22) reported weights in 1849 operatively excised stenotic valves in patients aged 21 to 91 years without concomitant mitral valve replacement or mitral stenosis. These authors found that the weight of the stenotic valves varied inversely with the number of aortic valve cusps (14). The unicuspid valves were the heaviest, the bicuspid valves the next heaviest, and the tricuspid aortic valves, the lightest. The men had heavier valves than did the women *(Figure 8)*, and the younger patients had heavier valves than did the older patients. The mean weights of the valves were similar in patients whose body mass index was <25, 25–30, and >30 kg/m^2. Mean valve weights also were heavier in the patients

Table 4. Underlying structure of the aortic valve in unoperated patients studied at necropsy with isolated aortic valve stenosis with or without associated aortic regurgitation (n = 192)

Variable	Unicuspid (n = 17) [9%]	Bicuspid (n = 89) [46%]	Tricuspid (n = 86) [45%]
Age (years): range (mean)	25–73 (46)	16–87 (62)	36–99 (64)
Males	16 (94%)	66 (74%)	57 (66%)
Symptomatic	15 (88%)	73/84 (87%)	57/78 (73%)
Total cholesterol (mg/dL)	216	203	173
Mode of death			
Sudden (outside hospital)	1 (6%)	15 (17%)	11 (13%)
Sudden (inside hospital)	1 (6%)	13 (15%)	6 (7%)
Nonsudden (cardiac)	14 (82%)	47 (53%)	45 (52%)
Vascular	0	2 (2%)	4 (5%)
Noncardiovascular	1 (6%)	12 (14%)	20 (23%)
Severity of stenosis			
1+	1 (6%)	11 (12%)	19 (22%)
2+	0	14 (16%)	17 (20%)
3+	16 (94%)	64 (72%)	50 (58%)
Coronary narrowing			
0	15 (88%)	57 (64%)	41 (48%)
≥1	2 (12%)	32 (36%)	45 (52%)
Mitral annular calcium			
0	12 (71%)	72 (81%)	40 (47%)
1+–3+	5 (29%)	17 (19%)	46 (53%)
Heart weight (g) (mean)	617	578	573
Left ventricular			
Fibrosis	8/15 (53%)	34/88 (39%)	28/85 (33%)
Necrosis	1/16 (6%)	8/87 (9%)	9/85 (11%)

who *did not* undergo simultaneous coronary artery bypass grafting than in those who did.

Table 5 shows various clinical findings in the 1849 patients whose stenotic aortic valves were studied by Roberts and colleagues (22). The patients underwent aortic valve replacement at three different institutions: NIH from 1963 to 1989, Georgetown University Medical Center (GUMC) from 1969 to 1992, and Baylor University Medical Center (BUMC) from 1993 to 2004. All 1849 operatively excised stenotic valves were examined and classified by WCR. Patients having simultaneous mitral valve replacement or mitral stenosis were excluded. The valves excised at NIH and at GUMC from 1963 to 1992 were heavier than the valves excised at BUMC from 1993 to 2004: men 4.05 ± 1.91 (NIH), 4.36 ± 1.83 (GUMC), and 3.11 ± 1.51 g (BUMC); women 2.80 ± 1.26 (NIH), 3.02 ± 1.26 (GUMC), and 1.89 ± 0.87 g (BUMC).

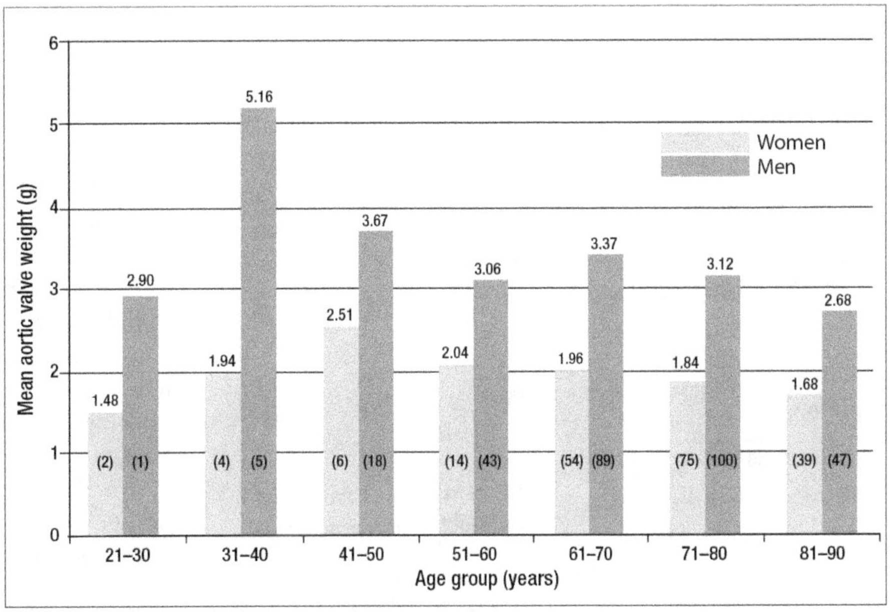

Figure 8. Aortic valve weights in men and women in each of 7 decades. All had aortic stenosis. Reproduced with permission from Roberts WC and Ko JM, 2003 (14).

Not only did the valve weights vary according to valve structure (unicuspid > bicuspid > tricuspid), but often there was variation in individual cusps among patients with bicuspid valves and among patients with tricuspid valves (15, 16). Of 200 operatively excised stenotic congenitally bicuspid valves, the two cusps in 152 patients (76%) differed in weight by >0.2 g, and in 48 patients (24%) the cusps were of similar weight (≤0.2 g difference) (15). In 161 of the 200 patients, a raphe was present in one of the two cusps: the raphe and nonraphe cusps differed in weight in 120 patients (74%) with the raphe cusps being heavier in 89 patients (55%), lighter in 31 patients (19%), and of similar weight in 41 (26%). Of the 39 patients without a raphe in one cusp, in 32 patients (82%) the two cusps were of different (>0.2 g) weight and in 7 patients (18%), similar in weight (≤0.2 g).

Of 260 operatively excised stenotic three-cuspid aortic valves, all three cusps differed (by >0.1 g) in weight in 71 patients (27%); all three cusps were similar (≤0.1 g difference) in weight in 33 patients (13%), and in 156 patients (60%) one cusp differed from either of the other two cusps which were similar in weight (16).

Why might cusps of operatively excised stenotic valves differ in weight? The most likely explanation seems to be that the cusps differ in size, that is, in surface area, from birth. The cusp with the largest surface area has, of course, a larger area on which calcium can be deposited, and the weight of a cusp is determined primarily by the amount of calcium deposited on its aortic surface.

Relation of aortic valve weight to transvalvular peak systolic pressure gradient

The best determinant of the magnitude of obstruction in patients with AS has been debated. Determinants considered have been aortic valve area or index, mean transvalvular systolic gradient, and peak transvalvular systolic gradients. Roberts and Ko (17) compared the weights of operatively excised stenotic

Table 5. Data in patients having isolated aortic valve replacement for aortic stenosis (± aortic regurgitation) at three different medical centers

Variable	NIH (1963–1989)	GUMC (1969–1992)	BUMC (1993–2004)
Valve structure			
Unicuspid			
Men	84/342 (25%)	56/255 (22%)	36/601 (6%)
Women	14/110 (13%)	24/145 (17%)	12/356 (4%)
Bicuspid			
Men	158/342 (46%)	129/255 (50%)	316/601 (53%)
Women	53/110 (48%)	68/145 (47%)	153/356 (43%)
Tricuspid			
Men	47/342 (14%)	63/255 (25%)	242/601 (40%)
Women	28/110 (25%)	48/145 (33%)	186/356 (52%)
Indeterminate			
Men	53/342 (15%)	7/255 (3%)	7/601 (1%)
Women	15/110 (14%)	5/145 (3%)	5/356 (1%)
Age (years): range (mean ± SD)			
Men	21–82 (54 ± 12)	24–88 (64 ± 11)	25–91 (69 ± 12)
Men ≥65	62/331 (19%)	124/251 (49%)	424/601 (71%)
Women	33–86 (57 ± 11)	22–89 (67 ± 12)	27–91 (70 ± 11)
Women ≥65	27/104 (26%)	94/142 (66%)	273/356 (77%)
Gender			
Men	342/452 (76%)	255/400 (64%)	601/957 (63%)
Women	110/452 (24%)	145/400 (36%)	356/957 (37%)
Aortic valve weight (g): range (mean ± SD)			
Men	0.70–10.2 (4.05 ± 1.91)	1.20–11.0 (4.36 ± 1.83)	0.89–11.30 (3.11 ± 1.51)
Women	0.55–5.50 (2.80 ± 1.26)	0.40–6.70 (3.02 ± 1.26)	0.45–4.97 (1.89 ± 0.87)
Left ventricular to aortic peak systolic gradient (mm Hg): range (mean ± SD)			
Men	10–145 (69 ± 30)	10–160 (69 ± 25)	10–141 (52 ± 23)
Women	10–165 (76 ± 34)	30–170 (81 ± 32)	10–133 (54 ± 28)
Aortic valve area (cm²): range (mean ± SD)			
Men	0.20–1.90 (0.66 ± 0.32)	0.27–1.97 (0.75 ± 0.31)	0.20–1.90 (0.78 ± 0.26)
Women	0.23–1.10 (0.53 ± 0.21)	0.20–1.30 (0.57 ± 0.21)	0.18–1.49 (0.67 ± 0.22)
Cardiac index (L/min/m²): range (mean ± SD)			
Men	1.10–5.00 (2.58 ± 0.72)	1.00–7.30 (2.87 ± 0.93)	–
Women	1.60–4.50 (2.68 ± 0.69)	1.60–6.20 (2.79 ± 0.81)	–
Simultaneous coronary bypass			
Men	21/238 (9%)	77/198 (39%)	332/601 (55%)
Women	6/74 (8%)	29/118 (25%)	167/356 (47%)

Reproduced with permission from Roberts WC et al, 2005 (22).

BUMC indicates Baylor University Medical Center; GUMC, Georgetown University Medical Center; NIH, National Institutes of Health.

aortic valves to peak transvalvular systolic pressure gradient and to aortic valve area. The results of these studies in 201 men and in 123 women with isolated AS are shown in *Table 6*. In both men and women the weights of the stenotic aortic valves increased significantly as the peak left ventricular-to-aortic systolic gradient increased, but valve weight had essentially no relation to aortic valve area. Women had significantly lower valve weights, with peak gradients similar to those in men. In men with valve weights from 1 to 2 g, the peak transvalvular gradient averaged 36 mm Hg and the valve areas, 0.86 cm²; in the men with valve weights >6 g, the peak gradients averaged 87 mm Hg, whereas the valve was 0.71 cm². In women with valve weights ≤1 g, the peak gradient averaged 28 mm Hg and valve area, 0.83 cm²; in women whose valve weighed from >3 to 4 g, the peak gradients averaged 85 mm Hg, and the valve area, 0.51 cm² (Table 6).

Relatively few operatively excised aortic valves in adults with AS are ≥5 g, and those reaching that weight are usually congenitally malformed. Of unicuspid valves, 37 (30%) of 124 valves in men and 5 (11%) of 44 in women reached this weight; of bicuspid valves, 96 (18%) of 521 valves in men and 4 (2%) of 236 valves in women reached this weight (unpublished data). In contrast, only 15 (4%) of 361 tricuspid valves in men and only 2 (0.7%) of 281 valves in women reached this weight. Of 1038 operatively excised stenotic aortic valves in men, 161 (16%) were ≥5 g, and of 571 valves in women, only 13 (2%) reached this weight. Seven operatively excised stenotic valves weighed ≥10 g: all were in men and all seven were either unicuspid or bicuspid and the peak pressure gradient across them ranged from 80 to 143 mm Hg (average, 101) (unpublished data).

Associated coronary arterial narrowing

Patients with operatively excised congenitally unicuspid and bicuspid valves have significantly less epicardial coronary arterial narrowing than do patients with tricuspid aortic valves *(Table 7)*. Concomitant coronary artery bypass grafting also varies according to the era during which the aortic valve replacement was done and the institution where it was done. Also, criteria for performing coronary artery bypass grafting in patients having aortic valve replacement have changed with time.

Relation to left bundle branch block and/or complete heart block

At one time, patients with AS and left bundle branch block or complete heart block were believed to have these conduction disturbances because of associated severe coronary arterial narrowing from atherosclerosis. Study at necropsy, however, of many patients with combined AS and left bundle branch block or complete heart block has indicated that the conduction disturbance was due not to associated coronary narrowing but to destruction of the left bundle branches or the atrioventricular bundle by calcific deposits that had extended caudally from the aortic valve (Roberts, unpublished data). Most of these patients had congenitally malformed aortic valves—not tricuspid valves—and severe degrees of hemodynamic obstruction as a result of the heavy calcific deposits.

Table 6. Age, body mass index, concomitant coronary artery bypass, left ventricular to aortic peak systolic gradients, and aortic valve areas in seven aortic valve weight groups in men and in women

AV weight (g)	No. of patients	Age (years): range (average)	BMI (kg/m^2): range (average)	AV weights (g): range (average)	LV–aorta PSG (mm Hg): range (average)	AV area (cm^2): range (mean)	Coronary bypass	UAV or BAV	Ejection fraction (%) No.	Range (mean)	No. (%) ≤40	No. (%) >40
Men												
≤1	0	–	–	–	–	–	–	–	–	–	–	–
>1–2	41	47–90 (72)	19–37 (27)	1.16–2.00 (1.64)	11–81 (36)	0.27–1.43 (0.86)	27 (66%)	11 (27%)	37	15–78 (48)	13 (35%)	24 (65%)
>2–3	60	29–87 (69)	20–43 (29)	2.01–3.00 (2.58)	15–97 (45)	0.42–2.25 (0.89)	32 (53%)	24 (40%)	52	10–85 (51)	14 (27%)	38 (73%)
>3–4	50	37–84 (69)	17–40 (27)	3.03–4.00 (3.40)	20–100 (56)	0.20–1.63 (0.75)	26 (52%)	30 (60%)	44	15–80 (53)	7 (16%)	37 (84%)
>4–5	29	42–87 (69)	18–45 (28)	4.01–4.84 (4.40)	20–108 (64)	0.32–1.06 (0.67)	11 (38%)	25 (86%)	26	15–70 (53)	5 (19%)	21 (81%)
>5–6	12	49–90 (70)	24–36 (28)	5.03–5.93 (5.60)	50–116 (71)	0.40–0.88 (0.60)	3 (25%)	10 (83%)	10	20–65 (43)	4 (40%)	6 (60%)
>6	9	38–84 (58)	21–38 (28)	6.24–11.30 (7.92)	35–141 (87)	0.39–1.23 (0.71)	2 (22%)	8 (89%)	8	15–70 (51)	2 (25%)	6 (75%)
Women												
≤1	10	55–85 (74)	21–44 (30)	0.69–0.95 (0.83)	15–62 (28)	0.34–1.28 (0.83)	7 (70%)	2 (20%)	9	30–70 (47)	4 (44%)	5 (56%)
>1–2	73	19–88 (71)	17–51 (29)	1.02–1.99 (1.46)	10–119 (49)	0.18–1.49 (0.72)	40 (55%)	14 (19%)	66	15–80 (56)	9 (14%)	57 (86%)
>2–3	29	30–87 (70)	18–50 (28)	2.04–3.00 (2.42)	26–113 (63)	0.27–1.09 (0.58)	15 (52%)	12 (41%)	23	30–80 (54)	4 (17%)	19 (83%)
>3–4	10	47–85 (73)	17–35 (26)	3.14–4.00 (3.42)	53–131 (85)	0.23–0.78 (0.51)	3 (30%)	9 (90%)	9	45–75 (53)	0	9 (100%)
>4–5	1	83	29	4.27	53	0.75	0	1 (100%)	1	50	0	1 (100%)
>5–6	0	–	–	–	–	–	–	–	–	–	–	–
>6	0	–	–	–	–	–	–	–	–	–	–	–

Reproduced with permission from Roberts WC and Ko JM, 2004 (17).

AV indicates aortic valve; BAV, bicuspid aortic valve; BMI, body mass index; LV, left ventricular; PSG, peak systolic gradient; UAV, unicuspid aortic valve.

PURE AORTIC REGURGITATION

There are two major causes of pure (no element of stenosis) AR: 1) conditions affecting primarily the valve, and 2) conditions affecting the aorta and only secondarily causing the valve to be incompetent. Roberts and Ko (25) recently reviewed the cause of pure AR in 268 patients having isolated aortic valve replacement at BUMC from 1993 to 2005. As shown in *Table 8*, conditions affecting primarily the valve were the cause of the AR in 122 patients (46%), and nonvalve conditions were the cause in 146 patients (54%). Among the former, the *congenitally bicuspid valve* unassociated with infective endocarditis was the problem in 59 patients, 22 (37%) of whom had resection of portions of the dilated ascending aorta. Eleven of the 22 patients with resected aortas had severe loss of medial elastic fibers. Infective endocarditis was the cause in 46 patients, 15 (33%) of whom had congenitally bicuspid aortic valves. Thus, of the 122 with valve conditions causing the AR, 74 (61%) had congenitally bicuspid aortic valves. Why one congenitally bicuspid aortic valve becomes stenotic (8, 26), another has pure regurgitation without superimposed infective endocarditis (27), another becomes severely dysfunctional only when

Table 7. Frequency of concomitant coronary artery bypass grafting among patients having isolated aortic valve replacement for aortic stenosis at three different institutions*

Valve structure	NIH (1963–1989) (n = 259)	GUMC (1969–1992) (n = 308)	BUMC (1993–2007) (n = 1351)
Unicuspid	2/61 (3%)	13/55 (24%)	13/83 (16%)
Bicuspid	13/140 (9%)	42/162 (26%)	280/646 (43%)
Tricuspid	10/58 (17%)	47/91 (52%)	390/622 (63%)

*Excludes cases in which the number of valve cusps was unclear (indeterminate).

BUMC indicates Baylor University Medical Center; GUMC, Georgetown University Medical Center; NIH, National Institutes of Health.

Table 8. Causes of aortic regurgitation in patients having isolated aortic valve replacement at Baylor University Medical Center (1993–2005)

Causes of aortic regurgitation	Total	Age (years) at operation: range (mean)	M	F	Acute	Chronic	SH	CABG	Portions of ascending aorta			BAV	Calcium deposits on AV cusps	Aortic valve weight (g): range (mean)	
									Excised	Examined histologically	CMN (3+, 4+)			Men	Women
Valve (n = 122; 46%)															
Congenital malformation without infective endocarditis															
Bicuspid	59 (22%)	22–77 (55)	49	10	0	59	39 (66%)	18 (31%)	22	22	11	59	31	0.52–2.99 (1.42)	0.68–1.80 (1.24)
Quadricuspid	2 (1%)	53, 79 (66)	0	2	0	2	0	1 (50%)	0	0	0	0	0	—	0.57, 1.13 (0.85)
Tricuspid	5 (2%)	33–48 (40)	3	2	0	5	2 (40%)	0	1	1	0	0	0	1.11–1.40 (1.23)	0.34, 0.66 (.050)
Infective endocarditis	46 (17%)	21–82 (45)	31	15	27	19	29 (63%)	7 (15%)	6	4	0	15	8	0.77–2.31 (1.53)	0.44–2.50 (0.98)
Rheumatic?	8 (3%)	25–63 (47)	6	2	0	8	6 (75%)	2 (25%)	0	0	0	0	3	1.10–2.45 (1.81)	1.31, 1.83 (1.57)
Miscellaneous	2 (1%)	24, 42 (33)	1	1	0	2	2 (100%)	1 (50%)	0	0	0	0	0	0.55	—
Nonvalve (n = 146; 54%)															
Aortic dissection	28 (10%)	25–78 (58)	20	8	21	7	22 (79%)	5* (17%)	28	20	5	3	4	0.51–1.19 (0.81)	0.37–0.90 (0.59)
Marfan or forme fruste	15 (6%)	21–71 (47)	9	6	0	15	10 (67%)	1† (7%)	15	13	13	0	2	0.73–1.01 (0.94)	0.35–0.85 (0.66)
Aortitis	12 (4%)	35–82 (66)	5	7	0	12	10 (83%)	5 (42%)	12	12	12	0	2	0.63–0.79 (0.70)	0.35–0.70 (0.54)
Etiology unclear	91 (34%)	50–84 (66)	58	33	0	91	83 (91%)	46 (51%)	7	7	0	0	26	0.48–2.13 (1.08)	0.31–1.74 (0.73)
Total	268 (100%)	21–84 (57)	182 (68%)	86 (32%)	48 (18%)	220 (82%)	203 (76%)	86 (32%)	91 (34%)	76	41	77 (29%)	76/263 (29%)	0.48–2.99 (1.22) 151‡	0.31–2.50 (0.81) 75‡

*Four other patients had CABG due to extension of the aortic dissection into a coronary artery.

†One additional patient had CABG due to extension of the aortic dissection into a coronary artery.

‡Number of cases with aortic valve weight.

Reproduced with permission from Roberts WC et al, 2006 (25).

AV indicates aortic valve; BAV, bicuspid aortic valve; CABG, coronary artery bypass grafting; CMN, "cystic medial necrosis" (magnitude of loss of elastic fibers in the aorta's media); F, female; M, male; SH, systemic hypertension.

infective endocarditis appears (28), and some function normally an entire lifetime is unclear (8). Of 85 patients, aged 15 to 79 years, with congenitally bicuspid aortic valves studied at autopsy by Roberts (8), 61 valves (72%) were stenotic, 2 (2%) had pure regurgitation without superimposed infective endocarditis, 9 (11%) had AR because of infective endocarditis, and 13 (15%) functioned normally during the patients' 23 to 59 years of life (mean, 45).

Rheumatic heart disease is a relatively infrequent cause of pure AR in patients with normally functioning mitral valves (9). All such patients (by our definition of rheumatic heart disease) have diffuse fibrosis of the mitral leaflets or at least diffuse thickening of the margins of these leaflets. In this circumstance mitral valve function would be normal despite the anatomic abnormality.

Infective endocarditis more commonly involves a three-cuspid aortic valve than a two-cuspid one because the tricuspid valve is so much more common than the bicuspid valve (28).

Rheumatoid arthritis is a rare cause of AR. The anatomic abnormality is specific for this condition and consists of rheumatoid nodules within the aortic valve cusps (29, 30).

Conditions affecting the ascending aorta and causing it to dilate cause AR more commonly than those conditions

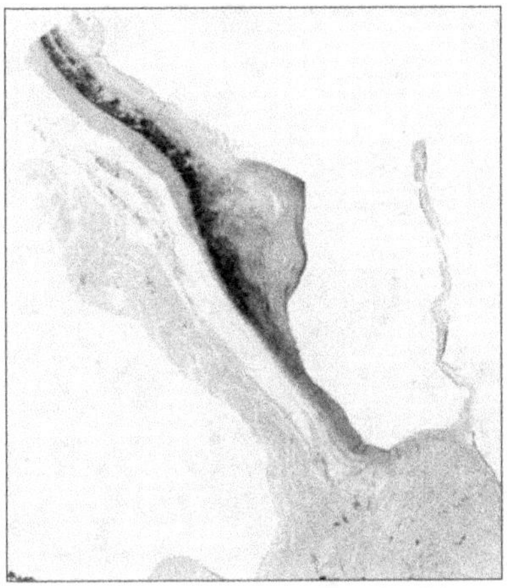

Figure 9. Cardiovascular syphilis. Photomicrographs of an aortic valve cusp, sinus portion of aorta (behind the cusp), and proximal tubular portion of ascending aorta, which is thickened by intimal and adventitial fibrous tissue. Many medial elastic fibers have been destroyed. The location of the process in the tubular portion of the aorta with sparing of the sinus portion of the aorta is characteristic of cardiovascular syphilis. Elastic tissue stain, ×4.5.

affecting primarily the aortic valve. Of 146 patients having pure AR and isolated aortic valve replacement, the cause of the AR was not determined after examination of the operatively excised aorta and aortic valve (25). Many of these patients had *systemic hypertension* but only mild dilation of the aorta, and all had normal or nearly normal three-cuspid aortic valves. It is likely that systemic hypertension in some way played a role in the AR (31, 32).

Aortic dissection usually produces acute AR due to the splitting of the aortic media behind the aortic valve commissures, resulting in prolapse of one or more cusps toward the left ventricular cavity (33).

Diffuse thickening of the tubular portion of the central ascending aorta with sparing of the aortic wall behind the sinuses is characteristic of *cardiovascular syphilis* (34). These patients generally undergo a cardiovascular operation because of diffuse aneurysmal dilatation of the tubular portion of ascending aorta, not as a rule because of severe AR. *Granulomatous (giant cell) aortitis* grossly mimics cardiovascular syphilis but is far less common. During the past 10 years, 15 patients have had resection of aneurysmally dilated syphilitic aortas with or without simultaneous aortic valve replacement at BUMC (unpublished). The characteristic histologic feature of cardiovascular syphilis is extensive thickening of the aortic wall due to fibrous thickening of the intima and adventitia *(Figure 9)*. The medial elastic fibers and smooth-muscle cells are also replaced focally by scars due to narrowings in the vasa vasora. Focal collections of plasma cells and lymphocytes are present in the adventitia. Giant cell aortitis is similar to syphilitic aortitis except for the presence of multinucleated giant cells.

The AR in patients with *the Marfan syndrome* and forme fruste varieties of it is the result of severe dilatation of the sinus portion and proximal tubular portion of the aorta (35). The consequence of the "aortic root" dilatation is stretching of the aortic valve cusps in roughly a straight line between the commissures, leading to a wide-open central regurgitant stream. In contrast to cardiovascular syphilis, the aortic wall in the Marfan syndrome is thinner than normal due to the massive loss of medial elastic fibers and lack of thickening of either the intima or the adventitia.

Ankylosing spondylitis causes AR by involving both the valve cusps and the portion of aorta behind and adjacent to the lateral attachments of the aortic valve cusps (36, 37). About 5% of patients with this form of arthritis develop AR. The bases of the aortic valve cusps become densely thickened by fibrous tissue, which is also present on the ventricular aspect of the anterior mitral leaflet and on the left ventricular aspect of the membranous ventricular septum. Varying degrees of heart block may result from this subaortic deposit of dense fibrous tissue. The AR associated with ankylosing spondylitis is usually severe, with diastolic pressures in both the aorta and the left ventricle often being similar. The histologic appearance of the aorta in ankylosing spondylitis is similar to that in syphilitis, but the syphilitic process never extends onto the aortic valve cusps or into the subvalvular area and rarely involves the wall of aorta behind the sinuses.

A diagram of the various conditions affecting the aortic valve is shown in *Figure 10*.

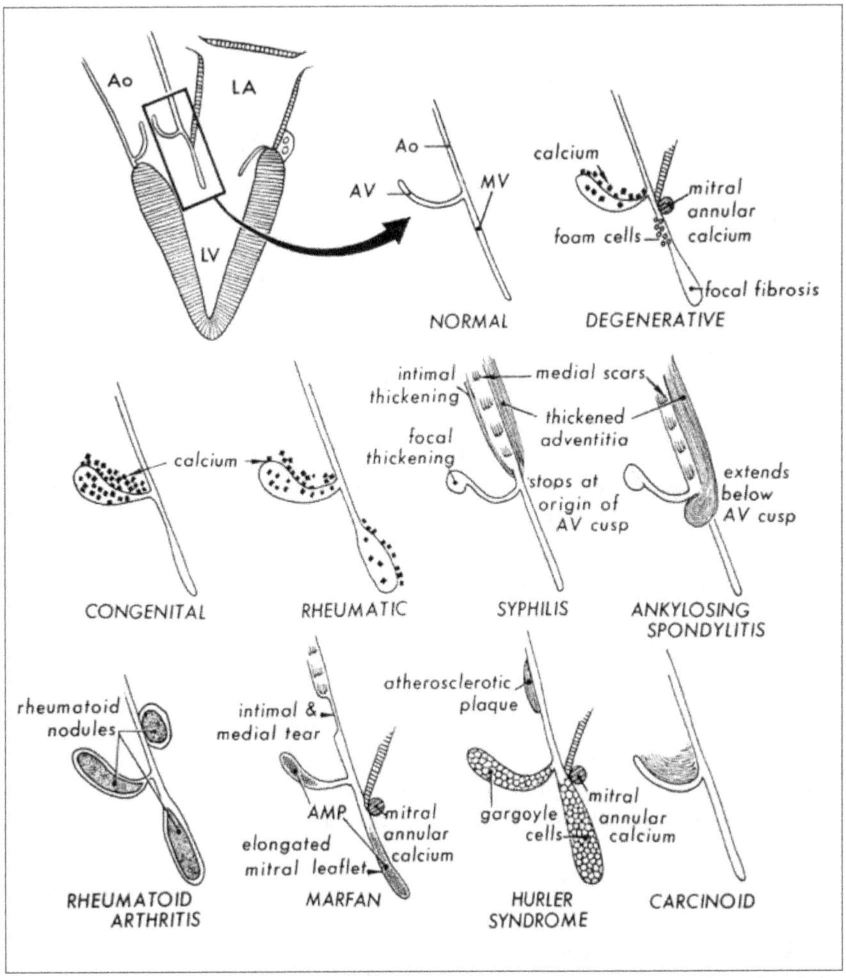

Figure 10. Some of the conditions affecting the aorta or aortic valve or mitral valve. Reproduced with permission from Roberts WC and Perloff JK, 1972 (38).

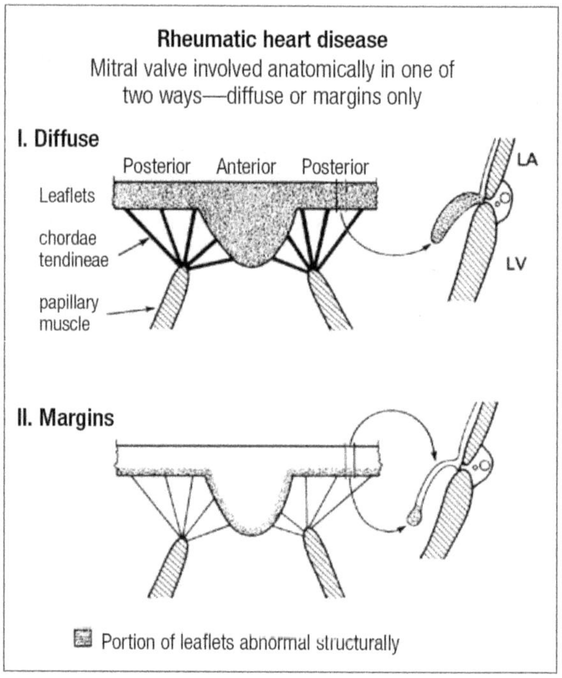

Figure 11. The two types of anatomic involvement of the mitral valve in rheumatic heart disease.

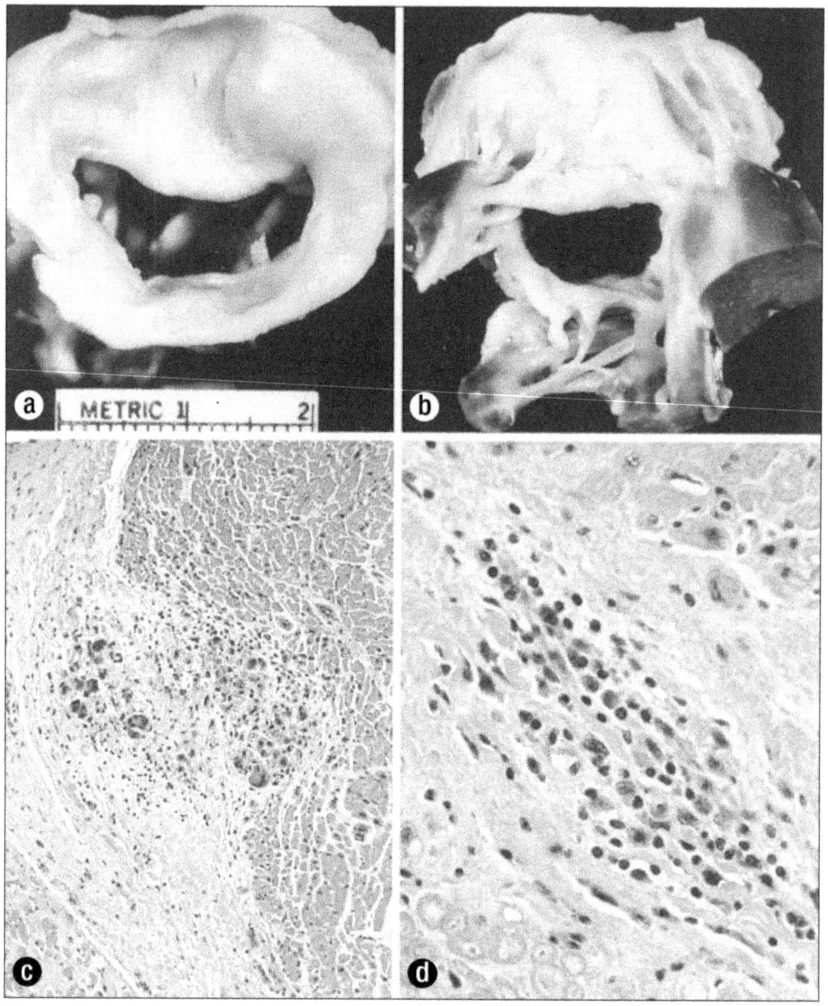

Figure 12. Acute rheumatic fever and mitral stenosis. Excised mitral valve in a 23-year-old Indian woman with mitral stenosis (13 mm Hg mean diastolic pressure gradient between pulmonary artery wedge and left ventricle) and regurgitation. She had had acute rheumatic fever initially at age 7 years and recurrence of migratory polyarthritis at age 22. During the early postoperative course after mitral valve replacement, she had swelling and pain in one knee and one ankle and erythema about two joints. Shown are the excised valves viewed from **(a)** the left atrium and **(b)** the left ventricle and **(c, d)** Aschoff bodies, which were numerous in both excised left ventricular papillary muscles. Hematoxylin and eosin stain, ×110 (c), ×400 (d). Reproduced with permission from Virmani R and Roberts WC, 1977 (41).

MITRAL STENOSIS

Of the 1010 patients aged ≥15 years with functionally severe valvular cardiac disease studied at necropsy by Roberts up to 1980, 434 (44%) had MS (1). MS occurred alone in 189 (44%) patients and in combination with other functional valve lesions in the other 245 patients (56%). MS was of rheumatic etiology in all 434 patients.

Rheumatic heart disease may be viewed as a disease of the mitral valve; other valves also may be involved both anatomically and functionally, but anatomically the mitral valve is always involved (38, 39) *(Figure 11). Aschoff bodies* have never been reported in hearts without anatomic disease of the mitral valve (39). Of the first 543 patients with severe valvular heart disease that Roberts and Virmani (40) studied at necropsy, 11 (2.7%) had Aschoff bodies, and all had anatomic mitral valve disease. The 11 patients ranged in age from 18 to 68 years (mean, 38), and 9 had a history of acute rheumatic fever; 9 had MS with or without dysfunction of one or more other cardiac valves; 1 had isolated AR; and 1 had both AR and MR. All 11 had diffuse fibrous thickening of the mitral leaflets, and all but one had diffuse anatomic lesions of at least two other cardiac valves. Thus, among patients with chronic valve disease, Aschoff bodies, the only anatomic lesion pathognomic of rheumatic heart disease, usually indicate diffuse anatomic lesions of one or more cardiac valves, and the most common hemodynamic lesion is MS ± MR.

Although rare at necropsy in patients with fatal chronic valve disease, Aschoff bodies are fairly common in the heart of patients having mitral commissurotomy for MS. Among 481 patients having various valve operations, Aschoff bodies were found by Virmani and Roberts (41) in 40 (21%) of 191 operatively excised left atrial appendages, in 4 (2%) of 273 operatively excised left ventricular papillary muscles, and in 1 (6%) of 17 patients in whom both appendage and papillary muscle were excised. Of these 45 patients with Aschoff bodies, 44 had MS *(Figure 12)* and only one, a 10-year-old boy, had pure MR. Sinus rhythm was present preoperatively in 38 (84%), and atrial fibrillation in 7 (16%).

Not only is rheumatic heart disease a disorder of the cardiac valves, it may also affect mural endocardium, epicardium, and myocardium. The atrial walls virtually always have increased amounts of fibrous tissue in both the myocardial interstitium and in the mural endocardium, atrophy of some and hypertrophy of other myocardial cells, and hypertrophy of smooth muscles in the mural endocardium. In all patients with rheumatic MS, the leaflets are diffusely thickened either by fibrous

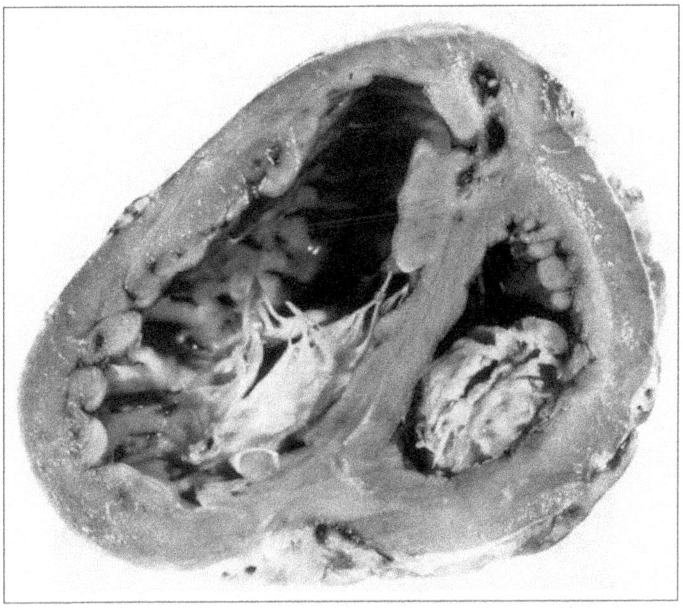

Figure 13. Mitral stenosis. Heart in a 16-year-old boy who had acute rheumatic fever at age 6 years and chronic heart failure beginning at age 10. He had severe mitral stenosis and tricuspid valve regurgitation. At cardiac catheterization 10 hours before death, the right ventricular pressure was 100/20 and the left ventricular pressure, 100/10 mm Hg. By left ventricular angiogram, the left ventricular cavity was of normal size and there was no mitral regurgitation. At necropsy, the heart weighed 450 g (patient weight, 43 kg). The right ventricular cavity was greatly dilated, and both ventricular walls were of similar thickness. Both mitral and tricuspid valve leaflets were diffusely thickened and free of calcific deposits. No Aschoff bodies were found. Reproduced with permission from Roberts WC, 1983 (39).

tissue or calcific deposits or both, the two commissures are usually fused, and the chordae tendineae are usually (but not always) thickened and fused *(Figures 13 and 14).*

The amount of calcium in the leaflets of stenotic mitral valves varies considerably *(Figure 15).* Generally, the calcific deposits are more frequent and in larger quantities in men than in women, in older than in younger patients, and in those with higher vs those with lower pressure gradients between the left atrium and left ventricle (Figure 14). The rapidity with which calcium develops also varies considerably: it is present at a younger age in men than in women. Lachman and Roberts (42) determined the presence or absence and the extent of calcific deposits in operatively excised stenotic mitral valves in 164 patients aged 26 to 72 years. The amount of calcific deposits in the stenotic mitral valves correlated with *sex* and the *mean transvalvular pressure gradient (Figure 16),* but it did not correlate with the patients' age (after 25 years), cardiac rhythm, pulmonary arterial or pulmonary arterial wedge pressure, previous mitral commissurotomy, presence of thrombus in the body or appendage of left ventricle, or the presence of disease in one or more other cardiac valves. Of the 164 patients, radiographs of the operatively excised valve showed no calcific deposits in 14 and only minimal deposits in 43. Of these 57 patients, however, 37 had moderate or severe MR. The remaining 20 in an earlier era would have been ideal or nearly ideal candidates for mitral commissurotomy (43).

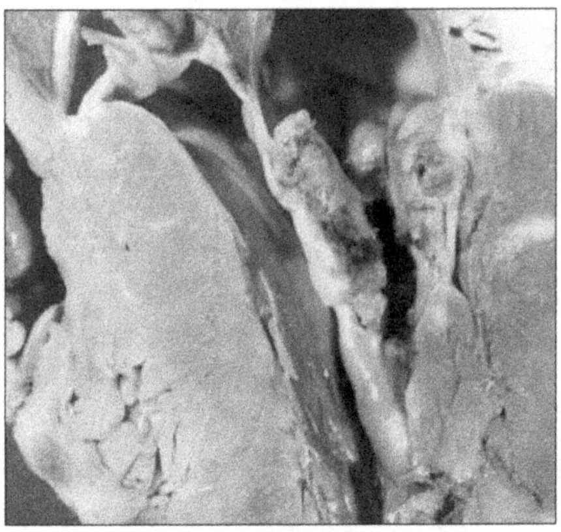

Figure 14. Mitral stenosis. Longitudinal view of a very narrow and thickened mitral valve in a 55-year-old man with equal peak systolic pressures in the right and left ventricles and no associated mitral regurgitation during cannulation of the aorta for planned mitral valve replacement. Both anterior and posterior mitral leaflets are heavily calcified. Reproduced with permission from Roberts WC, 1983 (39).

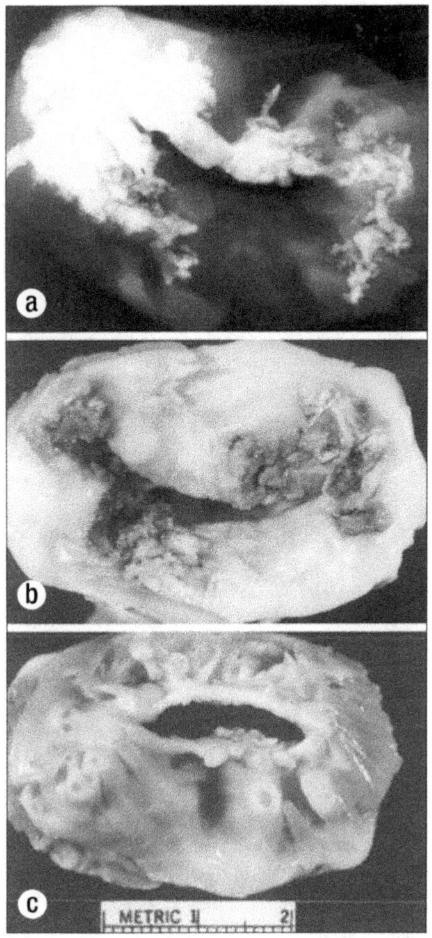

Figure 15. Mitral stenosis. Operatively excised heavily calcified stenotic mitral valve in a 57-year-old man with combined mitral stenosis (12 mm Hg mean transvalvular diastolic gradient) and aortic stenosis. **(a)** Radiograph of the excised valve. **(b)** View of valve from the left atrial aspect. Thrombi are present near and at the commissures. **(c)** View from the left ventricular aspect. The orifice is severely narrowed.

A major complication of MS is *thrombus formation in the left atrial cavity.* The thrombus may be limited to the atrial appendage (by far most common) or be located in both the appendage and body of the left atrium. Left atrial "body" thrombus was observed in 5% of the 1010 necropsy patients with fatal valvular heart disease studied by Roberts, and all had severe MS (unpublished data). Left atrial "body" thrombus was not found in any of the 165 patients with pure MR. All patients with left atrial "body" thrombus had atrial fibrillation. In contrast, of 46 patients with MS who had cardiotomy at the National Heart, Lung, and Blood Institute and had thrombus in the left atrial "body," 42 (91%) had atrial fibrillation and 4 (9%) had sinus rhythm. *Thrombus appears to occur in the body of the left atrium only in patients with MS, and atrial fibrillation in the absence of MS is incapable of forming thrombus in the left atrial body.*

Calcific deposits on the mural endocardium of the left atrium almost certainly are indicative of previous organization of left

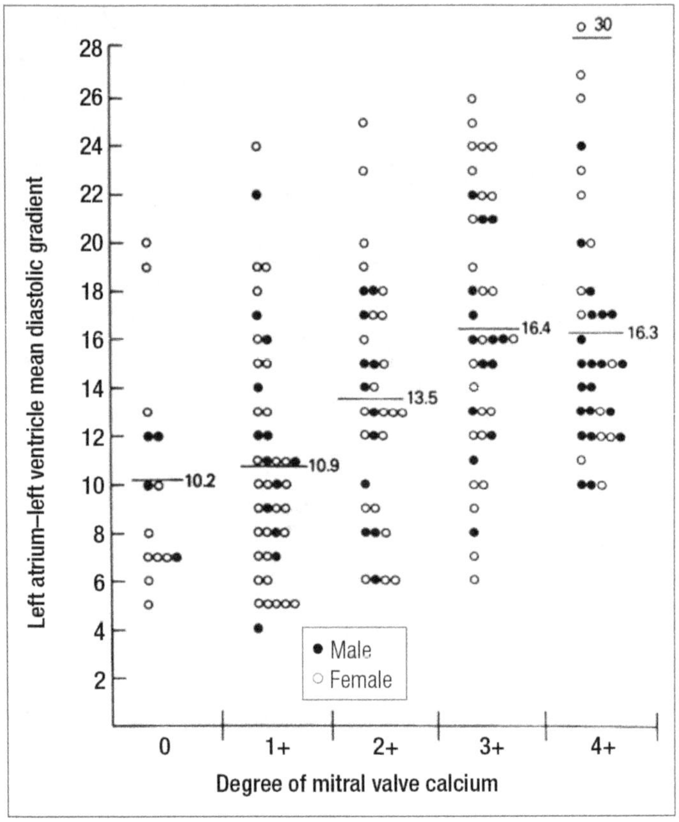

Figure 16. Mitral stenosis. Comparison of the relation of the mean left atrial–left ventricular diastolic gradient to the quantity of mitral valve calcium graded by radiograph of the operatively excised mitral valve. The greater the quantity of mitral calcium, the greater the transvalvular gradient. Reproduced with permission from Lachman AS and Roberts WC, 1978 (42).

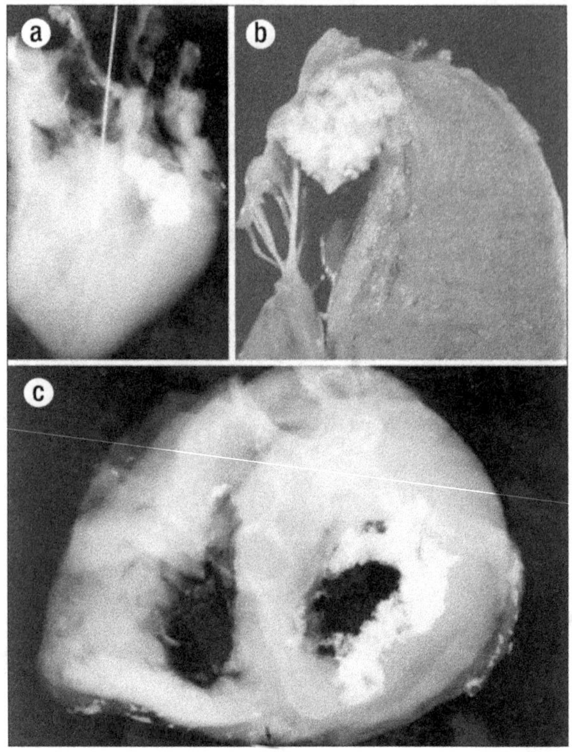

Figure 17. Mitral annular calcium. Heavily calcified mitral annulus in a 71-year-old woman with previous second-degree heart block and a pacemaker for 23 months. She died of acute myocardial infarction complicated by rupture of the left ventricular free wall. **(a)** Radiograph of the heart at necropsy showing mitral annular calcium and the pacemaker leads. **(b)** Longitudinal section showing heavy calcific deposits behind the posterior mitral leaflet. **(c)** Radiograph of the base of the heart (after removing its apical one-half) showing the circumferential extent of the mitral annular calcific deposits. Reproduced with permission from Roberts WC et al, 1973 (34).

atrial thrombi (44). Histologically, the "calcific thrombi" also contain cholesterol clefts and are identical to atherosclerotic plaques. The observation that left atrial thrombi can organize into lesions identical to atherosclerotic plaques supports the view that atherosclerotic plaques may in part be the result of organization of thrombi.

Nonrheumatic causes of MS include *congenital anomalies* (38, 39); *large mitral annular calcific deposits associated with left ventricular outflow obstruction* (45, 46) *(Figure 17); neoplasms* (particularly myxoma) protruding through the mitral orifice (47); *large vegetations from active infective endocarditis* (48); and of course a mechanical prosthesis or bioprosthesis used to replace a native mitral valve (49).

Histologic examination of sections of stenotic mitral valves when stained for elastic fibers shows the mitral leaflet to have lost most or all of its spongiosa element such that the leaflet itself consists entirely or nearly entirely of the fibrosa element. The leaflet (as are the chordae) is outlined by an elastic fibril (which stains black by an elastic tissue stain), and covering it on both atrial and ventricular aspects is dense fibrous tissue containing focally some vascular channels. Similar dense fibrous tissue surrounds the chordae, and the chordae themselves appear normal.

Patients with MS usually have distinct pulmonary vascular changes secondary to the pulmonary venous and arterial hypertension. These anatomic changes consist of thickening of the media of the muscular and elastic pulmonary arteries and focal intimal fibrous plaques. Plexiform lesions never occur in the lungs as a result of MS. The alveolar septa also thicken due to dilatation of the capillaries, proliferation of lining alveolar cells, and some increase of alveolar septal fibrous tissue.

PURE MITRAL REGURGITATION

Pure MR (no element of MS) is the most common dysfunctional cardiac valve disorder, and, in contrast to MS, it has many different causes. If patients with MR due to left ventricular dilatation from any cause (ischemic cardiomyopathy, idiopathic dilated cardiomyopathy, anemia, etc.) are excluded, the most common cause of MR treated operatively in the Western world today is *MVP (Figures 18 and 19)*. This condition, which was described initially in the 1960s by Barlow and colleagues (50) and by Criley and colleagues (51), is now recognized to occur in approximately 5% of adults, and, if one considers this condition a congenital deficiency of mitral tissues—which we do—it is the most common congenital cardiovascular disease. Among 97 patients having mitral valve replacement for pure MR from 1968 to 1981 at the National Heart, Lung, and Blood Institute, MVP was responsible in 60 patients (62%), papillary muscle dysfunction from coronary heart disease in 29 (30%), infective endocarditis in 5 (5%), and possibly rheumatic disease in 3 (3%) (52).

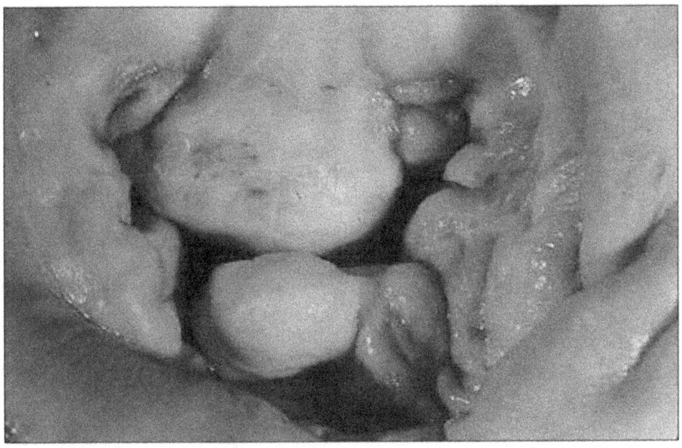

Figure 18. Mitral valve prolapse. View from above shows prolapse of both anterior and posterior cusps in a man who died from consequences of an acute myocardial infarction.

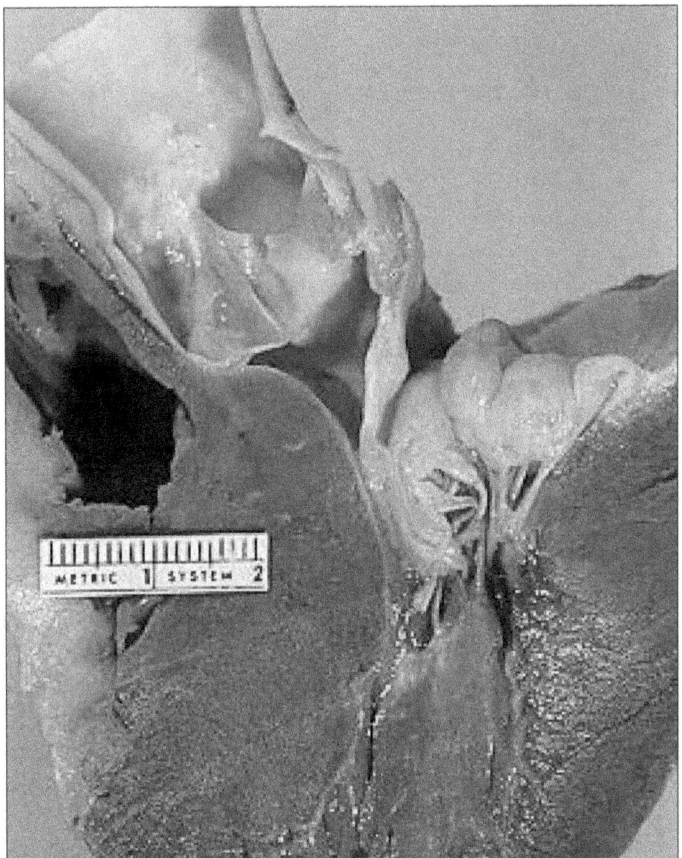

Figure 19. Mitral valve prolapse. View of prolapsed posterior leaflet in a 74-year-old woman who during life was found to have a precordial murmur but never had symptoms of cardiac dysfunction.

Although several authors have attempted to do so, defining MVP has not been easy (1). The following have proved useful in separating the valve affected by MVP from mitral valves affected by other conditions:

1. *Focal lengthening of the posterior and/or anterior mitral leaflets from their site of attachment to their distal margins.* Normally, the length of the posterior leaflet from its attachment to distal margin is about 1 cm. In MVP, this leaflet focally is often as long as the anterior leaflet (52).
2. *Elongation and thinning of chordae tendineae.*
3. *Focal thickening of the posterior and/or anterior leaflet.* This finding is particularly prominent on the portion of leaflet that prolapses toward or into the left atrium during ventricular systole. The atrial surface is uniformly smooth. The thickening of the leaflet produces a spongy feel.
4. *Increase in area, either focally or diffusely, of one or both mitral leaflets* (52).
5. *Loss of chordae tendineae on the ventricular aspect of the posterior mitral leaflet.* It is rare to actually see a ruptured chorda, but what is seen are areas where chordae should be attached but none are there. They presumably ruptured in the past and with time were matted down on the leaflets' ventricular aspect, giving this surface a "bumpy" appearance and feel. Chordae are nearly uniformly missing (previously ruptured) in portions of posterior mitral leaflet excised during mitral valve repair or during replacement. Indeed, MVP appears to be by far the most common cause of ruptured chordae tendineae. Infective endocarditis is the next most frequent cause (53).
6. *Dilatation of the mitral annulus.* Annular dilatation is probably the major cause of development of severe MR in the presence of MVP (52, 54). (The other is rupture of chordae tendineae.) Normally, the mitral annulus in adults averages about 9 cm in circumference. In patients with left ventricular dilatation from any cause, with or without MR, the mitral circumference usually dilates slightly, usually to about 11 cm or <25% above normal (55). Among patients with MVP associated with severe MR, this annular circumference generally increases >50% to 12 to 18 cm. Acute rupture of chordae tendineae may occur in patients with MVP in the absence of mitral annular dilatation.
7. *An increase in the transverse dimension of the mitral leaflets such that the length of the mitral circumference measured on a line corresponding to the distal margin of the posterior leaflet is much larger than the circumference measured at the level of the mitral annulus* (52). In the normal mitral valve, the two are the same. It is analogous to a skirt gathered at the waist. The leaflets of the opened normal mitral valve are flat or smooth on the atrial aspect (like the mucosa of the ileum) whereas those of the opened floppy mitral valve are undulating (like those of the duodenum or jejunum).
8. *Focal thickening of mural endocardium of the left ventricle behind the posterior mitral leaflet.* Salazar and Edwards (56) called these fibrous thickenings "friction lesions" to indicate that they are believed to result from friction between the overlying leaflets and chordae and the underlying left ventricular wall. Lucas and Edwards (57) observed these "friction lesions" in 77 (75%) of 102 necropsy cases of MVP, and Dollar and Roberts (58) found them in 23 (68%) of 34 necropsy cases of MVP.
9. *Fibrinous deposits on the atrial surface of the prolapsed portion of mitral leaflet and particularly at the angle formed between the prolapsed leaflet and left atrial wall* (mitral valve–left atrial angle). These fibrin deposits may be a source of emboli.

Histologically, the MVP valve is distinctive. Elastic tissue stains reveal that the mitral leaflet and chordae are surrounded by a single thick elastic fibril. The underlying leaflet generally—

Table 9. Reported necropsy cases of mitral valve prolapse

First author, year (reference)	Number with MVP	Age (years)	Male/female	MVP cause of death	No. of mitral leaflets prolapsed 1/2	MR	RCT	IE	SD	MS	ASD*	MAC	HW increased	DMA
Pomerance, 1969 (60)	35†	51–98 (mean 74)	23/12	4	12/23	8	2‡	2	1	0	1	9	13	–
Davies, 1978 (61)	90§	<40–100	44/46	6	69/21	23	–	9	13	0	0	3	8‖	6
Lucas, 1982 (57)	102¶	69 ± 12	62/40	4	34/68	18	7‡	7	0	1	3	–	–	–
Lucas, 1982 (57)	69**	–	–	–	–	–	19‡	7	16	20	9	–	–	–
Dollar, 1991 (58)	56**	16–70 (mean 48)	33/23	29	50/6	32	18‡	0	15	2	4	12	30††	40

*Secundum type atrial septal defect.
†Thirty cases from a single hospital (1% of autopsies).
‡Unassociated with infective endocarditis.
§Cases acquired from four different hospitals (4.5% of autopsies).
‖Heart weight >300 g.
¶Cases seen in a single community hospital (7% of autopsies).
**Cases "whose hearts had been sent to Edwards or Roberts for his opinion and interest."
††Heart weight >350 g in women and >400 g in men.
ASD indicates atrial septal defect; DMA, dilated mitral annulus; HW, heart weight; IE, infective endocarditis; MAC, mitral annular calcium; MR, mitral regurgitation; MS, the Marfan syndrome; MVP, mitral valve prolapse; RCT, ruptured chordae tendineae; SD, sudden death; –, no information available.

but not always—contains an excessive amount of the spongiosa element, and this causes the leaflet itself to be a bit thicker than normal. Most of the leaflet thickening, however, is due to superimposed fibrous tissue on both its atrial and ventricular aspects. The covering on the atrial side of the leaflet contains numerous elastic fibrils, whereas that on the ventricular aspect contains few or no elastic fibrils. Often on the ventricular aspect, previously ruptured and now "matted" chordae tendineae are covered by fibrous tissue. The spongiosa element within the leaflet itself appears normal—just increased in amount—and therefore the phrase "mucoid degeneration" appears inappropriate.

Ultrastructural studies of mitral valves grossly characteristic of MVP have disclosed alterations of the collagen fibers in the leaflets and in the chordae tendineae (59). These changes have included fragmentation, splitting, swelling, and course granularity of the individual collagen fibers, and also spiraling and twisting of the fibers. These alterations in the structure of the collagen are probably far more important than the excess acid mucopolysaccharide material in the leaflet in that they lead to focal weakness of the leaflets and chordae and their subsequent elongation. The left ventricular systolic pressure exerted against these weakened areas may account for the prolapse.

Just as the frequency of MVP varies clinically depending on the age and sex group being examined and in the clinical criteria employed for diagnosis (auscultatory, echocardiographic, angiographic), its frequency at necropsy is quite variable and the variation is determined by several factors: 1) age and sex group of the population being examined; 2) type of institution where necropsy is performed (general hospital, referral hospital for cardiovascular disease, or medical examiner's [coroner's] office); 3) expertise in cardiovascular disease of the physician performing the necropsy or reporting the findings; 4) percentage of total deaths having autopsies at the particular hospital; 5) presence or absence of evidence of cardiac disease before death; 6) whether the patient underwent mitral valve replacement or repair; and 7) whether the percentage of patients being examined had a high frequency of the Marfan syndrome, infective endocarditis, atrial septal defect, and so on.

No study shows better how bias alters the finding in necropsy studies than the one performed by Lucas and Edwards *(Table 9)* (57). These investigators, in one portion of their study, determined the frequency of and complications of floppy mitral valves observed at necropsy in one community (nonreferral) hospital for adults. Of 1376 autopsies performed, 7% or 102 patients had morphologically floppy mitral valves at necropsy. Their mean age at death was 69 ± 12 years; 62 (61%) were men and 40 (39%) were women. Of the 102 patients, MVP was the cause of death in only four. Of the 102 patients, one leaflet had prolapsed in 34 patients and two leaflets in 68. Only 18 had anatomic evidence of previous MR; 7 had infective endocarditis; 7 had ruptured chordae tendineae (without infection); 1 had the Marfan syndrome; and 3 had secundum atrial septal defect. No patient died suddenly. In contrast, in the other portion of their study, these authors described complications in 69 necropsy patients whose hearts had been sent to Edwards for his opinion and interest. Among these 69 patients, 16 (23%) had died suddenly and unexpectedly; 19 (28%) had ruptured chordae tendineae (without infection); 7 (10%) had infective endocarditis; 20 (29%) had the Marfan syndrome; and 9 (13%) had secundum-type atrial septal defect. Thus, in contrast to their infrequency in their community hospital series, most cases submitted to their cardiovascular registry from other institutions had ruptured chordae, infective endocarditis, sudden unexpected and unexplained death, or the Marfan syndrome.

The earlier studies by Pomerance (60) and by Davies and colleagues (61) can also be compared to the community hospital series of Lucas and Edwards (57) *(Table 9)*. The study by

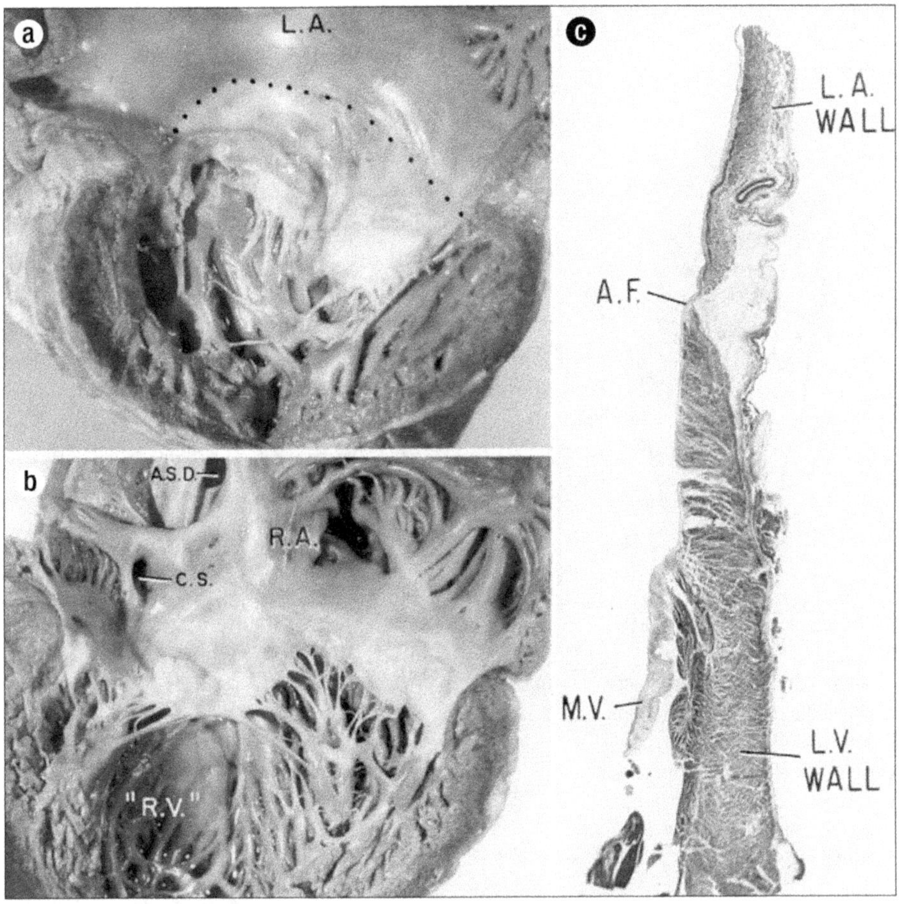

Figure 20. Corrected transposition of the great arteries and Ebstein's anomaly of the left-sided atrioventricular valve in a 38-year-old woman who was cyanotic from birth and in heart failure periodically all of her life. She also had severe pulmonic valve stenosis and ventricular septal defect. She died shortly after operative insertion of a conduit between the left subclavian and left main pulmonary arteries. **(a)** Opened left atrium (LA) and anatomic right ventricle. The normal annulus is shown by the dotted line. **(b)** Opened right atrium (RA) and anatomic left ventricle (RV). ASD indicates atrial septal defect; CS, ostium of coronary sinus. **(c)** Histologic section of left atrial and left ventricular (LV) walls showing the normal annulus fibrosis (AF) and insertion of the mitral valve (MV) considerably caudal to the annulus and directly across from the ventricular wall. Verhoeff-von Gieson stain, ×4. Reproduced with permission from Berry WB et al, 1964 (67).

Dollar and Roberts (58) is comparable to the study of Lucas and Edwards and their selected cases. These authors studied at necropsy 56 patients, aged 16 to 70 years (mean, 48), and compared findings in the 15 who died suddenly and unexpectedly with the other 41 who did not. Compared with the 34 patients without associated congenital heart disease and with non-MVP conditions capable in themselves of being fatal, the 15 patients who died suddenly with isolated MVP were younger (mean age, 39 vs 52 years), were more often women (67% vs 26%), had a lower frequency of MR (7% vs 38%), and were less likely to have ruptured chordae tendineae (29% vs 67%).

The frequency of atrial fibrillation is different in patients with MVP and those with MS immediately before a mitral valve replacement or "repair." Among 246 patients aged 21 to 84 years (mean, 61; men, 66%) who had mitral valve repair or replacement for MR secondary to MVP, Berbarie and Roberts (62) found only 37 patients (15%) (mean age, 60) with atrial fibrillation and 209 patients (88%) with sinus rhythm. In contrast, of 104 patients aged 33 to 80 years (12% men) with rheumatic MS severe enough or symptomatic enough to warrant mitral valve replacement, Sims and Roberts (63) found atrial fibrillation by electrocardiogram immediately preoperatively in 47 (45%) and sinus rhythm in 57 (55%).

Other causes of pure mitral regurgitation

Cleft anterior mitral leaflet. Partial atrioventricular "defect" includes a spectrum of five anatomic anomalies (64). Some patients have all five and others have only one or two. The five are the following: 1) defect in the lowermost portion of the atrial septum, so-called primum atrial septal defect; 2) defect in, or absence of, the posterobasal portion of the ventricular septum; 3) cleft anterior mitral leaflet; 4) anomalous chordae tendineae from the anterior mitral leaflet to the crest of the ventricular septum; and 5) partial or complete absence of the septal tricuspid valve leaflet. There are at least four potential functional consequences of these five anatomic anomalies: 1) shunt at the atrial level, 2) shunt at the ventricular level, 3) MR, and 4) obstruction to left ventricular outflow. Well over 95% of patients with partial atrioventricular defect have a primum-type atrial septal defect, and most of those without a primum defect have a shunt at the ventricular level. The occurrence of MR from a cleft in the anterior mitral leaflet unassociated with a defect in either atrial or ventricular septa is rare, but such has been the case in several reported patients (65).

Left-sided atrioventricular valve regurgitation associated with corrected transposition of the great arteries. Corrected transposition is an entity that has produced much confusion (66, 67). Corrected transposition and complete transposition are quite different; the only thing they have in common is the word "transposition." Complete transposition is essentially one defect: the great arteries are transposed, so that the aorta arises from the right ventricle and the pulmonary trunk from the left ventricle. In corrected transposition, the great arteries also are transposed, but in addition, the ventricles, atrioventricular valves, epicardial coronary arteries, and conduction system are inverted. Patients with complete transposition die because they have inadequate communications between the two circuits. Patients with corrected transposition theoretically should be able to live a full lifespan, but usually this is not the case because associated defects—namely, ventricular septal defect or regurgitation of the left-sided atrioventricular valve or both—cause the heart to function abnormally. The left-sided valve anatomically is a tricuspid valve (in the case of the situs solitus heart), and its most frequent abnormality is the Ebstein-type abnormality *(Figure 20).* Although most patients with corrected transpo-

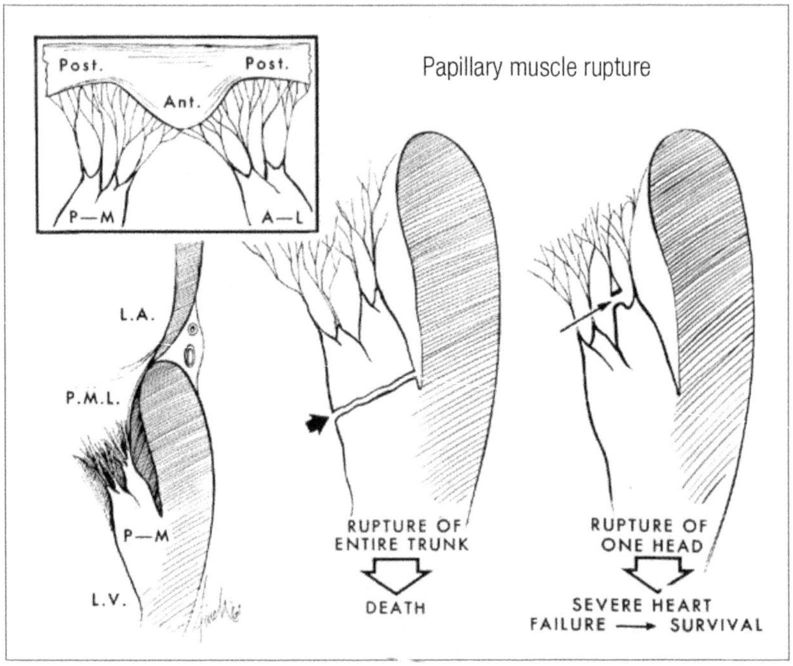

Figure 21. Papillary muscle rupture secondary to acute myocardial infarction. Representation of the possible consequences of papillary muscle rupture during acute myocardial infarction. Rupture of the entire trunk is incompatible with survival (left). With rupture of an apical "head" (right), survival depends on the extent to which function of the left ventricle has been impaired by the infarct. With severely impaired left ventricular function, the additional burden of even modest MR may be intolerable. If the left ventricle is less severely compromised, survival is possible for weeks or months, but heart failure will almost invariably develop. Modified with permission from Morrow AG et al, 1968 (72).

sition present with excessive pulmonary blood flow because of the left-to-right shunt via the ventricular septal defect, an occasional patient with corrected transposition has no defect in the cardiac septa and has evidence of pure "MR," occasionally mistaken for other causes of MR (68).

Infective endocarditis. The most common cardiac valve affected by infective endocarditis is the aortic valve, and the mitral valve is most commonly affected by vegetations growing down the anterior mitral leaflet from the regurgitant aortic valve causing mitral leaflet damage and chordal rupture (69, 70). Infection isolated to the mitral valve is far less common, and when this situation occurs the vegetations are on the atrial aspects of the mitral leaflets (71).

Coronary heart disease. The MR in patients with coronary heart disease is due to myocardial infarction, which may acutely cause necrosis of one or more left ventricular papillary muscles (usually the posteromedial one) with or without rupture of the entire muscle or, far more commonly, rupture of a portion of the "tip" of the papillary muscle (38, 72, 73) *(Figure 21).* Rupture, either partial or complete, of a papillary muscle during acute myocardial infarction is a far less common cause of acute MR than is necrosis of a papillary muscle and the free wall beneath it. When it occurs late after acute myocardial infarction, the MR is usually the result of dilatation of the left ventricular cavity and severe scarring of a papillary muscle, which tends to pull the mitral leaflets laterally, preventing proper coaptation of the two mitral leaflets during ventricular systole.

Cardiomyopathy. Most patients with idiopathic dilated cardiomyopathy (74), ischemic cardiomyopathy (75, 76), and hypertrophic cardiomyopathy (77) have MR at some time in their course. The first two conditions of course are associated with dilatation of the left ventricular cavity primarily in a lateral or right-to-left direction—not in a caudal-cephalad direction—and the consequence is abnormal papillary muscle "pull" on the mitral leaflets during ventricular systole with resulting incomplete coaptation of the mitral leaflets. Evidence that mitral annular dilatation is the prime cause of MR in patients with dilated cardiomyopathy is lacking (55). The cause of MR in patients with hypertrophic cardiomyopathy is entirely different from that in patients with dilated cardiomyopathy and results at least in part in anterior movement of the anterior mitral leaflet toward the ventricular septum during ventricular systole (77). Patients with chronic anemia, e.g., sickle cell anemia, usually also have MR from papillary muscle fibrosis and left ventricular cavity dilatation (78).

1. Roberts WC. Congenital cardiovascular abnormalities usually silent until adulthood. In Roberts WC, ed. *Adult Congenital Heart Disease.* Philadelphia: FA Davis, 1987:631–691.
2. Sprecher DL, Schaefer EJ, Kent KM, Gregg RE, Zech LA, Hoeg JM, McManus B, Roberts WC, Brewer HB Jr. Cardiovascular features of homozygous familial hypercholesterolemia: analysis of 16 patients. *Am J Cardiol* 1984;54(1):20–30.
3. Moura LM, Ramos SF, Zamorano JL, Barros IM, Azevedo LF, Rocha-Gonçalves F, Rajamannan NM. Rosuvastatin affecting aortic valve endothelium to slow the progression of aortic stenosis. *J Am Coll Cardiol* 2007;49(5):554–561.
4. Roberts WC, Perloff JK, Costantino T. Severe valvular aortic stenosis in patients over 65 years of age. A clinicopathologic study. *Am J Cardiol* 1971;27(5):497–506.
5. Stephan PJ, Henry AC 3rd, Hebeler RF Jr, Whiddon L, Roberts WC. Comparison of age, gender, number of aortic valve cusps, concomitant coronary artery bypass grafting, and magnitude of left ventricular-systemic arterial peak systolic gradient in adults having aortic valve replacement for isolated aortic valve stenosis. *Am J Cardiol* 1997;79(2):166–172.
6. Roberts WC, Morrow AG. Congenital aortic stenosis produced by a unicommissural valve. *Br Heart J* 1965;27:505–510.
7. Falcone MW, Roberts WC, Morrow AG, Perloff JK. Congenital aortic stenosis resulting from a unicommissural valve. Clinical and anatomic features in twenty-one adult patients. *Circulation* 1971;44(2):272–280.
8. Roberts WC. The congenitally bicuspid aortic valve. A study of 85 autopsy cases. *Am J Cardiol* 1970;26(1):72–83.
9. Roberts WC. Anatomically isolated aortic valvular disease. The case against its being of rheumatic etiology. *Am J Med* 1970;49(2):151–159.
10. Roberts WC, Ko JM. Clinical and morphologic features of the congenitally unicuspid acommissural stenotic and regurgitant aortic valve. *Cardiology* 2007;108(2):79–81.
11. Roberts WC. The senile cardiac calcification syndrome. *Am J Cardiol* 1986;58(6):572–574.
12. Hurwitz LE, Roberts WC. Quadricuspid semilunar valve. *Am J Cardiol* 1973;31(5):623–626.
13. Roberts WC, Ko JM, Filardo G, Henry AC, Hebeler RF Jr, Cheung EH, Matter GJ, Hamman BL. Valve structure and survival in *sexagenarians* having aortic valve replacement for aortic stenosis (± aortic regurgitation) with versus without coronary artery bypass grafting at a single US medical center (1993 to 2005). *Am J Cardiol* 2007;100(8):1286–1292.

14. Roberts WC, Ko JM. Weights of operatively-excised stenotic unicuspid, bicuspid, and tricuspid aortic valves and their relation to age, sex, body mass index, and presence or absence of concomitant coronary artery bypass grafting. *Am J Cardiol* 2003;92(9):1057–1065.
15. Roberts WC, Ko JM. Weights of individual cusps in operatively-excised congenitally bicuspid stenotic aortic valves. *Am J Cardiol* 2004;94(5):678–681.
16. Roberts WC, Ko JM. Weights of individual cusps in operatively-excised stenotic three-cuspid aortic valves. *Am J Cardiol* 2004;94(5):681–684.
17. Roberts WC, Ko JM. Relation of weights of operatively excised stenotic aortic valves to preoperative transvalvular peak systolic pressure gradients and to calculated aortic valve areas. *J Am Coll Cardiol* 2004;44(9):1847–1855.
18. Roberts WC, Ko JM. Frequency by decades of unicuspid, bicuspid, and tricuspid aortic valves in adults having isolated aortic valve replacement for aortic stenosis, with or without associated aortic regurgitation. *Circulation* 2005;111(7):920–925.
19. Roberts WC, Ko JM, Matter GJ. Isolated aortic valve replacement without coronary bypass for aortic valve stenosis involving a congenitally bicuspid aortic valve in a nonagenarian. *Am J Geriatr Cardiol* 2006;15(6):389–391.
20. Roberts WC, Ko JM, Garner WL, Filardo G, Henry AC, Hebeler RF Jr, Matter GJ, Hamman BL. Valve structure and survival in *octogenarians* having aortic valve replacement for aortic stenosis (± aortic regurgitation) with versus without coronary artery bypass grafting at a single US medical center (1993 to 2005). *Am J Cardiol* 2007;100(3):489–495.
21. Roberts WC, Ko JM, Filardo G, Henry AC, Hebeler RF Jr, Cheung EH, Matter GJ, Hamman BL. Valve structure and survival in *septuagenarians* having aortic valve replacement for aortic stenosis (± aortic regurgitation) with versus without coronary artery bypass grafting at a single US medical center (1993 to 2005). *Am J Cardiol* 2007;100(7):1157–1165.
22. Roberts WC, Ko JM, Hamilton C. Comparison of valve structure, valve weight, and severity of the valve obstruction in 1849 patients having isolated aortic valve replacement for aortic valve stenosis (with or without associated aortic regurgitation) studied at 3 different medical centers in 2 different time periods. *Circulation* 2005;112(25):3919–3929.
23. Roberts WC, Ko JM, Filardo G, Henry AC, Hebeler RF Jr, Cheung EH, Matter GJ, Hamman BL. Valve structure and survival in *quinquagenarians* having aortic valve replacement for aortic stenosis (± aortic regurgitation) with versus without coronary artery bypass grafting at a single US medical center (1993 to 2005). *Am J Cardiol* 2007;100(10):1584–1591.
24. Roberts WC, Ko JM, Filardo G, Kitchens BL, Henry AC, Hebeler RF Jr, Cheung EH, Matter GJ, Hamman BL. Valve structure and survival in *quadragenarians* having aortic valve replacement for aortic stenosis (± aortic regurgitation) with versus without coronary artery bypass grafting at a single US medical center (1993 to 2005). *Am J Cardiol* 2007;100(11):1683–1690.
25. Roberts WC, Ko JM, Moore TR, Jones WH 3rd. Causes of pure aortic regurgitation in patients having isolated aortic valve replacement at a single US tertiary hospital (1993 to 2005). *Circulation* 2006;114(5):422–429.
26. Roberts WC. The structure of the aortic valve in clinically isolated aortic stenosis: an autopsy study of 162 patients over 15 years of age. *Circulation* 1970;42(1):91–97.
27. Roberts WC, Morrow AG, McIntosh CL, Jones M, Epstein SE. Congenitally bicuspid aortic valve causing severe, pure aortic regurgitation without superimposed infective endocarditis. Analysis of 13 patients requiring aortic valve replacement. *Am J Cardiol* 1981;47(2):206–209.
28. Roberts WC, Oluwole BO, Fernicola DJ. Comparison of active infective endocarditis involving a previously stenotic versus a previously nonstenotic aortic valve. *Am J Cardiol* 1993;71(12):1082–1088.
29. Carpenter DF, Golden A, Roberts WC. Quadrivalvular rheumatoid heart disease associated with left bundle branch block. *Am J Med* 1967;43(6):922–929.
30. Roberts WC, Kehoe JA, Carpenter DF, Golden A. Cardiac valvular lesions in rheumatoid arthritis. *Arch Intern Med* 1968;122(2):141–146.
31. Waller BF, Zoltick JM, Rosen JH, Katz NM, Gomes MN, Fletcher RD, Wallace RB, Roberts WC. Severe aortic regurgitation from systemic hypertension (without aortic dissection) requiring aortic valve replacement: analysis of four patients. *Am J Cardiol* 1982;49(2):473–477.
32. Waller BF, Kishel JC, Roberts WC. Severe aortic regurgitation from systemic hypertension. *Chest* 1982;82(3):365–368.
33. Roberts WC. Aortic dissection: anatomy, consequences, and causes. *Am Heart J* 1981;101(2):195–214.
34. Roberts WC, Dangel JC, Bulkley BH. Nonrheumatic valvular cardiac disease: a clinicopathologic survey of 27 different conditions causing valvular dysfunction. *Cardiovasc Clin* 1973;5(2):333–446.
35. Roberts WC, Honig HS. The spectrum of cardiovascular disease in the Marfan syndrome: a clinico-morphologic study of 18 necropsy patients and comparison to 151 previously reported necropsy patients. *Am Heart J* 1982;104(1):115–135.
36. Bulkley BH, Roberts WC. Ankylosing spondylitis and aortic regurgitation. Description of the characteristic cardiovascular lesion from study of eight necropsy patients. *Circulation* 1973;48(5):1014–1027.
37. Roberts WC, Hollingsworth JF, Bulkley BH, Jaffe RB, Epstein SE, Stinson EB. Combined mitral and aortic regurgitation in ankylosing spondylitis. Angiographic and anatomic features. *Am J Med* 1974;56(2):237–243.
38. Roberts WC, Perloff JK. Mitral valvular disease. A clinicopathologic survey of the conditions causing the mitral valve to function abnormally. *Ann Intern Med* 1972;77(6):939–975.
39. Roberts WC. Morphologic features of the normal and abnormal mitral valve. *Am J Cardiol* 1983;51(6):1005–1028.
40. Roberts WC, Virmani R. Aschoff bodies at necropsy in valvular heart disease. Evidence from an analysis of 543 patients over 14 years of age that rheumatic heart disease, at least anatomically, is a disease of the mitral valve. *Circulation* 1978;57(4):803–807.
41. Virmani R, Roberts WC. Aschoff bodies in operatively excised atrial appendages and in papillary muscles. Frequency and clinical significance. *Circulation* 1977;55(4):559–563.
42. Lachman AS, Roberts WC. Calcific deposits in stenotic mitral valves. Extent and relation to age, sex, degree of stenosis, cardiac rhythm, previous commissurotomy and left atrial body thrombus from study of 164 operatively-excised valves. *Circulation* 1978;57(4):808–815.
43. Roberts WC, Lachman AS. Mitral valve commissurotomy versus replacement. Considerations based on examination of operatively excised stenotic mitral valves. *Am Heart J* 1979;98(1):56–62.
44. Roberts WC, Humphries JO, Morrow AG. Giant right atrium in rheumatic mitral stenosis. Atrial enlargement restricted by mural calcification. *Am Heart J* 1970;79(1):28–35.
45. Hammer WJ, Roberts WC, deLeon AC. "Mitral stenosis" secondary to combined "massive" mitral anular calcific deposits and small, hypertrophied left ventricles. Hemodynamic documentation in four patients. *Am J Med* 1978;64(3):371–376.
46. Theleman KP, Grayburn PA, Roberts WC. Mitral "annular" calcium forming a complete circle "O" causing mitral stenosis in association with a stenotic congenitally bicuspid aortic valve and severe coronary artery disease. *Am J Geriatr Cardiol* 2006;15(1):58–61.
47. Roberts WC. Neoplasms involving the heart, their simulators, and adverse consequences of their therapy. *Proc (Bayl Univ Med Cent)* 2001;14(4):358–376.
48. Roberts WC, Ewy GA, Glancy DL, Marcus FI. Valvular stenosis produced by active infective endocarditis. *Circulation* 1967;36(3):449–451.
49. Roberts WC, Bulkley BH, Morrow AG. Pathologic anatomy of cardiac valve replacement: a study of 224 necropsy patients. *Prog Cardiovasc Dis* 1973;15(6):539–587.
50. Barlow JB, Pocock WA, Marchand P, Denny M. The significance of late systolic murmurs. *Am Heart J* 1963;66:443–452.
51. Criley JM, Lewis KB, Humphries JO, Ross RS. Prolapse of the mitral valve: clinical and cine-angiocardiographic findings. *Br Heart J* 1966;28(4):488-496.
52. Waller BF, Morrow AG, Maron BJ, Del Negro AA, Kent KM, McGrath FJ, Wallace RB, McIntosh CL, Roberts WC. Etiology of clinically isolated, severe, chronic, pure mitral regurgitation: analysis of 97 patients over 30 years of age having mitral valve replacement. *Am Heart J* 1982;104(2 Pt 1):276–288.

53. Roberts WC, Braunwald E, Morrow AG. Acute severe mitral regurgitation secondary to ruptured chordae tendineae: clinical, hemodynamic, and pathologic considerations. *Circulation* 1966;33(1):58–70.
54. Roberts WC, McIntosh CL, Wallace RB. Mechanisms of severe mitral regurgitation in mitral valve prolapse determined from analysis of operatively excised valves. *Am Heart J* 1987;113(5):1316–1323.
55. Bulkley BH, Roberts WC. Dilatation of the mitral anulus. A rare cause of mitral regurgitation. *Am J Med* 1975;59(4):457–463.
56. Salazar AE, Edwards JE. Friction lesions of ventricular endocardium. Relation to chordae tendineae of mitral valve. *Arch Pathol* 1970;90(4):364–376.
57. Lucas RV Jr, Edwards JE. The floppy mitral valve. *Curr Probl Cardiol* 1982;7(4):1–48.
58. Dollar AL, Roberts WC. Morphologic comparison of patients with mitral valve prolapse who died suddenly with patients who died from severe valvular dysfunction or other conditions. *J Am Coll Cardiol* 1991;17(4):921–931.
59. Rentería VG, Ferrans VJ, Jones M, Roberts WC. Intracellular collagen fibrils in prolapsed ("floppy") human atrioventricular valves. *Lab Invest* 1976;35(5):439–443.
60. Pomerance A. Ballooning deformity (mucoid degeneration) of atrioventricular valves. *Br Heart J* 1969;31(3):343–351.
61. Davies MJ, Moore BP, Braimbridge MV. The floppy mitral valve. Study of incidence, pathology, and complications in surgical, necropsy, and forensic material. *Br Heart J* 1978;40(5):468–481.
62. Berbarie RF, Roberts WC. Frequency of atrial fibrillation in patients having mitral valve repair or replacement for pure mitral regurgitation secondary to mitral valve prolapse. *Am J Cardiol* 2006;97(7):1039–1044.
63. Sims JB, Roberts WC. Comparison of findings in patients with versus without atrial fibrillation just before isolated mitral valve replacement for rheumatic mitral stenosis (with or without associated mitral regurgitation). *Am J Cardiol* 2006;97(7):1035–1038.
64. Braunwald E, Ross RS, Morrow AG, Roberts WC. Differential diagnosis of mitral regurgitation in childhood: clinical pathological conference at the National Institutes of Health. *Ann Intern Med* 1961;54:223–242.
65. Barth CW 3rd, Dibdin JD, Roberts WC. Mitral valve cleft without cardiac septal defect causing severe mitral regurgitation but allowing long survival. *Am J Cardiol* 1985;55(9):1229–1231.
66. Schiebler GL, Edwards JE, Burchell HB, Dushane JW, Ongley PA, Wood EH. Congenital corrected transposition of the great vessels: a study of 33 cases. *Pediatrics* 1961;27(5 Suppl):849–888.
67. Berry WB, Roberts WC, Morrow AG, Braunwald E. Corrected transposition of the aorta and pulmonary trunk: clinical, hemodynamic and pathologic findings. *Am J Med* 1964;36:35–53.
68. Roberts WC, Ross RS, Davis FW Jr. Congenital corrected transposition of the great vessels in adulthood simulating rheumatic valvular disease. *Bull Johns Hopkins Hosp* 1964;114:157–172.
69. Buchbinder NA, Roberts WC. Left-sided valvular active infective endocarditis. A study of forty-five necropsy patients. *Am J Med* 1972;53(1):20–35.
70. Arnett EN, Roberts WC. Active infective endocarditis: a clinicopathologic analysis of 137 necropsy patients. *Curr Probl Cardiol* 1976;1(7):2–76.
71. Fernicola DJ, Roberts WC. Clinicopathologic features of active infective endocarditis isolated to the native mitral valve. *Am J Cardiol* 1993;71(13):1186–1197.
72. Morrow AG, Cohen LS, Roberts WC, Braunwald NS, Braunwald E. Severe mitral regurgitation following acute myocardial infarction and ruptured papillary muscle. Hemodynamic findings and results of operative treatment in four patients. *Circulation* 1968;37(4 Suppl):II124–II132.
73. Barbour DJ, Roberts WC. Rupture of a left ventricular papillary muscle during acute myocardial infarction: analysis of 22 necropsy patients. *J Am Coll Cardiol* 1986;8(3):558–565.
74. Roberts WC, Siegel RJ, McManus BM. Idiopathic dilated cardiomyopathy: analysis of 152 necropsy patients. *Am J Cardiol* 1987;60(16):1340–1355.
75. Virmani R, Roberts WC. Quantification of coronary arterial narrowing and of left ventricular myocardial scarring in healed myocardial infarction with chronic, eventually fatal, congestive cardiac failure. *Am J Med* 1980;68(6):831–838.
76. Ross EM, Roberts WC. Severe atherosclerotic coronary arterial narrowing and chronic congestive heart failure without myocardial infarction: analysis of 18 patients studied at necropsy. *Am J Cardiol* 1986;57(1):51–56.
77. Klues HG, Maron BJ, Dollar AL, Roberts WC. Diversity of structural mitral valve alterations in hypertrophic cardiomyopathy. *Circulation* 1992;85(5):1651–1660.
78. Berezowski K, Mautner GC, Roberts WC. Scarring of the left ventricular papillary muscles in sickle-cell disease. *Am J Cardiol* 1992;70(15):1368–1370.

Comparison of Interpretations of Valve Structure Between Cardiac Surgeon and Cardiac Pathologist Among Adults Having Isolated Aortic Valve Replacement for Aortic Valve Stenosis (± Aortic Regurgitation)

William Clifford Roberts, MD[a,b,c,*], Travis James Vowels[a], and Jong Mi Ko, BA[a]

Most studies concerning aortic valve structure in patients having aortic valve replacement have utilized the valve structure (unicuspid, bicuspid, tricuspid) as that called by the cardiac surgeon performing the operation. We determined valve structure of 744 operatively excised stenotic aortic valves submitted to the surgical pathology laboratory of a single hospital over a 6-year period and then compared valve structure determined by a single cardiac pathologist (WCR) with that recorded in the operative report dictated by the operating surgeon. Compared with that determined from examination of the operatively excised valve by the cardiac pathologist, valve structure determined at operation was *congruous* in 59% (440 of 744 patients), *incongruous* in 20% (152 of 744), of *uncertain* structure in 1% (9 of 744), and *not mentioned* in 19% (143 of 744). Valve structure was virtually always congruous (278 of 280 cases, 99%) in patients with 3-cuspid valves, less so with bicuspid valves (156 of 280, 56%), and infrequently so with unicuspid valves (6 of 41, 15%). In conclusion, in patients having isolated aortic valve replacement for aortic valve stenosis, the structure of the valve by the operating surgeon was similar (99%) to that described by 1 of us (WCR) when a 3-cuspid aortic valve was excised, but less so when a congenitally unicuspid (15%) or bicuspid (56%) valve was excised. **(Am J Cardiol 2009;103:1139–1145)**

It is useful in patients having aortic valve replacement (AVR) to determine the underlying valve structure, i.e., whether unicuspid, bicuspid, or tricuspid. The first 2 nearly always indicate that the patient has congenital heart disease, and the third that the valve dysfunction was acquired later. The accuracy of determining aortic valve structure at the time of AVR for patients with aortic stenosis (± aortic regurgitation) has not been investigated. To study the accuracy of its being determined at operation, aortic valve structure was determined by a single cardiac pathologist by examining the operatively excised aortic valve in patients having isolated AVR for aortic stenosis and that interpretation was compared with that described by the cardiac surgeon in the operative report.

Methods

From April 9, 2002, to May 31, 2008, a total of 749 operatively excised stenotic aortic valves (± aortic regurgitation) in patients having isolated AVR without associated mitral stenosis or mitral valve replacement were received in the surgical pathology department at Baylor University Medical Center (Dallas, Texas). All of these valves were examined and described by author WCR and all were photographed by author JMK. The April 2002 date was chosen because that was the time all operative reports were placed on the Baylor Physician Portal (Baylor electronic medical record). That the patients had isolated aortic valve disease was confirmed by examination of their preoperative cardiac catheterization and/or echocardiographic reports, which were also available on the Baylor Physician Portal. Patients were considered to have aortic valve stenosis if the peak transvalvular gradient between the left ventricle and ascending aorta was >10 mm Hg (this number was used because it indicates that the valve cusps are structurally abnormal). Patients with "pure" aortic regurgitation, i.e., no element of stenosis, were excluded. Also excluded were patients in whom the stenotic valve was excised in multiple pieces, a circumstance that prevents accurate determination of valve structure in the pathology laboratory. In addition, any patient having replacement of a cardiac valve other than the aortic valve was excluded from this analysis. Valve structure was determined by WCR who also weighed each operatively excised valve during the week that it was excised.

The interval (days) between AVR and dictation of the operative report by the operating surgeon was recorded for each of the 744 patients in whom the valve was intact or each cusp had been removed separately. The interval between the operation and the dictation of the operative note was compared for congruity/incongruity between the cardiac surgeon and cardiac pathologist. In addition, this interval was recorded for each of the 14 cardiac surgeons performing AVR in the 744 patients.

[a]Baylor Heart and Vascular Institute and Departments of [b]Pathology and [c]Internal Medicine, Division of Cardiology, Baylor University Medical Center, Dallas, Texas. Manuscript received December 11, 2008; revised manuscript received and accepted December 11, 2008.

*Corresponding author: Tel: 214-820-7911; fax: 214-820-7533.

E-mail address: wc.roberts@baylorhealth.edu (W.C. Roberts).

Table 1
Data demonstrating congruity/incongruity between a cardiac surgeon and a cardiac pathologist in patients having aortic valve replacement for aortic stenosis, whether or not valve structure was described in the operative report, and intervals between operation and dictation of the operative report

Variable	Cases (n = 744, 100%)	Aortic Valve Structure (determined by cardiac surgeon)			
		Congruous (n = 440, 5%)	Incongruous (n = 152, 59%)	Unclear (n = 9, 1%)	Not Mentioned (n = 143, 19%)
Aortic valve structure (determined by cardiac pathologist)					
Unicuspid	50 (7%)	6 (12%)	32 (64%)	3 (6%)	9 (18%)
Bicuspid	333 (45%)	156 (47%)	119 (36%)	5 (1%)	53 (16%)
Tricuspid	361 (48%)	278 (77%)	1 (<1%)	1 (<1%)	81 (22%)
Aortic valve weight (g)					
Range	0.43–18.38	0.43–18.38	0.67–8.08	1.28–5.44	0.74–6.44
Mean ± SD	2.59 ± 1.51	2.56 ± 1.62	2.89 ± 1.40	3.02 ± 1.49	2.33 ± 1.18
Interval (days) from AVR to dictation of operative report					
0	458 (62%)	299 (65%)	86 (19%)	4 (1%)	69 (15%)
1–7	171 (23%)	90 (53%)	41 (24%)	4 (2%)	36 (21%)
8–14	49 (6%)	21 (43%)	13 (26%)	1 (2%)	14 (29%)
>14	66 (9%)	30 (46%)	12 (18%)	0	24 (36%)

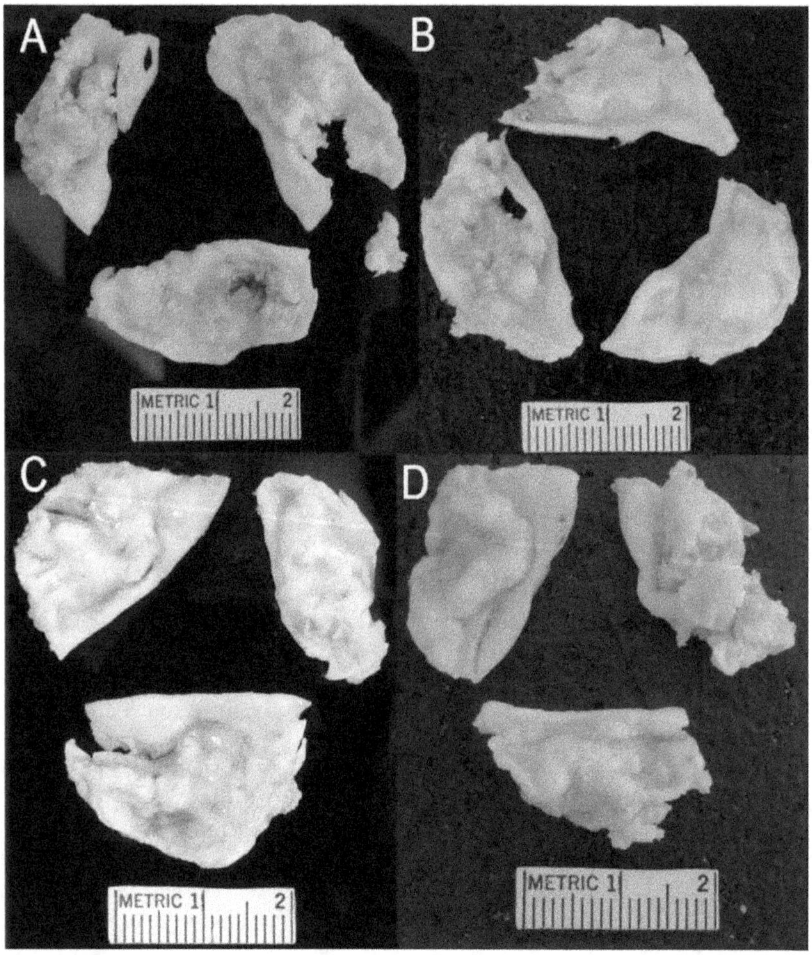

Figure 1. *Three-cuspid valves* in 4 men 71 to 88 years of age (mean 82). The surgeon called 3 (*A, C, D*) valves tricuspid, and the structure of B was not mentioned.

This study was approved by the institutional review board at Baylor University Medical Center.

Results

The major findings are presented in Table 1. Interpretation of aortic valve structure between the cardiac surgeon and cardiac pathologist was congruous in 59% of patients (440 of 744), incongruous in 20% (152 of 744), unclear in 1% (9 of 744), and aortic valve structure was not mentioned in the operative report in 19% (143). Relatively similar percentages were seen when men and women were analyzed separately.

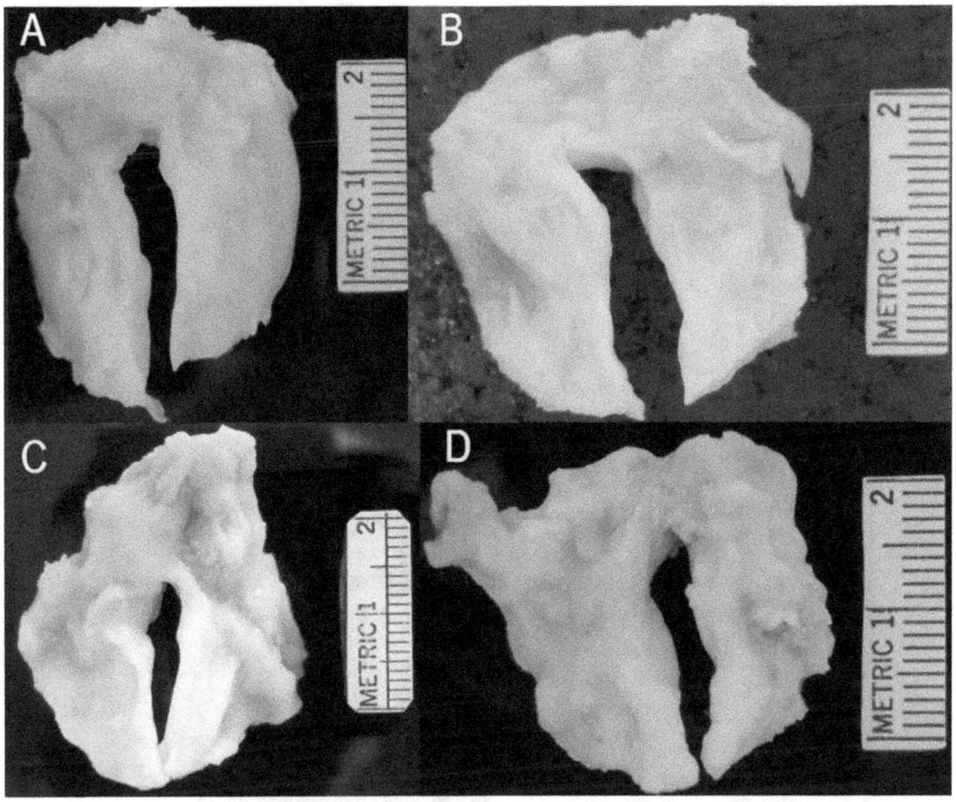

Figure 2. Congenitally unicuspid unicommissural valves in 4 patients 41 to 67 years of age. The cardiac surgeon called the valves bicuspid *(A, C)* and tricuspid *(B, D)*.

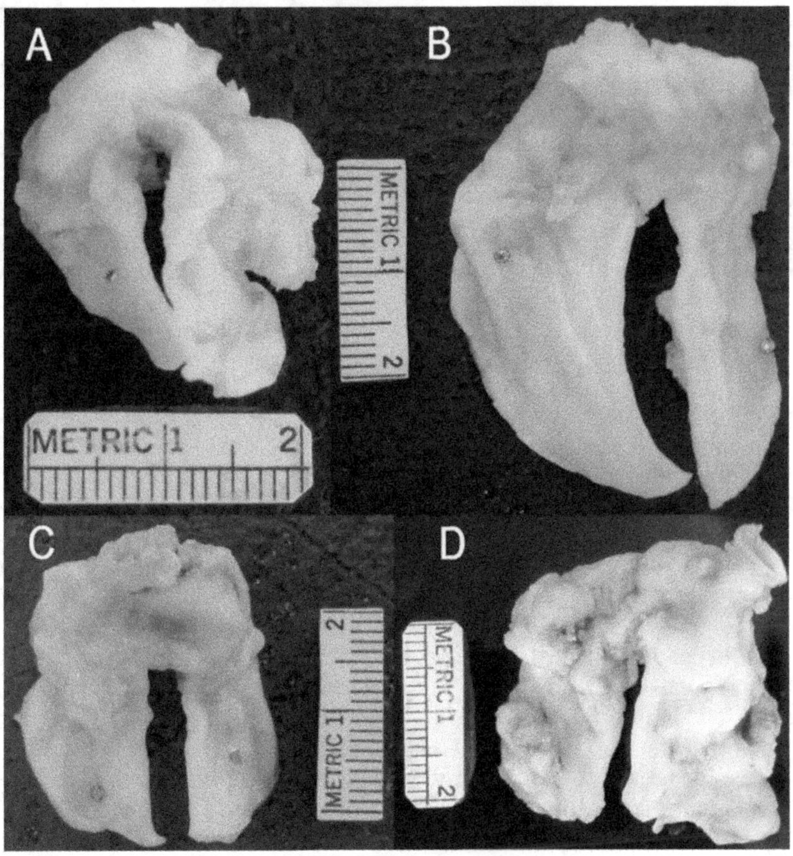

Figure 3. Congenitally unicuspid unicommissural valves in 4 patients 28 *(A)* to 51 *(D)* years of age. *(A, B, C)* Three were called unicuspid unicommissural by the surgeon and *(D)* 1 was called bicuspid.

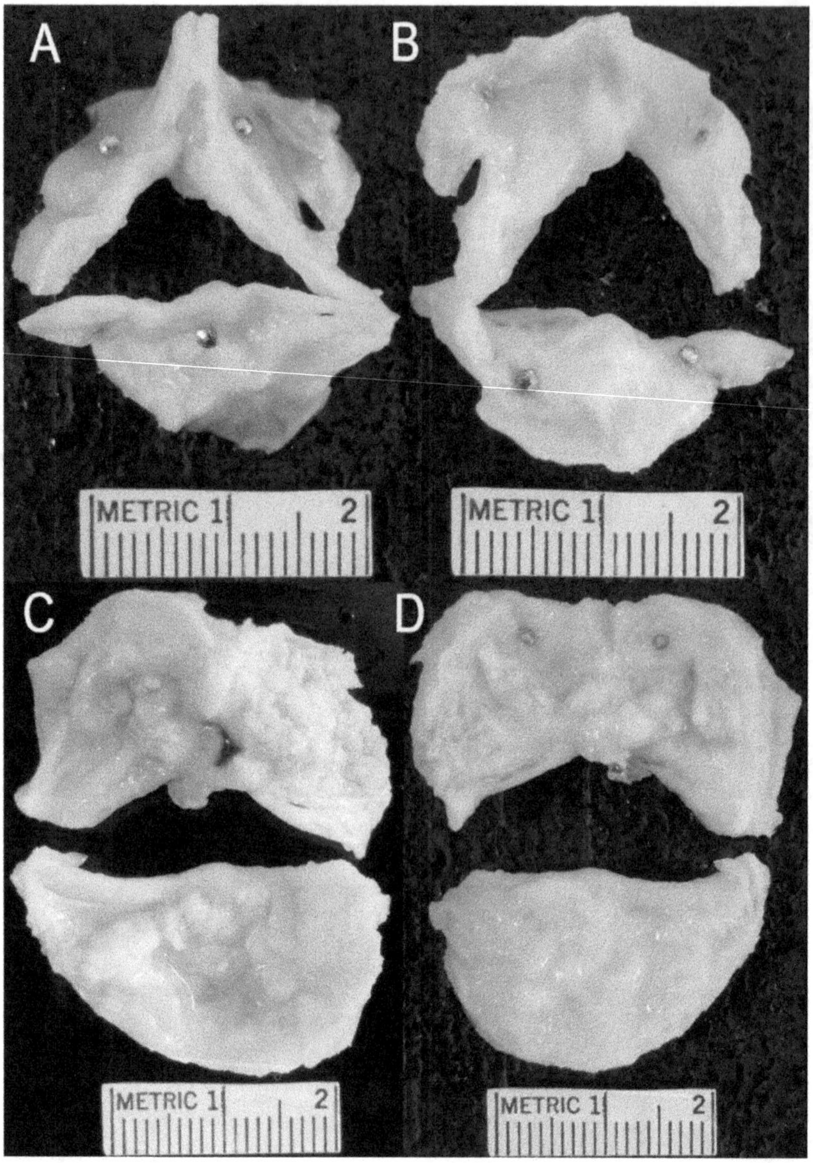

Figure 4. Congenitally bicuspid valves in 2 men 66 *(A, B)* and 67 *(C, D)* years of age showing the *(A, C)* aortic and *(B, D)* ventricular surfaces. The 2 valves were called tricuspid by the cardiac surgeon.

Number of aortic valve cusps was the major factor in determining congruity and incongruity. Excluding the cases in which valve structure was not mentioned in the operative report, in patients with 3-cuspid aortic valves, the cardiac surgeon and the cardiac pathologist were in agreement in 99% of cases (278 of 280). In nearly all of these cases, each of the 3 cusps was excised separately (Figure 1). Occasionally, 2 cusps were fused at a commissure but the length of the fusion was only 1 or 2 mm. In contrast, in the 41 patients with congenitally unicuspid aortic valves (Figures 2 and 3), congruity occurred in 6 (15%), and in the 280 patients with congenitally bicuspid valves, in which valve structure was mentioned in the operative note, congruity occurred in 156 (56%; Figures 4 to 7).

Valve weight appeared to affect valve congruity/incongruity, probably entirely because the unicuspid and bicuspid valves were heavier than the 3-cuspid aortic valves (Table 1). Valve weight did have some effect on whether valve structure was "clear" or "unclear" to the surgeon (Table 1).

The interval (days) between AVR and dictation of the operative report appeared to have some effect on the frequency of congruity/incongruity and unequivocal effect on whether or not the structure of the aortic valve was mentioned in the operative report (Table 1). Although the operative report was dictated on the day of operation in 458 of the 744 patients (62%) and within 1 week of operation in another 171 (23%), the report was dictated at later periods in 115 patients (15%), i.e., during the second week (49 patients, 6%) or later in 66 (9%). Although the mean interval ranged from 0 day to 133 days (mean ± SD 6 ± 15), the median was 0. The mean interval in the 440 patients in the congruous group was 4 ± 15 days, that in the incongruous group was 5 ± 14 days, and that in the 143 patients in whom valve structure was not mentioned in the operative report

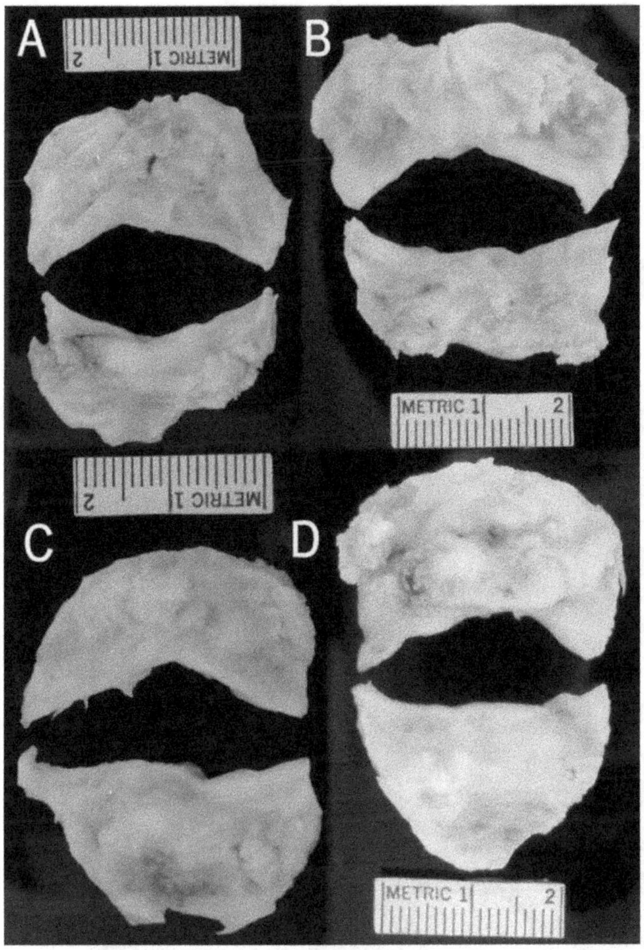

Figure 5. *Congenitally bicuspid valves* in 4 patients 50 to 69 years of age. *(A)* This valve was also called bicuspid by the surgeon; *(B, C, D)* these valves were called tricuspid by the surgeon.

was 9 ± 17 days. The mean interval from AVR to dictation in the patients with operatively excised unicuspid aortic valves was 4 ± 13 days, that in those with bicuspid valves was 6 ± 16 days, and that in those with tricuspid aortic valves was 5 ± 14 days.

Frequency of valve structure congruity/incongruity between the cardiac surgeon and cardiac pathologist, frequency of mention or nonmention of valve structure in the operative report, and interval from operation to dictation of the operative report *for each of the cardiac surgeons* is presented in Table 2.

Certain data in the 32 patients whose valves are displayed in Figures 1 to 7 are listed in Table 3.

Discussion

This study demonstrates for the first time that agreement regarding aortic valve structure in patients with aortic stenosis having isolated AVR is mainly dependent on the number of aortic valve cusps encountered at operation. In patients with a 3-cuspid aortic valve, there was virtually 100% agreement in number of valve cusps between the cardiac surgeon and cardiac pathologist. In patients with congenitally unicuspid and bicuspid valves, agreement was considerably less, 15% and 56%, respectively.

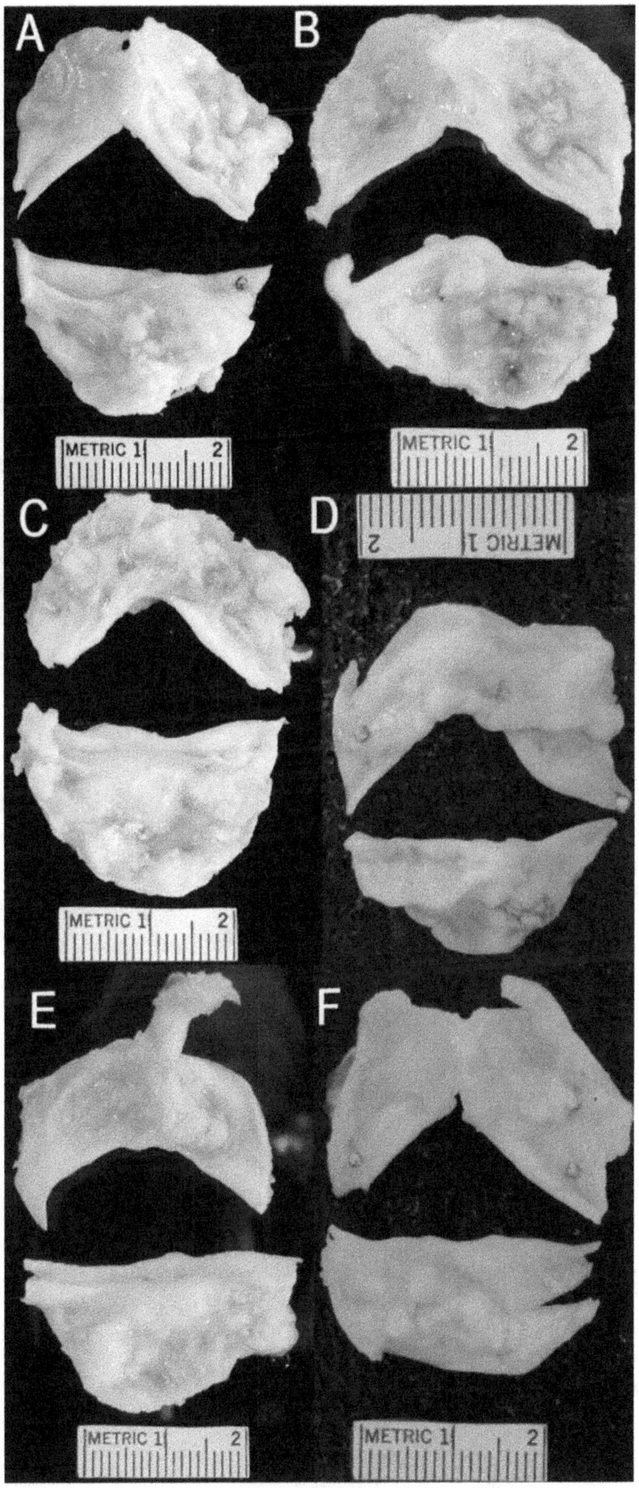

Figure 6. *(A to F) Congenitally bicuspid valves* in 6 men 56 to 75 years of age; each valve was called tricuspid by the cardiac surgeon.

With few exceptions, the congenitally unicuspid and bicuspid valves contain much heavier calcific deposits than do the tricuspid valves, and their structure often requires a bit more study than might be available at the operating table. A common confusion was the congenitally bicuspid valve when the free margins of the conjoined cusp (the cusp containing a raphe or false commissure) had a V-shaped

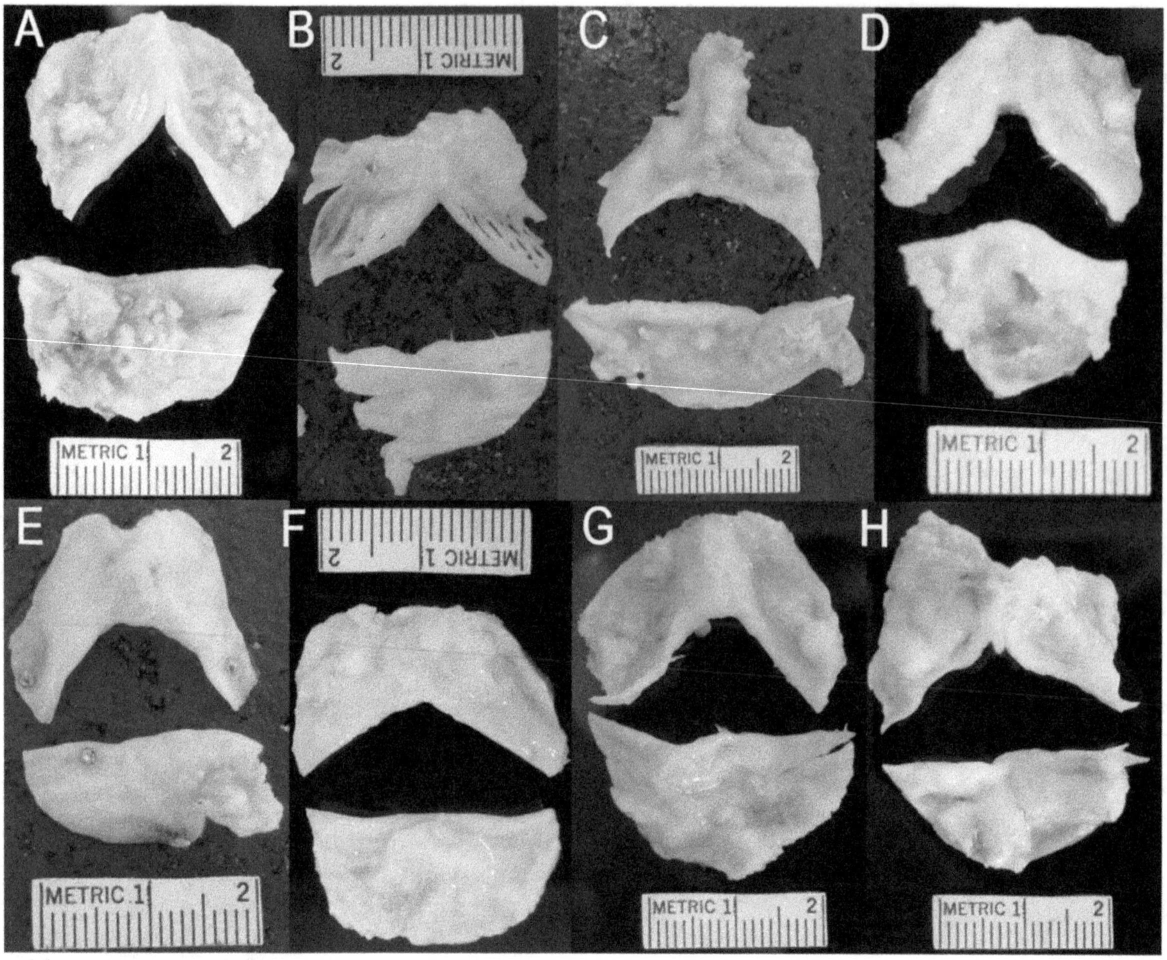

Figure 7. *(A to H)* Congenitally bicuspid valves in 8 patients 45 to 85 years of age. All 8 valves were called tricuspid by the cardiac surgeon.

Table 2
Data in individual surgeons demonstrating congruity/incongruity between a cardiac surgeon and a cardiac pathologist in patients having aortic valve replacement for aortic stenosis and interval from operation to dictation of the operative report

Surgeon	No. of Cases	Aortic Valve Structure				Interval (days) From AVR to Dictation of Operative Report
		Congruous	Incongruous	Unclear	Not Mentioned	Range/Mean ± SD/Median
A	208 (28%)	119 (57%)	44 (21%)	1 (<1%)	44 (21%)	0–82/3 ± 12/0
B	161 (22%)	118 (73%)	31 (19%)	0	12 (8%)	0–49/1 ± 6/0
C	124 (17%)	73 (59%)	13 (11%)	3 (2%)	35 (28%)	0–133/16 ± 28/3
D	119 (16%)	48 (40%)	35 (29%)	3 (3%)	33 (28%)	0–70/11 ± 10/7
E	54 (7%)	29 (54%)	17 (31%)	0	8 (15%)	0–5/0.3 ± 1/0
F	33 (4%)	27 (82%)	5 (15%)	0	1 (3%)	0–40/4 ± 8/2
G	20 (3%)	10 (50%)	4 (20%)	1 (5%)	5 (25%)	0–9/1 ± 2/0
H–N*	25 (3%)	16 (64%)	3 (12%)	1 (4%)	5 (20%)	0–3/0.1 ± 1/0
Totals	744 (100%)	440 (59%)	152 (21%)	9 (1%)	143 (19%)	0–133/6 ± 15/0

* There were 25 operations done by 7 different surgeons.

configuration with the apex of the V pointing to the raphe. In this circumstance, the free margins of the raphe cusp produce a concave configuration and the raphe is confused with a fused true commissure. These valves frequently were called "tricuspid" by the surgeon with "fusion of 1 of the 3 commissures." The undersurface or ventricular surface of the V-shaped raphe cusp is nearly always flattened rather than indented as occurs in acquired fusion of a 3-cuspid aortic valve at 1 commissure. When the raphe cusp has a concave configuration, the nonraphe cusp nearly always has a convex configuration.

Why might there be differences in the interpretation of congenitally malformed stenotic aortic valves between a cardiac surgeon and a cardiac pathologist? The following factors might be considered: (1) the cardiac surgeon may not be particularly concerned or focused on or interested in

Table 3
Data in the 32 patients whose operatively excised valves are shown in Figures 1 to 7

Figure No.	Label	Age (yrs)/Sex	No. Aortic Valve Cusps		Interval (days) From AVR to Operative Report Dictation	Aortic Valve Weight (g)	Figure No.	Label	Age (yrs)/Sex	No. Aortic Valve Cusps		Interval (days) From AVR to Operative Report Dictation	Aortic Valve Weight (g)
			Pathologist	Surgeon						Pathologist	Surgeon		
1	A	88/M	3	3	8	4.04	5	C	65/F	2	3	6	3.97
	B	79/M	3	—*	5	4.96		D	50/M	2	3	0	4.59
	C	71/M	3	3	0	3.06	6	A	74/M	2	3	6	2.49
	D	88/M	3	3	0	2.99		B	56/M	2	3	4	2.72
2	A	50/M	1	2	1	3.80		C	75/M	2	3	7	5.46
	B	60/F	1	3	11	2.60		D	59/M	2	3	1	1.96
	C	41/M	1	2	6	5.42		E	71/M	2	3	12	2.99
	D	67/F	1	3	0	4.53		F	65/M	2	3	0	2.26
3	A	28/M	1	1	0	2.73	7	A	78/F	2	3	7	2.54
	B	41/M	1	1	0	4.84		B	85/M	2	3	0	1.20
	C	33/M	1	1	0	3.14		C	57/M	2	3	6	3.38
	D	51/F	1	2	0	7.15		D	63/M	2	3	0	1.84
4	A, B	66/M	2	3	0	1.16		E	64/F	2	3	0	1.39
	C, D	67/M	2	3	27	4.29		F	63/F	2	3	0	1.55
5	A	66/M	2	2	0	1.95		G	45/M	2	3	0	2.26
	B	69/M	2	3	4	3.68		H	72/M	2	3	0	3.04

* No mention of valve structure in operative report.

valve structure[1,2]; (2) how to describe cardiac valve structure accurately was not a part of the surgeon's training[3]; (3) the surgeon does not excise enough stenotic aortic valves each year to become a student of aortic valve structure (the average cardiac surgeon in the United States performs about 10 valve operations/year); (4) the cardiac pathologist may be wrong in his/her interpretation; (5) there is no local or national requirement that valve structure be a part of the operative report or that the valve structure be described accurately; (6) criteria for a unicuspid or bicuspid may differ between the cardiac surgeon and cardiac pathologist; (7) the cardiac surgeon may not believe in the concept of a unicuspid or bicuspid aortic valve; and (8) the interval between the time of the AVR and the time the operative report was dictated may have been a bit long and the surgeon was unable to remember the valve's proper structure.

In most hospitals where cardiac valve replacement is performed, the surgical pathologist (often a first-year pathology resident) dictates the description of the operatively excised cardiac valve and then incises portions of it for preparation of histologic sections. As a consequence, the number of aortic valve cusps may never appear in the pathology report, and the description of the structure of the stenotic aortic valve accordingly is entirely dependent on the interpretation of the cardiac surgeon at operation. This responsibility should not be considered lightly. The Joint Commission of Accreditation of Healthcare Organizations expects the operative record to include an accurate description of "... any specimen(s) removed ...."[4]

The presence of a unicuspid or bicuspid aortic valve, of course, indicates that the patient has congenital heart disease. These patients usually have an abnormal media of ascending aorta that is prone to dilate much more than in patients of similar age with 3-cuspid aortic valves and similar types of valve dysfunction.[5] The aortic media in these patients tend to possess inadequate numbers of elastic fibers and adults with unicuspid and bicuspid aortic valves have aortic dissection (with a tear in the ascending aorta) 5 times more often than do patients with tricuspid aortic valves.[5] In addition, aortic isthmic aortic coarctation is a recognized accompaniment of congenitally unicuspid or bicuspid valves but is exceedingly uncommon in patients with 3-cuspid aortic valves. Moreover, if 1 family member has a congenitally unicuspid or bicuspid aortic valve, there is an increased chance that another family member may have the same valvular anomaly.[6–8] Indeed, Cripe et al,[7] Horne et al,[8] and Garg et al[9] have provided abundant evidence of the high heritability of the bicuspid aortic valve. Thus, this evidence demonstrates the importance of identifying the congenitally malformed aortic valve correctly, not only in the patient possessing the anomaly but also for other family members.

Acknowledgment: We thank Charles S. Roberts, MD, chief of the section of thoracic and cardiovascular surgery, Winchester Medical Center, Winchester, Virginia, for reading the report and providing thoughtful suggestions for improvement.

1. Baker MS, Baker BH. The operative report. *Int Surg* 1976;61:333–334.
2. Sing RF, Thomason MH, Dent TL. The dictated operative note. *Curr Surg* 1998;55:388–390.
3. Moore RA. The dictated operative note: important but is it being taught? *J Am Coll Surg* 2000;190:639–640.
4. JCAHO. Comprehensive Accreditation Manual for Hospitals: The Official Handbook. 2008:IM15–IM16.
5. Roberts CS, Roberts WC. Dissection of the aorta associated with congenital malformation of the aortic valve. *J Am Coll Cardiol* 1991;17:712–716.
6. Glick BN, Roberts WC. Congenitally bicuspid aortic valve in multiple family members. *Am J Cardiol* 1994;73:400–404.
7. Cripe L, Andelfinger G, Martin LJ, Shooner K, Benson DW. Bicuspid aortic valve is heritable. *J Am Coll Cardiol* 2004;44:138–143.
8. Horne BD, Camp NJ, Muhlestein JB, Cannon-Albright LA. Evidence for a heritable component in death resulting from aortic and mitral valve diseases. *Circulation* 2004;110:3143–3148.
9. Garg V, Muth AN, Ransom JF, Schluterman MK, Barnes R, King IN, Grossfeld PD, Srivastava D. Mutations in NOTCH1 cause aortic valve disease. *Nature* 2005;437:270–274.

Combined mitral and aortic stenosis of rheumatic origin with double-valve replacement in an octogenarian

William Clifford Roberts [a,b,d,*], Jong Mi Ko [d], John Ryan Schumacher [a], Albert Carl Henry III [c]

[a] *Department of Internal Medicine, Division of Cardiology, Baylor University Medical Center, Dallas, TX, United States*
[b] *Department of Pathology, Baylor University Medical Center, Dallas, TX, United States*
[c] *Department of Cardiothoracic Surgery, Baylor University Medical Center, Dallas, TX, United States*
[d] *Baylor Heart and Vascular Institute, Baylor University Medical Center, Dallas, TX, United States*

Received 29 October 2008; accepted 1 November 2008
Available online 30 November 2008

Abstract

We describe double valve replacement for rheumatic mitral and aortic stenosis in an 83-year-old woman, a very uncommon event in an octogenarian.

Keywords: Mitral stenosis; Aortic stenosis; Rheumatic heart disease; Octogenarians; Double valve replacement

Replacement of both mitral and aortic valves in octogenarians is infrequent especially for combined mitral stenosis (MS) and aortic stenosis (AS) of rheumatic etiology. Such was the case, however, in the patient to be described herein.

An 81-year-old woman, who was born on 23 September 1925, had increasing dyspnea for several years became of what was believed to be "pulmonary fibrosis," worse in the lower lobes than the upper lobes. In December 2004, she was placed on home oxygen, and in January 2005, on continuous oxygen by nasal cannula. She had never smoked and had no history of acute rheumatic fever. Because of rather dramatic worsening of her dyspnea, she was hospitalized at Baylor University Medical Center on 1 May 2007. Her body mass index was 20 kg/m^2. Precordial examination disclosed an apical diastolic murmur and a basal ejection type systolic murmur. Electrocardiogram disclosed prolonged P–R interval and increased voltage compatible with left ventricular hypertrophy. Telemetric monitoring disclosed runs of atrial fibrillation.

* Corresponding author. Department of Internal Medicine, Division of Cardiology, Baylor University Medical Center, Dallas, TX, United States.
E-mail address: wc.Roberts@baylorhealth.edu (W.C. Roberts).

Cardiac catheterization disclosed the following pressures in mm Hg: pulmonary artery wedge a-wave 21, v-wave 34, and mean 22; pulmonary artery, 68/26 (mean 39); left ventricle, 129/21 and aorta, 113/46; pulmonary arterial wedge — left ventricular mean diastolic gradient 8, and simultaneous left ventricular–aortic peak systolic gradient, 16. Cardiac index was 2.2 L/min/m^2. The calculated mitral valve area was 0.8 and the aortic valve area, 0.7 cm^2. Angiography disclosed insignificant coronary arterial narrowing.

On 4 May 2007, both left-sided cardiac valves (Fig. 1) were replaced with St. Jude Medical prostheses: mitral #29, and aortic #19. The postoperative course was relatively smooth. The pulmonary arterial pressure fell dramatically, and she was discharged to the Baylor Specialty Hospital on 14 May 2007 where she remained for 17 days.

Thereafter, she did well until about 1 January 2008, when she noted pedal edema which progressed to anasarca and a weight gain from 112 to 148 lb. She was rehospitalized on 4 February 2008. The blood hemoglobin was 9.8 g/L and the hematocrit, 30.3%. With diuretic therapy she lost 30 lb and returned home feeling much better. She was now in persistent atrial fibrillation. As of October 2008, she was doing well.

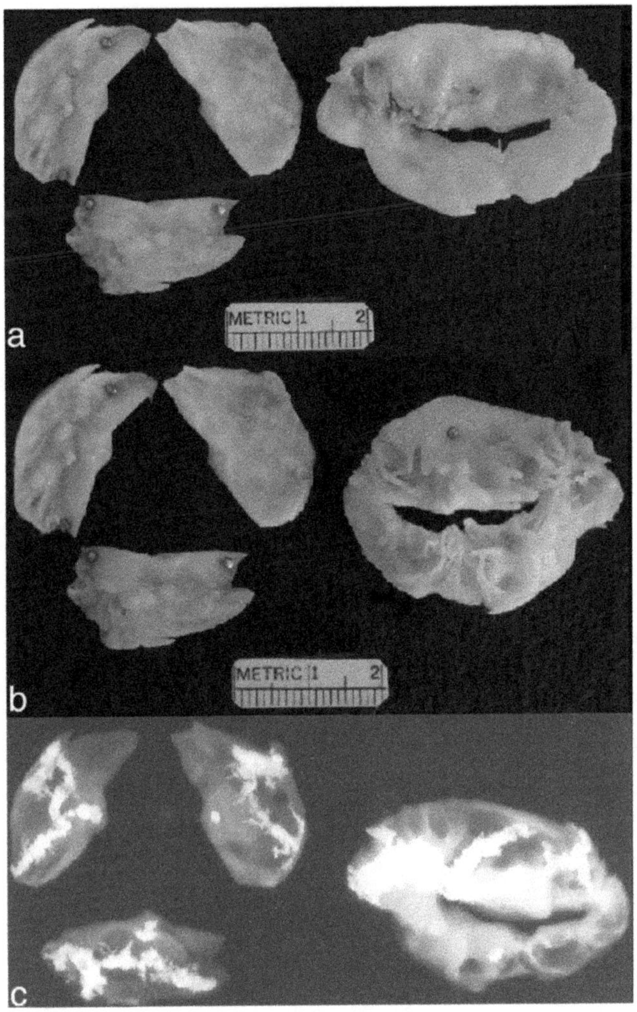

Fig. 1. Photographs of the operatively excised aortic valve (left) and mitral valve (right). The mitral valve is shown from the atrial aspect in a and from the ventricular aspect in b. Radiographs of each valve are shown in c.

Although now infrequent in the Western world, combined MS and AS of rheumatic origin was relatively common when acute rheumatic fever was far more prevalent. Roberts [1] collected 1010 cases at autopsy of valvular heart disease studied from approximately 1955 to 1980: isolated AS (with or without regurgitation) was the most frequent valve lesion (29%); isolated MS (with or without mitral regurgitation) was next (19%), and combined MS and AS was in third place (15%) (Table 1). None of the patients with combined MS and AS, however, was ≥80 years of age. In the last 3 decades, combined MS and AS of rheumatic etiology was infrequent in the Western world.

Combined MS and AS is particularly rare in octogenarians. Uricchio et al. [2] in 1959 reported 141 patients with combined MS and AS, all of whom had undergone both mitral and aortic commissurotomy: their ages ranged from 23 to 67 years. Katznelson et al. [3] studied 22 patients ranging in age from 23 to 61 years (mean 45); the average age of onset of symptoms of cardiac dysfunction was 40. Honey [4] studied 35 patients and their ages ranged from 24 to 54 years (mean 40). Reid et al. [5] studied 15 patients aged 26 to 48. Morrow et al. [6] studied 8 patients aged 20 to 48, all of whom had combined mitral and aortic valvulotomy. Zitnik et al. [7] studied 10 such patients who ranged in age from 34 to 55 (mean 42). Roberts and Sullivan [8] studied at necropsy 30 such patients who died within 60 days of double valve replacement for combined MS and AS: one was an octogenarian, aged 83, but the others were younger (mean age 57). Berman et al. [9] performed combined percutaneous mitral and aortic valvulotomy in 6 patients, aged 60 to 83. Thus, only 2 of the 267 patients in those studies with combined MS and AS were octogenarians.

Combined MS and AS is more common in women than in men. Of the 267 patients reported in the previously mentioned 8 studies [2–9], 171 (64%) were women.

Table 1
Functional and anatomic classification of valvular heart disease in 1010 necropsy patients aged >=15 years.[a]

Functional class	Patients	Anatomic class				
		AV	MV	MV-AV	TV-MV	TV-MV-AV
1. Aortic stenosis (AS)	292 (29%)	256 (88%)	0	35 (12%)	0	1 (0.3%)
2. Mitral stenosis (MS)	189 (19%)	0	117 (62%)	40 (21%)	13 (7%)	19 (10%)
3. MS+AS	152 (15%)	0	0	120 (79%)	0	32 (21%)
4. Aortic regurgitation (AR)[b]	119 (12%)	107 (90%)	0	10 (8%)	0	2 (2%)
5. Mitral regurgitation (MR)	97 (10%)	0	85 (88%)	8 (8%)	1 (1%)	3 (3%)
6. MS+AR	65 (6%)	0	52 (80%)	0	0	13 (20%)
7. MR+AR	45 (4%)	0	0	39 (87%)	0	6 (13%)
8. AS+MR	23 (2%)	0	0	21 (91%)	0	2 (9%)
9. Tricuspid stenosis+MS±AS	28 (3%)	0	0	0	4 (14%)	24 (86%)
Totals	1010 (100%)[c]	363 (36%)	254 (25%)	273 (27%)	18 (2%)	102 (10%)

AV = aortic valve; MV = mitral valve; TV = tricuspid valve.

Reproduced with permission from Elsevier and the author (Roberts WC. Am J Cardiol 1983;51:1005–1028).

[a] Excludes patients with mitral regurgitation secondary to coronary heart disease (papillary muscle dysfunction), carcinoid heart disease, hypertrophic cardiomyopathy, and those with infective endocarditis limited to 1 or both right-sided cardiac valves. Tricuspid valve regurgitation was present in many patients in most of the 9 functional groups. All patients were in functional class III or IV (New York Heart Association), and more than half had 1 or more cardiac operations.

[b] In many patients, the aortic valve cusps were normal or nearly normal and the regurgitation was the result of disease of the aorta (Marfan and Marfan-like syndrome, syphilis, systemic hypertension, healed aortic dissection).

[c] The hearts in all 1010 patients were examined and classified by WCR.

Several studies have examined cardiac hemodynamics in patients with combined MS and AS [2–9]. Although there are exceptions, the degree of AS when combined with MS is not as great (transvalvular peak systolic gradient) as in patients with isolated AS. Furthermore the MS, as emphasized by Zitnik et al. [7], can mask the presence of AS. If the AS is missed in this circumstance and mitral valve commissurotomy or replacement is performed and the downstream AS is neglected dire consequences can ensue. Obviously, it is best to diagnose both MS and AS preoperatively, but if one lesion is to be missed, it is far better to miss the upstream problem (MS) than the downstream problem (AS).

And finally, combined MS and AS can produce an operative challenge. First, the patients are most commonly women, some of whom, as in the present patient, are of small stature and, consequently, have relatively small hearts [8]. In combined MS and AS, neither the left ventricular cavity nor the ascending aorta is dilated, a circumstance which provides less space for either the mitral or the aortic mechanical prosthesis or bioprosthesis compared to the space provided in patients with isolated AS who often have congenitally bicuspid aortic valves and dilated ascending aortas.

Acknowledgment

The authors of this manuscript have certified that they comply with the Principles of Ethical Publishing in the International Journal of Cardiology [10].

References

[1] Roberts WC. Morphologic features of the normal and abnormal mitral valve. Am J Cardiol 1983;51:1005–28.

[2] Uricchio JF, Goldberg H, Sinha KP, Likoff W. Combined mitral and aortic stenosis: clinical and physiologic features and results of surgery. Am J Cardiol 1959;4:479–91.

[3] Katznelson G, Jreissaty RM, Levinson GE, Stein SW, Abelmann WH. Combined aortic and mitral stenosis. Am J Med 1960;29:242–56.

[4] Honey M. Clinical and haemodynamic observations on combined mitral and aortic stenosis. Brit Heart J 1961;23:545–55.

[5] Reid JM, Stevenson JG, Barclay RS, Welsh TM. Combined aortic and mitral stenosis. Brit Heart J 1962;24:509–15.

[6] Morrow AG, Awe WC, Braunwald E. Combined mitral and aortic stenosis. Brit Heart J 1962;24:606–12.

[7] Zitnik RS, Piemme TE, Messer RJ, Reed DP, Haynes FW, Dexter L. The masking of aortic stenosis by mitral stenosis. Am Heart J 1965;69:22–30.

[8] Roberts WC, Sullivan MF. Clinical and necropsy observations early after simultaneous replacement of the mitral and aortic valves. Am J Cardiol 1986;58:1067–84.

[9] Berman AD, Weinstein JS, Safian RD, Diver DJ, Grossman W, McKay RG. Combined aortic and mitral balloon valvuloplasty in patients with critical aortic and mitral valve stenosis: results in six cases. J Am Coll Cardiol 1988;11:1213–8.

[10] Coats AJ. Ethical authorship and publishing. Int J Cardiol 2009;131:149–50.

Massive acute infarction of the right ventricular wall without or only minimal infarction of the left ventricular wall after aortic valve replacement with or without simultaneous replacement of the ascending aorta

William Clifford Roberts[a,b,c,*], Brent Andrew Patterson[c], Jong Mi Ko[a], Rebecca Anne Sager[b], Jason Andrew Clark[b], Joseph Manuel Guileyardo[b]

[a]*Baylor Heart and Vascular Institute, Baylor University Medical Center, Dallas, TX 75246, USA*
[b]*Department of Pathology, Baylor University Medical Center, Dallas, TX 75246, USA*
[c]*Department of Internal Medicine (Cardiology), Baylor University Medical Center, Dallas, TX 75246, USA*

Received 1 October 2008; received in revised form 17 November 2008; accepted 16 December 2008

Abstract

Certain clinical and cardiac morphologic findings are presented in two men who developed massive right ventricular (RV) infarction with only minimal or no left ventricular infarction early after aortic valve replacement. The ostium of the right coronary artery was severely narrowed in one patient by the ring of the bioprosthesis, and in the other patient the right coronary artery was completely severed at the time of valve replacement without insertion of a coronary bypass conduit. Such massive infarction of the RV free wall has not been reported previously.

Keywords: Acute infarction; Right ventricular wall; Left ventricular wall; Aortic valve replacement; Ascending aorta

Acute infarction of the right ventricular (RV) wall usually occurs in the setting of acute infarction of the left ventricular wall and ventricular septum [1]. The left ventricular infarct in this circumstance is virtually always limited to the posterior wall of the left ventricle and the posterior portion of the ventricular septum, and the RV infarct is usually limited to its posterior wall. On occasion, the RV infarct involves a small portion of the anterior wall of the right ventricle. This report was prompted by observing near-complete acute infarction of the RV free wall with either no or minimal acute infarction of the left ventricular free wall in each of two patients who died early after aortic valve replacement (AVR) with or without replacement of the ascending aorta.

Funding: No grant was used to support this investigation.

Conflict of interest disclosures: The authors have no conflicts of interest.

* Corresponding author. Baylor Heart and Vascular Institute, Baylor University Medical Center, Dallas, TX 75246, USA. Tel.: +1 214 820 7911; fax: +1 214 820 7533.

E-mail address: wc.roberts@baylorhealth.edu (W.C. Roberts).

1. Patients studied

Some findings in each of the two patients are summarized in Table 1. Patient 1 had had mitral valve replacement for papillary muscle dysfunction and coronary arterial bypass grafting (CABG) at age 60 and repeat CABG with AVR (aortic valve stenosis with a three-cuspid aortic valve) with a bioprosthesis at age 67, 32 days before death. The postoperative period was characterized by evidences of low cardiac output syndrome despite prolonged inotropic support, intraaortic balloon pump, prolonged ventilator support, hemodialysis, and severe jaundice. At necropsy, the heart weighed 665 g. A healed myocardial infarct involved the posterior wall of the left ventricle (Fig. 1). The RV wall was acutely infarcted as was the ventricular septum

Table 1
Certain clinical and necropsy finding in the two men having massive acute RV infarction early after aortic valve replacement

Variable	Patient 1	Patient 2
Age (years) at death	67	35
Age (years) at first operation	60	30
Coronary bypass	+	0
Mitral valve replacement	+	0
Aortic valve replacement	0	+
Ascending aorta excised	0	0
Age (years) at second operation	67	35
Coronary bypass	+	0
Mitral valve replacement	0	0
Aortic valve replacement	+	+
Ascending aorta excised	0	+
Aortic dissection, healed	0	+
Blockage or severance, ostium, RCA	+	+
Low cardiac output PO	++++	++++
Body mass index (kg/m^2)	28	34
Heart weight (g)	665	550
Healed MI (posterior)	+	0
Acute MI (LV posterior)	0	+
Acute MI, RV (huge)	+	+
RCA dominant	+	+
Atrial septal defect	0	+

MI=myocardial infarct; PO=postoperatively; RCA=right coronary artery; LV=left ventricle; RV=right ventricle.

focally. The ostium of the right coronary artery was partially obliterated by the ring of the bioprosthesis which was in the aortic valve position (Fig. 1). Additionally, several pledgets with sutures surrounded the right coronary artery about 1 cm from its ostium and they also severely narrowed the lumen of this artery. Although both an "old" and a new conduit (saphenous vein) had been placed to the distal posterior descending coronary artery, the lumen of the native artery just distal to the anastomotic sites was extremely small. The atrial septum was devoid of a defect.

Patient 2 had AVR with a mechanical prosthesis (St. Jude Medical) at age 30 for a dysfunctional congenitally bicuspid aortic valve. At age 35, 4 days before death, computed tomography showed the ascending aorta to be aneurysmal (10 cm in diameter) and a second operation was performed. The mechanical prosthesis was replaced with another similar prosthesis, the ascending aorta was replaced with a composite graft, and the left main coronary artery was grafted into the conduit. At operation, the ostium of the right coronary artery was not found by the surgeon who concluded that the patient had a single coronary artery arising from the aorta. The postoperative period also was characterized by evidences of low cardiac output, severe systemic arterial desaturation, excessive bleeding, cardiac arrest (ventricular fibrillation), and repeated seizures. The operatively excised ascending aorta had a healed tear beginning just distal to the previous aortotomy. The proximal 1 cm of the right coronary artery was present on the aorta, and its ostium, although patent, was small. Histologic examination of the aortic wall showed massive loss of medial elastic fibers (grade 4/4, "cystic medial necrosis"). The two discs of the St. Jude Medical prosthesis moved normally. The heart weighed

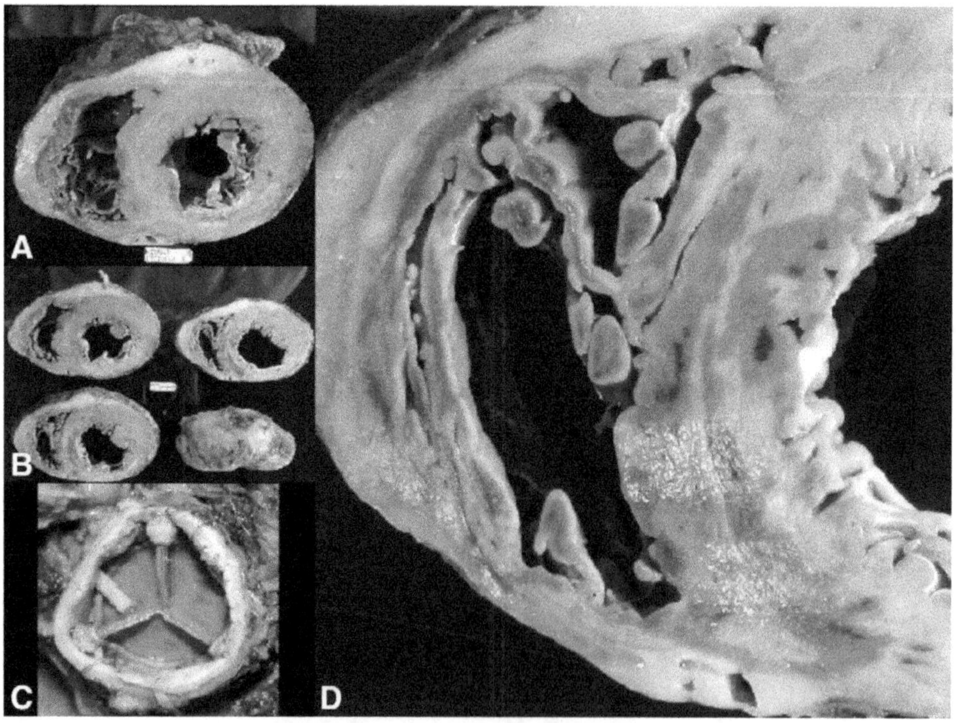

Fig. 1. Patient 1. (A) Base of heart showing necrosis of most of the RV wall and dilated RV cavity. (B) Ventricular "slices" showing healed posterior wall left ventricular (LV) infarct and dilated LV cavity. The RV free wall measures up to 1 cm in thickness. (C) View of the bioprosthesis in the aortic valve position. The wooden stick is in the ostium of the right coronary artery. The ostium is severely narrowed, however, by the base of the bioprosthesis. The stick has been tilted cephalad to become visible. Otherwise, it would have been blocked by the ring of the prosthesis. (D) Close-up of the necrotic RV wall with necrosis also in the ventricular septum.

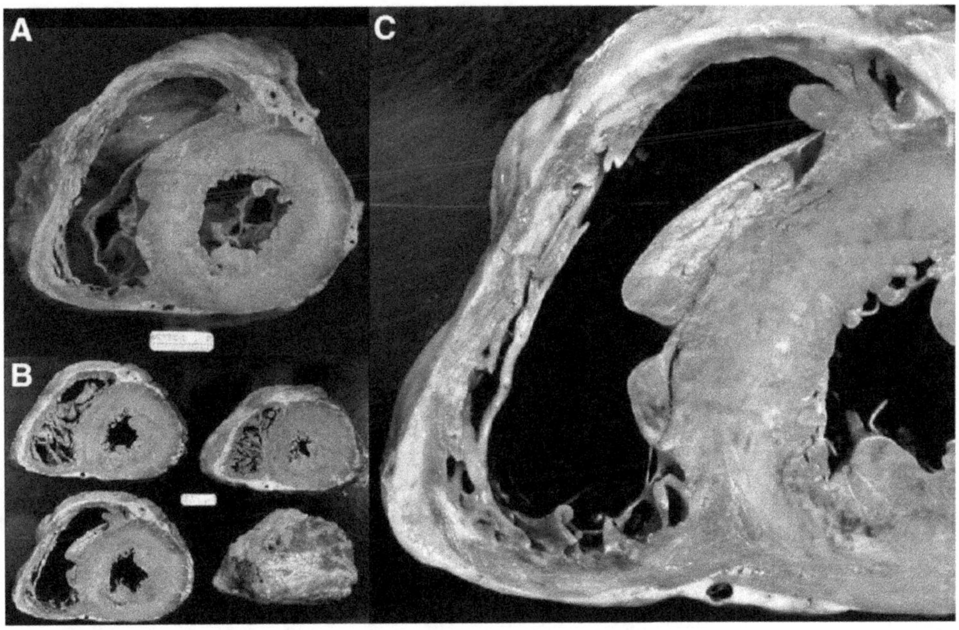

Fig. 2. Patient 2. (A) Base of heart showing acutely infarcted RV wall and very dilated RV cavity. (B) Ventricular "slices" at different levels. (C) Close-up view of the acutely infarcted RV wall and a small acute infarct involving the posterior LV wall. The RV free wall measures up to 6 mm in thickness.

550 g. The entire RV wall was necrotic, and a small acute infarct involved the posterior portion of the ventricular septum and left ventricular free wall (Fig. 2). The RV cavity was markedly dilated. The fossa ovale membrane was aneurysmal and four defects (atrial septal defect) were present at the junction of the fossa ovale membrane and muscular portion of the atrial septum.

2. Discussion

The common feature in each of the two patients described herein was the presence of massive acute infarction of the RV free wall with mild or no necrosis of the left ventricular free wall. The cause was total disruption of the dominant right coronary artery from the aorta in one patient (no. 2), and interference with flow through the right coronary artery due to impingement of the cloth ring of the bioprosthesis in the aortic valve position and also to pledgeted sutures surrounding the right coronary artery with impingement on its lumen just after its origin from the aorta. Patient 2 lived just 4 days postoperatively. Right ventricular dysfunction was not apparent after discontinuation of cardiopulmonary bypass probably because of the four defects in the atrial septum which allowed sizable right-to-left shunting as evidenced by low systemic arterial saturation postoperatively. Patient 1 probably was able to survive 32 days postoperatively because the right coronary artery, although very narrowed, was not totally occluded and, additionally, a saphenous venous conduit had been inserted into the distal portion of the posterior descending coronary artery. Neither patient had pulmonary parachymal nor pulmonary vascular disease.

Near total acute infarction of the RV free wall is an extremely rare event. One of us (WCR) has examined approximately 20,000 hearts at necropsy in patients with fatal heart disease, and the two patients described herein are the only two in whom the RV free wall in its near entirety was acutely infarcted.

Review of previous published reports of massive RV infarction disclosed reports of two such patients. Zaus and Kearns [2] in 1952 described a 69-year-old man with "massive" RV necrosis associated with small foci of necrosis and fibrosis in the left ventricular free wall posteriorly and in the posterior portion of the adjacent ventricular septum. A diagram of the areas of infarction was presented. The infarction was attributed to coronary arterial disease. The dominant right coronary artery was totally occluded over 8 cm by a thrombus beginning 0.5 cm from its ostium.

In 1982, Kircher and Moothart [3] described a 68-year-old man with "isolated right ventricular infarction with massive dilation" who presented with atrial flutter and symptoms of heart failure. Coronary angiogram showed a nondominant right coronary artery which was "partially occluded at its origin and 80% narrowed in the proximal third..." The left anterior descending and left circumflex were narrowed ≤40% (presumably in cross-sectional area). Because of repeated sustained episodes of poorly tolerated arrhythmias, a pacemaker was inserted via thoracotomy. The RV cavity was very dilated and its wall, thin. A year later, he had a cardiac arrest while shopping, resuscitation was initially successful but he never regained consciousness and he died 5 days later. At necropsy, "the entire [RV] wall demonstrated old infarction." Although the authors described the left side of the heart as "normal", a photograph of both cardiac ventricles in our view shows considerable infarction of both the ventricular septum and left ventricular free wall. The coronary arteries at necropsy were similar to those described at angiogram a year earlier.

References

[1] Isner JM, Roberts WC. Right ventricular infarction complicating left ventricular infarction secondary to coronary heart disease. Frequency, location, associated findings and significance from analysis of 236 necropsy patients with acute or healed myocardial infarction. Am J Cardiol 1978;42:885–94.

[2] Zaus EA, Kearns WM. Massive infarction of the right ventricle and atrium. Report of a case. Circulation 1952;6:593–8.

[3] Kircher T, Moothart R. Isolated right ventricular infarction with massive dilation. Acquired Uhl's disease? Arch Pathol Lab Med 1982;106: 385–7.

Prophylactic Replacement of a Dilated Ascending Aorta at the Time of Aortic Valve Replacement of a Dysfunctioning Congenitally Unicuspid or Bicuspid Aortic Valve

Recently, I examined a beautifully excised severely stenotic congenitally bicuspid aortic valve in a 64-year-old man who, at the same operation, had undergone excision of the ascending aorta, which, by preoperative imaging studies, had a maximal diameter of 4.3 cm. Histologically, the wall of the aorta was normal. Although the aortic valve replacement (AVR) was clearly appropriate, was excision of the ascending aorta justified on a prophylactic basis? I would argue that the latter should be reconsidered.

Before the 1990s, relatively few patients with stenotic or purely regurgitant congenitally malformed aortic valves also underwent concomitant resection of the dilated ascending aorta. During the 1990s, some prominent and persuasive cardiac surgeons began advocating prophylactic concomitant ascending aortic resection in these circumstances, mainly for 3 reasons. First, to prevent postoperative dilation of the ascending aorta in a previously normal sized aorta or to prevent additional dilation in an already dilated aorta; second, to prevent aortic dissection, which is recognized to occur more commonly in patients with congenitally unicuspid and bicuspid aortic valves than in patients with tricuspid aortic valves[1,2]; and, finally, to prevent rupture of the ascending aorta late postoperatively. The latter reason was because it is recognized that the media of the ascending aorta in patients with congenitally bicuspid aortic valves can be depleted of certain elements (elastic fibers, smooth muscle cells, collagen) and can be repleted with certain other elements (mucopolysaccharide material) compared to the aorta's structure in adults with tricuspid aortic valves[3] (except in those patients with the Marfan syndrome and the forme fruste variety of it,[4] cardiovascular syphilis,[5–7] and ankylosing spondylitis,[8] and giant-cell aortitis[9]).

But how often do these potential aortic complications (additional dilation, dissection, rupture) occur in patients who have had AVR because of a dysfunctioning congenitally malformed aortic valve (either unicuspid or bicuspid) without concomitant resection of the dilated ascending aorta? The answer is infrequently. The best data (largest number of patients and longest follow-up) supporting that view comes from an analysis of 1,286 patients (1,180 [92%] with aortic stenosis [AS], 85 [7%] with aortic regurgitation [AR], and 20 [1%] aortic valve dysfunction type not stated) who had undergone AVR at the Mayo Clinic from 1960 to 1995 because of a dysfunctioning bicuspid aortic valve, without concomitant resection of the ascending aorta, irrespective of its size.[10] The mean age at operation was 58 years (72% men). The follow-up period was 0 to 38 years (median 12). During that postoperative period (excluding the 36 who died early [2.8%] and the 26 lost to follow-up [2.6%]), documented aortic dissection occurred in 13 (1%) and additional aortic dilation (ascending aorta diameter reached ≥5.0 cm or >1.0 from that at the time of AVR) occurred in 127 (9.9%). Additionally, 11 (0.08%) of the 1,227 patients not dying early or lost to follow-up later underwent resection of the ascending aorta; in 9 of the 11, however, it was at the time of replacement of a malfunctioning mechanical prosthesis or a bioprosthesis in the aortic valve position.

Although 151 events affecting the ascending aorta occurred during the long follow-up period, 127 (84%) consisted of dilation of the aorta, something that can occur after any aortotomy, irrespective of the structure of the aortic valve, and dilation of the ascending aorta after an aortotomy in and of itself infrequently produces clinical consequences. Indeed, the 15-year all-cause survival was greater in the patients with "enlarged" aortas than in those with normal-size aortas at the time of AVR (56% vs 50%). Although the ascending aorta was later excised in 11 patients, that aortic resection probably would not have been done in 9 if excision of a dysfunctioning prosthesis or bioprosthesis had not been required. Additionally, aortotomy, performed with isolated AVR, causes proliferation of fibrous tissue around the aorta, making the aorta thicker than normal, and the resulting thicker wall almost surely is more difficult to rupture than an aortic wall of normal or less than normal thickness. Furthermore, any type of interruption of the wall of ascending aorta (be it for insertion of a saphenous vein conduit or arterial cannula or incision for AVR or for resection of an aortic tear in aortic dissection) increases the risk of late dissection or rupture, be it in patients with unicuspid, bicuspid or tricuspid aortic valves.[11]

Similar long-term follow-up after isolated AVR in patients with dysfunctioning tricuspid aortic valves without concomitant resection of ascending aorta was recently presented by Gaudino et al.[12] They described 93 consecutive patients (mean age 67 years; 74% men) undergoing isolated AVR for AS at their institution (Catholic University Rome) from January 1990 to December 2000. Preoperatively, the maximal diameter of the ascending aorta ranged from 5.0 to 5.9 cm (mean 5.6). The diagnosis of tricuspid aortic valve was confirmed in each patient at operation by visual inspection. The ascending aorta was neither replaced nor plicated. The 92 patients surviving the operation were followed up for a mean of 14.7 ± 4.8 years. During that period, 16 patients died (17%). In no case was death attributed to an aortic event. Indeed, no patient during the long follow-up experienced an acute ascending aortic rupture, dissection, or pseudoaneurysm formation. Also, during the follow-up, no patient required reoperation for thoracic aortic complications. Additionally, the diameter of the ascending aorta during the 10 years after AVR changed insignificantly (56 ± 2 mm preoperatively vs 57 ± 11 mm at the end of follow-up). The mean expansion rate of the ascending aorta was 0.3 ± 0.2 mm/year. Patients with connective tissue disorders such as the Marfan syndrome were excluded from their study. The report by Gaudino et al[12] included the largest number of patients with dilated ascending aortas and stenotic 3-cuspid aortic valves undergoing AVR alone and followed up for ≥10 years. The frequency of late ascending aortic complications is lacking in patients who have had combined AVR for dysfunctioning unicuspid, bicuspid, or tricuspid aortic valves and resection of the dilated ascending aortas with similarly long (10 to 15 years) follow-up.

Adding ascending aortic resection to AVR usually significantly increases the operative mortality. Data from the Society of Thoracic Surgeons database indicate that ascending aortic resection increases the operative risk by a factor of 2.78 compared to AVR alone.[13] I agree with McKeller et al[10] from the Mayo Clinic who stated: "The widespread adoption of an aggressive attitude toward [aortic] root replacement, therefore, may create more problems than it solves."

Another recent report also provides some evidence that prophylactic resection of the ascending aorta is probably performed too frequently (unnecessarily) in patients undergoing AVR for dysfunctioning congenitally malformed aortic valves.[14] The evidence is provided by a histologic study of operatively excised dilated (>4.5-cm) aortas in patients undergoing AVR for dysfunctioning unicuspid or bicuspid aortic valves. My colleagues and I examined histologically the operatively excised ascending aortas in 58 patients undergoing AVR for AS involving a congenitally unicuspid or bicuspid aortic valve and in 38 patients undergoing AVR for pure AR involving a bicuspid aortic valve.[14] All 96 patients by preoperative imaging studies had ascending aortas with diameters >4.5 cm. We found that dividing the patients into those with AS and those with pure AR, something that had not been done previously, was helpful in predicting whether the structure of the ascending aorta was likely to be normal, in which case its resection probably was not indicated, or abnormal, in which case its resection probably was indicated. In the 58 patients with AS, the structure of the aortic media was normal or nearly normal (consistent with aging) in all 14 patients with unicuspid aortic valves and in 39 (87%) of the 44 patients with bicuspid valves. In contrast, of the 38 patients with purely regurgitant congenitally bicuspid aortic valves (none had unicuspid valves), the aortic media was normal in 20 (53%) and abnormal in 18 (47%). These findings suggest that among patients with preoperative imaging studies showing the ascending aorta to have a diameter >4.5 cm, it is unlikely the ascending aorta requires resection if the congenitally malformed aortic valve is stenotic. However, aortic resection will be necessary in about 1/2 of the patients with purely regurgitant congenitally bicuspid valves. Unfortunately, among the patients with pure AR, no preoperative features were found to distinguish those with normal from those with abnormal aortic media histologically (judged exclusively by the degree, if any, of the loss of medial elastic fibers).

In summary, it is likely that too many dilated ascending aortas are being excised prophylactically in patients with aortic valve dysfunction involving a congenitally unicuspid or bicuspid aortic valve. The rates of late postoperative occurrence of aortic dissection and/or rupture are extremely low, and additional dilation of the ascending aorta after AVR infrequently produces deleterious clinical events. The histologic structure of the dilated ascending aorta is usually normal in patients with stenotic congenitally unicuspid or bicuspid aortic valves. In contrast, the aortic histologic structure is often (about 50%) abnormal in patients with dilated ascending aortas and purely regurgitant congenitally bicuspid aortic valves.

William Clifford Roberts, MD
Baylor Heart and Vascular Institute
Baylor University Medical Center
Dallas, Texas

1. Roberts CS, Roberts WC. Dissection of the aorta associated with congenital malformation of the aortic valve. *J Am Coll Cardiol* 1991;17:712–716.
2. Roberts CS, Roberts WC. Morphologic aspects of aortic dissection. In: Ernst CB, Stanley JC, eds. *Current Therapy in Vascular Surgery*. Philadelphia: B.C. Decker; 1991:245–151.
3. Fazel SS, Mallidi HR, Lee RS, Sheehan MP, Liang D, Fleishman D, Herfkens R, Mitchell RS, Miller DC. The aortopathy of bicuspid aortic valve disease has distinctive patterns and usually involves the transverse aortic arch. *J Thorac Cardovasc Surg* 2008;135:901–907.
4. Roberts WC, Honig HS. The spectrum of cardiovascular disease in the Marfan syndrome: a clinico-morphologic study of 18 necropsy patients and comparison to 151 previously reported necropsy patients. *Am Heart J* 1982;104:115–135.
5. Roberts WC, Ko JM, Vowels TJ. Natural history of syphilitic aortitis. *Am J Cardiol* 2009;104:1578–1587.
6. Roberts WC, Bose R, Ko JM, Henry AC, Hamman BL. Identifying cardiovascular syphilis at operation. *Am J Cardiol* 2009;104:1588–1594.
7. Roberts WC, Lensing FD, Kourlis H Jr, Ko JM, Newberry JW, Smerud MJ, Burton EC, Hebeler RF Jr. Full blown cardiovascular syphilis with aneurysm of the innominate artery. *Am J Cardiol* 2009;104:1595–1600.
8. Bulkley BH, Roberts WC. Ankylosing spondylitis and aortic regurgitation. Description of the characteristic cardiovascular lesion from study of eight necropsy patients. *Circulation* 1973;48:1014–1027.
9. Roberts WC, MacGregor RR, DeBlanc HJ Jr, Beiser GD, Wolff SM. The prepulseless phase of pulseless disease, or pulseless disease with pulses: a newly recognized cause of cardiac disease, monoclonal gammopathy and "fever of unknown origin." *Am J Med* 1969;46:313–324.
10. McKeller SH, Michelena HI, Li Z, Schaff HV, Sundt TM III. Long-term risk of aortic events following aortic valve replacement in patients with bicuspid aortic valves. *Am J Cardiol* 2010;106:1626–1633.
11. Muna WF, Spray TL, Morrow AG, Roberts WC. Aortic dissection after aortic valve replacement in patients with valvular aortic stenosis. *J Thorac Cardiovasc Surg* 1977;74:65–69.
12. Gaudino M, Anselmi A, Morelli M, Pragliola C, Tsiopoulos V, Glieca F, Possati G. Aortic expansion rate in patients with dilated post-stenotic ascending aorta submitted only to aortic valve replacement: long-term follow-up. *J Am Coll Cardiol* 2011;58:581–584.
13. Rankin JS, Hammill BG, Ferguson TB Jr, Glower DD, O'Brien SM, DeLong ER, Peterson ED, Edwards FH. Determinants of operative mortality in valvular heart surgery. *J Thorac Cardiovasc Surg* 2006;131:547–557.
14. Roberts WC, Vowel TJ, Ko JM, Filardo G, Hebeler RF Jr, Henry AC, Matter GJ, Hamman BL. Comparison of the structure of the aortic valve and ascending aorta in adults having aortic valve replacement for aortic stenosis versus for pure aortic regurgitation and resection of the ascending aorta for aneurysm. *Circulation* 2011;123:896–903.

Accuracy of Two-Dimensional Echocardiography in Determining Aortic Valve Structure in Patients >50 Years of Age Having Aortic Valve Replacement for Aortic Stenosis

Ramy Fouad Ayad, MD[a], Paul Arthur Grayburn, MD[a,c], Jong Mi Ko, BA[c], Giovanni Filardo, PhD, MPH[d,e], and William Clifford Roberts, MD[a,b,c,*]

We sought to measure the accuracy of 2-dimensional transthoracic echocardiography in determining aortic valve structure in patients with aortic stenosis (AS) undergoing aortic valve replacement (AVR). Few studies have compared aortic valve structure determined by echocardiogram to that determined by examination of the operatively excised stenotic aortic valve. Two-dimensional echocardiograms were reviewed and interpreted by an expert echocardiographer in blinded fashion in 100 patients >50 years of age (mean 70) who had undergone AVR for isolated AS ± aortic regurgitation and the aortic valve structure (unicuspid, bicuspid, tricuspid) was compared to that from examination of the operatively excised stenotic valve. After excluding 14 cases in which echocardiograms were uninterpretable because of heavy calcium and/or poor image quality, congenitally malformed valves were present in 44 patients (51%) and tricuspid valves in 42 of the 86 patients (49%). Ten of the 14 patients (71%) with uninterpretable echocardiograms had congenitally malformed valves. Valve structure by echocardiogram was concordant with morphologic interpretation in 57 of 86 patients (66% accuracy, kappa = 0.33). Accuracy trended toward improvement as degree of AS decreased. In patients with valve areas similar to those enrolled in the recent transcatheter aortic valve implantation trial (PARTNER; 0.7 ± 0.2 cm^2), aortic valve structure was accurately determined by echocardiography in 21 of 35 patients (60%). In conclusion, aortic valve structure was interpretable by transthoracic echocardiogram in 86 of 100 patients and accurate in 57 of these 86 patients (66%). **(Am J Cardiol 2011;108:1589–1599)**

Determining the number of aortic valve cusps is essential in patients with aortic stenosis (AS) who are considered for transcatheter aortic valve implantation without replacement because the presence of a congenitally malformed valve is a relative contraindication to this procedure.[1] At least 4 previously published studies have compared the accuracy of aortic valve structure determined by transthoracic echocardiography to that determined by the surgeon at the time of aortic valve replacement (AVR) or by examination of the excised stenotic valve.[2–5] Each of these 4 studies had deficiencies that limited their usefulness such as including only patients <50 years of age,[2] including patients with pure aortic regurgitation (AR) of those with AS,[2,3] or relying entirely on interpretation of valve structure by the cardiac surgeon.[4,5] We compared aortic valve morphology determined by 2-dimensional echocardiography in patients >50 years of age with AS to that determined by examining the operatively excised valve.

Methods

From December 21, 2004 to May 27, 2010, 687 operatively excised stenotic aortic valves (± AR) in patients having isolated AVR (± coronary bypass) without associated mitral stenosis or mitral valve replacement were received in the surgical pathology department at Baylor University Medical Center (BUMC). The valve was weighed and its structure was determined by W.C.R. in all cases during the week that the valve was excised. Any patient having replacement of a cardiac valve other than the aortic valve was excluded from the study.

Patients' isolated aortic valve disease was confirmed by examination of their preoperative cardiac catheterization and/or echocardiographic reports, which were available on the Baylor Physician Portal and/or cardiovascular computer database (Apollo Advance C/S 4.2.13, LUMEDX Corp., Oakland, California). Patients were considered to have AS if the peak systolic transvalvular gradient was >10 mm Hg. Aortic valve gradient and valve area were obtained from the cardiac catheterization report.

The December 2004 date was chosen because that was the time the echocardiograms were available on the Cardiology Consultants of Texas computerized database and/or on the Baylor Physician Portal (Baylor electronic medical record).

[a]Departments of Internal Medicine (Division of Cardiology) and [b]Pathology and [c]Baylor Heart and Vascular Institute, Baylor University Medical Center, Dallas, Texas; [d]Institute for Health Care Research and Improvement, Baylor Health Care System, Dallas, Texas; [e]Department of Statistical Science, Southern Methodist University, Dallas, Texas. Manuscript received September 8, 2011; revised manuscript received and accepted September 10, 2011.

The study was funded by Baylor Health Care System Foundation, Dallas, Texas.

*Corresponding author: Tel: 214-820-7911; fax: 214-820-7533.

E-mail address: wc.roberts@baylorhealth.edu (W.C. Roberts).

Table 1
Comparison of demographics, hemodynamics, and valve morphology in all study patients and in patients with different echocardiographic interpretations (P.A.G.) of aortic valve structure

Factor	All	Echocardiographic Interpretation of Aortic Valve Structure					
	(n = 100)	Interpretable (n = 86)	Uninterpretable (n = 14)	p Value*	Concordant† (n = 57, 66%)	Discordant† (n = 29, 34%)	p Value‡
Age (years), range (mean ± SD)	51–91 (70 ± 10)	51–91 (71 ± 10)	54–78 (69 ± 8)	0.481	51–91 (71 ± 10)	52–88 (69 ± 9)	0.421
Men:women	61:39	54:32	7:7	0.365	41:16	13:16	0.112
Body mass index (kg/m^2), range (mean ± SD)	19.7–47.1 (29.0 ± 5.8)	19.7–47.1 (29.3 ± 6.1)	20.2–35.3 (27.2 ± 4.0)	0.404	19.7–38.9 (28.7 ± 5.0)	21.4–47.1 (30.4 ± 7.7)	0.455
Aortic valve morphology (tricuspid:bicuspid:unicuspid)§	46:51:3	42:42:2	4:9:1	0.221	28:29:0	14:13:2	0.538
Aortic valve weight (g), range (mean ± SD)	0.81–18.38 (3.03 ± 2.11)	0.81–18.38 (2.99 ± 2.17)	1.15–6.32 (3.24 ± 1.72)	0.691	0.81–18.38 (3.18 ± 2.46)	0.82–7.17 (2.63 ± 1.44)	0.265
Peak systolic transvalvular gradient (mm Hg), range (mean ± SD)	11–125 (49 ± 22)	11–125 (47 ± 21)	38–113 (61 ± 22)	0.122	11–96 (45 ± 18)	17–125 (53 ± 27)	0.241
Aortic valve area (cm^2), range (mean ± SD)	0.25–1.69 (0.81 ± 0.29)	0.25–1.69 (0.82 ± 0.29)	0.48–1.33 (0.76 ± 0.26)	0.577	0.42–1.69 (0.89 ± 0.29)	0.25–1.34 (0.68 ± 0.23)	0.023
Coronary bypass	44 (44%)	41 (47%)	3 (21%)	0.101	27 (47%)	14 (48%)	0.941

* Corrected (Bonferroni) p value for significance between interpretable and uninterpretable groups and the given factor.
† In echocardiograms that were interpretable for aortic valve structure (n = 86), echocardiographic interpretations (P.A.G.) were concordant or discordant with morphologic interpretations (W.C.R.).
‡ Corrected (Bonferroni) p value for significance between concordant and discordant groups (excluding 14 uninterpretable cases) and the given factor.
§ Determined by W.C.R.

Of the 687 patients, 100 were >50 years of age at the time of AVR and had preoperative echocardiograms available on the Cardiology Consultants of Texas computerized database and/or on the Baylor Physician Portal. Echocardiograms were recorded from 2 to 1,460 days (mean 89, median 36) before AVR. Of 100 echocardiograms, 80 were recorded <120 days before AVR. At least 1 parasternal long-axis and 1 parasternal short-axis view of the aortic valve were available in each patient.

Echocardiograms were interpreted by a staff cardiologist (P.A.G.) who was blinded to the surgical, pathological, and echocardiographic reports. His interpretations were the primary focus of our analysis. Echocardiograms were also independently reviewed and interpreted by a second cardiologist (R.F.A.) who is a fellow in training (third year) and these interpretations were used to measure interobserver agreement.

Aortic valve structure was interpreted as unicuspid, bicuspid, tricuspid, or indeterminate. The latter was because of heavy calcium and/or because of poor image quality. A valve was considered bicuspid if 2 of 3 echocardiographic criteria were present: (1) elliptical or slitlike orifice in ventricular systole in the parasternal short-axis view, (2) cuspal doming in ventricular systole, or (3) an asymmetrical closure line in the parasternal long-axis view. There were no prespecified echocardiographic criteria for unicuspid or tricuspid valves.

We also reviewed echocardiographic reports made at the time the echocardiograms had originally been recorded. In addition, we reviewed the surgeons' interpretations of the aortic valve structure from the operative reports. We used the echocardiographic report closest to the date of AVR.

Associations between various factors (demographic, clinical, and anatomic) and echocardiographic interpretations of aortic valve structure (uninterpretable, interpretable, concordant with morphologic interpretation, and discordant with morphologic interpretation) were tested with a Wilcoxon (for continuous factors) or a chi-square (for categorical factors) test. A Bonferroni correction was employed to account for multiplicity. Kappa tests, specificity, and sensitivity were used to assess agreement between echocardiographic and morphologic interpretations of aortic valve structure.

This study was approved by the institutional review board at BUMC.

Results

Table 1 presents demographics and pertinent cardiac findings in all patients, those with interpretable versus uninterpretable echocardiograms for aortic valve structure, and those with concordant versus discordant echocardiographic (P.A.G.) and morphologic (W.C.R.) interpretations. Patients' age ranged from 51 to 91 years (mean 70 ± 10); 61 were men and 39 were women. Body mass index ranged from 19.7 to 47.1 kg/m^2 (mean 29.0 ± 5.8, median 27.5). There were 3 unicuspid, 51 bicuspid, and 46 tricuspid valves as determined morphologically (W.C.R.).

Aortic valve weights ranged from 0.81 to 18.38 g (mean 3.03 ± 2.11). Peak systolic transvalvular gradients (by cardiac catheterization) ranged from 11 to 125 mm Hg (mean 49 ± 22). Aortic valve area (by cardiac catheterization) ranged from 0.25 to 1.69 cm^2 (mean 0.81 ± 0.29). Sixteen

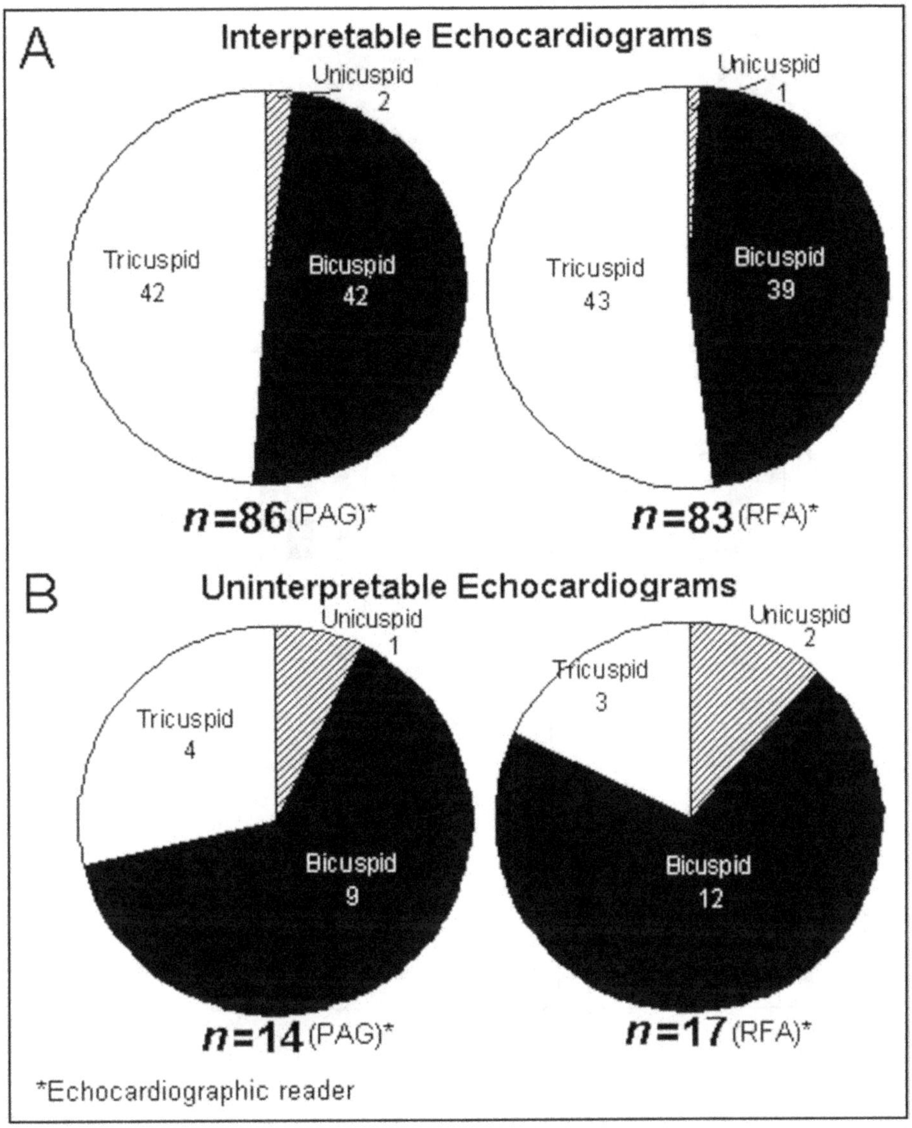

Figure 1. Each pie chart displays echocardiograms in which each echocardiographic reader (P.A.G. or R.F.A.) could *(A)* or could not *(B)* interpret aortic valve structure. In each chart, the morphologic interpretations (W.C.R.), not echocardiographic interpretations, of valve structure are shown. Most valves that were uninterpretable (P.A.G. or R.F.A.) were congenitally malformed valves (10/14 [71%] and 14/17 [82%], respectively). *Echocardiographic reader.

valves had areas >1 cm^2 but only 2 of these 16 valves had valve areas >1 cm^2 when measured by echocardiogram. Of these 16 patients, peak systolic gradients ranged from 19 to 96 mm Hg (mean 40 ± 18), mean transvalvular gradients ranged from 14 to 77 mm Hg (mean 31 ± 15), and aortic valve weights ranged from 1.47 to 6.33 g (mean 3.22 ± 1.43, normal aortic valve weight ≤0.50 g).

Of the 100 patients, 86 had echocardiograms that were interpretable for aortic valve structure (P.A.G.). In 57 of these 86 patients (66%), echocardiographic interpretation was concordant with morphologic interpretation (kappa test = 0.33). Aortic valve structure in patients with interpretable compared to uninterpretable echocardiograms is shown in Figure 1. Ten of the 14 patients (71%) who had echocardiograms that were uninterpretable (P.A.G.) had congenitally malformed valves (Figure 1).

Graphical comparisons of echocardiographic interpretability and concordance of echocardiographic (P.A.G.) and morphologic (W.C.R.) interpretations of aortic valve structure in different groups according to valve weight, gender, age at time of AVR, body mass index, peak systolic gradient, and valve area are shown in Figures 2 to 5. Unadjusted associations between these factors and echocardiographic interpretability and accuracy are presented in Table 1.

At heavier valve weights (>4 g in men and >3 g in women), stenotic valve structure was less interpretable (71% vs 90%) but equally accurate (66%) by echocardiogram compared to lighter weights (<4 g in men and <3 g in women; Figure 2). Frequency of congenitally malformed valves in these heavier valves was also higher than in the lighter valves (90% vs 44%; Figure 2).

Men had higher mean valve weights (quantity of calcium) than women (3.76 ± 2.36 vs 1.86 ± 0.69 g; Figure 2). Aortic valve structure was similarly interpretable by echocardiography (82% vs 88%) but less accurately interpreted (48% vs 76%) in women than in men (Figure 2).

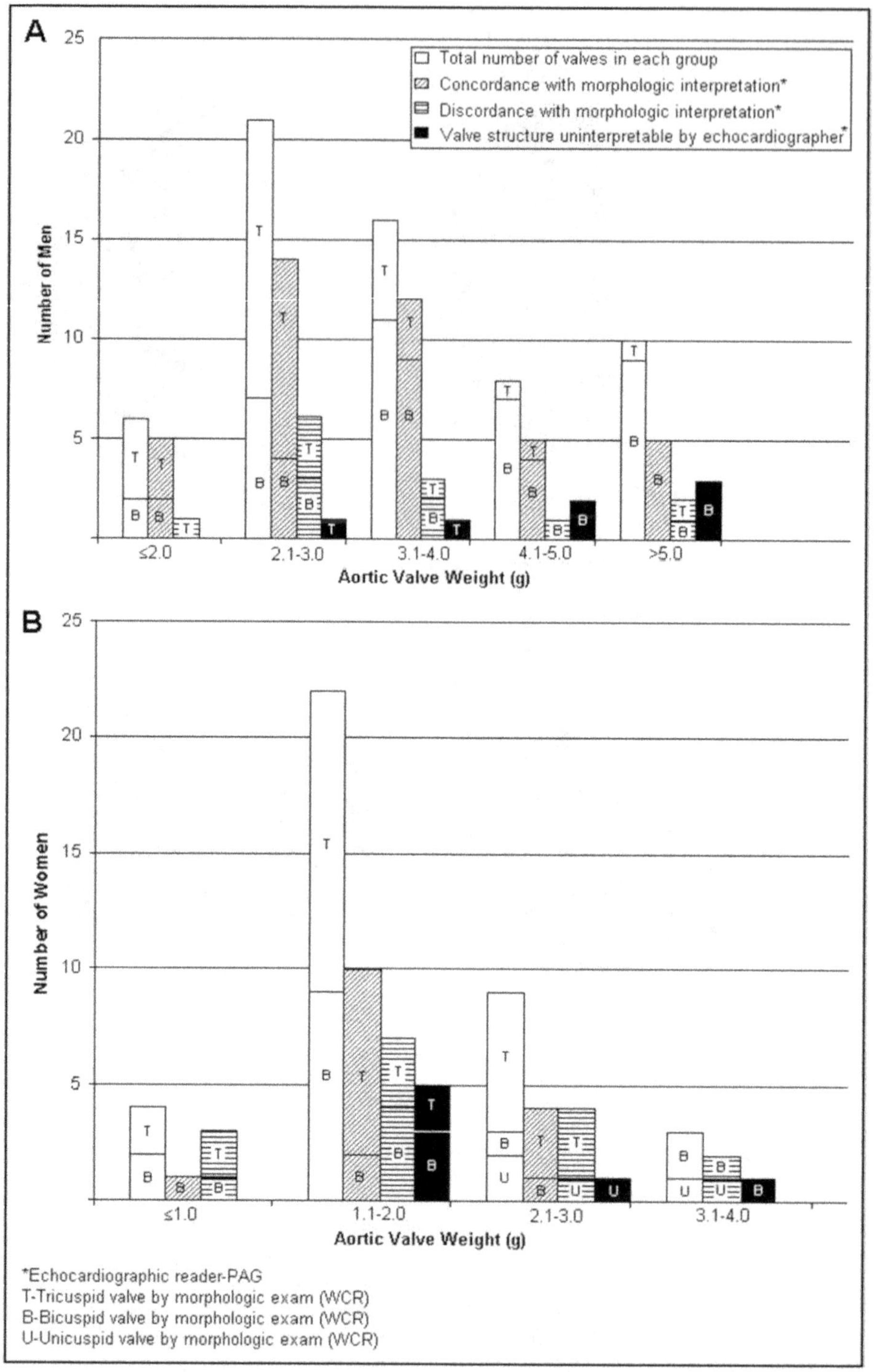

Figure 2. In each weight group of men *(A)* and women *(B)*, the total number of patients *(white bar)* and the number of patients in whom the echocardiographic reader was able to interpret valve structure (concordant) *[diagonal hatched bar]* or discordant *[horizontal hatched bar]* with that of the morphologic reader [W.C.R.]) or unable to interpret valve structure *(black bar)* are shown. Numbers of tricuspid (T), bicuspid (B), and unicuspid (U) aortic valves (determined by W.C.R.) in each group are displayed. Valve weight was determined primarily by quantity of calcium in valve cusps. Frequency of congenitally malformed valves was higher (90% vs 44%) in patients with heavier valves (>4 g in men and >3 g in women) compared to lighter valves (<4 g in men and <3 g in women). Echocardiographic interpretability was lower (71% vs 90%) but echocardiographic accuracy was identical (66%) in patients with heavier valves compared to lighter valves. Men had heavier valves than women (3.76 ± 2.36 vs 1.86 ± 0.69 g). Echocardiographic interpretability was similar (88% vs 82%) but echocardiographic accuracy was higher (76% vs 48%) in men than women. *Echocardiographic reader (P.A.G.).

Echocardiographic interpretability appeared higher in patients >80 years old (100% vs 84%) than in patients ≤80 years old at time of AVR (Figure 3). Echocardiographic accuracy was similar in the 2 age groups (73% vs 65%; Figure 3). Older patients (>80 years old) had a lower frequency of heavily calcified valves (weight >4 g in men

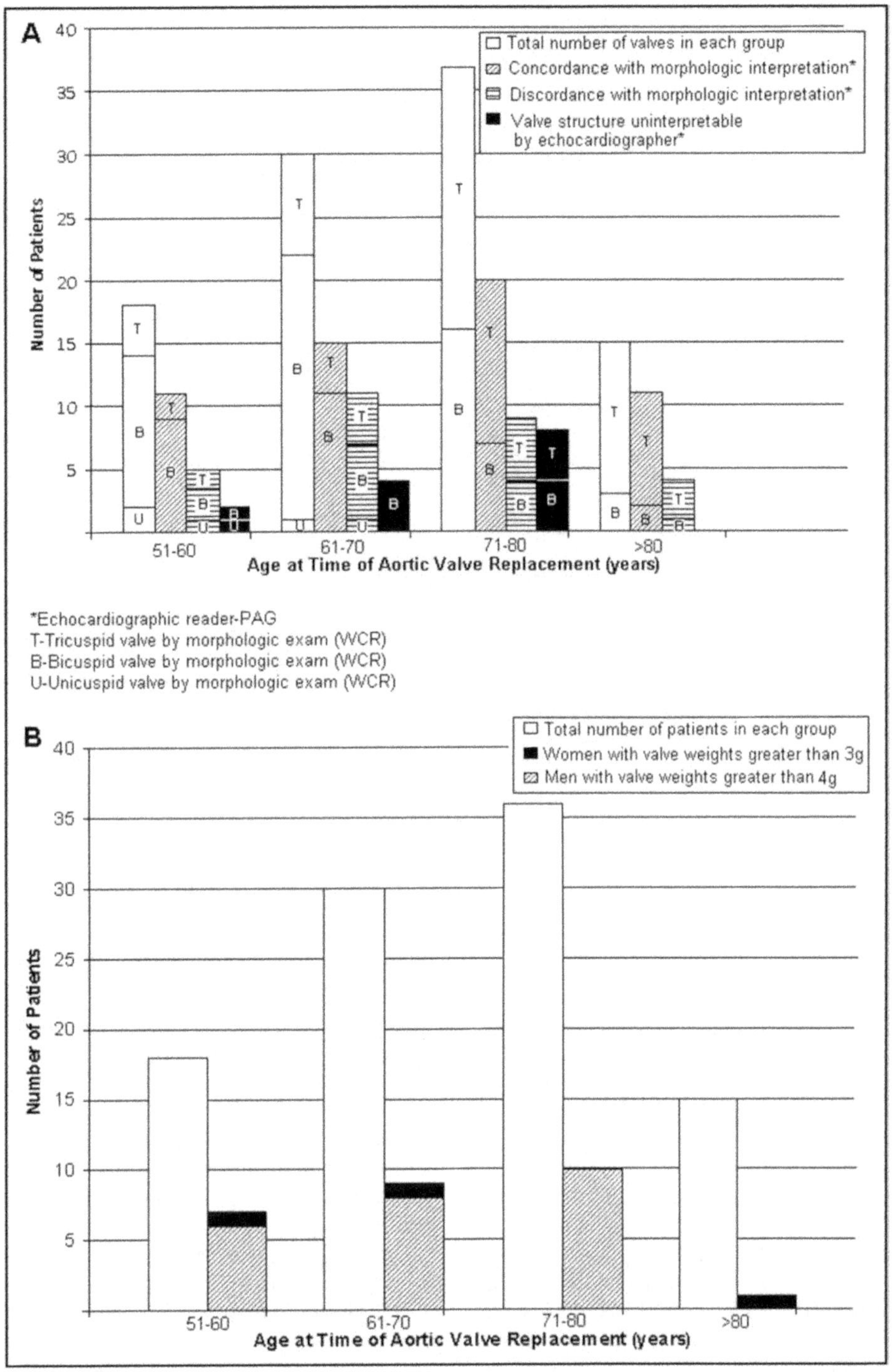

Figure 3. *(A)* In each age group, the total number of patients *(white bar)* and the number of patients in whom the echocardiographic reader was able to interpret valve structure (concordant *[diagonal hatched bar]* or discordant *[horizontal hatched bar]* with that of the morphologic reader [W.C.R.]) or unable to interpret valve structure *(black bar)* are shown. Numbers of tricuspid, bicuspid, and unicuspid aortic valves (determined by W.C.R.) in each group are displayed. Echocardiographic interpretability was higher (100% vs 84%) in patients >80 than in patients ≤80 years of age at time of aortic valve replacement. Frequency of tricuspid valves was higher in patients >80 years old (80%) than in patients ≤80 years (33%). Echocardiographic accuracy was similar in the 2 age groups (73% vs 65%). *(B)* In each age group, the number of heavily calcified valves (men with valves weighing >4 g *[diagonal hatched bar]* and women with valves weighing >3 g *[black bar]*) are shown. Seven percent of patients >80 years old had heavily calcified valves versus 37% of patients ≤80 years. *Echocardiographic reader (P.A.G.). Abbreviations as in Figure 2.

and >3 g in women) than younger patients (<80 years old, 7% vs 37%; Figure 3). Older patients also had a higher frequency of tricuspid valves than younger patients (80% vs 33%; Figure 3).

Overall, echocardiographic interpretability and accuracy did not change with body mass index (Figure 4). Nevertheless, comparison of the largest and smallest body mass index groups showed differences. Of the 12 patients with body mass index

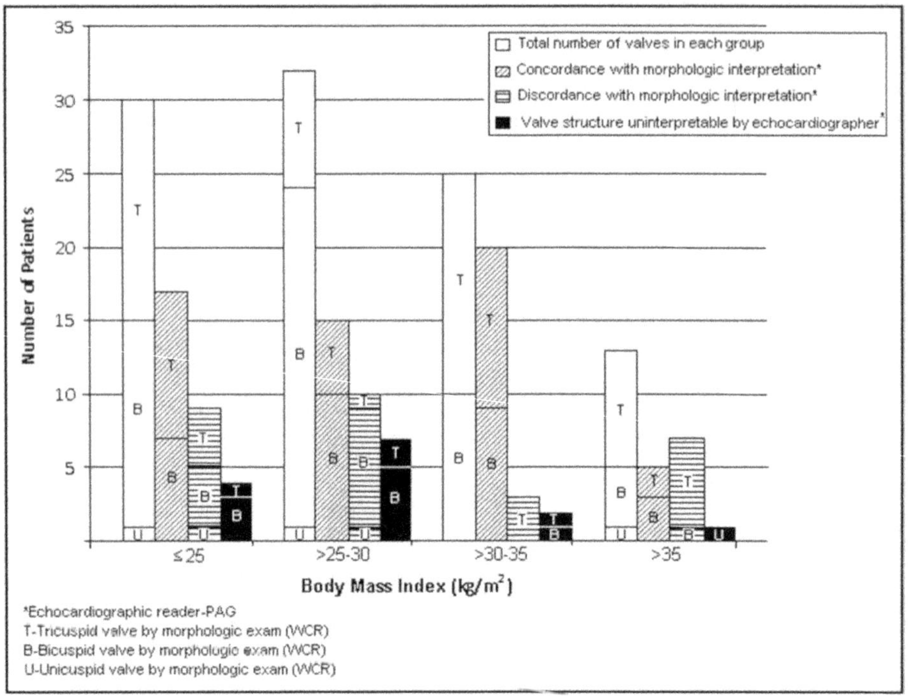

Figure 4. In each body mass index group, the total number of patients *(white bar)* and the number of patients in whom the echocardiographic reader was able to interpret valve structure (concordant *[diagonal hatched bar]* or discordant *[horizontal hatched bar]* with that of the morphologic reader [W.C.R.]) or unable to interpret valve structure *(black bar)* are shown. Numbers of tricuspid, bicuspid, and unicuspid aortic valves (determined by W.C.R.) in each group are displayed. Of the 12 patients with body mass index >35 kg/m^2, in only 5 (42%) was the echocardiogram interpretable and accurate; in contrast, of the 33 patients with body mass index ≤25 kg/m^2, in 17 (52%) the echocardiogram was interpretable and accurate. *Echocardiographic reader (P.A.G.). Abbreviations as in Figure 2.

>35 kg/m^2, in only 5 (42%) was the echocardiogram interpretable and accurate; in contrast, of the 33 patients with body mass index ≤25 kg/m^2, in 17 (52%) the echocardiogram was interpretable and accurate.

Echocardiographic interpretability and accuracy decreased slightly (86% vs 94% and 59% vs 68%, respectively) with higher peak systolic transvalvular gradient (>50 vs ≤50 mm Hg; Figure 5). In patients with valve area ≤0.7 compared to >0.7 cm^2, echocardiographic accuracy was lower (50% vs 80%), but interpretability was similar (86% vs 91%; Figure 5).

Comparisons of aortic valve structure determined by echocardiogram by the 2 readers to each other and to that determined by examination of the operatively excised stenotic valve are presented in Table 2. Sensitivity and specificity of echocardiography (P.A.G.) were 69% and 67% for detection of a bicuspid and 67% and 69% for detection of a tricuspid aortic valve, respectively. Neither echocardiographic reader accurately identified any of the 3 unicuspid valves. Both readers accurately identified 28 (61%) of the 46 tricuspid valves. P.A.G. accurately identified 29, and the fellow in training (R.F.A.), 24 of the 51 bicuspid valves (57% vs 47%). P.A.G. and R.F.A. were concordant with morphologic findings in 69% and 63% of bicuspid valves, respectively, that were interpretable by echocardiography. Of tricuspid valves interpretable by echocardiography, their rates of concordance were 67% and 65%, respectively. In 62% of interpretable echocardiograms, the 2 readers agreed in their interpretation of aortic valve structure (kappa test = 0.20).

Original echocardiographic and operative reports were available in 97 and 100 of patients. The 97 echocardiograms were originally interpreted by 12 different attending physicians at the Cardiology Consultants of Texas or BUMC at the time of the study. AVR was performed by 7 different cardiac surgeons at BUMC. Number of aortic valve cusps was mentioned in 13 (13%) of the 97 echocardiographic reports and in 79 (79%) of the 100 operative reports. The surgeon agreed with the cardiac pathologist (W.C.R.) in 29 (63%) of the 46 congenitally malformed valves (unicuspid and bicuspid) and in 31 (94%) of the 33 tricuspid valves in which the number of cusps were mentioned. In 84 (87%) echocardiograms and in 21 (21%) operative reports, the valve was described as stenotic, calcific, or thickened, but the number of valve cusps was not mentioned.

Representative echocardiographic images and photographs of corresponding excised valves are shown in Figures 6 and 7 with the Video Supplement.

Discussion

Of our patients with AS ± AR, transthoracic echocardiography had limited accuracy (57 of 86 patients with interpretable echocardiograms, 66%) in determining aortic valve structure. Echocardiograms were uninterpretable in 14 patients and 10 of these patients (71%) had congenitally malformed valves. Compared to less calcified valves, heavily calcified valves (weight >4 g in men and >3 g in women) were more commonly congenitally malformed (90% vs 44%), had echocardiographic images that were less frequently interpretable (71% vs 90%), but echocardiographic interpretations were equally accurate (66%). These observations suggest that increasing valve weight (quantity of

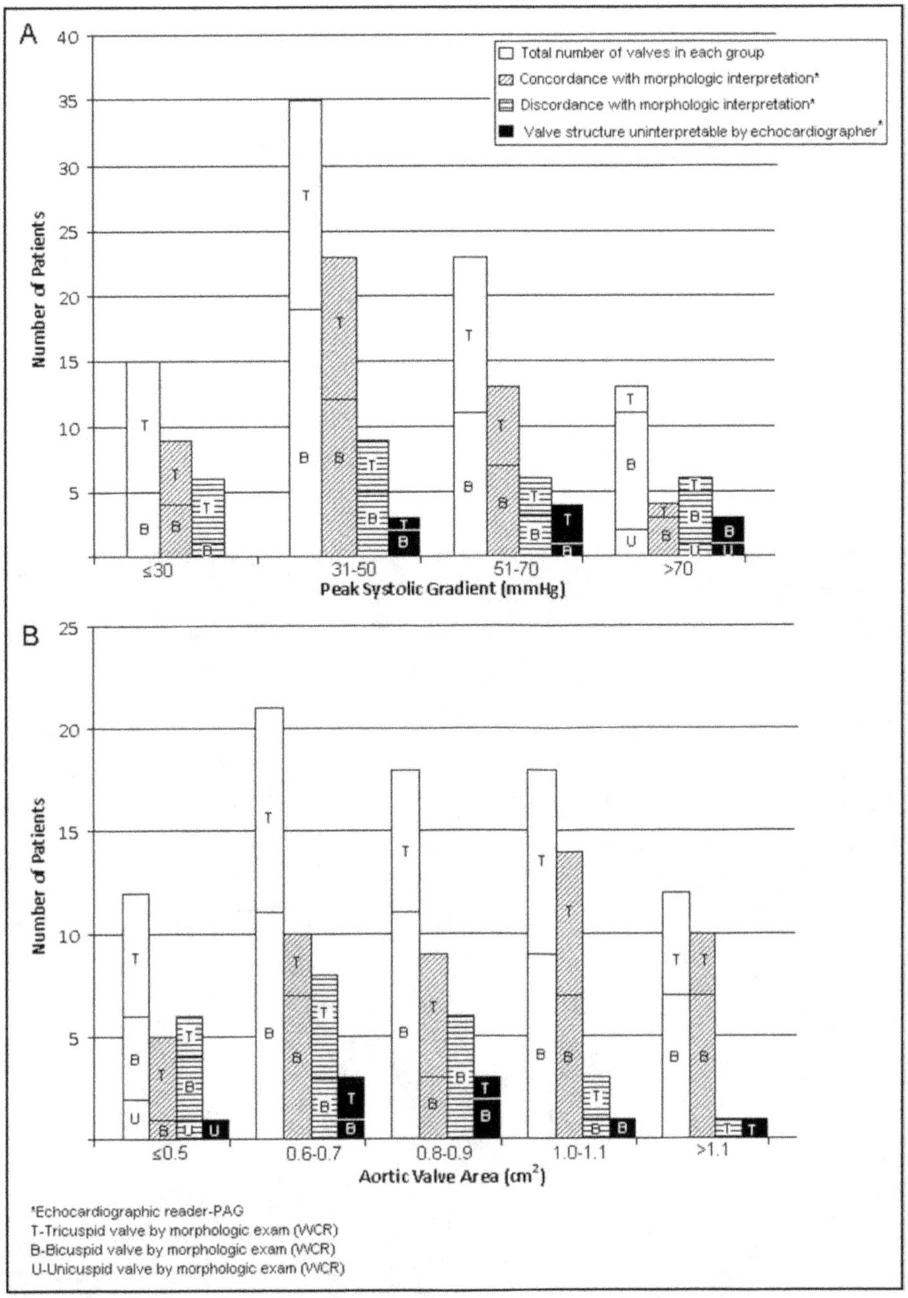

Figure 5. In each peak systolic gradient group *(A)* and valve area group *(B)*, the total number of patients *(white bar)* and the number of patients in whom the echocardiographic reader was able to interpret valve structure (concordant *[diagonal hatched bar]* or discordant *[horizontal hatched bar]* with that of the morphologic reader [W.C.R.]) or unable to interpret valve structure *(black bar)* are shown. Numbers of tricuspid, bicuspid, and unicuspid aortic valves (determined by W.C.R.) in each group are displayed. Echocardiographic interpretability and accuracy decreased slightly (86% vs 94% and 59% vs 68%, respectively) with higher peak systolic transvalvular gradient (>50 vs ≤50 mm Hg). In patients with valve area ≤0.7 compared to >0.7 cm^2, echocardiographic accuracy was lower (50% vs 80%), but interpretability was similar (86% vs 91%). *Echocardiographic reader (P.A.G.). Abbreviations as in Figure 2.

calcium) decreases the interpretability (by obscuring visualization of the valve orifice) but not the accuracy of echocardiography in determining aortic valve structure. Hence, the location of the calcium, not necessarily its quantity (weight), may be the more important factor affecting echocardiographic accuracy in determining aortic valve structure.

Despite men having higher mean valve weights (quantity of calcium) than women (3.76 vs 1.86 g), aortic valve structure was similarly interpretable by echocardiography (82% vs 88%) but less accurately interpreted (48% vs 76%) in women than in men. Overall, echocardiographic interpretability and accuracy did not change with body mass index. Breast tissue, more than quantity of valve calcium or total adipose tissue, may significantly decrease echocardiographic accuracy.

We observed a high interobserver variability (the 2 readers agreed in their interpretation of aortic valve structure in 62% of interpretable echocardiograms) and a trend toward an inverse association between degree of valve stenosis and accuracy of echocardiographic interpretation of valve struc-

Table 2
Comparison of aortic valve structure determined by echocardiogram by the two readers to each other and to that determined by examination of operatively excised stenotic aortic valves (n = 100)

Echocardiographic Interpretation	Morphologic Interpretation*								
	Unicuspid (n = 3)			Bicuspid (n = 51)			Tricuspid (n = 46)		
	P.A.G.†	R.F.A.†	P.A.G. = R.F.A.‡	P.A.G.†	R.F.A.†	P.A.G. = R.F.A.‡	P.A.G.†	R.F.A.†	P.A.G. = R.F.A.‡
Bicuspid	1			29	24	15	14	15	6
Tricuspid	1	1	1	13	15	5	28	28	18
Indeterminate–heavily calcified	1	2	1	7	6	2	4	2	
Indeterminate–poor image quality				2	6	1		1	

Kappa test = 0.334 between echocardiographic (P.A.G.) and morphologic (WCR) interpretations, 0.259 between echocardiographic (R.F.A.) and morphologic (WCR) interpretations, and 0.201 between echocardiographic interpretations (P.A.G. and R.F.A.).

* Determined by W.C.R.

† Echocardiographic reader.

‡ Readers agreed in their interpretations.

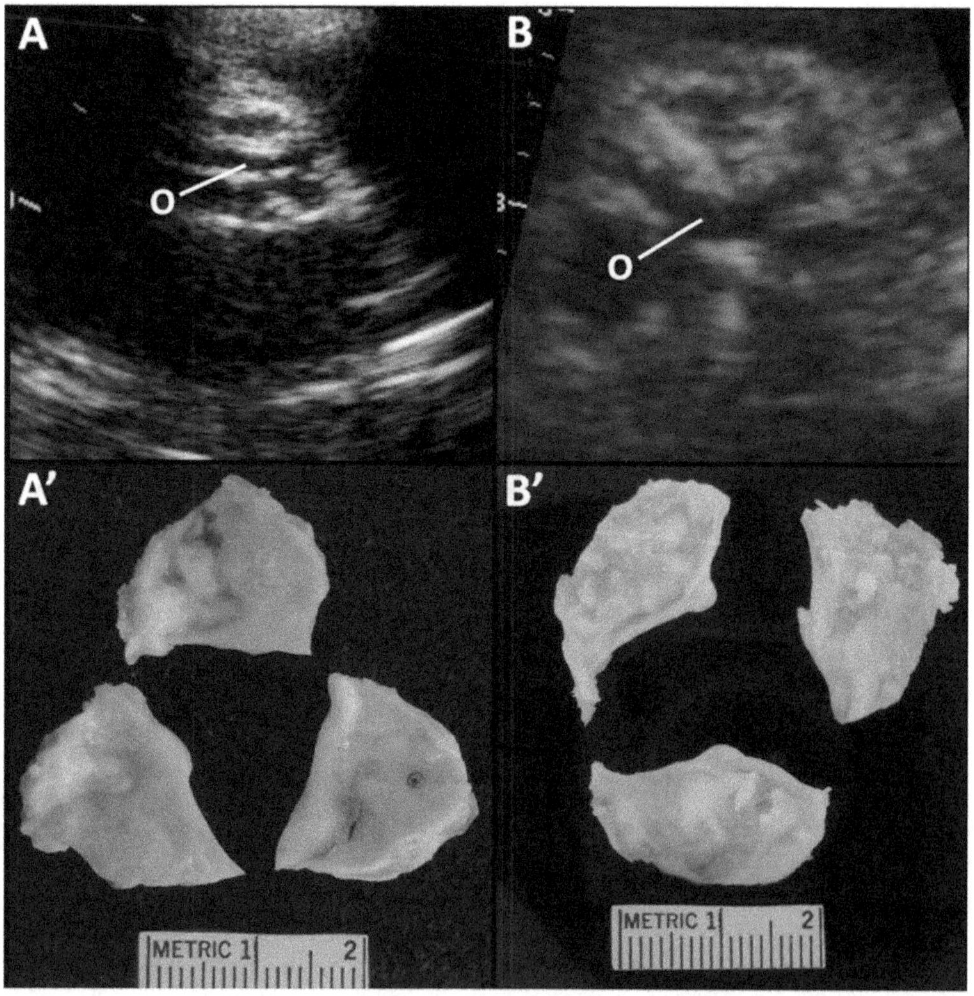

Figure 6. Parasternal short-axis echocardiographic views in ventricular systole *(A, B)* and excised specimens *(A', B')* from 2 patients with tricuspid aortic valves. The valve orifice (O) in *A* appears slitlike in contrast to the V-shape in *B* (Video 6A and 6B). The 2 echocardiographic readers interpreted valve *A* as bicuspid (discordant with actual morphology) and valve *B* as tricuspid (concordant with actual morphology). *(A)* Patient is a 67-year-old man whose operatively excised valve weighed 1.5 g. *(B)* Patient is an 80-year-old woman whose operatively excised valve weighed 1.7 g.

ture. An elliptical-shaped orifice in ventricular systole, the chief criterion of the bicuspid configuration, is not easily or consistently appreciated in stenotic aortic valves, especially the severely narrowed valves. Inaccuracy of 2-dimensional echocardiography in determining aortic valve structure in patients with AS is almost certainly attributable to inherent

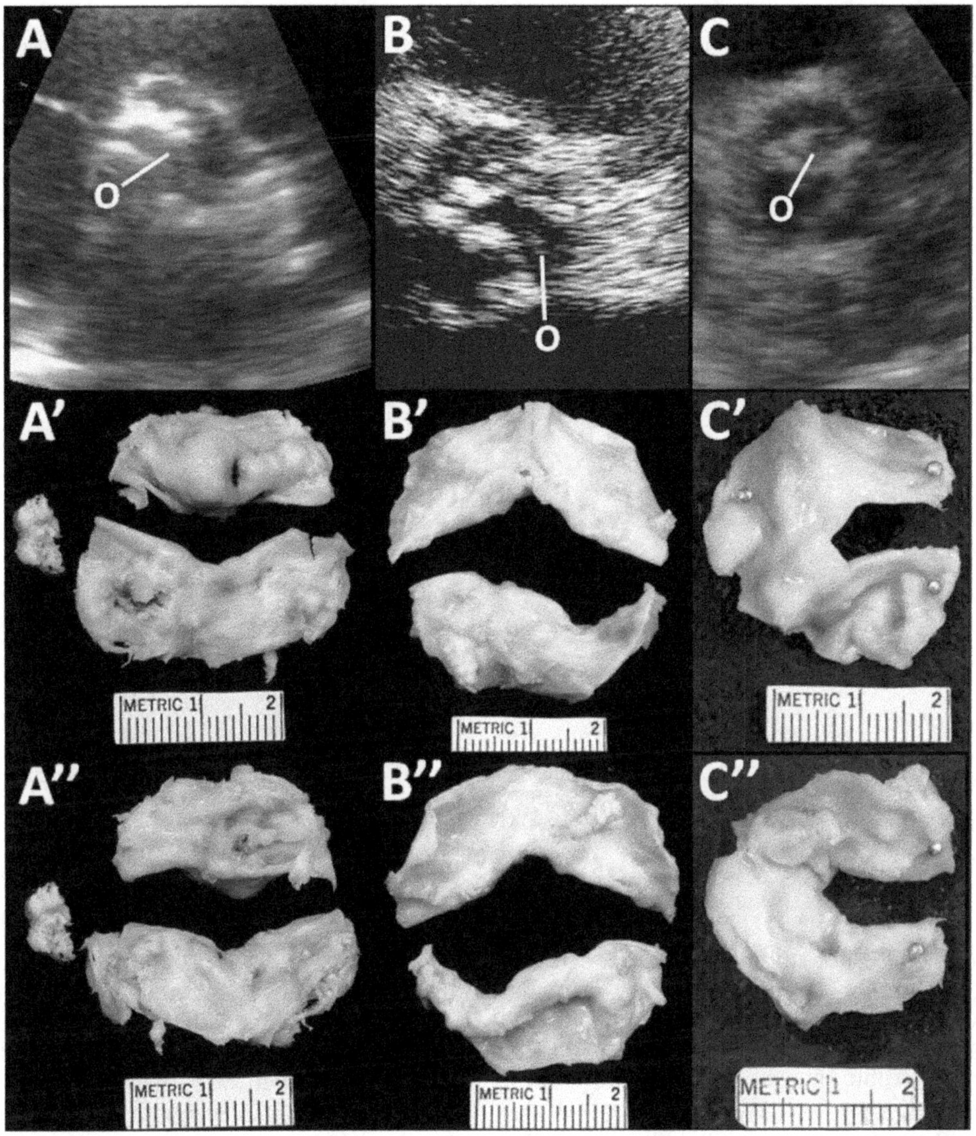

Figure 7. Parasternal short-axis echocardiographic views in ventricular systole *(A, B, C)* and excised specimens seen from an aortic aspect *(A', B', C')* and a ventricular aspect *(A'', B'', C'')* from 2 patients with bicuspid aortic valves *(A, B)* and from 1 patient with a unicuspid aortic valve *(C)*. The valve orifice is elliptical in the bicuspid valves *(A, B)* and difficult to discern in the unicuspid valve *(C)* (Video 7A, 7B, and 7C). The 2 echocardiographic readers interpreted valves in *A* and *B* as bicuspid (concordant with actual morphology) and valve in *C* as tricuspid (discordant with actual morphology). *(A)* Patient is a 57-year-old man whose operatively excised valve weighed 3.9 g. *(B)* Patient is a 58-year-old man whose operatively excised valve weighed 3.2 g. *(C)* Patient is a 66-year-old woman whose operatively excised valve weighed 2.5 g. Abbreviation as in Figure 6.

limitations of the imaging method rather than to incorrect interpretation.

The bicuspid aortic valve was frequently present in our older patients: of our 52 patients >70 years of age, 19 (37%) had a congenitally bicuspid valve, a fact important in selecting candidates for transcatheter aortic valve implantation. In our patients with valve areas similar to those enrolled in the recent transcatheter aortic valve implantation trial (PARTNER; 0.7 ± 0.2 cm^2), aortic valve structure was accurately determined by 2-dimensional echocardiography in only 21 of 35 patients (60%).[1] Transesophageal echocardiography is more precise in determining aortic valve structure in patients with AS.[6]

Table 3 presents summary findings in 4 previously published studies examining the accuracy and interpretability of 2-dimensional transthoracic echocardiography in determining aortic valve structure in patients with AS compared to a surgical or morphologic gold standard.[2–5] These studies differ from our study in several important ways: (1) *patient age* (1 study included only patients <50 years of age, range 2 months to 50 years, a group much younger than most patients with AS[2]), (2) *type of valve dysfunction* (2 studies included patients with pure AR intermixed with those with AS[2,3]; 1 of these studies showed that echocardiographic interpretability and accuracy was much greater in patients with pure AR [83% and 93%, respectively] compared to those with isolated AS [69% and 70%, respectively][2]), (3) *rate of echocardiographic interpretability* (1 study accurately measured valve structure by echocardiography in only 58% of study patients because of inadequate image

Table 3
Comparison of previously published studies measuring the accuracy and interpretability of two-dimensional transthoracic echocardiography in determining aortic valve structure in patients with aortic stenosis

Variable	First Author (year of publication)			
	Brandenburg First Author[2] (1983) (n = 115)	Chan First Author[3] (1999) (n = 178)	Tanaka First Author[4] (2010) (n = 50)	Joziasse First Author[5] (2011) (n = 80)
Clinical diagnosis				
Aortic stenosis ± aortic regurgitation	62	—*	50	80
Pure aortic regurgitation	53	—*	0	0
Age (years), range (mean)	1–50 (32)	— (64)	43–83 (70)	56–74 (69)
Men:women	83:32	118:60	23:27	54:26
Diagnostic gold standard				
Surgeon's view	29	0	50	80
Pathologist's view	86	178	0	0
Interpretable echocardiograms	86 (75%)	104 (58%)	40 (80%)	58 (73%)
Aortic valve structure				
Tricuspid	60 (52%)†	111 (62%)	33 (66%)	48 (60%)
Bicuspid	50 (43%)	66 (37%)	17 (34%)	32 (40%)
Unicuspid	4 (3%)	1 (1%)	0	0
Peak systolic transvalvular gradient (mm Hg), range (average)	—	—	— (102)	— (78)
Aortic valve area (cm^2), range (mean)	—	—	— (0.66)	— (0.76)
Accuracy‡				
All valves	88%	94%	83%	66%
Tricuspid valves only	96%	96%	77%	91%
Bicuspid valves only	78%	92%	93%	54%

* Included patients who underwent aortic valve replacement for any indication.
† One patient had a quadricuspid valve.
‡ In patients with interpretable echocardiograms.
— = information was not available.

quality, a much lower rate of interpretability than observed by us and others[3]), (4) *source of echocardiographic interpretations* (1 study used echocardiographic interpretations from preoperative echocardiographic reports, not from a review of echocardiographic images by study investigators[3]; our data show that cardiologists reading echocardiograms at our institution, and undoubtedly at many others, often do not adequately and consistently describe aortic valve morphology [only 13 of 97 reports, 13%, mentioned the number of aortic valve cusps]), and (5) *diagnostic gold standard* (2 studies used cardiac surgeons' intraoperative determination, not by examination by a cardiac pathologist, as their diagnostic gold standard[4,5]; 1 study compared surgical assessment of valve structure to pathologic assessment and found that interpretations differed in 33% of cases of bicuspid valves[5]; in our present study, the surgeons' operative description agreed with that of the pathologist [W.C.R.] in 94% of tricuspid valves and in 63% of unicuspid and bicuspid valves, and these findings are similar to those of a larger study also at BUMC where valve structure at operation in patients with AS was very accurate for tricuspid valves [99% of surgeons' operative descriptions agreed with that of the pathologist, i.e. W.C.R.], but highly inaccurate for unicuspid and bicuspid valves [15% and 56%, respectively][7]). Other reported studies were not included in Table 3 because they included only very young patients, included cases with functionally normal valves, or examined interpretability (not accuracy) of echocardiography.[8–10]

The positive features of our study are the following: it is the first to compare accuracy of 2-dimensional echocardiography in patients with AS >50 years of age to morphologic examination by an experienced cardiac pathologist. It is also the first to quantitate the effect of valve calcium (measured by valve weight), gradient, and area on echocardiographic interpretability and accuracy. Each study was reviewed by 2 independent readers with different levels of experience and proficiency. Previous studies used only a single reader's interpretation. We have shown for the first time that determining the accuracy of echocardiography in determining aortic valve structure is more complex than simply measuring the accuracy of 1 reader's interpretations. Although our 2 readers had similar accuracy overall, the interobserver variability in interpretation was substantial.

Our study has limitations. We cannot exclude the possibility that retrospective review and interpretation of echocardiograms by study investigators introduced potential bias because our investigators were aware that study patients had undergone AVR for AS and were focused specifically on interpreting aortic valve structure. There was a wide range of intervals (2 to 1,460 days) between the dates echocardiograms were recorded and AVR. The interval, however, did not appear to affect our results because echocardiographic interpretability and accuracy were almost identical in the 20 studies recorded ≥120 days (17/20 [85%] and 10/17 [59%], respectively) or <12 days (18/20 [90%] and 10/18 [56%], respectively) before AVR.

Supplementary data

Supplementary data associated with this article can be found, in the online version, at doi:10.1016/j.amjcard.2011.09.006.

1. Smith CR, Leon MB, Mack MJ, Miller DC, Moses JW, Svensson LG, Tuzcu EM, Webb JG, Fontana GP, Makkar RR, Williams M, Dewey T, Kapadia S, Babaliaros V, Thourani VH, Corso P, Pichard AD, Bavaria JE, Herrmann HC, Akin JJ, Anderson WN, Wang D, Pocock SJ; PARTNER Trial Investigators. Transcatheter versus surgical aortic-valve replacement in high-risk patients. *N Engl J Med* 2011;364:2187–2198.
2. Brandenburg RO, Tajik AJ, Edwards WD, Reeder GS, Shub C, Seward JB. Accuracy of 2-dimensional echocardiographic diagnosis of congenitally bicuspid aortic valve: echocardiographic-anatomic correlation in 115 patients. *Am J Cardiol* 1983;51:1469–1473.
3. Chan KL, Stinson WA, Veinot JP. Reliability of transthoracic echocardiography in the assessment of aortic valve morphology: pathological correlation in 178 patients. *Can J Cardiol* 1999;15:48–52.
4. Tanaka R, Yoshioka K, Niinuma H, Ohsawa S, Okabayashi H, Ehara S. Diagnostic value of cardiac CT in the evaluation of bicuspid aortic stenosis: comparison with echocardiography and operative findings. *AJR Am J Roentgenol* 2010;195:895–899.
5. Joziasse IC, Vink A, Cramer MJ, van Oosterhout MF, van Herwerden LA, Heijmen R, Sieswerda GT, Mulder BJ, Doevendans PA. Bicuspid stenotic aortic valves: clinical characteristics and morphological assessment using MRI and echocardiography. *Neth Heart J* 2011;19:119–125.
6. Espinal M, Fuisz AR, Nanda NC, Aaluri AR, Mukhtar O, Sekar PC. Sensitivity and specificity of transesophageal echocardiography for determination of aortic valve morphology. *Am Heart J* 2000;139:1071–1076.
7. Roberts WC, Vowels TJ, Ko JM. Comparison of interpretations of valve structure between cardiac surgeon and cardiac pathologist among adults having isolated aortic valve replacement for aortic valve stenosis (+/− aortic regurgitation). *Am J Cardiol* 2009;103:1139–1145.
8. Zema MJ, Caccavano M. Two dimensional echocardiographic assessment of aortic valve morphology: feasibility of bicuspid valve detection. Prospective study of 100 adult patients. *Br Heart J* 1982;48:428–433.
9. Fowles RE, Martin RP, Abrams JM, Schapira JN, French JW, Popp RL. Two-dimensional echocardiographic features of bicuspid aortic valve. *Chest* 1979;75:434–440.
10. Alegret JM, Palazón O, Duran I, Vernis JM. Aortic valve morphology definition with transthoracic combined with transesophageal echocardiography in a population with high prevalence of bicuspid aortic valve. *Int J Cardiovasc Imaging* 2005;21:213–217.

Presence of a Congenitally Bicuspid Aortic Valve Among Patients Having Combined Mitral and Aortic Valve Replacement

William Clifford Roberts, MD[a,b,d,*], Kaitlin Georgeanne Janning[d,e], Travis James Vowels[d,f], Jong Mi Ko, BA[d], Baron Lloyd Hamman, MD[c], and Robert Frederick Hebeler, Jr., MD[c]

Although bicuspid aortic valve occurs in an estimated 1% of adults and mitral valve prolapse in an estimated 5% of adults, occurrence of the 2 in the same patient is infrequent. During examination of operatively excised aortic and mitral valves because of dysfunction (stenosis and/or regurgitation), we encountered 16 patients who had congenitally bicuspid aortic valves associated with various types of dysfunctioning mitral valves. Eleven of the 16 patients had aortic stenosis (AS): 5 of them also had mitral stenosis, of rheumatic origin in 4 and secondary to mitral annular calcium in 1; the other 6 with aortic stenosis had pure mitral regurgitation (MR) secondary to mitral valve prolapse in 3, to ischemia in 2, and to unclear origin in 1. Of the 5 patients with pure aortic regurgitation, each also had pure mitral regurgitation: in 1 secondary to mitral valve prolapse and in 4 secondary to infective endocarditis. In conclusion, various types of mitral dysfunction severe enough to warrant mitral valve replacement occur in patients with bicuspid aortic valves. A proper search for mitral valve dysfunction in patients with bicuspid aortic valves appears warranted. **(Am J Cardiol 2012;109:263–271)**

In 1994 Fernicola and Roberts[1] described morphologic features of operatively excised aortic and mitral valves in 12 patients who had undergone combined aortic and mitral valve replacement for dysfunctioning congenitally bicuspid aortic valves (aortic stenosis [AS] in 8 and pure aortic regurgitation [AR] in 4) and dysfunctioning mitral valves (mitral regurgitation [MR] in 11 and congenital mitral stenosis [MS] in 1). The 12 patients (10%) were from 115 having combined mitral and aortic valve replacement. The present report examines at another institution 16 patients who had undergone combined aortic and mitral valve replacement for dysfunctioning congenitally bicuspid aortic valves and dysfunctioning mitral valves to demonstrate again the relative frequency of structural mitral disease in patients with dysfunctioning congenitally bicuspid aortic valves.

Methods

At Baylor University Medical Center (BUMC) at Dallas from March 3, 1993 to July 8, 2011, 3,054 native valve replacement operations were performed (Figure 1). Of that number, 2866 (94%) involved a single valve (aortic in 2,174, mitral in 677, and tricuspid in 15) and 169 (6%) the replacement of >1 cardiac valve (mitral and aortic valves in 180 and tricuspid plus ≥1 other valve in 8). Of the 180 who had left-sided double valve replacements, 16 (9%) were in patients having a stenotic or purely regurgitant congenitally bicuspid aortic valve and a stenotic or purely regurgitant mitral valve. These 16 patients are the subject of this report. All 32 valves from these 16 patients were examined in the cardiovascular pathology laboratory of BUMC at Dallas, a part of the surgical pathology department, by 1 of us (W.C.R.). Photographs of the operatively excised valves were taken by 1 of us (J.M.K.). Histologic sections after the gross photographs were prepared from the valves that were the sites of infective endocarditis and from the mitral valves considered on gross examination to be characteristic of mitral valve prolapse. Stenotic valves were not studied histologically.

Medical records and available echocardiographic, hemodynamic, and angiographic reports were acquired on all 16 patients. Records of death were obtained from the Social Security Death Index. Intervals from the time of combined mitral and aortic valve replacement to June 30, 2011, were calculated.

Results

Pertinent findings in the 16 patients are presented in Tables 1 and 2 and illustrated in 13 patients in Figures 2 through 14. Of the 16 patients, 12 were men age 24 to 77 (mean 57) and 4 were women age 53 to 84 (mean 67). Fifteen were white (94%) and 1 was Hispanic (6%, case 2).

Patients were divided into 3 major groups: (1) those with combined AS (with or without AR) and MS (cases 1 to 5; Tables 1 and 2), (2) those with AS and pure MR (cases 6 to 11; Tables 1 and 2), and (3) those with combined pure AR

[a]Departments of Internal Medicine (Cardiology), [b]Pathology, and [c]Cardiothoracic Surgery and [d]Baylor Heart and Vascular Institute, Baylor University Medical Center, Dallas, Texas; [e]Furman University, Greenville, South Carolina; [f]University of Texas at Austin, Austin, Texas. Manuscript received August 16, 2011; revised manuscript received and accepted September 2, 2011.

*Corresponding author: Tel: 214-820-7911; fax: 214-820-7533.

E-mail address: wc.roberts@baylorhealth.edu (W.C. Roberts).

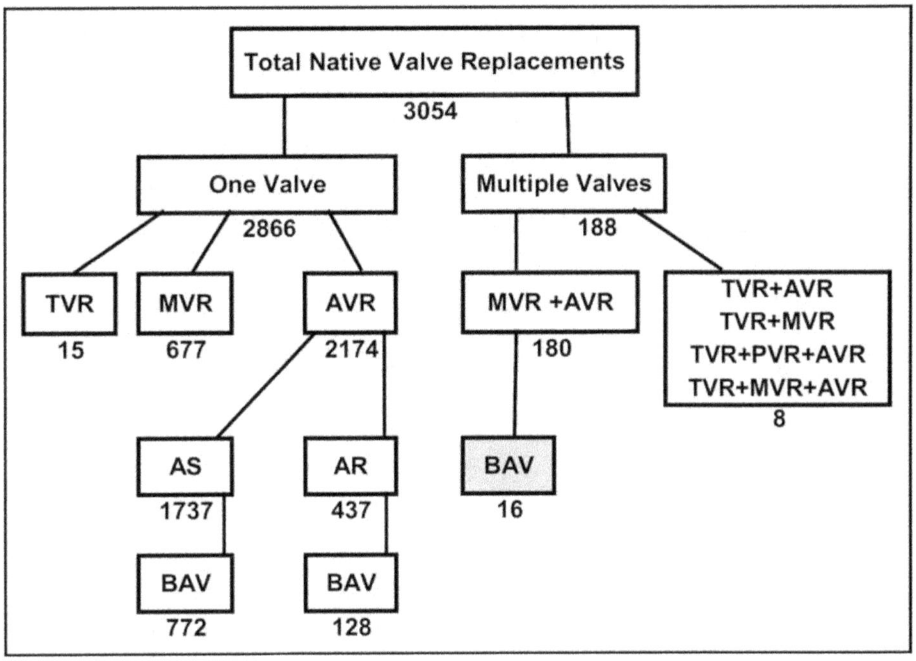

Figure 1. Flow chart of types of cardiac valve replacement operations at Baylor University Medical Center at Dallas from March 3, 1993 through July 8, 2011. AR = aortic regurgitation; AS = aortic stenosis; AVR = aortic valve replacement; BAV = bicuspid aortic valve; MVR = mitral valve replacement; PVR = pulmonary valve replacement; TVR = tricuspid valve replacement.

Table 1
Pertinent clinical findings in patients with bicuspid aortic valves and dysfunctioning mitral valves with replacement of the two

Case Number (figure number)	Age (years)/ Sex	AVR to Discharge (days)	AVR to Death (days)	CABG	AS	AR	MS	MR	IE	RHD	IMR	MVP	MAC	Preoperative AF	BMI (kg/m^2)
1 (2)	53/F	5	alive (5,264)	0	+	0	+	0	0	+	0	0	0	0	34
2	50/M	9	3,704	+	+	0	+	0	0	+	0	0	0	0†	27
3 (3)	46/M	4	2,534	0*	+	0	+	0	0	+	0	0	0	+	26
4 (4)	74/F	13	4,856	0	+	0	+	0	0	+	0	0	0	+	21
5 (5)	71/M	12	alive (1,162)	+	+	0	+	0	0	0	0	0	+	0	35
6 (6)	84/F	18	3,858	+	+	0	0	+	0	0	+	0	0	0	29
7 (7)	77/M	7	867	+	+	0	0	+	0	0	+	0	0	0†	22
8 (8)	58/F	6	alive (1,301)	0	+	0	0	+	0	0	0	0	0	0	42
9 (9)	68/M	6	1,540	0	+	0	0	+	0	0	0	+	0	0	23
10 (10)	67/M	6	alive (1,267)	0	+	0	0	+	0	0	0	+	0	0†	24
11 (11)	66/M	7	472	0	+	0	0	+	0	0	0	+	0	0	27
12	48/M	56	alive (6,096)	+	0	+	0	+	0	0	0	+	0	+	—
13 (12)	66/M	6	alive (1,252)	0	0	+	0	+	+	0	0	0	0	0	23
14 (13)	47/M	5	674	0	0	+	0	+	+	0	0	0	0	0	36
15	24/M	14	alive (2,017)	0	0	+	0	+	+	0	0	0	0	0	20
16 (14)	50/M	11	alive (1,127)	0	0	+	0	+	+	0	0	0	0	0	23

AF = atrial fibrillation; AR = aortic regurgitation; AS = aortic stenosis; AVR = aortic valve replacement; BMI = body mass index; CABG = coronary artery bypass grafting; F = female; IE = infective endocarditis; IMR = ischemic mitral regurgitation; M = male; MAC = mitral annular calcium; MR = mitral regurgitation; MS = mitral stenosis; MVP = mitral valve prolapse; RHD = rheumatic heart disease.

* Previous resection of aortic isthmic coarctation.

† Developed atrial fibrillation postoperatively after double-valve replacement.

Table 2
Hemodynamic findings, valve weights, and substitute valves employed in 16 patients with bicuspid aortic valves, mitral dysfunction, and replacement of two left-sided valves

Case Number (figure number)	Pressures (mm Hg)								AV Area (cm^2)	MV Area (cm^2)	MR (0–4+)	AR (0–4+)	EF (%)	AV Weight (g)	MV Weight (g)	Type (size [mm]) Substitute Valve	
	LV (s/d)	Ao (s/d)	LV-Ao (psg)	LV-Ao (msg)	LV-MV (mdg)	RV (s/d)	RA (Mean)	PW (Mean)								AV	MV
1 (2)	—	—	—	—	—	—	—	—	0.9	1.8	—	—	—	—	—	P (20)	P (27)
2	173/40	146/88	27	30	25	56/18	13	39	1.0	1.28	2+	1+	50	—	—	P (21)	P (27)
3 (3)	139/17	133/88	6	54	15	48/18	13	26	0.46	0.95	—	2+	55	1.37	3.44	P (23)	P (31)
4 (4)	226/19	195/85	31	129	14	79/17	54	33	0.53	0.95	0	2+	60	—	—	P (21)	P (29)
5 (5)	159/27	140/65	19	—	6	57/21	20	22	1.1	2.33	—	—	20	2.54	3.70	B (27)	B (29)
6 (6)	163/17	124/56	39	46	14	99/28	18	36	0.39	—	—	1+	70	0.90	1.00	P (19)	P (25)
7 (7)	180/8	148/63	32	40	—	—	—	—	0.77	—	4+	2+	70	2.40	0.90	P (25)	P (29)
8 (8)	234/	110/	124	—	—	44/17	12	18	0.5	1.0	—	—	60	2.39	0.40	P (23)	P (27)
9 (9)	149/38	118/64	31	21	—	34/13	5	16	—	—	4+	—	60	2.81	4.66	P (25)	P (33)
10 (10)	154/24	94/63	60	41	—	73/24	9	29	0.52	—	4+	—	20	5.86	0.52	B (27)	B (29)
11 (11)	—	125/79	—	—	—	49/12	7	21	—	—	1+	4+	—	5.20	5.09	P (24)	P (33)
12	142/8	134/78	8	—	—	58/14	—	—	—	—	4+	2+	40	—	—	P (—)	P (—)
13 (12)	—	130/60*	—	—	—	—	—	—	—	—	4+	4+	—	1.55	0.67	P (25)	P (29)
14 (13)	—	116/61	—	—	—	28/11	6	8	—	—	—	3+	60	1.30	1.28	P (25)	P (31)
15	—	100/60*	—	—	—	—	—	—	—	—	—	—	60	—	—	B (25)	B (29)
16 (14)	—	120/60*	—	—	—	—	—	—	—	—	—	—	—	1.02	2.01	B (23)	B (31)

Ao = aorta; AR = aortic regurgitation; AV = aortic valve; B = bioprosthesis; EF = ejection fraction; LV = left ventricular; mdg = mean diastolic gradient; msg = mean systolic gradient; MV = mitral valve; P = prosthesis; psg = peak systolic gradient; PW = pulmonary wedge; RA = right atrial; RV = right ventricular; s/d = peak systolic/end-diastolic.

* Indirect pressure.

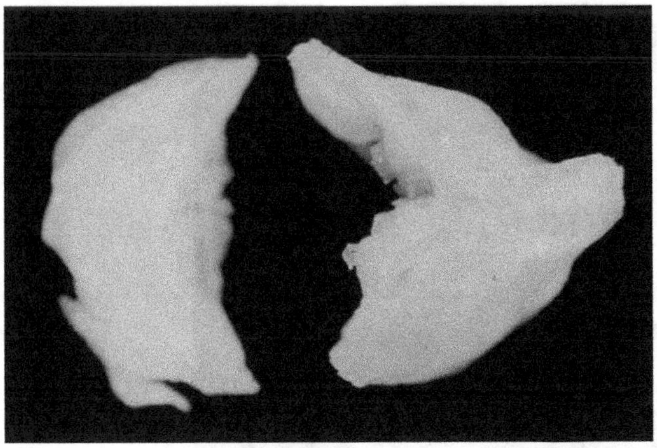

Figure 2. Case 1. Bicuspid aortic valve in a 53-year-old woman with combined mitral and aortic valve stenosis. The mitral valve was diffusely thickened by fibrous tissue and was devoid of calcified deposits; it was excised in multiple pieces. The aortic valve, in contrast, contained calcific deposits covered by thick fibrous tissue.

and pure MR (no element of stenosis, cases 12 to 16; Tables 1 and 2).

Of the 5 patients with combined AS and MS, the cause of MS appeared to be rheumatic heart disease in 4 and "massive" mitral annular calcium in 1 (case 5).[2] Of the 6 patients with AS and pure MR, the latter was attributed to mitral valve prolapse in 3 (cases 9, 10, and 11), to ischemic origin in 2 (concomitant coronary artery bypass grafting also was performed, cases 6 and 7), and in case 8 the cause of MR was unclear, possibly "functional." The latter patient (case 8) had severe AS with a peak left ventricular pressure of 234 mm Hg and a body mass index of 42 kg/m^2. Whether either finding or the 2 findings played a role in MR is unclear.

In the 5 patients with combined AR and MR, the cause of MR in 1 patient was mitral valve prolapse (case 12), and in the other 4, infective endocarditis (cases 13 to 16). In each of these latter 4 patients examination of noninfected portions of the cusps suggested that function of the aortic and mitral valves before the onset of active infective endocarditis was probably normal.

Weights of most operatively excised mitral and aortic valves are listed in Table 2. All patients had excision of the

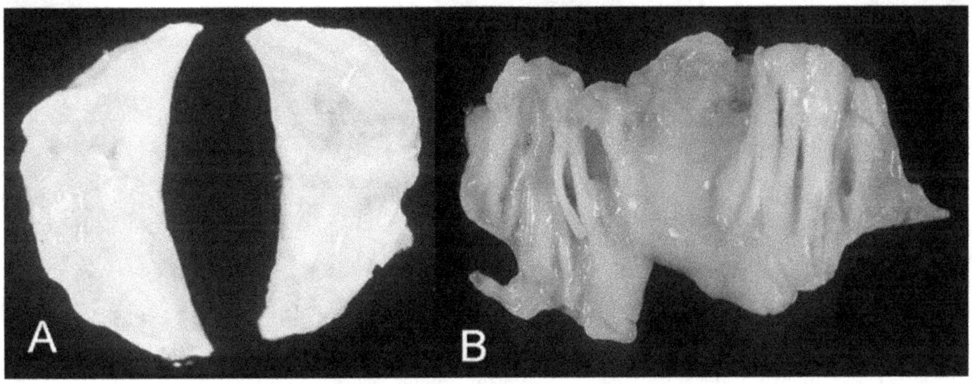

Figure 3. Case 3. Bicuspid stenotic aortic valve *(A)* and thickened mitral valve *(B)* in a 46-year-old man. The mitral valve is consistent with rheumatic stenosis. The aortic valve weighed 1.37 g (normal <0.50 g) and the excised anterior mitral leaflet weighted 3.44 g.

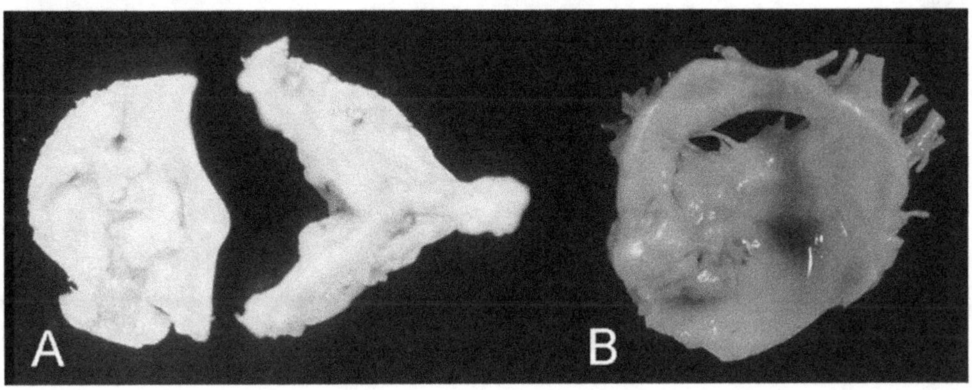

Figure 4. Case 4. Bicuspid stenotic valve *(A)* and stenotic mitral valve *(B)*. The 2 valves were excised entirely intact.

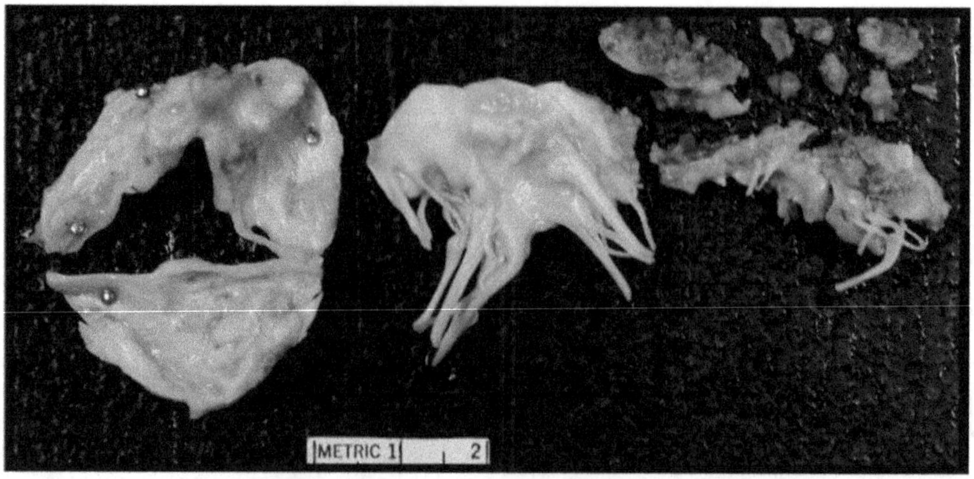

Figure 5. Case 5. Congenitally bicuspid aortic valve, ventricular aspect of anterior mitral leaflet, and portions of posterior leaflet with calcific fragments from the mitral annulus in a 71-year-old man with combined aortic stenosis and mitral stenosis. The latter was the result of heavy calcific deposits on the mitral annular region.

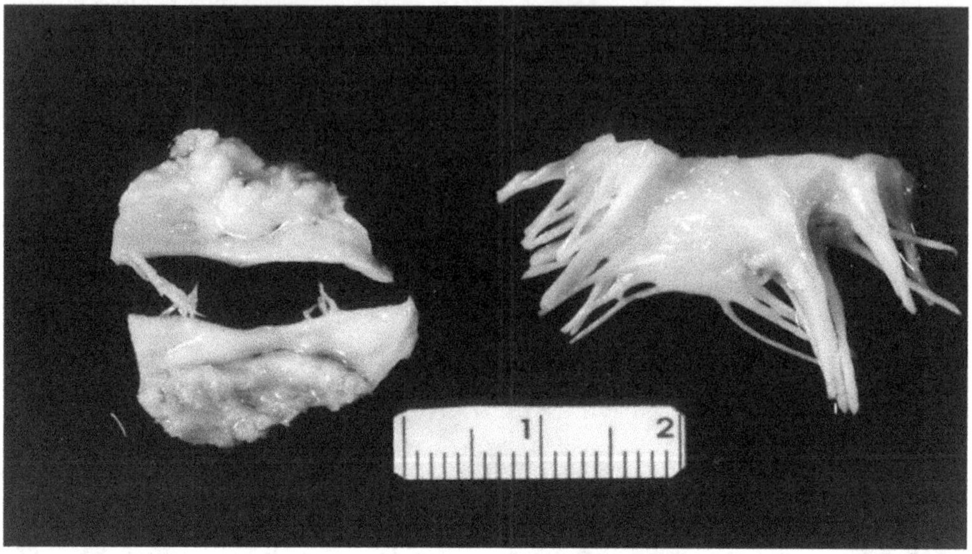

Figure 6. Case 6. Bicuspid aortic valve and anterior mitral leaflet (ventricular aspect) in an 84-year-old woman. The aortic valve is calcified (weight 0.90 g) and stenotic. The mitral leaflet is focally thickened as seen typically in ischemic mitral regurgitation.

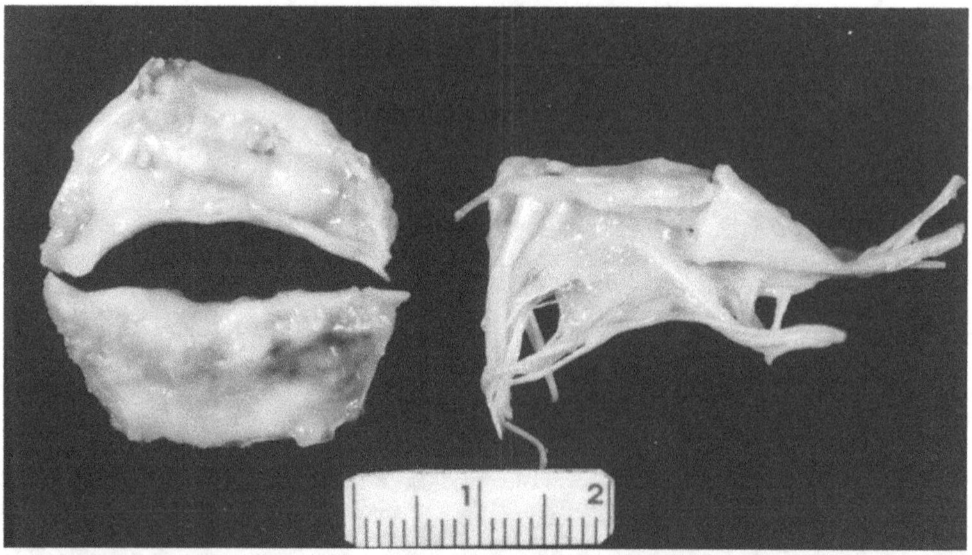

Figure 7. Case 7. Bicuspid aortic valve *(left)* and ventricular aspect of anterior mitral leaflet *(right)* in a 77-year-old man with aortic stenosis, mitral regurgitation, and severe coronary artery disease necessitating concomitant coronary artery bypass grafting. The mitral valve shows changes consistent with ischemic mitral regurgitation.

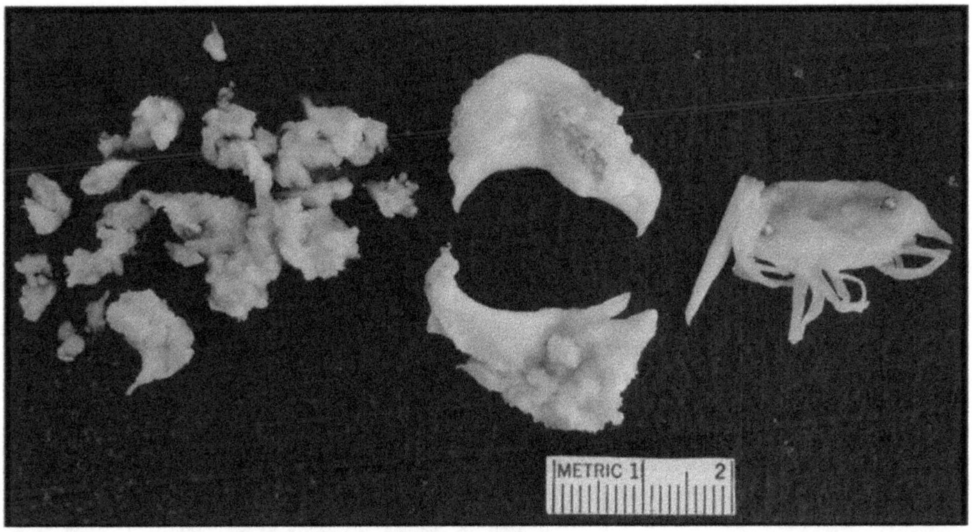

Figure 8. Case 8. Calcific fragments from aortic valve *(left)*, 2 aortic valve cusps *(middle)*, and atrial aspect of anterior mitral leaflet *(right)* in a 58-year-old woman with aortic stenosis and pure mitral regurgitation, the latter of uncertain origin. The coronary arteries angiographically were normal and there were no calcific deposits in the mitral annular region.

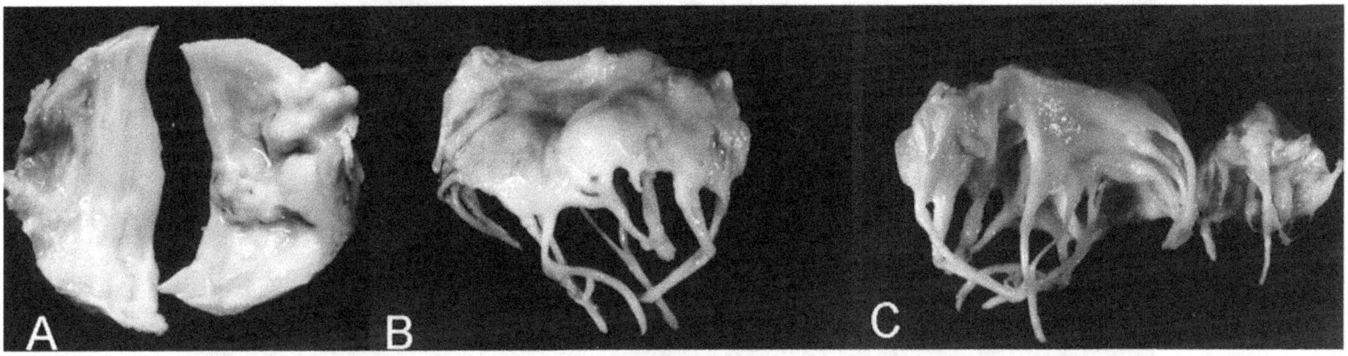

Figure 9. Case 9. Congenitally bicuspid and stenotic aortic valve *(A)*, atrial aspect of anterior mitral leaflet displaying a scallop *(B)*, and ventricular aspect of anterior mitral leaflet and a portion of posterior leaflet *(C)* in a 68-year-old man. The mitral changes are characteristic of mitral valve prolapse.

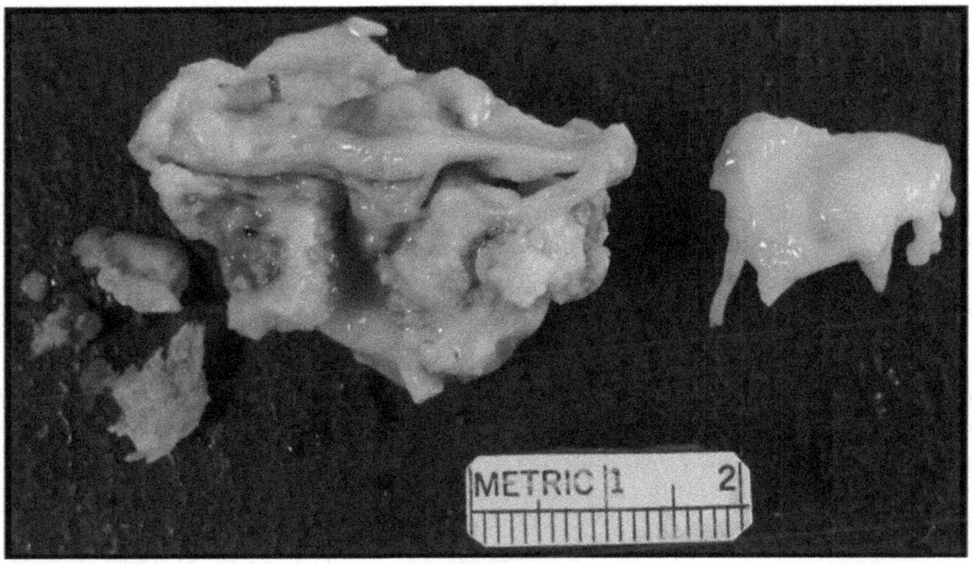

Figure 10. Case 10. Heavily calcified (5.86 g) congenitally bicuspid aortic valve *(left)* and fragment of posterior mitral leaflet *(right)* in a 67-year-old man with severe aortic stenosis and pure mitral regurgitation, the consequence of mitral valve prolapse.

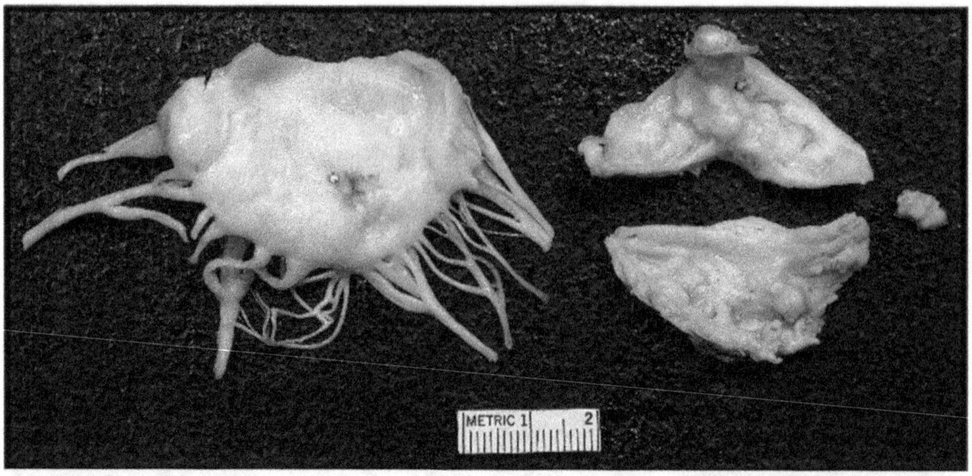

Figure 11. Case 11. Atrial aspect of anterior mitral leaflet *(left)* and heavily calcified (weight 5.86 g) congenitally bicuspid aortic valve *(right)* in a 66-year-old man. The mitral valve was purely regurgitant because of mitral valve prolapse and the aortic valve was severely stenotic.

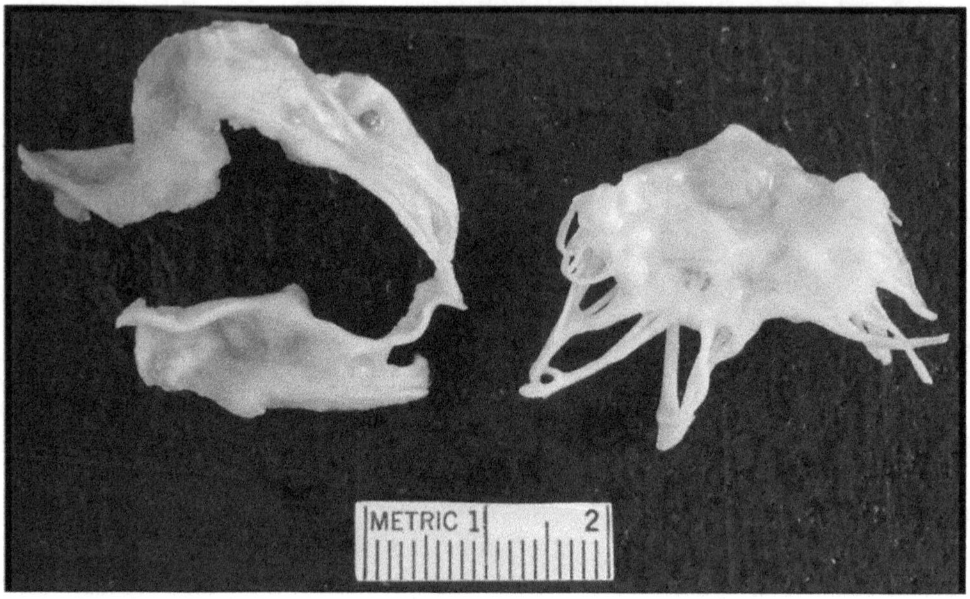

Figure 12. Case 13. Congenitally bicuspid aortic valve *(left)* and atrial aspect of anterior mitral leaflet *(right)* in a 66-year-old man with pure aortic regurgitation and pure mitral regurgitation secondary to *Streptococcus bovis* endocarditis, which is healing. Histologic sections of the valves disclosed fibrin, collections of polymorphonuclear leukocytes, but no microorganisms. He had been receiving antibiotics.

anterior mitral leaflet, and 3 (cases 4, 5, and 9) also had excision of the posterior mitral leaflet.

Type of substitute cardiac valve employed in the 16 patients also is presented in Table 2: in 12 patients a mechanical prosthesis was used in the 2 valve positions and in the other 4 patients (cases 5, 10, 15, and 16) a bioprostheses was used in the 2 valve positions. Various sizes of the prostheses and bioprostheses employed also are presented in Table 2. The interval from valve replacement to hospital discharge in the 16 patients varied from 4 to 56 days (mean 12, median 7). Eight of the 16 patients have died. Intervals from valve replacement to death ranged from 1.3 to 13.3 years (mean 6.3, median 5.6). The other 8 patients are alive (as of June 30, 2011) and their intervals from valve replacement have ranged from 1.8 to 16.7 years (mean 7.2, median 4.5).

Discussion

This study demonstrates that some patients with congenitally bicuspid aortic valves have dysfunctioning mitral valves that lead not only to replacement of the aortic valve but also to replacement of the mitral valve. Of 162 patients having replacement of the 2 left-sided valves at BUMC in Dallas during the previous 17 years, 16 (10%) had congenitally bicuspid aortic valves and malfunctioning mitral valves. In 11 of the 16 patients, the aortic valve was stenotic: in 5 of them, the mitral valve was also stenotic, the apparent result of rheumatic heart disease in 4 and mitral annular calcium in 1; in the other 6 patients with AS, MR was the result of mitral valve prolapse in 3, of ischemic disease in 2, and from uncertain cause in 1. All 5 patients with pure AR also had pure MR, the consequence of mitral

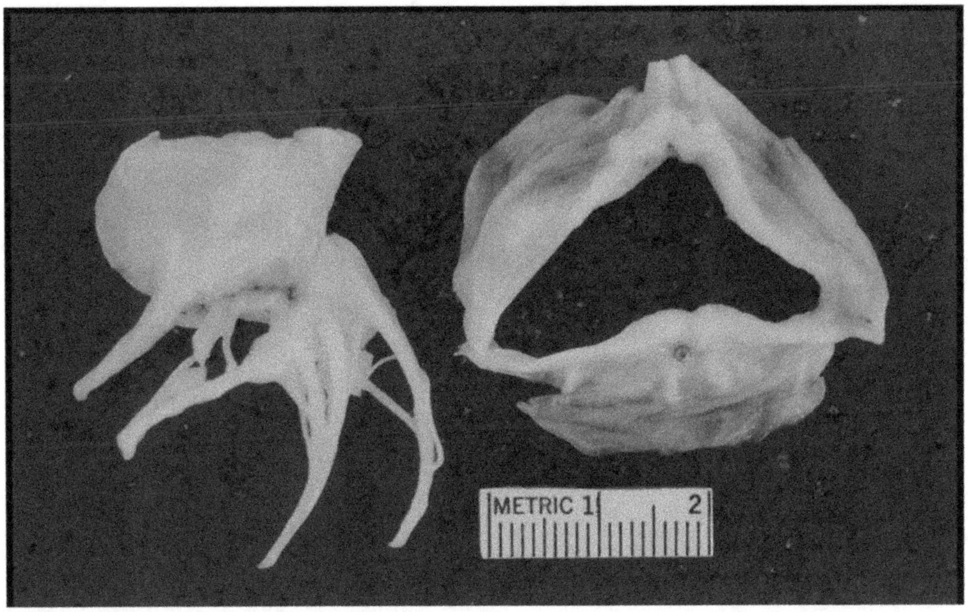

Figure 13. Case 14. Fragment of anterior mitral leaflet *(left)* and congenitally bicuspid aortic valve *(right)* in a 47-year-old man who had had 2 episodes of *Streptococcus viridans* before double-valve replacement for pure mitral regurgitation and pure aortic regurgitation.

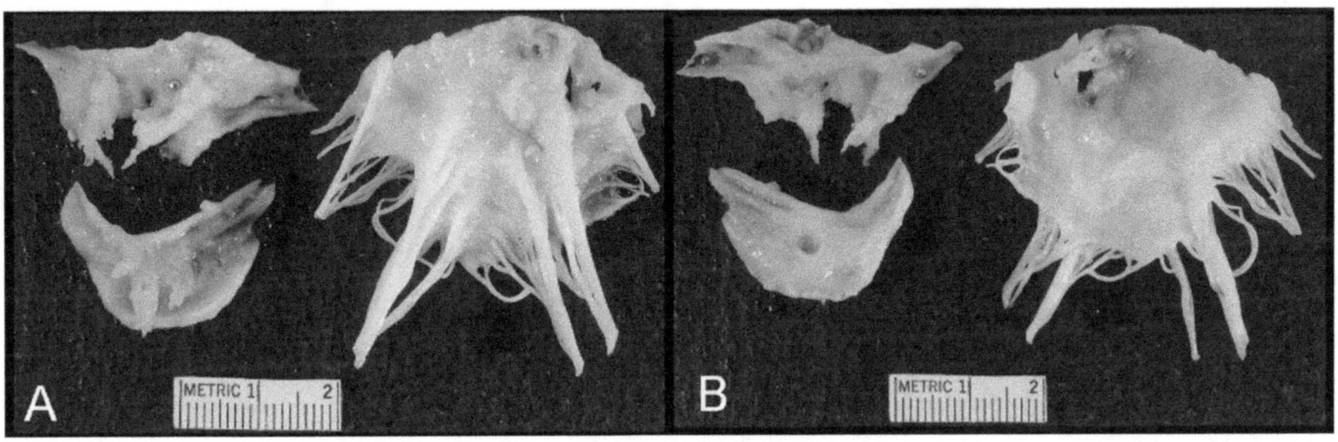

Figure 14. Case 16. Infected congenitally bicuspid aortic valve and anterior mitral leaflet in a 50-year-old with pure aortic and mitral regurgitation secondary to *Streptococcus viridans* endocarditis. *(A)* Aortic aspect of the aortic valve and ventricular aspect of the anterior mitral leaflet. *(B)* Ventricular aspect of the aortic valve cusps and atrial aspect of the anterior mitral leaflet again showing the perforations.

valve prolapse in 1 and infective endocarditis in 4. It is well recognized that infection on the aortic valve often extends to involve the mitral valve, causing regurgitation in each.[3]

The occurrence of 2 different types of congenital heart disease in the same heart is a common occurrence but not so for bicuspid aortic valve and mitral valve prolapse as occurred in 4 of our 16 patients. If mitral valve prolapse occurs in about 5% of the United States population (roughly 15 million people) and if bicuspid aortic valve occurs in 1% of this population (roughly 3 million people), it should not be surprising that the 2 conditions might occur periodically in the same patient. One of our patients (case 3) also had aortic isthmic coarctation, a well-recognized coexisting congenital lesion in patients with congenitally bicuspid aortic valves.[4]

The present report is not the first to describe mitral valve prolapse in patients with bicuspid aortic valves. Fernicola and Roberts[1] in 1994 described 11 men age 25 to 77 who had aortic and mitral valve replacements for dysfunctioning congenitally bicuspid aortic valves (AS in 7, pure AR in 4) associated with pure MR (secondary to mitral valve prolapse in 6 and to infective endocarditis in 5). Schaefer et al[5] in 2002 found by echocardiogram "myxomatous mitral valve" in 9 of 192 adults (5%) with bicuspid aortic valves, most of which apparently functioned normally or were purely regurgitant. Lad et al[6] described first-time operations for MR secondary to "myxomatous degeneration" in 1,595 patients and operations for congenitally bicuspid aortic valves in 1,820 patients; of the 3,415 patients, 29 (1%) had a congenitally bicuspid aortic valve and "degenerative disease" of the mitral valve. Of the 29 patients, 8 (28%) had AS and 21 (72%) had AR. Of these 29 patients, the mitral valve was repaired in 24 and replaced in 5; the bicuspid aortic valve was repaired in 10 patients and replaced in 19. The mitral annulus was dilated in all but 1 of their 29 patients and the anterior mitral leaflet was elongated in 22 of these 29 patients.

1. Fernicola DJ, Roberts WC. Pure mitral regurgitation associated with a malfunctioning congenitally bicuspid aortic valve necessitating combined mitral and aortic valve replacement. *Am J Cardiol* 1994;74:619–624.
2. Hammer WJ, Roberts WC, deLeon AC Jr. "Mitral stenosis" secondary to combined "massive" mitral anular calcific deposits and small, hypertrophied left ventricles. Hemodynamic documentation in four patients. *Am J Med* 1978;64:371–376.
3. Buchbinder NA, Roberts WC. Left-sided valvular active infective endocarditis. A study of forty-five necropsy patients. *Am J Med* 1972;53:20–35.
4. Glancy DL, Morrow AG, Simon AL, Roberts WC. Juxtaductal aortic coarctation. Analysis of 84 patients studied hemodynamically, angiographically, and morphologically after age 1 year. *Am J Cardiol* 1983; 51:537–551.
5. Schaefer BM, Lewin MB, Stout KK, Gill E, Prueitt A, Byers PH, Otto CM. The bicuspid aortic valve: an integrated phenotypic classification of leaflet morphology and aortic root shape. *Heart* 2008;94:1634–1638.
6. Lad V, David TE, Vegas A. Mitral regurgitation due to myxomatous degeneration combined with bicuspid aortic valve disease is often due to prolapse of the anterior leaflet of the mitral valve. *Ann Thorac Surg* 2009;87:79–82.

Cardiac Transplantation in Adults With Aortic Valve Disease With Focus on the Bicuspid Aortic Valve

William Clifford Roberts, MD[a,b,d,*], Carey Camille Roberts[d,e], Jong Mi Ko, BA[d], Shelley Anne Hall, MD[a,d], and John Edward Capehart, MD[c]

The frequency of congenitally bicuspid aortic valves in patients having cardiac transplantation (CT) is unknown. We reviewed 243 explanted hearts in patients having CT at Baylor University Medical Center, Dallas from June 1997 through November 2011 to determine the frequency of a bicuspid aortic valve in this population. Of the 243 explanted hearts, 7 (2.9%) were found to have a congenitally bicuspid aortic valve: 3 had severe aortic valve stenosis and before CT had had the aortic valve replaced; the other 4 had normally functioning bicuspid valves and underwent CT for cardiomyopathy (ischemic in 1, idiopathic in 2, and hypertrophic in 1). Review of previously published reports of CT and aortic valve disease disclosed that 4 patients had had aortic valve replacement (AVR) from 2 to 8 years before CT, 3 had AVR or aortic valve repair of the donor heart at the time of CT, and 4 had AVR or transcatheter aortic valve implantation from 1 to 14 years after CT. Some of these aortic valve replacements, before, at the time of, or after CT were in patients with congenitally bicuspid aortic valves. In conclusion, congenitally bicuspid aortic valves were found in 7 of 243 explanted hearts in patients having CT at a single medical center in a 14-year period: 4 had functioned normally and 3 were severely stenotic. Previous reports of patients having AVR or repair before, during, and after CT were reviewed. **(Am J Cardiol 2012;109:1212–1214)**

Cardiac transplantation (CT) is performed mainly in patients with ischemic or idiopathic dilated cardiomyopathy and infrequently in patients with valvular heart disease. This report describes the frequency of finding a bicuspid aortic valve in patients undergoing CT at a single medical center in a 14-year period and reviews previously published reports of patients having aortic valve replacement (AVR) or repair before, at the time of, and after CT.

Methods

From June 1997 through November 2011, CT was performed at Baylor University Medical Center, Dallas in 243 patients and in each the recipient heart was submitted to the cardiovascular division of the surgical pathology department. Each heart was examined and described by 1 of the authors (W.C.R.) and photographed. Among the 243 hearts studied, 9 had structural (primary) cardiac valve disease: 1 had had mitral valve replacement 2 times, originally for rheumatic mitral stenosis; 1 had replacement of both mitral and aortic valves for pure regurgitation secondary to radiation therapy for Hodgkin's disease many years previously; and the remaining 7 patients had congenitally bicuspid aortic valves, 3 stenotic valves had been replaced and the other 4 were functionally normal (Table 1).

This study was approved by the institutional review board at Baylor University Medical Center and informed consent was waived.

Results

Pertinent data in each of the 7 patients—all men—are presented in Table 1. Four of the 7 patients (cases 1 to 4) had normally functioning congenitally bicuspid aortic valves discovered during examination of the recipient heart: 2 of these patients had idiopathic dilated cardiomyopathy,[1] 1 had hypertrophic cardiomyopathy, and 1 had ischemic cardiomyopathy.

The remaining 3 patients (cases 5 to 7) had had AVR for aortic valve stenosis and all 3 had congenitally bicuspid aortic valves (Figure 1). Case 7 also had coronary artery bypass grafting at the time of AVR. The interval from AVR to CT in these 3 patients was 8, 4.7, and 5.2 years, respectively. During the interval from AVR to CT, heart failure persisted and eventually progressed in each to New York Heart Association class IV without evidence of significant dysfunction of the mechanical prosthesis or the bioprosthesis in the aortic valve position. Case 6 had a left ventricular assist device inserted 5 months before CT. All 3 patients had left ventricular ejection fractions during the months before CT of ≤20%. All 3 patients are alive as of October 28, 2011. The hearts in each of the 3 patients who had CT after AVR had very dilated left ventricular cavities (maximum internal diameter 5.5, 6.0, and 7.5 cm, respectively), hearts of increased weight (650, 730, and 615 g, respectively, not including the portion of the atrial walls to which the donor heart was connected), and 2 had transmural left ventricular

Departments of [a]Internal Medicine (Division of Cardiology), [b]Pathology, [c]Cardiothoracic Surgery, and [d]Baylor Heart and Vascular Institute, Baylor University Medical Center, Dallas, Texas; [e]Junior, The University of Georgia, Athens, Georgia. Manuscript received November 29, 2011; revised manuscript received and accepted December 1, 2011.

The study was funded by the Baylor Health Care System Foundation, Dallas, Texas.

*Corresponding author: Tel: 214-820-7911; fax: 214-820-7533.

E-mail address: wc.roberts@baylorhealth.edu (W.C. Roberts).

Table 1
Pertinent data in seven men having cardiac transplantation and congenitally bicuspid aortic valves with or without aortic valve replacement

Patient Number	Age at CT (years)	Diagnosis	AVR	Year of AVR	Interval (years) AVR → CT	LVAD	BMI (kg/m²)	LVEF (%)	Date of CT	HW (g)	LV Diameter (cm)	RV Diameter (cm)	CABG	CABG Date	LV Scar
1	35	HC	0	—	—	+	28.2	5	10/13/2011	435	6.0	1.0	0	—	0
2	46	IDC	0	—	—	+	29.9	15	12/23/2001	565	5.0	2.5	0	—	0
3	47*	IDC	0	—	—	+	30.3	10	4/25/2001	705	5.0	3.0	0	—	0
4	60	IC	0	—	—	0	27.5	7	7/1/2011	635	8.0	5.0	+	2005	+
5	30	AS	+ (SJM)	1991	8	0	25.0	10	10/14/1999	650	5.5	2.8	0	—	+
6	56	AS	+ (Bio)	2002	4.7	+	28.3	5	7/1/2007	730	6.0	4.0	0	—	0
7	65	AS	+ (SJM)	1997	5.2	0	18.4	20	1/16/2003	615	7.5	3.0	+	1997	+

— = not applicable; AS = aortic stenosis; AVR = aortic valve replacement; Bio = bioprosthesis; BMI = body mass index; CABG = coronary artery bypass grafting; CT = cardiac transplantation; HC = hypertrophic cardiomyopathy; HW = heart weight; IC = ischemic cardiomyopathy; IDC = idiopathic dilated cardiomyopathy; LV = left ventricular; LVAD = left ventricular assist device; LVEF = left ventricular ejection fraction; RV = right ventricular; SJM = St. Jude Medical mechanical prosthesis.

* Died March 22, 2011, or 10 years after cardiac transplantation.

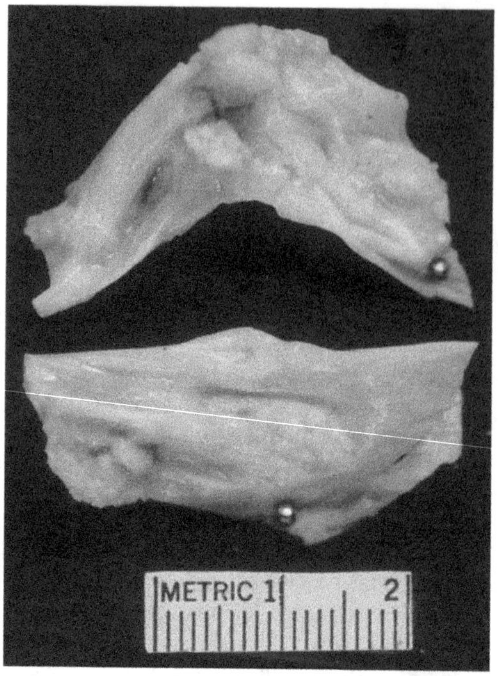

Figure 1. Case 6 (Table 1). Operatively excised severely stenotic congenitally bicuspid aortic valve.

scars, only 1 (case 7) of whom had narrowed coronary arteries. Case 6 had focally thickened left ventricular mural endocardium (possibly the consequence of the left ventricular assist device inserted 5 months previously).

Discussion

A common denominator in each of the heretofore described men was the presence of a congenitally malformed bicuspid aortic valve. In 4, the malformed valve functioned normally and was unrecognized during life. CT was performed in 2 of them because of idiopathic dilated cardiomyopathy, in 1 for ischemic cardiomyopathy, and in 1 for hypertrophic cardiomyopathy.

The remaining 3 patients had AVR for aortic stenosis superimposed on their malformed valve and of them 1 had concomitant coronary bypass grafting. The decision to do CT in these 3 patients rather than repeat AVR was based on the presence of progressively worsening heart failure without evidence of dysfunction of the mechanical prosthesis or bioprosthesis in the aortic valve position, extremely dilated left ventricular cavities (≥5 cm) in ventricular systole, and extremely low left ventricular ejection fractions (≤20%). These 3 patients may have had underlying dilated cardiomyopathy in addition to aortic stenosis.

The frequency of congenitally malformed aortic valves is unclear but probably is about 1% of the population, an involvement of about 3 million Americans.[2] In the present study, 7 congenitally malformed valves were found in 243 patients undergoing CT.

The present report is not the first to describe aortic valve disease and CT (Figure 2). Park et al[3] described a 33-year-old man who underwent orthotopic CT after 2 previous valve replacements for active infective endocarditis involving the native mitral and aortic valves followed by infection

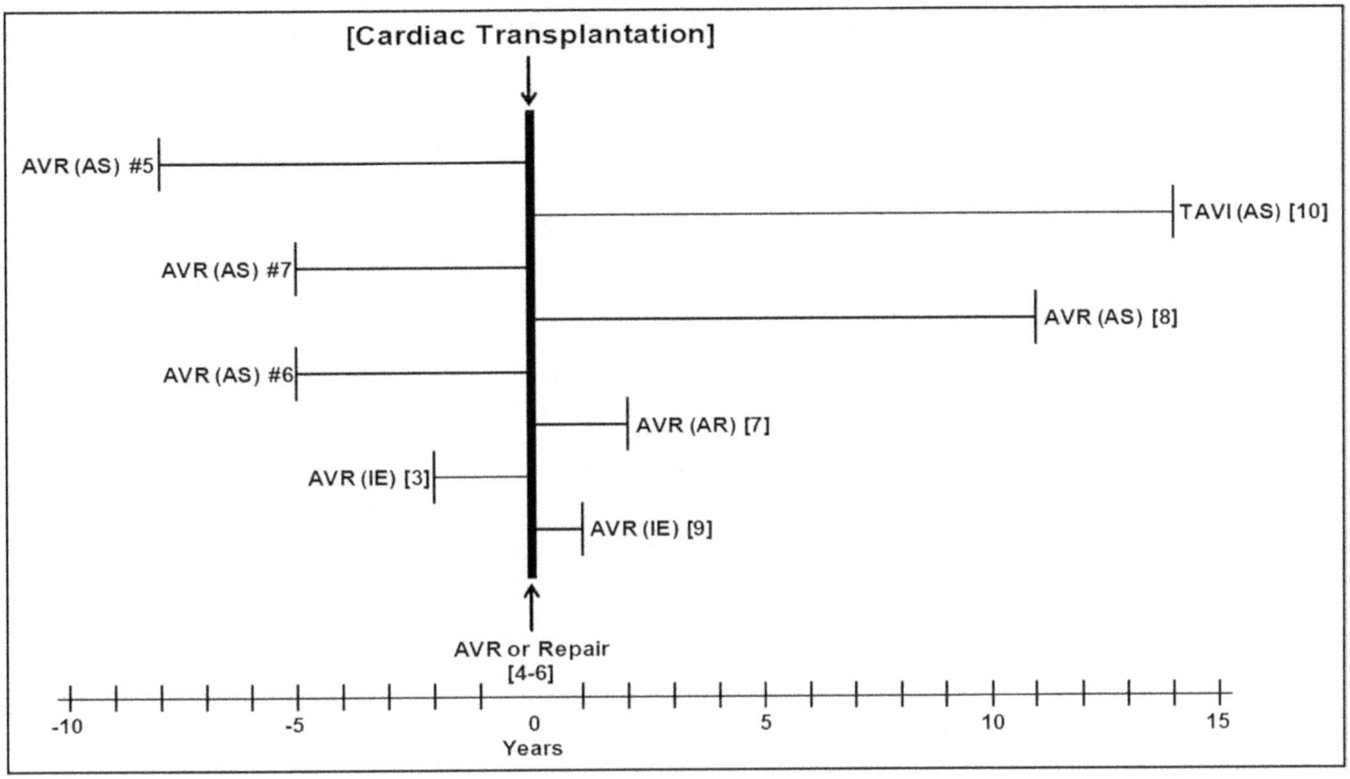

Figure 2. This diagram shows the present cases (5 to 7) and the previously reported patients *(reference in brackets)* having cardiac transplantation and aortic valve replacement or repair, before, at the time of, or after cardiac transplantation. Time in years *(horizontal axis)* is presented before (minus), at the time of, and after cardiac transplantation for aortic stenosis (AS) and/or regurgitation (AR). Several patients clearly had malfunctioning congenitally bicuspid aortic valves. IE = infective endocarditis; TAVI = transcatheter aortic valve implantation (without replacement).

involving the prosthetic aortic valve. Navia et al[4] repaired a purely regurgitant aortic valve in the donor heart before using it for CT. Rao et al[5] and Larobina et al[6] found a donor's heart to have a very stenotic aortic valve and replaced it before CT. Goenen et al[7] found a donor heart to have a mildly regurgitant congenitally bicuspid aortic valve, used the heart for CT, but 2 years after CT did AVR in the donor heart because of development of severe aortic regurgitation. Joyce et al[8] described severe aortic stenosis involving a congenitally bicuspid aortic valve in a donor heart 11 years after CT with successful AVR. Sayeed et al[9] performed AVR for infective endocarditis in a donor heart a year after CT. And finally, Seiffert et al[10] performed successfully transcatheter aortic valve implantation (without replacement) in a 67-year-old heart transplant recipient for severe symptomatic aortic stenosis 14 years after CT.

1. Roberts WC, Siegel RJ, McManus BM. Idiopathic dilated cardiomyopathy: analysis of 152 necropsy patients. *Am J Cardiol* 1987;60: 1340–1355.
2. Roberts WC. The congenitally bicuspid aortic valve. A study of 85 autopsy cases. *Am J Cardiol* 1970;26:72–83.
3. Park SJ, Sullivan HJ, Lonchyna V, Hinkamp TJ, Pifarre R. Heart transplantation for complicated and recurrent early prosthetic valve endocarditis. *J Heart Lung Transplant* 1993;12:802–803.
4. Navia JL, Atik FA, Marullo A, Starling RC, Garcia M, Vega PR, Smedira NG, McCarthy PM. Bench repair of donor aortic valve with minimal access orthotopic heart transplantation. *Ann Thorac Surg* 2005;80:313–315.
5. Rao JN, Prendergast B, Dark JH. Orthotopic heart transplantation with concurrent aortic valve replacement and coronary artery bypass grafting. *J Heart Lung Transplant* 2000;19:897–899.
6. Larobina ME, Mariani JA, Rowland MA. Aortic valve replacement for aortic stenosis during orthotopic cardiac transplant. *Ann Thorac Surg* 2008;86:1979–1982.
7. Goenen MJ, Jacquet L, De Kock M, Van Dyck M, Schoevardts JC, Chalant CH. Aortic valve replacement thirty-one months after orthotopic heart transplantation. *J Heart Lung Transplant* 1991;10:604–607.
8. Joyce DL, Russell SD, Conte JV, Cattaneo SM. Aortic valve replacement in a diseased bicuspid valve eleven years after transplantation. *Interact Cardiovasc Thorac Surg* 2009;8:594–595.
9. Sayeed R, Drain AJ, Sivasothy PS, Large SR, Wallwork J. Aortic valve replacement for late infective endocarditis after heart-lung transplantation. *Trans Proc* 2005;37:4537–4539.
10. Seiffert M, Meyer S, Franzen O, Conradi L, Baldus S, Schirmer J, Deuse T, Costard-Jaeckle A, Reichenspurner H, Treede H. Transcatheter aortic valve implantation in a heart transplant recipient: a case report. *Trans Proc* 2010;42:4661–4663.

Effect of Coronary Bypass and Valve Structure on Outcome in Isolated Valve Replacement for Aortic Stenosis

William Clifford Roberts, MD[a,b,d,*], Carey Camille Roberts[d,g], Travis James Vowels[d,h], Jong Mi Ko, BA[d], Giovanni Filardo, PhD, MPH[e,f], Baron Lloyd Hamman, MD[c], Gregory John Matter, MD[c], Albert Carl Henry III, MD[c], and Robert Frederick Hebeler, Jr., MD[c]

Reports differ regarding the effect of concomitant coronary artery bypass grafting (CABG) in patients who undergo aortic valve replacement (AVR) for aortic stenosis (AS), and no reports have described the effect of aortic valve structure in patients who undergo AVR for AS. A total of 871 patients aged 24 to 94 years (mean 70) whose AVR for AS was their first cardiac operation, with or without first concomitant CABG, were included. Patients who underwent mitral valve procedures were excluded. In comparison with the 443 patients (51%) who did not undergo CABG, the 428 (49%) who underwent concomitant CABG were significantly older, were more often male, had lower transvalvular peak systolic pressure gradients and larger valve areas, had lower frequencies of congenitally malformed aortic valves, had lighter valves by weight, had higher frequencies of systemic hypertension, and had longer stays in the hospital after AVR. Early and late (to 10 years) mortality were similar by propensity-adjusted analysis in patients who did and did not undergo concomitant CABG. Congenitally unicuspid or bicuspid valves occurred in approximately 90% of those aged 21 to 50, in nearly 70% in those aged 51 to 70 years, and in just over 30% in those aged 71 to 95 years. Unadjusted and adjusted survival was significantly higher in patients with unicuspid or bicuspid valves compared to those with tricuspid valves. In conclusion, although concomitant CABG had no effect on the adjusted probability of survival, the type of aortic valve (unicuspid or bicuspid vs tricuspid) significantly affected the unadjusted and adjusted probability of survival. **(Am J Cardiol 2012;109:1334–1340)**

Adults with isolated (no mitral valve disease) aortic stenosis (AS) (with or without aortic regurgitation) frequently have associated narrowing of ≥1 major (right, left main, left anterior descending, or left circumflex) epicardial coronary arteries. In reported patients who undergo aortic valve replacement (AVR) for AS, the effect of concomitant coronary artery bypass grafting (CABG) on early and late mortality has been variable. The aim of this study was to compare among patients with isolated AS the outcomes of AVR in patients with versus without CABG and also the effect of aortic valve structure (unicuspid or bicuspid vs tricuspid) on the probability of long-term survival after AVR for AS.

Methods

The surgical pathology files of the cardiovascular laboratory, a part of the pathology department at Baylor University Medical Center (BUMC) in Dallas, were searched for patients having operatively excised aortic valves without simultaneous replacement of the mitral valve or evidence of mitral stenosis. From January 2002 through June 2010 (102 months [8.5 years]), a total of 1,040 operatively excised stenotic aortic valves were submitted to the cardiovascular laboratory at BUMC. Each was described, and the surgical report was prepared by W.C.R. and photographed by J.M.K. The valve structure in each was determined by W.C.R from examination of the operatively excised aortic valve. This study was approved by the Institutional Review Board at BUMC on May 5, 2010, and the requirement for individual patient consent was waived.

Included in the present study were 871 adults whose AVR for AS was their first cardiac operation, with or without first simultaneous CABG. Patients who underwent isolated AVR for AS and later in a second operation underwent CABG or vice versa were excluded.

Clinical records, including admission note, discharge summary, echocardiographic and cardiac catheterization reports, and operative records, were sought from the patients' medical charts and/or BUMC Apollo cardiovascular database (Apollo Advance c/s version 4.2.13; LUMEDX Corporation, Oakland, California). (The Apollo system became operational at BUMC in January 2002.)

Echocardiographic and hemodynamic data were obtained from the cardiovascular computer database. Whether simultaneous CABG was performed at the time

Departments of [a]Internal Medicine (Division of Cardiology), [b]Pathology, and [c]Cardiothoracic Surgery and the [d]Baylor Heart and Vascular Institute, Baylor University Medical Center; [e]Institute for Health Care Research and Improvement, Baylor Health Care System; [f]Department of Statistical Science, Southern Methodist University, Dallas Texas; [g]University of Georgia, Athens, Georgia; and [h]University of Texas at Austin, Austin, Texas. Manuscript received December 5, 2011; revised manuscript received and accepted December 8, 2011.

*Corresponding author: Tel: 214-820-7911; fax: 214-820-7533.

E-mail address: wc.roberts@baylorhealth.edu (W.C. Roberts).

Table 1
Frequency of concomitant coronary artery bypass grafting in patients who underwent isolated aortic valve replacement for aortic stenosis (n = 871)

Variable	Coronary Artery Bypass Grafting		
	Yes (n = 428 [49%])	No (n = 443 [51%])	p Value
Age group (years)			<0.001
21–50	12 (3%)	54 (12%)	
51–70	139 (32%)	201 (45%)	
71–95	277 (65%)	188 (42%)	
Gender			<0.001
Male	289 (68%)	233 (53%)	
Female	139 (32%)	210 (47%)	
Race			0.953
White	354 (83%)	367 (83%)	
Black	24 (6%)	22 (5%)	
Hispanic	16 (4%)	19 (4%)	
Other or unknown	34 (8%)	35 (8%)	
Number of major coronary arteries narrowed ≥50%	(n = 205)	(n = 272)	<0.001
0	32 (16%)*	246 (90%)	
1	60 (29%)	20 (7%)	
2	68 (33%)	5 (2%)	
3	34 (17%)	1 (<1%)	
4	11 (5%)	0	
LV-aorta peak systolic gradient (mm Hg) (n = 475), range (mean) [median]	10–119 (46) [41]	11–154 (54) [52]	<0.001
Aortic valve area (cm^2) (n = 474), mean ± SD	0.85 ± 0.31	0.76 ± 0.25	0.008
Aortic valve structure			<0.001
Unicuspid	11 (3%)	49 (11%)	
Bicuspid	142 (33%)	243 (55%)	
Tricuspid	275 (64%)	151 (34%)	
Aortic valve weight (g)			<0.001
Unicuspid, range (mean) [median]	1.20–4.78 (2.89) [2.71]	1.19–7.15 (3.47) [3.28]	
Bicuspid, range (mean) [median]	0.67–18.38 (3.11) [2.62]	0.81–9.68 (3.11) [2.91]	
Tricuspid, range (mean) [median]	0.43–6.40 (2.00) [1.84]	0.55–5.63 (2.11) [1.98]	
Systemic hypertension by history	324 (76%)	292 (66%)	0.015
Body mass index (kg/m^2)			0.872
≤25	148 (35%)	140 (32%)	
>25–30	156 (37%)	136 (31%)	
>30–40	104 (24%)	141 (32%)	
>40	18 (4%)	22 (5%)	
Range (mean ± SD)	15–69 (28 ± 6)	15–61 (29 ± 6)	
Days in hospital postoperatively in patients living >30 days, range (mean) [median]	3–53 (10) [8]	3–71 (8) [6]	0.001
Died ≤30 days postoperatively	29/427 (7%)	18/437 (4%)	0.179
Ascending aorta replaced	11 (3%)	26 (6%)	0.159
Implanted valve type			<0.001
Mechanical	64 (16%)	140 (32%)	
Bioprosthetic	355 (84%)	289 (67%)	
Ross procedure	1 (<1%)	6 (1%)	

* These patients had significant narrowing of a branch of ≥1 major coronary artery.

of AVR was also obtained from either the computer database or from the medical records. Information regarding the death of any patient was obtained from 3 sources: (1) the medical records in the deaths during the hospitalization at the time of AVR, (2) the Society of Thoracic Surgeons National Database, and (3) the Social Security Death Index for posthospitalization deaths. Echocardiographic data preoperatively were available for 426 patients (49%). Cardiac catheterization data preoperatively were available for 561 patients (64%).

Means, standard deviations, and percentages were calculated to describe the study cohort (n = 871). Differences in demographic, clinical, and morphologic details were tested using Wilcoxon's tests (for continuous variables) or chi-square tests (for categorical variables). Bonferroni's correction was used to account for multiplicity. Unadjusted p values, odds ratios, hazard ratios, 95% confidence intervals (CIs), and log-rank statistics were estimated to describe 30-day and long-term mortality. Kaplan-Meier plots were used to describe unadjusted survival in patients who underwent concomitant CABG compared to those who did not and in patients with unicuspid or bicuspid valves compared to those with tricuspid valves.

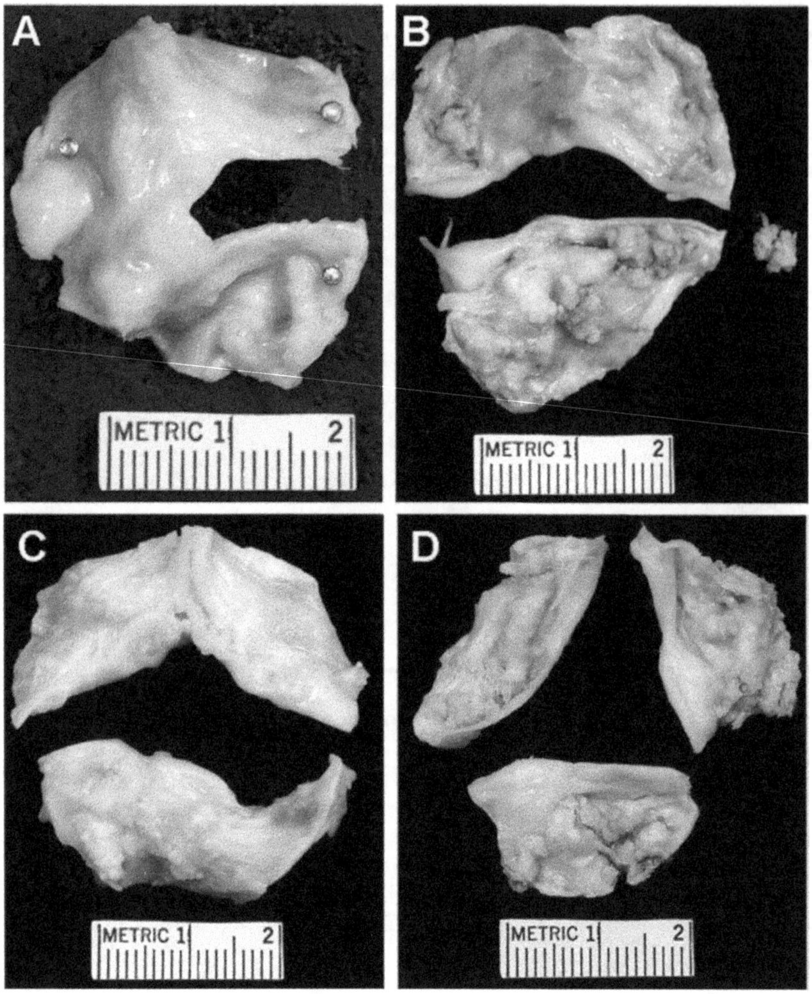

Figure 1. Photographs of operatively excised stenotic aortic valves in 4 patients. *(A)* Congenitally unicuspid unicommissural valve in a 66-year-old patient. *(B)* Congenitally bicuspid valve in an 81-year-old man. *(C)* Congenitally bicuspid valve in a 58-year-old man. *(D)* Tricuspid aortic valve in a 79-year-old woman. CABG was performed also in patients whose valves are shown in *(B)* and *(D)*. Valve weights were 2.48 g *(A)*, 3.55 g *(B)*, 3.19 g *(C)*, and 2.71 g *(D)*.

A propensity score approach was used to assess the adjusted association between undergoing concomitant CABG (vs not) and 30-day and long-term mortality.[1,2] To estimate the propensity score, we used a logistic regression model with receiving concomitant CABG (vs not) as the dependent variable and age, gender, race, body mass index, aortic valve structure, valve weight, systemic hypertension, ascending aorta replaced, and type of implanted valve as independent variables. Restricted cubic splines were used for all continuous variables.[3,4] Multiple imputation via predictive mean matching was used to account for missing data regarding the independent variables in this model.[1] Estimates from the aforementioned propensity model were then used to adjust the effect of concomitant CABG on 30-day mortality in a logistic regression model and on long-term mortality in a Cox proportional-hazards model. Possible effect modification by gender and age was investigated for the 2 models and ruled out. The Grambsch and Therneau test statistic was used to test for proportionality of hazards in the Cox model.[5]

The same approach, controlling for the same confounding factors except that valve structure was replaced by concomitant CABG, was used to assess the adjusted association between valve structure (unicuspid or bicuspid vs tricuspid valve structure) and 30-day and long-term mortality.

Statistical analyses were performed using SAS version 9.2 (SAS Institute Inc., Cary, North Carolina) and R software version 2.12.1 (R Project for Statistical Computing, Vienna, Austria).

Results

Demographic, clinical, and morphologic findings in the 871 patients included in the present study and their comparison between those with versus without concomitant CABG are listed in Table 1. Of the 871 patients, 428 (49%) underwent concomitant CABG, and 443 (51%) did not. In comparison to the group that did not undergo CABG, those who underwent concomitant CABG were significantly older, were more often male, had lower transvalvular peak systolic pressure gradients and larger valve areas, had higher frequencies of tricuspid aortic

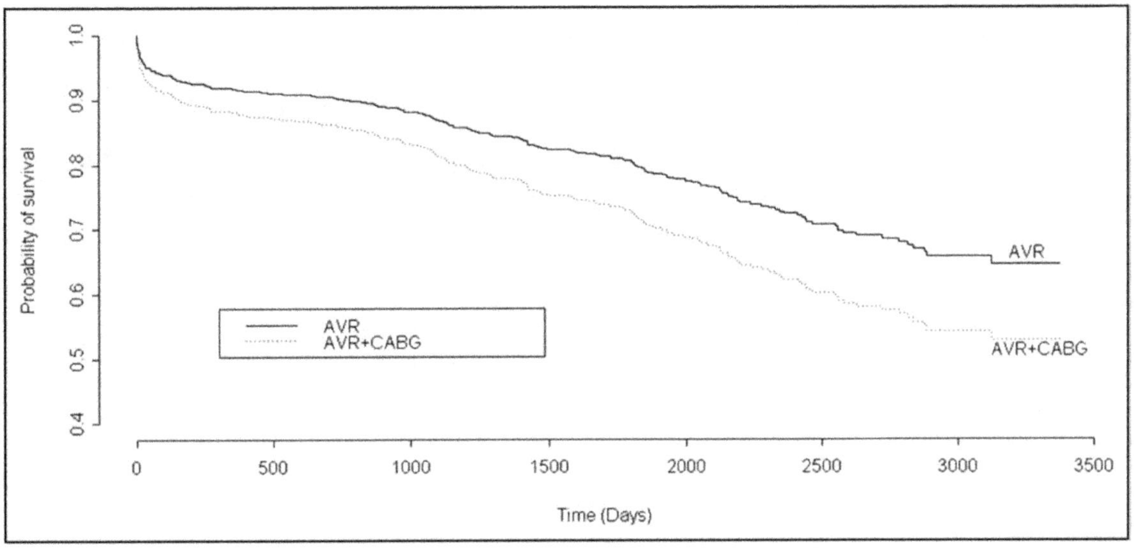

Figure 2. Unadjusted (Kaplan-Meier) curves depicting the probability of long-term survival in the patients who underwent compared to those who did not undergo concomitant coronary artery bypass grafting with the aortic valve replaced for stenosis (unadjusted hazard ratio 1.46, 95% CI 1.12 to 1.91, log-rank p = 0.005).

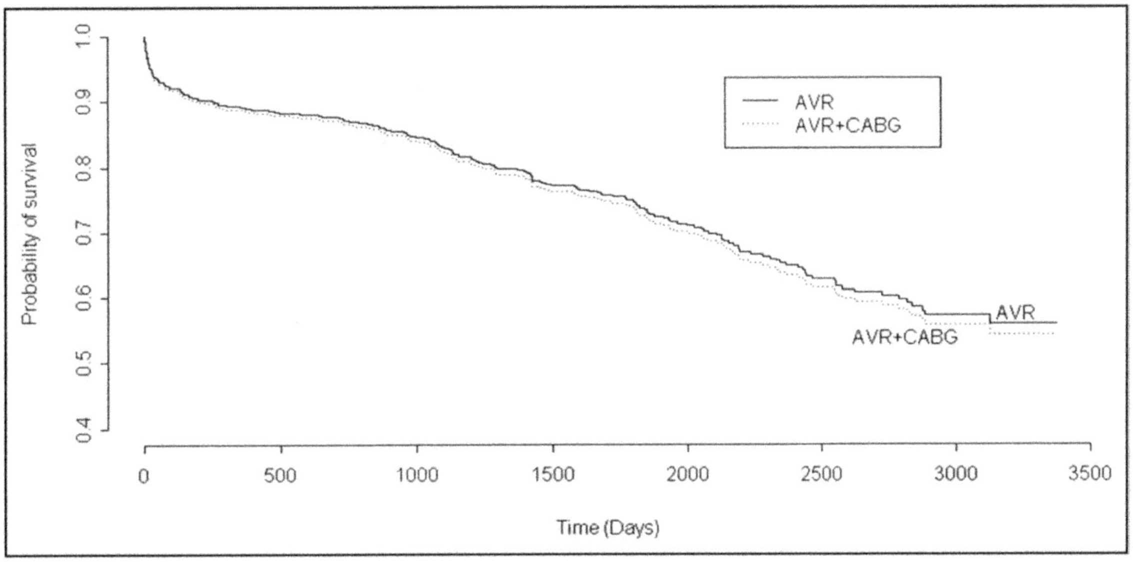

Figure 3. Adjusted (proportional-hazards model) curves depicting no significant difference in long-term survival in those who underwent compared to those who did not undergo concomitant coronary artery bypass grafting. The propensity-adjusted model included the following risk factors: age, gender, race, body mass index, aortic valve structure, valve weight, systemic hypertension, ascending aorta replaced, and type of implanted valve (adjusted hazard ratio 1.01, 95% CI 0.74 to 1.34, adjusted p = 0.976).

valves and lower frequencies of congenitally malformed aortic valves (Figure 1), had lighter aortic valves by weight, had higher frequencies of systemic hypertension, and had longer stays in the hospital after AVR (Table 1). Unadjusted early mortality (30 days) was not significantly (odds ratio 1.59, 95% CI 0.89 to 2.85) different between those who underwent (29 deaths [7%]) and those who did not undergo (18 deaths [4%]) simultaneous CABG. The length of stay for patients surviving >30 days and long-term survival (up to 10-year follow-up) were significantly higher in those who underwent concomitant CABG (median length of stay 8 days vs 6 days for patients who did not undergo concomitant CABG, p = 0.001; unadjusted hazard ratio for survival 1.46, 95% CI 1.12 to 1.91, log-rank p = 0.005). The unadjusted survival curves are depicted in Figure 2. However, after adjustment for possible confounders (age, gender, race, body mass index, aortic valve structure, valve weight, systemic hypertension, ascending aorta replaced, and type of implanted valve), neither early mortality (30 days; adjusted odds ratio 1.69, 95% CI 0.87 to 3.29) nor long-term mortality (10-year follow-up; adjusted hazard ratio 1.01, 95% CI 0.74 to 1.34) was different between those who did and did not undergo simultaneous CABG. The adjusted long-term survival curves are depicted in Figure 3.

Table 2
Comparison of aortic valve structure in patients who underwent isolated aortic valve replacement for aortic stenosis with or without concomitant coronary artery bypass grafting (n = 871)

Variable	Aortic Valve Structure			p Value
	Unicuspid (n = 60 [7%])	Bicuspid (n = 385 [44%])	Tricuspid (n = 426 [49%])	
Age group (years)				<0.001
21–50	31 (52%)	29 (8%)	6 (1%)	
51–70	24 (40%)	206 (54%)	110 (26%)	
71–95	5 (8%)	150 (39%)	310 (73%)	
Gender				0.169
Male	36 (60%)	252 (65%)	234 (55%)	
Female	24 (40%)	133 (35%)	192 (45%)	
Race				0.274
White	47 (78%)	324 (84%)	350 (82%)	
Black	2 (3%)	12 (3%)	32 (8%)	
Hispanic	4 (7%)	18 (5%)	13 (3%)	
Other	7 (12%)	31 (8%)	31 (7%)	
Coronary artery bypass grafting	11 (18%)	142 (37%)	275 (65%)	<0.001
Number of major coronary arteries narrowed ≥50%	(n = 29)	(n = 212)	(n = 236)	<0.001
0	23 (79%)	143 (67%)	102 (43%)	
1	3 (10%)	34 (16%)	52 (22%)	
2	2 (7%)	23 (11%)	49 (21%)	
3	1 (3%)	8 (4%)	26 (11%)	
4	0	4 (2%)	7 (3%)	
LV-aorta peak systolic gradient (mm Hg) (n = 475), range (mean) [median]	20–154 (64) [63]	11–130 (55) [51]	11–119 (45) [41]	<0.001
Aortic valve area (cm^2) (n = 474), mean ± SD	0.80 ± 0.34	0.78 ± 0.25	0.83 ± 0.30	0.139
Aortic valve weight (g), range (mean) [median]	1.19–7.15 (3.37) [3.17]	0.67–18.38 (3.11) [2.79]	0.43–6.40 (2.04) [1.92]	<0.001
Systemic hypertension by history	27 (45%)	260 (68%)	329 (77%)	<0.001
Body mass index (kg/m^2)				0.863
≤25	24 (41%)	119 (31%)	145 (34%)	
>25–30	21 (36%)	130 (34%)	141 (33%)	
>30–40	13 (22%)	111 (29%)	121 (29%)	
>40	1 (2%)	22 (6%)	17 (4%)	
Range (mean ± SD)	17–44 (27 ± 5)	16–66 (29 ± 7)	15–69 (29 ± 6)	
Days in hospital postoperatively in patients living >30 days, range (mean) [median]	3–32 (7) [6]	3–43 (8) [6]	3–71 (10) [8]	<0.001
Died ≤30 days postoperatively	0/59	20/380 (5%)	27/425 (6%)	0.222
Ascending aorta replaced	9 (15%)	25 (6%)	3 (1%)	<0.001
Implanted valve type				<0.001
Mechanical	41 (68%)	118 (31%)	53 (12%)	
Bioprosthetic	17 (28%)	264 (69%)	371 (87%)	
Ross procedure	2 (3%)	3 (<1%)	2 (<1%)	

The valve structure in the 871 patients is listed in Table 2. The 426 patients (49%) with tricuspid aortic valves, compared to the 445 patients (51%) with either congenitally unicuspid or bicuspid valves, were significantly older (p <0.001), had much higher frequencies of concomitant CABG (p <0.001), had higher likelihoods of having ≥1 major epicardial coronary artery being narrowed >50% in diameter on angiogram (p <0.001), had lower transvalvular peak systolic pressure gradients (p <0.001), had lighter aortic valves by weight (p <0.001), had higher frequencies of systemic hypertension (p <0.001), had more days in the hospital after AVR (p <0.001), and had higher late (>30 days) mortality rates after AVR. Unadjusted early mortality (30 days) was not significantly (odds ratio 1.16, 95% CI 0.56 to 2.42) different between patients with unicuspid or bicuspid versus tricuspid valves. Both unadjusted and adjusted survival, however, were significantly higher in patients with unicuspid or bicuspid valves compared to patients with tricuspid aortic valves (adjusted hazard ratio 0.70, 95% CI 0.50 to 0.97; Figures 4 and 5).

Coronary angiographic data were available for 477 of the 871 patients (55%). Compared to the 278 patients (58%) in whom none of the major coronary arteries was narrowed to this degree, the 199 patients (42%) with ≥1 coronary artery narrowed >50% were significantly older (p = 0.012), were more often male (p = 0.005), had much higher frequencies of concomitant CABG (p <0.001), had smaller peak systolic transvalvular pressure gradients (p = 0.010) and larger valve areas (p = 0.002), had higher frequencies of tricuspid aortic valves and lower frequencies of congenitally malformed valves (p <0.001), and had smaller aortic valves by weight (p = 0.030).

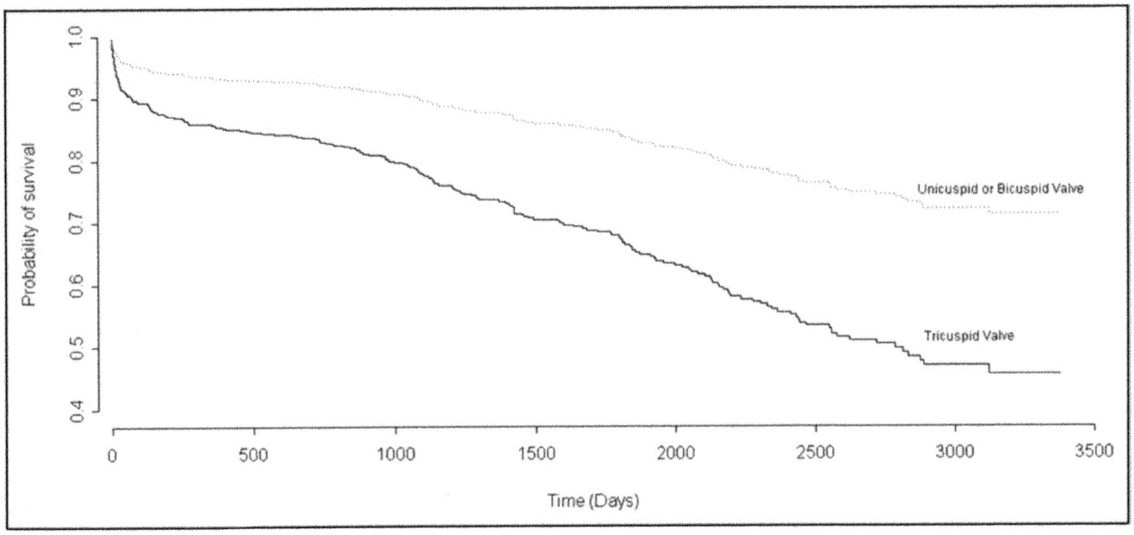

Figure 4. Unadjusted (proportional-hazards model) curves depicting significantly different survival in patients with unicuspid or bicuspid valves compared to those with tricuspid valves, all of whom underwent AVR (unadjusted hazard ratio 0.43, 95% CI 0.32 to 0.57, unadjusted p <0.001).

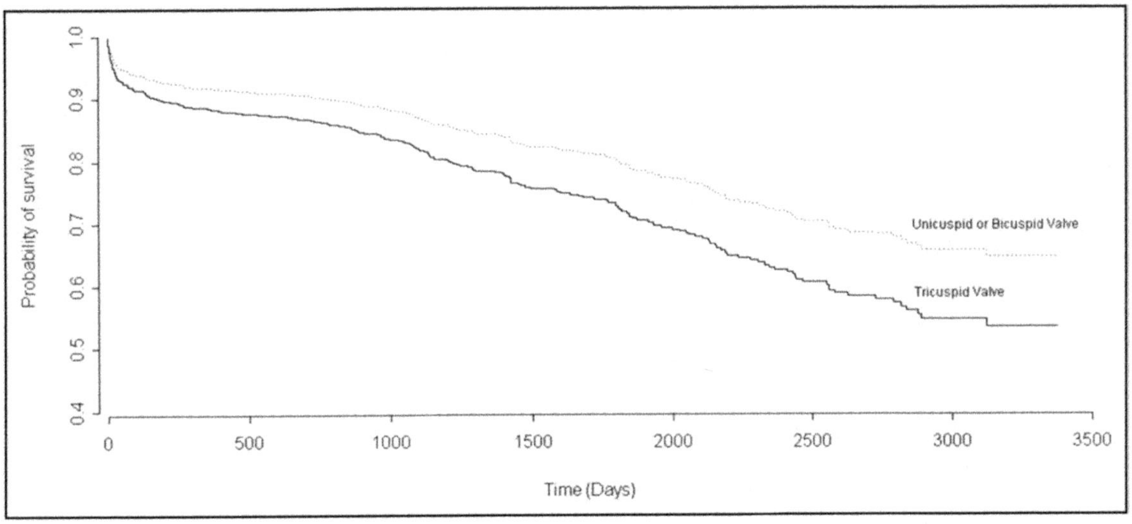

Figure 5. Adjusted (proportional-hazards model) curves depicting significantly different survival in those with unicuspid or bicuspid aortic valves compared to those with tricuspid valves, all of whom underwent AVR (adjusted hazard ratio 0.70, 95% CI 0.50 to 0.97, adjusted p = 0.031). The propensity-adjusted model included the following risk factors: age, gender, race, body mass index, concomitant CABG, valve weight, systemic hypertension, ascending aorta replaced, and type of implanted valve.

Discussion

The present study of patients who underwent AVR for AS (with or without aortic regurgitation) examined whether simultaneous CABG (vs not) and aortic valve structure (unicuspid or bicuspid vs tricuspid) affected short- and long-term survival. Although the patients who underwent simultaneous CABG compared to those who did not were significantly older, were more often male, had smaller transvalvular peak systolic pressure gradients and larger valve areas, most often had tricuspid aortic valves and much less frequently congenitally malformed valves, had higher frequencies of systemic hypertension, and had longer hospital stays, the adjusted probability of long-term survival was no different in those with versus without concomitant CABG. The unadjusted p value regarding the association between concomitant CABG (vs not) and long-term survival was 0.005, while the adjusted p value was 0.976.

None of the previously published reports of patients who underwent AVR for AS with or without simultaneous CABG focused on the structure of stenotic aortic valve.[6–13] In the present study, aortic valve structure was determined by the same investigator (W.C.R.) from examination of the operatively excised valve. We found in a previous study that congruence between cardiac surgeons and cardiac pathologists regarding aortic valve structure is virtually 100% when the structure of the aortic valve is tricuspid but that it is only 56% in the case of congenitally bicuspid valves and only 15% in the case of unicuspid valves.[14] Thus, uniformity of determination of valve structure results in far more accurate information compared to valve structure determined by several different surgeons, each of whom may have varying expertise in describing aortic valve structure or even mentioning valve structure in the operative note. Additionally, the intervals between AVR and dictation of the operative note were quite variable among surgeons, whose memories also might be quite variable.[14] The present study found that among the 426 patients with tricuspid aortic valves, 65% underwent concomitant CABG, whereas among the 60 patients with unicuspid valves and the 385 with congenitally bicuspid valves, concomitant CABG was far less frequently performed (18% and 37%, respectively). Both unadjusted and adjusted survival was significantly better in the patients with unicuspid or bicuspid aortic valves compared to those with tricuspid aortic valves.

A bit surprising to many students of aortic valve disease was the relatively high frequency of the congenitally malformed valves in all 3 age groups examined. Among the 66 patients aged 21 to 50 years, 60 (91%) had congenitally malformed aortic valves (unicuspid in 31 and bicuspid in 29); of the 340 patients aged 51 to 70 years, 230 (68%) had congenitally malformed valves (unicuspid in 24 and bicuspid in 206); and of the 465 patients aged 71 to 95 years, 155 (33%) had congenitally malformed valves (unicuspid in 5 and bicuspid in 150).

That CABG was significantly more frequent in the group with tricuspid aortic valves partly supports the view that AS in older patients with tricuspid aortic valves is the result of "atherosclerosis" involving the aortic valve. Patients with rheumatic heart disease were presumably excluded from the present study on the basis of having excluded all patients with mitral stenosis and those who underwent any operative procedure on the mitral valve (either repair or replacement).

There were limitations to the present study. Echocardiographic and hemodynamic data were not available in all patients. Not all patients with narrowing >50% in diameter of ≥1 major coronary artery underwent CABG. Many patients who underwent concomitant CABG and AVR would not have undergone AVR unless ≥1 of the coronary arteries had not been quite narrowed by preoperative angiogram. A major strength of the present study is that it is the first to compare long-term survival after AVR for AS (with or without aortic regurgitation) according to the underlying valve structure (unicuspid, bicuspid, or tricuspid).

1. Harrell FE Jr. Regression Modeling Strategies: With Application to Linear Models, Logistic Regression, and Survival Analysis. *New York, New York: Springer-Verlag*; 2001.
2. D'Agostino RB Jr. Propensity score methods for bias reduction in the comparison of a treatment to a non-randomized control group. *Stat Med* 1998;17:2265–2281.
3. Filardo G, Hamilton C, Hamman B, Ng HK, Grayburn P. Categorizing BMI may lead to biased results in studies investigating in-hospital mortality after isolated CABG. *J Clin Epidemiol* 2007;60:1132–1139.
4. Filardo G, Hamilton C, Hamman B, Grayburn P. Obesity and stroke after cardiac surgery: the impact of grouping body mass index. *Ann Thorac Surg* 2007;84:720–722.
5. Grambsch PM, Therneau T. Proportional hazards tests and diagnostics based on weighted residuals. *Biometrika* 1994;81:515–526.
6. Jones EL, Weintraub WS, Craver JM, Guyton RA, Shen Y. Interaction of age and coronary disease after aortic valve replacement: implications for valve selection. *Ann Thorac Surg* 1994;58:378–385.
7. Akins CW. Long-term results with the Medtronic-Hall valvular prosthesis. *Ann Thorac Surg* 1996;61:806–813.
8. Litmathe J, Boeken U, Feindt P, Gams E. Concomitant CABG procedures in elderly patients undergoing aortic valve replacement. *Z Kardiol* 2003;92:947–952.
9. Gillinov AM, Garcia MJ. When is concomitant aortic valve replacement indicated in patients with mild to moderate stenosis undergoing coronary revascularization? *Curr Sci* 2005;7:101–104.
10. Kuduvalli M, Grayson AD, Au J, Grotte G, Bridgewater B, Fabri BM. A multi-centre additive and logistic risk model for in-hospital mortality following aortic valve replacement. *Eur J Cardiothorac Surg* 2007;31:607–613.
11. Kobayashi KJ, Williams JA, Nwakanma L, Gott VL, Baumgartner WA, Conte JV. Aortic valve replacement and concomitant coronary artery bypass: assessing the impact of multiple grafts. *Ann Thorac Surg* 2007;83:969–978.
12. Gulbins H, Malkoc A, Ennker J. Combined cardiac surginal procedures in octogenarians: operative outcome. *Clin Res Cardiol* 2008;97:176–180.
13. Likosky DS, Sorensen MJ, Dacey LJ, Baribeau YR, Leavitt BJ, DiScipio AW, Hernandez F Jr, Cochran RP, Quinn R, Helm RE, Charlesworth DC, Clough RA, Malenka DJ, Sisto DA, Sardella G, Olmstead EM, Ross CS, O'Connor GT. Long-term survival of the very elderly undergoing aortic valve surgery. *Circulation* 2009;120:127–133.
14. Roberts WC, Vowels TJ, Ko JM. Comparison of interpretations of valve structure between cardiac surgeon and cardiac pathologist among adults having isolated aortic valve replacement for aortic valve stenosis (± aortic regurgitation). *Am J Cardiol* 2009;103:1139–1145.

Frequency of Congenitally Bicuspid Aortic Valves in Patients ≥80 Years of Age Undergoing Aortic Valve Replacement for Aortic Stenosis (With or Without Aortic Regurgitation) and Implications for Transcatheter Aortic Valve Implantation

William Clifford Roberts, MD[a,b,d,*], Kaitlin Georgeanne Janning[d,e], Jong Mi Ko, BA[d], Giovanni Filardo, PhD, MPH[f,g], and Gregory John Matter, MD[c]

The purpose of the present report was to determine the frequency of a congenitally bicuspid aortic valve in patients ≥80 years of age old with aortic stenosis (AS) severe enough to warrant aortic valve replacement. Transcatheter aortic valve implantation (TAVI) has traditionally been reserved for patients ≥80 years of age with severe AS involving a 3-cuspid aortic valve. Traditionally, AS involving a 2-cuspid aortic valve has been a contraindication to TAVI. We examined operatively excised stenotic aortic valves in 364 patients aged ≥80 years to determine the frequency of an underlying congenitally bicuspid aortic valve. Of the 347 octogenarians and 17 nonagenarians, 78 (22%) and 3 (18%) had stenotic congenitally bicuspid aortic valves, respectively. In conclusion, because the results of TAVI are less favorable in patients with stenotic congenitally bicuspid valves than in patients with stenotic tricuspid aortic valves, proper identification of the underlying aortic valve structure is important when considering TAVI as a therapeutic procedure for AS in older patients. **(Am J Cardiol 2012;109:1632–1636)**

It is generally believed that older patients with isolated aortic stenosis (AS) (with or without aortic regurgitation [AR]) infrequently have congenitally bicuspid aortic valves, the presence of which has been considered in most institutions to be a contraindication for transcatheter aortic valve implantation (TAVI) without replacement.[1] Most patients undergoing TAVI are ≥80 years of age, and most, of course, do not have a bicuspid aortic valve. Our purpose was to describe the frequency of congenitally bicuspid aortic valves in patients ≥80 years of age having had aortic valve replacement (AVR) for AS at Baylor University Medical Center (BUMC), Dallas, in the past 2 decades and to examine their survival in relation to valve structure.

Methods

From March 2, 1993 to July 8, 2011, a total of 1,725 operatively excised native stenotic aortic valves (with or without AR) in patients aged >20 years having isolated AVR (with or without coronary artery bypass grafting [CABG]) were received in the surgical pathology department at BUMC. The excised valve was weighed beginning in 1998.[2] Its structure in all cases was determined by one of us (W.C.R.) during the week that the valve was excised. Of the 1,725 patients, 364 (21%) were ≥80 years of age at the time of AVR. These 364 patients were the subject of the present report (Figure 1). Any patient undergoing replacement of a cardiac valve other than the aortic valve, any patient with previous aortic valvulotomy or replacement, and any patient with mitral stenosis were excluded from the study. The AVR in the patients included was their first cardiac operation.

That the patients had AS (with or without AR) was confirmed by examination of their preoperative cardiac catheterization and/or echocardiographic reports, which were available from the Baylor Physician Portal, BUMC electronic medical records, and/or the cardiovascular computer database (Apollo Advance C/S, version 4.2.13, LUMEDX, Oakland, California). The patients were considered to have AS if the peak systolic transvalvular gradient was >10 mm Hg. The aortic valve gradients and valve areas were obtained from the cardiac catheterization reports.

Cardiac catheterization data were available to us in most patients: peak transvalvular pressure gradients in 198 patients (57%), mean transvalvular pressure gradients for 193 (56%), aortic valve areas in 204 patients (59%), and left ventricular ejection fractions in 100 patients (29%). Most patients in whom cardiac catheterization data were not available were referred directly to a cardiovascular surgeon. The patients without cardiac catheterization data available to us underwent coronary angiographic studies before being referred to BUMC; however, the results of these studies were not available to us.

The mean ± standard deviation and percentages were

Departments of [a]Internal Medicine (Division of Cardiology), [b]Pathology, [c]Cardiacthoracic Surgery, and [d]Baylor Heart and Vascular Institute, Baylor University Medical Center, Dallas, Texas; [e]Furman University, Greenville, South Carolina; [f]Institute for Health Care Research and Improvement, Baylor Health Care System, Dallas, Texas; and [g]Department of Statistical Science, Southern Methodist University, Dallas, Texas. Manuscript received January 10, 2012; revised manuscript received and accepted January 11, 2012.

The study was funded by the Baylor Health Care System Foundation, Dallas, Texas.

*Corresponding author: Tel: (214) 820-7911; fax: (214) 820-7533.

E-mail address: wc.roberts@baylorhealth.edu (W.C. Roberts).

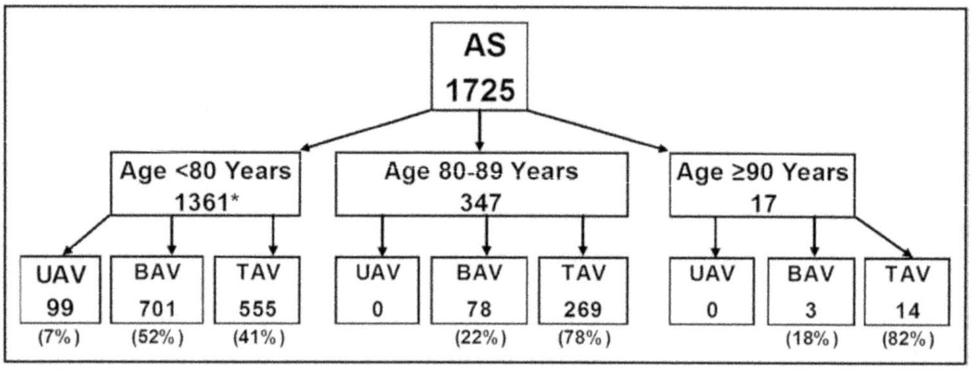

Figure 1. Ages and valve structure in the 1,725 patients having aortic valve replacement for aortic stenosis are included in the present study. Of the patients <80 years of age, 59% had a congenitally malformed valve (unicuspid aortic valve [UAV] in 7% and bicuspid [bicuspid aortic valve [BAV] in 52%); of these 80 to 89 years, 22% had a BAV and of those ≥90 years of age 18% had a BAV. TAV = tricuspid aortic valve. *Valve structure in 5 was indeterminate and in 1, quadricuspid.

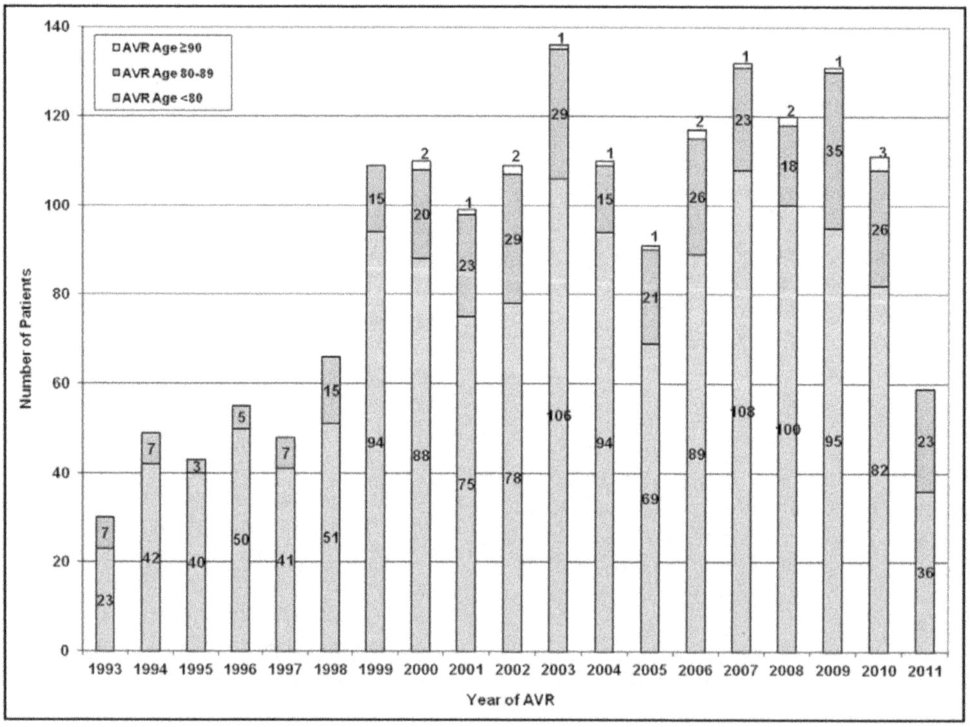

Figure 2. Bar graph displays the number of patients having aortic valve replacement for aortic stenosis during each of 19 years (1993 to 2011) at BUMC, Dallas. *Yellow* represents number of patients aged ≥90 years, *pink*, the number of patients aged 80 to 89 years, and *blue*, the number of patients aged <80 years.

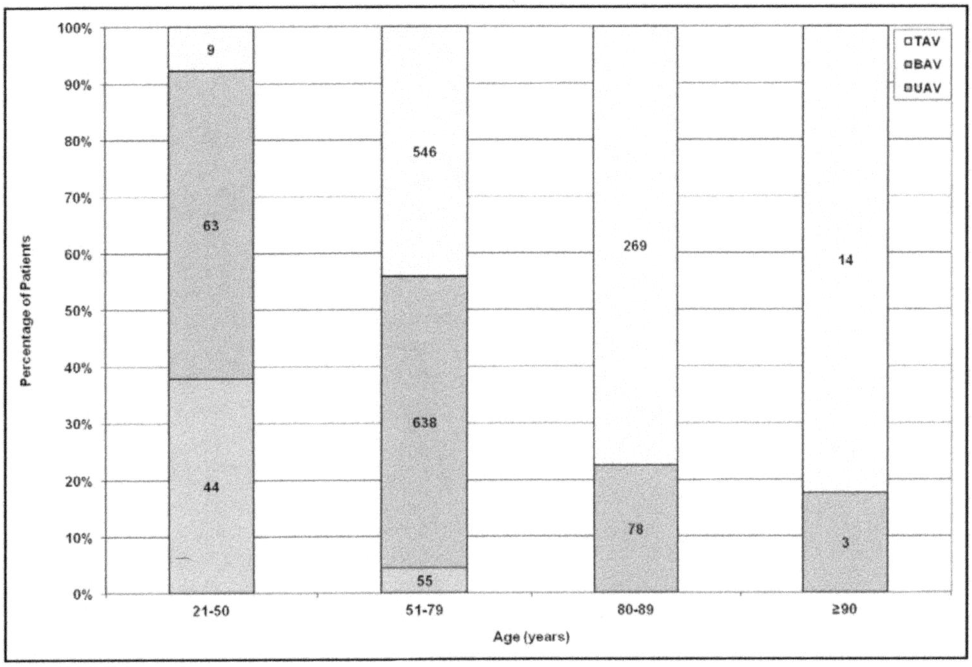

Figure 3. Bar graph illustrates the percentage of 1,725 patients having aortic valve replacement for aortic stenosis and the frequency of tricuspid *(yellow)* (tricuspid aortic valve [TAV]), bicuspid *(pink)* (bicuspid aortic valve [BAV]), and unicuspid *(blue)* (unicuspid aortic valve [UAV]) valves in each of the 4 groups. *One quadricuspid valve in age group 51 to 79, and 5 valves of indeterminate from the age group 51 to 79 were excluded.

calculated to describe the study cohort. The hazard ratios and 95% confidence intervals were estimated to describe survival. Kaplan-Meier plots were used to describe the unadjusted survival in patients with bicuspid valve disease—versus—tricuspid valve disease. A Cox proportional hazards model was used to assess the adjusted association between undergoing concomitant bicuspid valve disease (vs tricuspid valve disease) and survival. The model was adjusted by age, gender, and concomitant CABG. Restricted cubic splines were used for age.[3] Possible effect modification by gender and age was investigated and ruled out. The Grambsch and Therneau test statistic was used to test for proportionality of hazards in the Cox model.[4] Statistical analyses were performed using SAS, version 9.2 (SAS Institute, Cary, North Carolina) and R software, version 2.13.0.

Results

The frequency of AVR for AS with or without AR in the octogenarians and nonagenarians among the 1,725 patients during each year of the study years (1993 to 2011) is displayed in Figure 2. The frequency of aortic valve structure stratified by 3 age groups is displayed in Figures 2 and 3 and stratified by 4 age groups in all 1,725 patients is displayed in Figure 3. Of the 116 patients aged 21 to 50 years, 107 (92%) had either a congenitally unicuspid or bicuspid aortic valve. Of the 1,245 patients aged 51 to 79 years, 693 (56%) had a congenitally malformed valve (unicuspid in 55 and bicuspid in 638). Of the 364 octogenarians and nonagenarians, none had a unicuspid valve. Of the 347 octogenarians, 78 (22%) had bicuspid valves, and of the 17 nonagenarians, 3 (18%) had a bicuspid aortic valve (Figure 3).

The characteristics of the 347 octogenarians and 17 nonagenarians are listed in Table 1. Concomitant CABG was performed in 208 (60%) of the 347 octogenarians. Of the 347 octogenarians, survival data were available for 340. A total of 133 (39%) died either during the operation or during follow-up (≤14 years after AVR). The interval from AVR to death ranged from 0 to 14 years (median 4.3). Of these 347 octogenarians, 78 patients (22%) had bicuspid aortic valves and 269 (78%) had tricuspid aortic valves; 150 (43%) were women and 197 (57%) were men. The operatively excised bicuspid aortic valves in the men weighed from 0.81 to 7.84 g (mean 3.61), and in the women, from 0.79 to 4.90 g (mean 2.62). The operatively excised tricuspid aortic valves in the men ranged from 1.00 to 6.60 g (mean 2.31), and in the women, from 0.45 to 6.40 g (mean 1.64).

Of the 17 patients aged ≥90 years, 5 (29%) were women and 12 (71%) were men. Concomitant CABG was performed in 13 (76%) of these 17 patients. Of the 16 patients with long follow-up, 6 (37%) died during the operation or later (≤7 years after AVR). The interval from AVR to death ranged from 0 to 7 years (median 3.3). The operatively excised bicuspid aortic valves in the 3 men weighed 4.20, 5.73, and 9.75 g, respectively.

The complications postoperatively in the patients undergoing AVR from January 1, 2004 to June 3, 2011 are summarized in Table 2.

Patients with stenotic bicuspid valves had better (but not significantly) survival than patients with tricuspid aortic valves (adjusted hazard ratio 0.71, 95% confidence intervals 0.48 to 1.06). Figures 4 and 5 depict the unadjusted and adjusted survival curves in those having bicuspid—versus—tricuspid valves.

Table 1
Patient characteristics

Characteristic	Patients	Octogenarians	Nonagenarians
Total (n)	364	347	17
Mean age (years)	—	83	91
Men	209 (57%)	197 (57%)	12 (71%)
Women	155 (43%)	150 (43%)	5 (29%)
Bicuspid aortic valve	81 (22%)	78 (22%)	3 (18%)
Weight (g)			
Men			
Range		0.81–7.84	4.20, 5.73, 9.75
Mean		3.61	6.56
Women			
Range		0.79–4.90	—
Mean		2.62	
Tricuspid aortic valve	283 (78%)	269 (78%)	14 (82%)
Weight (g)			
Men			
Range		1.00–6.60	1.08–4.43
Mean		2.31	2.30
Women			
Range		0.45–6.40	0.43–2.22
Mean		1.64	1.27
Preoperative hemodynamics			
Left ventricular peak systole (mm Hg)	195		
Range		96–266	95–237
Mean		187	179
Left ventricular end diastole (mm Hg)	193		
Range		2–56	14–32
Mean		22	22
Aorta peak systole (mm Hg)	233		
Range		75–200	64–168
Mean		143	129
Aorta end diastole (mm Hg)	233		
Range		34–101	28–76
Mean		62	54
Left ventricular aortic peak systolic gradient (mm Hg)	205		
Range		11–130	20–69
Mean		47	49
Left ventricular aortic mean gradient (mm Hg)	203		
Range		9–89	25–57
Mean		39	42
Aortic valve area (cm^2)	214		
Range		0.18–1.84	0.41–1.07
Mean		0.73	0.66
Ejection fraction (%)	96		
Range		10–80	15–70
Mean		51	39
Concomitant coronary bypass grafting	221 (61%)	208 (60%)	13 (76%)
Hospital stay* (days)	344		
Range		3–38	4–25
Mean		11.1	10.1

* Aortic valve replacement to discharge, excluding preoperative days.

Table 2
Postoperative complications

Complications	Total (n = 187)
Operative	
Reoperation for bleeding	17 (9%)
Reoperation for valve dysfunction	1 (<1%)
Reoperation for graft occlusion	1 (<1%)
Reoperation for other cardiac	1 (<1%)
Perioperative myocardial infarction	0
Infection	
Septicemia	6 (3%)
Sternum-deep	0
Thoracotomy	0
Leg	1 (<1%)
Arm	0
Pulmonary	
Pneumonia	5 (3%)
Pulmonary embolism	0
Pulmonary insufficiency or ventilator >24 hours	35 (19%)
Neurologic	
Stroke, permanent >24 hours	5 (3%)
Stroke, transient ischemic attack	0
Renal	
Renal failure (creatinine >2 and 2 times baseline)	21 (11%)
Dialysis (newly required)	8 (4%)
Other	
Heart block (permanent pacemaker)	7 (4%)
Anticoagulant event	0
Gastrointestinal event	9 (5%)
Multisystem failure	7 (4%)
Tamponade	0
Cardiac arrest	7 (4%)
Atrial fibrillation	66 (35%)
Other complication	18 (10%)
Pleural effusion requiring thoracentesis	2 (1%)

Discussion

The purpose of the present study was to demonstrate the frequency of congenitally bicuspid aortic valves in patients ≥80 years of age who had undergone AVR for AS (with or without AR) and with or without concomitant CABG. Knowledge of the frequency of the bicuspid condition obviously is important in the present era of TAVI. Most patients considered for TAVI are ≥80 years of age, and the presence of a bicuspid aortic valve has been considered by most to be a contraindication to this percutaneous or transapical procedure.[1] In the present study of 364 patients ≥80 years of age, 81 (22%) had a congenitally bicuspid aortic valve.

How accurate is the 2-dimensional echocardiogram in distinguishing a congenitally bicuspid stenotic aortic valve from a stenotic tricuspid valve? In a recent report in which a world-renowned echocardiographer reviewed blindly echocardiograms of 100 patients >50 years of age with AS severe enough to warrant AVR, the accuracy of determining the number of aortic valve cusps in these patients was 66%.[5] After excluding 14 patients in which the echocardiograms were uninterpretable because of heavy calcium and/or poor image quality (10 of whom had unicuspid or bicuspid valves), congenitally malformed valves were present in 44 patients (51%), and tricuspid valves in 42 patients (49%). The valve structure on the echocardiogram was concordant with morphologic interpretation in only 57 of the 86

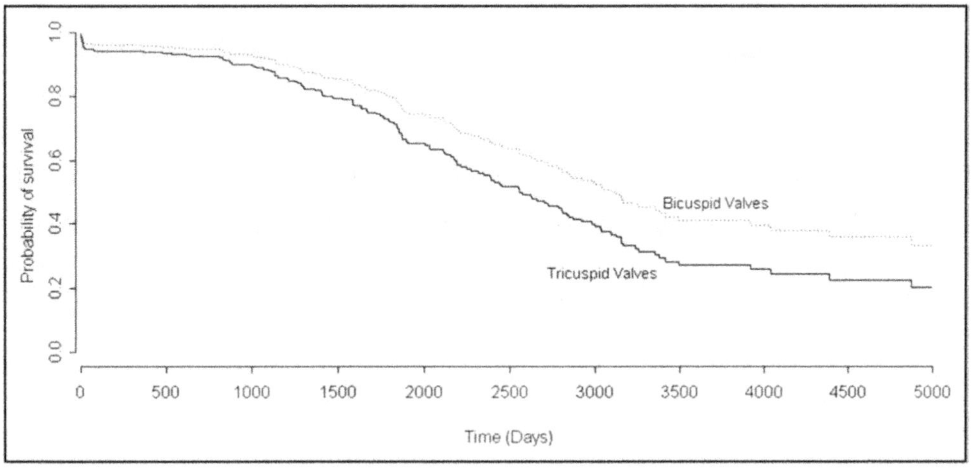

Figure 4. This curve depicts the probability of long-term survival in the group having bicuspid valves versus the group with tricuspid valves. p Value = 0.064; unadjusted hazard ratio = 0.69 (95% confidence intervals: 0.46, 1.02).

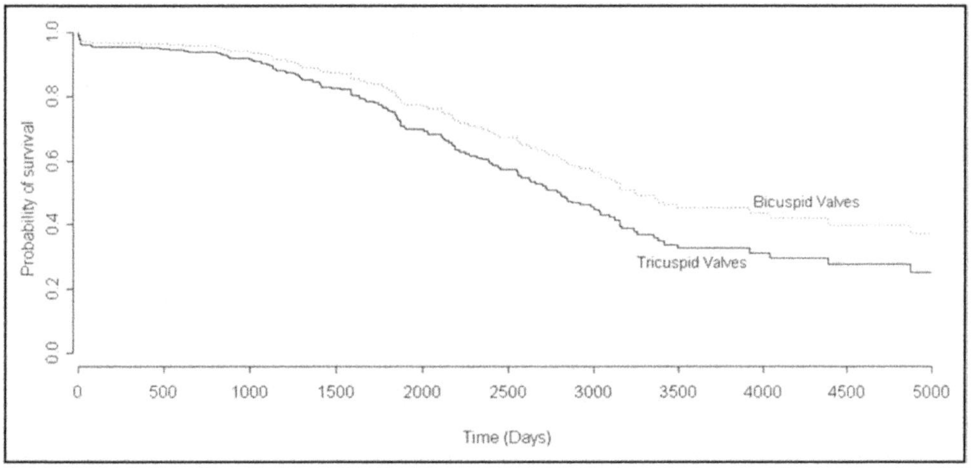

Figure 5. This curve depicts long-term survival in those having bicuspid valves versus tricuspid valves. The propensity-adjusted model includes the following risk factors: age, gender, and concomitant coronary artery bypass graftting. Adjusted p value = 0.095; adjusted hazard ratio = 0.71 (95% confidence intervals: 0.48, 1.06).

patients (66% accuracy). In the patients with valve areas similar to those enrolled in the recent TAVI trial (Placement of AoRTic TraNscathetER Valve Trial [PARTNER]; 0.7 ± 0.2 cm^2), the aortic valve structure was accurately determined by echocardiography in only 21 (60%) of 35 patients.[1,5]

The positive features of the present study included that the aortic valve structure in all patients was determined by the same individual (W.C.R.) by examination of the operatively excised valve,[6] the degree of AS in most patients was known, and the follow-up period was relatively long.

The present study was limited by the absence of hemodynamic and echocardiographic data in all patients and by the availability of postoperative complications in only 51%.

1. Smith CR, Leon MB, Mack MJ, Miller DC, Moses JW, Svensson LG, Tuzcu EM, Webb JG, Fontana GP, Makkar RR, Williams M, Dewey T, Kapadia S, Babaliaros V, Thourani VH, Corso P, Pichard AD, Bavaria JE, Herrmann HC, Akin JJ, Anderson WN, Wang D, Pocock SJ; PARTNER Trial Investigators. Transcatheter versus surgical aortic-valve replacement in high-risk patients. *N Engl J Med* 2011;364:2187–2198.
2. Roberts WC, Ko JM. Weights of operatively-excised stenotic unicuspid, bicuspid, and tricuspid aortic valves and their relation to age, sex, body mass index, and presence or absence of concomitant coronary artery bypass grafting. *Am J Cardiol* 2003;92:1057–1065.
3. Filardo G, Hamilton C, Hamman B, Ng HK, Grayburn P. Categorizing BMI may lead to biased results in studies investigating in-hospital mortality after isolated CABG. *J Clin Epidemiol* 2007;60:1132–1139.
4. Grambsch PM, Therneau T. Proportional hazards tests and diagnostics based on weighted residuals. *Biometrika* 1994;81:515–526.
5. Ayad RF, Grayburn PA, Ko JM, Filardo G, Roberts WC. Accuracy of two-dimensional echocardiography in determining aortic valve structure in patients >50 years of age having aortic valve replacement for aortic stenosis. *Am J Cardiol* 2011;108:1589–1599.
6. Roberts WC, Vowels TJ, Ko JM. Comparison of interpretations of valve structure between cardiac surgeon and cardiac pathologist among adults having isolated aortic valve replacement for aortic valve stenosis (+/− aortic regurgitation). *Am J Cardiol* 2009;103:1139–1145.

Natural History of Adults With Congenitally Malformed Aortic Valves (Unicuspid or Bicuspid)

William Clifford Roberts, MD, Travis James Vowels, BBA, and Jong Mi Ko, BA

Abstract: Appreciation of the frequency of the congenitally malformed aortic valve has come about during the last 50 years, a period during which aortic valve replacement became a predictably successful operation. Study of patients at necropsy with either a congenitally unicuspid (1 true commissure) or bicuspid (2 true commissures) valve in whom no aortic valve operation has been performed has not been conducted during these 50 years, to our knowledge. We studied 218 patients at necropsy with congenitally malformed aortic valves: 28 (13%) had a unicuspid valve and 190 (87%), a bicuspid valve. Their ages at death ranged from 21 to 89 years (mean, 55 yr), and 80% were men. Of the 218 adults, the aortic valve functioned normally during life in 54 (25%) and abnormally in 164 (75%): aortic stenosis in 142 (65%), pure aortic regurgitation without superimposed infective endocarditis (IE) in 2 (1%), and IE superimposed on a previously normally functioning aortic valve in 20 (9%). IE occurred in a total of 31 (14%) of the 218 patients: involving a previously normally functioning valve in 20 (65%) and a previously stenotic valve in 11 (35%). Of the 218 patients, at least 141 (65%) died as a consequence of aortic valve disease (124 patients) or ascending aortic tears with or without dissection (17 patients). An estimated 1% of the population, maybe higher in men, has a congenitally malformed aortic valve. Data from this study suggest that about 75% of them will develop a major complication. Conversely, and encouragingly, about 25% will go through life without a complication.

(*Medicine* 2012;91: 287–308)

Abbreviations: AR = aortic regurgitation, AS = aortic stenosis, CABG = coronary artery bypass grafting, IE = infective endocarditis, NHLBI = National Heart, Lung, and Blood Institute.

INTRODUCTION

The frequency of the congenitally malformed aortic valve at birth remains unclear but the best estimates are that it is present in 1% of live births,[22,50,58] probably a bit higher in males. That frequency translates into 3,130,000 persons in the United States having a congenitally malformed aortic valve. If systemic hypertension is excluded, complications of the malformation of this valve may be the second most common cardiac cause of death (after coronary heart disease) if untreated.

The frequency of the malformed aortic valve has not been properly appreciated until relatively recent decades. Paul Dudley White, the most prominent cardiologist in the United States in the first half of the 20th century, wrote in the 4th edition (1951) of his book *Heart Disease*, "Serious congenital aortic valve lesions, stenosis and atresia, are very rare, but congenital bicuspid aortic valves are found occasionally and are likely to be the site of subacute bacterial endocarditis...".[101] Paul Wood, the most prominent cardiologist in the United Kingdom during his lifetime, wrote in the 3rd edition (1968) of his book *Diseases of the Heart and Circulation*, "Apart from its association with [aortic] coarctation, bicuspid aortic valve is clinically important for four reasons: 1) it may leak spontaneously or as a result of acquired hypertension; 2) about one-quarter of all cases become infected sooner or later; 3) an associated weakness of the sinuses of Valsalva may lead to aneurysmal dilatation or rupture; 4) an insidious sclerosing process may lead to calcified aortic stenosis in middle age...".[103] And in the 3rd edition (1968) of *Pathology of the Heart and Blood Vessels* edited by S. E. Gould, only 2 of 1162 pages were devoted to aortic stenosis (AS), and bicuspid aortic valve was mentioned in only 1 of 9 paragraphs.[28] It is notable that successful aortic valve replacement had been a reality for 8 years, since 1960.[48]

The congenitally bicuspid aortic valve has captured the interest of many prominent physicians and one illustrious artist.[98,99] Leonardo da Vinci (1452–1519) appears to have been the first to draw and publish a congenitally bicuspid aortic valve and indeed to appreciate its clear difference from a tricuspid aortic valve.[34] Sir James Paget (1814–1899) described at necropsy 3 patients with stenotic bicuspid aortic valves.[52] Sir Thomas Peacock (1812–1882) also described and illustrated 3 patients studied at necropsy with stenotic congenitally bicuspid aortic valves.[54] A number of reports followed (Table 1), describing mainly patients studied at necropsy with valvular AS.[1,2,6,7,9,10,12–15,17,18,20,24,25,29,31,33,35,37–41,47,50,52,54,56,57,91,92,100] Many authors considered the AS to be the result of rheumatic heart disease,[2,7,9,13–15,17,18,29,31,33,37,57] but several authors provided illustrations of the stenotic aortic valve showing it clearly to be a congenitally bicuspid valve.[2,6,7,9,12,14,18,20,24,33,40,54,91,92] Roberts in 1970 provided a strong case against a rheumatic etiology for AS in patients with anatomically normal mitral valves.[59,60] Maude Abbott (1868–1940) demonstrated that most patients (about 75%) with coarctation of the aorta have congenitally bicuspid aortic valves,[1] and many authors later supported that view.[6,26,57,58,92] Roberts and colleagues[82] opined that 100% of patients with complete interruption of the aortic arch have bicuspid aortic valves. Authors after 1950 describing patients with AS commonly described and illustrated underlying congenitally bicuspid valves (see Table 1).[6,10–12,20,24,32,36,49,55,58–61,64,92]

Although Carl Rokitansky (1804–1878) had earlier identified bacteria in vegetations in patients with infective endocarditis (IE), Osler (1849–1919) in his 1885 Gulstonian Lectures[51] called

From the Departments of Internal Medicine (Division of Cardiology) and Pathology (WCR), and Baylor Heart and Vascular Institute (WCR, TJV, JMK), Baylor University Medical Center, Dallas, Texas.
Travis James Vowels is currently a medical student at The University of Texas Medical School at Houston, Houston, Texas.
This work was supported by the Baylor Heart and Vascular Institute, Cardiovascular Research Review Committee, the Cardiovascular Research Fund of the Baylor Health Care System Foundation.
The authors have no conflicts of interest to disclose.
Reprints: Dr. William Clifford Roberts, Baylor Heart and Vascular Institute, Baylor University Medical Center, 3500 Gaston Avenue, Dallas, TX (e-mail: wc.roberts@baylorhealth.edu).

ISSN: 0025-7974
DOI: 10.1097/MD.0b013e3182764b84

TABLE 1. Reported Necrospy Cases (Before 1970) of Aortic Stenosis and/or Bicuspid Aortic Valves in Adults Without Anatomic Disease of the Mitral Valve

Year of Publication	Author(s) (Reference)	Number of Cases						Etiology of Aortic Valve Disease
		Total	Bicuspid Aortic Valve	Aortic Stenosis	Infective Endocarditis	Coarctation of Aorta	Photos (BAV)*	
1844	Paget[52]	6	3	3	0	0	0	C
1865	Peacock[54]	3	3	3	0	0	+(3/3)†	C
1886	Osler[50]	18	18	6‡	8	0	0	C
1904	Mönckeberg[47]	32	0	32	0	0	0	D
1923	Lewis, Grant[39]	13	13	0	13	0	0	C
1926	Cabot[9]	28	2	23	5	0	+(2/3)	R
1926	Clawson, Bell, Hartzell[14]	13	—	13	6	0	+(1/1)	R
1928	Wauchope[100]	52	52	0	7	2	0	C
1928	Abbott[1]	200	51	0	13	200§	0	C
1931	Christian[13]	21	0	21	0	0	0	R
1931	Margolis, Ziellessen, Barnes[40]	42	20	42	0	0	+(3/4)¶	U
1933	Laws, Levine[37]	11	—	11	2	0	0	R
1934	McGinn, White[41]	35	4	35	1	0	0	U
1934	Bishop, Bishop, Trubek[7]	9	9	2	1	1	+(2/2)	R
1935	Gibbs[25]	12	0	12	0	0	0	A
1936	Sohval, Gross**[24,91]	15	1	15	0	0	+(1/4)	NR
1937	Gross[29]	16	2	16	—	—	+	R
1938	Lesnick, Schlesinger[38]	17	0	17	0	0	0	NR
1938	Clawson, Noble, Lufkin[15]	132	0	97	0	0	0	R
1939	Dry, Willius[18]	15	1	15	0	0	+(2/4)	R
1940	Cohen, Gray, Nash, Fink[17]	7	1	7	0	0	0	R
1941	Koletsky[35]	7	7	4	1	1	0	C
1945	Reich[56]	22	0	22	0	0	0	—
1947	Karsner, Koletsky[33]	119	16	119	0	0	+(2/8)	R
1947	Reifenstein, Levine, Gross[57]	104	58	11	23	104	0	C, R
1948	Horan, Barnes[31]	100	—	100	6	0	0	R
1952	Anderson, Kelsey, Edwards[2]	49	—	49	0	0	+(2/4)‖	C, R
1953	1953 Campbell, Kauntze[12]	4	4	4	0	0	+(4/4)#	C
1955	Smith, Matthews[92]	27	20	27	0	7	+(2/2)	C
1959	Bacon, Matthews[6]	28	28	19	0	4	+(6/6)	C
1961	Edwards[20]	10	8	9	0	0	+(8/10)	C
1968	Campbell[10]	46	16	46	0	0	0	C

Abbreviations: A = atherosclerotic, C = congenital, D = degenerative, NR = non-rheumatic, R = rheumatic, U = uncertain.

*The second number in this vertical column represents the number of gross illustrations of the aortic valve.

†Drawings.

‡Osler described only 1 of these 6 cases as having aortic stenosis ("The two segments from their position obstruct and narrow the orifice") but the description of the valves make it likely that the orifices were stenotic.

§Rupture of ascending aorta in 33 and cerebral hemorrhage in 25.

‖One of the 2 is unicuspid.

¶One of the 3 is unicuspid.

#Three of the 4 are unicuspid. All are drawings.

**Clinical features in the cases were reported by Friedberg and Sohval.

attention to the congenitally bicuspid aortic valve's extreme propensity to be the site of IE. Whether Osler realized that stenosis was also a complication of the bicuspid condition is less clear; if he did, he did not write about that possibility. Mensah and Friesinger[44] believed that Osler missed entirely "the link" between the bicuspid valve and AS. The reason they suggested was that the average age of death in the United States in 1900 was 47 years, and most patients with stenosis superimposed on a bicuspid aortic valve are older than that. Osler described 18 patients with congenitally bicuspid aortic valves that he studied at autopsy, and although the aortic valve "was invariably thickened and the seat of sclerotic changes," clear AS was seen in only 1 of the 18 patients. During the 20th century a number of other authors stressed the frequent connection between IE and the congenitally malformed aortic valve.[3–5,8,22,23,58,63]

That pure aortic regurgitation (AR) without superimposed IE may be a consequence of the bicuspid condition was not reported, to our knowledge, until 1981 when Roberts and colleagues[83] described 13 such patients who had undergone aortic valve replacement. Today, the bicuspid valve without superimposed IE is recognized as one of the most common causes of pure (no element of stenosis) AR severe enough to warrant aortic valve replacement.[65,80,83,88]

An association between aortic valve disease and "cystic medial necrosis" of the ascending aorta appears to have been first described by McKusick (1921–2008) and colleagues[43] in 1957. Although the structure of the valve was not known in their 4 cases, the severity of stenosis and the lack of associated mitral valve disease makes congenital malformation of the aortic valve highly likely, and that association has been reported often since then.[30,42,86,88,95,97,104] Not only is the ascending aorta dilated in patients with stenotic and/or purely regurgitant congenitally bicuspid aortic valves, but tears in the ascending aorta with or without dissection also is a recognized complication.[86,88] Roberts and Roberts[86] found aortic dissection to be 5 times more frequent in patients with bicuspid compared to those with tricuspid aortic valves. Although the ascending aorta may be dilated in patients with AS or pure AR, Roberts and associates[88] found that aortic-medial-elastic-fiber loss was absent or minimal in 90% of their patients undergoing aortic valve replacement for stenotic unicuspid or bicuspid aortic valves, but in only

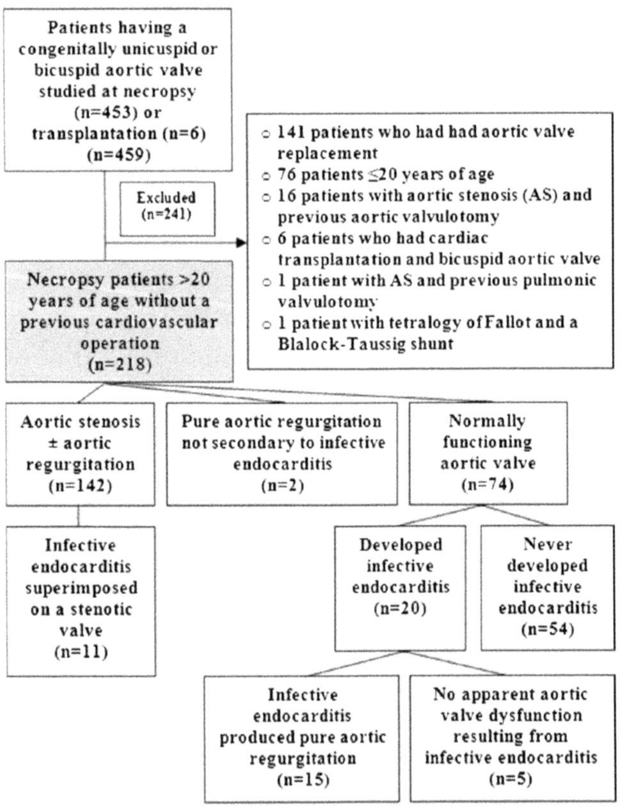

FIGURE 1. Flow chart showing our experience with patients having a congenitally malformed aortic valve. Of the total 453 patients with unicuspid or bicuspid aortic valves studied at necropsy, 241 (53%) were eliminated from this analysis mainly because of an operative intervention on the aortic valve. (In addition, we have examined 276 operatively excised congenitally unicuspid and 1330 operatively excised congenitally bicuspid aortic valves, but these 1606 cases were not included in the present analysis.)

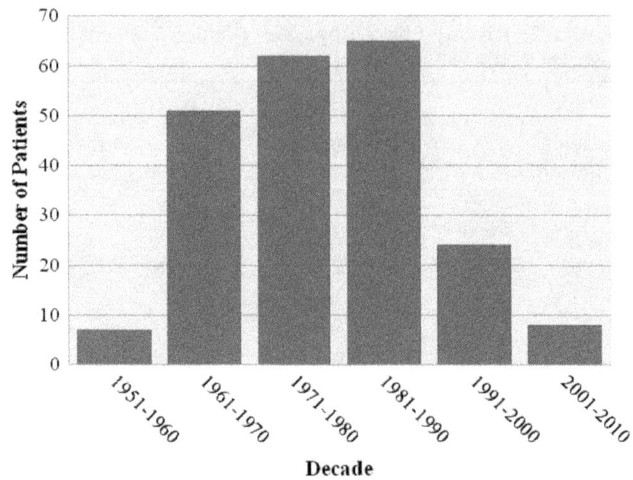

FIGURE 2. Decades during which the 218 patients were studied.

50% of patients with purely regurgitant bicuspid aortic valves. This observation suggests that the type of aortic valve dysfunction may be a major determinant of whether the ascending aorta needs to be resected at the time of aortic valve replacement, an occurrence that has become quite common in the last 2 decades.[95,96,104]

To our knowledge, the concept of the unicuspid aortic valve was first proposed by Edwards[19] (1911–2008) in 1958. He described a unicuspid unicommissural stenotic aortic valve as having only 1 true commissure and a slit-like orifice resembling an exclamation point. He opined that the unicuspid unicommissural aortic valve was stenotic from the time of birth, and that this valve structure was the structure most commonly seen in infants and very young children with severe AS. In contrast, he believed that the bicuspid aortic valve was not stenotic at birth but became so as fibrous tissue and calcific deposits developed on its cusps. Several reports on consequences of the unicuspid unicommissural aortic valve followed.[21,70,78,81,88] Probably most surgeons and pathologists call the unicuspid unicommissural aortic valve a congenitally bicuspid valve.[87] In 2007, Roberts and associates[71] described 4 patients whose operatively excised stenotic aortic valves had no true commissures and similar degrees of "commissural" fusion resulting in a central symmetrical triangular-shaped orifice. The authors called the valve congenitally unicuspid acommissural.

In the last 20 years most morphologic studies of stenotic, purely regurgitant, and infected congenitally malformed aortic valves have been of operatively excised valves, because the frequency of autopsy in patients dying in hospitals in the United States has dropped to <10% in most institutions, and operative intervention is now common and usually successful.[48,53,66–80,88,90,93,94] Nevertheless, multiple studies of operatively excised valves have demonstrated that the unicuspid ones contain the most calcium and therefore are the heaviest and the most stenotic,[69] that the bicuspid valves are the next most calcified, and that the stenotic tricuspid valves have the least calcific deposits and therefore are the lightest and the least stenotic.[66,69,70,72,78,84] Additionally, these studies have shown that men have significantly heavier valves than women, and that the stenotic valves are far heavier than the purely regurgitant valves with or without superimposed active IE.[66,69,70,72,78,80,88]

Although the natural history of patients having congenitally unicuspid or bicuspid aortic valves has received attention during the last 50 years, most reports included some patients

TABLE 2. Comparison of Various Variables Among Patients With Unicuspid vs Bicuspid Aortic Valves (n = 218)

Variable	Total, n = 218 (100%)	Aortic Valve Structure: Unicuspid, n = 28 (13%)	Aortic Valve Structure: Bicuspid, n = 190 (87%)
Age at death (years)			
Mean ± SD [median]	55 ± 15 [57]	48 ± 15 [53]*	56 ± 15 [57]*
(Range)	(21–89)	(25–77)	(21–89)
Gender†			
Men	169 (80%)	26 (93%)	143 (78%)
Women	43 (20%)	2 (7%)	41 (22%)
Aortic valve function (before infective endocarditis)			
Normal	74 (34%)	0	74 (39%)
Stenosis	142 (65%)	27 (96%)	115 (61%)
Pure regurgitation	2 (1%)	1 (4%)	1 (<1%)
Infective endocarditis‡			
Active	25 (11%)	2 (7%)	23 (12%)
Healed	6 (3%)	1 (4%)	5 (3%)
Infective endocarditis superimposed on a:			
Previously normally functioning valve	20 (9%)	0	20 (11%)
Previously stenotic valve	11 (5%)	3 (11%)	8 (4%)
Previously purely regurgitant valve	0	0	0
Heart weight (g)			
Mean ± SD [median]	558 ± 162 [530]	603 ± 143 [605]§	551 ± 164 [520]§
(Range)	(170–1050)	(320–880)	(170–1050)

*-*p - value = 0.0109.

†Data missing on 6 patients.

‡Of the 25 patients with active infective endocarditis, 16 had a normally functioning aortic valve prior to infection and 9 had a previously stenotic valve; of the 6 patients with healed infective endocarditits, 4 had a previously normal aortic valve and 2 had infection superimposed onto a stenotic valve.

§-§p - value = 0.1428.

TABLE 3. Comparison of Various Variables According to Type of Function of the Congenitally Malformed Aortic Valve (n = 218)

Variable	Aortic Valve Function Prior to Infective Endocarditis: Normal, n = 74 (34%)	Stenosis, n = 142 (65%)	Pure Regurgitation, n = 2 (1%)
Age at death (years)			
Mean ± SD [median]	48 ± 16 [48]*	59 ± 14 [59]*	32, 42
(Range)	(21–82)	(23–89)	
Gender†			
Men	57 (78%)	110 (80%)	2
Women	16 (22%)	27 (20%)	0
Valve structure			
Unicuspid	0	27 (19%)	1
Bicuspid	74	115 (81%)	1
Infective endocarditis			
Active	16 (22%)	9 (6%)	0
Healed	4 (5%)	2 (1%)	0
Aortic valve orientation			
Anterior/posterior	43/63 (68%)	62/89 (70%)	1
Right/left	20/63 (32%)	27/89 (30%)	0
Raphe present	46/57 (81%)	66/78 (85%)	1
Heart weight (g)			
Mean ± SD [median]	477 ± 148 [450]‡	598 ± 152 [573]‡	470, 920
(Range)	(170–1010)	(300–1050)	

-, ‡-‡p - value = <0.0001.

†Data missing on 6 patients.

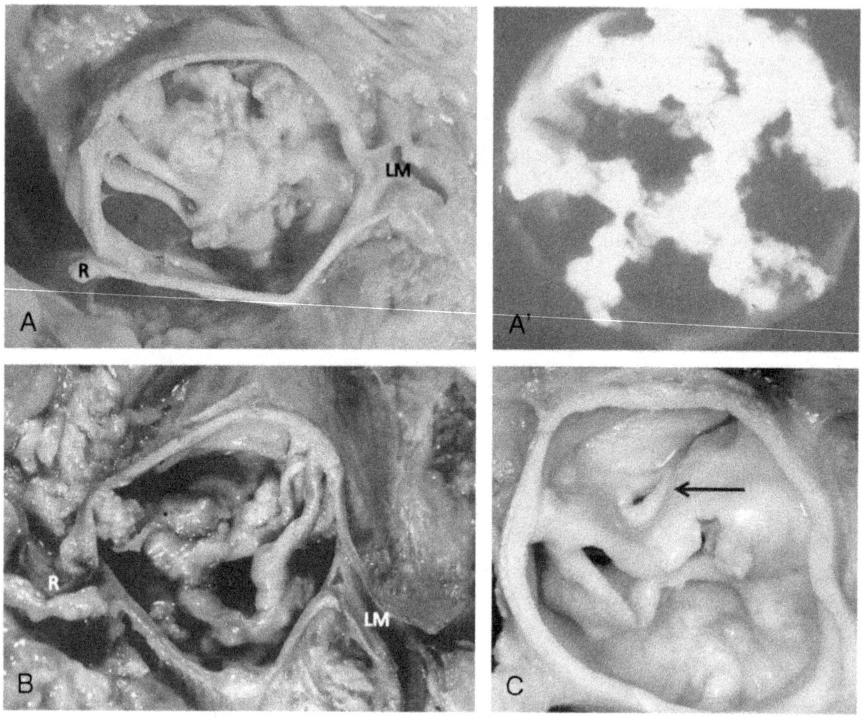

FIGURE 3. Unicuspid aortic valves in 3 patients. A and A′ (radiograph), Valve of a 48-year-old man who had been well until 5 months before death when signs and symptoms of heart failure began and progressed. Terminally, he developed pneumonia, which prevented cardiac catheterization and cardiac valve replacement. The heart weighed 750 g. LM = left main coronary artery; R = right coronary artery. B, Valve of a 31-year-old man who had been a splendid 3-letter athlete and had won his country club golf championship several days before dying quickly of severe acute heart failure. The heart failure was the first he had ever had. The peak systolic pressure difference between left ventricle and aorta was 11 mm Hg. The patient also had considerable AR with similar diastolic pressures in both left ventricle and aorta (50 and 60 mm Hg respectively). He was deemed too sick to undergo aortic valve replacement in 1969. His heart at necropsy weighed 880 g. C, Valve of a 26-year-old man who died suddenly while dancing in a disco. According to some friends, he had no known medical ailments and was not taking any medications. Prior to the sudden collapse there were apparently no complaints of feeling ill. The heart weighed 760 g. A cuspal perforation (arrow) is present, suggesting previous IE that had healed.

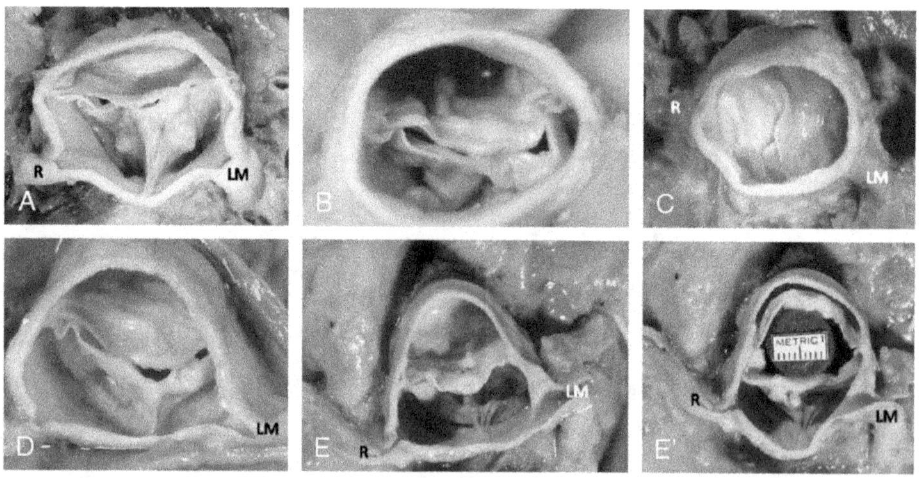

FIGURE 4. Congenitally bicuspid normally functioning aortic valves in 5 different patients, none of whom had clinical evidence of aortic valve disease. In 4 of the 5 patients the cusps are situated anterior-to-posterior, and in 1 patient (C), right-to-left. A, Valve in a 36-year-old man who died suddenly while watching television. He was a habitual alcoholic and he had a fatty liver that weighed 2900 g. The heart weighed 405 g and the coronary arteries were clean. The right coronary artery was dominant. He was found dead by fellow residents in a shelter home. LM = left main coronary artery; R = right coronary artery. B, Valve in a 63-year-old man who had undergone 2 coronary bypass grafting operations. The second operation was performed 17 days before death. The heart weighed 590 g. There are a few calcific deposits on each cusp but each cusp was freely mobile. C, Valve in a 60-year-old man who died of cancer of the pancreas. His heart weighed 470 g and he had systemic hypertension. D, Valve in a 71-year-old woman who died from Parkinson disease. She was cachexic. The heart weighed 290 g. E and E′, Valve shown in both ventricular diastole (E) and ventricular systole (E′) in a 72-year-old woman who died after a fall. The heart weighed 300 g. Small calcific deposits were present in each cusp.

who also had aortic valve replacement or repair, and thus their "natural history" was interrupted by this therapeutic event, or they included only children or young adults, or patients were followed not until death, but just for a few years.[11,16,22,32,45,46,55,89] In the present report we focus on 218 patients with congenitally malformed aortic valves all studied at necropsy by the same investigator (WCR) during the last 50 years. Our purpose is to determine the natural history of patients with this valvular abnormality without operative intervention on the aortic valve at any time.

METHODS

The cases included in the current study came from 37 different institutions including 34 cases from the National Heart, Lung, and Blood Institute (NHLBI), Bethesda, MD; 133 cases from 12 different hospitals in the Washington, DC, area, including 31 from Georgetown University Hospital; 27 from medical institutions in Dallas, TX, and the remaining 24 from 22 different medical centers excluding those in the Washington, DC, and Dallas, TX, areas. The cases from the Washington, DC, area were obtained as follows: WCR gave a conference for nearly 25 years on cardiovascular pathology at 11 or 12 hospitals each month (at Georgetown University Hospital weekly) and after conference the specimens were brought to the Pathology Branch, NHLBI, and described and photographed. Both the reports and photographs were sent to the submitting institutions. Some specimens were received via mail from more distant institutions. All hearts were examined and classified by WCR, and most were photographed or drawn or both.

The clinical records were provided by the Clinical Center of the National Institutes of Health (34 cases) or Baylor University Medical Center at Dallas (16 cases) or by the submitting hospital. Cardiac catheterization and echocardiographic data were sought in all patients. The symptomatic status of each patient was determined from the clinical records. The severity of the aortic valve dysfunction, if present, was determined by the cardiac catheterization reports for patients having that procedure. For the few cases with echocardiograms, we used that examination to determine severity, and if a patient had both an echocardiogram and a left-sided cardiac catheterization, we used the catheterization data. Photographs of stenotic aortic valves in patients in whom cardiac catheterization had been performed were compared to valves in patients in whom no cardiac catheterization was performed to show that the degrees of severity by anatomic examination were similar. All patients included were aged >20 years at the time of death. We excluded patients who had undergone aortic valvulotomy, aortic valve replacement, or replacement of another cardiac valve. Additionally, patients with mitral stenosis irrespective of the structure of the aortic valve were excluded. Patients with diffuse fibrous thickening of the mitral valve leaflets irrespective of the function of the mitral valve

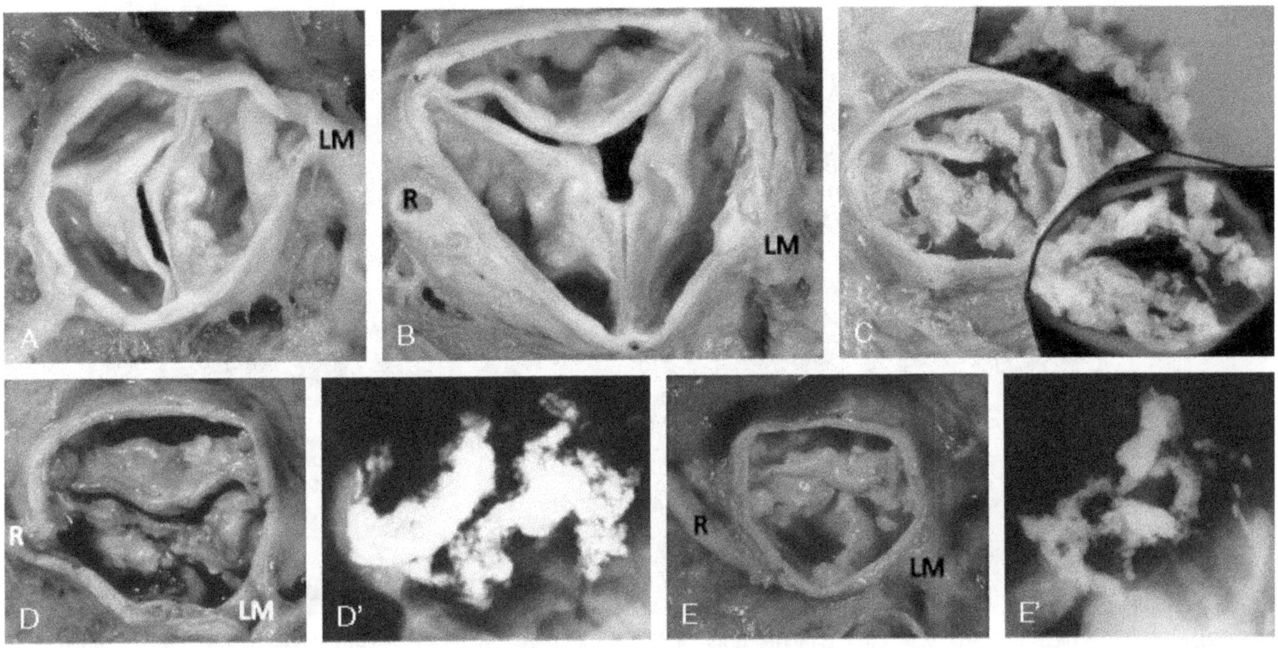

FIGURE 5. Stenotic bicuspid aortic valves in 5 patients, all of whom had undergone cardiac catheterization. The 2 cusps in the valve shown in (A) are located right and left, and all of the others are located anterior and posterior. Heavy calcific deposits are present in each valve. A, Valve belonging to a 65-year-old woman who died from cancer of the breast. She never had evidence of cardiac dysfunction. The heart at necropsy weighed 410 g. The transvalvular peak systolic pressure gradient was 25 mm Hg. LM = left main coronary artery. B, Valve in a 77-year-old man who had evidence of severe heart failure. The peak transvalvular systolic pressure gradient was 50 mm Hg. The left main coronary artery was severely narrowed, and the left ventricular ejection fraction was 40%. The heart weighed 570 g and the left ventricular wall was free of foci of necrosis and fibrosis. R = right coronary artery. C, Valve in a 37-year-old man who died suddenly in a cardiac clinic of a major hospital. He had periodic chest pain and exertional dyspnea for nearly 2 years. The peak transvalvular systolic pressure gradient was 50 mm Hg. Not only was the aortic valve heavily calcified, but also the mitral annulus was as well. The coronary arteries were insignificantly narrowed. D and D′, Heavily calcified aortic valve in a 67-year-old man who had severe angina pectoris and a 72 mm Hg peak systolic pressure gradient across the aortic valve. He had cardiac arrest the night before planned aortic valve replacement. At necropsy, the heart weighed 680 g and the heart was devoid of foci of necrosis and fibrosis. E and E′, Heavily calcified valve in a 61-year-old man who died suddenly. Earlier, the peak transvalvular systolic pressure gradient was 100 mm Hg. The heart weighed 530 g.

also were excluded. The origin of the 218 patients included in the present study is shown in the flow chart of Figure 1. The decades in which the patients were studied at necropsy are shown in Figure 2.

Means, standard deviations, and percentages were calculated to describe the study cohort. Differences in demographic, clinical, and morphologic details were tested using a 2-tailed t-test with equal variance in Microsoft Excel 2007 (Microsoft, Redmond, WA).

RESULTS

Frequency of Unicuspid and Bicuspid Aortic Valves

Of the 218 patients, 28 (13%) had unicuspid aortic valves and 190 (87%) had bicuspid aortic valves (Table 2). The men (80% of the total) at death ranged in age from 21 to 89 years (mean, 54 ± 15 yr) and the women (20% of the total), from 21 to 87 years (mean, 59 ± 15 yr). Of the 28 unicuspid valves, 26 (93%) were in men and 2 (7%) were in women; of the 190 bicuspid aortic valves, 78% were in men and 22% were in women. Thus, of the congenitally malformed aortic valves in men, 85% were bicuspid and 15% were unicuspid; in the women, 95% were bicuspid and 5% were unicuspid.

Age and Race

The ages of patients with unicuspid and bicuspid aortic valves differed significantly ($p < 0.02$): 48 ± 15 years in the unicuspid group and 56 ± 15 years in the bicuspid group (Table 2). The mean age of patients with stenotic valves was greater than that of patients with normally functioning valves before IE occurred (age 59 ± 14 yr vs. 48 ± 16 yr, respectively; $p < 0.0001$) (Table 3). Of the total patients, 89% were white, 8% were black, and 3%, other.

Aortic Valve Function

Of the 28 patients with unicuspid valves, 27 (96%) were stenotic and 1 (4%) was purely regurgitant (no apparent evidence of stenosis) (Figure 3, Table 3). Of the 190 bicuspid valves, 74 (39%) appeared to have functioned normally (until IE appeared and caused AR in 15 [20%] of the 74 patients) (Figure 4); 115 (61%) were clearly stenotic as judged morphologically (Figures 5–8); and 1 (<1%) was purely regurgitant without evidence at any time of IE. Thus, none of the 28 unicuspid valves appeared to have functioned normally, whereas 74 (39%) of the bicuspid valves (at least before IE altered that status) appeared to have functioned normally; only 2 valves (1 unicuspid, 1 bicuspid) were purely regurgitant (neither having

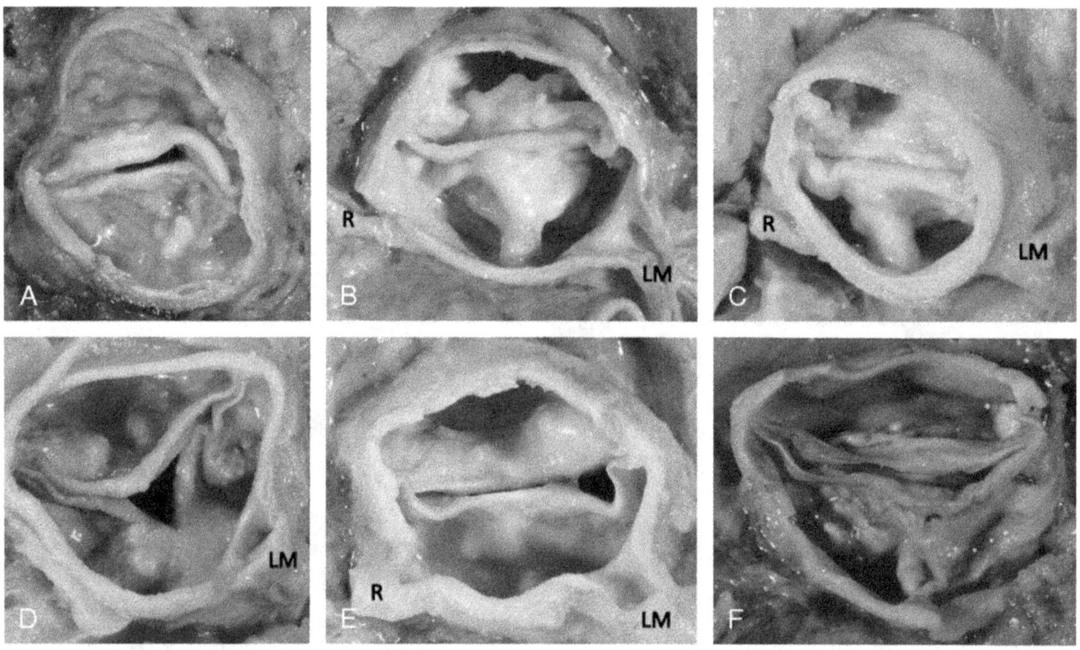

FIGURE 6. Stenotic bicuspid aortic valves in 6 patients, none of whom had undergone cardiac catheterization. At autopsy, the left ventricular walls in each were free of foci of necrosis and fibrosis. The cusps in each of these 6 patients are located anterior and posterior. A, Valve in a 69-year-old woman who died suddenly while driving. Necropsy disclosed a tear in the ascending aorta and an aortic dissection limited to the ascending and arch portions. The heart weighed 400 g. Both right and left circumflex coronary arteries were narrowed by atherosclerotic plaque. B, Valve in a 57-year-old woman in whom aortic valve stenosis was never diagnosed clinically. She presented to the hospital in severe pulmonary edema, and precordial examination did not disclose a murmur because of the chest noise. The coronary arteries were insignificantly narrowed. LM = left main coronary artery; R = right coronary artery. C, Valve in a 56-year-old woman who died suddenly after running up a flight of stairs. Previously she had fainted on 2 occasions during exertion, the first time was 10 months before she died. She never went to a physician and was not known to have medical problems. At autopsy, the heart weighed 380 g. D, Valve in a 62-year-old man who had nonfatal cardiac arrest 5 months before death and severe acute heart failure beginning 14 days before death, which progressively worsened. The patient weighed >135 kg and had considerable pulmonary hypertension (pulmonary artery pressure was 70/30 mm Hg). He also developed ventricular tachycardia. His heart weighed 900 g. E, Valve in a 48-year-old man who died suddenly while eating. At autopsy, there was no evidence of aspiration. The heart weighed 540 g. F, Valve in a 56-year-old man who had evidence of heart failure during his last 3 years of life. He died suddenly. The heart weighed 670 g and the coronary arteries were devoid of atherosclerotic plaques.

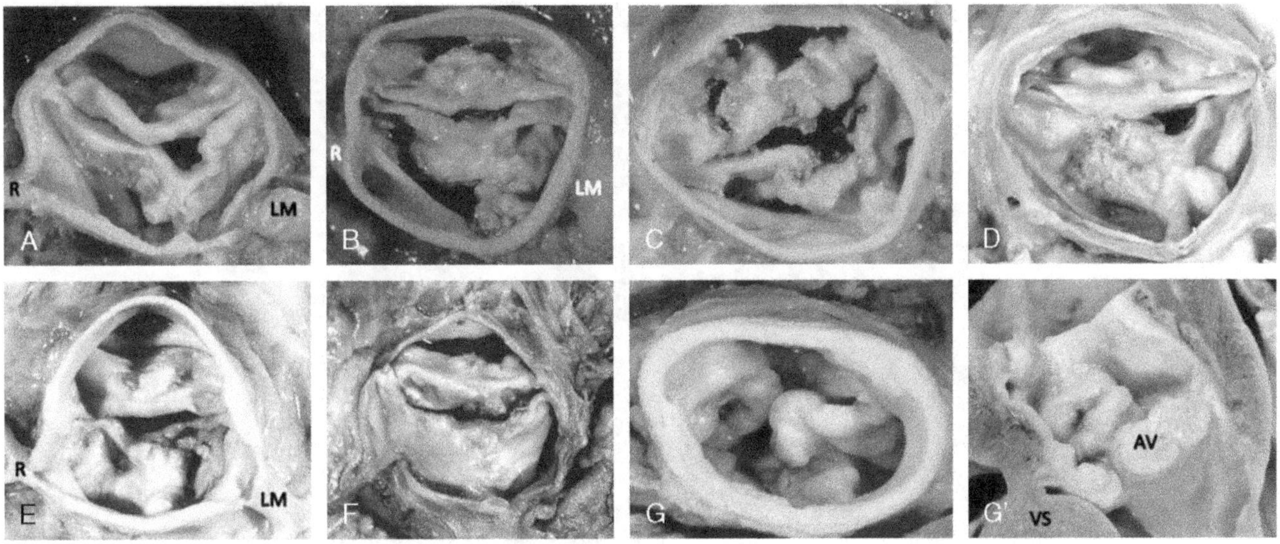

FIGURE 7. Stenotic aortic valves in 7 patients, none of whom had cardiac catheterization but all of whom had morphologic evidence of severe aortic valve stenosis. A, Valve in a 66-year-old man who died suddenly but also had severe coronary disease. A healed myocardial infarct was present in the left ventricular wall. LM = left main coronary artery; R = right coronary artery. B, Valve in an 81-year-old man who also had considerable coronary disease, a healed left ventricular myocardial infarct, and severe angina pectoris. The heart weighed 750 g. C, Valve in a 60-year-old man who died of heart failure. Heavy calcific deposits were found in the aortic valve cusps, the mitral valve annulus, and the major epicardial coronary arteries. At necropsy, he had both a healed and an acute myocardial infarct. His coronary arteries were severely narrowed. His heart weighed 1050 g. D, Valve in a 64-year-old woman who developed exertional dyspnea 4 months before death and the heart failure progressed. At necropsy the coronary arteries were essentially devoid of atherosclerotic plaques and there were no foci of necrosis or fibrosis in the ventricular walls. The heart weighed approximately 500 g. Additionally, the patient had evidence of pulmonary fibrosis. E, Heart in a 51-year-old man who died suddenly while taking a shower. At necropsy, the heart weighed 800 g, the coronary arteries were devoid of plaques, and the ventricular walls were free of foci of necrosis or fibrosis. F, Valve in a 69-year-old woman who had evidence of heart failure intermittently for 2 years but never chest pain or syncope. She was hospitalized for evaluation and found to have AS but she refused to have cardiac catheterization or operation and died of worsening heart failure. At necropsy, the aortic valve, mitral annulus, and epicardial coronary arteries were heavily calcified. The coronary arteries were severely narrowed but the left ventricular wall was devoid of foci of necrosis or fibrosis. G and G′, Aortic valve from above and from the side in a 23-year-old man who died suddenly while walking home after playing tennis for 2 hours. The heart weighed 590 g and a small scar was present near the apex of the left ventricle. The coronary arteries were devoid of plaques. AV = aortic valve; VS = ventricular septum.

IE). Thirty-four percent of the men and 37% of the women had normally functioning aortic valves; 65% of the men and 63% of the women had stenotic valves, and 2 men and no women had intrinsically purely regurgitant valves.

Frequency of IE

Of the 25 patients with active IE, 16 (64%) involved a previously normally functioning aortic valve (Figures 9–13) and 9 (36%), a previously stenotic valve (Figures 14–18, Table 4).

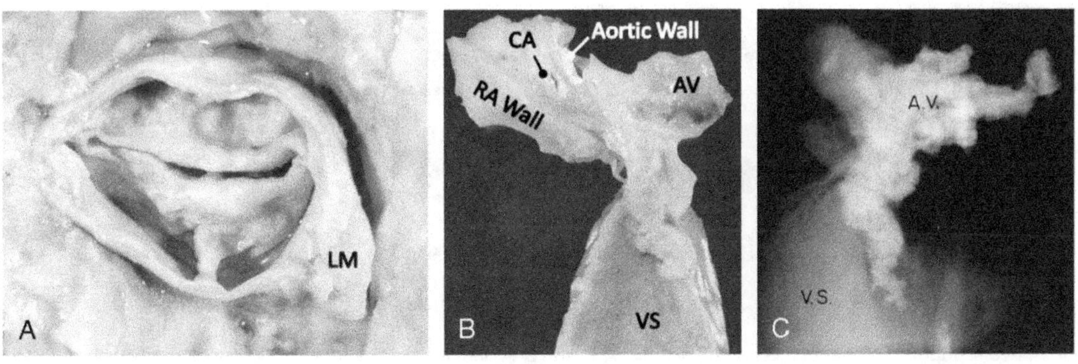

FIGURE 8. Stenotic bicuspid aortic valve. A, Aortic valve from above in a 59-year-old man who died of heart failure. The left ventricular peak systolic pressure gradient across the aortic valve was 45 mm Hg by catheterization. A raphe is present in the anterior cusp. LM = left main coronary artery. B, Longitudinal section through the right atrial (RA) wall, coronary artery (CA), aortic valve (AV), and ventricular septum (VS) showing heavy calcific deposits in the aortic valve and in the apex of the muscular ventricular septum obliterating the AV bundle and also the left bundle branch. C, Radiograph of the same longitudinal section showing heavy calcific deposits again in the aortic valve, membranous ventricular septum, and in the area of the AV bundle and left bundle branch. An electrocardiogram showed complete heart block.

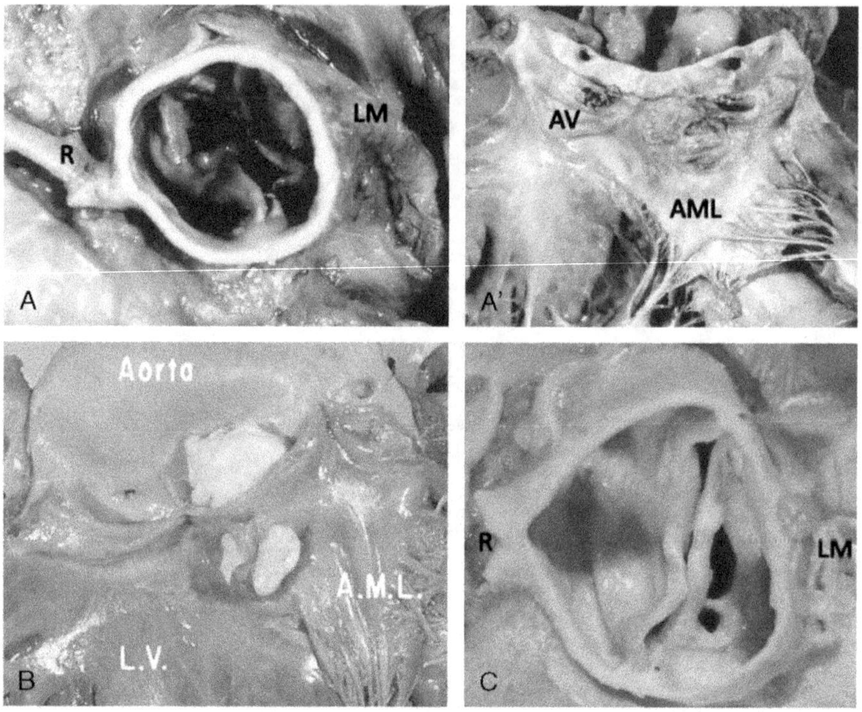

FIGURE 9. Infective endocarditis involving a bicuspid valve. A and A′, Aortic valve from above and after opening showing perforations in each of the 2 cusps and vegetative material on the ventricular surface of each cusp and bordering the perforations. The patient was a 39-year-old man who died suddenly on the golf course. His heart weighed 1010 g and he had evidence of severe AR. In addition to evidence of both active and healed infection on the aortic valve, several chordae tendineae from the mitral valve had ruptured due to dislodgment of vegetative material from the aortic valve. The ventricle, despite its severe dilatation, was devoid of foci of necrosis and fibrosis in its wall. Three months before his sudden death he underwent cardiac catheterization. The left ventricular pressure was 140/20 and simultaneous aortic pressure, 140/38 mm Hg. AML = anterior mitral leaflet; AV = aortic valve; LM = left main coronary artery; R = right coronary artery. B, Valve opened in a 33-year-old man who had had IE that healed and left severe AR thereafter. Cotton has been placed in the posterior (noncoronary) cusp. One of the 2 cusps was perforated by the infection, and heart failure was the consequence. He died of severe heart failure, becoming emaciated. The heart weighed 430 g. No foci of ventricular wall necrosis or fibrosis were present at autopsy. LV = left ventricle. C, Valve in a 47-year-old man who had active IE in the past that had healed. He died suddenly from a skull fracture when a horse kicked him in the head. In addition to the bicuspid aortic valve he had a congenitally bicuspid pulmonic valve that had functioned normally. His heart weighed 590 g. The regurgitation was due mainly to the perforations in 1 of the 2 cusps.

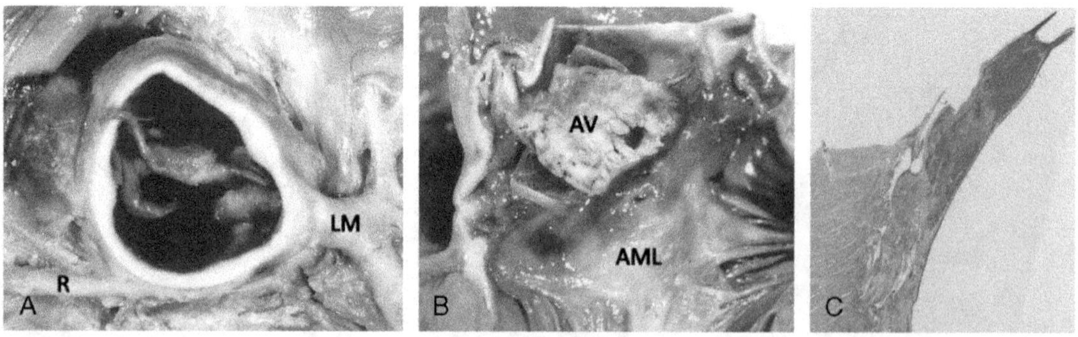

FIGURE 10. Active IE superimposed on a congenitally bicuspid valve. A, Valve from above in a 22-year-old man, an opiate addict who developed *Staphylococcus epidermidis* endocarditis several weeks before death. The cusps are located anterior and posterior. The infection involves mainly the anterior cusp which is perforated by the vegetative material. LM = left main coronary artery; R = right coronary artery. B, Longitudinal view of the vegetation that has spread to the aortic wall causing a ring abscess in it. AML = anterior mitral leaflet; AV = aortic valve. C, Photomicrograph of a histology section of a left ventricular papillary muscle that is completely necrotic. The epicardial coronary arteries were entirely normal. The patient developed severe AR with resulting severe heart failure. At necropsy, the heart weighed 670 g. A mycotic aneurysm also developed in the membranaceous portion of the ventricular septum protruding into the right side of the heart. (Hematoxylin and eosin stain, 5× magnification.)

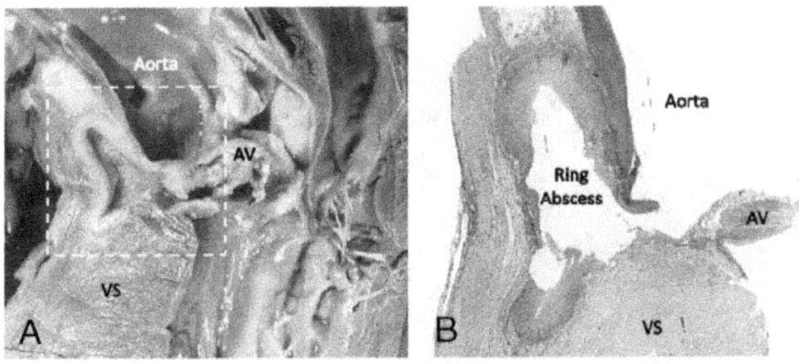

FIGURE 11. Active IE superimposed on a previously normally functioning bicuspid aortic valve. A, Longitudinal view of an aortic valve showing massive destruction of the cusps with a ring abscess adjacent to the aorta within the ventricular septum in a 41-year-old man. The valve was made severely incompetent by the infection. AV = aortic valve; VS = ventricular septum. B, Photomicrograph showing an incompetent aortic valve cusp, wall of aorta and ring abscess that separates the aorta from the left ventricle. VS = ventricular septum. The valve cusps were oriented right and left. This patient developed alpha streptococcus IE following a dental procedure approximately 2 months before the onset of symptoms or approximately 4 months before death. During the infection he developed evidence of severe AR. When hospitalized 20 days before death his blood pressure was 100/0 mm Hg and he was in pulmonary edema. He died the night before scheduled aortic valve replacement, which almost certainly would have been fruitless. His heart weighed 500 g. The residual aortic valve cusps contained minimal calcific deposits. (Movat stain, 5 × magnification.)

Additionally, 6 patients had both histories of and morphologic residual damage from active IE that had healed. Of the 31 total cases of IE, 3 (10%) involved a unicuspid valve (3 [11%] of the 28 unicuspid valves) and 28 (90%) involved a bicuspid valve (28 [15%] of the 190 bicuspid valves). Of the 31 cases, 26 (84%) were men (15% of total men), and 5 (16%) were women (12% of total women). Various clinical and morphologic findings in the 31 patients with active and healed IE are summarized in Table 4.

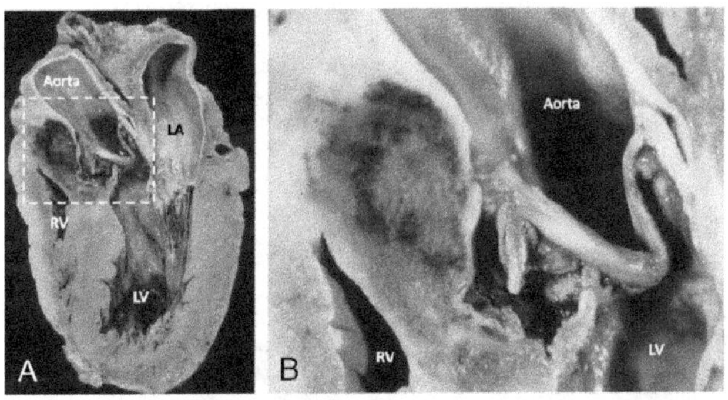

FIGURE 12. Active IE involving a bicuspid aortic valve that had probably functioned normally before the infection. A, Longitudinal view of a heart showing a huge ring abscess anteriorly in a 36-year-old woman who had multiple myeloma and Turner syndrome. LA = left atrium; LV = left ventricle; RV = right ventricle. B, Close-up of the ring abscess. The cusps are slightly thickened by fibrous tissue and were oriented right and left. The patient was in her usual state of health until approximately 6 weeks before death, when she developed abdominal pain and was found to have a large spleen. A bone marrow biopsy was done and it was consistent with multiple myeloma. Several days before death she lost consciousness and was hospitalized. Blood cultures grew alpha streptococcus. She died shortly thereafter. At autopsy, the cardiac infection was limited to the aortic valve and adjacent para-aortic areas. The spleen weighed 1850 g and the liver, 2600 g. The heart weighed 460 g and was devoid of myocardial lesions except in the area adjacent to the aortic valve.

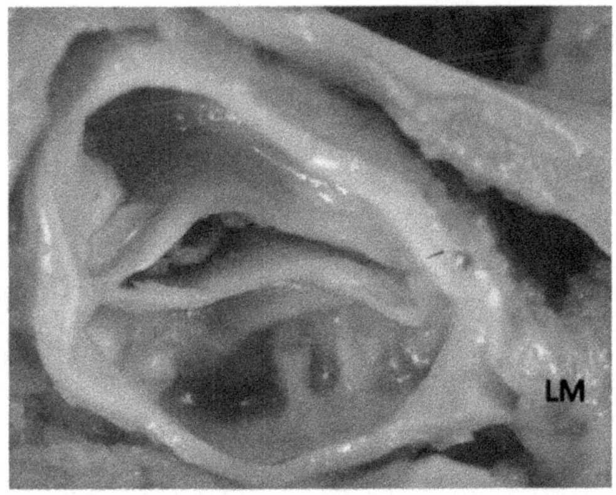

FIGURE 13. Active IE involving a normally functioning bicuspid aortic valve. View of the aortic valve from above showing vegetation between the 2 cusps but no vegetative material on the aortic aspect of either cusp. The patient was a 52-year-old man who had undergone bone marrow transplantation 1 month before death because of myelodysplastic syndrome. After the bone marrow transplant he never left the hospital. Infective endocarditis was never diagnosed clinically. Necropsy disclosed vegetation on each of the 2 cusps of the bicuspid valve, and the cusps were located anterior and posterior. The heart weighed 610 g. LM = left main coronary artery.

Hemodynamic Data

Of the 218 patients, hemodynamic data were available in 36 patients (17%): 34 had AS, with peak transvalvular gradients ranging from 11 to 148 mm Hg (mean, 69; median, 69 mm Hg).

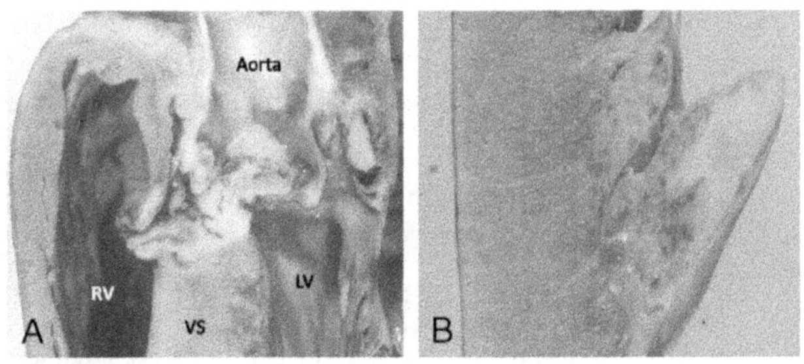

FIGURE 14. Active IE. A, Longitudinal cut of the aortic valve and adjacent structures showing severe destruction of the aortic valve cusps and large ring abscesses both anteriorly burrowing into the right ventricle (RV) and posteriorly pushing toward the left atrium in a 30-year-old man who was a habitual fingernail biter to the extent that his fingernail area would bleed. X-ray of the heart at necropsy showed calcific deposits in the aortic valve. LV = left ventricle. VS = ventricular septum. B, A left ventricular papillary muscle that is necrotic due to extremely diminished profusion of the left ventricle. The epicardial coronary arteries were normal. The patient was hospitalized 16 days before death because of fever, chills, malaise, and myalgia. Several blood cultures grew *Staphylococcus aureus*. He developed several signs typical of active IE. An electrocardiogram showed right bundle branch block, and an echocardiogram suggested a bicuspid aortic valve. The heart at autopsy weighed 560 g.

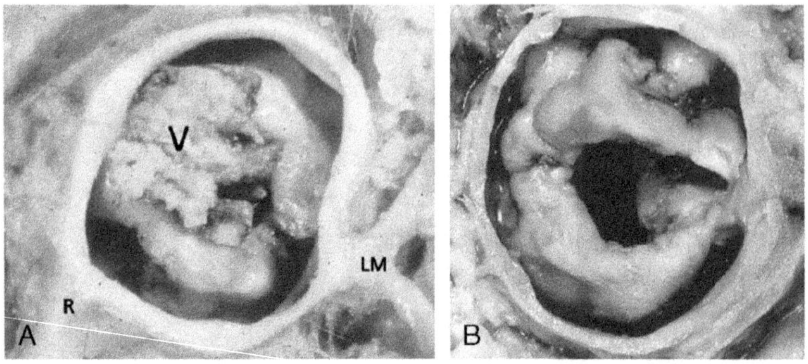

FIGURE 15. Active IE superimposed on a stenotic unicuspid unicommissural aortic valve. A, View of the valve from above showing vegetation (V) further narrowing the orifice. LM = left main coronary artery; R = right coronary artery. B, View of the valve after excising the vegetation showing the underlying stenotic valve with heavy calcific deposits. The patient was a 35-year-old man, an opiate addict who became ill 6 weeks before death, including the last 4 weeks in a hospital. Despite septic emboli in the kidneys and spleen, blood cultures throughout his hospitalization were negative. At necropsy, the heart weighed 550 g.

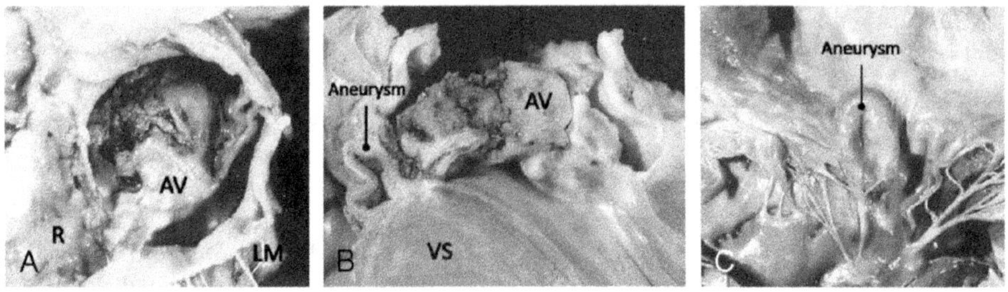

FIGURE 16. Active IE superimposed on a stenotic bicuspid aortic valve. A, Aortic valve from above showing vegetation superimposed on the right cusp of a congenitally bicuspid aortic valve in a 67-year-old man who was known to have AS and had some evidence of heart failure for at least a year before his final illness, which was rapidly progressing heart failure. Calcific deposits are present in both right and left cusps but the vegetative material involves the right cusp much more than the left. AV = aortic valve; LM = left main coronary artery; R = right coronary artery. B, Longitudinal section across the aortic valve showing the large vegetation involving mainly the right cusp with rather heavy calcific deposits in the left cusp. A ring abscess is also present in the base of the aorta. VS = ventricular septum. C, View of the tricuspid valve, right atrium, and right ventricle showing an aneurysm of the membranaceous ventricular septum bulging into the right side of the heart. Blood cultures were all positive for alpha hemolytic streptococcus, and the patient was treated with penicillin. During the infection his electrocardiogram changed from prolonged P-R interval to complete heart block. Not only did he have evidence of AS, but mitral regurgitation also developed during the infection. This is an example of IE superimposed on a heavily calcified stenotic aortic valve. The infection rapidly spread to the soft tissue both above and below the valve creating a ring abscess of the aorta and an aneurysm of the membranaceous ventricular septum.

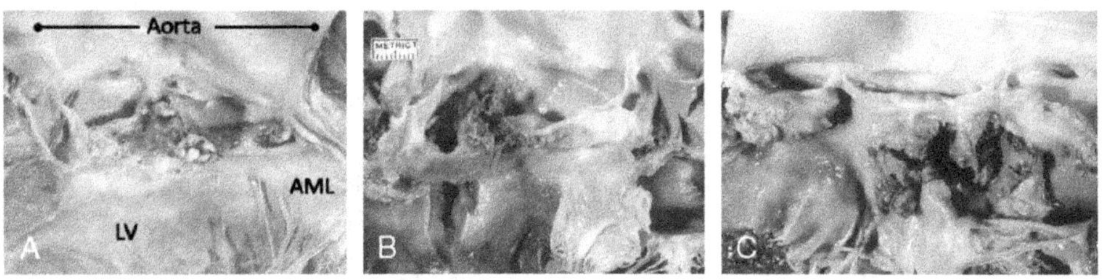

FIGURE 17. Active IE: opened aortic valves exposing vegetations that have destroyed the 2 aortic valve cusps to varying degrees. A, Valve in a 35-year-old man who had alpha streptococcus IE with a ring abscess and severe AR. This patient was an opiate addict who probably had infection in the past that healed because the heart at necropsy weighed 760 g. The cusps are located anterior and posterior, and a raphe is present in the anterior cusp. The infection caused severe AR. AML = anterior mitral leaflet; LV = left ventricle. B, Valve in a 60-year-old man. The cusps are located anterior and posterior, and vegetative material is particularly heavy in the area of the raphe. This patient had the triad of active IE, meningitis, and pneumonitis. The vegetative material had burrowed into the aortic wall causing a large ring abscess and complete heart block. The patient was a habitual alcoholic. The last episode of IE produced acute symptoms beginning 7 days before death. Blood cultures grew *Streptococcus pneumoniae.* Complete heart block developed 2 days before death. Six months before death he had undergone cardiac catheterization because of severe AR: an 11 mm Hg peak transvalvular pressure gradient and severe AR were found. C, Bicuspid valve in a 45-year-old man with pre-existing aortic valve stenosis who was hospitalized 12 days before death because of confusion, fever, and leukocytosis. Echocardiogram showed vegetation on the aortic valve, and blood cultures grew *Streptococcus milleri.* Computed tomogram (CT) disclosed multiple cerebral infarcts. The patient weighed >135 kg. At autopsy, the heart weighed 920 g. The 2 aortic valve cusps were calcified. The vegetative material had burrowed into the right ventricular cavity. Emboli were present in the brain. Additionally, there was diffuse fibrinous pericarditis. Both left ventricular papillary muscles were necrotic in the absence of significant coronary disease. Both aortic valve cusps were perforated by the vegetation.

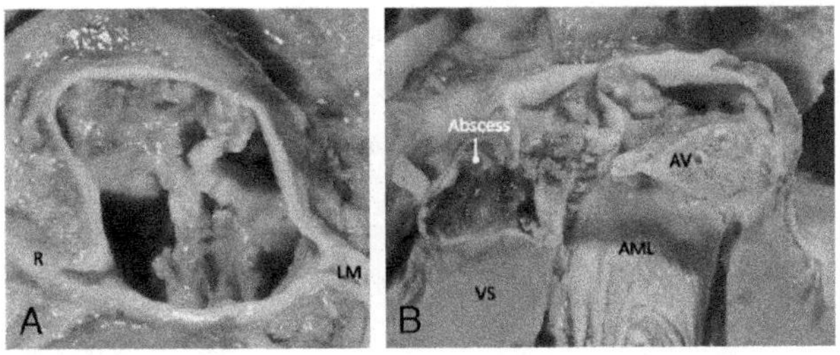

FIGURE 18. Active IE superimposed on a heavily calcified stenotic bicuspid aortic valve. A, Valve from above with vegetative material involving the cuspal margins with underlying heavy calcific deposits. The cusps are located right and left. LM = left main coronary artery; R = right coronary artery. B, Longitudinal cut of the aortic valve area showing destruction by vegetative material of 1 cusp with extension into the ventricular septum (VS) producing a large ring abscess. The aortic valve (AV) is heavily calcified and was quite stenotic. At autopsy, the heart weighed 850 g. The patient was a 54-year-old man who was known to have a precordial murmur for at least 10 years. He developed exertional dyspnea 2 years before death. Cardiac catheterization 2 months before death disclosed severe AS. The aortic valve could not be crossed by the catheter, and he was discharged to have his carious teeth extracted before planned aortic valve replacement. He developed alpha streptococcus endocarditis with onset of symptoms 23 days before death. While being treated on the ward he had sudden fatal cardiac arrest. Both left ventricular papillary muscles were necrotic. AML = anterior mitral leaflet.

TABLE 4. Patients Having Infective Endocarditis (IE) on a Unicuspid or Bicuspid Aortic Valve (n = 31)

	Infective Endocarditis	
Variable	Active n = 25 (81%)	Healed n = 6 (19%)
Unicuspid aortic valve	2	1
Bicuspid aortic valve	23	5
Aortic valve function before IE		
Normal	16	4
Stenosis ± regurgitation	9	2
Pure regurgitation	0	0
Aortic valve function after IE		
Normal	5	0
Stenosis ± regurgitation	9	2
Pure regurgitation*	11	4
Predisposing factors		
Intravenous opiate use	5	0
Alcoholism	4	1
Dental procedure	4	1
Stepped on a nail	1†	0
Habitual fingernail biter	1	0
Heart block		
First degree	1	0
Right bundle branch	1	0
Complete	2	0
Infected aneurysm		
Cerebral	3	0
Aorta	4	2

*The 15 patients with pure aortic regurgitation as a result of infective endocarditis had normally functioning aortic valves prior to infection.

†Patient is also an alcoholic.

TABLE 5. Men With Bicuspid Aortic Valves and Coronary Artery Bypass Grafting (n = 12)

Patient	Aortic Valve Function*	Age (Years)	Total Number of CABG Procedures	Total Number of Distal Anastamoses	Interval From Last (First) CABG to Death (Months)	Heart Weight (g)	Cause of Cardiac Death
1	Normal	43	1	3	0	530	CABG
2	Normal	62	1	4	<1	470	CABG
3	Normal	63	1	4	110	690	CAD-IC
4	Normal	63	2	—	<1 (—)	590	CABG
5	Normal	69	1	2	108	700	CAD-IC
6	Normal	71	2	7	<1 (84)	650	CABG
7	Stenotic	49	1	2	96	525	CAD-IC
8	Stenotic	53	2	3	0 (132)	460	CABG
9	Stenotic	56	1	2	17	475	AS-SD
10	Stenotic	58	1	—	2	—	CABG
11	Stenotic	68	1	4	17	550	CAD-IC
12	Stenotic	69	2	4	48 (132)	760	CAD-SD

Abbreviations: AS = aortic stenosis, CABG = coronary artery bypass grafting, CAD = coronary artery disease, IC = ischemic cardiomyopathy, SD = sudden death, — = no information available.

*Prior to infective endocarditis.

TABLE 6. Causes or Modes of Death in Patients Studied at Necropsy Having a Unicuspid or Bicuspid Aotic Valve (n = 218)

	Aortic Valve Function Prior to Infective Endocarditis				
Variable	**Normal n = 74 (34%)**	**Stenosis n = 142 (65%)**	**Pure Regurgitation n = 2 (1%)**	**Total n = 218 (100%)**	
Cardiac					
Aortic valve disease					
Heart failure	0	62		62	124 (57%)
Infective endocarditis					
Active	16*	9		25	
Healed	4†	2‡		6	
Sudden	0	21	1§	22	
Cardiac catheterization	0	7		7	
Anesthesia induction for aortic valve replacement	0	1		1	
Ruptured sinus of Valsalva aneurysm	1	0		1	
Coronary artery disease					
Acute myocardial infarction	2	5		7	25 (11%)
Ischemic cardiomyopathy	3	2		5	
Sudden	3	4		7	
Early post coronary bypass¶	4	2		6	
Other					
Hypertrophic cardiomyopathy (sudden)	1	0		1	
SUBTOTAL	34	115	1	150 (69%)	
Non-cardiac vascular					
Ascending aortic tear (±dissection)	12**	4	1	17	
Cerebrovascular accident	0	1		1	
Pulmonary embolism	1	0		1	
Early postop after vascular surgery	0	3‖		3	
SUBTOTAL	13	8	1	22 (10%)	
Non-cardiac non-vascular					
Cancer	14	3		17	
Suicide	2	0		2	
Trauma	3#	0		3	
Renal failure	1	3		4	
Pancreatitis (alcoholism)	1	0		1	
Gastrointestinal hemorrhage	0	1		1	
Food aspiration	0	1		1	
Hypothermia	0	1		1	
Cirrhosis	1	0		1	
Parenchymal lung disease	1	1		2	
Parkinson's disease	1	0		1	
Early postop after bowel surgery	0	2		2	
SUBTOTAL	24	12	0	36 (17%)	
Cause unclear					
Sudden death outside hospital, cause unclear	2	0		2	
Unknown	1	7		8	
SUBTOTAL	3	7	0	10 (5%)	

*The aortic valve appeared to have been normal before the active infective endocarditis (IE) appeared. Of the 16 patients, all but 1 died of the active infection; the remaining patient developed IE after a bone marrow transplant for myelodysplastic syndrome, and the aortic valve appeared funtionally normal despite the infection.

†The IE caused perforation in 1 or both aortic valve cusps in 3 of these 4 patients leading to severe aortic regurgitation (AR) in each. The remaining patient had no cuspal perforations, but had a prolapsed aortic valve, several ruptured chords of anterior mitral leaflet, and a saccular aneurysm of ascending aorta causing residual AR from IE; he died suddenly; he also had coarctation of the aorta.

‡The degree of stenosis probably was worsened by the superimposed IE which healed in each.

§Patient had massive cardiomegaly: heart weight 920 g. Of the 218 patients, 5 (2%) had hearts weighing >900 g. One had AR secondary to healed cuspal perforation from IE; 3 others had severely stenotic aortic valves, and of these 3, 1 had superimposed IE.

‖One patient died 1 day after resection of abdominal aortic aneurysm; 1 patient died 3 days after femoral-popliteal bypass grafting; 1 patient died 6 hours after axillo-femoral bypass grafting.

¶A total of 12 patients (6%) had coronary artery bypass grafting (CABG): 6 died within 2 months of the last CABG operation and are included here; of the other 6 patients having had CABG, all died late: 2 with ischemic cardiomyopathy (IC) and a normally functioning aortic valve; 2 with IC and a stenotic aortic valve; 1 died suddenly secondary to aortic stenosis, and 1 with a stenotic aortic valve died suddenly secondary to coronary artery disease.

#One patient, a habitual alcoholic, died from injuries in a single-car accident; the other 2 from broken necks from falls. None had significant coronary disease.

**One patient died during operative repair of ascending aortic dissection, and another, 3 weeks after operative repair for dissection.

The peak transvalvular gradient was ≤50 mm Hg in 12 patients (35%) and >50 mm Hg in 22 patients (65%). Neither of the 2 patients with normally functioning aortic valves had a gradient across the valve. The heart weights in the patients with hemodynamically confirmed AS ranged from 410 to 880 g (mean, 629; median, 655 g).

Coronary Artery Bypass Grafting

Twelve (6%) (all men) of the 218 patients had coronary artery bypass grafting (CABG), in 4 patients on 2 occasions (Table 5). In none of the 16 CABG operations on those 12 patients was a procedure performed on the aortic valve. At necropsy, the bicuspid aortic valve appeared to have functioned normally in 6, and to be stenotic in the other 6. Two of the latter 6 had CABG twice. The presence of AS in these latter 6 patients was either not diagnosed at the time of CABG or the degree of AS was not considered severe enough to warrant aortic valve replacement at the time of CABG.

Causes of Death

Causes of death are divided into 4 major groups: cardiac, noncardiac vascular, noncardiac and nonvascular, and cause unclear (Table 6). Of the 218 patients, death was attributed to aortic valve disease in 124 patients (57%), to the consequences of coronary arterial atherosclerosis in 25 (11%), and to hypertrophic cardiomyopathy in 1. Thus, death was attributed to cardiac disease in 150 (69%) of the 218 patients. Death in 22 patients (10%) was attributed to noncardiac vascular causes, and in 36 patients (17%) to neither cardiac nor vascular causes. Among the 22 patients with noncardiac vascular causes of death, 17 (8% of the total) died of tears in the ascending aorta with resulting fatal hemopericardium; 14 had tears with dissection and 3 had tears without dissection[86] (Table 7; Figure 19).

Reasons Aortic Valve Operation Was Not Performed

We considered the reasons an aortic valve operation was not performed in these patients (Table 8). Of the 131 patients with AS without superimposed IE, 25 patients (19%) died suddenly outside the hospital, and most of them previously were asymptomatic. Another 32 patients (24%) died before 1970, a period when aortic valve replacement essentially was limited to only those with severe symptoms and severe AS. Most patients with acute IE were not operated on because their physicians believed aortic valve replacement to be fruitless in the circumstances.

Heart Weight and Its Relation to Aortic Valve Structure, Valve Function, and Sex

Heart weight data were available in 178 (82%) of the 218 patients (Tables 2, 3, and 9). The mean heart weights were greater in patients with unicuspid aortic valves than in those with bicuspid aortic valves (603 ± 143 g vs. 551 ± 164 g, respectively; $p = 0.14$); in patients with stenotic compared to those with normally functioning valves (598 ± 152 g vs. 477 ± 148 g, respectively; $p < 0.0001$); and in men compared to women (586 ± 156 g [270–1050 g] vs. 433 ± 136 g [170–730], respectively; $p < 0.0001$).

Orientation of the 2 Cusps and Presence of a Raphe Among Patients With Bicuspid Valves and Relation to Valve Complication

In 69% of the valves, 1 cusp was located anterior, and the other posterior, such that both coronary arteries arose from the anterior cusp; in 31% of cases, 1 cusp was right and the other, left, such that 1 coronary artery arose from 1 cusp and the other

TABLE 7. Patients Studied at Necropsy Having a Unicuspid or Bicuspid Aortic Valve and Tear in Ascending Aorta (n = 17)

Patient	Aortic Valve Function*	Age (Years)	Gender	Heart Weight (g)	Number of Aortic Valve Cusps	Aortic Valve Orientation	Raphe Present	SH
Aortic Tear With Dissection								
1	Normal	21	M	450	2	A/P	+	+
2	Normal	30	M	410	2	A/P	+	—
3†	Normal	48	M	—	2	A/P	+	+
4	Normal	52	M	530	2	A/P	+	+
5†	Normal	57	M	—	2	A/P	+	+
6	Normal	62	M	690	2	A/P	0	—
7	Normal	67	M	—	2	R/L	+	+
8	Normal	69	F	—	2	A/P	+	0
9	Normal	71	F	430	2	A/P	+	—
10	Regurgitant	32	M	470	1	—	—	—
11	Stenotic	25	M	610	1	—	—	—
12	Stenotic	69	F	400	2	A/P	0	—
13	Stenotic	70	M	390	2	R/L	+	+
14	Stenotic	82	M	590	2	A/P	+	+
Aortic Tear Without Dissection								
15	Normal	21	M	450	2	A/P	+	—
16	Normal	32	F	310	2	A/P	+	—
17	Normal	32	M	510	2	A/P	0	—

Abbreviations: — = no information available or not applicable, 0 = absent, + = present, A/P = anterior/posterior, R/L = right/left, SH = systemic hypertension by history.

*Prior to infective endocarditis.

†Patient had operative intervention for acute aortic dissection.

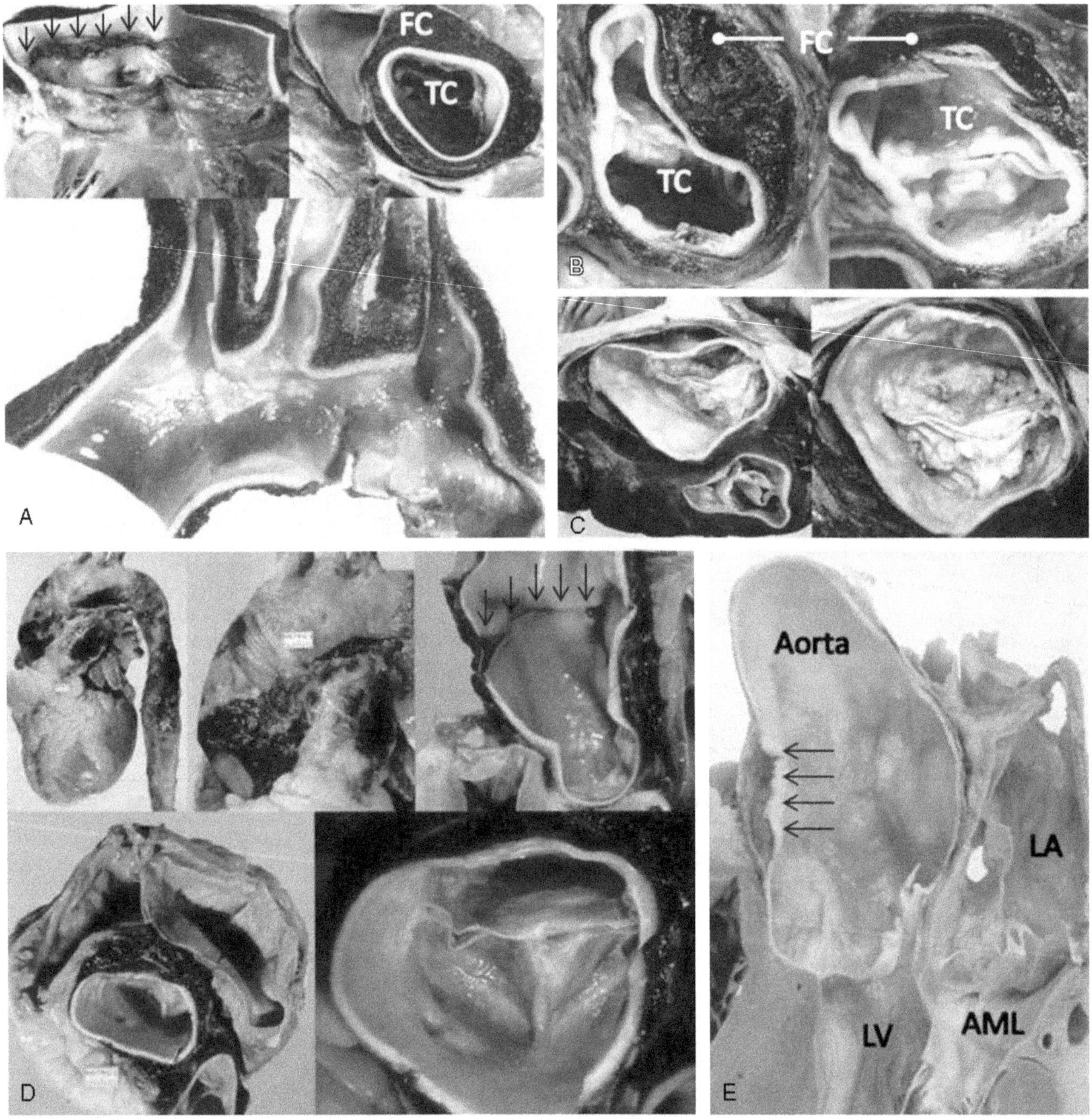

FIGURE 19. Acute aortic dissection with tear (arrows) in ascending aorta in 5 patients with congenitally bicuspid aortic valves. All patients died from rupture of the false channel (FC) into the pericardial sac. A, Views of the opened bicuspid aortic valve and a transverse tear just above that with hematoma in the false channel of ascending aorta and in the false channel of each of the arch arteries and in a portion of descending thoracic aorta. This woman had Turner syndrome. The aortic valve had functioned normally. The heart weighed 310 g. The medial dissection of aorta extended into its adventitia and then into the adventitia of the pulmonary trunk, which shares a common adventitia with the aorta. TC = true channel. B, Two views of hematoma in the false channel just above the aortic valve (left) and at the level of the aortic valve (right). The true channel is indented by the hematoma in the false channel. The bicuspid valve is calcified and stenotic. The heart weighed 385 g. C, Stenotic bicuspid valve with a hematoma in the false channel and fatal rupture into the pericardial sac. The valve is stenotic. Symptoms of the acute dissection began 36 hours before death. The dissection was limited to ascending aorta. A large tear was present in the distal ascending aorta. The heart weighed 585 g. D, Bicuspid valve that functioned normally in a 69-year-old woman who developed chest and neck pain a few hours before dying suddenly in the hospital. The dissection was limited to ascending aorta. The dissection extended into the adventitia of aorta and then into the adventitia of pulmonary trunk. E, Longitudinal view of ascending aorta, left atrium (LA), and left ventricle (LV) showing a false channel in the anterior of the aorta just above the 1 aortic valve commissure. The patient had an aortic isthmus coarctation that had been resected earlier in life. The proximal ascending aorta had a diameter of 8.5 cm. The heart weighed 690 g. The bicuspid aortic valve was devoid of calcium and appeared to have functioned normally. AML = anterior mitral leaflet.

TABLE 8. Reasons Patients With Aortic Stenosis or Pure Aortic Regurgitation Did Not Undergo Aortic Valve Replacement (Excludes 74 Patients With Normally Functioning Aortic Valves With or Without Superimposed Infective Endocarditis)

Variable	AS (n = 142)	AR Without IE (n = 2)
Not diagnosed during life	43	1
Active infective endocarditis	9	0
Diagnosed clinically but		
Died before 1962 (before AVR established)	5	0
Severe heart failure/too sick to have AVR	23	0
Another condition preventing AVR	8	0
AVR planned but died before operation	10	1
Refused AVR	7	0
Refused cardiac catheterization	1	0
Death in the cardiac catheterization lab	7	0
AS not severe enough to warrant AVR or severity of AS not appreciated clinically	12	0
Reason unclear/died suddenly	5	0
Unknown	12	0

Abbreviations: AR = aortic regurgitation, AS = aortic stenosis, AVR = aortic valve replacement, IE = infective endocarditis.

TABLE 9. Comparison of Heart Weights According to Gender, and Structure and Function of the Congenitally Malformed Aortic Valve (n = 178*)

Variable	Heart Weight (g) Mean ± SD [Median] (Range), Number (%) of Enlarged Hearts†
Total	
Men (n = 146)	586 ± 156 [570] (270–1050), n = 127 (87%)
Women (n = 32)	433 ± 136 [413] (170–730), n = 21 (66%)
Valve structure	
Unicuspid	
Men (n = 23)	607 ± 144 [610] (320–880), n = 21 (91%)
Women (n = 1)	510, n = 1 (100%)
Bicuspid	
Men (n = 123)	582 ± 159 [550] (270–1050), n = 106 (86%)
Women (n = 31)	431 ± 138 [410] (170–730), n = 20 (65%)
Aortic valve function	
Aortic stenosis	
Men (n = 95)	622 ± 149 [610] (320–1050), n = 88 (93%)
Women (n = 20)	491 ± 130 [478] (300–730), n = 17 (85%)
Pure aortic regurgitation secondary to IE	
Men (n = 12)	583 ± 175 [545] (405–1010), n = 12 (100%)
Women (n = 3)	350, 400, 460, n = 2 (67%)
Unassociated with IE	
Men (n = 2)	920, 470, n = 2 (100%)
Women (n = 0)	—
Functionally normal	
Men (n = 37)	487 ± 120 [470] (270–700), n = 25 (68%)
Women (n = 9)	314 ± 81 [310] (170–430), n = 2 (22%)
Infective endocarditis	
Active	
Men (n = 21)	571 ± 147 [540] (375–920), n = 20 (95%)
Women (n = 4)	363 ± 93 [375] (240–460), n = 2 (50%)
Healed	
Men (n = 4)	670 ± 245 [620] (430–1010), n = 4 (100%)
Women (n = 1)	510, n = 1 (100%)

— = not applicable.

*Heart weights were only available in 178 (82%) of the 218 patients included in this study.

†Hearts weighing >350 g in women and >400 g in men.

coronary artery from the other cusp (Tables 3 and 10). A raphe (false commissure) was present in at least 83%: if the configuration of the cusps was anterior and posterior, the raphe, if present, was always in the anterior cusp; if the cusps were configured right and left, the raphe, if present, was always in the right cusp.

Associated Congenital Cardiovascular Anomalies

Six patients had aortic isthmic coarctation, with operative excision in 2 early in life; 5 patients had a congenitally bicuspid pulmonic valve, and 1 had a quadricuspid pulmonic valve, all of which functioned normally and otherwise were structurally normal; 1 patient had a parachute mitral valve or single papillary muscle syndrome (Shone syndrome); 2 patients had Turner syndrome; and 4 had a congenital coronary anomaly (Table 11). None of the coronary anomalies was clinically important.

DISCUSSION

We describe here the findings in 218 patients studied at necropsy with congenitally unicuspid (n = 28) or bicuspid (n = 190) aortic valves. Of the 4 major complications of this congenital anomaly—valve stenosis, pure valve regurgitation, valve infection, and aortic dilatation—most (142 [65%]) had AS including 27 (96%) of the 28 patients with unicuspid valves and 115 (61%) of the 190 patients with bicuspid valves. Of the 17 with pure AR, 15 developed it as a consequence of IE and 2 as a consequence of the aortic valve malformation without superimposed IE; of these 17 patients, 1 had a unicuspid valve and 16 (94%) had a bicuspid valve. Possibly the most intriguing observation in this study was the finding of 59 patients (27%) (aged 21–82 yr; mean, 51 ± 16 yr) with congenitally bicuspid valves that appeared to have functioned normally during their entire lifetimes. Although 31 (14%) of the 218 patients developed IE at some time, the infection was superimposed on an already stenotic valve in 11, and on a previously normally functioning valve in 20. Of the latter 20 patients, 15 developed AR as a consequence of IE; of the other 5, all of whom died during the active infection, none apparently had AR during life as a consequence of IE.

Although several studies have discussed the natural history of AS, particularly of congenital origin,[11,16,21,22,32,45,46,55,58,59,84,89] to our knowledge only 4 reports have described the natural history of patients with bicuspid aortic valve. Roberts[58] in 1970 described at necropsy 85 patients in whom he found a congenitally bicuspid aortic valve, but only 42 (19% of 218) of them are included in the present study because the other 43 patients underwent operative therapy for AS (n = 40) or pure AR (n = 3). Nevertheless, as far as we know it was the first study to separate the patients into those with AS, pure AR, and IE. Nearly all of the AS patients had severe AS (peak transvalvular gradient ranging from 12 to 165 mm Hg [mean, 92 mm Hg]).

Fenoglio and colleagues[22] in 1977 described 152 patients with congenitally bicuspid aortic valves studied at autopsy. Of their 43 patients with AS, 23 (53%) had "died with congestive heart failure or during attempted surgical repair of the stenotic aortic valve." Therefore, their "natural history" was also interrupted by this iatrogenic event, namely aortic valve surgery. Nevertheless, their study is the closest to the present study, and some similarities and differences are shown in Table 12. The percentage of patients with AS and pure AR, for reasons unclear, is quite different between the 2 studies. It appears that their study was based on examination of observations recorded in autopsy reports prepared by a number of different prosectors.

TABLE 10. Comparison of Various Variables Among Patients With Bicuspid Aortic Valves Oriented Right to Left vs Anterior to Posterior (n = 153)

	Aortic Valve Orientation	
Variable	**Right/Left, n = 47 (31%)**	**Anterior/Posterior, n = 106 (59%)**
Age at death (years)		
Mean ± SD [median]	53 ± 16 [57]*	56 ± 15 [59]*
(Range)	(23–82)	(21–89)
Gender†		
Men	38 (84%)	79 (75%)
Women	7 (16%)	26 (25%)
Aortic valve function (before infective endocarditis)		
Normal	20 (43%)	43 (41%)
Stenosis	27 (57%)	62 (58%)
Pure regurgitation	0	1 (1%)
Infective endocarditis		
Active	11 (23%)	7 (7%)
Healed	2 (4%)	3 (3%)
Infective endocarditis superimposed on a:		
Previously normally functioning valve	10 (21%)	7 (7%)
Previously stenotic valve	3 (6%)	3 (3%)
Previously purely regurgitant valve	0	0
Heart weight (g)		
Mean ± SD [median]	545 ± 163 [505]‡	535 ± 165 [510]‡
(Range)	(320–1010)	(170–1050)

*-*p - value = 0.27

† Data missing on 3 patients.

‡-‡p - value = 0.76.

TABLE 11. Patients Studied at Necropsy Having a Unicuspid or Bicuspid Aortic Valve and Other Congenital Cardiovascular Malformations (n = 19)

Congenital Abnormality	Aortic Valve Function*	Age (Years)	Gender	Number of AV Cusps	Aortic Valve Orientation	Raphe Present	Infective Endocarditis		Heart Weight (g)
							Active	Healed	
Coarctation of aorta									
1†,‡	Normal	21	M	2	A/P	+	0	0	450
2	Normal	30	M	2	A/P	+	0	0	410
3	Normal	36	M	2	A/P	+	+	0	500
4	Stenotic	39	M	2	—	—	0	0	1000
5†	Normal	46	M	2	A/P	0	0	+	650
6	Normal	62	M	2	A/P	0	0	0	690
Coronary anomalies									
Hypoplasia									
RCA and LMCA									
7	Stenotic	26	M	1	—	—	0	0	760
High takeoff									
LMCA									
8	Normal	29	M	2	A/P	+	+	0	500
LMCA and RCA									
9	Normal	40	M	2	A/P	+	0	0	320
RCA									
10	Normal	52	M	2	—	—	+	0	610
Pulmonic valve									
Bicuspid									
11	Stenotic	34	M	1	—	—	0	0	570
12	Stenotic	37	M	2	R/L	+	0	0	860
13	Stenotic	47	F	2	R/L	+	0	0	340
14	Normal	47	M	2	R/L	+	0	+	590
15	Stenotic	66	M	2	R/L	+	0	0	—
Quadricuspid									
16	Normal	57	F	2	A/P	0	0	0	—
Shone syndrome									
17	Normal	30	M	2	R/L	+	0	0	395
Turner syndrome									
18	Normal	32	F	2	A/P	+	0	0	310
19	Normal	36	F	2	R/L	+	+	0	460

Abbreviations: — = not applicable or no information available, 0 = absent, + = present, A/P = anterior/posterior, AV = aortic valve, LMCA = left main coronary artery, RCA = right coronary artery, R/L = right/left.

*Prior to infective endocarditis.

†Early operative intervention for isthmic coarctation.

‡Patient also has a separate left main and circumflex coronary ostia.

TABLE 12. Comparison of the Present Necropsy Study to the Earlier Study (1977) by Fenoglio et al

Aortic Valve Function (After Infective Endocarditis)	Fenoglio Series (n = 152)	Roberts Series (n = 218)
Aortic stenosis	43 (28%)	142 (65%)
Age (year) (mean)	28–89 (55)	23–89 (59)
Men	40 (93%)	110 (77%)
Infective endocarditis		
Acute	5 (12%)	9 (6%)
Healed	4 (9%)	2 (1%)
Coarctation of aorta	5 (12%)	1 (1%)
Heart weight (g) (mean)	320–900 (603)	300–1050 (598)
Unicuspid aortic valves	0	27 (19%)
Aortic valve calcium	43 (100%)	142 (100%)
Pure aortic regurgitation	61 (40%)	17 (8%)
Age (year) (mean)	21–69 (35)	22–52 (37)
Men	61 (100%)	14 (82%)
Infective endocarditis		
Acute	28 (46%)	11 (65%)
Healed	19 (31%)	4 (24%)
Coarctation of aorta	6 (10%)	1 (6%)
Heart weight (g) (mean)	310–1300 (611)	350–1010 (569)
Unicuspid aortic valves	0	1 (6%)
Aortic valve calcium	25 (41%)	4 (24%)
Functionally normal	48 (32%)	59 (27%)
Age (year) (mean)	20–81 (48)	21–82 (51)
Men	41 (85%)	45 (76%)
Infective endocarditis*		
Acute	5 (10%)	5 (8%)
Healed	0	0
Coarctation of aorta	7 (15%)	4 (7%)
Heart weight (g) (mean)	200–675 (386)	170–700 (453)
Unicuspid aortic valves	0	0
Aortic valve calcium	7 (15%)	15 (25%)

*Infective endocarditis on a previously normally functioning aortic valve resulting in no valvular dysfunction.

Mills and associates[46] in 1978 described 41 patients with "non-invasive" evidence of a bicuspid aortic valve and followed them for 5–25 years (mean, 11 yr). Two patients underwent an aortic valve operation for severe AS; 2 developed pure AR; 3 developed IE resulting in AR in 2 and death in 1; 5 developed mild AS; 3 died (none as a consequence of aortic valve disease); and the clinical status did not change in the remaining 26.

The study by Michelena and colleagues[45] in 2008 from the Mayo Clinic was an analysis of 212 asymptomatic patients (mean age, 32 ± 20 yr) in whom a bicuspid aortic valve was found by echocardiogram. Survival 20 years after diagnosis was 90% ± 3%. The natural history centered on the status (operated, unoperated, dead, symptomatic, asymptomatic) 20 years after diagnosis.

We found only 1 study that included any natural history information on patients with unicuspid aortic valves, the study by Falcone and colleagues[21] in 1971 who described at necropsy 21 patients with stenotic unicuspid aortic valves, 3 of whom had undergone an aortic valve operation. Their ages (17 males) ranged from 16 to 62 years (mean, 44 yr). The transvalvular peak gradients (13 patients) ranged from 15 to 158 mm Hg (mean, 87 mm Hg). The heart weights ranged from 400 to 800 g (mean, 590 g).

Today, most congenitally malformed aortic valves are encountered by echocardiogram, computed tomography, or magnetic resonance imaging and not at operation or autopsy.[62] Although prophylactic use of antibiotics to prevent infectious endocarditis has not been recommended,[102] the identification of a congenitally malformed aortic valve allows patients and physicians to have a heightened awareness for symptoms that may suggest valve infection. Further, noninvasive imaging can help determine the need for, and proper timing of, valve surgery, and can identify aortic dilatation, which often occurs without causing symptoms. Because aortic valve malformations may occur in families, the finding in 1 family member should probably suggest a search in other family members.[27]

It is also well to keep in mind that another malformation of the aortic valve, namely aortic valve atresia, is the worst known cardiac condition because it allows the shortest lifespan. Indeed, aortic valve atresia is the most common cause of death in the first week of life.[85]

Some positive features of the present study include the following: 1) a large number of unoperated cases were collected during the 50 years in which aortic valve commissurotomy and replacement operations were available; 2) all cases were studied by a single investigator (WCR) and data were not simply retrieved from autopsy protocols prepared by a variety of physicians with varying expertise in cardiovascular disease; 3) most of the patients appeared to have had severe AS or AR; and 4) natural history data were presented on patients with unicuspid aortic valves.

Deficiencies or limitations of the present study include the following: 1) hemodynamic and echocardiographic data were available in a minority of patients; 2) 12 (6%) of the 218 patients studied had had CABG but no aortic valve surgery (possibly considered a "contaminant"); and 3) despite an extensive examination of a large number of patients, all studied at necropsy, the reason that some patients with bicuspid valves developed AS, some developed IE, a few developed AR without superimposed IE, and some (59 [31%] of the 190 with bicuspid valves) never developed an aortic valve complication, was not forthcoming.

Conclusion

In conclusion, the current study highlights several important findings in patients with congenitally malformed aortic valves. A patient with a unicuspid or bicuspid aortic valve 1) may go through life without ever developing dysfunction of the valve (27% of the total); 2) will most likely develop AS as a result of the congenital malformation (65% of the total); 3) is most likely male (80% of the total); 4) appears to be highly susceptible to IE (14% of the total); 5) is at a relatively high risk of developing aortic dissection or tears in the ascending aorta (8% of the total); and 6) is at an increased risk of dying from complications related to the aortic valve (57% of the total).

REFERENCES

1. Abbott ME. Coarctation of the aorta of the adult type. II. A statistical study and historical retrospect of 200 recorded cases, with autopsy, of stenosis or obliteration of the descending arch in subjects above the age of two years. *Am Heart J.* 1928;3:574–628.
2. Anderson MW, Kelsey JR Jr, Edwards JE. Clinical and pathological considerations in cases of calcific aortic stenosis. *JAMA.* 1952;149:9–15.

3. Arnett EN, Roberts WC. Active infective endocarditis: a clinicopathologic analysis of 137 necropsy patients. *Curr Probl Cardiol*. 1976;1:1–76.

4. Arnett EN, Roberts WC. Valve ring abscess in active infective endocarditis. Frequency, location, and clues to clinical diagnosis from the study of 95 necropsy patients. *Circulation*. 1976;54:140–145.

5. Arnett EN, Roberts WC. Pathology of active infective endocarditis: a necropsy analysis of 192 patients. *Thorac Cardiovasc Surg*. 1982;30:327–335.

6. Bacon APC, Matthews MB. Congenital bicuspid aortic valves and the aetiology of isolated aortic valvular stenosis. *Q J Med*. 1959;28:545–560.

7. Bishop LF, Bishop LF Jr, Trubek M. Aortic stenosis of inflammatory origin with a differential study of the acquired or congenital origin of a bicuspid aortic valve. *Am J Med Sci*. 1934;188:506–510.

8. Buchbinder NA, Roberts WC. Left-sided valvular active infective endocarditis. A study of forty-five necropsy patients. *Am J Med*. 1972;53:20–35.

9. Cabot RC. *Facts on the Heart*. Philadelphia: WB Saunders; 1926.

10. Campbell M. Calcific aortic stenosis and congenital bicuspid aortic valves. *Br Heart J*. 1968;30:606–616.

11. Campbell M. The natural history of congenital aortic stenosis. *Br Heart J*. 1968;30:514–526.

12. Campbell M, Kauntze R. Congenial aortic valvular stenosis. *Br Heart J*. 1953;15:179–194.

13. Christian HA. Aortic stenosis with calcification of the cusps. A distinct clinical entity. *JAMA*. 1931;97:158–161.

14. Clawson BJ, Bell ET, Hartzell TB. Valvular diseases of the heart. With special reference to the pathogenesis of old valvular defects. *Am J Pathol*. 1926;2:193–234.

15. Clawson BJ, Noble JF, Lufkin NH. The calcified nodular deformity of the aortic valve. *Am Heart J*. 1938;15:58–76.

16. Cohen LS, Friedman WF, Braunwald E. Natural history of mild congenital aortic stenosis elucidated by serial hemodynamic studies. *Am J Cardiol*. 1972;30:1–5.

17. Cohen L, Gray I, Nash PI, Fink H. Calcareous aortic stenosis; report of nine cases with autopsy findings. *Ann Intern Med*. 1940;13:2091–2103.

18. Dry TJ, Willius FA. Calcareous disease of the aortic valve. A study of two hundred twenty-eight cases. *Am Heart J*. 1939;17:138–157.

19. Edwards JE. Pathologic aspects of cardiac valvular insufficiencies. *AMA Arch Surg*. 1958;77:634–649.

20. Edwards JE. Calcific aortic stenosis: pathologic features. *Proc Staff Meet Mayo Clin*. 1961;36:444–451.

21. Falcone MW, Roberts WC, Morrow AG, Perloff JK. Congenital aortic stenosis resulting from a unicommissural valve. Clinical and anatomic features in twenty-one adult patients. *Circulation*. 1971;44:272–280.

22. Fenoglio JJ Jr, McAllister HA Jr, DeCastro CM, Davia JE, Cheitlin MD. Congenital bicuspid aortic valve after age 20. *Am J Cardiol*. 1977;39:164–169.

23. Fernicola DJ, Roberts WC. Clinicopathologic features of active infective endocarditis isolated to the native mitral valve. *Am J Cardiol*. 1993;71:1186–1197.

24. Friedberg CK, Sohval AR. Nonrheumatic calcific aortic stenosis. *Am Heart J*. 1939;17:452–469.

25. Gibbs AJ. Aortic stenosis: its etiology and morbid anatomy. *Guy's Hosp Rep*. 1935;85:275–288.

26. Glancy DL, Morrow AG, Simon AL, Roberts WC. Juxtaductal aortic coarctation. Analysis of 84 patients studied hemodynamically, angiographically and morphologically after age 1 year. *Am J Cardiol*. 1983;51:537–551.

27. Glick BN, Roberts WC. Congenitally bicuspid aortic valve in multiple family members. *Am J Cardiol*. 1994;73:400–404.

28. Gould SE. *Pathology of the Heart and Blood Vessels*. 3rd ed. Springfield, IL: Charles C Thomas; 1968.

29. Gross L. So-called congenital bicuspid aortic valve. *Arch Pathol*. 1937;23:350–362.

30. Guntheroth WG. A critical review of the American College of Cardiology/American Heart Association practice guidelines on bicuspid aortic valve with dilated ascending aorta. *Am J Cardiol*. 2008;102:107–110.

31. Horan MJ Jr, Barnes AR. Calcareous aortic stenosis and coronary artery disease. *Am J Med Sci*. 1948;215:451–455.

32. Hossack KF, Neutze JM, Lowe JB, Barratt-Boyes BG. Congenital valvular aortic stenosis. Natural history and assessment for operation. *Br Heart J*. 1980;43:561–573.

33. Karsner HT, Koletsky S. *Calcific Disease of the Aortic Valve*. Philadelphia: JB Lippincott; 1947.

34. Keele KD. *Leonardo da Vinci on Movement of the Heart and Blood*. London: Harvey and Blythe; 1952.

35. Koletsky S. Congenital bicuspid aortic valves. *Arch Intern Med*. 1941;67:129–176.

36. Lander SR, Taylor JE, Roberts WC. Observations on the heart—congenitally bicuspid stenotic aortic valves in octogenarians. *Am J Geriatr Cardiol*. 1999;8:304–306.

37. Laws CL, Levine SA. Clinical notes on rheumatic heart disease with special reference to the cause of death. *Am J Med Sci*. 1933;186:833–849.

38. Lesnick G, Schlesinger MJ. Calcareous aortic valve stenosis. With particular reference to its etiology. *Am Heart J*. 1938;16:43–50.

39. Lewis T, Grant RT. Observations relating to subacute infective endocarditis. *Heart*. 1923;10:21–99.

40. Margolis HM, Ziellessen FO, Barnes AR. Calcareous aortic valvular disease. *Am Heart J*. 1931;6:349–374.

41. McGinn S, White PD. Clinical observations on aortic stenosis. *Am J Med Sci*. 1934;188:1–15.

42. McKusick VA. Association of congenital bicuspid aortic valve and Erdheim's cystic medial necrosis. *Lancet*. 1972;1:1026–1027.

43. McKusick VA, Logue RB, Bahnson HT. Association of aortic valvular disease and cystic medial necrosis of the ascending aorta. *Circulation*. 1957;16:188–194.

44. Mensah GA, Friesinger GC. Calcific aortic valve stenosis and the congenitally bicuspid aortic valve: did Osler miss the link? *Am J Cardiol*. 1996;77:417–419.

45. Michelena HI, Desjardins VA, Avierinos JF, Russo A, Nkomo VT, Sundt TM, Pellikka PA, Tajik AJ, Enriquez-Sarano M. Natural history of asymptomatic patients with normally functioning or minimally dysfunctional bicuspid aortic valve in the community. *Circulation*. 2008;117:2776–2784.

46. Mills P, Leech G, Davies M, Leatham A. The natural history of a non-stenotic bicuspid aortic valve. *Br Heart J*. 1978;40:951–957.

47. Monckeberg JG. Der normale histologische Bau und die Sklerose der Aortenklappen. *Virchows Arch Pathol Anat Physiol*. 1904;176:472–514.

48. Morrow AG, Austen G, Braunwald E. The surgical treatment of calcific aortic stenosis: operative methods and the results of the pre- and postoperative hemodynamic assessments. *Ann Surg*. 1963;158:936–951.

49. Morrow AG, Roberts WC, Ross J Jr, Fisher RD, Behrendt DM, Mason DT, Braunwald E. Obstruction to left ventricular outflow. Current concepts of management and operative treatment. *Ann Intern Med*. 1968;69:1255–1286.

50. Osler W. The bicuspid condition of the aortic valve. *Trans Assoc Am Physicians*. 1886;1:185–192.

51. Osler W. The Gulstonian Lectures, on malignant endocarditis. *Br Med J*. 1885;1:467–470.

52. Paget J. On obstructions of the branches of the pulmonary artery. *Med Chir Trans*. 1884;27:162–188.

53. Passik CS, Ackerman DM, Pluth JR, Edwards WD. Temporal changes in the causes of aortic stenosis: a surgical pathologic study of 646 cases. *Mayo Clin Proc*. 1987;62:119–123.

54. Peacock TB. *On Malformations, & c., of the Human Heart With Original Cases*. London: John Churchill; 1865.

55. Peckham GB, Keith JD, Evans JR. Congenital aortic stenosis: some observations on the natural history and clinical assessment. *Can Med Assoc J*. 1964;91:639–643.

56. Reich NE. Calcific aortic valve stenosis: a clinicopathologic correlation of 22 cases. *Ann Intern Med*. 1945;22:234–251.

57. Reifenstein GH, Levine SA, Gross RE. Coarctation of the aorta. A review of 104 autopsied cases of the "adult type," 2 years of age or older. *Am Heart J*. 1947;33:146–168.

58. Roberts WC. Tzhe congenitally bicuspid aortic valve. A study of 85 autopsy cases. *Am J Cardiol*. 1970;26:72–83.

59. Roberts WC. The structure of the aortic valve in clinically isolated aortic stenosis. An autopsy study of 162 patients over 15 years of age. *Circulation*. 1970;42:91–97.

60. Roberts WC. Anatomically isolated aortic valvular disease. The case against its being of rheumatic etiology. *Am J Med*. 1970;49:151–159.

61. Roberts WC. The 2 most common congenital heart diseases. *Am J Cardiol*. 1984;53:1198.

62. Roberts WC. Living with a congenitally bicuspid aortic valve. *Am J Cardiol*. 1989;64:1408–1409.

63. Roberts WC, Buchbinder NA. Healed left-sided infective endocarditis: a clinicopathologic study of 59 patients. *Am J Cardiol*. 1977;40:876–888.

64. Roberts WC, Dangel JC, Bulkley BH. Non-rheumatic valvular cardiac disease: a clinicopathologic survey of 27 different conditions causing valvular dysfunction. *Cardiovasc Clin*. 1973;5:333–446.

65. Roberts WC, Day PJ. Electrocardiographic observations in clinically isolated, pure, chronic, severe aortic regurgitation: analysis of 30 necropsy patients aged 19 to 65 years. *Am J Cardiol*. 1985;55:432–438.

66. Roberts WC, Ko JM. Weights of operatively-excised stenotic unicuspid, bicuspid, and tricuspid aortic valves and their relation to age, sex, body mass index, and presence or absence of concomitant coronary artery bypass grafting. *Am J Cardiol*. 2003;92:1057–1065.

67. Roberts WC, Ko JM. Weights of individual cusps in operatively-excised congenitally bicuspid stenotic aortic valves. *Am J Cardiol*. 2004;94:678–681.

68. Roberts WC, Ko JM. Weights of individual cusps in operatively-excised stenotic three-cuspid aortic valves. *Am J Cardiol*. 2004;94:681–684.

69. Roberts WC, Ko JM. Relation of weights of operatively excised stenotic aortic valves to preoperative transvalvular peak systolic pressure gradients and to calculated aortic valve areas. *J Am Coll Cardiol*. 2004;44:1847–1855.

70. Roberts WC, Ko JM. Frequency by decades of unicuspid, bicuspid, and tricuspid aortic valves in adults having isolated aortic valve replacement for aortic stenosis, with or without associated aortic regurgitation. *Circulation*. 2005;111:920–925.

71. Roberts WC, Ko JM. Clinical and morphologic features of the congenitally unicuspid acommissural stenotic and regurgitant aortic valve. *Cardiology*. 2007;108:79–81.

72. Roberts WC, Ko JM, Filardo G. Comparison of heavier versus lighter operatively excised stenotic aortic valves in adults with aortic stenosis and implications for percutaneous aortic valve implantation without replacement. *Am J Cardiol*. 2009;104:393–405.

73. Roberts WC, Ko JM, Filardo G, Henry AC, Hebeler RF Jr, Cheung EH, Matter GJ, Hamman BL. Valve structure and survival in septuagenarians having aortic valve replacement for aortic stenosis (±aortic regurgitation) with versus without coronary artery bypass grafting at a single US medical center (1993 to 2005). *Am J Cardiol*. 2007;100:1157–1165.

74. Roberts WC, Ko JM, Filardo G, Henry AC, Hebeler RF Jr, Cheung EH, Matter GJ, Hamman BL. Valve structure and survival in sexagenarians having aortic valve replacement for aortic stenosis (±aortic regurgitation) with versus without coronary artery bypass grafting at a single US medical center (1993 to 2005). *Am J Cardiol*. 2007;100:1286–1292.

75. Roberts WC, Ko JM, Filardo G, Henry AC, Hebeler RF Jr, Cheung EH, Matter GJ, Hamman BL. Valve structure and survival in quinquagenarians having aortic valve replacement for aortic stenosis (±aortic regurgitation) with versus without coronary artery bypass grafting at a single US medical center (1993 to 2005). *Am J Cardiol*. 2007;100:1584–1591.

76. Roberts WC, Ko JM, Filardo G, Kitchens BL, Henry AC, Hebeler RF Jr, Cheung EH, Matter GJ, Hamman BL. Valve structure and survival in quadragenarians having aortic valve replacement for aortic stenosis (±aortic regurgitation) with versus without coronary artery bypass grafting at a single US medical center (1993 to 2005). *Am J Cardiol*. 2007;100:1683–1690.

77. Roberts WC, Ko JM, Garner WL, Filardo G, Henry AC, Hebeler RF Jr, Matter GJ, Hamman BL. Valve structure and survival in octogenarians having aortic valve replacement for aortic stenosis (±aortic regurgitation) with versus without coronary artery bypass grafting at a single US medical center (1993 to 2005). *Am J Cardiol*. 2007;100:489–498.

78. Roberts WC, Ko JM, Hamilton C. Comparison of valve structure, valve weight, and severity of the valve obstruction in 1849 patients having isolated aortic valve replacement for aortic valve stenosis (with or without associated aortic regurgitation) studied at 3 different medical centers in 2 different time periods. *Circulation*. 2005;112:3919–3929.

79. Roberts WC, Ko JM, Matter GJ. Aortic valve replacement for aortic stenosis in nonagenarians. *Am J Cardiol*. 2006;98:1251–1253.

80. Roberts WC, Ko JM, Moore TR, Jones WH III. Causes of pure aortic regurgitation in patients having isolated aortic valve replacement at a single US tertiary hospital (1993 to 2005). *Circulation*. 2006;114:422–429.

81. Roberts WC, Morrow AG. Congenital aortic stenosis produced by a unicommissural valve. *Br Heart J*. 1965;27:505–510.

82. Roberts WC, Morrow AG, Braunwald E. Complete interruption of the aortic arch. *Circulation*. 1962;26:39–59.

83. Roberts WC, Morrow AG, McIntosh CL, Jones M, Epstein SE. Congenitally bicuspid aortic valve causing severe, pure aortic regurgitation without superimposed infective endocarditis. Analysis of 13 patients requiring aortic valve replacement. *Am J Cardiol*. 1981;47:206–209.

84. Roberts WC, Perloff JK, Costantino T. Severe valvular aortic stenosis in patients over 65 years of age. A clinicopathologic study. *Am J Cardiol*. 1971;27:497–506.

85. Roberts WC, Perry LW, Chandra RS, Myers GE, Shapiro SR, Scott LP. Aortic valve atresia: a new classification based on necropsy study of 73 cases. *Am J Cardiol*. 1976;37:753–756.

86. Roberts CS, Roberts WC. Dissection of the aorta associated with congenital malformation of the aortic valve. *J Am Coll Cardiol.* 1991;17:712–716.

87. Roberts WC, Vowels TJ, Ko JM. Comparison of interpretations of valve structure between cardiac surgeon and cardiac pathologist among adults having isolated aortic valve replacement for aortic valve stenosis (±aortic regurgitation). *Am J Cardiol.* 2009;103:1139–1145.

88. Roberts WC, Vowels TJ, Ko JM, Filardo G, Hebeler RF Jr, Henry AC, Matter GJ, Hamman BL. Comparison of the structure of the aortic valve and ascending aorta in adults having aortic valve replacement for aortic stenosis versus for pure aortic regurgitation and resection of the ascending aorta for aneurysm. *Circulation.* 2011;123:896–903.

89. Ross J Jr, Braunwald E. Aortic stenosis. *Circulation.* 1968;38:61–67.

90. Sabet HY, Edwards WD, Tazelaar HD, Daly RC. Congenitally bicuspid aortic valves: a surgical pathology study of 542 cases (1991 through 1996) and a literature review of 2,715 additional cases. *Mayo Clin Proc.* 1999;74:14–26.

91. Sohval AR, Gross L. Calcific sclerosis of the aortic valve (Monckeberg type). *Arch Pathol.* 1936;22:477–494.

92. Smith DE, Matthews MB. Aortic valvular stenosis with coarctation of the aorta. With special reference to the development of aortic stenosis upon congenital bicuspid valves. *Br Heart J.* 1955;17:198–206.

93. Stephan PJ, Henry AC III, Hebeler RF Jr, Whiddon L, Roberts WC. Comparison of age, gender, number of aortic valve cusps, concomitant coronary artery bypass grafting, and magnitude of left ventricular-systemic arterial peak systolic gradient in adults having aortic valve replacement for isolated aortic valve stenosis. *Am J Cardiol.* 1997;79:166–172.

94. Subramanian R, Olson LJ, Edwards WD. Surgical pathology of pure aortic stenosis: a study of 374 cases. *Mayo Clin Proc.* 1984;59:683–690.

95. Tadros TM, Klein MD, Shapira OM. Ascending aortic dilatation associated with bicuspid aortic valve. Pathophysiology, molecular biology, and clinical implications. *Circulation.* 2009;119:880–890.

96. Tzemos N, Therrien J, Yip J, Thanassoulis G, Tremblay S, Jamorski MT, Webb GD, Siu SC. Outcomes in adults with bicuspid aortic valves. *JAMA.* 2008;300:1317–1325.

97. Vallely MP, Semsarian C, Bannon PG. Management of the ascending aorta in patients with bicuspid aortic valve disease. *Heart Lung Circ.* 2008;17:357–363.

98. Vaslef SN, Roberts WC. Early descriptions of aortic valve stenosis. *Am Heart J.* 1993;125:1465–1474.

99. Vaslef SN, Roberts WC. Early descriptions of aortic regurgitation. *Am Heart J.* 1993;125:1475–1483.

100. Wauchope GM. The clinical importance of variations in the number of cusps forming the aortic and pulmonary valves. *Q J Med.* 1928;21:383–406.

101. White PD. *Heart Disease.* 4th ed. New York: MacMillan; 1951.

102. Wilson W, Taubert KA, Gewitz M, Lockhart PB, Baddour LM, Levison M, Bolger A, Cabell CH, Takahashi M, Baltimore RS, Newburger JW, Strom BL, Tani LY, Gerber M, Bonow RO, Pallasch T, Shulman ST, Rowley AH, Burns JC, Ferrieri P, Gardner T, Goff D, Durack DT. Prevention of infective endocarditis: guidelines from the American Heart Association: a guideline from the American Heart Association Rheumatic Fever, Endocarditis, and Kawasaki Disease Committee, Council on Cardiovascular Disease in the Young, and the Council on Clinical Cardiology, Council on Cardiovascular Surgery and Anesthesia, and the Quality of Care and Outcomes Research Interdisciplinary Working Group. *Circulation.* 2007;116:1736–1754.

103. Wood P. *Diseases of the Heart and Circulation.* 3rd ed. London: Eyre & Spottiswoode; 1968.

104. Yasuda H, Nakatani S, Stugaard M, Tsujita-Kuroda Y, Bando K, Kobayashi J, Yamagishi M, Kitakaze M, Kitamura S, Miyatake K. Failure to prevent progressive dilatation of ascending aorta by aortic valve replacement in patients with bicuspid aortic valve: comparison with tricuspid aortic valve. *Circulation.* 2003;108(Suppl 1):II291–II294.

Necropsy Findings Early After Transcatheter Aortic Valve Implantation for Aortic Stenosis

William C. Roberts, MD[a,b,d,*], Robert C. Stoler, MD[b], Paul A. Grayburn, MD[b,c,d], Robert F. Hebeler, Jr., MD[c], Jong M. Ko, BA[d], David L. Brown, MD[e], William T. Brinkman, MD[f], Michael J. Mack, MD[f], and Joseph M. Guileyardo, MD[a]

Although transcatheter aortic valve implantation has been available for 10 years, reports of cardiovascular morphologic studies after the procedure are virtually nonexistent. The investigators describe such findings in 2 patients, both 86 years of age, who died early (hours or several days) after transcatheter aortic valve implantation. Although the prosthesis in each was seated well, and each of the 3 calcified cusps of the native aortic valves was well compressed to the wall of the aorta, thus providing a good bioprosthetic orifice, the ostium of the dominant right coronary artery in each was obliterated by the native right aortic valve cusp. Atherosclerotic plaques in the common iliac artery led to a major complication in 1 patient, who later died of hemorrhagic stroke. The other patient developed fatal cardiac tamponade secondary to perforation of the right ventricular wall by a pacemaker catheter. **(Am J Cardiol 2013;111:448–452)**

Although transcatheter aortic valve implantation (TAVI) was first introduced by Cribier and colleagues[1] in 2002, virtually no studies have appeared describing cardiovascular morphologic findings in patients who have had fatal consequences early after the procedure. This report describes necropsy findings in 2 patients who had this procedure several hours or days earlier.

Case Descriptions

Pertinent findings in the 2 patients are listed in Table 1. Both were 86 years of age, 1 woman and 1 man. Both had evidence of heart failure. Neither had had chest pain. By coronary angiography, both had "luminal irregularities," but neither had significant narrowings, even though patient 2 had had a stent placed in the right coronary artery 17 years earlier, when 69 years of age. Both patients had decreased renal function: patient 2 had had a unilateral nephrectomy, apparently for cancer, many years earlier. The cardiac index in case 1 was 3.0 L/min/m^2 and in case 2 was 2.4 L/min/m^2; the left ventricular ejection fraction in each patient was 40%. A Medtronic CoreValve (Medtronic, Inc., Minneapolis, Minnesota) was used in case 1 and an Edwards SAPIEN valve (Edwards Lifesciences, Irvine, California) in case 2. Before insertion of the bioprostheses, each had balloon

Table 1
Pertinent clinical and morphologic findings in the 2 patients having transcatheter aortic valve implantation for aortic stenosis

Variable	Patient 1	Patient 2
Age (yrs)	86	86
Gender	Female	Male
Heart failure class (0–4+)	3+	1+
Co-morbidities		
Peripheral neuropathy	+	0
Chronic kidney disease	+	+*
Body mass index (kg/m^2)	25.4	26.1
LV ejection fraction	40%	40%
Pressures (mm Hg)		
Left ventricle	178/21	172/20
Aorta	114/37	107/70
LV-aorta peak systolic gradient	64	65
Pulmonary artery wedge mean	14	9
Cardiac index (L/min/m^2)	3.0	2.4
Coronary arteries narrowed	0	0†
Aortic valve area (cm^2)	0.62	0.77
Aortic valve area index (cm^2/m^2)	0.38	0.50
Type of bioprosthesis used	CoreValve (Medtronic)	SAPIEN (Edwards)
Heart weight (g)	390	470
Mitral annular calcium (0–4+)	2+	3+
Aorta calcium (0–4+)	2+	4+
Coronary calcium (0–4+)	1+	3+
Aortic valve calcium (0–4+)	3+	3+
Dilated left ventricle	0	0
Dilated right ventricle	+	+
Obliteration of the ostium of the right coronary artery by the native right aortic valve cusp compressed against aorta	+	+
Interval TAVI to death	6 days	3 hours
Cause of death	Stroke	Tamponade

LV = left ventricular.
* Unilateral nephrectomy.
† Stent placed in right coronary artery years earlier.

[a]Department of Pathology; [b]Department of Internal Medicine, Division of Cardiology; and [c]Department of Cardiothoracic Surgery; [d]Baylor Heart and Vascular Institute, Baylor University Medical Center, Dallas, Texas; and [e]Departments of Internal Medicine (Cardiology); and [f]Cardiothoracic Surgery, The Heart Hospital Baylor Plano, Plano, Texas. Manuscript received September 19, 2012; revised manuscript received and accepted September 30, 2012.

See page 452 for disclosure information.

*Corresponding author: Tel: 214-820-7911; fax: 214-820-7533.
E-mail address: wc.roberts@baylorhealth.edu (W.C. Roberts).

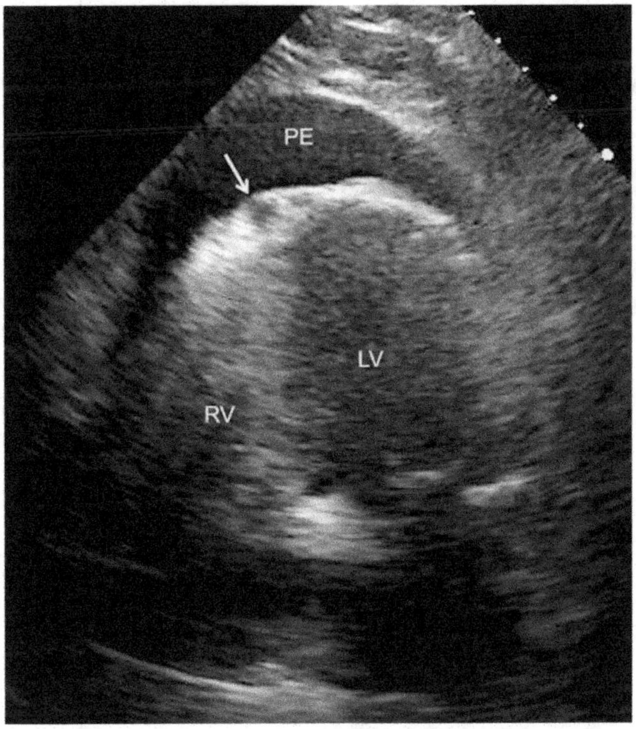

Figure 1. Case 2. Four-chamber echocardiogram obtained during cardiac arrest. A large pericardial effusion (PE) is present. The *arrow* points to a perforation in the subepicardial adipose tissue above the right ventricular apex. The right ventricular cavity (RV) is collapsed, and the left ventricular cavity (LV) is of normal size.

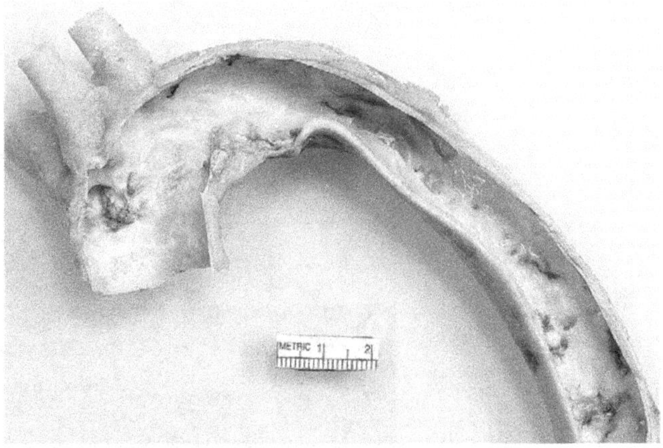

Figure 2. Case 1. Aortic arch and descending thoracic aorta showing focal but fairly heavy calcific deposits.

aortic valvuloplasty. The bioprostheses reduced the peak systolic transvalvular pressure gradient from 64 to 0 mm Hg in patient 1 and from 65 to 23 mm Hg in case 2, and neither patient developed more than minimal aortic regurgitation after insertion of the bioprosthesis.

During the procedure, a common iliac artery was transected in patient 1, and as a consequence, this artery was operatively ligated, and a right-to-left femoral-to-femoral artery bypass was performed. Eight transfusions were given, and manual chest compression was applied (for 15 minutes). Although appearing to be recovering from this complication, 7 days post procedure, she suddenly deteriorated mentally: computed tomography disclosed a large hematoma in the left frontal lobe. She died 2 days later. Several hours after completion of the procedure on patient 2, bradycardia suddenly appeared, followed by shock and loss of electrical activity. Echocardiogram (Figure 1) disclosed a huge pericardial effusion and right ventricular diastolic collapse. Resuscitative efforts were unsuccessful. Necropsy disclosed that the pacemaker catheter had extended through the wall of the right ventricle with extensive extravasation of blood into the subpericardial adipose tissue with eventual rupture of the visceral epicardium leading to pericardial tamponade.

Photographs of the heart in patient 1 are shown in Figures 2–4 and in patient 2 in Figures 5–8. In both patients, each of the 3 calcified aortic valve cusps was displaced well laterally, and the cusps of the bioprosthesis appeared to open and close well. In both patients, the calcified right aortic cusp displaced laterally obliterated the ostium of the right coronary

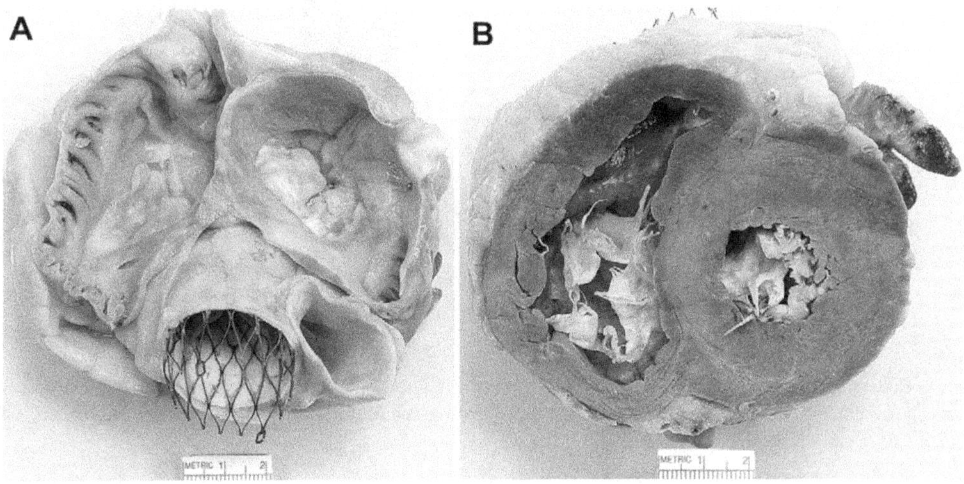

Figure 3. Case 1. *(A)* Photograph exposing the right and left atria, aorta with the bioprosthesis, and pulmonary trunk. *(B)* View of both ventricles and atrioventricular valves. The left ventricular cavity is of normal size. The quantity of subepicardial adipose tissue is large. Calcium is present in the mitral annular region and in the left anterior descending coronary artery. The right ventricular cavity is dilated, and its wall is thickened.

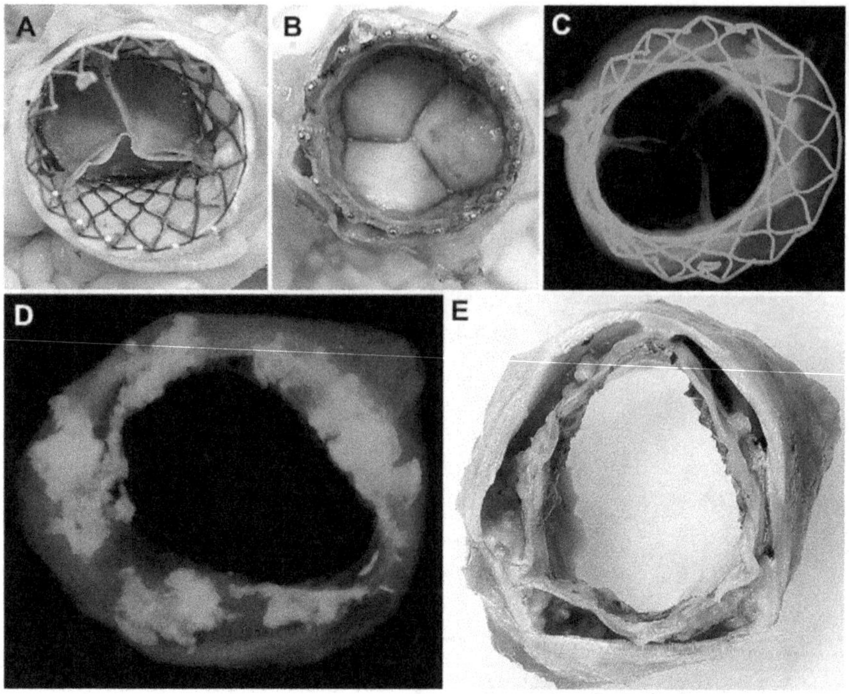

Figure 4. Case 1. Multiple views of the aortic valve area with the bioprosthesis in place *(A to C)* and after removal of the bioprosthesis. The 3 calcified aortic valve cusps are compressed against the aortic wall, providing a large central bioprosthetic orifice *(E)*. The 2 radiographs of the aortic valve area *(C,D)* show heavy calcific deposits in each native cusps.

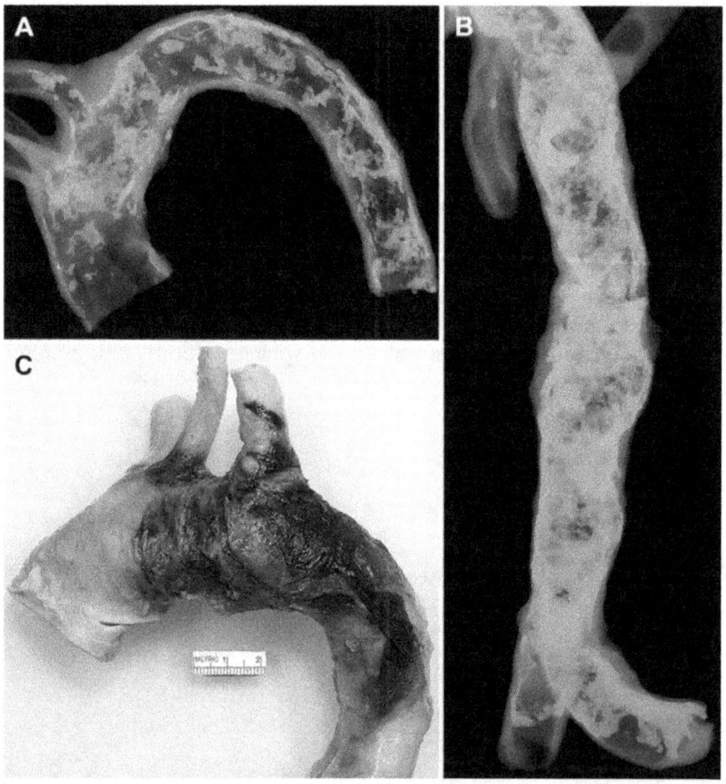

Figure 5. Case 2. Aorta. *(A)* Radiograph of arch and descending thoracic aorta showing focal but extensive calcific deposits. *(B)* Radiograph of abdominal aorta and common iliac arteries showing massive near diffuse calcific deposits. *(C)* Photograph of the aortic arch and descending thoracic aorta showing adventitial blood, the source of which was not determined.

artery. In patient 2, however, heavy calcific deposits surrounded the ostium of this artery, and even after removal of the bioprosthesis, a 0.5-mm-diameter probe could not be placed into the right coronary artery via its ostium. In both patients, the ostium of the left main coronary artery was unobstructed.

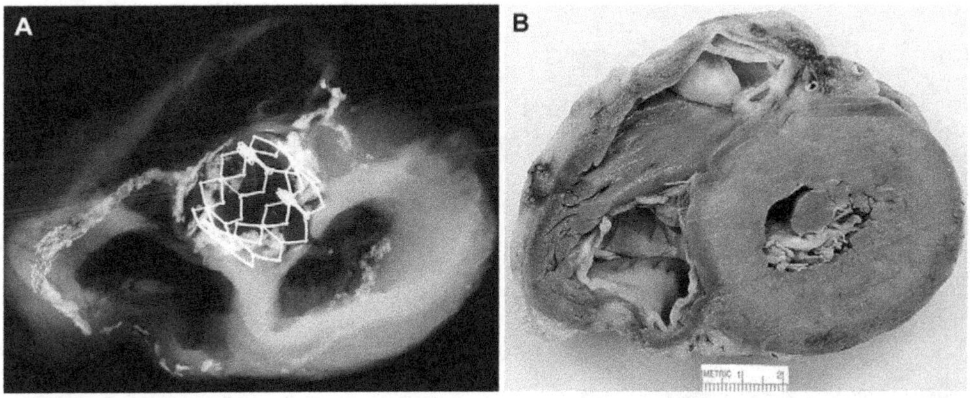

Figure 6. Case 2. *(A)* Radiograph of the base of the heart at autopsy showing the metallic cage of the bioprosthesis and calcific deposits and stent in the right coronary artery and focal calcific deposits in the left main, left anterior descending, and left circumflex coronary arteries and in the mitral annular area. *(B)* Photograph of the base of the heart showing a normal-sized left ventricular cavity and a dilated right ventricular cavity. The anterior mitral leaflet is thickened, probably due to the small space within the left ventricular cavity.

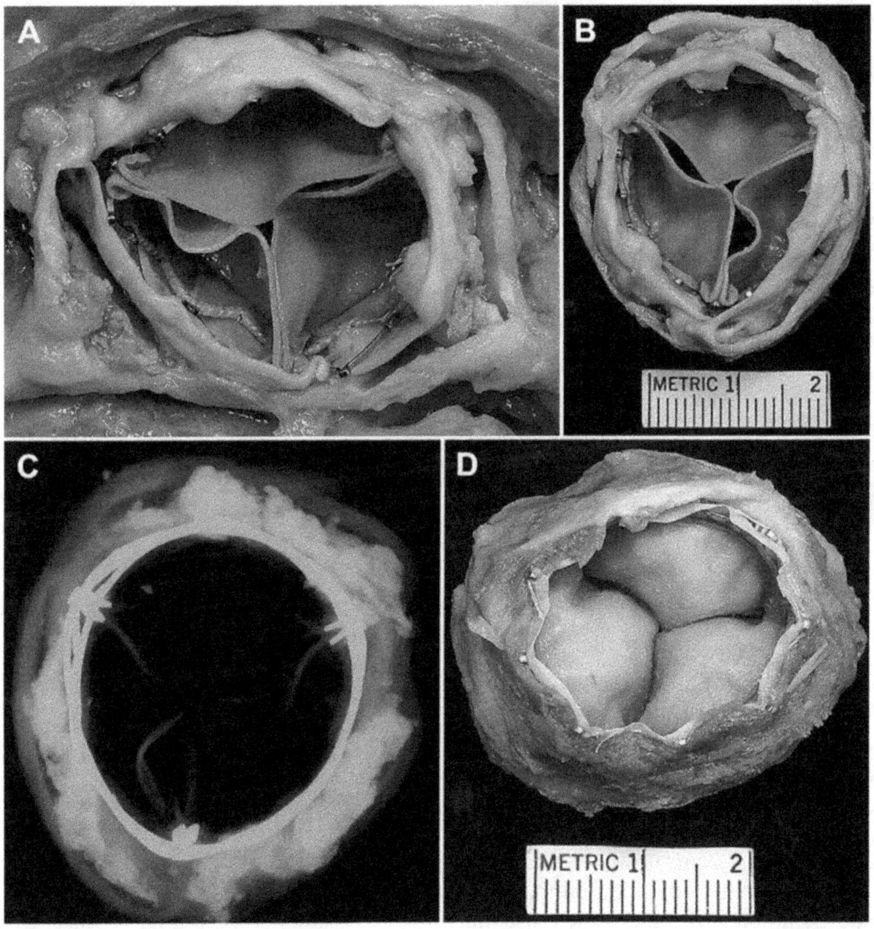

Figure 7. Case 2. Aortic valve area. *(A)* View from above with the bioprosthesis in place and the 3 calcified cusps pushed laterally. The ostium of the right coronary artery is directly behind the right aortic valve cusp. The ostium of the left main coronary artery is just cephalad to the free margin of the left aortic valve cusp. *(B)* View more caudal than the one in *(A)*. There is plenty of room for the bioprosthetic orifice. *(C)* Radiograph of the bioprosthesis and calcified aortic valve cusps after removal from the heart. *(D)* View of the bioprosthetic cusps from the left ventricular aspect.

Comments

Review of several major reports describing the techniques and results of TAVI disclosed that none illustrated morphologic cardiovascular observations early after TAVI.[2–8] Study of the 2 patients described herein shows that each of the 2 bioprostheses inserted was well seated and

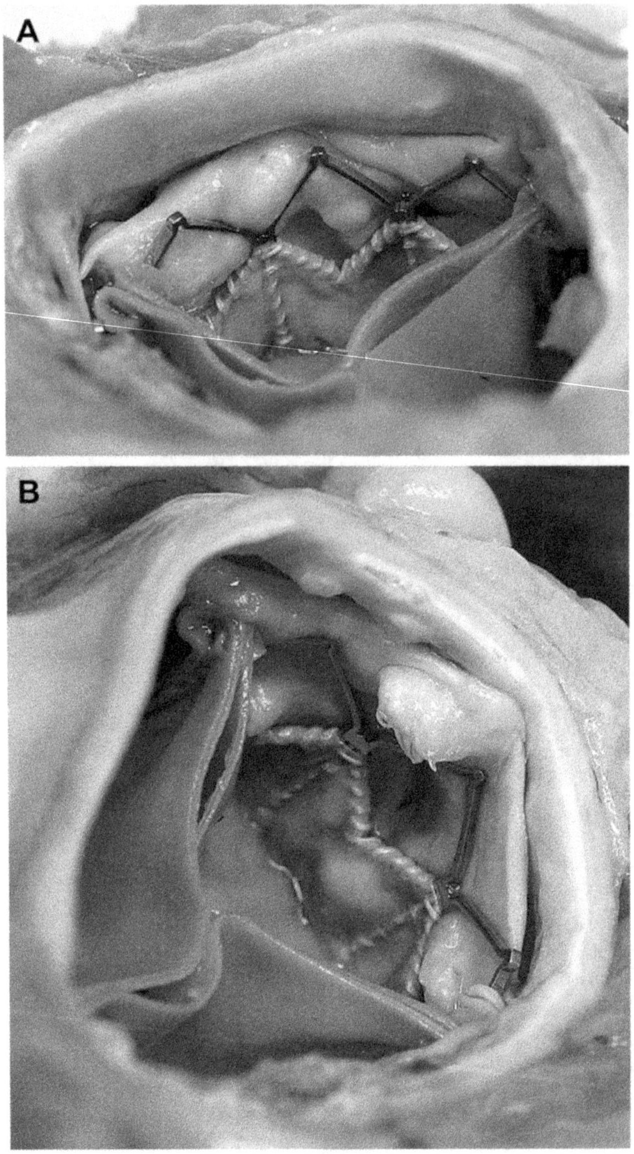

Figure 8. Case 2. *(A,B)* Close-up views of the metallic struts of the bioprosthesis compressing the calcified native aortic valve cusps against the aortic wall.

that each compressed the 3 native calcified aortic cusps well against the aortic wall, providing very adequate aortic orifices for the bioprostheses. The right native aortic valve cusp, however, obliterated the orifice of the right coronary artery in each patient. In neither patient, however, was this obliterated orifice the cause of death. Although both patients had extensive aortic and common iliac atherosclerosis, the patient with the smaller quantity of atherosclerosis (patient 1) was the one who developed a peripheral arterial tear resulting in ligation and femoro-femoral right-to-left bypass. This patient, however, died of a stroke 6 days later. In patient 1, a 1.0 sheath to femoral artery ratio with circumferential calcific deposits was present by computed tomography before the TAVI procedure. This combination has been described as a risk factor for vascular complications of TAVI.[9] A recent analysis of the Placement of Aortic Transcatheter Valves (PARTNER) trial data showed that the only predictor of a major vascular complication on multivariate analysis was female gender.[10] A major vascular complication was associated with a fourfold increase in 30-day mortality. Thorough evaluation of the extent of atherosclerosis in these peripheral arteries obviously is essential before TAVI.[11]

Disclosures

The authors have no conflicts of interest to disclose.

1. Cribier A, Eltchaninoff H, Bash A, Borenstein N, Tron C, Bauer F, Derumeaux G, Anselme F, Laborde F, Leon MB. Percutaneous transcatheter implantation of an aortic valve prosthesis for calcific aortic stenosis: first human case description. *Circulation* 2002;106:3006–3008.
2. Webb JG, Chandavimol M, Thompson CR, Ricci DR, Carere RG, Munt BI, Buller CE, Pasupati S, Lichtenstein S. Percutaneous aortic valve implantation retrograde from the femoral artery. *Circulation* 2006;113:842–850.
3. Piazza N, Grube E, Gerckens U, den Heijer P, Linke A, Luha O, Ramondo A, Ussia G, Wenaweser P, Windecker S, Laborde JC, de Jaegere P, Serruys PW. Procedural and 30-day outcomes following transcatheter aortic valve implantation using the third generation (18 Fr) CoreValve Revalving System: results from the multicentre, expanded evaluation registry 1-year following CE mark approval. *Eurointervention* 2008;4:242–249.
4. Webb JG, Altwegg L, Boone RH, Cheung A, Ye J, Lichtenstein S, Lee M, Masson JB, Thompson C, Moss R, Carere R, Munt B, Nietlispach F, Humphries K. Transcatheter aortic valve implantation: impact on clinical and valve-related outcomes. *Circulation* 2009;119:3009–3016.
5. Masson JB, Kovac J, Schuler G, Ye J, Cheung A, Kapadia S, Tuzcu ME, Kodali S, Leon MB, Webb JG. Transcatheter aortic valve implantation: review of the nature, management, and avoidance of procedural complications. *JACC Cardiovasc Interv* 2009;2:811–820.
6. Leon MB, Smith CR, Mack M, Miller DC, Moses JW, Svensson LG, Tuzcu EM, Webb JG, Fontana GP, Makkar RR, Brown DL, Block PC, Guyton RA, Pichard AD, Bavaria JE, Herrmann HC, Douglas PS, Petersen JL, Akin JJ, Anderson WN, Wang D, Pocock S; PARTNER Trial Investigators. Transcatheter aortic-valve implantation for aortic stenosis in patients who cannot undergo surgery. *N Engl J Med* 2010;363:1597–1607.
7. Baan J Jr, Yong ZY, Koch KT, Henriques JP, Bouma BJ, Vis MM, Cocchieri R, Piek JJ, de Mol BA. Factors associated with cardiac conduction disorders and permanent pacemaker implantation after percutaneous aortic valve implantation with the CoreValve prosthesis. *Am Heart J* 2010;159:497–503.
8. Van Mieghem NM, Nuis RJ, Piazza N, Apostolos T, Ligthart J, Schultz C, de Jaegere PP, Serruys PW. Vascular complications with transcatheter aortic valve implantation using the 18 Fr Medtronic CoreValve system: the Rotterdam experience. *Eurointervention* 2010;5:673–679.
9. Hayashida K, Lefèvre T, Chevalier B, Hovasse T, Romano M, Garot P, Mylotte D, Uribe J, Farge A, Donzeau-Gouge P, Bouvier E, Cormier B, Morice MC. Transfemoral aortic valve implantation new criteria to predict vascular complications. *J Am Coll Cardiol Intv* 2011;4:851–858.
10. Généreux P, Webb JG, Svensson LG, Kodali SK, Satler LF, Fearon WF, Davidson CJ, Eisenhauer AC, Makkar RR, Bergman GW, Babaliaros V, Bavaria JE, Velazquez OC, Williams MR, Hueter I, Xu K, Leon MB; PARTNER Trial Investigators. Vascular complications after transcatheter aortic valve replacement: insights from the PARTNER (Placement of Aortic Transcatheter Valve) trial. *J Am Coll Cardiol* 2012;60:1043–1052.
11. Sinning JM, Horack M, Grube E, Gerckens U, Erbel R, Eggebrecht H, Zahn R, Linke A, Sievert H, Figulla HR, Kuck KH, Hauptmann KE, Hoffmann E, Hambrecht R, Richardt G, Sack S, Senges J, Nickenig G, Werner N. The impact of peripheral arterial disease on early outcome after transcatheter aortic valve implantation: results from the German Transcatheter Aortic Valve Interventions Registry. *Am Heart J* 2012;164:102–110.

Congenitally bicuspid aortic valve in brothers: coarctation of the aorta with a normally functioning aortic valve in one and no coarctation but severe aortic stenosis in the other

Saleha Zafar, MD, and William C. Roberts, MD

Described herein are two brothers, both with a congenitally bicuspid aortic valve—one of which was stenotic and one of which functioned normally—and one with associated aortic isthmic coarctation. Summarized also are previously reported families with more than one member with a congenitally bicuspid aortic valve.

The occurrence of a congenitally bicuspid aortic valve (BAV) in more than one family member has been described in several published reports (1–7). Of the 47 family members in whom the BAV was confirmed at the time of aortic valve replacement or at necropsy, the valve was stenotic in at least 27 of them, and none had associated aortic isthmic coarctation. In this report we describe two brothers with a congenitally BAV—stenotic in one and functionally normal in the other—and aortic coarctation in one of them *(Figure)*.

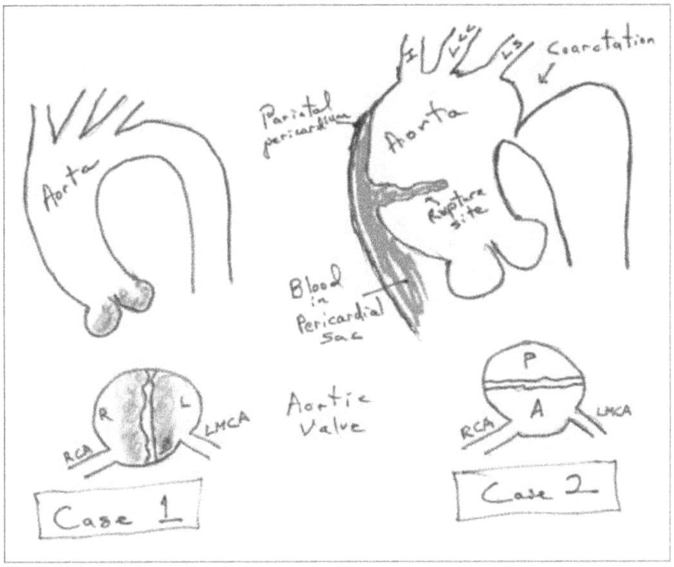

Figure 1. Diagram showing the cardiovascular features of each of the two patients. Both had congenitally bicuspid aortic valves. In case 1, the valve was severely stenotic, and there was no coarctation of the aorta. In case 2, the valve functioned normally, and there was a severe coarctation of the aorta. A indicates anterior aortic valve cusp; I, innominate artery; L, left; LCC, left common carotid; LMCA, left main coronary artery; LS, left subclavian; P, posterior aortic valve cusp; R, right aortic valve cusp; RCA, right coronary artery.

PATIENT DESCRIPTIONS

Case 1

A 16-year-old white boy had been well until about a month before hospitalization when he had an episode of severe dizziness followed by progressive breathlessness. He was hospitalized for "pneumonia" but never had any microorganisms cultured from sputum. When the chest radiograph cleared, cardiac catheterization disclosed the following pressures in mm Hg: pulmonary artery wedge a wave 34, v 32, and mean 32; pulmonary trunk 55/38; right ventricle 57/29; left ventricle 133/36 and aorta 77/66, yielding a peak systolic pressure gradient of 56 mm Hg; and mean systolic gradient 39 mm Hg. The calculated aortic valve area was 0.6 cm^2, and the cardiac output was 4.6 L/min/m^2. A cardiac operation was performed, and he died 2 weeks later.

Case 2

This 21-year-old white man had been well until he was found dead in the bathroom at home, shortly after taking an amphetamine. He apparently never had evidence of cardiac dysfunction. Necropsy disclosed the pericardial sac to be filled with blood (550 mL). The ascending aorta had a 5-cm long tear without dissection with a through-and-through perforation. The ascending aorta was quite dilated. At the aortic isthmus (that portion of aorta just distal to the origin of the left subclavian artery), a severe coarctation was found. The aortic valve was congenitally bicuspid but the cusps were very pliable and noncalcified. Thus, the aortic valve function was considered to have been normal. A fibrous, nonstenotic ring was located in the left ventricular outflow tract about 1 cm below the base of the aortic valve cusps. The mitral valve was normal. The left main coronary artery ostium was located about 1 cm cephalad to the sinotubular junction.

From the Baylor Heart and Vascular Institute (Zafar, Roberts) and the Departments of Internal Medicine (Division of Cardiology) and Pathology (Roberts), Baylor University Medical Center at Dallas.

Corresponding author: William C. Roberts, MD, Baylor Heart and Vascular Institute, 621 North Hall Street, Dallas, TX 75226 (e-mail: wc.roberts@BaylorHealth.edu).

Table. Previously published reports of patients with a familial congenitally bicuspid aortic valve with aortic valve replacement or necropsy

Year of publication	First author	Family	Case number	Patient age (yrs) at AVR	Patient age (yrs) at death	Patient relation	Bicuspid aortic valve AR	AS	Functionally normal
1972	McKusick	I	1	44	46	Father	+	–	–
			2	–	19	Son	+	–	–
1977	Gale	I	3	38	–	Brother	–	+	–
			4	44	–	Brother	+	+	–
1978	Emanuel*	I	6	–	62	Uncle	–	+	–
			7	–	–	Mother	–	–	–
			8	20	–	Son	–	–	–
		II	9	–	–	Mother	–	–	–
			10	41	–	Son	–	+	–
		III	11	–	–	Mother	–	–	–
			12	–	–	Son	–	+	–
			13	–	–	Niece	+	+	–
			14	–	–	Nephew	–	+	–
			15	–	68	Grandfather	–	+	–
		IV	16	–	–	Mother	–	–	–
			17	16	–	Son	–	+	–
		V	18	93	–	Mother	–	+	–
			19	–	–	Son	–	–	–
		VI	20	–	97	Mother	–	+	–
			21	–	–	Son	–	–	–
1987	Godden	I	22	57	–	Brother	–	+	–
			23	57	61	Brother	+	+	–
1989	McDonald	I	24	–	19	Brother	–	+	–
			25	23	–	Brother	–	+	–
			26	26	–	Brother	+	+	–
1994	Glick	I	27	58	58	Father	0	+	–
			28	–	–	Daughter	+	0	–
		II	29	44	58	Father	+	+	–
			30	26	26	Son	+	0	–
		III	31	53	60	Sister	–	+	–
			32	72	–	Brother	+	+	–
			33	–	70	Sister	–	+	–
		IV	34	21	–	Brother	+	0	–
			35	26	26	Brother	+	0	–
			36	–	–	Sister	–	–	–
			37	–	–	Sister	–	–	–
			38	–	–	Brother	–	–	–
		V	39	70	80	Brother	–	+	–
			40	69	73	Brother	–	+	–
		VI	41	78	–	Mother	–	+	–

continues

Table. Continued.

Year of publication	First author	Family	Case number	Patient age (yrs) at AVR	Patient age (yrs) at death	Patient relation	Bicuspid aortic valve		
							AR	AS	Functionally normal
			42	65	–	Daughter	–	+	–
			43	–	–	Daughter	–	+	–
1996	Clementi	I	44	–	47	Brother	–	+	–
			45	42	–	Brother	+	–	–
			46	–	–	Sister	+	–	–
		II	46	–	–	Mother	+	–	–
			47	–	–	Son	+	0	+

*The bicuspid nature of the aortic valve was "surgically proven" in all patients listed here.

AR indicates aortic regurgitation; AS, aortic stenosis; AVR, aortic valve replacement; –, no information or not applicable.

DISCUSSION

The *Table* lists previously published reports (1–7) describing a BAV in more than one family member with study of the valve at either aortic valve replacement or at necropsy. In the 18 families, 47 members had a congenitally BAV: 11 families had 2 members, 5 families had 3 members, and 2 families had 5 members with a BAV. Of the involved family members, 3 were fathers, 8 were mothers, 20 were sons, 8 were daughters, and the remaining were siblings or other relatives. Of the 47 family members, 30 (64%) were male and 17 (36%) were female. Twenty-three family members had aortic valve replacement; their ages ranged from 16 to 93 years (mean 47). Sixteen family members had died, 9 after aortic valve replacement. In the 18 families, all with BAVs were male in 3 families, all were female in 1 family, and both males and females were represented in 14 families.

In addition to the studies where the bicuspid structure of the aortic valve was confirmed morphologically, an echocardiographic study (8) described 11 families in whom 28 members had a BAV, 3 (11%) of whom had associated coarctation of the aorta.

1. McKusick VA. Association of congenital bicuspid aortic valve and Erdheim's cystic medial necrosis. *Lancet* 1972;1(7758):1026–1027.
2. Gale AN, McKusick VA, Hutchins GM, Gott VL. Familial congenital bicuspid aortic valve: secondary calcific aortic stenosis and aortic aneurysm. *Chest* 1977;72(5):668–670.
3. Emanuel R, Withers R, O'Brien K, Ross P, Feizi O. Congenitally bicuspid aortic valves. Clinicogenetic study of 41 families. *Br Heart J* 1978;40(12):1402–1407.
4. Godden DJ, Sandhu PS, Kerr F. Stenosed bicuspid aortic valves in twins. *Eur Heart J* 1987;8(3):316–318.
5. McDonald K, Maurer BJ. Familial aortic valve disease: evidence for a genetic influence? *Eur Heart J* 1989;10(7):676–677.
6. Glick BN, Roberts WC. Congenitally bicuspid aortic valve in multiple family members. *Am J Cardiol* 1994;73(5):400–404.
7. Clementi M, Notari L, Borghi A, Tenconi R. Familial congenital bicuspid aortic valve: a disorder of uncertain inheritance. *Am J Med Genet* 1996;62(4):336–338.
8. Huntington K, Hunter AG, Chan KL. A prospective study to assess the frequency of familial clustering of congenital bicuspid aortic valve. *J Am Coll Cardiol* 1997;30(7):1809–1812.

Natural History of Unoperated Aortic Stenosis During a 50-Year Period of Cardiac Valve Replacement

William C. Roberts, MD[a,b,c,d,*], Travis J. Vowels, BBA[a], Giovanni Filardo, PhD, MPH[e,f], Jong M. Ko, BA[a], Raj P. Mathur, MD[d], and Jamshid Shirani, MD[d]

Although a number of publications have described the natural history of patients with aortic stenosis (AS), the definition of "natural history" varies widely. Those describing a large number of patients with AS without operative therapy with necropsy findings are rare. Two hundred sixty patients >15 years of age with AS were studied at necropsy over a 50-year period by the same investigator. Of the 260 patients, the valve in 37 (14%) was congenitally unicuspid, in 123 (47%), congenitally bicuspid, and in 100 (38%), tricuspid. Aortic valve structure varied with age of death (in years; unicuspid 52 ± 17, bicuspid 63 ± 12, and tricuspid 70 ± 14 years); gender (men/women: unicuspid 95%/5%, bicuspid 78%/22%, and tricuspid 63%/37%), and frequency of calcium in the mitral valve annulus and epicardial coronary arteries. The patients with cardiac-related symptoms compared with those without were more likely to have a congenitally malformed valve (unicuspid 17% vs 12%; bicuspid 51% vs 29%; tricuspid 31% vs 60%; unadjusted p = 0.013), to die from cardiac disease (86% vs 54%; unadjusted p = 0.001), and to have larger hearts (mean cardiac weight 606 ± 138 g vs 523 ± 121 g; unadjusted p = 0.009) and a larger quantity of calcium in the aortic valve cusps. In conclusion, the length of survival in adults with AS is related to valve structure, gender, presence of cardiac-related symptoms, cardiac mass, and quantity of calcium in the aortic valve cusps.
(Am J Cardiol 2013;112:541–553)

During the past 80 years or so, a number of reports describing the natural history of patients with valvular aortic stenosis (AS) have been published. Before 1970, most focused on patients with AS studied at necropsy, and most centered on the cause of the AS.[1] After predictably successful aortic valve replacement became a reality in the early 1960s, more reports appeared on the natural history of AS, but "natural history" meant something different in most studies. In some studies, it meant what happened when patients were followed for a specified period of time. In others, the term focused on the survival duration of symptomatic or asymptomatic patients until either an aortic valve operation was performed or death. A few included only subjects who had cardiac catheterization or echocardiography performed such that the severity of the AS was accurately known. No study in the past 50 years has focused on a large group of adults with AS studied at necropsy in whom an aortic valve operation during life had never been performed. Such is the purpose of this report.

Methods

From January 1956 until July 2012, 260 patients with AS unassociated with mitral stenosis were studied at necropsy either at the National Institutes of Health (Pathology Branch, National Heart, Lung, and Blood Institute, Bethesda, Maryland) or at Baylor University Medical Center, Dallas, Texas; they are the subject of this study. All hearts were examined and classified by one of us (WCR). Many hearts had been submitted from other hospitals, particularly those in the Washington, DC, and surrounding areas. To be included in this study, at the time of necropsy, patients had to be >15 years of age, have a nonstenotic mitral valve, and had no operative procedure at any time on any cardiac valve. The aortic valve morphologically had to be clearly stenotic, that is, contain enough calcific deposits such that mobility of the aortic valve cusp or cusps was clearly diminished. The underlying structure of the stenotic aortic valve (i.e., unicuspid, bicuspid, or tricuspid) was determined in all cases by the same observer (WCR). The major epicardial coronary arteries were examined for obstructions, and the left ventricular walls were examined for foci of necrosis and fibrosis. Myocardial necrosis/fibrosis was confirmed by study of histologic sections of these areas. The medical records were sought and received from the hospitals submitting the heart

[a]Baylor Heart and Vascular Institute, [b]Department of Internal Medicine, Division of Cardiology, and [c]Department of Pathology, Baylor University Medical Center, Dallas, Texas; [d]Pathology Branch, National Heart, Lung, and Blood Institute, National Institutes of Health, Bethesda, Maryland; [e]Institute for Health Care Research and Improvement, Baylor University Medical Center; and [f]Department of Statistical Science, Southern Methodist University, Dallas, Texas. Manuscript received March 21, 2013; revised manuscript received and accepted April 3, 2013.

TJV is a first year medical student at the University of Texas Medical School at Houston, TX.

Present address (RPM): 106 Irving NW St Suite 218, Washington, DC 20010.

Present address (JS): St. Luke's University Health Network Cardiology, 801 Ostrum Street, Bethlehem, PA 18015.

This work was supported by grants from the Baylor Heart and Vascular Institute Cardiovascular Research Review Committee and Baylor Health Care System Foundation.

See page 552 for disclosure information.

*Corresponding author: Tel: (214) 820-7911; fax: (214) 820-7533.

E-mail address: wc.roberts@baylorhealth.edu (W.C. Roberts).

Table 1
Morphologic and clinical variables, and modes of death in 260 patients with valvular aortic stenosis according to aortic valve structure

Variable	Unicuspid	Bicuspid	Tricuspid	Unadjusted* p Value
	n = 37 (14%)	n = 123 (47%)	n = 100 (38%)	
Age in years: range (n = 254)	16–87	23–89	36–99	0.001
(Mean ± SD)	(52 ± 17)	(63 ± 12)	(70 ± 14)	
95% CI	47,56	60,65	67,72	
Men/Women (n = 257)	35/2	93/27	63/37	0.005
	95%/5%	78%/22%	63%/37%	
Symptoms[†] (n = 260)				0.013
Symptomatic	30 (81%)	89 (72%)	54 (54%)	
Asymptomatic	6 (16%)	15 (12%)	31 (31%)	
Unknown	1 (3%)	19 (16%)	15 (15%)	
Mode of death (n = 260)				0.511
Cardiac				
Sudden	6 (16%)	29 (24%)	26 (26%)	
Non-sudden	28 (76%)	66 (54%)	47 (47%)	
Vascular	1 (3%)	5 (4%)	2 (2%)	
Noncardiac, nonvascular	2 (5%)	20 (16%)	25 (25%)	
Unknown	0	3 (2%)	0	
Heart weight (g): range (n = 231)	320–880	340–1,050	305–960	0.127[‡]
(Mean ± SD)	(633 ± 136)	(591 ± 148)	(552 ± 132)	
95% CI	585,681	564,618	523,581	
Men	320–880	385–1,050	380–960	
	(637 ± 137)	(620 ± 147)	(603 ± 115)	
Women	510	340–730	305–710	
	—	(496 ± 119)	(458 ± 108)	
Number of enlarged hearts[§] (n = 215 of 231)	31 of 33 (94%)	100 of 106 (94%)	84 of 92 (91%)	0.689
Narrowing of ≥1 major coronary arteries >75% (n = 96/234)	6 (17%)	43 (41%)	47 (51%)	0.018
Left ventricular (n = 260)				0.513
Necrosis only	1 (3%)	8 (7%)	6 (6%)	
Fibrosis only	15 (41%)	44 (36%)	25 (25%)	
Both	2 (5%)	7 (6%)	5 (5%)	
Neither	19 (51%)	64 (52%)	64 (64%)	
Calcium				
Aortic valve (n = 251)				0.404
0	1 (3%)	1 (1%)	1 (1%)	
1+	5 (14%)	9 (8%)	7 (7%)	
2+	2 (5%)	15 (13%)	18 (18%)	
3+	10 (27%)	27 (23%)	30 (31%)	
4+	19 (51%)	64 (55%)	42 (43%)	
Mitral annulus (n = 89 of 245)	7 (19%)	22 (20%)	60 (61%)	0.001
Coronary arteries (n = 121 of 232)	11 (31%)	43 (41%)	67 (73%)	0.001

* Multiplicity accounted for.
† Symptoms include heart failure, angina pectoris, and syncope, or any combination of the 3.
‡ Unicuspid versus tricuspid p value = 0.051.
§ Hearts weighing >350 g in women and >400 g in men.

specimens. Most stenotic aortic valves were photographed at either the Pathology Branch, National Heart, Lung, and Blood Institute, or in the Cardiovascular Laboratory at Baylor University Medical Center.

Means, SDs, and percentages were calculated to describe the study cohort (n = 260). Differences in demographic, clinical, and morphologic details were tested with a Wilcoxon (for continuous factors) or a chi-square (for categorical factors) test. Unadjusted p values and 95% confidence intervals (CIs) were also estimated. A Bonferroni correction was used to account for multiplicity. A multivariable logistic regression model was used to assess the adjusted-association between patients having symptoms (heart failure, angina pectoris, and/or syncope) and cause of death (e.g., cardiac or vascular).[2] Covariates included gender, valve structure, heart weight (in grams), degree of coronary narrowing, foci of left ventricular necrosis and/or fibrosis, presence of calcium in the coronary arteries (in ≥1 coronary arteries). Likewise, 2 multivariable logistic regression models were used to assess the adjusted-association between age and (1) congenital valve disease and (2) presence of calcium in the coronary arteries. Covariates included patient having symptoms (heart failure, angina pectoris, and/or syncope), gender, valve structure (for calcium model only), heart weight (in grams), degree of coronary narrowing, foci of left ventricular necrosis and/or fibrosis, and presence of calcium in the coronary arteries (congenital valve model only). Restricted cubic splines were used for all continuous variables, and multiple imputation via

Table 2
Morphologic and clinical variables, and modes of death in 257 patients with valvular aortic stenosis according to gender

Variable	Men	Women	Unadjusted* p Value
	n = 191 (74%)	n = 66 (26%)	
Age in years: range (n = 254)	16–99	32–90	0.001
(Mean ± SD)	(61 ± 15)	(70 ± 13)	
95% CI	59,64	66,73	
Aortic valve structure (n = 257)			0.005
Unicuspid	35 (18%)	2 (3%)	
Bicuspid	93 (49%)	27 (41%)	
Tricuspid	63 (33%)	37 (56%)	
Symptoms† (n = 257)			0.973
Symptomatic	129 (68%)	44 (67%)	
Asymptomatic	38 (20%)	14 (21%)	
Unknown	24 (12%)	8 (12%)	
Mode of death (n = 257)			0.558
Cardiac			
Sudden	45 (24%)	16 (24%)	
Non-sudden	109 (57%)	32 (48%)	
Vascular	6 (3%)	2 (3%)	
Noncardiac, nonvascular	30 (16%)	16 (24%)	
Unknown	1 (1%)	0	
Heart weight (g): range (n = 231)	320–1,050	305–730	0.001
(Mean ± SD)	(617 ± 135)	(474 ± 112)	
95% CI	598,636	440,509	
Number of enlarged hearts‡ (n = 215 of 231)	167 of 175 (95%)	48 of 56 (86%)	0.129
Coronary narrowing >75%§ (n = 95 of 233)	74 (43%)	21 (35%)	0.292
Left ventricular (n = 257)			0.829
Necrosis only	11 (6%)	4 (6%)	
Fibrosis only	69 (36%)	14 (21%)	
Both	11 (6%)	2 (3%)	
Neither	100 (52%)	46 (70%)	
Calcium			
Aortic valve (n = 249)			0.385
0	3 (2%)	0	
1+	17 (9%)	4 (6%)	
2+	27 (15%)	8 (12%)	
3+	51 (28%)	14 (22%)	
4+	86 (47%)	39 (60%)	
Mitral annulus (n = 88 of 243)	51 (28%)	37 (59%)	0.001
Coronary arteries (n = 120 of 231)	85 (49%)	35 (61%)	0.100

* Multiplicity accounted for.
† Symptoms include heart failure, angina pectoris, and syncope, or any combination of the 3.
‡ Hearts weighing >350 g in women and >400 g in men.
§ In cross-sectional area.

predictive mean matching was used to account for missing data regarding the independent variables in this model. The adjusted p values, odds ratios, and 95% CIs were also estimated.[2,3]

The study protocol was approved by the Institutional Review Board of Baylor University Medical Center.

Results

The findings in the present study are summarized in Tables 1 through 7. Table 1 displays data according to aortic valve structure, Table 2 according to gender, Table 3 according to symptomatic status, Table 4 according to age group at death, Table 5 according to heart weight, and Table 6 according to degree of coronary narrowing. Table 7 provides findings in the 37 patients who had left-sided cardiac catheterization. Table 8 lists findings in the 29 patients whose stenotic aortic valves are illustrated in Figures 1 through 4. Figure 5 illustrates the length of survival after onset of symptoms: angina pectoris, heart failure, syncope, and various combinations of these. Figure 6 shows the length of survival after onset of any cardiac symptom: angina pectoris, heart failure, syncope, or any combination of these. Figure 7 displays the relation of age to the probability of having a congenitally malformed aortic valve (unicuspid or bicuspid) and calcium in ≥1 coronary arteries.

Of the 260 patients, the aortic valve was *unicuspid* in 37 (14%; Figure 1), *bicuspid* in 123 (47%; Figures 2 and 3), and *tricuspid* in 100 (38%; Figure 4; Table 1). The fewer the number of aortic valve cusps, the higher the frequency of males (95% with unicuspid valves, 78% with bicuspid valves, and 63% with tricuspid valves, unadjusted p = 0.005). The

Table 3
Morphologic and clinical variables, and modes of death in 260 patients with valvular aortic stenosis according to the presence or absence of symptoms*

Variable	Symptomatic n = 173 (67%)	Asymptomatic n = 52 (20%)	Unknown n = 35 (13%)	Unadjusted† p Value
Age in years: range (n = 254)	16–92	23–89	37–99	0.854
(Mean ± SD)	(64 ± 14)	(64 ± 17)	(62 ± 15)	
95% CI	62,66	60,68	57,68	
Men/Women (n = 257)	129/44	38/14	24/8	0.973
	75%/25%	73%/27%	75%/25%	
Aortic valve structure (n = 260)				0.013
Unicuspid	30 (17%)	6 (12%)	1 (3%)	
Bicuspid	89 (51%)	15 (29%)	19 (54%)	
Tricuspid	54 (31%)	31 (60%)	15 (43%)	
Mode of death (n = 260)				0.001
Cardiac				
Sudden	38 (22%)	14 (27%)	9 (26%)	
Non-sudden	111 (64%)	14 (27%)	16 (46%)	
Vascular	4 (2%)	4 (8%)	0	
Noncardiac, nonvascular	20 (12%)	20 (38%)	7 (20%)	
Unknown	0	0	3 (9%)	
Heart weight (g): range (n = 231)	320–1,050	305–920	310–1,000	0.009
(Mean ± SD)	(606 ± 138)	(523 ± 121)	(563 ± 173)	
95% CI	584,628	484,561	511,608	
Men	320–1,050	340–920	420–1,000	
	(638 ± 131)	(543 ± 115)	(633 ± 147)	
Women	370–730	305–650	310–500	
	(499 ± 106)	(465 ± 123)	(381 ± 72)	
Number of enlarged hearts‡ (n = 215 of 231)	148 of 152 (97%)	43 of 50 (86%)	24 of 29 (83%)	0.015
Narrowing of ≥1 major coronary arteries >75% (n = 96 of 234)	67 (41%)	15 (33%)	14 (56%)	0.161
Left ventricular (n = 260)				0.449
Necrosis only	9 (5%)	4 (8%)	2 (6%)	
Fibrosis only	64 (37%)	9 (17%)	11 (31%)	
Both	12 (7%)	0	2 (6%)	
Neither	88 (51%)	39 (75%)	20 (57%)	
Calcium				
Aortic valve (n = 251)				0.038
0	2 (1%)	1 (2%)	0	
1+	10 (6%)	6 (12%)	5 (17%)	
2+	19 (11%)	13 (25%)	3 (10%)	
3+	40 (23%)	15 (29%)	12 (41%)	
4+	100 (58%)	16 (31%)	9 (31%)	
Mitral annulus (n = 89 of 245)	59 (35%)	18 (36%)	12 (43%)	0.745
Coronary arteries (n = 121 of 232)	80 (49%)	24 (52%)	17 (71%)	0.147

* Symptoms include heart failure, angina pectoris, and syncope, or any combination of the 3.
† Multiplicity accounted for.
‡ Hearts weighing >350 g in women and >400 g in men.

frequency of angina pectoris, heart failure, and/or syncope was similar in patients with unicuspid and bicuspid valves and less in those with tricuspid valves (83% vs 86% vs 64%, unadjusted p = 0.013). Men had mean heart weights larger than women in all 3 valve-structure groups; the patients with unicuspid valves had larger hearts than those with tricuspid aortic valves (633 vs 552 g, unadjusted p = 0.051). Calcific deposits in the coronary arteries and in the mitral annulus were less frequent in those with unicuspid and bicuspid valves than in those with tricuspid valves (19% vs 20% vs 61%, unadjusted p = 0.001, and 31% vs 41% vs 73%, unadjusted p = 0.001, respectively). Coronary narrowing >75% in cross-sectional area by atherosclerotic plaques was less the fewer the number of aortic valve cusps (17% vs 41% vs 51%, unadjusted p = 0.018). No significant differences were observed in modes of death, frequency of foci of left ventricular wall necrosis or fibrosis, or both or neither.

Differences among the 8 variables analyzed between *men* and *women* are summarized in Table 2. The mean ages, number of aortic valve cusps, heart weight, and calcium in the mitral annular region were significantly different between genders. No significant differences were observed between men and women in the frequency of cardiac symptoms, mode of death, frequency of severe (>75%) coronary narrowing or foci of left ventricular necrosis and/or fibrosis, and quantity of calcium in the aortic valve and in the coronary arteries.

Table 3 summarizes differences in the various variables in the *symptomatic versus the asymptomatic patients*. Of the symptomatic patients, 69% had a unicuspid or bicuspid valve and 31%, a tricuspid valve; of the asymptomatic patients, 40%

Table 4
Morphologic and clinical variables, and modes of death in 254 patients with valvular aortic stenosis according to age group

Variable	Age Groups (years)			Unadjusted* p Value
	16–35	36–65	>65	
	n = 11 (4%)	n = 119 (47%)	n = 124 (49%)	
Men/Women (n = 254)	10/1 91%/9%	97/22 82%/18%	81/43 65%/35%	0.069
Aortic valve structure (n = 254)				0.001
Unicuspid	9 (82%)	22 (18%)	6 (5%)	
Bicuspid	2 (18%)	64 (54%)	52 (42%)	
Tricuspid	0	33 (28%)	66 (53%)	
Symptoms[†] (n = 254)				0.229
Symptomatic	6 (55%)	83 (70%)	84 (68%)	
Asymptomatic	5 (45%)	17 (14%)	30 (24%)	
Unknown	0	19 (16%)	10 (8%)	
Mode of death (n = 254)				0.380
Cardiac				
Sudden	3 (27%)	32 (27%)	26 (21%)	
Non-sudden	6 (55%)	68 (57%)	64 (52%)	
Vascular	1 (9%)	2 (2%)	5 (4%)	
Noncardiac, nonvascular	1 (9%)	16 (13%)	29 (23%)	
Unknown	0	1 (1%)	0	
Heart weight (g): range (n = 230)	480–880	305–1,050	310–860	0.107[‡]
(Mean ± SD)	(622 ± 116)	(609 ± 157)	(554 ± 126)	
95% CI	538,706	582,636	527,580	
Men	480–880 (633 ± 116)	320–1,050 (638 ± 148)	380–860 (593 ± 117)	
Women	510	305–730 (483 ± 133)	310–710 (468 ± 103)	
Number of enlarged hearts[§] (214 of 230)	11 of 11 (100%)	99 of 108 (92%)	104 of 111 (94%)	0.547
Narrowing of ≥1 major coronary arteries >75% (n = 95/232)	0	41 (37%)	54 (48%)	0.069
Left ventricular (n = 254)				0.502
Necrosis only	2 (18%)	5 (4%)	7 (6%)	
Fibrosis only	4 (36%)	38 (32%)	41 (33%)	
Both	0	8 (7%)	5 (4%)	
Neither	5 (45%)	68 (57%)	71 (57%)	
Calcium				
Aortic valve (n = 248)				0.101
0	1 (9%)	1 (1%)	1 (1%)	
1+	0	11 (9%)	10 (8%)	
2+	3 (27%)	18 (16%)	14 (12%)	
3+	5 (45%)	27 (23%)	33 (27%)	
4+	2 (18%)	59 (51%)	63 (52%)	
Mitral annulus (n = 88 of 242)	0	36 (32%)	52 (44%)	0.059
Coronary arteries (n = 119 of 230)	1 (10%)	34 (33%)	84 (71%)	0.001

* Multiplicity accounted for.
† Symptoms include heart failure, angina pectoris, and syncope, or any combination of the 3.
‡ Age groups 36 to 65 versus >65 p value = 0.042.
§ Hearts weighing >350 g in women and >400 g in men.

had either a unicuspid or bicuspid valve and 60%, a tricuspid valve (unadjusted p = 0.013). The symptomatic patients had larger hearts than the asymptomatic ones (606 vs 523 g, unadjusted p = 0.009), more left ventricular wall scarring (46% vs 18%), and a larger quantity of calcific deposits in the aortic valve cusps (unadjusted p = 0.038). No significant differences were observed between the symptomatic and asymptomatic groups in age, gender, frequency of severe coronary narrowing, frequency of foci of left ventricular necrosis, or the frequency of calcific deposits in the mitral annulus or coronary arteries. However, the adjusted analysis showed that patients having symptoms (heart failure, angina pectoris, and/or syncope) were more likely to die from cardiac causes than asymptomatic patients (adjusted odds ratio = 3.61; 95% CI: 1.85, 7.05, p <0.001).

Findings according to *age group* (16 to 35, 36 to 65, and >65 years) are summarized in Table 4. All 11 patients aged 16 to 35 had unicuspid (n = 9) or bicuspid (n = 2) valves; 72% of the 119 patients aged 36 to 65 had unicuspid (n = 22) or bicuspid (n = 64) valves, and 47% of the 124 patients aged >65 years had unicuspid (n = 6) or bicuspid (n = 52) valves (unadjusted p = 0.001; Figure 6). The frequency of calcium in either the coronary arteries or mitral annulus was least in the younger age group and greatest in

Table 5
Morphologic and clinical variables, and modes of death in 234 patients with valvular aortic stenosis according to heart weight

Variable	Heart Weight (g)			Unadjusted* p Value
	≤400	401–600	>600	
	n = 26 (11%)	n = 108 (46%)	n = 100 (43%)	
Age in years: range (n = 230)	47–90	23–99	16–89	0.021
(Mean ± SD)	67 ± 11	66 ± 15	59 ± 15	
Men/Women (n = 231)	8/18	76/29	91/9	0.001
	31%/69%	72%/28%	91%/9%	
Aortic valve structure (n = 234)				0.202
Unicuspid	2 (8%)	11 (10%)	20 (20%)	
Bicuspid	11 (42%)	53 (49%)	45 (45%)	
Tricuspid	13 (50%)	44 (41%)	35 (35%)	
Symptoms† (n = 234)				0.031
Symptomatic	12 (46%)	62 (57%)	78 (78%)	
Asymptomatic	8 (31%)	31 (29%)	11 (11%)	
Unknown	6 (23%)	15 (14%)	11 (11%)	
Mode of death (n = 234)				0.659
Cardiac				
Sudden	9 (35%)	21 (19%)	23 (23%)	
Non-sudden	8 (31%)	57 (53%)	62 (62%)	
Vascular	2 (8%)	2 (2%)	3 (3%)	
Noncardiac, nonvascular	7 (27%)	26 (24%)	11 (11%)	
Unknown	0	2 (2%)	1 (1%)	
Narrowing of ≥1 major coronary arteries >75% (n = 92/213)	11 (42%)	43 (40%)	38 (38%)	0.922
Left ventricular (n = 234)				0.729
Necrosis only	1 (4%)	10 (9%)	3 (3%)	
Fibrosis only	9 (35%)	28 (26%)	42 (42%)	
Both	0	6 (6%)	8 (8%)	
Neither	16 (62%)	64 (59%)	47 (47%)	
Calcium				
Aortic valve (n = 229)				0.261
0	0	0	3 (3%)	
1+	4 (15%)	8 (8%)	6 (6%)	
2+	3 (12%)	20 (19%)	10 (10%)	
3+	7 (27%)	29 (28%)	27 (27%)	
4+	12 (46%)	47 (45%)	53 (54%)	
Mitral annulus (n = 80/223)	11 (42%)	35 (32%)	34 (34%)	0.558
Coronary arteries (n = 110/211)	16 (62%)	55 (51%)	39 (39%)	0.578

* Multiplicity accounted for.
† Symptoms include heart failure, angina pectoris, and syncope, or any combination of the 3.

the oldest age group (0% vs 32% vs 44%, p = 0.059, and 10% vs 33% vs 71%, unadjusted p = 0.001) (Figure 6). No significant differences were observed among the 3 age groups in gender, symptomatic status, mode of death, heart weight, frequency of severe coronary narrowing, or left ventricular necrosis or fibrosis.

Findings according to 3 *heart weight* groups are summarized in Table 5. Women had smaller hearts than men, and 69% of the smaller hearts (≤400 g) belonged to women; of the 100 hearts weighing >600 g, 91 (91%) belonged to men (unadjusted p = 0.001). Of the 33 patients with unicuspid aortic valves, 31 (94%) weighed >400 g and 20 (61%) weighed >600 g, and of the 92 patients with tricuspid aortic valves, 79 (86%) weighed >400 g, but only 35 (38%) weighed >600 g. No significant differences were observed in the 3 age groups in aortic valve structure, mode of death, percent with severe (>75%) coronary narrowing or left ventricular necrosis or fibrosis, or presence of calcium in the aortic valve, mitral annulus, or coronary arteries.

Findings according to whether *coronary narrowing* >75% in cross-sectional area occurred is summarized in Table 6. Those with severe coronary narrowing were more likely to be older, to have a tricuspid aortic valve, to have calcific deposits in the coronary arteries and foci of left ventricular necrosis and/or fibrosis than those with lesser degrees of coronary narrowing (unadjusted p = 0.001).

Pertinent findings in the 37 patients who underwent *left-sided cardiac catheterization* are summarized in Table 7.

Discussion

This study of 260 adult patients with unoperated AS followed to death and autopsy demonstrated that patients with unicuspid or bicuspid valves (congenital origin) as

Table 6
Morphologic and clinical variables, and modes of death in 234 patients with valvular aortic stenosis according to coronary artery narrowing

Variable	Coronary Narrowing (Cross-Sectional Area)		Unadjusted* p Value
	>75%	<75%	
	n = 96 (41%)	n = 138 (59%)	
Age in years: range (n = 232)	42–99	16–90	0.001
(Mean ± SD)	68 ± 12	61 ± 15	
Men/Women (n = 233)	74/21	99/39	0.292
	78%/22%	72%/28%	
Aortic valve structure (n = 234)			0.018
Unicuspid	6 (6%)	30 (22%)	
Bicuspid	43 (45%)	63 (46%)	
Tricuspid	47 (48%)	45 (33%)	
Symptoms[†] (n = 234)			0.161
Symptomatic	67 (69%)	96 (70%)	
Asymptomatic	15 (16%)	31 (22%)	
Unknown	14 (15%)	11 (8%)	
Mode of death (n = 234)			0.245
Cardiac			
Sudden	26 (27%)	31 (22%)	
Non-sudden	47 (49%)	80 (58%)	
Vascular	5 (5%)	2 (1%)	
Noncardiac, nonvascular	17 (18%)	25 (18%)	
Unknown	1 (1%)	0	
Heart weight (g): range (n = 212)	305–1,050	310–960	0.222
(Mean ± SD)	566 ± 137	590 ± 142	
Men	320–1,050	380–960	
	593 ± 132	630 ± 130	
Women	305–730	310–710	
	472 ± 118	473 ± 105	
Number of enlarged hearts[‡] (n = 197 of 212)	85 of 91 (93%)	112 of 121 (93%)	0.813
Left ventricular (n = 234)			0.001
Necrosis only	7 (7%)	5 (4%)	
Fibrosis only	49 (51%)	28 (20%)	
Both	8 (8%)	4 (3%)	
Neither	32 (33%)	101 (73%)	
Calcium			
Aortic valve (n = 234)			0.464
0	0	3 (2%)	
1+	10 (10%)	9 (7%)	
2+	13 (14%)	22 (16%)	
3+	22 (23%)	35 (25%)	
4+	51 (53%)	69 (50%)	
Mitral annulus (n = 81/231)	39 (41%)	42 (30%)	0.112
Coronary arteries (n = 111/221)	64 (67%)	47 (34%)	0.001

* Multiplicity accounted for.
[†] Symptoms include heart failure, angina pectoris, and syncope, or any combination of the 3.
[‡] Hearts weighing >350 g in women and >400 g in men.

opposed to those with tricuspid valves (acquired origin) had a younger age of death, a greater likelihood of being male, a higher likelihood of having cardiac-related symptoms, heavier hearts, larger quantities of calcium in the aortic valve cusps, but a lower frequency of calcium in the epicardial coronary arteries and in the mitral annulus.

Although a number of reports before 1960 described clinical and/or necropsy findings in patients with AS, the structure of the aortic valve and the severity of AS were infrequently mentioned.[1] The morphologic data in most studies were garnered from autopsy protocols prepared by a number of prosectors with varying expertise in cardiovascular disease. Additionally, few contained photographs of the stenotic valves, or the number was quite limited, preventing the reader's being assured of the severity of the AS. Moreover, some studies of patients with AS also included patients with mitral stenosis, highly prevalent before World War II. Indeed, many of the morphologic studies concluded that rheumatic heart disease was the origin of AS in most patients.[1] The present study excluded patients with mitral stenosis in an attempt to exclude rheumatic heart disease as a cause of the AS in any of our 260 patients.[4]

Table 7

Clinical and morphologic findings in 37 patients seen at necropsy having valvular aortic stenosis and a left heart catheterization within 2 years of death

Patient	Age (Years)	Gender	Number of AV Cusps	AV Calcium	Interval from Cath to Death (Days)	Left Ventricle		Aorta		PSG (mm Hg)	Heart Weight (g)
						Systolic (mm Hg)	Diastolic (mm Hg)	Systolic (mm Hg)	Diastolic (mm Hg)		
1	32	F	1	4+	34	172	26	82	66	90	510
2	33	M	1	3+	24	135	50	120	60	15	880
3	34	M	1	3+	37	184	36	92	68	92	570
4	39	M	1	4+	40	162	25	96	66	66	750
5	57	M	1	4+	670	202	18	122	72	80	630
6	60	M	1	1+	30	—	—	—	—	60	—
7	16	M	2	3+	11	230	8	105	75	125	680
8	37	M	2	4+	365	146	37	96	74	50	750
9	42	F	2	2+	10	240	12	115	65	125	420
10	52	M	2	3+	30	—	—	—	—	80	630
11	52	F	2	4+	1	230	30	100	70	130	700
12	54	M	2	4+	30	238	37	90	70	148	850
13	54	M	2	4+	2	192	10	63	34	129	700
14	56	M	2	3+	30	191	24	104	61	87	—
15	58	M	2	1+	60	—	—	—	—	20	—
16	59	M	2	4+	720	200	12	155	60	45	580
17	59	M	2	2+	1	—	—	—	—	35	470
18	60	F	2	4+	15	—	—	—	—	110	680
19	61	M	2	4+	2	165	40	111	—	54	630
20	67	M	2	2+	730	202	7	175	95	27	—
21	67	M	2	4+	30	—	35	—	—	55	740
22	67	M	2	4+	90	—	8	—	—	72	680
23	68	M	2	1+	522	123	20	112	59	11	550
24	75	F	2	4+	1	—	—	—	—	125	—
25	77	M	2	4+	2	—	—	—	—	50	570
26	44	M	3	4+	9	—	—	—	—	82	590
27	49	M	3	4+	12	188	20	114	48	74	710
28	51	M	3	2+	720	—	—	—	—	20	960
29	62	M	3	3+	1	—	—	—	—	15	500
30	66	M	3	4+	30	182	40	120	60	62	655
31	71	M	3	2+	570	—	—	—	—	20	800
32	76	F	3	4+	1	—	—	—	—	60	—
33	77	F	3	3+	90	180	4	115	—	65	380
34	79	M	3	3+	8	150	10	120	80	30	505
35	61	M	2	4+	90	—	—	—	—	100	530
36	60	M	2	—	180	197	12	186	72	11	540
37	70	M	2	—	92	—	—	—	—	93	—

AV = aortic valve; Cath = catheterization; F = female; M = male; PSG = peak systolic pressure gradient; — = no information available.

Beginning in approximately 1960, a number of clinical studies focused on the "natural history" of patients with AS.[5–20] Early on the focus was mainly in children and young adults with congenital AS and, by the 1980s, most studies centered on older adults. An early article by Ross and Braunwald[21] delineated the average length of survival in patients with AS after onset of symptoms (angina pectoris, heart failure, and/or syncope) based on earlier studies, and their predictions have subsequently proven to be quite accurate. Cohen and colleagues[2] in 1972 reported on 15 initially asymptomatic children with congenital AS studied at cardiac catheterization at an average age of 8.5 years and then again at an average age of 15.1 years and showed that there was in general a poor correlation among the presence of symptoms, the electrocardiographic and radiographic findings, and the severity of the AS. Frank and colleagues[8] in 1973 studied 15 adults with the degree of AS documented hemodynamically and no aortic valve operation performed. During follow-up of 10 years, 13 of the 15 had died. Subsequently, many reports of "natural history" of symptomatic and asymptomatic AS have appeared with the severity of AS documented by cardiac catheterization or by echocardiogram with the patients followed for a specific period of time after hemodynamic or echocardiographic documentation or until death or aortic valve operation. Most confirmed the dire predictions of Ross and Braunwald. None of the reports of "natural history" of AS in the past 50 years have focused on adults with AS studied at necropsy.

The strong point of the present study is that it includes a large group of patients with AS unassociated with mitral stenosis and each case at necropsy was studied by a single individual over a period of more than 50 years. No patient had an aortic valve operation, and all were followed to death with subsequent autopsy. All attempts were made in this

Table 8
Clinical and morphologic findings in 29 patients whose stenotic aortic valves are illustrated in Figures 1 through 4

Figure	Age (Years)	Gender	Number of AV Cusps	Year of Death	AS Diagnosed During Life	Cause of Death	Symptomatic			Duration of Symptoms (Months)	Left Ventricular		CAD	MAC	PSG (mm Hg)	Heart Weight (g)
							Heart Failure	Syncope	Angina Pectoris		Necrosis	Fibrosis				
1A	68	M	1	1963	—	NC	0	0	+	—	+	+	0	0	—	750
1B	77	M	1	1971	+	C (NS)	+	0	0	1	0	0	0	0	—	495
1C	83	M	1	1978	—	C (NS)	+	0	0	48	0	0	0	0	—	805
1D	54	M	1	1961	+	C (NS)	+	0	0	108	0	+	0	0	129	700
1E	54	M	1	1966	—	C (NS)	+	0	0	36	0	0	0	0	—	—
1F	59	M	1	1969	+	C (NS)	+	+	0	11	0	0	0	0	—	650
1G	34	M	1	1966	+	C (NS)	+	0	+	180	0	+	0	+	92	570
1H	48	M	1	1968	+	C (NS)	+	0	0	132	0	+	0	+	—	750
1I	60	M	1	1971	+	C (NS)	+	0	0	12	0	+	0	+	—	700
2A	49	M	2	1985	+	C (NS)	+	0	+	96	0	+	+	0	—	525
2B	59	M	2	1964	+	C (NS)	+	0	0	42	0	0	0	0	45	580
2C	77	M	2	1989	+	C (NS)	+	0	0	1	0	0	+	0	50	570
2D	56	F	2	1970	+	C (NS)	—	—	—	—	0	+	+	0	—	375
2E	66	M	2	1984	—	C (NS)	+	0	0	11	0	+	+	0	—	500
2F	81	F	2	1980	—	C (NS)	+	0	0	12	0	0	0	0	—	550
2G	66	M	2	1968	—	C (NS)	+	0	0	336	0	+	0	+	—	800
2H	71	M	2	1969	—	C (NS)	+	0	0	36	0	+	+	+	—	650
2I	87	M	2	1970	—	C (NS)	+	0	+	1	0	+	+	0	—	625
2J	52	F	2	1968	+	C (NS)	+	0	0	36	0	0	0	+	130	700
2K	59	M	2	1984	0	C (S)	0	+	0	2	0	+	+	0	—	575
2L	65	F	2	1991	0	NC	+	0	0	3	0	0	0	0	—	440
3A, A′	54	F	2	1969	—	C (S)	+	0	0	48	0	0	0	+	—	430
3B–B‴	60	M	2	1971	—	C (NS)	+	0	+	8	+	+	+	+	—	1,050
4A	75	F	3	1980	—	C (NS)	+	0	0	48	0	+	+	+	—	520
4B	77	F	3	1969	—	C (NS)	0	+	0	12	+	0	+	+	—	380
4C	79	M	3	1988	+	NC	0	0	0	—	0	0	0	+	30	505
4D	81	F	3	1970	—	C (S)	0	0	+	12	0	0	0	0	—	400
4E	87	F	3	1970	—	C (S)	+	0	+	72	0	0	0	0	—	430
4F	90	F	3	1981	—	C (NS)	—	—	—	—	0	0	0	+	—	345

AS = aortic stenosis; AV = aortic valve; C = cardiac; CAD = coronary artery disease; Cath = catheterization; F = female; M = male; MAC = mitral annular calcium; NC = noncardiac; NS = non-sudden; PSG = peak systolic pressure gradient; S = sudden; — = no information available/not applicable.

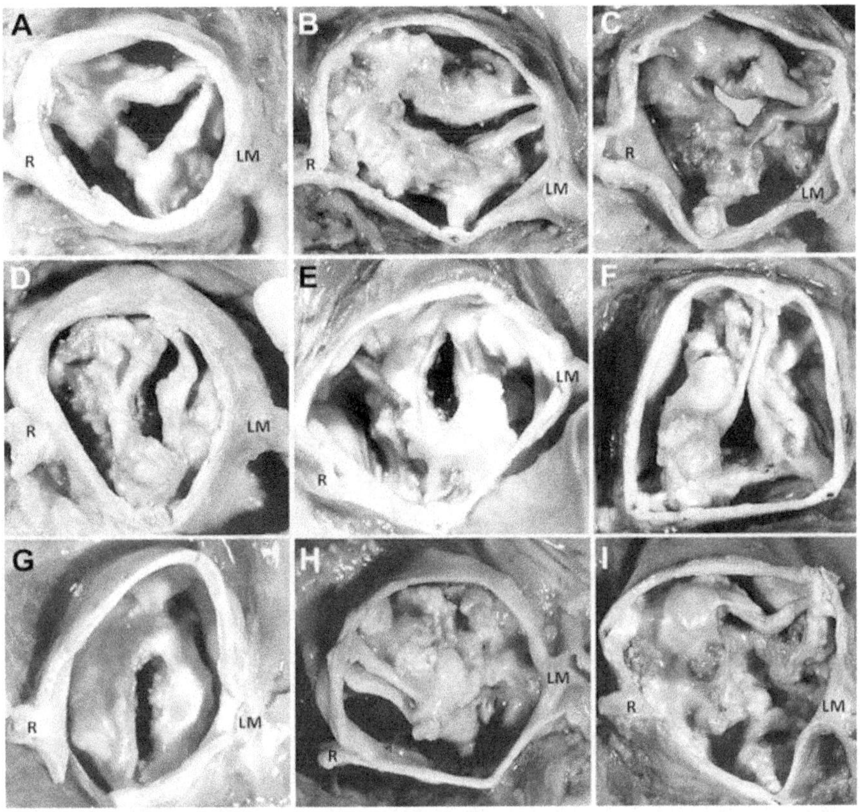

Figure 1. Unicuspid stenotic aortic valves from above. See Table 8 for clinical data on each patient. LM = left main coronary artery; R = right coronary artery. (Figure 1H was reproduced with permission from Roberts WC, Vowels TJ, Ko JM. Natural history of adults with congenitally malformed aortic valves (unicuspid or bicuspid). *Medicine* 2012;91:287–308.)

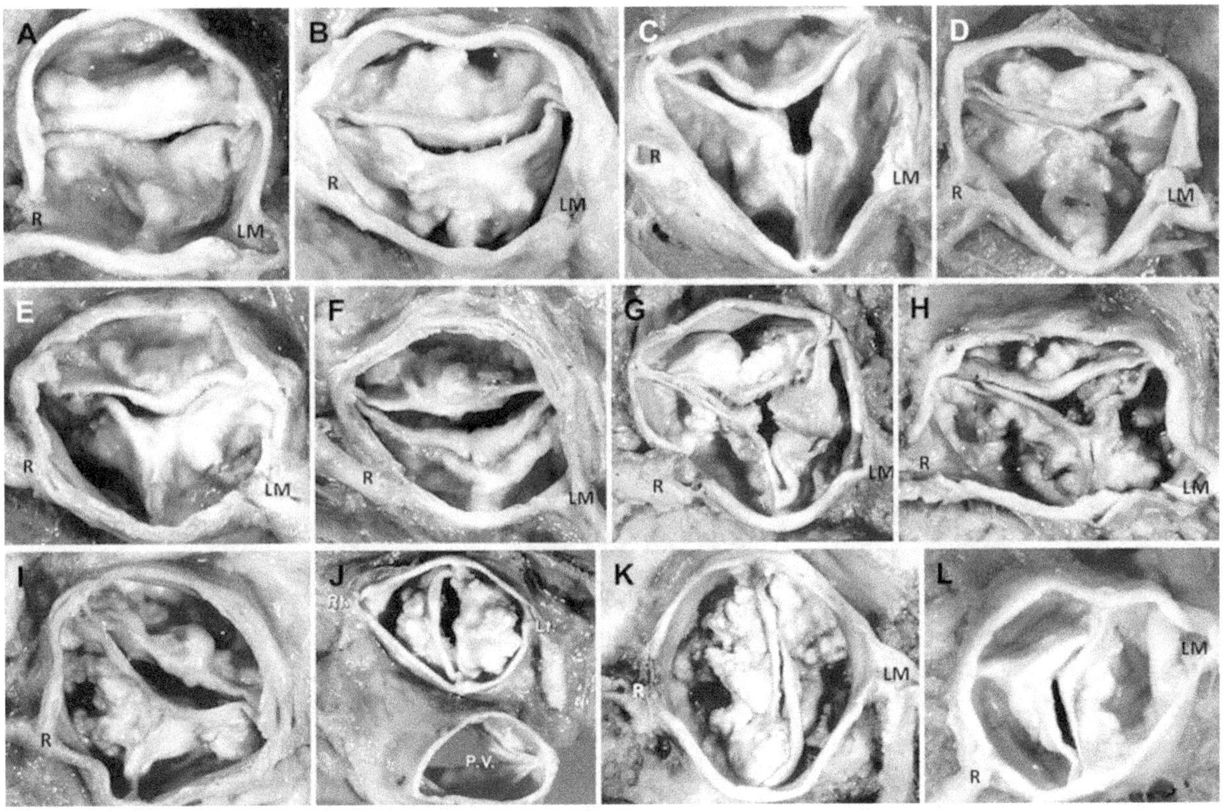

Figure 2. Bicuspid stenotic aortic valves from above orientated anterior-posterior *(A–F, H, I)* such that both coronary ostia arise from behind the anterior cusp, and right-left *(G, J–L)* such that each coronary ostium arises from behind a separate cusp. See Table 8 for clinical data on each patient. LM = left main coronary artery; PV = pulmonic valve; R = right coronary artery. (Figure 2C and 2I were reproduced with permission from Roberts WC, Vowels TJ, Ko JM. Natural history of adults with congenitally malformed aortic valves (unicuspid or bicuspid). *Medicine* 2012;91:287-308.)

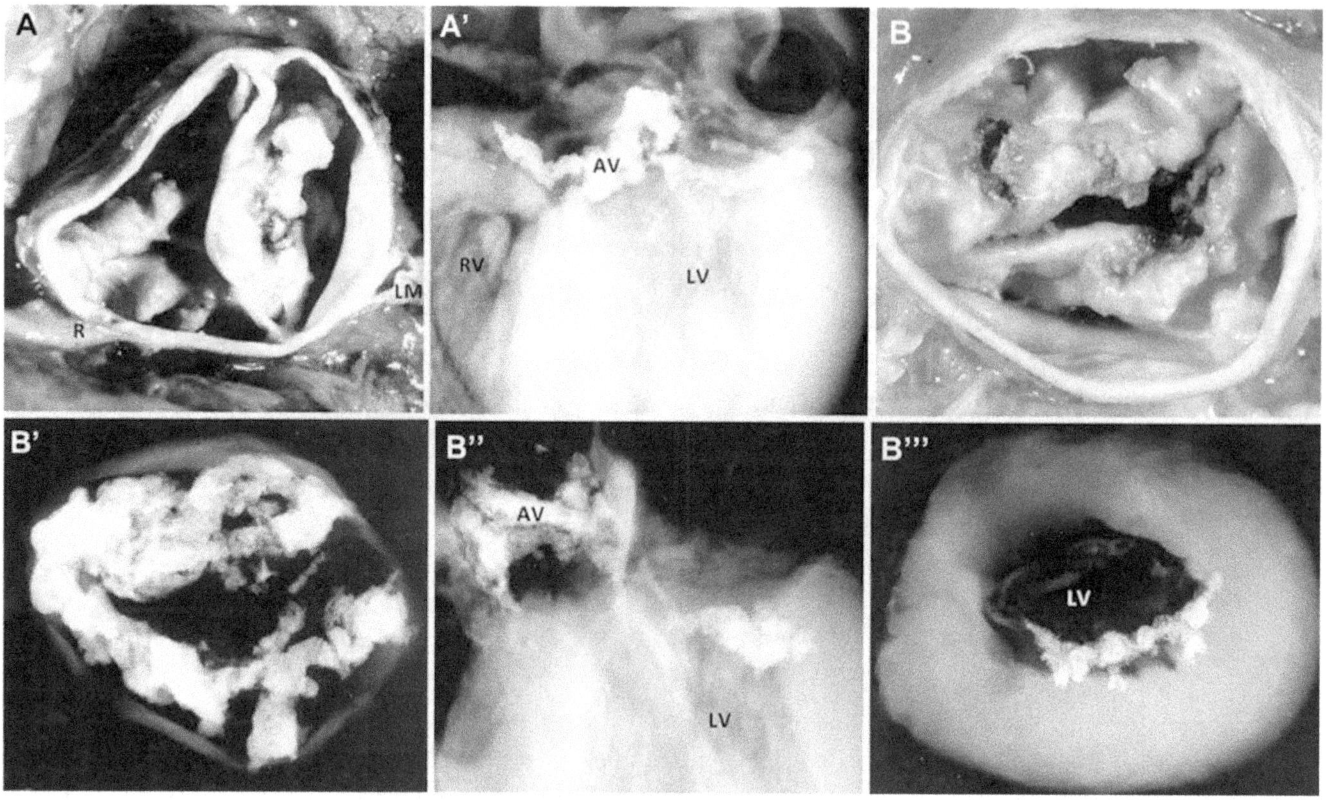

Figure 3. Bicuspid stenotic aortic valves from above *(A* and *B)* and radiographs showing calcific deposits on the aortic valve and mitral annulus (A', $B'-B'''$). See Table 8 for clinical data on each patient. AV = aortic valve; LM = left main coronary artery; LV = left ventricle; R = right coronary artery; RV = right ventricle.

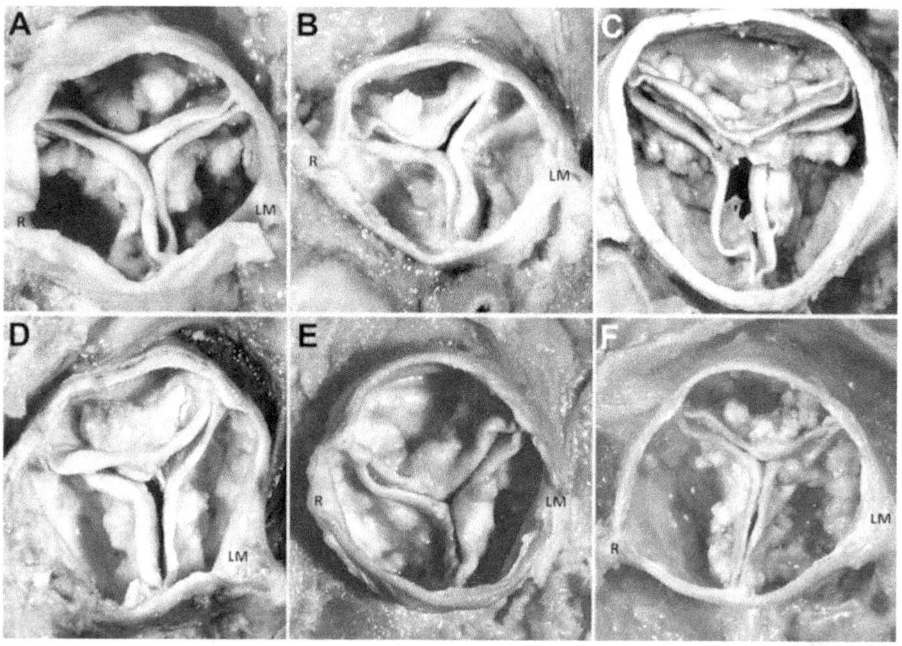

Figure 4. Tricuspid stenotic aortic valves from above. See Table 8 for clinical data on each patient. LM = left main coronary artery; R = right coronary artery.

study to exclude rheumatic heart disease as a cause of the AS by excluding any patient with associated mitral stenosis.

The present study, like virtually all studies, has limitations. The severity of the AS was determined mainly by morphologic means, that is, the degree of rigidity of the aortic valve cusps as a result of calcific deposits, and not by hemodynamic or echocardiographic means. Only 37 patients (14%) had left-sided cardiac catheterization or at least had that data

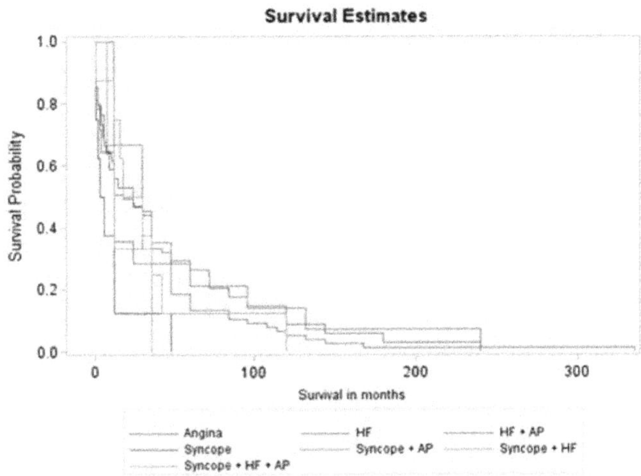

Figure 5. This graph displays survival from the onset of symptoms (heart failure, angina pectoris, and/or syncope) in patients having aortic valve stenosis.

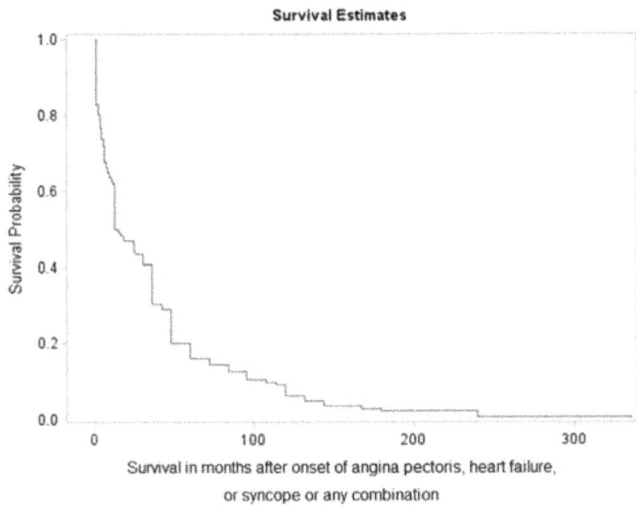

Figure 6. This graph displays survival from onset of symptoms (heart failure, angina pectoris, or syncope or any combination) in patients having aortic valve stenosis.

available to us. Four of these 37 patients had peak systolic pressure gradients between left ventricle and aorta in the teens, but all 4 had rather rigid aortic valve cusps at autopsy, and all 4 had hearts weighing ≥500 g. The interval from catheterization to death was relatively long in 2 of the 4 patients. The appearance of the aortic valves at necropsy in the patients who did not have left-sided cardiac catheterization were similar to those who did undergo cardiac catheterization. Most patients included died between 1960 and 1980, a period when the echocardiogram was unavailable or rarely used, but it was also a period when autopsies were more commonly performed than in the past 3 decades.

The causes of death in the older patients were complicated by their higher frequency of associated coronary arterial narrowing compared with the younger patients. The older patients (>65 years of age) had high frequencies of tricuspid aortic valves, and the etiology of the AS in them

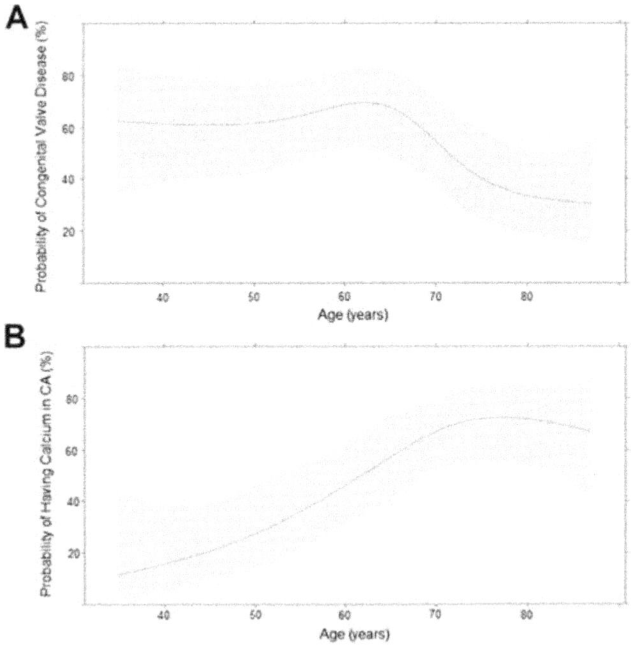

Figure 7. These graphs display the propensity-adjusted probability of having a unicuspid or bicuspid aortic valve *(A)* ($p = 0.007$) or calcium in ≥1 coronary arteries *(B)* ($p = 0.001$) by age. The propensity models were adjusted for patient having symptoms (heart failure, angina pectoris, and/or syncope), gender, valve structure (for calcium model only), heart weight (g), degree of coronary narrowing, foci of left ventricular necrosis and/or fibrosis, and presence of calcium in the coronary arteries (congenital valve model only).

was attributed to atherosclerosis. Most patients ≤65 years of age had congenitally malformed valves.

Disclosures

The authors have no conflicts of interest to disclose.

1. Roberts WC, Vowels TJ, Ko JM. Natural history of adults with congenitally malformed aortic valves (unicuspid or bicuspid). *Medicine* 2012;91:287–308.
2. Harrell FE Jr. Regression Modeling Strategies: With Application to Linear Models, Logistic Regression, and Survival Analysis. New York: Springer-Verlag, 2001.
3. Filardo G, Hamilton C, Hamman B, Ng HK, Grayburn P. Categorizing BMI may lead to biased results in studies investigating in-hospital mortality after isolated CABG. *J Clin Epidemiol* 2007;60:1132–1139.
4. Roberts WC. Anatomically isolated aortic valvular disease: the case against its being of rheumatic etiology. *Am J Med* 1970;49:151–159.
5. Peckham GB, Keith JD, Evans JR. Congenital aortic stenosis: some observations on the natural history and clinical assessment. *Can Med Assoc J* 1964;91:639–643.
6. Campbell M. The natural history of congenital aortic stenosis. *Br Heart J* 1968;30:514–526.
7. Cohen LS, Friedman WF, Braunwald E. Natural history of mild congenital aortic stenosis elucidated by serial hemodynamic studies. *Am J Cardiol* 1972;30:1–5.
8. Frank S, Johnson A, Ross J Jr. Natural history of valvular aortic stenosis. *Br Heart J* 1973;35:41–46.
9. Mills P, Leech G, Davies M, Leatham A. The natural history of a non-stenotic bicuspid aortic valve. *Br Heart J* 1978;40:951–957.
10. Hossack KF, Neutze JM, Lowe JB, Barratt-Boyes BG. Congenital valvar aortic stenosis: natural history and assessment for operation. *Br Heart J* 1980;43:561–573.
11. Chizner MA, Peale DL, deLeon AC Jr. The natural history of aortic stenosis in adults. *Am Heart J* 1980;99:419–424.

12. Horstkotte D, Loogen F. The natural history of aortic valve stenosis. *Eur Heart J* 1988;9(Suppl E):57–64.
13. Pellikka PA, Nishimura RA, Bailey KR, Tajik AJ. The natural history of adults with asymptomatic, hemodynamically significant aortic stenosis. *J Am Coll Cardiol* 1990;15:1012–1017.
14. Kennedy KD, Nishimura RA, Holmes DR Jr, Bailey KR. Natural history of moderate aortic stenosis. *J Am Coll Cardiol* 1991;17:313–319.
15. Livanainen AM, Lindroos M, Rilvis R, Heikkilä J, Kupari M. Natural history of aortic valve stenosis of varying severity in the elderly. *Am J Cardiol* 1996;78:97–101.
16. Christensen KL, Ivarsen HR, Thuesen L, Kristensen BO, Egeblad H. Aortic valve stenosis: fatal natural history despite normal left ventricular function and low invasive peak-to-peak pressure gradients. *Cardiology* 2004;102:147–151.
17. Rosenhek R, Klaar U, Schemper M, Scholten C, Heger M, Gabriel H, Binder T, Maurer G, Baumgartner H. Mild and moderate aortic stenosis: natural history and risk stratification by echo-cardiography. *Eur Heart J* 2004;25:199–205.
18. Pai RG, Kapoor N, Bansal RC, Varadarajan P. Malignant natural history of asymptomatic severe aortic stenosis: benefit of aortic valve replacement. *Ann Thorac Surg* 2006;82:2116–2122.
19. Michaelena HI, Desjardins VA, Avierinos JF, Russo A, Nkomo VT, Sundt TM, Pellikka PA, Tajik AJ, Enriquez-Sarano M. Natural history of asymptomatic patients with normally functioning or minimally dysfunctional bicuspid aortic valve in the community. *Circulation* 2008;117:2776–2784.
20. Rosenhek R, Zilberszac R, Schemper M, Czerny M, Mundigler G, Graf S, Bergler-Klein J, Grimm M, Gabriel H, Maurer G. Natural history of very severe aortic stenosis. *Circulation* 2010;121: 151–156.
21. Ross J Jr, Braunwald E. Aortic stenosis. *Circulation* 1968;38: V61–V67.

Infective endocarditis superimposed on a massively calcified severely stenotic congenitally bicuspid aortic valve

Syed Sarmast, MD, Jeffrey M. Schussler, MD, Jong M. Ko, BA, and William C. Roberts, MD

We describe a 55-year-old man who presented with a stroke resulting from active infective endocarditis (IE) involving a heavily calcified bicuspid aortic valve. The case highlights the infrequency of IE involving a heavily calcified valve, the inability of the infection to penetrate the calcific deposits, and the ability of the infection to spread to the adjacent soft tissues, leading to ring abscess and its multiple complications.

The aortic valve is the most common site for one or more vegetations to form in infective endocarditis (IE) (1). Since the introduction of corticosteroids and the increased frequency of immunotherapy and intravenous drug addiction, infection involving the aortic valve has most commonly involved a previously structurally normal valve. The next most common aortic valve to be involved by IE was a congenitally malformed bicuspid aortic valve that had functioned normally or had only mild dysfunction (2). IE involving a previously calcified valve is unusual and particularly so when the aortic valve is massively calcified. The present report was prompted by study of a patient who developed IE on a previously heavily calcified, severely stenotic aortic valve.

CASE DESCRIPTION

A 55-year-old white man, on chronic hemodialysis for end-stage renal disease believed to be secondary to diabetes mellitus, was hospitalized because of the sudden onset of confusion. Diabetes mellitus was diagnosed when he was 43 years old (2001), requiring insulin therapy by age 49. Systemic hypertension was diagnosed at age 50. He had a sedentary lifestyle and was obese (body mass index 35 kg/m^2). Twelve months earlier, hemodialysis had been initiated; 7 months earlier, a malfunctioning right arm arteriovenous fistula had been repaired; and 1 month earlier, he presented with fever, nausea, vomiting, and abdominal pain. Methicillin-resistant *Staphylococcus aureus* bacteremia related to a right internal jugular PermaCath infection was diagnosed. During that admission, a grade 2/6 precordial systolic ejection murmur was heard. Echocardiography revealed a calcified stenotic bicuspid aortic valve with trace aortic regurgitation, and a small mobile mass attached to the aortic valve was seen. An aortic root abscess also was seen. He was discharged home to receive intravenous vancomycin for 6 weeks and then returned because of confusion. Repeat blood cultures again grew *Staphylococcus aureus*. He was treated with daptomycin.

On July 31, 2010, the aortic valve (bioprosthesis) and proximal portion of the ascending aorta were replaced (the latter was a homograft), the paravalvular abscess was debrided, and the coronary ostial sites were implanted into the homograft. The excised stenotic and infected aortic valve weighed 8.36 g and was congenitally bicuspid *(Figure 1)*. Culture of the excised valve grew methicillin-resistant *Staphylococcus aureus*. The patient's early postoperative course was complicated by episodes of paroxysmal atrial fibrillation and nonsustained ventricular tachycardia.

One month following the operation, the patient was back at home and continuing his hemodialysis treatments 3 times a week. A successful renal transplant was performed on September 13, 2012, and hemodialysis was discontinued. As of October 2013, he remains active and exercises 30 minutes a day at least 3 times a week. He is currently unemployed and on disability.

DISCUSSION

The patient described herein with end-stage renal disease requiring chronic hemodialysis had a heavily calcified stenotic congenitally bicuspid aortic valve and developed superimposed IE initiated as a result of infection at the percutaneous dialysis entry site. The infection, unable to grow well in the calcified valve, rapidly spread to the adjoining soft tissue, producing a ring abscess.

The unusual feature of the present patient is the development of IE on a massively calcified aortic valve. The normal aortic valve weighs about 0.4 g. Thus, the valve in the present patient (8.36 g) was 20 times heavier than normal, and most of that excessive weight was the result of the calcific deposits, not the superimposed vegetative material. Roberts and Ko (3) initially reported weights of operatively excised stenotic aortic valves in 2003 and from January 1998 to August 2013 had

From the Division of Cardiology, Department of Internal Medicine, Baylor University Medical Center at Dallas and the Jack and Jane Hamilton Heart and Vascular Hospital, Dallas, Texas.

Corresponding author: Syed Sarmast, MD, Baylor Heart and Vascular Hospital, 621 N. Hall Street, Dallas, TX 75226 (e-mail: Syed.Sarmast@BaylorHealth.edu).

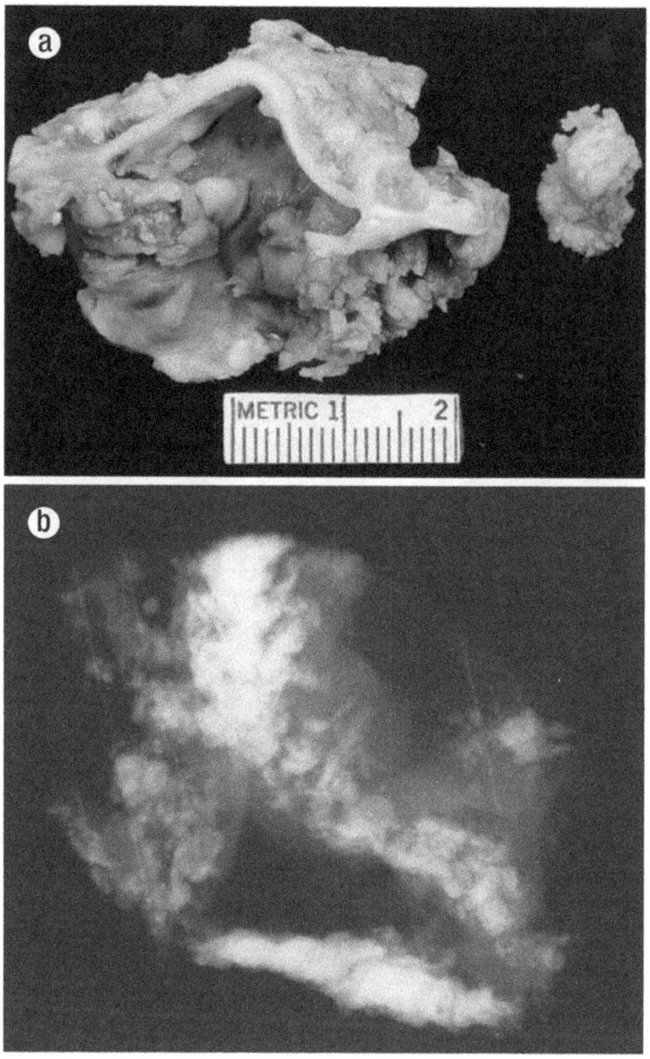

Figure 1. (a) Photograph of the operatively excised stenotic aortic valve and **(b)** radiograph of the valve in the patient described.

weighed 1726 stenotic aortic valves: only 12 (0.7%) weighed >8 g, and none of the other 11 patients had IE. Indeed, the lighter the aortic valve, the greater the likelihood of its being complicated by IE (2).

IE involving a stenotic aortic valve is far less common than IE involving a nonstenotic aortic valve. Fernicola and Roberts (4) studied at necropsy 96 patients with active IE involving the aortic valve: 25 (26%) had underlying stenosis and 71 (74%) had an underlying nonstenotic valve. Of the 25 with underlying stenosis, 21 (84%) had a ring abscess and 10 (40%) had an underlying congenitally bicuspid valve; of the 71 with a nonstenotic aortic valve, 37 (52%) had a ring abscess ($P = 0.005$) and 21 (30%), a congenitally bicuspid valve (ns).

The patient described had two reasons for having a heavily calcified aortic valve: 1) the underlying bicuspid condition (2), and 2) the presence of end-stage renal disease with chronic hemodialysis (5).

1. Arnett EN, Roberts WC. Pathology of active infective endocarditis: a necropsy analysis of 192 patients. *Thorac Cardiovasc Surg* 1982;30(6):327–335.
2. Roberts WC, Vowels TJ, Ko JM. Natural history of adults with congenitally malformed aortic valves (unicuspid or bicuspid). *Medicine (Baltimore)* 2012;91(6):287–308.
3. Roberts WC, Ko JM. Weights of operatively-excised stenotic unicuspid, bicuspid, and tricuspid aortic valves and their relation to age, sex, body mass index, and presence or absence of concomitant coronary artery bypass grafting. *Am J Cardiol* 2003;92(9):1057–1065.
4. Roberts WC, Oluwole BO, Fernicola DJ. Comparison of active infective endocarditis involving a previously stenotic versus a previously nonstenotic aortic valve. *Am J Cardiol* 1993;71(12):1082–1088.
5. Roberts WC, Taylor MA, Shirani J. Cardiac findings at necropsy in patients with chronic kidney disease maintained on chronic hemodialysis. *Medicine (Baltimore)* 2012;91(3):165–178.

Relation of left ventricular free wall rupture and/or aneurysm with acute myocardial infarction in patients with aortic stenosis

Irtiza N. Sheikh, BS, and William C. Roberts, MD

This minireview describes 6 previously reported patients with left ventricular free wall rupture and/or aneurysm complicating acute myocardial infarction (AMI) in patients with aortic stenosis. The findings suggest that left ventricular rupture and/or aneurysm is more frequent in patients with AMI associated with aortic stenosis than in patients with AMI unassociated with aortic stenosis, presumably because of retained elevation of the left ventricular peak systolic pressure after the appearance of the AMI.

In 1983, one of us (WCR) reported a patient with severe aortic stenosis (AS) and a healed left ventricular (LV) apical aneurysm (1). The authors speculated that LV aneurysm and LV free wall rupture would be more frequent in patients with acute myocardial infarction (AMI) associated with severe AS than in patients with AMI without AS. Herein, we summarize findings in 5 subsequently reported patients with LV rupture and/or aneurysm with AMI associated with severe AS.

Table 1. Reported cases of acute myocardial infarction in patients with aortic valve stenosis with left ventricular free wall rupture or aneurysm

	Reported cases: First author, year of publication					
	1	2	3	4	5	6
Variable	Roberts 1983	Duke 1984	Connary 1994	Kadri 1994	Ikeda 2002	Tanaka 2006
1. Age (years) at AMI	62	57	62	58	69	74
2. Sex	M	M	F	F	F	F
3. LV free wall rupture	0	+	+*	+	+	+
4. LV aneurysm	+	0	+	0	+	0
5. Days from AMI onset to rupture	–	6	?30	10	20	2
6. Previous hypertension (history)	+	0	–	+	–	+
7. ECG location of the infarct	–	Ant	Ant	Ant	–	Ant
8. Apical location of the infarct	+	+	0*	+	+	–
9. LV-SA psg (mm Hg)	–	–	50	105	70†	177†
10. Aortic valve area (cm^2)	–	–	0.4	–	0.7†	0.3†
11. Systemic artery (s/d) (mm Hg)	–	110/70	100/60	150/90	–	116/85
12. Heart weight (g)	630	610	–	–	–	–

*False left ventricular aneurysm.
†By echocardiogram.
AMI indicates acute myocardial infarction; Ant, anterior; ECG, electrocardiographic; LV, left ventricular; psg, peak systolic gradient; SA, systemic artery; s/d, peak systole/end diastole.

METHODS

An initial PubMed search was conducted to locate publications of "cardiac rupture or aneurysm in patients with acute myocardial infarction complicated by aortic stenosis." A second search was made for publications of "myocardial infarction in patients with aortic stenosis."

RESULTS

Since the report by Roberts and colleagues (1) in 1983, we found 5 additional case reports of patients with AMI complicated by LV free wall rupture and/or aneurysm in patients with AS (2–6). The findings in them are summarized in the *Table 1,* which also includes the initial report by Roberts et al (1). No reported cases were found in the search for AMI associated with AS irrespective of whether an LV free wall rupture and/or aneurysm was present. At the time of AMI, the 6 patients ranged in age from 57 to 74 years (mean 64); 4 were women and 2 were men. The rupture site in all patients was the LV free wall, leading to hemopericardium. The interval from onset of AMI to rupture ranged from 1 to possibly 30 days. The AS appeared to be severe in all patients: the peak LV systolic gradients (reported in 4 patients) ranged from 50 to 177 mm Hg.

DISCUSSION

When AMI occurs in patients with systemic hypertension, the systemic arterial and LV pressures generally return to or toward normal if the AMI is fairly large. Several reports have demonstrated that systemic hypertension unassociated with

From the Baylor Heart and Vascular Institute and the Departments of Internal Medicine and Pathology, Baylor University Medical Center at Dallas (Roberts); and Texas College of Osteopathic Medicine, Fort Worth, Texas (Sheikh).

Corresponding author: William C. Roberts, MD, Baylor Heart and Vascular Institute, Baylor University Medical Center at Dallas, 3500 Gaston Avenue, Dallas, TX 75246 (e-mail: william.roberts1@bswhealth.org).

AS in patients with AMI is not a risk factor for LV free wall rupture and/or aneurysm formation (2, 3). When AMI occurs in patients with significant AS, however, the LV systolic pressure remains elevated and the continuation of this elevation appears to increase the likelihood of LV rupture and/or aneurysmal formation, particularly when the AMI involves the LV apical wall, which normally is several times thinner than the LV basal wall.

There is some data on the frequency of AS in older populations and on the frequency of AMI and sudden cardiac death among patients with AS. In an autopsy study, Roberts and Shirani (7) found severe AS to be present in 43 (11%) of 391 patients aged 80 to 89 years, in 8 (9%) of 93 patients aged 90 to 99 years, and in 0 of 6 patients aged ≥100 years, or in 51 (10%) of the total 490 patients aged 80 years or over. Of the 490 autopsied patients, 229 (47%) had acute and/or healed myocardial infarcts. Aronow and colleagues (8) studied by echocardiogram 1797 older patients (mean age 82 years) and found AS in 301 (17%)—severe in 40, moderate in 96, and mild in 165. Among their 301 patients with AS, 158 (52%) had had an earlier AMI that healed, and 217 (72%) had a new AMI or died suddenly. There was no mention of LV free wall rupture or LV aneurysm. There have been at least 2 case reports of AMI in patients with AS and normal epicardial coronary arteries (9, 10). Neither had LV free wall rupture or aneurysm.

The major limitation of this minireview is that the number of patients with AMI associated with AS without LV free wall rupture or LV aneurysm is entirely unknown. Conversely, the reported cases of LV free wall rupture and/or aneurysm complicating AMI in patients with AS may represent, of course, the tip of the iceberg.

1. Roberts WC, Arnett EN, Aisner SC, Techlenberg P. Aortic valve stenosis and left ventricular apical aneurysm and/or rupture: real or potential complications of persistent left ventricular systolic hypertension after acute myocardial infarction. *Am Heart J* 1983;105(3):513–514.
2. Duke M. Aortic stenosis, myocardial infarction and cardiac rupture: an unusual triad. *Tex Heart Inst J* 1984;11(1):96–97.
3. Connery CP, Dumont HJ, Dervan JP, Hartman AR, Anagnostopoulos CE. Transmural myocardial infarction with coexisting critical aortic stenosis as an etiology for early myocardial rupture. *J Cardiovasc Surg (Torino)* 1994;35(1):53–56.
4. Kadri MA, Kakadellis J, Campbell CS. Survival after postinfarction cardiac rupture in severe aortic valve stenosis. *Eur Heart J* 1994;15(1):140–142.
5. Ikeda M, Ohashi H, Tsutsumi Y, Kawai T, Ohnaka M. Endoventricular circular patch plasty with aortic valve replacement for post-infarction cardiac rupture complicated with aortic valve stenosis: case report. *Circ J* 2002;66(10):974–976.
6. Tanaka M, Goto Y, Suzuki S, Morii I, Otsuka Y, Miyazaki S, Nonogi H. Postinfarction cardiac rupture despite immediate reperfusion therapy in a patient with severe aortic valve stenosis. *Heart Vessels* 2006;21(1):59–62.
7. Roberts WC, Shirani J. Comparison of cardiac findings at necropsy in octogenarians, nonagenarians, and centenarians. *Am J Cardiol* 1998;82(5):627–631.
8. Aronow WS, Ahn C, Shirani J, Kronzon I. Comparison of frequency of new coronary events in older persons with mild, moderate, and severe valvular aortic stenosis with those without aortic stenosis. *Am J Cardiol* 1998;81(5):647–649.
9. Jondeau G, Dubourg O, Partovian C, Dib JC, Lacombe P, Chikli F, Bourdarias JP. Acute myocardial infarction in a patient with severe aortic stenosis and normal coronary arteries. *Eur Heart J* 1994;15(5):715–717.
10. Lin CF, Chu KC. Acute myocardial infarction in an elderly patient with severe aortic stenosis and angiographically normal coronary arteries. *Int J Gerontol* 2010;4(3):157–160.

Combined mitral and aortic valve stenosis caused by two different etiologies, rheumatic and congenital

William C. Roberts, MD, and Joshua K. Dodderer, BS

Table 1. Pertinent findings in the five patients with stenotic congenitally bicuspid aortic valves and stenotic rheumatic mitral valves

Case number	Age at VR (years)	Sex	BMI (kg/m²)	Pressures (mm Hg) PAW (mean)	RV (s/d)	RA (mean)	LV (s/d)	Ao (s/d)	LV-Ao (psg)	PAW-LV (mdg)	AV area (cm²)	MV area (cm²)	AV weight (g)	MV weight (g)
1	44	M	26	21	86/19	16	126/14	108/66	18	16	–	1.54	0.9	3.8
2	46	M	26	26	48/18	13	139/17	133/88	28	15	0.46	0.95	1.37	3.44
3	50	M	27	39	56/18	13	173/40	146/88	27	25	1.0	1.28	–	–
4	53	F	34	–	–	–	–	–	–	–	0.9	1.8	–	–
5	74	F	21	33	79/17	54	226/19	195/85	31	–	0.53	0.95	–	–

Ao indicates aorta; AV, aortic valve; BMI, body mass index; LV, left ventricular; mdg, mean diastolic gradient; MV, mitral valve; PAW, pulmonary artery wedge; psg, peak systolic gradient; RA, right atrium; RV, right ventricular; s/d, peak systole/end diastole; VR, valve replacement.

Described herein are five patients who had double left-sided cardiac valve replacement for mitral and aortic valve stenosis resulting from two different etiologies: rheumatic heart disease, the cause of the mitral stenosis, and congenital heart disease (bicuspid valve), the underlying cause of the aortic stenosis.

Combined mitral and aortic valve stenosis in the same patient today in the Western world is relatively uncommon. Worldwide, its most common cause is rheumatic heart disease. Today in native Europeans and in European Americans, the most common cause of this combination appears to be massive mitral annular calcification (probably the consequence of atherosclerosis) as the cause of the mitral stenosis and either congenital (unicuspid or bicuspid aortic valve) or nonrheumatic causes (tricuspid aortic valve) as the cause of the aortic stenosis (atherosclerotic etiology) (1). On very rare occasions, the mitral stenosis may be the result of rheumatic heart disease and the aortic stenosis, the result of an underlying congenital heart disease (unicuspid or bicuspid aortic valve). Such was the case in the five patients described herein.

METHODS

Shown in *Table 1* are pertinent findings in the five patients with combined rheumatic mitral stenosis and aortic stenosis superimposed on a congenitally bicuspid aortic valve. Photographs of the operatively excised valves are shown in *Figures 1 and 2*. Only Case 1 is still alive. Cases 2 to 5 survived from 6.9 to 14.4 years (mean 11.2) after the double valve replacement.

DISCUSSION

The patients described here had two different causes for the two stenotic valves on the left side of the heart: rheumatic heart disease for the mitral stenosis and congenital heart disease (bicuspid aortic valve) for the aortic stenosis. Relatively few such combinations have been reported previously. McReynolds and associates (2) in 1976 described an 18-year-old man with a purely regurgitant congenitally bicuspid aortic valve (without commissioned fusion) and a diffusely fibrotic nonstenotic mitral valve proven to be of rheumatic etiology by the presence of Aschoff nodules in the left atrial wall. Tejada and associates (3) in 2001 described a 60-year-old woman who had a noncalcified congenitally bicuspid aortic valve and percutaneous valvuloplasty for a typical rheumatic stenotic mitral valve. Muthiah (4) in India in 2016 described by echocardiogram a

From the Baylor Heart and Vascular Institute and the Departments of Internal Medicine (Division of Cardiology) and Pathology, Baylor University Medical Center, Dallas, Texas (Roberts); and Texas Tech University Health Sciences Center Paul L. Foster School of Medicine, El Paso, Texas (Dodderer).

Corresponding author: William C. Roberts, MD, Baylor Heart and Vascular Institute, Baylor University Medical Center at Dallas, 621 North Hall Street, Dallas, TX 75226 (e-mail: william.roberts1@bswhealth.org).

41-year-old man with a "congenitally malformed" stenotic aortic valve and a stenotic mitral valve that appeared to be of rheumatic origin.

On occasion, in patients with rheumatic mitral stenosis, the aortic valve may have fusion of one of its three commissures, simulating a congenitally bicuspid aortic valve. In these circumstances, however, the ventricular aspect of the fusion appears as a V-shaped indention, producing some space below the fusion. In contrast, with a congenitally bicuspid aortic valve, the ventricular aspect of the raphe area, which some may interpret as fusion of the two cusps, is flat, such that there is no space beneath the fusion. Such was the case in each of the five patients described herein, indicating that the aortic valve in each was congenitally malformed and not the result of rheumatic heart disease.

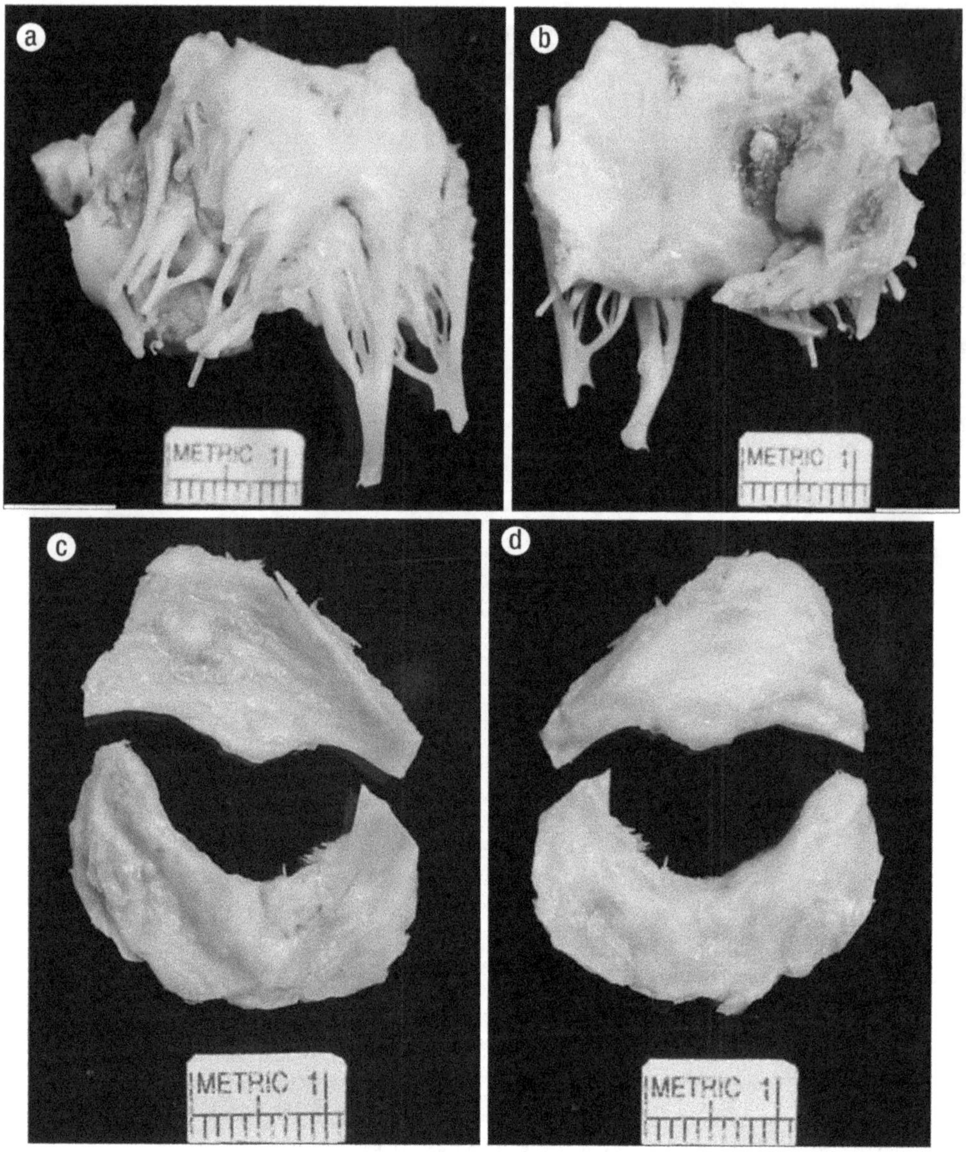

Figure 1. Case 1. Mitral valve as viewed from the **(a)** ventricular aspect and **(b)** atrial aspect. Aortic valve as viewed from the **(c)** aortic aspect and **(d)** ventricular aspect.

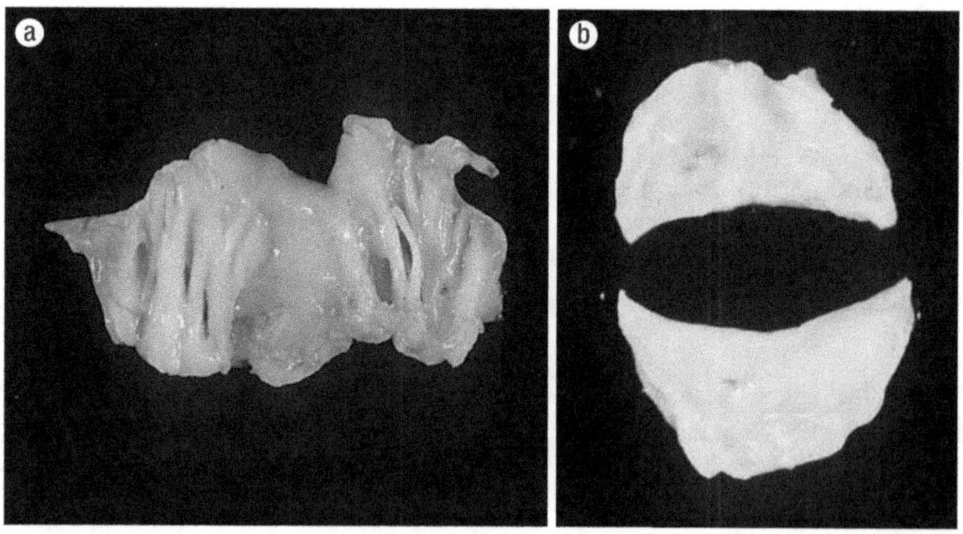

Figure 2. Case 2. **(a)** Thickened mitral valve and **(b)** bicuspid aortic valve.

1. Theleman KP, Grayburn PA, Roberts WC. Mitral "annular" calcium forming a complete circle "O" causing mitral stenosis in association with a stenotic congenitally bicuspid aortic valve and severe coronary artery disease. *Am J Geriatr Cardiol* 2006;15(1):58–61.
2. McReynolds RA, Ali N, Cuadra M, Roberts WC. Combined acute rheumatic fever and congenitally bicuspid aortic valve: a hitherto unconfirmed combination. *Chest* 1976;70(1):98–100.
3. Tejada JG, Albarran A, Hernandez F, Jimenez S, Tascon JC. Anomalous coronary artery origin associated with bicuspid aortic valve in a patient with rheumatic mitral stenosis: a case report. *Angiology* 2001;52(9):649–652.
4. Muthiah R. Rheumatic aortic valve disease with mitral stenosis—a case report. *J Clin Med Case Rep* 2016;5(8):268–295.

Perforation of a Stenotic Congenitally Bicuspid Aortic Valve Cusp by Heavy Calcium in the Other Cusp

William C. Roberts, MD[a,b,*], Ishani Kale[c], and Charles S. Roberts, MD[d]

On occasion in patients with stenotic congenitally bicuspid aortic valves (BAVs), the quantity of calcium in one of the cusps is considerably greater than in the other cusp. We examined operatively excised stenotic congenitally BAVs in 630 patients having isolated aortic valve replacement (No other cardiac valve was replaced, and none had had infective endocarditis.) Of the 630 valves, 3 contained a perforation in the mildly calcified cusp due to a large calcific "spur" extending across the orifice from a heavily calcified cusp. In conclusion, heavy calcific deposits in 1 of 2 BAVs may extend across the orifice causing a perforation in the noncalcified portion of the opposing cusp. **(Am J Cardiol 2020;125:299–301)**

In 1987, 32 years ago, Roberts and colleagues[1] reported 3 patients who had cuspal perforations in heavily calcified stenotic aortic valves without associated infective endocarditis or significant aortic regurgitation. Two of the patients were men aged 62 and 64 years of age with congenitally bicuspid aortic valves (BAVs). Subsequently, there have been no reports describing similar patients. In this report, we describe for the first time the weights of the perforated and nonperforated cusps in 3 additional patients with stenotic congenitally BAVs in an attempt to better understand the mechanism of the cuspal perforation.

Methods

All operatively excised valves at Baylor University Medical Center are submitted to the surgical pathology section of the department of pathology. Since 1993, one of us (WCR) has examined all of the valves and submitted the official medical reports. All operatively excised valves were weighed by WCR after removing formaldehyde/water on the cusps by gently patting them with paper towels. Their medical records thereafter were examined for pertinent clinical data. A total of 1,445 operatively excised stenotic aortic valves were received and examined from 2004 through July 2018: 94 were congenitally unicuspid; 630 were congenitally bicuspid, and 721 were tricuspid. Patients who had associated mitral valve replacement were not included in these numbers.

[a]Baylor Scott & White Heart and Vascular Institute, Baylor University Medical Center, Baylor Scott & White Health, Dallas, Texas; [b]Departments of Internal Medicine (Division of Cardiology), Baylor University Medical Center, Baylor Scott & White Health, Dallas, Texas; [c]Sophomore, Case Western University, Cleveland, Ohio; and [d]Department of Cardiac Surgery, Baylor University Medical Center, Baylor Scott & White Health, Dallas, Texas. Manuscript received October 8, 2019; revised manuscript received and accepted October 24, 2019.

*Corresponding author: Tel:(214) 820-7911; fax: (214) 820-7533.

E-mail address: william.roberts1@bswhealth.org (W.C. Roberts).

Results

Of the 94 stenotic congenitally unicuspid aortic valves examined during the 15-year period, none had cuspal perforations; of the 630 stenotic congenitally BAVs, 3 had perforations in 1 cusp due to calcium's penetrating from the opposing cusp, and of the 721 stenotic tricuspid aortic valves, none had a cuspal perforation.

Pertinent clinical and morphologic data in the 3 patients with a cuspal perforation in 1 of the 2 cusps are tabulated in Table 1 and illustrated in Figures 1–3. The total aortic valve weights in the 3 patients were 2.20, 4.50, and 4.68 grams, respectively, and the nonperforated cusps comprised 76%, 72%, and 70%, respectively, of the weight of the combined 2 cusps.

Comments

Described herein are 3 men, aged 40, 58, and 63 years, respectively, with stenotic congenitally BAVs in which 1 cusp weighed 3 times that of the opposing cusp leading to a spur of calcium in the heavily calcified cusp causing perforation in the less calcified cusp. The 2 previously reported patients with heavily calcified stenotic congenital BAVs with a perforation in the opposing cusp also were men.[1] Men tend to have heavier stenotic aortic valves than do women.[2] Stenotic BAVs also tend to be heavier than stenotic tricuspid aortic valves even though the patients with tricuspid valves tend to be older. Stenotic unicuspid aortic valves, which tend to be heavier than the stenotic congenitally BAVs, did not have perforations in any portion of these valves, possibly because the number of patients with stenotic unicuspid valves was far less than the number of patients with stenotic congenitally BAVs and because the orifice is slit-like and fixed.[1] The weight of the operatively excised stenotic aortic valves is primarily dependent on the quantity of calcium present on the cusps.[2]

Although 2 of the patients described herein had some degree of aortic regurgitation, the major functional derangement in each of the 3 patients was stenosis, despite a perforation in 1 of 2 cusps.

Table 1
Certain clinical and aortic valvular observations in the three men

	Age (yrs)	Race	Total weight AV cusps (g)	Weight of nonperforated cusp (g)	Weight of perforated cusp (g)	BMI (kg/m^2)	LVEF (%)	Pressures (mm Hg) LV (s/d)	Aorta (s/d)	Peak LV-Ao gradient (psg)	Mean LV - Ao gradient (msg)	CAD by Angio	AR (0-3+)	Diameter ascending aorta (cm)	HF	AP	S	DM
1	40	Hispanic	2.20.	1.69 (76%)	0.53 (24%)	29	25	—	98/52 (I)	30 (E)		0	2+	*	+	O	O	+
2	58	White	4.50.	3.26 (72%)	1.25 (28%)	40	40	165/8 (C)	116/68 (C)	49 (C)	42 (C)	0	0	4.7	+	+	0	+
3	63	White	4.68	3.68 (70%)	0.99 (21%)	27	55	—	110/65 (I)	60 (E)	30 (E)	0	1+	4.6	0	+	0	0

Ao = aorta; AP = angina pectoris; Angio = coronary angiography; AR = aortic regurgitation; AV = aortic valve; BMI = body mass index; C = cardiac catheterization; CAD = coronary artery disease; cm = centimeters; DM = diabetes mellitus; E = echocardiogram, g = grams; HF = heart failure; I = indirect; LV = left ventricular; LVEF = left ventricular ejection fraction; msg = mean systolic gradient; psg = peak systolic gradient; S = syncope; s/d = peak systole and end diastole; * = not dilated at operation.

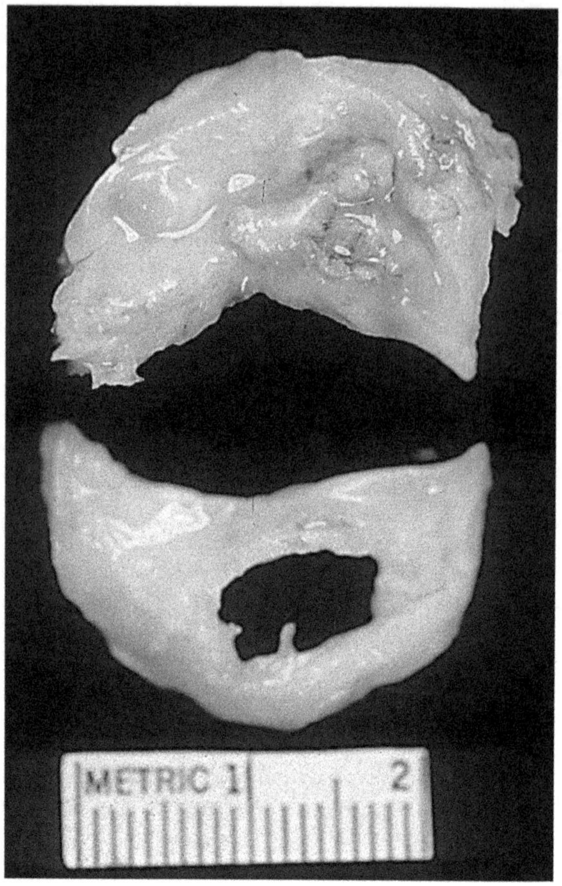

Figure 1. (Case #1, Table 1). Photograph of the 2 cusps showing heavy calcific deposits in 1 cusp (*top*) and the absence of calcific deposits in the other cusp (*bottom*) which contains a large hole.

A previous study describing the weights of 200 stenotic congenitally BAVs demonstrated that the weights of each cusp differed by >0.2 in 74% and were of similar weight (≤0.2 g difference) in 26%. Of the patients without raphes

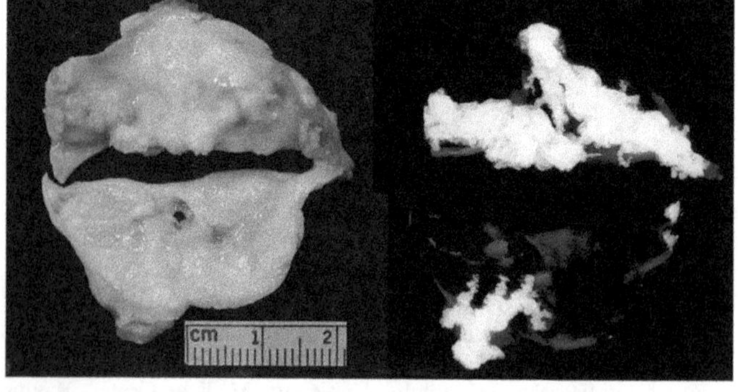

Figure 2. (Case #2, Table 1). Photograph of the aortic valve (*left*) and radiograph of the valve (*right*) showing heavy calcific deposits in 1 cusp and a small perforation in the opposing cusp with only a small calcific deposit in it.

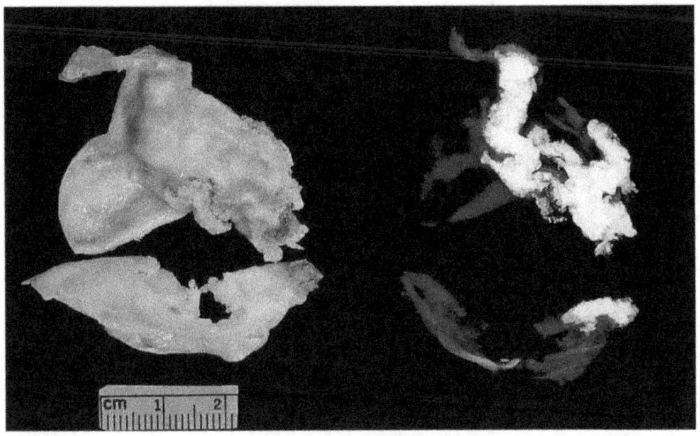

Figure 3. (Case #3, Table 1). Photograph of the aortic valve (*left*) and radiograph of the valve (*right*) showing heavy calcific deposit in one cusp and only a small calcific deposit near the perforation.

in either cusp, the 2 cusps differed in weight (>0.2 g) in 82% and were similar in weight in 18%.

In summary, a perforation of 1 aortic valve cusp in each of the 3 patients resulted from trauma engendered by a calcific nodule in 1 cusp protruding into and finally perforating a noncalcified portion of the opposing cusp. The perforated cusp weighed only a quarter as much as the nonperforated cusp.

1. Roberts WC, McIntosh CL, Wallace RB. Aortic valve perforation with calcific aortic valve stenosis and without infective endocarditis or significant aortic regurgitation. *Am J Cardiol* 1987;59:476–478.
2. Roberts WC, Ko JM. Weights of individual cusps in operatively-excised stenotic congenitally bicuspid aortic valves. *Am J Cardiol* 2004;94:678–681.

www.ingramcontent.com/pod-product-compliance
Lightning Source LLC
LaVergne TN
LVHW062135200926
848484LV00007B/1815